Textbook of
Oral and Maxillofacial Surgery

Textbook of
Oral and Maxillofacial Surgery

Editor

Rajiv M Borle MDS FAOMSI
Professor
Oral and Maxillofacial Surgery
Sharad Pawar Dental College and Hospital

Director
Smile Train Project, Acharya Vinoba Bhave Rural Hospital

Registrar
Datta Meghe Institute of Medical Sciences (Deemed University)
Wardha, Maharashtra, India

Foreword

GE Ghali

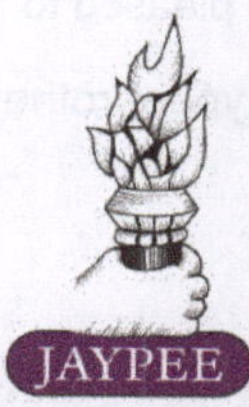

JAYPEE BROTHERS MEDICAL PUBLISHERS
The Health Sciences Publisher
New Delhi | London

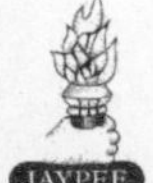

Jaypee Brothers Medical Publishers (P) Ltd

Headquarters
EMCA House
23/23-B, Ansari Road, Daryaganj
New Delhi 110 002, India
Landline: +91-11-23272143, +91-11-23272703
+91-11-23282021, +91-11-23245672
E-mail: jaypee@jaypeebrothers.com

Corporate Office
4838/24, Ansari Road, Daryaganj
New Delhi 110 002, India
Phone: +91-11-43574357
Fax: +91-11-43574314
E-mail: jaypee@jaypeebrothers.com

Overseas Office
J.P. Medical Ltd
83, Victoria Street, London
SW1H 0HW (UK)
Phone: +44-2031708910
E-mail: info@jpmedpub.com

EU GPSR Authorised Representative
Logos Europe, 9 rue Nicolas Poussin
17000, La Rochelle, France
Phone: +33 (0) 6 67 93 73 78
E-mail: contact@logoseurope.eu

Website: www.jaypeebrothers.com
Website: www.jaypeedigital.com

Inquiries for bulk sales may be solicited at: jaypee@jaypeebrothers.com

Textbook of Oral and Maxillofacial Surgery

First Edition: 2014
Reprint : **2026**

ISBN 978-93-5152-009-2

Printed in India

Dedicated to

My Parents

Mrs Malati and Dr Mukund Borle

My Patients

Who volunteered themselves and provided me opportunities to learn.

My Patron

Honorable Shri Datta Meghe
Chancellor, Datta Meghe Institute of Medical Sciences (Deemed University)
Who provided me facilities, opportunities and infrastructure to work.

Contributors

Agni Nishit MDS (Oral and Maxillofacial Surgery)
Associate Professor
Vaidik Dental College and Research Center
Nani Daman (Union Territory)
India

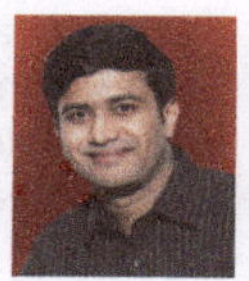

Arora Aakash MDS (Oral and Maxillofacial Surgery)
Associate Professor
Department of Oral and Maxillofacial Surgery
Subharti Dental College
Swami Vivekanand Subharti University
Meerut, Uttar Pradesh, India

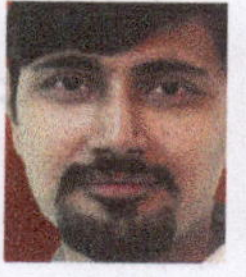

Borle Rajiv M MDS FAOMSI
Professor
Oral and Maxillofacial Surgery
Sharad Pawar Dental College and Hospital
Director
Smile Train Project, Acharya Vinoba Bhave Rural Hospital
Registrar
Datta Meghe Institute of Medical Sciences (Deemed University), Wardha
Maharashtra, India

Agrawal Poonam MDS (Oral and Maxillofacial Surgery)
Associate Professor
Saraswati Dental College
Lucknow, Uttar Pradesh, India

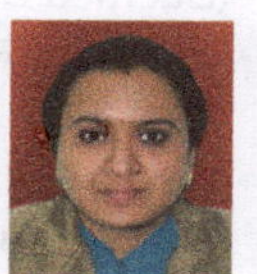

Bhola Nitin MDS (Oral and Maxillofacial Surgery)
Associate Professor and Head
Sharad Pawar Dental College and Hospital
Datta Meghe Institute of Medical Sciences (Deemed University)
Sawangi (M), Wardha, Maharashtra, India

Gadbail Amol MDS (Oral and Maxillofacial Pathology)
Associate Professor
Sharad Pawar Dental College and Hospital
Datta Meghe Institute of Medical Sciences (Deemed University)
Wardha, Maharashtra, India

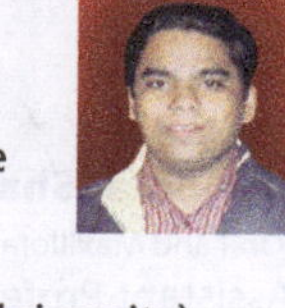

Angik Richa MDS (Oral and Maxillofacial Surgery)
Associate Professor
Awadh Dental College and Hospital
Jamshedpur, Jharkhand, India

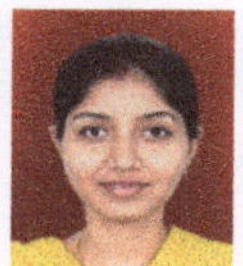

Bhoyar Anjali MDS (Prosthodontics)
Postgraduate Diploma in Clinical Research
Hospital and Health Care Management
Professor and Vice Dean
Peoples' College of Dental Sciences and Research Center
Bhopal, Madhya Pradesh, India

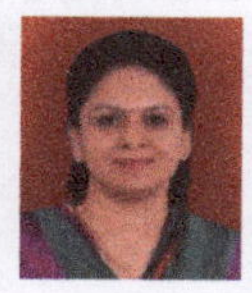

Gaidhane Abhay MD (Community Medicine)
Professor
Community Medicine
Associate Dean
Global Health Jawaharlal Nehru Medical College
Datta Meghe Institute of Medical Sciences (Deemed University)
Wardha, Maharashtra, India

Anjankar AJ MD (Forensic Medicine)
Professor and Head
Forensic Medicine
Jawaharlal Nehru Medical College
Datta Meghe Institute of Medical Sciences (Deemed University)
Wardha, Maharashtra, India

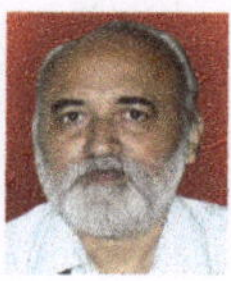

Bora Smriti MDS (Oral and Maxillofacial Surgery)
Assistant Professor
Nair Hospital Dental College
Mumbai, Maharashtra, India

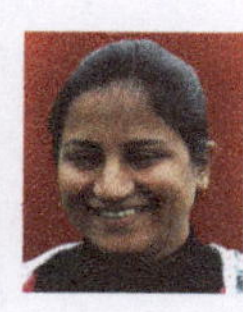

Garg Ketan MDS (Oral and Maxillofacial Surgery)
Consultant Maxillofacial Surgeon
Nagpur, Maharashtra, India

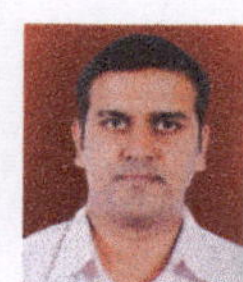

Garg Rajat MDS (Oral and Maxillofacial Surgery)
Consultant Maxillofacial Surgeon
Panipat, Haryana, India

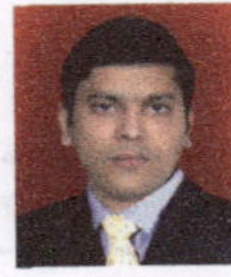

Nimonkar Pranali V MDS (Oral and Maxillofacial Surgery)
Associate Professor
VSPM Dental College and Hospital
Nagpur, Maharashtra, India

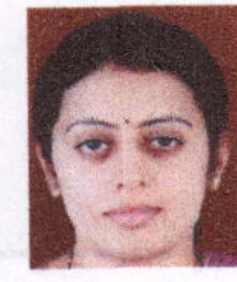

Sachdeva Sachin Dev MDS (Oral and Maxillofacial Surgery)
Associate Professor
Mithila Minority Dental College and Hospital
Darbhanga, Bihar, India

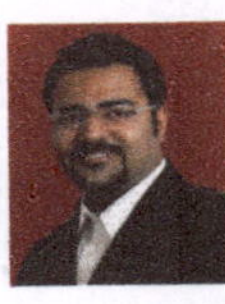

Singh Divya BDS (Oral and Maxillofacial Surgery)
Resident Surgeon
Sharad Pawar Dental College and Hospital
Datta Meghe Institute of Medical Sciences (Deemed University)
Wardha, Maharashtra, India

Jajoo Suhas N MS MCh (Plastic Surgery)
Professor
Jawaharlal Nehru Medical College
Datta Meghe Institute of Medical Sciences (Deemed University)
Wardha, Maharashtra, India

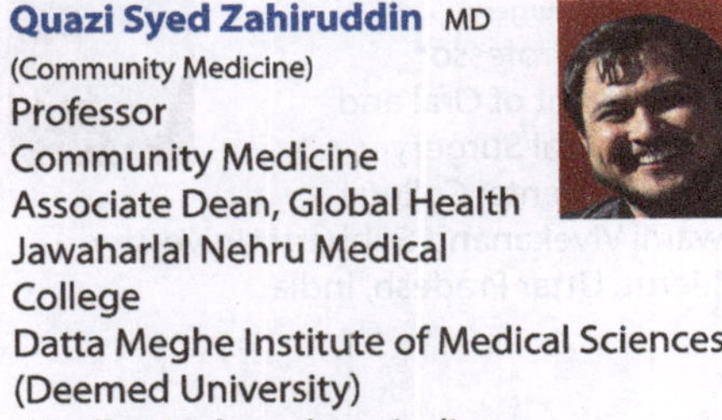

Quazi Syed Zahiruddin MD (Community Medicine)
Professor
Community Medicine
Associate Dean, Global Health
Jawaharlal Nehru Medical College
Datta Meghe Institute of Medical Sciences (Deemed University)
Wardha, Maharashtra, India

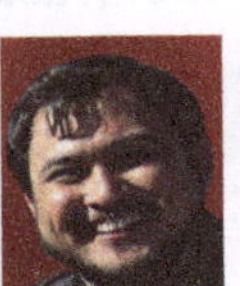

Vibhute Pawan J MDS (Orthodontics and Dentofacial Orthopedics)
Associate Professor
Sharad Pawar Dental College and Hospital
Datta Meghe Institute of Medical Sciences (Deemed University)
Wardha, Maharashtra, India

Magarkar Shashwat D MDS (Oral and Maxillofacial Surgery)
Assistant Professor
Government Dental College and Hospital
Nagpur, Maharashtra, India

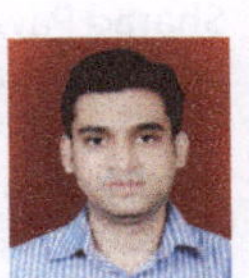

Rai Anshul MDS (Oral and Maxillofacial Surgery)
Assistant Professor
Department of Trauma and Emergency Medicine
All India Institute of Medical Sciences, Bhopal, Madhya Pradesh, India

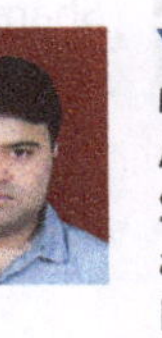

Yadav Abhilasha MDS (Oral and Maxillofacial Surgery)
Assistant Professor
Sharad Pawar Dental College and Hospital
Datta Meghe Institute of Medical Sciences (Deemed University)
Wardha, Maharashtra, India

Foreword

The depth and scope of this book provides the reader a contemporary guide to the knowledge and procedures undertaken in any leading-edge oral and maxillofacial training program. This work is attractive to me for many reasons, not the least of which is its completeness and contemporary nature. This work by Dr Borle is of such a quality that, if need be, it could even be utilized as a curriculum guideline for oral and maxillofacial surgery education and development.

Additionally, the value and meticulous organization of this work, embracing the entire scope of oral and maxillofacial surgery, is remarkable not only for its enormous content but also because it introduces an entirely new cohort of highly qualified contributors to our specialty. The editor has done a fabulous job and should be commended for bringing these young talents forward for all to be exposed to in a scholarly venue. There is even a thorough section devoted to such scholarly, but often over-looked, exercises such as trainee thesis writing.

Beyond the traditional surgery and conditions that are commonplace in the Western world, there is a valuable and needed section devoted to the management of submucous fibrosis and another on temporomandibular joint ankylosis with expert coverage of there inherent management difficulties. There is much to appreciate in this solid address of conditions that rarely exist in the Western world but remain persistent to many of our colleagues.

My mentor, the late RV Walker, often emphasized: "There was always more to learn in the world of oral and maxillofacial surgery than any single person has the time to achieve or do." With this new century comes an ever-expanding frontier of technology pertinent to our wonderful specialty that is so vast that more than one lifetime would be needed to barely scratch the body of knowledge or attempt to master the skills at hand. Well, these are but a few of the reasons why a treatise of the kind compiled by Dr Borle, with the help of his contributors, is so comforting as a go-to resource of all that is contemporary and germane to oral and maxillofacial surgery.

Once again, I commend Dr Borle for this ambitious and monumental project that will surely appeal to a wide readership, both nationally and internationally, which will forever be captivated by our specialty.

GE Ghali DDS MD FACS
President, American Board of Oral
and Maxillofacial Surgery (2013–2014)
Gamble Professor and Chairman
Department of Oral and Maxillofacial Surgery/
Head and Neck Surgery
Louisiana State University School of Medicine
Shreveport, Louisiana, USA

Preface

This book is not just a compilation of literature but personal experiences of the authors, especially while working in the rural circumstances have also been incorporated. Clinical pictures of various clinical conditions and photographic depictions of the surgical procedures have been added for better understanding. Certain diseases such as temporomandibular ankylosis and oral submucous fibrosis, which are predominantly seen in our subcontinent, have been discussed in details. The experiences in the management of oral cancer, where patients often report with advanced diseases and with varied presentation, are shared. The topics such as management of burns, management of soft tissue trauma and medico-legal aspects of injury, which are not routinely covered in the textbook, have been introduced for better readership. While writing the text, care has been taken to give explanations based on basics for better understanding to the beginners. At the same time, the surgical anatomy relevant to the topic has also been discussed.

Some chapters such as Basic Principles of Surgery and Incisions in Maxillofacial Surgery are the highlights of the book and it is sincerely hoped that not only the undergraduates but also the postgraduate students will be benefitted. The aspects of instrumentations, commonly used antiseptics, and aseptic technique have been explained in details. One chapter is dedicated to suture material and technique and plenty of information has been incorporated. The salient features in the individual chapters are highlighted by inserting text boxes.

All the incorporations have been authenticated by giving necessary bibliography (references) at the end of each chapter and the appropriate source of information has been acknowledged.

The overall patient care is needed in surgery; and, hence, to generate understanding in postoperative care, airway management, care of patient under general anesthesia, emergencies, their identification and management, fluid and electrolyte balance and derangements of the same with management thereof have been discussed to make the information comprehensive and elaborate.

This is the first edition of the book and lapses, if any, on my part, will be taken care of in the subsequent edition based on the feedback received from the peers, experts in the field and all other stakeholders, more important the readers.

Rajiv M Borle

Acknowledgments

I consider myself to be lucky to get proper opportunities at proper time to work and learn. Staying in small town like Wardha, Maharashtra, India, and joining a rural institute was considered to be a setback but it was proved fruitful as I came in contact with great personalities who encouraged me, helped me, admired me, and taught me. I am indebted to my teachers who not only selflessly taught me but also ensured that I do not loose way. I am grateful to my patients who trusted a stranger like me and provided me opportunity to learn and sharpen my surgical skills.

My sincere thanks are due to my family members, friends and well-wishers for their support, encouragement and constructive criticism.

I shall be unreasonable if I do not mention my gratitude to my staff and students for their help and for teaching me computer applications.

I wish to express my sincere gratitude to the contributors, my departmental colleagues and postgraduate students, who are more computer savvy, and helped me in writing the book.

I shall be failing in my duty if I do not acknowledge my teachers Late Dr SR Johrapurkar, MS, Former Professor Emeritus of Surgery, Datta Meghe Institute of Medical Sciences (Deemed University), Sawangi (M), Wardha, Maharashtra; Dr JN Khanna, MDS, Professor Emeritus of Maxillofacial Surgery, Mahatma Gandhi Mission's Dental College, Navi Mumbai, Maharashtra, India, and pioneering maxillofacial surgeon of the international fame; Dr DS Gupta, MDS, Former Professor of Maxillofacial Surgery, Government Dental College, Nagpur, Maharashtra, India; and my postgraduate guides, who have been my mentors, teachers and role models.

In my professional career, I have come across many great personalities who not only taught me but also most importantly constructively criticized me; and because of them, I could learn not only basics but also advances in maxillofacial surgery. To name some of them Dr SV Golhar, MS; Ex-Professor of ENT, Jawaharlal Nehru Medical College; Dr SN Jajoo, MS, MCH, Plastic Surgery and Professor, Jawaharlal Nehru Medical College; and Dr R Narang, Professor Emeritus, Mahatma Gandhi Institute of Medical Science, Sewagram, Wardha, Maharashtra, India. I wish to acknowledge these great personalities with deep sense of humility and gratitude.

I would like to express my sincere gratitude to Shri Jitendar P Vij (Group Chairman), Mr Ankit Vij (Managing Director), Mr Tarun Duneja (Director-Publishing), Mrs Samina Khan (PA to Director), Mr KK Raman (Production Manager); Mr Sunil Kumar Dogra (Production Executive), Mr Neelambar Pant (Production Coordinator), Mr Akhilesh Kumar Dubey (Proofreader), Mr Ashutosh Pathak (Proofreader), Mr Manoj Pahuja (Graphic Designer), Mr Vijay Singh (Graphic Designer), Mr Dilip Kumar (Typesetter), Dr Shyam Chaudhary (Commissioning Editor, Nagpur office) and staff of M/s Jaypee Brothers Medical Publishers (P) Ltd, New Delhi, India, for expressing personal interest to bring the book in the present form.

Last but not least, I am indebted to Datta Meghe Institute of Medical Sciences (Deemed University), its Chancellor and office bearers, for showing faith in me and providing me suitable environments, facilities, support and encouragement to progress.

Contents

Section 1: Principles of Surgery

Section 6: Infections of Maxillofacial Region

Section 7: Maxillofacial Trauma

Section 8: Facial Deformities

Section 9: Temporomandibular Joint

Section 10: Neoplastic Conditions of Head, Neck and Face

Section 1

Principles of Surgery

- Basic Principles of Surgery
- Sutures
- Incisions in Maxillofacial Surgery
- Fluid, Electrolyte Balance and Acid-base Equilibrium
- Shock
- Medical Emergencies in the Clinical Practice
- Management of Airway in Maxillofacial Surgery
- Biomedical Waste Management

1 Basic Principles of Surgery

Borle Rajiv M, Rai Anshul, Yadav Abhilasha

INTRODUCTION

The basic principles of surgery remain same to any branch of surgery, including the oral and maxillofacial surgery. A surgeon must have apt knowledge of anatomy, applied physiology, pathological conditions and more importantly, a very sound technique and skills. The skills are acquired through extensive practice. A correct diagnosis is the key to successful treatment. There can be a variety of treatment modalities for a single disease, but the diagnosis has to be single and accurate. Hence, sincere and thorough approach to history taking and clinical examination is required and there cannot be a shortcut to these procedures. A surgeon must train his eyes, fingers and mind and should believe in them rather than relying totally on investigations. The investigations are of great importance in making proper diagnosis, but they cannot be a substitute for the clinical methodology and skills. Even for ordering the relevant investigations a clinical diagnosis is required. Every case should be considered as a new challenge as the patient's response to a given pathology and treatment could be different. A surgeon must have regard for asepsis, sterilization, tissue respect and for all the basic principles of surgery to achieve good results, because, the result of a good surgery can get spoiled due to infection and sometimes it may prove fatal. The antibiotics are a great help in controlling the infection, but they are not a substitute for aseptic principle. Similarly, tissue respect is also of immense importance in achieving the desirable outcome of surgery.

ASEPSIS AND STERILIZATION

The surgical procedures have been revolutionized from the antiseptic methods of Joseph Lister (1865), to the aseptic technique of today. Every effort is made to prevent the entry of germs into a surgical wound by sterilization of instruments, material used for surgery and preparation of the environments. The success of surgery including the quality of healing of the wound, the amount of local and constitutional reaction, morbidity to the patient following the surgery depends upon not only the surgical skill but also upon the care exercised by the surgeon and his team during the patient care.

ASEPTIC TECHNIQUE

The word 'asepsis' means absence of sepsis (infection). The aseptic technique accurately describes the series of practices employed to prepare environment, the personnel and the patient before the surgery. It is impossible to sterilize the air and personnel in the operating room. The term sterilization describes the procedures employed to prepare the instruments, supplies and certain other inanimate objects (motor, hand piece, etc.) used to perform surgical procedure. These practices are designed to achieve total absence of all living microorganisms and are referred to as 'sterile technique'.

STERILIZATION

Sterilization is a procedure by which we make an instrument or surface free from all vegetative bacteria, spores, fungi, including the viruses. This can be achieved by:

- **Physical methods:** Dry heat, moist heat, UV light, ionizing radiations, etc.
- **Chemical methods**: Formaldehyde, phenolics, quaternary ammonium compounds, chlorhexidine, sodium hypochlorite, ethylene dioxide, glutaraldehyde, etc.

Dry Heat Sterilization

Heat is the most reliable method of sterilization. The moist heat is more effective than dry heat.

Open Flaming

The instruments are held over the open spirit flame. This method is simple, not requiring any special equipment. It is particularly useful in villages, domiciliary services or in emergency when other methods are not available. The large instrument trays, surgical trolley tops can be

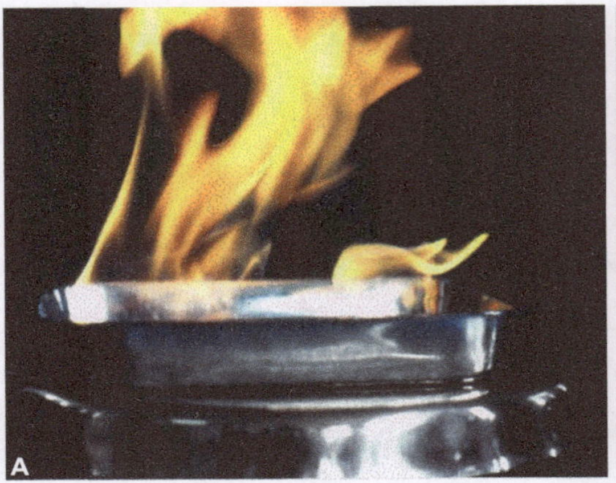

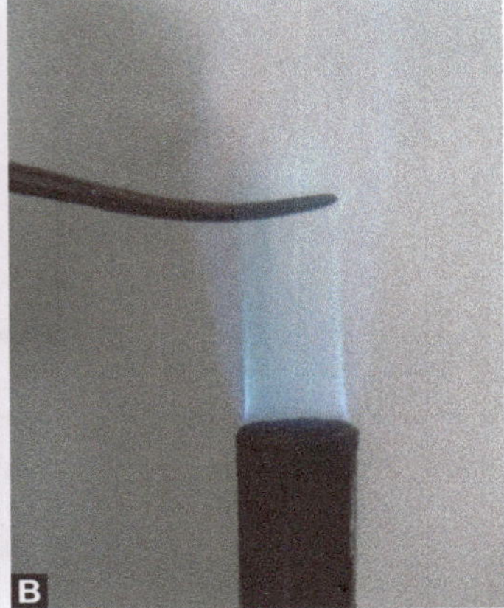

Figs 1.1A and B: Open flaming

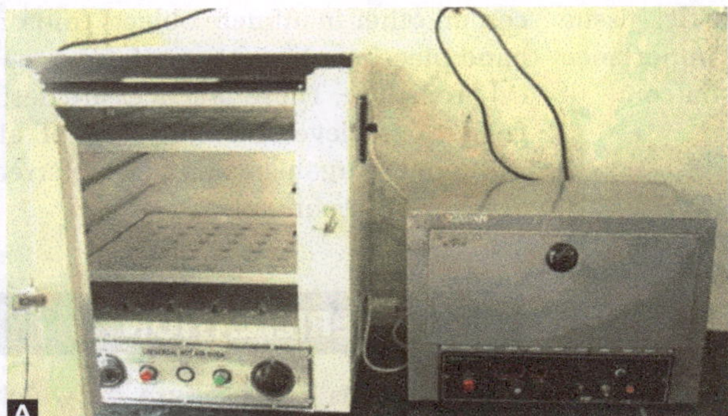

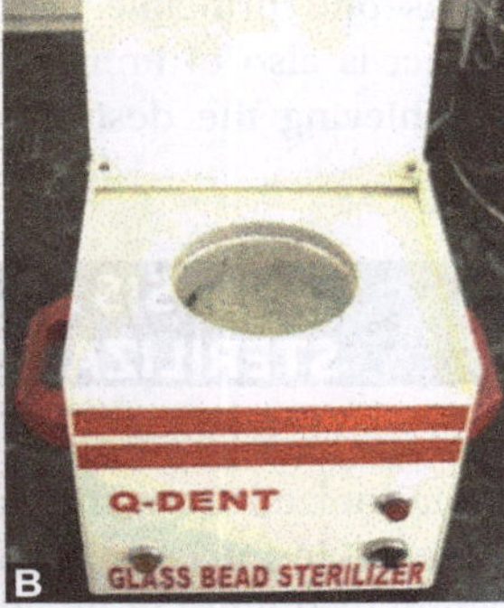

Figs 1.2A and B: Hot air oven and glass bead sterilizer

disinfected with this means. However, it is no more practiced in the clinical practice due to its unreliability (Figs 1.1A and B).

Hot Air Oven

This is the means of dry heat sterilization (Figs 1.2A and B). This method is widely used for the articles like anhydrous oils, petroleum products, talcum powder, etc. which cannot be penetrated by steam. The conventional ovens are electrically heated and a blower forces the hot air in motion around the items to hasten up the heating and to ensure uniform temperature in all the corners of the oven. The early models attained the temperature of 160° to 170°C for 2 hours. The fast table top models attain the temperature of 190° to 204°C with a total cycle time of 6 minutes for unwrapped items and 12 minutes for the wrapped items.

The temperature cycles for dry heat sterilization are as shown in Table 1.1.

Table 1.1: Time, temperature cycle in an oven

Temperature	Time
121°C	6–12 hours
140°C	3 hours
150°C	2½ hours
160°C	2 hours
170°C	1 hours

Articles that can be sterilized

Metallic instruments, powders, oils, greases, culture media and glass articles.

Advantages

- Does not corrode the instruments.
- It is simple.

Disadvantages

- It is time consuming
- Sharp instruments are rendered dull and brittle
- Rubber gloves, plastic, PVC rubber articles cannot be sterilized.

Moist Heat Sterilization

The moist heat is more effective means of sterilization than the dry heat. The methods of using moist heat as a means of sterilization are:

Boiling

The temperature of boiling water does not rise above 100°C (212°F) and thus, only vegetative microorganisms are killed and the bacterial spores may survive this procedure. Before the instruments are put in a boiler, it is desirable to clean all the instruments of dried, crusted secretions, blood and rust as they tend to prevent the penetration of the heat and thus, render the process of sterilization ineffective. It is achieved by thorough cleansing of the instruments by washing, scrubbing, use of fat solvents and ultrasonic cleaning.

The instruments to be sterilized are dipped in boiling water for a period of one hour. Sodium carbonate (2%) may be added to the water for alkalinization which elevates the boiling point of water, reduces sterilization time and prevents corrosion of instruments by reducing O_2 content of water. Earlier boiling was a method of choice, however, it must be remembered that it is only intermediate level disinfection and its reliability is doubtful in this era of HIV and Hepatitis.

Articles that can be sterilized

- Surgical instruments
- Catheters
- Syringes, needles.

Advantage

It is simple and economical.

Disadvantages

- Not reliable
- Instruments tend to get corroded
- Time consuming
- Sharp instruments tend to get dull.

Autoclaving

This is the means of moist heat sterilization. It is a method of choice for sterilization of instruments as it reliably eliminates even resistant, spore forming microorganisms, fungi, viruses, along

Table 1.2: Time, temperature and pressure cycle in an autoclave

Pressure	Temperature	Time
15 psi	121°C	30 minutes
20 psi	134°C	3–5 minutes (Flash method)

with vegetative microorganisms. It works on the principle of 'steam under pressure'. It provides moist heat in the form of saturated steam under pressure. The pressure increases the boiling point of water. Roughly for every 5 lbs. pressure, the boiling point of water rises by 10°C by increasing the latent heat of energy for boiling of water. Hence, at 15 lbs. pressure the boiling point of water rises to 121°C.

The temperature pressure and sterilization time cycle is as shown in Table 1.2.

Mechanism of action

The steam is the mixture of heat and water vapor. When it comes in contact with any cool surface, it gets condensed and heat is released from water. This heat is taken up by the surface it comes in contact with. The heat goes on penetrating in the deeper layers of the object. Hence, the steam must come in contact with the objects that are to be sterilized and thus, the objects must not be sealed in plastic wrappers or in the non-porous metallic containers. The steam and the air move in vertical direction and therefore the movement will be quicker and thereby the penetration of the steam into the material will also be better if the articles are placed vertically in the autoclave.

Procedure

The clinician must be well acquainted with the various parts of the autoclave and their operation. The autoclaves can be vertically or horizontally loading (Figs 1.3A and B). High speed autoclaves capable of producing more pressure and the temperature thus, completing the cycle in less time are available. The articles to be sterilized are first thoroughly cleaned with tap water, spirit and solvents like ether. All the blood stains, rust should be cleaned meticulously. The instruments should be wrapped in muslin, paper or linen pouches, commercially available autoclaving pouches, porous cassettes or gauze before putting them in surgical drum. The articles should be kept loosely in the chamber/drum to facilitate proper circulation of the steam. The articles/material which require more time for sterilization must be kept on the upper part of the drum since steam penetration starts earlier in the upper part than the lower part. The muffler of the drum is eased and the perforated body of the drum (steam inlets) is exposed to facilitate the entry of steam into the drum (Figs 1.4A and B). Once the heating source is started, all the air in the autoclave should be allowed to escape by opening the outlet valve as the heated air becomes lighter it escapes through the open valve readily and the autoclave gets filled with pure, saturated steam. The saturated steam is more lethal to the microorganisms than the mixture of air and steam. The air is a bad conductor of the heat and if it surrounds the article/instruments in the drum the penetration of the heat will be adversely affected. Once the desirable pressure is achieved then the

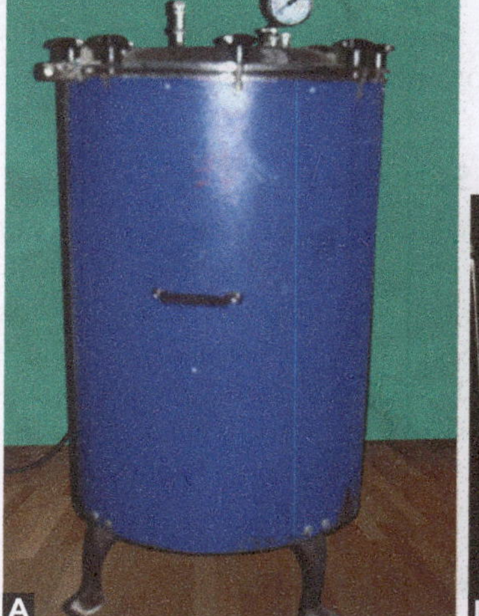

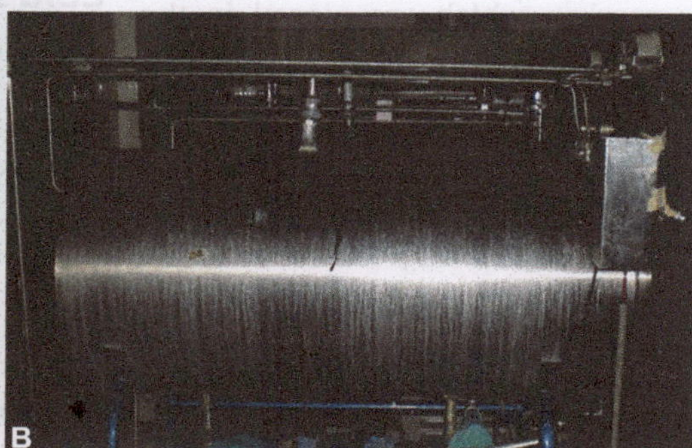

Figs 1.3A and B: (A) Vertical loading autoclaves; (B) Front loading autoclaves

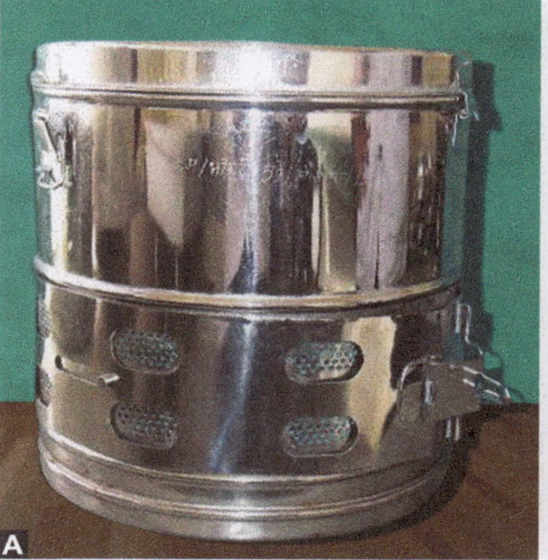

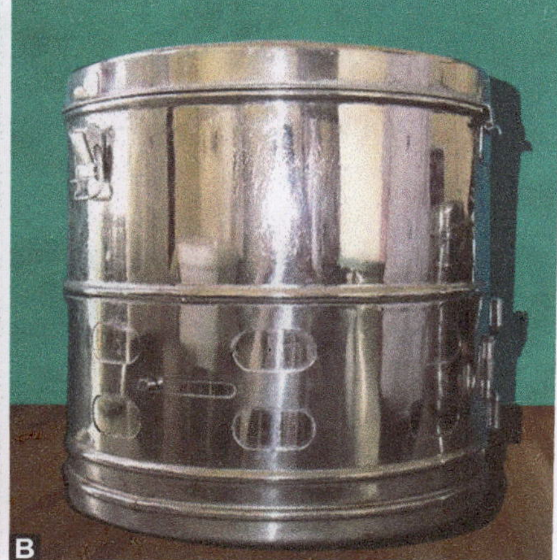

Figs 1.4A and B: (A) Dressing drum with open muffler showing perforations in the body of the drum for entry of the steam; (B) Muffler is closed covering the perforated area of the drum to prevent contamination

time should be counted and depending on pressure the autoclaving should be continued till the prescribed time is completed. The autoclave lid must be closed tightly and it should not be opened until the steam is evacuated and the inside pressure is brought down to normal by opening the escape/ release valve, after completion of the procedure to prevent accidental blowing of lid. The muffler of the drum should be immediately closed after the autoclaving is over, to prevent the entry of microorganisms in the sterile drum. During the autoclaving care should be taken to prevent entry of boiling water into the drum, as it tends to corrode the instruments. To achieve full quality of sterilization the temperature, pressure and time must be followed. Nowadays autoclaving indicators (chemical and biological indicators) are available in the market, which are placed in the drums during autoclaving, their color change is an indicator of complete sterilization (Fig. 1.5). These indicator strips may be preserved and pasted in the autoclave registers as a record and proof of autoclaving for medicolegal purpose. The autoclaved drums must be handled by aseptic care. Normally, the contents of sterile drum remain sterile for about 48 hours, however with increased handling this time decreases rapidly.

Articles that can be sterilized

Instruments, gauze, cotton, linen, needles, syringes, catheters, drains, autoclavable hand pieces, gloves, etc.

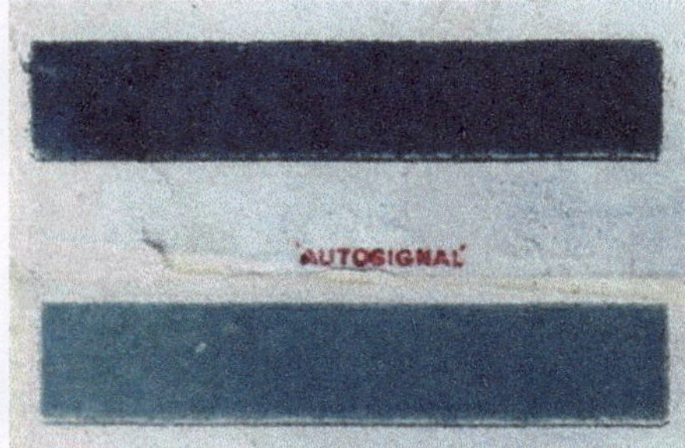

Fig. 1.5: Chemical indicator strips, showing the color change from green to black

Articles that cannot be sterilized

Powders, oils, greases, thermolabile material like electrical cords of micro-motors, fiberoptic cable, etc.

Advantages

- Simple
- Economical
- Reliable.

Disadvantages

- Tends to corrode the instruments
- Makes sharp instruments dull.

Chemiclaving

It is also called chemical vapor sterilization. A combination of formaldehyde, alcohols, acetone, ketones and steam at 138 KPa (combination available commercially) is used.

Cold Sterilization

Articles to be sterilized are immersed in the chemicals for achieving sterilization. The commonly used agents for chemical sterilization are absolute alcohol, carbolic acid 2 percent, glutraldehyde 2 percent (Cidex), formaldehyde, chlorhexidine gluconate, ethylene trioxide (ETO), etc.

Articles that can be sterilized

Sharp instruments like scissors, blades and suturing needles.

The following articles can be sterilized in ETO chamber, as immersion in liquids may spoil them.

- Splints
- Templates
- Handpieces
- Fibrooptic cables
- Micromotor cords, etc.

Articles that cannot be sterilized

Gauze, cotton, gloves, indwelling catheters, syringes, hypodermic needles, etc.

Advantages

- Simple
- Thermolabile articles can be sterilized
- Does not make sharp instruments dull.

Disadvantages

- It is not cost effective
- It tends to corrode the instruments
- It is time consuming.
- The residue of chemicals may be carried to the tissues along with the instruments during the surgery, which can evoke undesirable tissue reactions.

ANTISEPTIC SOLUTIONS

Relative Terms in Disinfection Level

Antisepsis

It is the process to kill pathogenic organisms in the environment of the patient. The process may be either bactericidal or bacteriostatic.

Disinfection

It is the process to kill pathogenic organisms from inanimate objects such as surgical instruments.

Antiseptic agent

It is a chemical which either kills pathogenic organisms or inhibits their growth so long as there is contract between the agent and microbe. In general, the term 'antiseptic' is reserved for agents applied to the living body surfaces.

Asepsis

It is the process by which environment of the patient is protected from contact with infective organisms.

Disinfectant

It is a germicidal chemical substance used on inanimate objects (non-living objects) to kill pathogenic micro-organisms but not necessarily all others.

Various Commercially Available Products

Korsolex®

- Gluteraldehyde–7 g
- 1,6 dihydroxy 2,5 dioxahexane–8.2 g (chemically bound formaldehyde)
- Polymethyl urea derivatives–17.6 g
- Rust inhibitors (trade secrets).

Prepared solution remains effective (viable) for 15 days.

For disinfection—5 percent for 30 minutes.

For sterilization—10 percent for 5 hours.

Sterillium

Alcoholic rub—it is used as a hand disinfectant.

Composition

- 2-Propanolol: 45 g
  1-Propanolol: 30 g
- Ethyl hexa decyl dimethyl ammonium ethyl sulphate: 0.2 g
- Skin protecting substances.

It is available in calibrated dispensers. For the hand disinfection 3 mL solution to be rubbed for 30 seconds.

Dettol®

Composition

- Chloroxylenol : 4.8 percent
- Terpineol : 9 percent
- Absolute alcohol: 13.1 percent

It is commonly used as a disinfectant in the clinics and for the household purposes. In a lesser strength it is used as an antiseptic solution.

Lysol®,[1] (Concentrated Cresol Solution)

Color

Dark brown.

Dilution and use

1:100 in water. It is used for sterilization of sharp instruments, e.g. suturing needles, knives, scissors, etc.

Time

Thirty minutes for 100 percent solution (i.e. undiluted) and 1 to 2 hours for 1:100 solution.

Special remarks

Lysol is an irritant chemical and causes burns when it comes in contact with the skin. Instruments should be cleansed with sterile water before use.

Weak Iodine Solution

Composition

Iodine tincture IP	66.2 percent
Alcohol	65 percent to 48 percent v/v

Use

Preoperative painting (preparation) of the skin.

Special remarks

- Iodine should be wiped with spirit after 2 minutes of painting.
- Idiosyncrasy may occur in sensitive patient.
- Alcohol increases the permeability of the iodine.
- Savlon decreases iodine's efficiency due to its detergent action.
- Iodine-spirit is the best preparation for painting.
- It kills 90 percent of skin bacteria in one and a half minutes.

Savlon®,[2] (Hospital Concentrate)

Composition

Chlorhexidine gluconate	7.5% v/v
Strong cetrimide	16% w/v
Isopropyl alcohol	6.8% v/v.

Color

Tartrazine (yellow).

Properties and effects

Germicide and detergent.

Dilution and uses

1:100 (aqueous) solution

10 mL of Savlon is made up to 1 liter with water.

Uses

- Cleaning and disinfection of the equipment in the vicinity of the patient
- Storage of previously sterilized instrument
- Cleaning and disinfection of the postoperative wounds
- Swabbing in obstetrics, gynecology and urology
- Aseptic management of burns
- Scrubbing
- Cleaning and disinfection of the instrument (Immerse for 30 minutes)
- Prolonged storage of clinical thermometer.

1:30 (aqueous) solution

35 mL of Savlon is made up to 1 liter with water.

Uses

- Cleaning and disinfection of physically dirty wounds where extra detergent (action) is required
- Cleaning and disinfection of used catheters and appliances.

1:30 in 70 percent alcohol solution

35 mL of Savlon is mixed with 200 mL water and made up to 1 liter with 95 percent alcohol.

Uses

- Skin disinfection (preoperative and other invasive procedures)
- Emergency disinfection of clean instruments and equipment (immerse for 2 minutes)
- Disinfection of clinical thermometers.

Remarks

- Sodium nitrate (4% or four 1 g tablets per liter) should be added to the solution to prevent rusting.
- The solution should be changed weekly.
- Syringes and needles that have been immersed in the Savlon solution should be rinsed very carefully with sterile water before use.
- Instruments containing mirrors or other cemented glass components should not be immersed in Savlon solution.
- Prolonged immersion of rubber appliances in Savlon is not recommended.

Phenol®

Composition

0.5 percent carbolic acid.

Properties and effects

It is dark pink in color and a strong irritant and caustic. Pure form may cause skin burns.

Uses

- Disinfection of sharp instruments. In 100 percent solution, the instruments should be immersed for 2 to 3 hours and in 20 percent solution for 24 hours.
- Disinfection during cholera epidemic for disposal of excreta.
- Chemical sympathetic block (phenol in almond oil is used)
- Diluted solution is used for disinfection of dog bite wounds.
- Carbolization (cauterization) of appendicular stump and polyps.
- Phenol has antipruritic potential, so it is used in certain skin lotions.
- Phenol in almond oil is used as an injection treatment for the first degree of internal piles.
- Two percent carbolic acid solution is used to carbolize (disinfect) the objects in the OR and wards like trolleys, OR table, Boyle's machine, etc.

Hydrogen Peroxide (H_2O_2)

Composition

Twenty volume hydrogen peroxide (one volume of 20 volume hydrogen peroxide solution releases 20 volume of nascent oxygen).

Properties and effects

It is not an antiseptic but a cleansing agent.

Mechanism of action and uses

- It destroys anaerobic organisms by releasing nascent oxygen and therefore used for cleaning the wounds infected or contaminated with anaerobes.
- It produces frothing and brings out debris from the depth of the wound.
- It produces heat when it comes in contact with the tissues. So it prevents capillary oozing and hence it is used as hemostatic solution whenever there is capillary oozing, e.g. after incision and drainage. However, it is also believed that the infection passes to deeper tissue planes due to frothing.
- Used in cleaning wounds, bleaching, boils and as a throat spray and mouth wash. Very diluted form is used in ear syringing to remove wax and foreign body.
- Used to remove blood stains from clothes.

Spirit

Composition

Methyl alcohol (optimum concentration of 70 percent alcohol is highly effective).

Uses

- Disinfection of skin before intramuscular and intravenous injections.
- As a solvent for the removal of iodine in preparation of skin for operation.
- Cleaning the stiched wound.
- Cleaning the skin of the surrounding ulcer or open wounds.
- As it dissolves the greasy material, 50 percent spirit in water (gutta spirit) is used as ear drops.
- Used along with other disinfectants such as iodine-spirit and Cetavlon-spirit, for painting the parts before operation.

Formalin Solution

Composition

30 percent aldehyde plus 10 percent methane.

Concentration

38 to 40 percent w/v solution.

Uses

- Ten percent solution in water is used as preservative for biopsy specimens.[3]
- Operation theater sterilization (fumigation 40% solution).
- Two to five percent solution is used for sterilization of surgical gloves and instruments.
- Tablets of formalin are available, which are used in a chamber for the sterilization of thermolabile articles.

Eusol® (Edinburgh University Solution (BP)

Composition

1.25 g of boric acid, 1.25 g of bleaching powder (chlorinated lime), sterile water up to 100 mL.

Mechanism

It releases nascent chlorine and becomes useless after 24 hours.

Uses

- To separate slough from infected wounds, ulcers, bed-sores and burn wounds.[4]
- Acidic in pH, therefore it is very useful in wounds infected with pseudomonas bacteria.

Cidex®

Composition

Glutaraldehyde, 2 percent acidic solution.

Properties

It kills all pathogens. It is bactericidal, tuberculocidal, pseudomonacidal, viricidal and fungicidal.

Time

Complete disinfection in 10 minutes, sporicidal within 4 hours.

Uses

- Tray system of sterilization with cidex for large instruments, fiberoptic endoscopes with lenses.
- Sterilization of small and sharp instruments, catheters and thermometers.
- Sterilization of equipment of anesthesia and of inhalation therapy.

Special remarks

- Best disinfectant with rapid action.
- Cidex is effective even in the presence of protein material.
- Recommended time is 10 hours to take care of the deep crevices in the instruments.

Glycerine Magsulf Solution

Composition

Saturated solution of magnesium sulphate ($MgSO_4$) crystals and glycerine (sterile), the solution is boiled for a few minutes and then cooled.

Properties and uses

Since magnesium sulphate is hygroscopic, it pulls out the fluid from the edematous tissue across the skin or the mucosa, which acts as a semipermeable membrane and the mixture is exothermic producing vasodilatation which facilitates reabsorption of interstitial fluid from the edematous in the tissue thereby reducing edema. It is used to reduce edema in:

- Prolapsed thrombosed piles } Local applications
- Cellulitis } Local applications
- Paraphimosis and } Local applications
- This solution is used to give magnesium sulphate enema in order to reduce intracranial pressure.
- Glycerine has soothening action.

Turpentine IP

Properties

It is a highly irritant mineral oil.

Uses

- Diluted form is used to bring out and kill the maggots from the wounds and ears.[5]
- Used as a solvent to remove the zinc paste of sticking plaster from the skin.

Ether

Properties

It is evaporable, highly inflammable. It makes the surface cool.

Uses

- As surface and the inhalation anesthesia.
- Used to clean the dirty skin as it removes the greasy substances by dissolving them.
- Used as a solvent to remove the zinc paste of sticking plaster from the skin.

Gentian Violet

Concentration

Dilution of 1:100 and 1:1,000 are generally used.

Properties and effects

It coagulates the serous discharge on oozing surface and makes the ulcer dry.

Uses

To dress eczematous lesion with copious seropurulent discharge.

Undesirable effects

It colors the ulcer, so the progress of the healing becomes difficult to judge.

Acriflavine

Properties

It is available in crystals. It is yellow in color.

Concentration

0.5 to 2 percent solution made with sterile water.

Uses

- It is a mild antiseptic and astringent on ulcers with purulent discharge.
- Effective on wounds with gram negative bacteria.
- Acriflavine dressing on raw area is left after hemorrhoidectomy.

Potassium Permanganate ($KMnO_4$)

It has oxidizing effect. It is available in crystal form. 1:5000 to 1:10000 solution is made with water.

Uses

- Used as mouth wash, e.g. after tonsillectomy and in stomatitis. (Condy's gargles).
- Used for urinary bladder irrigation and wash.

Mercurochrome

Concentration

0.5 to 2 percent solution is made with water; it is available in crystal form.

Properties and effects

It is an inhibitor of 5-hydroxytryptamine (5-HT). Strong solution kills white blood cells (WBCs) and damages the granulation tissue. It has an astringent action.

Uses

- Used for bed sore dressing.
- Diluted solution is applied on wounds with healthy granulation.
- Strong solution is applied on wounds with hypergranulation.
- Applied on exomphalos awaiting surgery.
- Not used on non-healing ulcer, because it stains floor of the ulcer and hence makes it difficult to judge the progress of the healing ulcer.
- Diluted solution is used as eye drops.

Silver Nitrate ($AgNO_3$)

Concentration

Solutions with dilutions ranging from 1:100 to 1:10000 are available.

Special remarks

Impregnated cotton sticks are kept in dark container because, on exposure to light, silver nitrate gets destroyed.

Uses

- Chemical cauterization of warts and hyper/granulation tissue.
- Used for dressing burns (silver sulfadiazine)
- Useful in bladder irrigation in cases of hematuria, due to its cauterizing effect.

Chlorhexidine[6] (Hibitane® Concentrate)

Composition

Contains chlorhexidine gluconate, 5 percent w/v (equivalent to chlorhexidine gluconate solution, 25% v/v) (Table 1.3).

Table 1.3: Mechanism of action of different antiseptics (Ref–McDonnell and Russell. Antiseptic and disinfectants. Clin microbial Rev. 1999;12:148-58)

Name of antiseptic	Target	Mechanism of action
Aldehydes- • Gluteraldehyde	Cell wall, outer membrane	• Gram +ve bacteria and fungi—cross linking of proteins, Gram –ve bacteria—removal of Mg^{2+}, release of some phospholipids Virus—Inhibition of DNA synthesis
• Formaldehyde	DNA	• Reacts with carboxyl, sulfhydril and hydroxyl group also reacts with nucleic acids thus inhibit RNA and DNA synthesis by cross linking of proteins
• Chlorhexidine and quaternary ammonium compounds (cetrimide),	Cytoplasmic membrane	• Generalized membrane damage involving phospholipid bilayers. Low conc. affects membrane integrity and high conc. cause congealing of cytoplasm
• Phenols	Cytoplasmic membrane	• Leakage of K^{+} and other intracellular constituents, uncoupling of oxidative phosphorylation causing irreversible cell damage
• Halogen—chlorine releasing (hypochlorites, bleaching powder)	DNA	Inhibition of DNA synthesis
H_2O_2	DNA	Causes DNA strand breakage
Iodines	Proteins	Exact action unknown, enters the cell and attacks proteins (cysteine and methionine), nucleotides and fatty acids leading to cell death
Alcohol	Cell membrane	Rapid denaturation of proteins, interference with cell metabolism, leading to cell lysis

Color

Poceau 4R, red.

Dilution and uses

1:250 aqueous solution.

Uses

- Disinfection of equipment, furniture and fittings in the vicinity of the patient.
- Storage of sterile instruments.

Antiseptic Technique

Apply liberally the diluted solution on the surface of the article to be disinfected with clean (sterile) swab or cloth. Store sterile instruments by immersing in the diluted solution up to 8 hours; rinse with sterile water before use.

Dilution and uses

1:100 aqueous solution.

Disinfection of wounds and burns, skin swabbing in obstetric patients, washing of hands and scrubbing.

Technique

Apply the diluted solution liberally on the surface to be disinfected with a sterile swab.

1:10 solution in 70 percent alcohol.

Uses

- Preparative skin disinfection.
- Emergency disinfection of instruments.

Technique

Apply the diluted solution liberally on the surface to be disinfected with a sterile swab. Clean the instruments under running water. Immerse them in the solution for 2 minutes. Rinse in sterile water before use.

Cetavlon®

Composition

Cetrimide 0.5 percent w/v, rectified spirit equivalent to 62 to 68 percent v/v of absolute alcohol.

Color

Carmoisine + erythrosin (pink).

Precautions

It should not come in contact with brain, meninges or middle ear.

Dilution and uses

As per chlorhexidine—it should not be used in open wounds and burns because it contains spirit which is an irritant.

The other important use is as a scolicidal agent in the operation of hydatid cysts[7] of liver. After evacuating the cyst, 0.5 to 1 percent of cetrimide solution is instilled into the residual host cavity and left for 5 minutes. Then it is sucked out. Other scolicidal agents used are;

- Ten percent povidone-iodone (providex).
- Formalin solution–no longer used.
- Hypertonic saline.

Povidone–Iodine[8] (Betadine®)

Povidone-iodine (PVP-I) is a stable chemical complex of polyvinylpyrrolidone (povidone, PVP) and elemental iodine. It contains from 9.0 to 12.0 percent available iodine, calculated on a dry basis.

Products available

Povidone-iodine (5 and 10%) topical solutions, surgical scrub (7.5% w/v) mouthwash (gargle), povidone-iodine ointment, povidone-iodine vaginal pessaries.

Properties and effect

Iodine is recognized as an effective and useful germicide. It is very effective against a variety of microorganisms such as viruses, bacteria, protozoa, yeast and fungi. However, its frequent use is contraindicated because of its insolubility, instability and its staining and irritating properties.

Many of these undesirable qualities of iodine could be eliminated by combining it with polyvinylpyrrolidone (Povidon). This organic polymer is water-soluble. When it is combined with iodine, a complex is formed in which iodine's toxic properties are lost without its bactericidal activity being affected. This complex, povidone-iodine (polyvinylpyrrolidone iodine, abbreviated as PVP-1), has been used effectively as a surface disinfectant.

Povidone is an effective germicide. High dilutions are active in destroying organisms within 15 seconds. Color loss is accompanied by the weakening germicidal activity.

Advantages

- Broad spectrum of action with fungistatic action.
- Non-antibiotic
- Immediate action—nonselective
- Film forming
- Extremely safe.

Uses

- As mouth rinse and gargle for dryness of mouth and minor irritation and infections.
- As a local antiseptic and for wound dressing.
- Used for irrigation of bladder, wound (subcutaneous) pyothorax and intraperitoneal cavity.

CARE OF ANTISEPTIC SOLUTION

Do's

- Always use recommended dilutions before use, as directed.
- Always prepare dilutions in small volumes, preferably not more than 1 liter.
- Always use all diluted solutions within 8 hours and discard the remaining solution at the end of the working day.
- Always ensure that the mouth of the bottle is not touched by hands or other materials while pouring.

Do not's

- Never mix up old diluted solutions with the freshly prepared ones.
- Never leave diluted solutions for more than one working day.
- Never use corks for sealing the bottles.
- Never leave bottles open.

Precautions

- Instruments with glass or metal components should not be disinfected with hibitane.
- Sodium nitrate (0.1% w/v, i.e. 1 g tablet per liter) is added to instrument storage solutions to prevent rusting. The solution should be changed at weekly intervals.
- Instruments, especially syringes and needles that have been immersed in hibitane, should be thoroughly rinsed in sterile water before use.
- Prolonged immersion of rubber appliances in hibitane is undesirable.
- Hibitane concentrate (chlorhexidine) should not come in contact with brain, meninges or middle ear.

Ethylene Oxide (EO) Gas Sterilization[9]

Composition

- CFC-12 (12/88).
- HCFC-124 (OXYFUME 2000).
- 100 percent EO (67–134 g).
- EO/CO_2 (10/90).

Temperature (85–145°F)

Humidity (30–80%)

Advantages of EO Sterilization

- Heat sensitive articles can be sterilized
- Moisture sensitive articles can be sterilized
- Automatic control
- Leaves no film on the surface
- Permeates porous packaging material.

Disadvantages of EO Sterilization

- Slow process
- Expensive
- Hazardous with repeated use
- Vesicant and burns
- EO gas is mucosal irritant
- Potential carcinogen and mutagen
- Highly flammable and explosive.

EO Gas Sterilizer

The EO sterilizer has following components:

- Capacity of chamber (12 × 12 × 24 inches to 28 × 67 × 78 inches).
- Automatic control.
- Vacuum pumps.
- Steam ejector.
- Digital printer.
- Sterilizer and aerator.

Preparing Items for EO Gas

- Clean and dry.
- Disassemble detachable parts.
- Remove lubricant.
- Lensed instruments, cameras and films can also be sterilized.

Packaging material used for EO gas sterilizer are:

- Woven fabric.
- Non-woven fabric.
- Peel packs and pouches.

Hydrogen Peroxide Plasma Sterilization

Advantages of H_2O_2

- Dry and non-toxic
- Byproducts safely evacuated
- Aeration not required
- Low temperature
- Simple design of sterilizer
- Non-corrosive

Disadvantages of H_2O_2

- Metal tray block radiofrequency waves
- Not compatible with cellulose
- Nylon becomes brittle.

Ozone Gas Sterilization

Advantages of Ozone Gas Sterilizer

- Simple and inexpensive to operate
- Heat and moisture sensitive
- Safe with titanium, chromium, silicon and teflon
- Low temperature

- No aeration
- Leaves no residue-converts to O_2.

Disadvantages of Ozone Gas Sterilization

- Corrosive
- Oxidizes steel, brass, copper and aluminum
- Destroys natural rubber, latex, natural fibers and some plastics
- Stearothermophilus biologic indicators are required to assess the sterilization.
- Cycle time may be up to 60 minutes after which ozone is converted back to oxygen safely released in room air.

Handling of the Sterilized Instruments

The autoclaved instruments kept in the dressing drum need to be handled carefully to prevent contamination of the instruments and preserve the sterile environments inside the drum. The drum should be in good condition and the lid should be airtight. The drum should not be opened frequently and the lid should be closed immediately after removing the sterile instruments. The more the frequency of opening the lid the lesser the time for which the inside environments of the drum are likely to be sterile. The instruments must be removed using a sterile chital forceps. The chital forceps must be sterilized daily and must be preserved properly. A sterilized chital forceps must be kept in a sterilized container/bottle, which is long enough to cover at least two-third the length of the chital forceps as while picking up the sterile instruments from the sterile drum, about 2/3rd the length of the forceps will enter the depth of the drum and only the handle shall stay out (Figs 1.6A and B). The container should contain a sterile antiseptic solution (2% gluteraldehide or savlon, 1:100 (aqueous) solution (10 mL of Savlon is made up to 1 liter with water) When the glass bottles are used to store the sterile chital forceps, cotton wool is often added to the bottle containing the disinfectant solution. The cotton wool will soak the solution and settle at the bottom of the bottle. This is done because most of the times the chital forceps is just dropped in the bottle which hits the base of the bottle and may break it. The presence of cotton wool will prevent this and also prevent noise. The container should be sterilized daily and fresh solution should be prepared daily. The water used as solvent for the antiseptic solution should be boiled and then allowed to cool to the room temperature before the antiseptic agent is added, to avoid its precipitation.

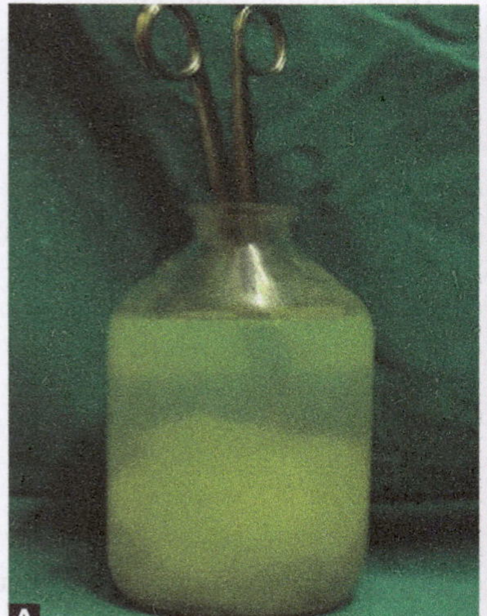

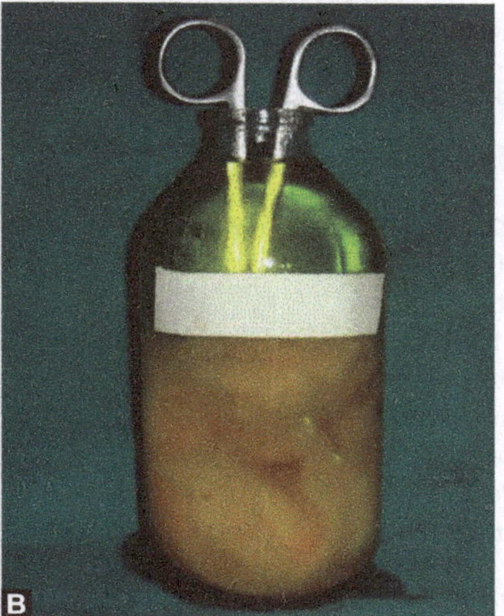

Figs 1.6A and B: The sterile chital forceps are immersed in sterile bottles containing antiseptic solution. Care should be taken to use longer bottles to ensure that 2/3rd length of the forceps is submerged

ASEPTIC TECHNIQUE

The word 'Asepsis' means lack of sepsis. It is the series of practices undertaken to prevent the entry of germs in the wound. This topic will be discussed under following heads:

- Planning and design of operating room.
- Preparation of environments in the operating room.
- Preparation of personnel.
  - Preparation of patient.
  - Preparation of surgical team.
- Disposal of hospital waste.

Planning and Design of Operating Room[10,11]

The location of operating room should be such that it is isolated from rest of the hospital units so that to and fro movement of the public is minimized. The air circulation and water supply must be separate. Separate overhead water tanks and separate pipelines should be laid for the operating room to prevent retrograde, cross infection from toilets and other units of hospital. The operating room (OR) should be constructed in such a way that it is divided into unrestricted (non-critical), semi-restricted (semi-critical) and restricted (critical) area (Box 1.1). This division prevents direct access into the operating room thus brings down the chances of infection. The unrestricted area is a barrier between the outside environments and the semi-restricted area. This unrestricted area harbors the preanesthetic room, office, changing rooms, etc. The outside clothing and foot wear is changed in this area before advancing into the semi- restricted area as the outside wears harbor lot of dust and germs. The personnel must change to sterile scrub suit and change the outside foot wear to the OR foot wear made up of rubber or plastic, which is easily washable and can be disinfected.

Box 1.1: Distribution of various zones in operating room

Non-restricted area
Pre-anesthetic room
Offices
Store
Toilets
Changing areas
Semi-restricted area
Surgeon rooms
Anesthetist rooms
Nurses room
Recovery rooms
Endoscopy room
Minor OR
Restricted area
Operating room (OR)
Scrub area
Sterile storage room
Surgical ICU

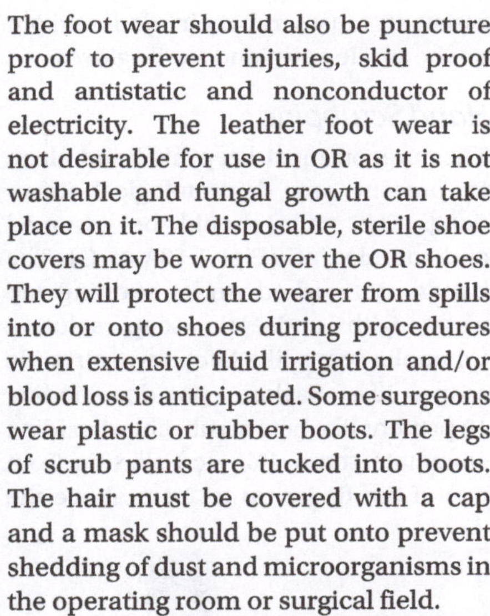

The foot wear should also be puncture proof to prevent injuries, skid proof and antistatic and nonconductor of electricity. The leather foot wear is not desirable for use in OR as it is not washable and fungal growth can take place on it. The disposable, sterile shoe covers may be worn over the OR shoes. They will protect the wearer from spills into or onto shoes during procedures when extensive fluid irrigation and/or blood loss is anticipated. Some surgeons wear plastic or rubber boots. The legs of scrub pants are tucked into boots. The hair must be covered with a cap and a mask should be put onto prevent shedding of dust and microorganisms in the operating room or surgical field.

The non-restricted (non-critical) area of the operating room (OR) is where the patients are shifted from the ward on a stretcher to the preanesthetic room for the surgery. The outside stretcher should never cross beyond this area to enter into the semi-restricted area. In the preanesthetic room, the patient's feet are covered with foot covers (leggings) and hair are also covered with caps, before shifting into semi-restricted or restricted area. The patient is essentially shifted on another stretcher, which plies between the restricted area and the non-restricted area and in no case goes out of the OR complex.

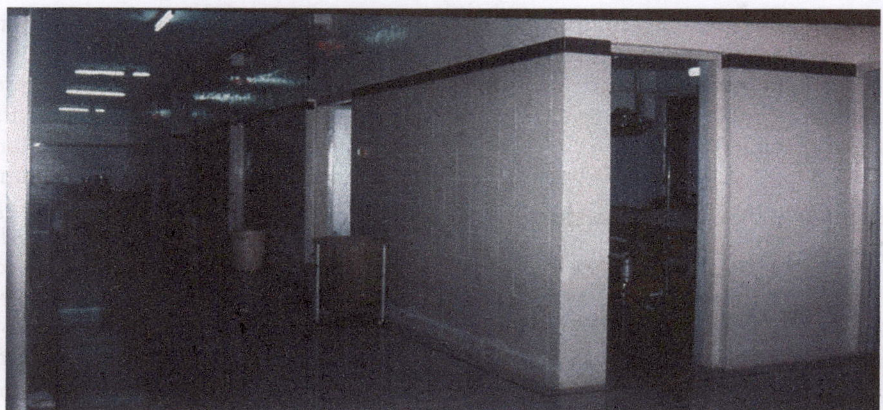

Fig. 1.7A: Inside of the operating room

The semi-restricted (semi-critical) area contains endoscopy rooms, sterilization rooms and sterile store room, postoperative recovery, etc. and serves as a barrier between the unrestricted and restricted area.

The restricted area is a critical area where actual operating rooms are present. Scrub rooms for scrubbing the hands and areas for putting on the sterile gowns and gloves are located outside the main operating room in the critical area.

Designing of an Operating Room

The size of the operating room should be adequate for housing all the equipment and accessories. It should allow free movement of the surgical team members. Ideally the size of the OR should not be less than 500 sq ft. The operating room should be designed in such a way that the floors and walls should be absolutely plain and easily cleanable (Fig. 1.7A). They must not harbor dust, dirt and microorganisms. The material selected for making floor should have smooth finish and should have minimum and neatly made or no joints. The material used for the flooring should be non-porous, scratch proof, antiskid and antistatic (epoxy resin flooring). The walls should also be covered with smooth material like granite with minimum joints. The ideal OR room walls should be of stainless steel without sharp line angles and the corners should be molded round. The ceilings should be painted with oil paints, which give smooth finish. The walls and the floor should be washable. No offsets or projections are permitted in OR. All the electrical fittings and water pipelines in the OR must be concealed. Ceiling fans are not permitted as the blades of the fan harbor dust and when they are switched on the dust gets splashed in the surgical field. The use of exhaust fans in the OR is prohibited and if they are used they should have unidirectional air ducts to prevent entry of dust in the OR. The OR should have airconditioning and use of pedestal fans should be avoided.

The OR complex should have only one entry and all the windows should be air tight. This prevents multi-directional air flow and entry of dust in the OR. The doors of the operation theater complex which exist between critical area, semi-critical and non-critical area must not be in single line to break the air velocity. The operating room must have unidirectional air flow (desirably lamellar air flow with micro and HEPA filters) with air flow velocity of 2 meters/minute, as greater air velocity facilitates transport of light dust particles. The temperature in the OR must be maintained to around 20°C and relative humidity should be less than 40 percent. Higher temperature and humidity facilitates the growth of microorganism and fungi. If the environments are unpleasant, hot and humid they are tiring to the surgeon and his team. More importantly, it also tends to desiccate the exposed tissue during the surgery. It is impossible to sterilize the air, however, efforts must be made to prevent entry and restrict the growth of microorganism, both vegetative and spore forming (Box 1.1).

Preparation of Operating Room

Before commissioning the operating complex a thorough washing and dusting is required. All the walls and inanimate objects are carbolized with 2 percent carbolic acid solution. The operating room is fumigated with the help of 40 percent formaldehyde (350 mL) added with $KMnO_4$ (174 g) for a room measuring 1,000 cu Ft. This mixture procedures an exothermic reaction and should be kept in a stainless steel bowl in the OR. The fumes rapidly spread in the OR and kill the microorganisms. The OR should be closed in an air tight manner during this procedure and sealed from outside to prevent leakage of fumes. When it is done for the first time the OR should be kept closed for 48 hours and for repeated weekly fumigation it can be kept closed for 24 hours. Mechanical fumigators are also available in which 500 mL of 40 percent formaldehyde and 500 mL of water is used for a room measuring thousand cubic feet (Fig. 1.7B). The machine is switched on and kept operating overnight. When the formaldehyde and $KmNO_4$ solution is used, it should not be kept near bottles of ether, spirit or any other inflammable substance as this exothermic reaction can precipitate accidents due to fire. After the OR is opened the fumes are allowed to settle by opening the vents of the airconditioning system (aeriation time) and then swabs are taken from different sites like floor, walls, operating table. Trolleys, etc. of OR (two from each site) and these swabs are subjected to microbiology lab for aerobic and anaerobic culture to detect dreadful microorganism like *pseudomonas, Clostridium tetani, Clostridium welchii.* The OR can be commissioned only after obtaining the negative report from microbiology laboratory. If the OR is found to be contaminated with these dreaded organisms the OR should be closed and rewashing, fumigation and disinfection of the OR should be done. Periodic maintenance of the OR should be done by daily dusting swabbing and weekly washing and fumigation. The swabs used for cleaning the OR should be earmarked for the OR and in no case should be used for swabbing other areas. Similarly the outside swabs should never be permitted in the OR. The floor of the OR should be washed with soap and antiseptic solution like sodium hypochlorite of any other disinfectant like phenolics (phenyl).

Fig. 1.7 B: Mechanical fumigator

Preparation of Personnel

It is impossible to disinfect personnel and their entry in the OR. However, the precautions are taken to minimize the contamination due to personnel in the OR. As mentioned earlier the outside clothing and foot wear must be change to a scrub suit and OR footwear and the hair and nose, mouth should be covered with the cap and mask respectively before entering into the critical area of the OR. The specification for the cloth to be used for making the masks, gowns and drapes is that it should be made up of cotton having a thread count of 240/sq inch to 270/sq inch for the reusable stuff and spunbond oleifin for disposables ones. The colors is usually green for better visibility (Figs 1.8A and B). The special scrub suit to be worn as a part of universal precaution kit consists of water resistant material and has double-layered protection (Fig. 1.9). Before performing the surgery the surgeon and assistants must scrub their hands and put on the sterile gown and sterile gloves.

Hand Scrubbing

The surgeon must keep his hand clean to prevent any dermatological infections. The nails should be trimmed and rounded off (Figs 1.10A to C). The hands are washed under running tap water with antiseptic soap solution (phenolic soaps like Lifebuoy, cetrimide soaps like Savlon, povidon iodine 10 percent like beta scrub, chlorhexidine gluconate scrub 4%, etc.) starting from tips of the finger up to 2 cm above the

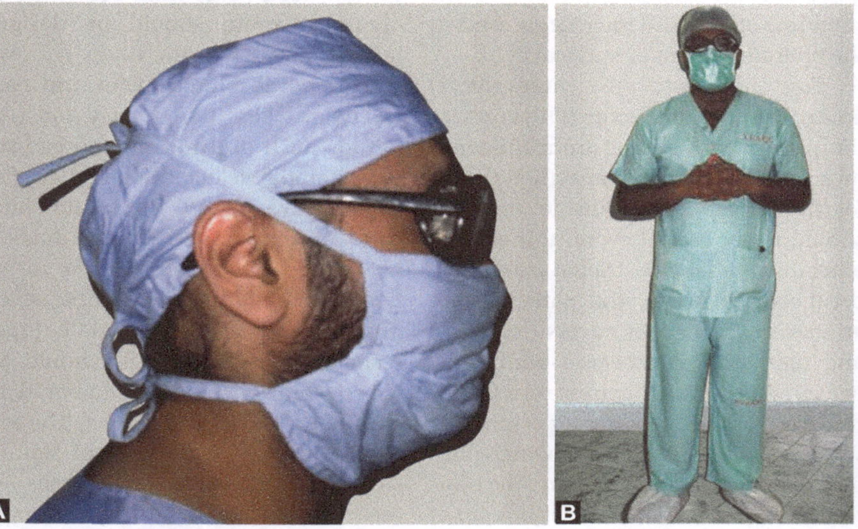

Figs 1.8A and B: Cap, mask, eye wear and scrub suit

elbow (Figs 1.11A to F). Foam is generated by vigorous scrubbing the nail beds and clean with soft brush kept in a sterile container containing antiseptic solutions. The method followed for the hand scrubbing is the "Time-Stroke method". The time is about 3 minutes and the strokes applied at different sites of the palm (Fig. 1.11) range between 20 to 30 strokes at each site. The purpose of this exercise is to make the hands surgically clean by removing dirt and colonies of vegetative microorganisms from the skin creases, hair and nail beds thus reducing the count of microorganism as it is impossible to sterilize the hands (Fig. 1.12A). During this whole exercise, hands are held at a higher level than the elbow to prevent the water from contaminated arms to roll back on the cleaned forearms and hands (*see* Fig. 1.10).

Fig. 1.9: The universal precaution suit

The scrub area sink should be wide enough to facilitate easy scrubbing without touching anywhere and it should have depth of about 3 feet, which prevents splashing of rebound water onto the clean hands (Fig. 1.12B). The scrub sinks are fitted with doctors' taps (Fig. 1.12B) rather than ordinary taps, to facilitate its operation with the help of arms to prevent contamination of scrubbed hands during closing the tap. The peddle operated taps are ideal in scrub areas as it permits hand

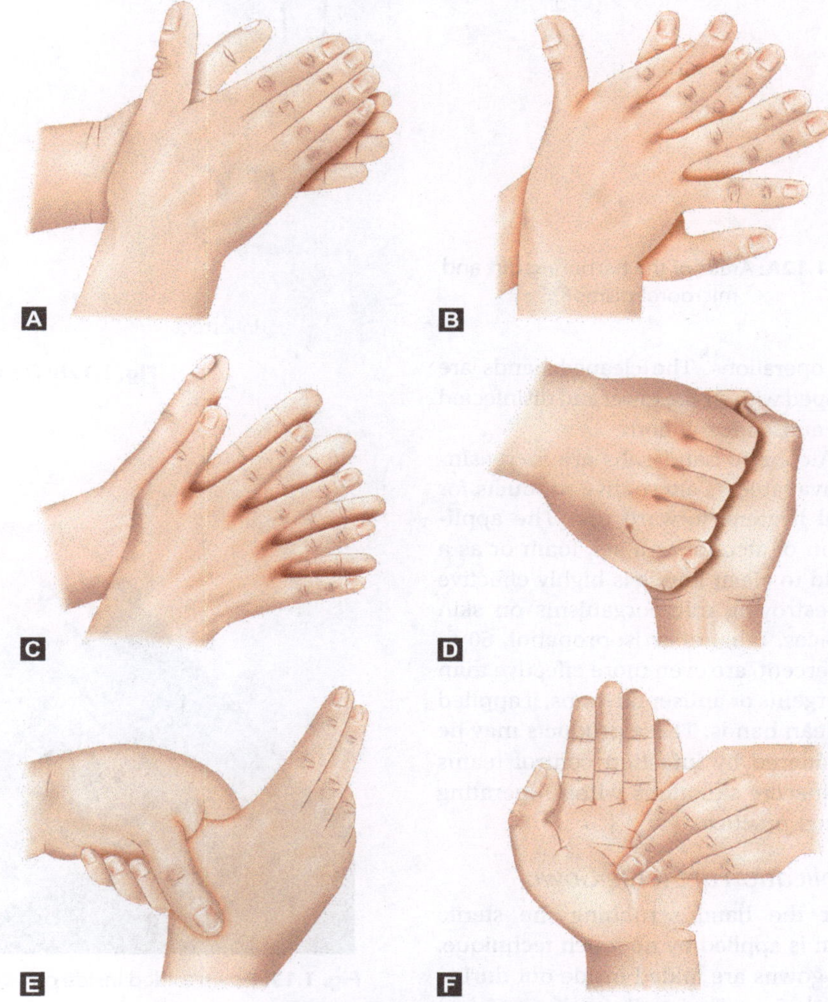

Figs 1.11A to F: Strokes during hand scrubbing

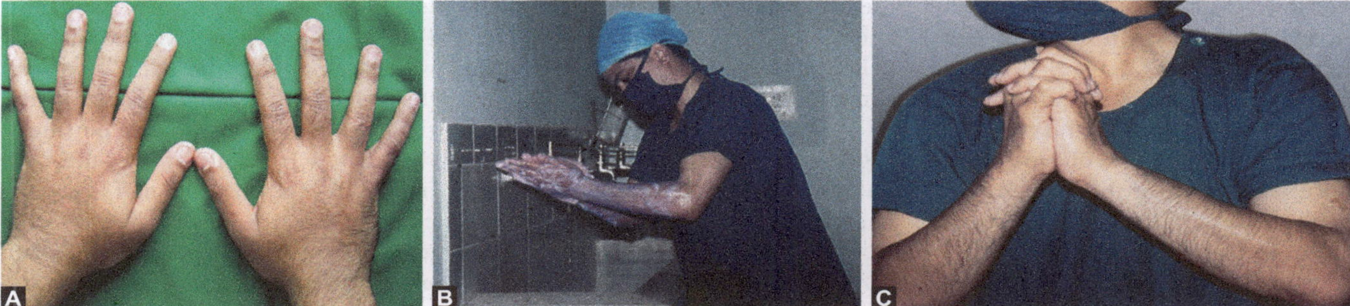

Figs 1.10A to C: (A) Watch the hands, nails trimmed and rounded off; (B) Surgical scrub; (C) Holding the hands up so that the water trickles down the elbows

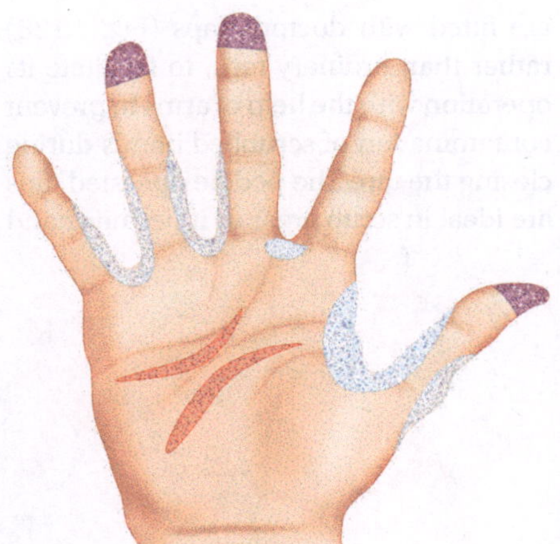

Fig. 1.12A: Areas of the harboring dirt and microorganisms

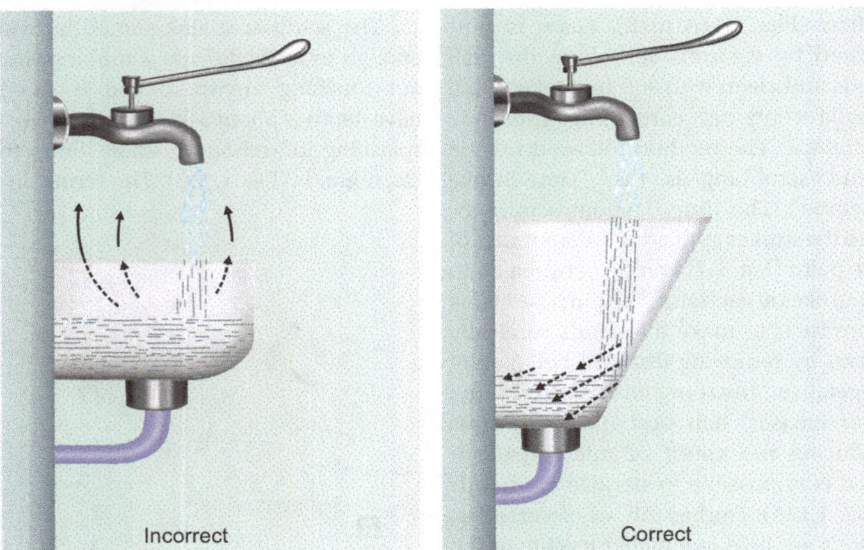

Fig. 1.12B: Design of the washing sink

free operations. The cleaned hands are mopped with sterile towel and disinfected with antiseptic solution.

Alcoholic hand rubs are increasingly available as alternative products for hand hygiene forward use. The application of alcohol as a gel, foam or as a liquid to clean hands is highly effective at destroying microorganisms on skin surfaces. Ethanol or isopropanol, 60 to 80 percent, are even more effective than detergents or antiseptic soaps, if applied to clean hands. These products may be considered by infection control teams for specific situations within operating theater practice.

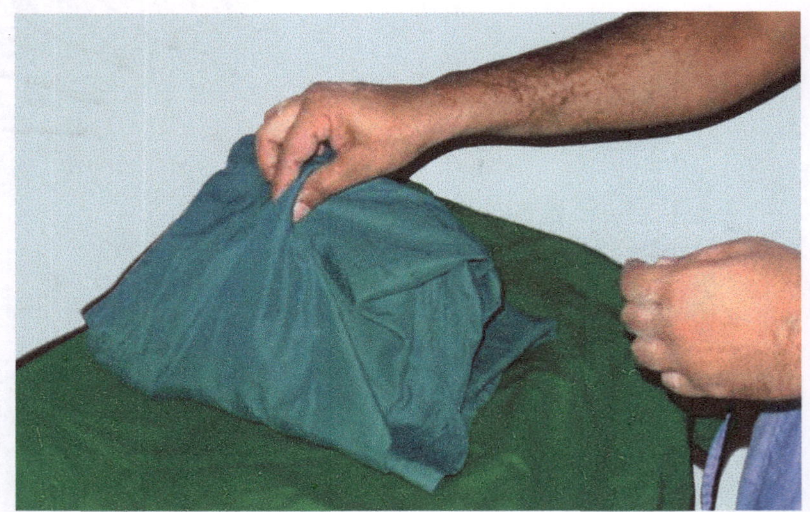

Fig. 1.13: Gown folded inside out, surgeon touches the inside of the gown with scrubbed hands

Application of Sterile Gown

After the hand scrubbing the sterile gown is applied by no touch technique. The gowns are folded inside out during autoclaving. The sterile gown is picked up by the assistant with the help of sterile chital forceps. The surgeon holds the gown with clean hands touching the inside of the gown which is folded outside (Fig. 1.13).

He opens the gown and slides the gown over his hands and the body without touching the outside of the gown. The straps of the gown are tied by the assistant at the back and the straps of the gown are tightened by the surgeon himself around his wrists (Figs 1.14A and B). The front portion of the gown between the chest and the waist is considered to be sterile and should always face the operating field and sterile trolley on which sterile surgical equipment are kept.

Putting on Gloves

The gloves are pre-powdered and folded in such a way that the inside of the cuff faces outside during autoclaving. The surgeon applies sterile gloves powder over his scrubbed hands and then picks up the left glove with bare right hand, touching the inside out folded cuff only. He slides the left glove over the left hand without unfolding the cuff. Then with the gloved left hand he picks up the right glove touching only the outside of right glove. He slides it over the right hand and unfolds the cuff over the cuff of the sterile gown. Then with the gloved right hand he unfolds the cuff of left glove over the cuff of gown of the left hand, touching only out side of left glove. This is called as 'open method' of gloving. The surgeon is now prepared to undertake the surgical procedure (Figs 1.15, 1.16, 1.17).

Preparation of Patient

The preparation of patient is divided into two phases:

1. Preparation of patient in the ward and
2. Preparation of the part on table.

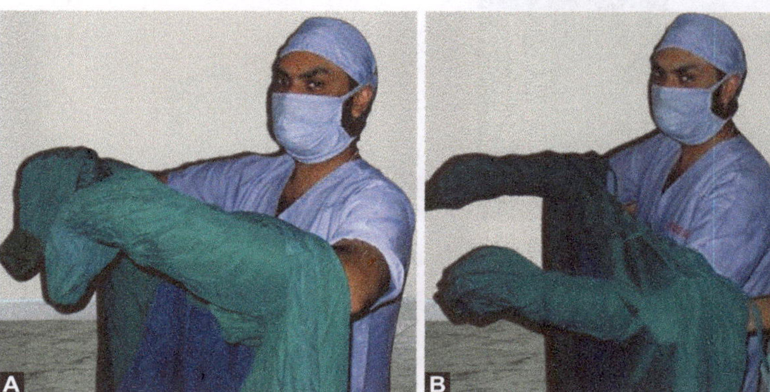

Figs 1.14A and B: Gowning without touching the outside of the gown

Fig. 1.15: Sterile gloves—cuffs folded inside out

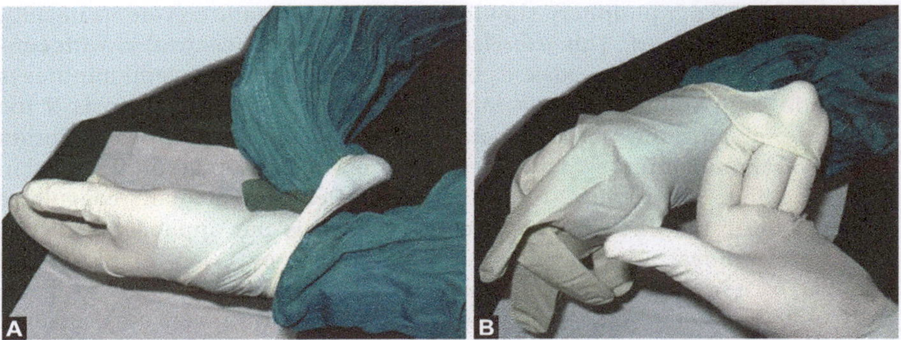

Figs 1.16A and B: Closed gloving technique—note the left glove is slided over the hand with the right hand overed by sterile gown. The right cuff is then adjusted with gloved left hand and the right glove is slided using left gloved hand without touching the outside of the gloves with bare hands

Preparation of Patient in the Ward

In Indian circumstances the patient are often poor, illiterate, ignorant about personnel hygiene. Thus, they require a good preparation before shifting to the operating room. The preparation comprises of:

- Hospitalization 2 to 3 days prior to surgery for acclimatization to the hospital environment for preoperative and to relieve anxiety.
- **Bath:** The patients should be asked to take a good bath to clean all the dirt from the body.
- **Clothing:** The outside clothing should be discarded and the patient should be provided clean hospital clothing.
- When the patient is unable to do these things of his own due to illness good nursing care should be provided to him to complete this job.
- **Preparation of part:** The part to be operated should be washed thoroughly with soap and water. The hair should be removed by shaving at least 12 hours prior to the surgery as on time shaving can produce scratches on the skin, which breaks the barrier and facilitates the entry of microorganism in the operating area. The clean and shaved part is vigorously scrubbed with antiseptic solution like Savlon, chlorhexidine or povidon iodine and mopped with sterile gauge. The cleaned part is painted with solution like mercury chrome or 2 percent picric acid, covered with sterile pad and sealed with adhesive taps to isolate it and prevent contamination from fomites.
- **Preparation of oral cavity:** In maxillofacial surgery preparation of oral cavity is very important to prevent wound infection. The oral cavity should be thoroughly inspected for any septic foci, calculus, tarter,

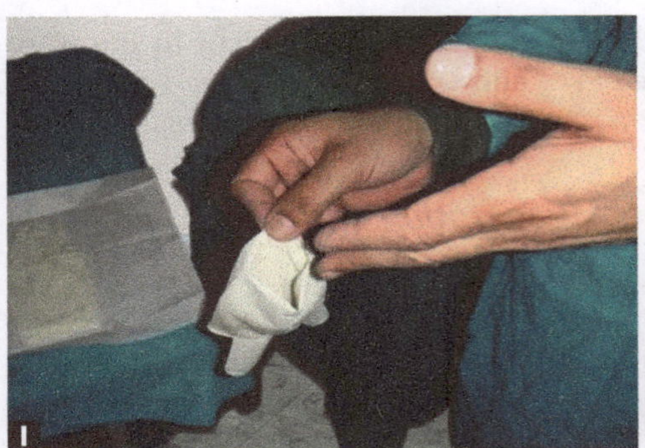

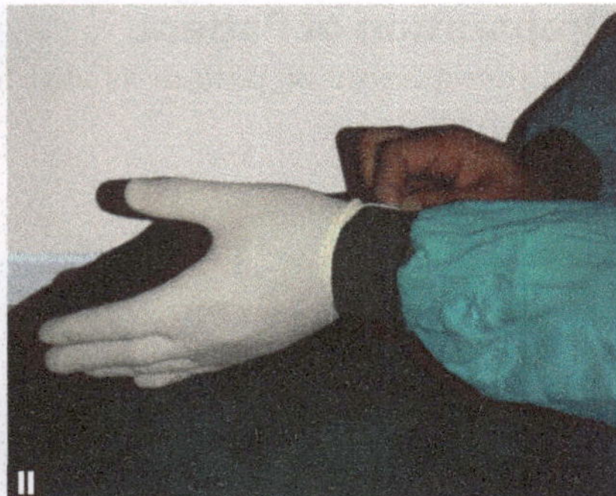

Fig. 1.17A: Open method of gloving: Left glove is picked up with bare, scrubbed right hand, touching its inside and slided over left hand without uncuffing it

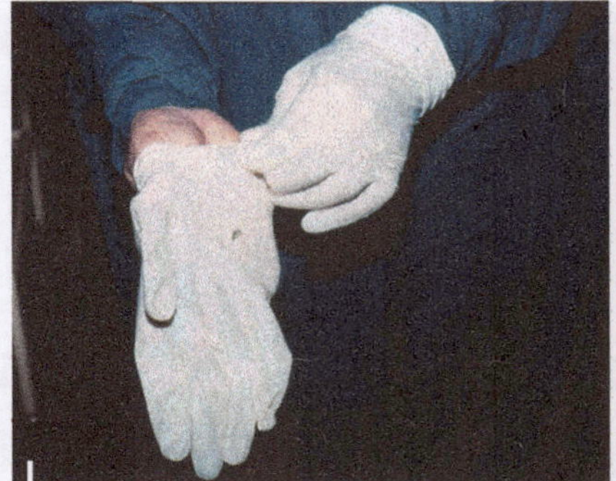

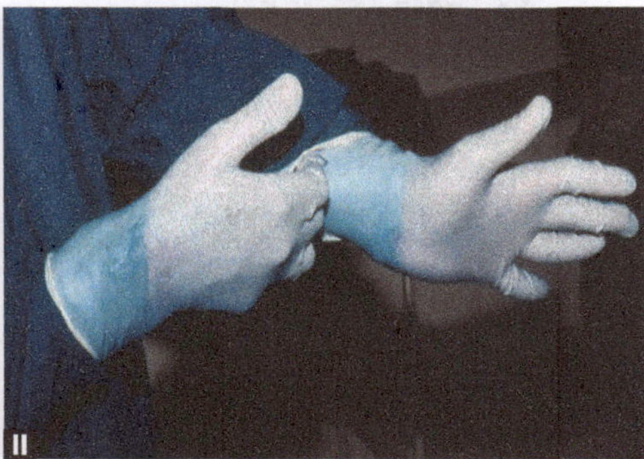

Fig. 1.17B: The right glove is picked up with gloved left hand touching only its outside. It is uncuffed over the cuff of the gown. Then with the gloved right hand the left glove is uncuffed. Note that during the entire procedure the out side of the gloves was not touched by bare hands

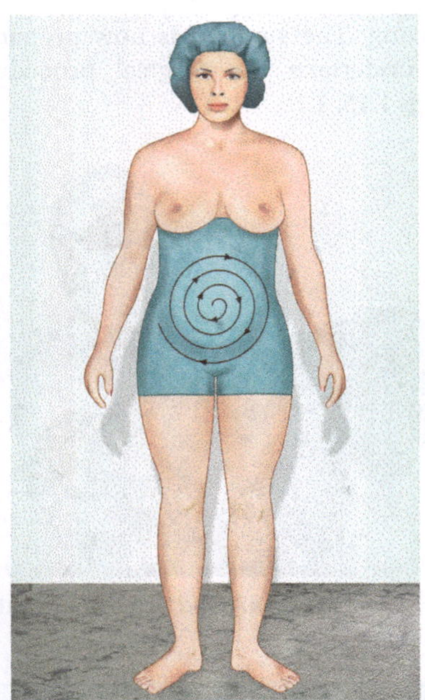

Fig. 1.18: Preparation of the part starts fron center to periphery

infected carious teeth, infected periodontal pockets, etc. and they should be treated/removed. Antiseptic mouth washes should be prescribed (chlorhexidine, povidon, iodine, etc.) for periodic mouth rinsing to reduce the count of microorganism. Loose teeth should be extracted as they may come in the way of intubations of patient and may get knocked out and aspirated during the intubation.

Preparation of Part on Operation Table

The part which is preliminary prepared in the ward preoperatively is finally prepared on the table before the surgery is started. The part on which the surgery is to be performed and its adjoining area is scrubbed vigorously using a sterile swab holding forceps with a no touch technique, i.e. the surgeon does not touch the swab or any other area with his gloved hands. The scrubbing is started from the center and goes to periphery and the swab is discarded (Fig. 1.18). In no case the swab from periphery should touch the central area. This exercise is first done with swab soaked in antiseptic soap solution like savlon, cetrimide or povidon iodine (beta scrub) for about 2 minutes. The detergent facilitates reduction of surface tension of the dirt particles and their easy removal. The mechanical removal of microbiological colonies and reducing their count of due to antiseptic action is achieved by scrubbing. The area is then mopped with dry sponge or sponge soaked in sterile normal saline to remove the residue of the antiseptic agent and detergent, which could be irritating or harmful to the exposed deeper tissue during surgery. Finally the area is painted with 5 percent povidon iodine solution and this should not be wiped off because microbial activity is sustained by release of free iodine as the agent dries and color fades from skin. It should remain on skin for at least 2 minutes. To hasten drying of skin, alcohol may be painted on the area without friction before a self-adhering drape is applied. Isopropyl and ethyl alcohol are broad spectrum agents that denature proteins in cells. A 70 percent concentration with continuous contact for several minutes is satisfactory for skin antisepsis if the surgeon prefers a colorless solution that permits observation of true skin color. Because alcohol coagulates protein, it is not applied to mucous membranes or used on an open wound. Isopropyl alcohol is more effective fat solvent than ethyl alcohol. Both are volatile and flammable. They must not pool around or under the patient, especially if an electrosurgical unit or laser will be used.

The oral cavity should be prepared again with chlorexidine or povidon iodine 5 percent solution to achieve maximum antisepsis and prevent wound contamination.

The prepared area is the surgical area/field and needs to be isolated from rest of the body area and environments to prevent cross contamination. Hence, the area is isolated by draping the other parts with the help of sterile surgical towels exposing only the surgical field (Figs 1.19A and B).

Removing Gown

The gown is always removed before the gloves at the end of the surgical procedure.

The circulator unfastens the neck and back closures of the gown so the

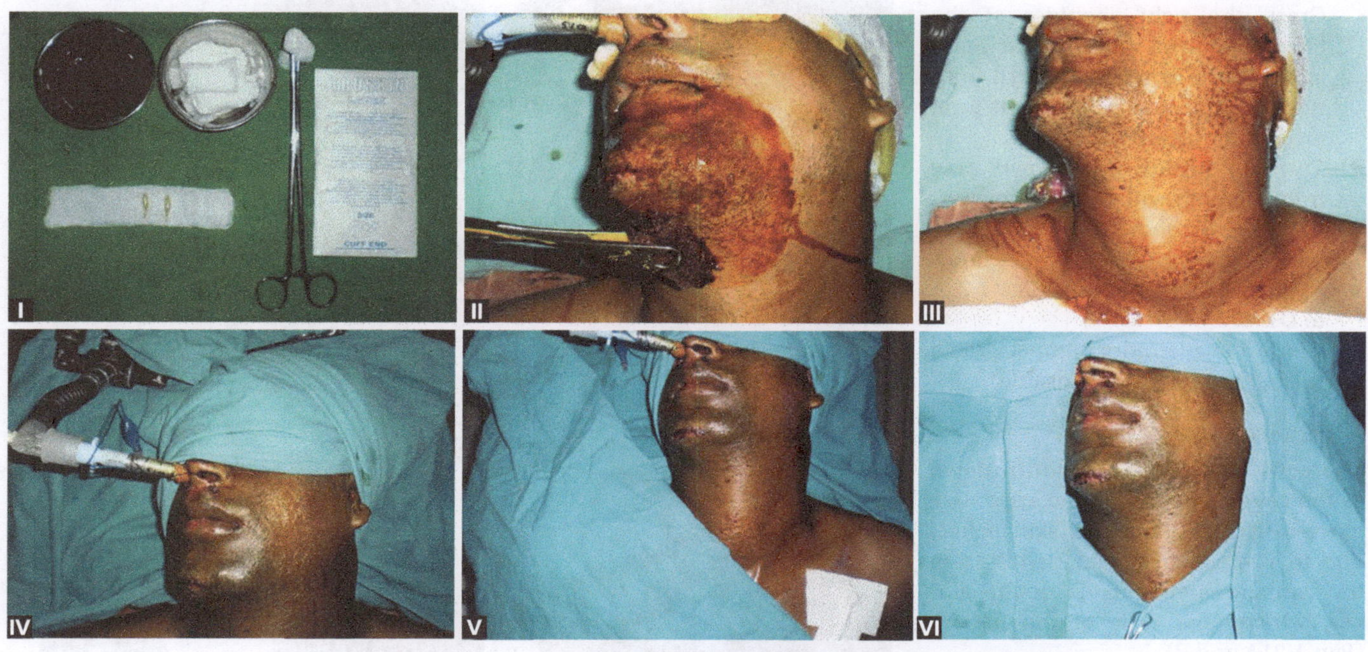

Fig. 1.19A: Part preparation set and sequential part preparation and draping

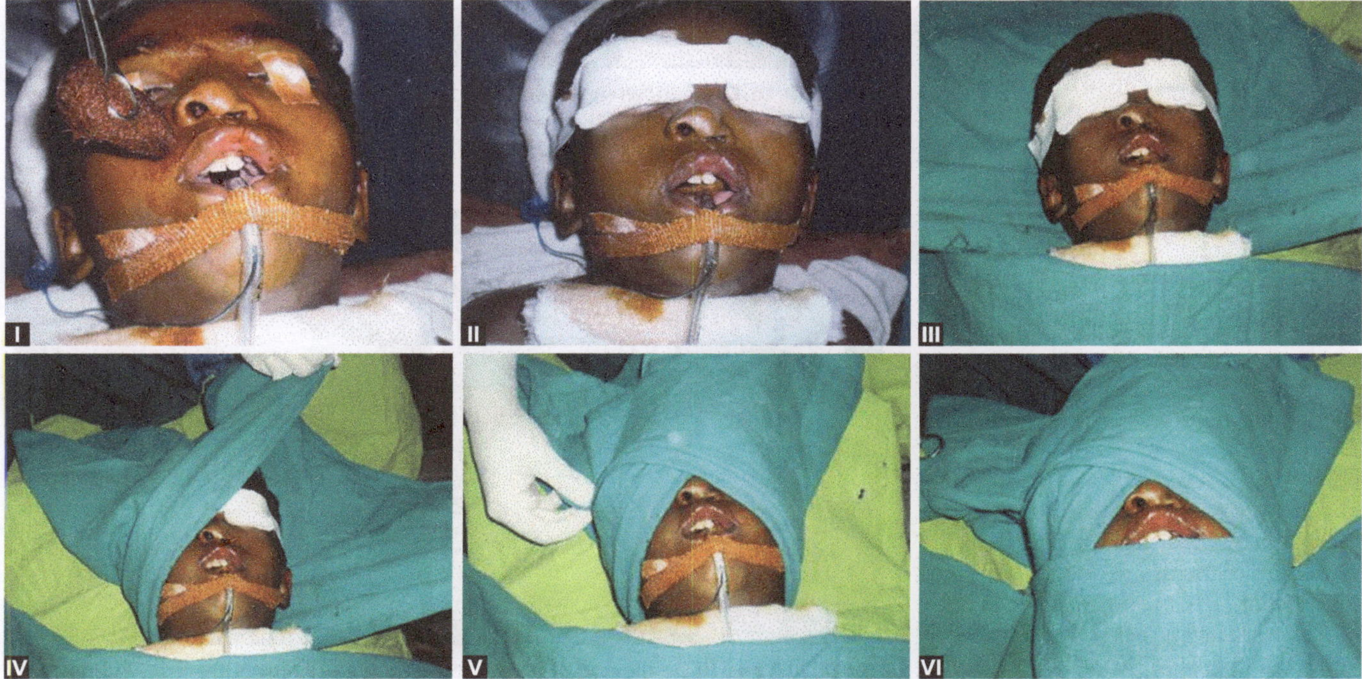

Fig. 1.19B: Sequential part preparation and draping, note the eyes are well protected by applying chloromycetin eye applicaps to prevent drying and covered with sterile pads to prevent the antiseptic solution from entering in eyes to cause chemical injuries

wearer does not contaminate his or her scrub suit. If wearing a wrap around gown, the wearer unfastens the waist closure in front. The gown is always removed inside out to protect the arms and scrub suit from contaminated outside of the gown. To remove:

- Grasp the right shoulder of the loosened gown with the left hand and pull the gown downward from the shoulder and of the right arm, turning the sleeve inside out.
- Turn the outside of the gown away from the body with flexed elbows.
- Grasp the left shoulder with the right hand and remove the gown entirely, pulling it off inside out (Figs 1.20A to D).
- Discard in a laundry hamper or in a trash receptacle (if disposable).

Removing Gloves

The cuffs of gloves usually turn down as the gown is pulled off the arms. Use glove-to-glove, then skin-to skin technique to protect the clean hands from the contaminated outside of the gloves, which bear cells of the patient (Figs 1.21A and B).

- Grasp the cuff of the left glove with gloved fingers of the right hand and pull it off inside out.
- Slip the ungloved fingers of the left hand under the cuff of the right glove and slip it off inside out.
- Discard gloves in a trash receptacle.
- Wash the hands thoroughly using antiseptic soap.

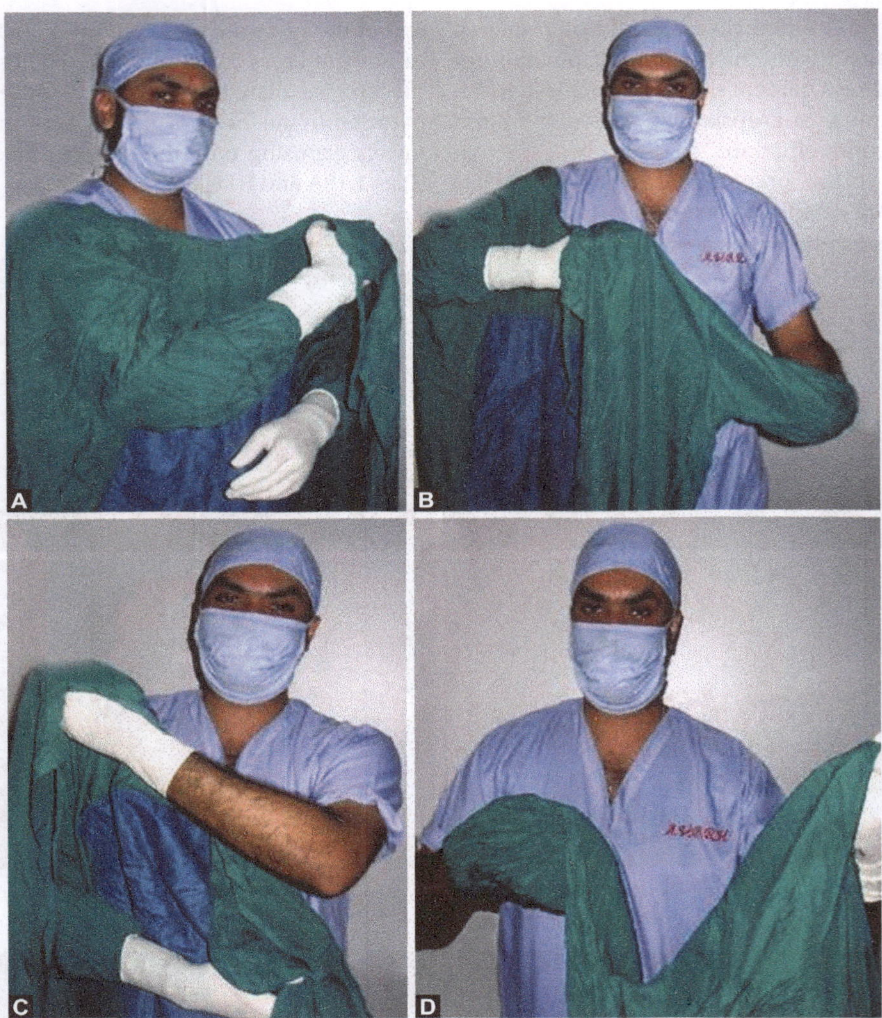

Figs 1.20A to D: De-gowning process, note that the gown is removed first without removing glove, the inside of the gown is not touched with contaminated gloves. Gown is always removed first and then gloves are removed

Tissue Handling and Tissue Respect

"Respect the tissue and it will reward you by providing uncomplicated healing". The gentle handling of the tissue during the surgery is of paramount importance for uneventful wound healing and achieving desirable results out of the surgical procedure. The forceful retraction of the tissue, rough handling, injudicious dissection, excessive use of electrocautery, using dull scissors/ knife for incision and allowing the tissue to desiccate during the surgery

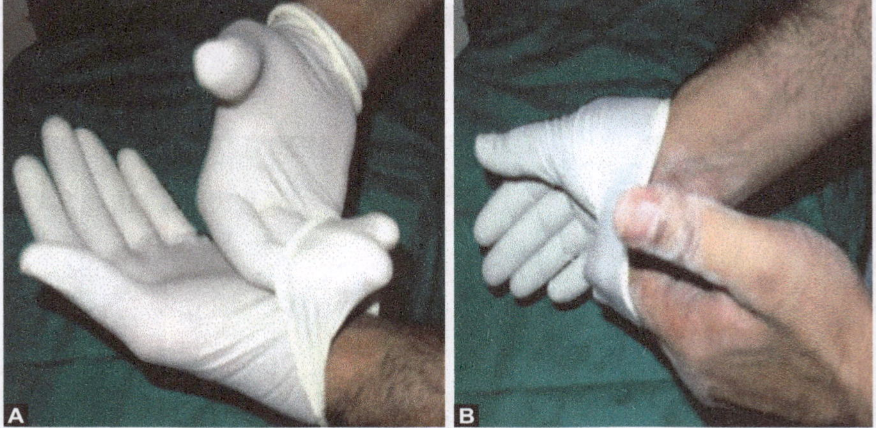

Figs 1.21A and B: De-gloving process, the contaminated gloves are removed without touching the outside of the glove with bare hands

amount to tissue insult, which is bound to be reacted with more tissue reaction (inflammation) delayed healing, tissue necrosis and thus, chances of infection. The surgeon should handle the tissue minimally and exercise sound discipline and principles to avoid tissue insult (injudicious handling). The 'tissue respect' can be optimized and the chances of wound related complications can be significantly minimized if the precautions are taken during each step of the surgery as mentioned below.

Incision

During the surgery the tissue needs to be incised for creating an access. The incision is made with sharp Bard-Parker knife. In oral and maxillofacial surgery, the commonly used BP handled number 3 to 5 on which 15 blade is mounted. Stab knife (No. 11 blade) is used for incision and drainage of abscess, inserting drains or taking gingival crevicular incisions (Figs 1.22A and B). The skin incisions are not made with electro cautery knife as there are chances of tissue necrosis and impaired healing however, the deeper tissues and the mucosal incisions can be made using it. During taking the incision following principles must be followed:

- Always mark the incision with marking ink first to avoid mistakes (Figs 1.23A and B).
- The incision should be taken in normal skin folds or along the Langer's lines to prevent tension across the incision line, to ensure good quality of healing and a cosmetic scar, to prevent dehiscence of the wound due to tension and to camouflage the scar.
- The incision should be long enough to facilitate easy passive access to the deeper structures. This avoids tissue trauma due to forceful retraction in case of short incision, which subsequently leads to more tissue reactions and inflammation. It is a false notion that short incision heals faster however the healing along the incision is a simultaneous process and is independent of the length of the incision.
- While taking incision, precautions must be taken to avoid injury to vital structures like major blood vessels and nerves.
- The cross serrations (cross hatching) are marked across the incision with the blunt side of knife blade by scratching superficially, which serves as guidance for proper approximation of the skin during closer especially when the skin is likely to be lax following the surgery.
- The knife is held with a pen grip and the hand is given proper rest to have a better control over the knife (Figs 1.24A and B).
- The knife blade is held perpendicular to the tissues to be incised unless indicated otherwise.
- Controlled, uniform pressure is applied during making an incision depending on the consistency of

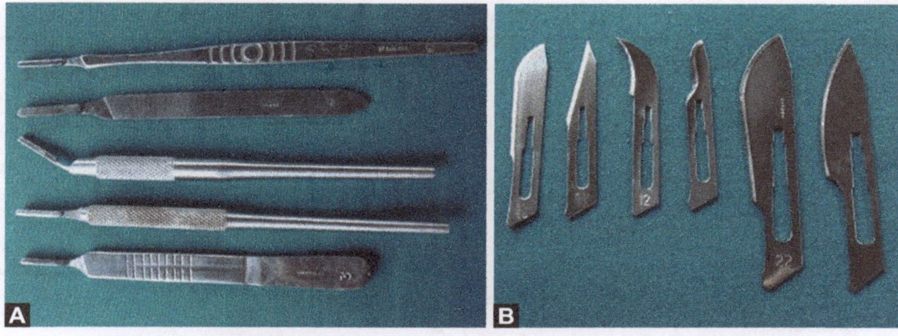

Figs 1.22A and B: Different types of Bard-Parker handles and blades

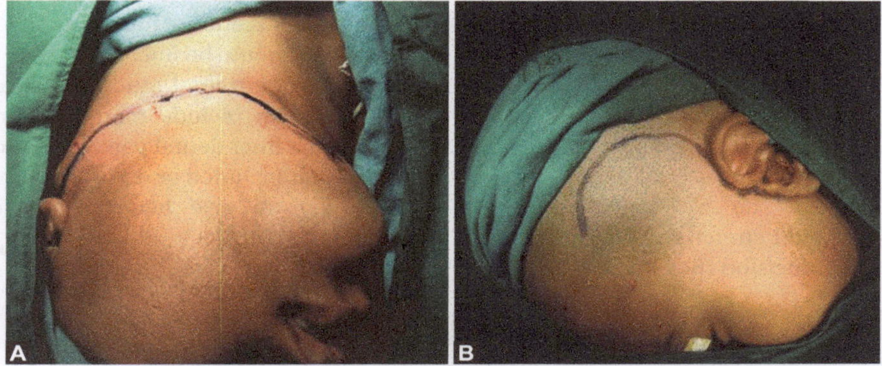

Figs 1.23A and B: Marking the incision with ink

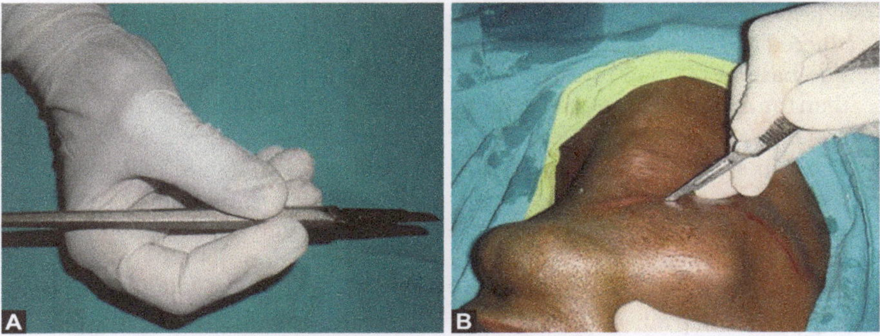

Figs 1.24A and B: Pen grip

Box 1.2: Guide lines for making incision

- Mark incision with ink
- Cross hatching
- Avoid damage to vital structures
- Place it in Langerhan's lines or skin folds
- Hold the knife with pen grip for better control and support
- Blade perpendicular to tissue
- Assistant should stretch the skin
- Incise in one stroke applying moderate pressure

Box 1.3: Ideal requirements of the flap

- Base should be wider than apex for good vascularity
- Wide enough to facilitate proper access and cover the surgical defect
- Should be raised Full thickness
- Include or exclude gingival papilla
- The edges must lay on healthy bone at the time of closure.

the structure to be incised and the structure should be incised to its full thickness is one and single stroke, as repeated incisions may lacerate the edges of the wound which would subsequently compromise the healing process. While the surgeon makes an incision the assistant should stretch the skin to facilitate the incision (Box 1.2).

Flap Designing

Whenever a flap is required to be reflected during the surgery for creating an access to the surgical site following basic principles of flap designing must be adhered to:

- The base of the flap must be wider than the apex to ensure good afferent and efferent vascularity (Fig. 1.25).
- The flap should be wide enough to facilitate free, passive and direct access and should cover the surgical defect adequately.
- In case of mucoperiosteal flaps the edges of the flap must not lie on bony defects as the flap is unsupported from below and tends to collapse to create dehiscence of the wound.
- The flap should be full thickness.
- In case of intraoral mucoperiosteal flaps which include marginal gingival, the inter dental papilla should be either included or excluded from the flap to give better cosmetic results (Box 1.3).

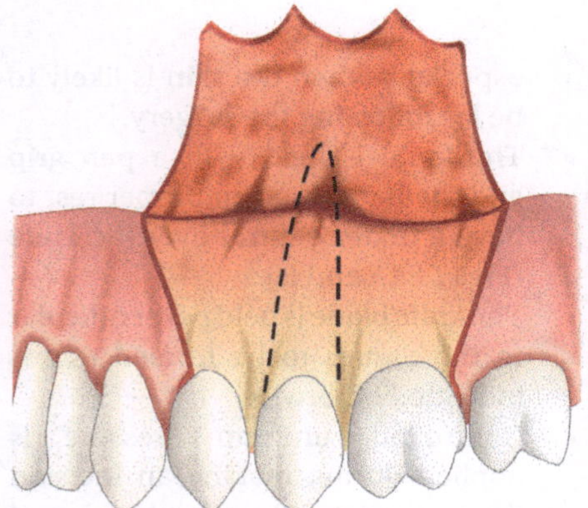

Fig. 1.25: Base of the flap wider than the apex

Dissection of Tissue

The tissues are dissected by two ways:

1. By blunt dissection or
2. By sharp dissection.

The sharp dissection is less traumatic and is preferred for tough and tenacious tissues. It should be avoided when vital structures are in vicinity and can get traumatized. The blunt dissection is preferred in the tissues which are soft, fragile and friable and where there is anatomical proximity with the vital structures. The sharp dissection is done with the help of knife. The sharp dissection is less traumatic to tissues than the blunt dissection as there is less tissue handling. Further, the cutting of the tissue with knife is less traumatic than the cutting with the help of scissors, as the latter crushes the tissue while cutting. The blunt dissection is done with the help of non-cutting edge of scissors, blades by opening action or with the help of opening action of the hemostat tips. The tips of the dissecting scissors used for blunt dissection should be preferably rounded and appropriate curvature of scissors should be selected to gain proper access. Cautery tips can also be used for the dissection, its advantage is that it incises the tissue and simultaneously coagulates the smaller blood vessels to provide dry surgical field. The disadvantage with the cautery dissection is that it inflicts more tissue necrosis due to heat and compromises the quality of healing.

Tissue Retraction

The tissues are required to be retracted during the surgery to facilitate good visibility and access to the surgical site. Soft, friable tissues tend to get lacerated if retracted forcefully or using traumatic retractors like Allie's forceps or cat's paw retractor. Instead atraumatic retractors like Langenbeck's (L) retractor should be used. Tough, tenacious tissues should be retracted with retractors like Allie's forceps or cat's paw retractor (e.g. skin, tendons, periosteum, muscle, etc.) While applying the Allie's forceps to the skin it should never be applied on the outer surface of the skin but, should be applied to the inner surface of the skin flap to avoid ugly bite marks on skin. The slippery, glandular structures are held with the help of Babcock's gland holding forceps (lymph nodes, salivary glands). During fine plastic surgical work on the skin the tiny edges of flaps should be retracted using skin hooks. The same can be used for stretching the edges of the incision during the suturing for better approximation of skin edges. A nerve is retraced with the help of blunt nerve hooks. During intraoral procedures the mouth is kept open using a mouth prop or a self-retaining Doyen's, Hyster's or Dingman's mouth gag (Figs 1.26A and B, 1.27, 1.28A and B). During laparotomies or thoracotomy the edges of abdominal incision or the ribs are retracted with the help of self-retaining retractors. Some special retractors are designed for different sites and surgeries. Some commonly used retractors in oral and maxillofacial surgery are condylar retractor (for condylectomy), mastoid retractor (self-retaining), copper malleable retractor for the retraction of the eyeball, coronoid retractor (forked L retractor) for coronoidectomy of ramal osteotomies, chin retractor for the genioplasty, channel retractor during osteotomies and the Austin's retractor during third molar surgeries, etc. (Figs 1.29 to 1.41).

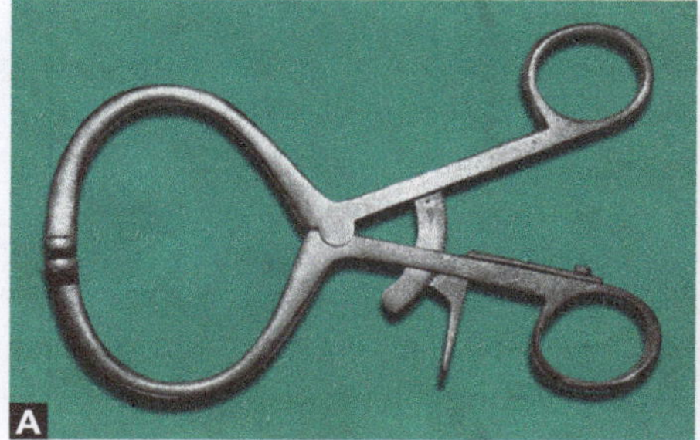
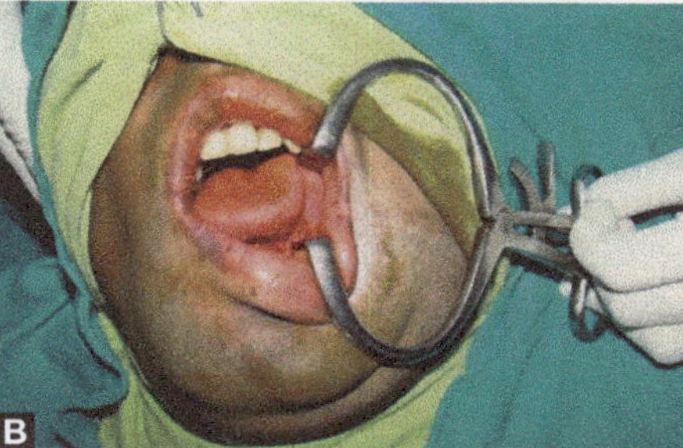

Figs 1.26A and B: Doyen's mouth gag

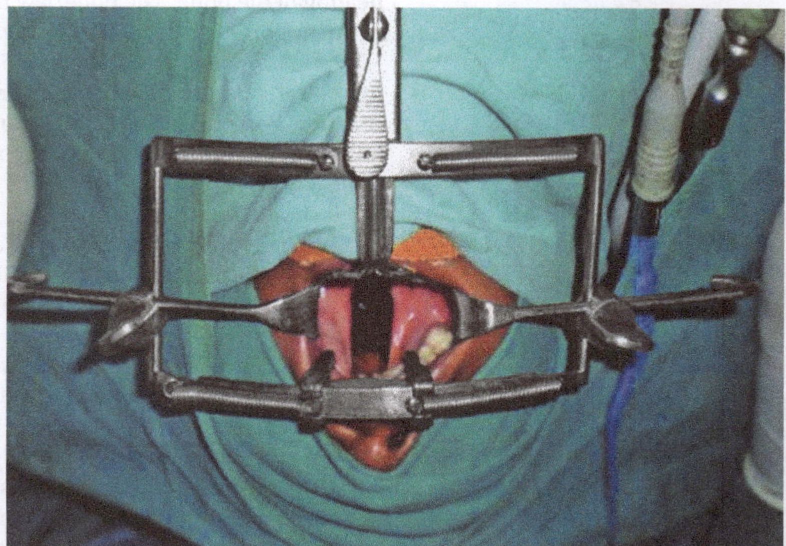

Fig. 1.27: Dingman's mouth gag

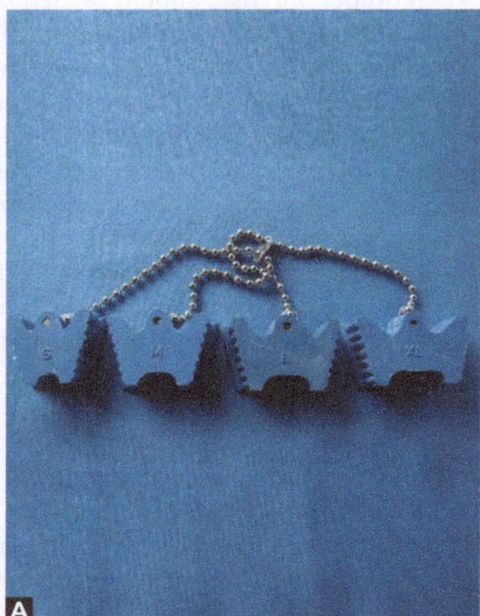
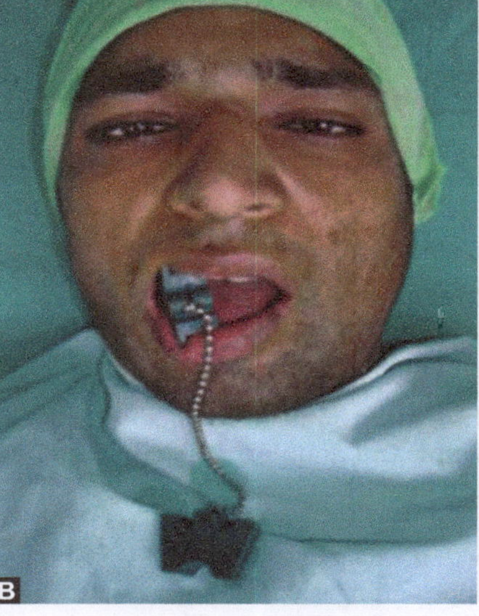

Figs 1.28A and B: Mouth props

Bone Removal

In oral and maxillofacial surgery bone removal is often required for gaining access, osteotomies or during resections of jaw. This can be done with the help of:

- Rotary instruments like motor and bur.
- Osteotomes.
- Chisel and mallet.
- Gigli saw.
- Power saw having reciprocating, oscillating and sagittal blades.
- Bone cutter, rongeur/nibbler, etc.

The rotary instruments include motor and burs. While doing bone cutting with these instruments, care should be taken to avoid excessive heat generation by avoiding very high speed and by doing copious irrigation with cold normal saline. The ideal speed of the bur should be 20,000 RPM. The outline of the bony incision should be marked by drilling serial holes with a round bur (post-stamp incision) which are later joined by using flat fissure bur (Figs 1.42A to D). The incision should be started with a round bur as it gets good purchase on the bone and does not slip and injure the adjoining soft tissue. The bur should be sharp, as dull burs produce more frictional heat. If the temperature rises above 40°C, alkaline phosphatase is released from the osteoblasts and bone necrosis takes place. The bur should be made up of either stainless steel or carbide as they cut the bone with cutting edges unlike the diamond bur, which does abrasive cutting and tends to generate more heat. The diamond burs may be used for odontectomy rather than bone cutting. While doing bone cutting with a rotary instruments precaution should be taken not to keep any cotton wool or gauze piece in the vicinity to prevent accidental entangling and tissue injury. The soft tissue should be protected from accidental injury due to slipping of the bur by proper retraction and keeping a guard. The operator must use protective eye glasses as the saline used during the bone cutting may get splashed in the eyes.

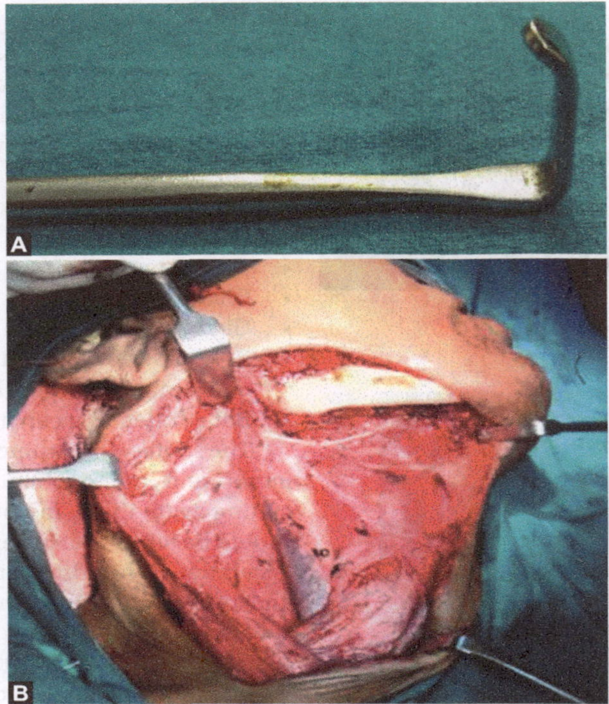

Figs 1.29A and B: Langenback's retractor

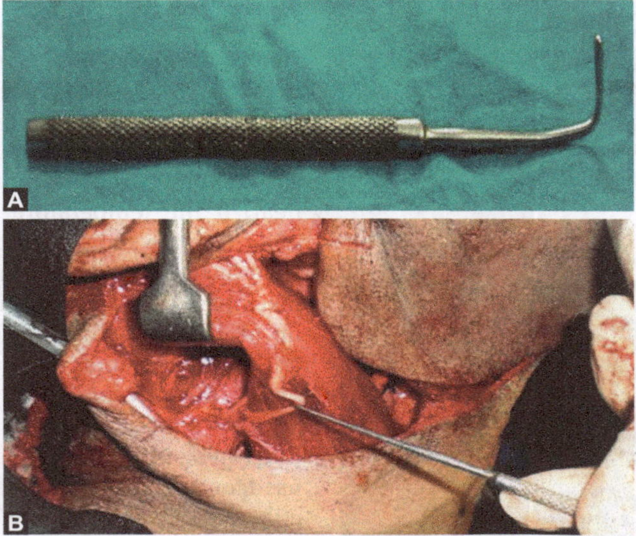

Figs 1.30A and B: Nerve hook

The power saws have different types of handpieces and blades like oscillating, reciprocating and sagittal which are useful in different indications. They often produce more precise and fine cuts.

The bone cutting with the help of bone cutter requires a sharp instrument or else the bone tends to get crushed.

The nibbler takes out small bites of thin, sharp bone. It is available as single action and double action and with fine and heavy beaks.

A gigli saw is a wire saw and it is held with the help of gigli saw holders and the bone cutting is done by a see saw action. During the cutting, constant irrigation with the cold normal saline is done to dissipate the heat. While cutting the bone with gigli saw care should be taken to ensure that the saw slides smoothly, long strokes are applied so that the entire length of the saw is used for cutting rather than a limited area, as it can lead to make that portion dull and the saw breaks. While cutting the bone with the gigli saw the adjoining soft tissue should be retracted and guarded and copious saline irrigation should be done to avoid over heating of the bone. The bone/jaw needs to be supported during bone cutting.

An osteotome splits the bone and the chisel cuts the bone in a controlled manner. Following precautions must be taken while the bone with a chisel or osteotome.

- It should be sharp.
- Too heavy blows should not be applied as it may result into a fracture.
- The action of mallet should be with wrist movement.
- A mallet with appropriate weight should be selected (200 Oz, 500 Oz) depending upon the density of bone to be cut.
- The vertical stop cuts must be marked before actual bone removal as the bone tends to get split along with bone grains.
- The bone/jaw must be well-supported to prevent fracture or dislocation.
- A proper purchase should be created for engaging the chisel or else it will slip and injure the soft tissue or vital structures. The soft tissue should be adequately retraced and guard should be kept to prevent its laceration. After the bone cutting all the sharp bone ends should be rounded off, using a bone rasp/bone file. The bone file is used in a pull motion only as the serrations facilitate filling in this direction. To and fro motion leads to clogging of the bone and causes necrosis.

Drains

A drain is the material that acts as a channel for escape of fluid. It is the material used to drain fluids (exudates, transudate, hematoma, pus, blood, etc.) from the tissue dead spaces or cavities.

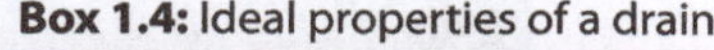

Purpose

- Prophylactic.
- To prevent accumulation of fluid (bile, lymph, blood, exudates).
- To encourage the obliteration of the dead space otherwise the accumulated fluid acts as a separating agent and prevents the collapse of raw surfaces.
- Therapeutic.

To promote escape of the fluid already collected, e.g. blood, exudates, pus (Box 1.4).

The drain is kept *in situ* (indwelling) to facilitate free, passive and uninterrupted drainage of fluids along it. When the abscess is drained, to allow the drainage of pus a drain is used.

Box 1.4: Ideal properties of a drain

- It should be non-toxic.
- It should be non-antigenic.
- It should resist bio-degradation.
- It should not have capillarity and should facilitate free drainage along it.
- It should be sterilizable.

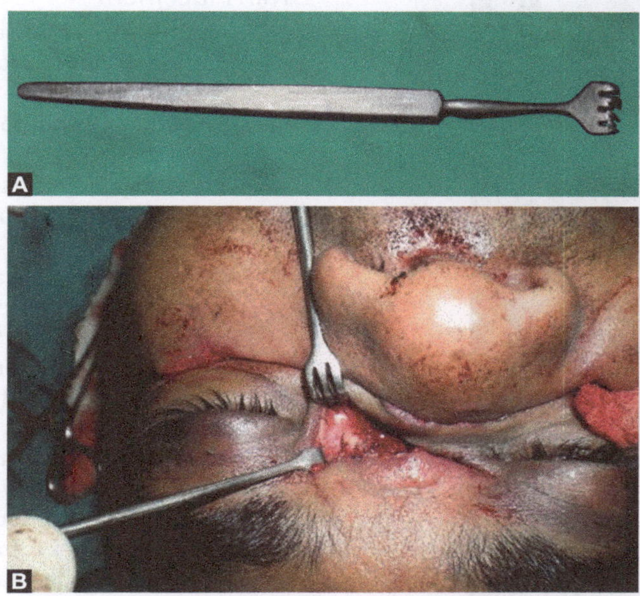

Figs 1.31A and B: Cat's paw retractor

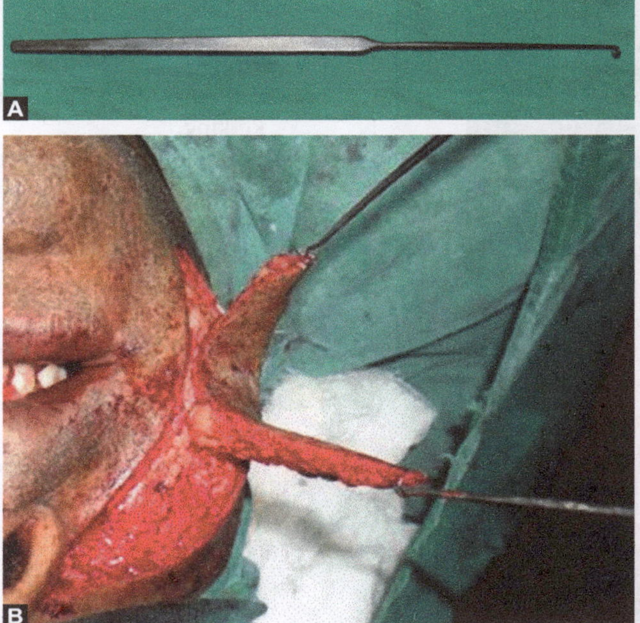

Figs 1.32A and B: Skin hook

After removal of tumors, the dead space existing in the tissue is drained with a drain, as exudates, blood accumulates in this dead space and can lead to hematoma and wound infection. The vacuum drain exerts negative pressure and facilitates very good drainage even if the drain is placed at a non-gravity dependent site. The corrugated rubber dam or PVC (portex), drains are required to be kept at a gravity dependent site to be more effective. The corrugations prevent it from getting clogged and permit free drainage. The gauze drains are not ideal as they have capillarity and absorb fluids, swell in size and obstruct the drainage. They are suitable only for packing the cavities for achieving hemostasis (e.g. abscess cavity, cystic cavity which heals by secondary intention). The tube drains also facilitate irrigation of the cavity.

The time for removal of the drain is not fixed it should be left in place till the drainage from the wound stops completely. It is advisable to displace the drain first, when the soakage becomes negligible, as there could be blockage of the drain due to the thick exudates or slough, before it is finally removed. If the drain is kept unduly long or if the aseptic precautions are not taken the infection can travel into the wound along it.

Advantages

- Drainage of the collected fluid removes the nidus of infection.
- It helps in monitoring the hemorrhage or leakage at the suture line, thus, gives warning of future complications.
- It obliterates the tissue dead space and removes the separating fluid and allows the raw surfaces to collapse and come in contact so that the healing is faster.

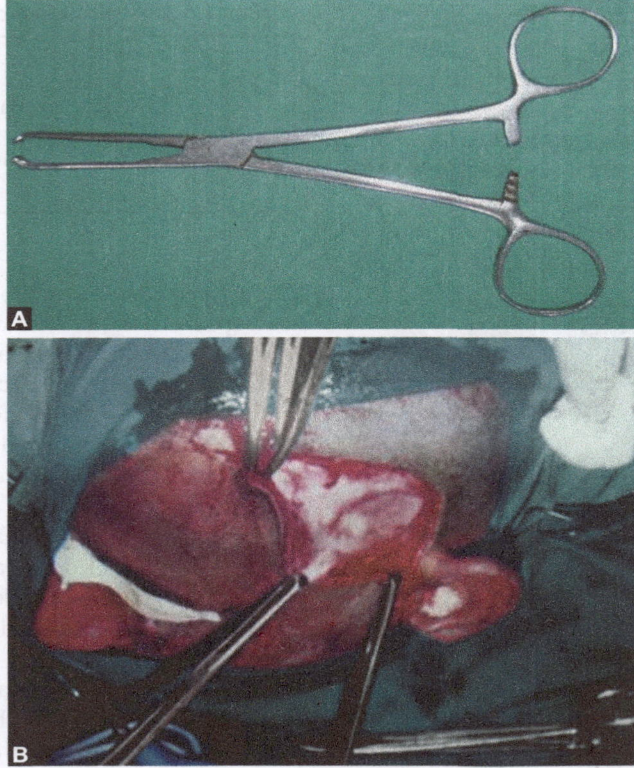

Figs 1.33A and B: Allie's tissue holding forceps

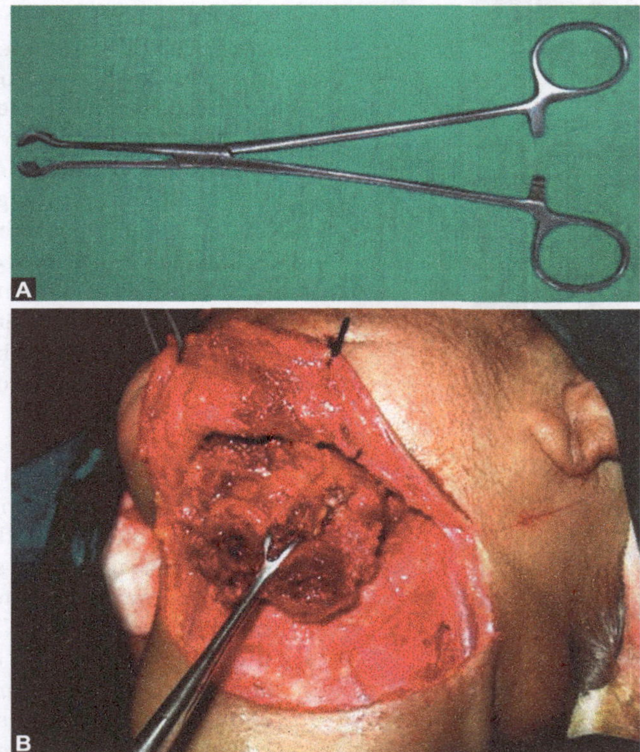

Figs 1.34A and B: Babcock's forcep, atraumatic forcep used to hold glandular tissue

Disadvantages

- It forms portal of entry for infection.
- It can delay the healing.
- It can lead to breakdown of the suture line thus used judiciously.
- It can initiate tissue reaction.
- It can get blocked and become no functional.

Drain Placement

- The drain used should be
  - Soft, so as not to erode the surrounding tissues,
  - Smooth, so as not to permit fibrin to cling to it.
  - Preferably radio-opaque or having radio-opaque line along the tube.
  - Made up of a material that will not disintegrate and leave foreign bodies in the wound.
  - Be brought out through a separate stab wound and fixed properly and
  - It should be non-irritant.
- The stab wound that gives access to the drainage cavity should be large enough to permit free drainage.
- The drain must be placed in the dependent position if gravity alone is to accomplish drainage. Sump tube must be used to remove drainage 'uphill', i.e. against the force of gravity.
- The drain should be brought out through the shortest route to avoid kinking.
- Proper daily dressing of the drainage site should be done to prevent infection.
- When prosthesis is present, closed tube system should be used to lessen the risk of infection.
- It should not damage the nerve or blood vessel.
- The inner end should not be placed near the suture lines.
- The drain should be secured properly.

Precautions

- Drains act as two-way conduits. The benefits of prophylactic use of a drain must be weighed against

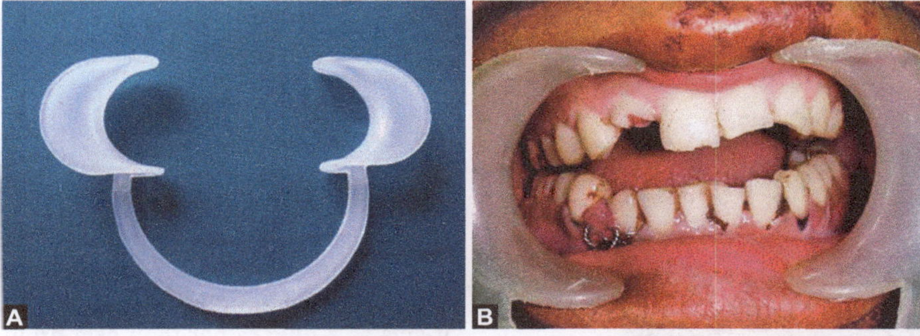

Figs 1.35A and B: Cheek retractor

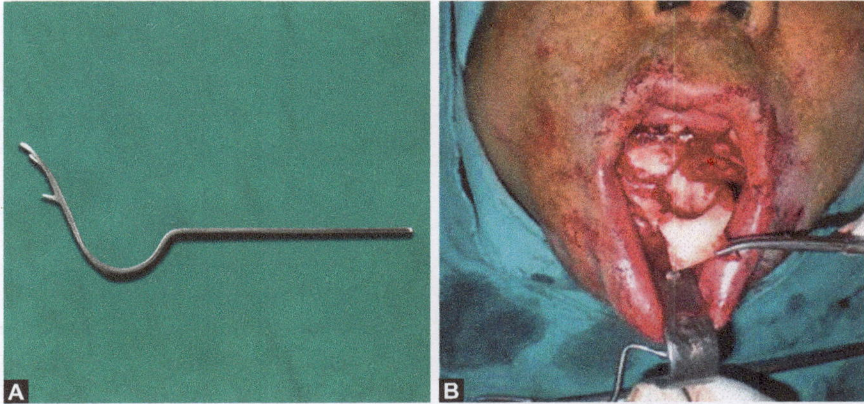

Figs 1.36A and B: Chin retractor

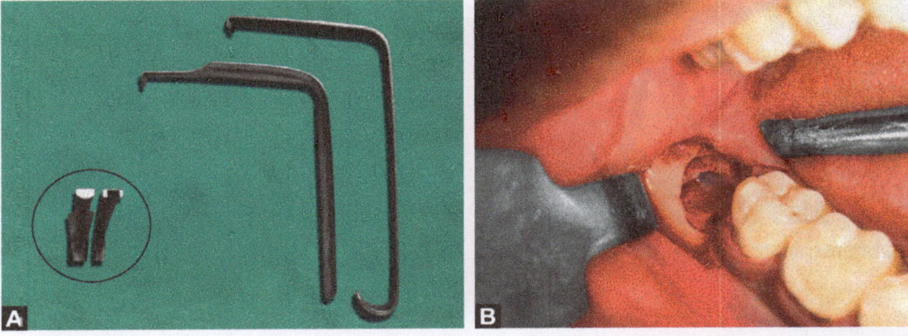

Figs 1.37A and B: Austin's retractor, traumatic and atraumatic, retractor in use during third molar surgery

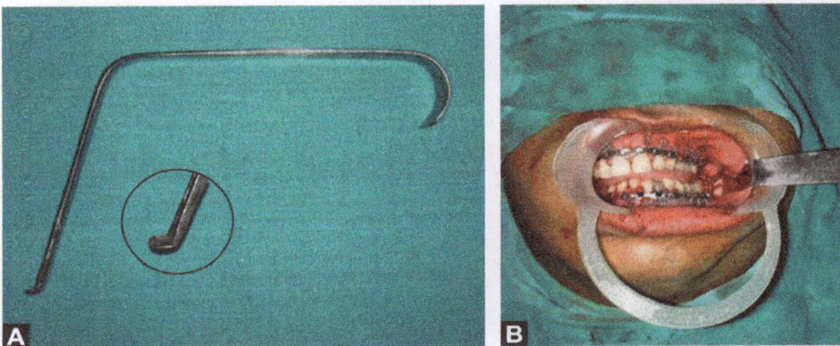

Figs 1.38A and B: Channel retractor has a groove which facilitates use of rotary instruments along with retraction, used for ramal osteotomies

possible ensuing infection. Careful dressing of the wound and drain should be removed as soon as the purpose is over. It reduces the likelihood of significant infection.

- It should never be brought out through the operative incision, but through separate stab incision. If drain is brought out through the operative wound, it not only permits bacterial ingress and infection of the operative wound but also prevents its closure.
- Fix the drain properly with skin stitches. If it is detached from skin surface, refix it. Otherwise, it may come out or disappear into the drainage cavity.
- A drain should not be placed through an area where fibrosis will cause impairment of function, e.g. across the joint or near tendon sheaths, etc.
- Do not drain bowel/vascular anastomotic suture line, since this may increase chances of anastomotic leak.
- Too hard or stiff drain may cause pressure necrosis of the surrounding tissues, especially one near a large blood vessel, tendon, nerve or solid organ.

Removal of Drain

- The prophylactically placed drain should be removed as soon as drainage has subsided, usually after 48 hours.
- The therapeutically placed drain is kept in position until the drainage subsides. The lack of drainage could be due to blockade of the pores due to tissue contact or fibrinous plug, in such cases before removing the drain it should be displaced to observe if any drainage is still present. If the drainage is not present then it is removed gradually, a 3 to 4 cm of drain is withdrawn each day and refixed to allow closure of the drainage tract from its depth, thus preventing pocketing.
- Tube drains are removed when drainage output is minimal or ceased.

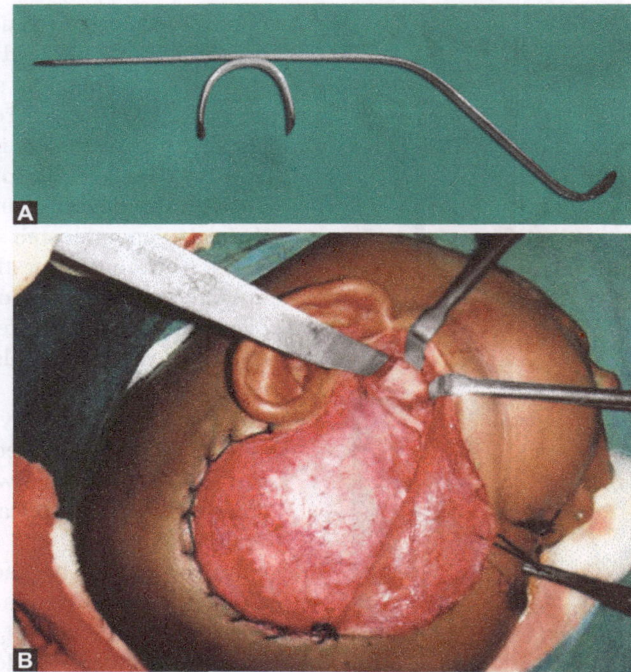

Figs 1.39A and B: Condylar retractor used during TMJ surgery as a guard

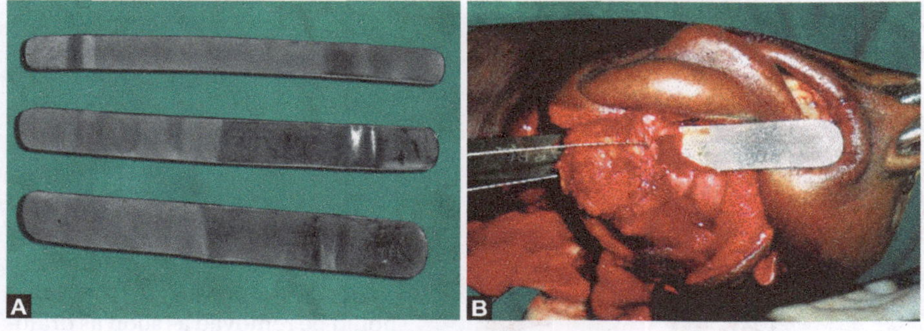

Figs 1.40A and B: Malleable retractor

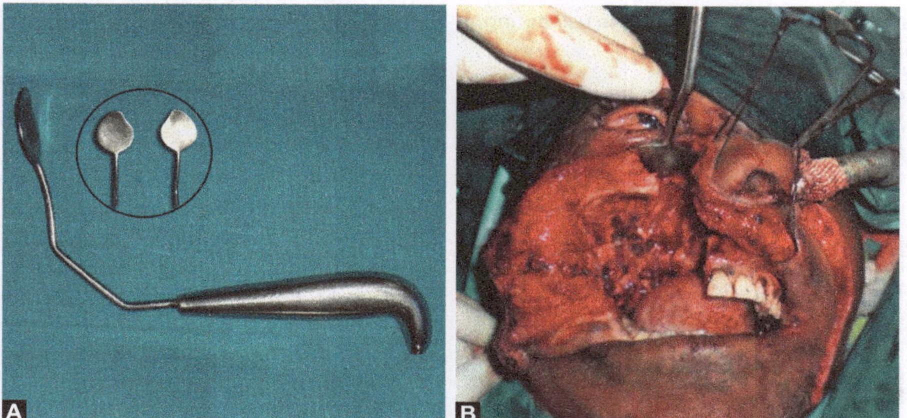

Figs 1.41A and B: Eyeball retractor

- Corrugated drains are usually removed on the third day or when there is cessation of discharge.

Types of Drains

Cotton gauze

Gauze acts as a drain by capillary action in the fabric, which absorbs the fluid (Fig. 1.43). Once it becomes saturated, it acts as a plug rather than as a drain, hence, it should be changed twice every 24 hours.

Uses

To pack a cavity to prevent its closure and allow healing from floor or to control diffused oozing, e.g. after incision and drainage of:

- Injection abscess in gluteal or deltoid region.
- Breast abscess, enucleated and infected odontogenic cysts, etc.

The gauze drain can also be inserted in an abscess cavity as a pack cum drain if the oozing of blood is present for achieving hemostasis. However, it must be remembered that gauze has an undesirable property of capillarity which impedes the patent drainage and thus, it should be replaced by corrugated rubber dam drain once the purpose of hemostasis is achieved, to facilitate proper drainage.

Advantage

It acts as a temporary drainage.

Disadvantages

- Gets soaked rapidly.
- Gets sealed within 6 hours by fibrin network.
- When soaked it acts as a moist channel for the penetration of bacteria.
- When a soaked gauze is removed, it is often followed by a gush of accumulated fluid from the cavity.
- When a pack is left in contact with the raw surfaces, it damages the raw surfaces since it becomes adherent to it. When gauze is soaked in liquid paraffin the damage to the raw surface can be avoided, but it decreases the absorption capacity.

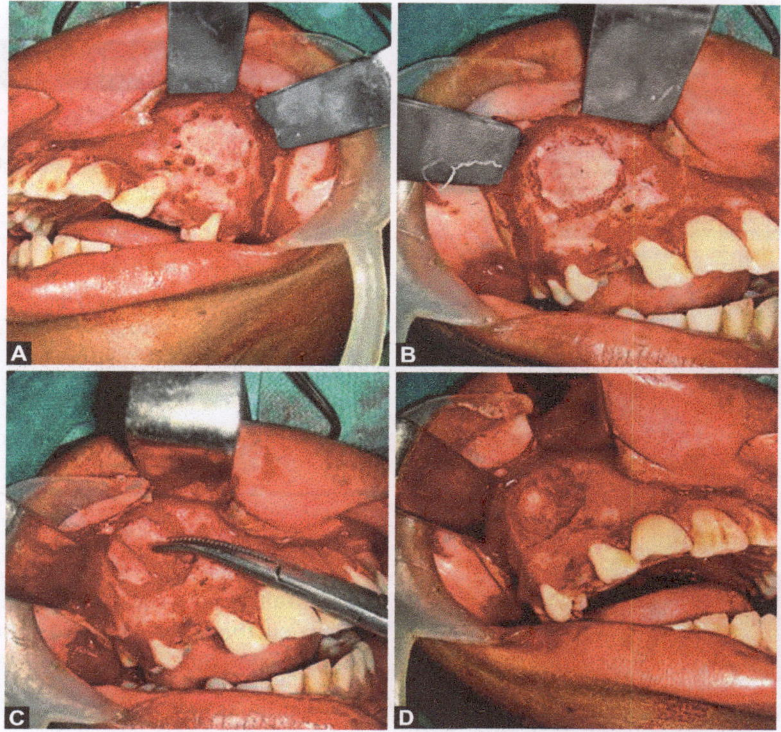

Figs 1.42A to D: Poststamp incision for controlled bone removal

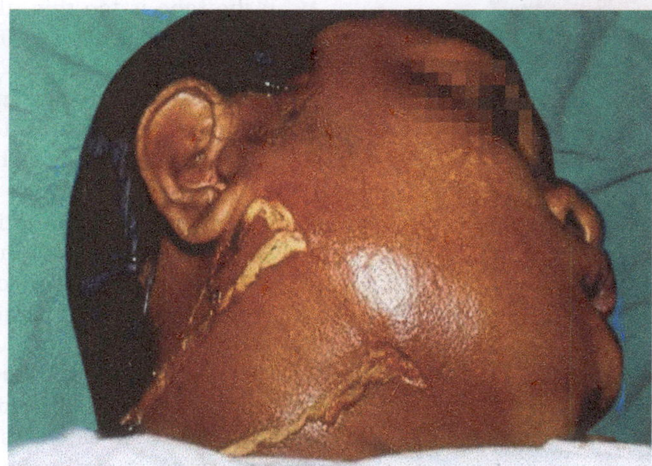

Fig. 1.43: Wick drain

Wicks

The wick is formed from gauge or threads of ligatures or suture material twisted together or bound loosely. Where the source of drainage cannot be brought to the surface, then a wick can be passed down to it.

Advantages

- When the oozing of the blood is present from the abscess cavity due to presence of friable granulation tissue, wicks can be packed in the cavity to achieve hemostasis. The wick can be replaced by corrugated drain after 24 hours.
- The wick can be impregnated with antiseptic solution or antibiotics to ensure local drug delivery in adequate concentration.
- It is economical and easily available and can be made of a required size in the OT.

Disadvantages

- It becomes soaked by the fluid.
- When a wick is made of folded gauze, it swells upon soaking which will obstruct the tract.
- It can adhere to the surface.
- It requires frequent change because it becomes ineffective due to the soaking.

Red rubber corrugated drain (sheet drain)

It is made up of red rubber which is available in the form of unsterile sheets, from which the strips of required length and breadth are cut and sterilized by autoclaving. With this drain, fluid reaches the surface by gravity hence it must be covered with the gauze pad (Figs 1.44A and B).

Advantages

- Drainage of the fluid occurs along the grooves of the drain, so chances of blockage are less.
- Red rubber is an irritant. It forms a fibrous tract around itself, which is advantageous.
- This drain is used only when there is minimal amount of discharge.

Disadvantages

If it is used for a prolonged period and removed at a time, the track of the drain will start healing from superficial and deep aspects while the middle part remains infected. This leads to sinus formation or pocket formation. Prolonged insertion leads to release of sulfur from red rubber drain evoking adverse tissue reactions.

Being a tough material, it can injure intestine and can cause fistula, if kept for a longer period, because when the drain is in the vicinity of the suture line, it may break up the suture line.

It might be sucked into the wound when it is not fixed properly to the surface or not removed carefully.

Currently portex drain is used instead of red rubber drain as it is less irritant than the red rubber and it also has a radio opaque line which helps in detecting the drain radiographically in case the drain is lost in the cacity (Fig. 1.45).

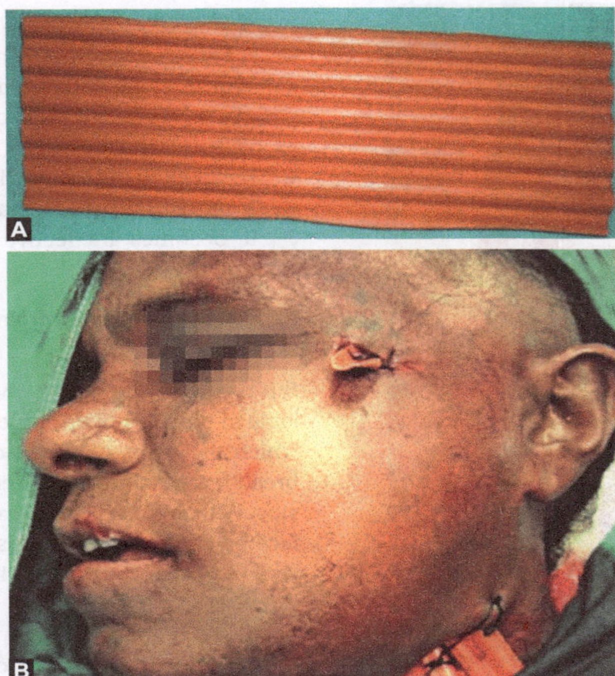

Figs 1.44A and B: (A) Corrugated rubber dam drain; (B) Drains *in situ*, fixed with sutures

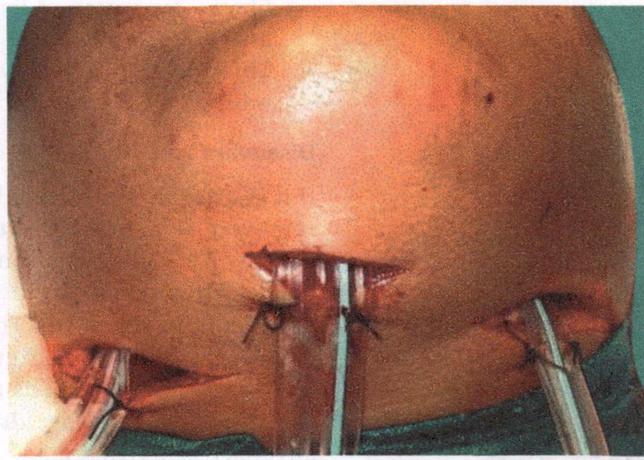

Fig. 1.45: Corrugated portex drain

Uses

- Drainage of the peritoneal cavity after an operation is done for any of the following: enteric perforation, perforated appendicitis, biliary surgery and sever peritonitis (Table 1.4).
- Drainage of perirenal areas after pyelolithotomy.
- Drainage of large abscess cavity, e.g. after incision and drainage of the submandibular space abscess.
- To drain retropubic space after surgery on the bladder, e.g. cystolithotomy, suprapubic prostatectomy.
- To drain subcutaneous tissue after removal of multiple enlarged nodes in neck, groin, etc.
- After mastectomy, removal of tumors.
- **Tube Drain:** When the fluid enters the tube, it can be guided into a collecting apparatus.

Table 1.4: Site-wise preference of the drain

Site	Preferable drain
Subcutaneous	Gauze wicks, corrugated sheet glove drain, soft tube drain
Subfascial	Tube drain
Intramuscular	Tube drain
Extraperitoneal	Tube drain or corrugated sheet
Intraperitoneal	Soft drain
Cysts	Closed tube drain
Abscess	Corrugated rubber drain

Advantage

Tube drain forms the closed drainage system so that raw surface cannot be contaminated due to entry of bacteria.

Disadvantages

- It drains only in the direction of the gravity.
- If the tube is too thin, the force of capillarity tends to retard the free flow of fluid through it.
- It cannot drain viscous fluid.
- It drains the fluid only when the tube is larger; so the fluid can be replaced by the air.
- When continuous negative suction is applied to a tube drain, the tissue is drawn into the inner hole.

The types of tube drains are as follows:

Catheters (Red rubber catheter, Malecot's catheter and Foley's catheter): Use of catheters is similar to that of sheet drain, but they are used particularly when the amount of drainage is high.

Advantage

Catheters can be directly connected to the apparatus, so that the contamination on wound with the drainage is less.

Disadvantage

The inner end of a catheter can be blocked, due to the obstruction caused by the draining material.

Uses

- To drain large abscess cavity.
- To drain pyogenic abscess.
- To drain the infected hydatid cyst of the liver (drain should be put near the incision on liver and not in the cavity itself).
- To drain retropubic area after prostatectomy. This prevents the soiling of the skin, if leakage persists.
- To drain after thoracocentesis, cholecystostomy, cecostomy, cystostomy.
- To drain pelvic abscess.
- To drain peritoneal abscesses.
- To drain bladder after Freyer's prostatectomy to give an alternative pathway, if clot retention occurs.

Portex drainage tube: It is made up of soft portex material. It is elastic and has side holes as well as terminal holes at the tip. It causes least irritation, therefore can be used for a prolonged period. It has a radio-opaque line along its length. Presterilized tubes are available.

Uses

- To drain pleural cavity in:
  - Empyema
  - Hydropneumothorax
  - Pneumothorax
  - Hemothorax.
- To drain postoperatively after an operation on heart or lungs.

Precaution

Portex intercostals drainage tube should be connected to underwater seal bottle by extension tubing.

Penrose drain

It is a hollow tube of latex rubber with thin wall, and can be made by cutting the finger stall of surgical glove. Its tip is cut so that both the ends are open.

Uses

- As a cigarette drain.
- As a simple drain.
- For sump drainage of the peripancreatic retroperitoneal tissue in patients with infected pancreatic abscess. For this, special drain is made as follows:
  No. 24 or 22 Foley's catheter is taken, bulb and the valve of balloon channel are cut. Multiple side holes are made on half the length of the catheter. Two or three layers of ribbon gauze are placed around it and then it is put in penrose drain after cutting side holes onto it.

Cigarette drain: Penrose drain that has a gauze within it is called a cigarette drain in cigarette drain; the ooze exists along and not through the gauze. The rubber acts as conduit.

Advantages and uses are same as for penrose drain.

Disadvantages

- Secretions cannot be collected in bags, so they cannot be measured.
- Chances of infection are more than in penrose but less than those in corrugated rubber drain.
- Skin irritation and excoriation may occur due to seepage of irritant effluent.

Vacuum drain/suction drain (redivac drain, romovac drain)

Principle: Active suction is applied in a continuous manner. So it does not allow the secretions to collect inside and also maintains patency of the drainage tube; it does not allow the secretions to dry and occlude the drain site (Figs 1.46A to C).

Purposes

It serves two purposes:

1. The provision of access for accumulated pus or intestinal contents.
2. The prophylactic removal of any fluid within the peritoneal cavity (e.g. bile) before its presence can lead to complications. This prophylactic drainage may be best accomplished by the use of close wound suction drainage. As, it is more important where small amount of drainage and non-dependent drainage is required.

Advantages

- Less irritating to the tissues.
- Less likely to cause infection because it is a closed system.
- It is particularly effective under large skin flaps, e.g. after radical neck dissection, modified radical mastectomy.
- Closed suction drainage decreases the incidence of infection that occurs secondary to contamination of the drain itself and is mandatory in the presence of a foreign body.
- It can be placed at a non-dependent site.

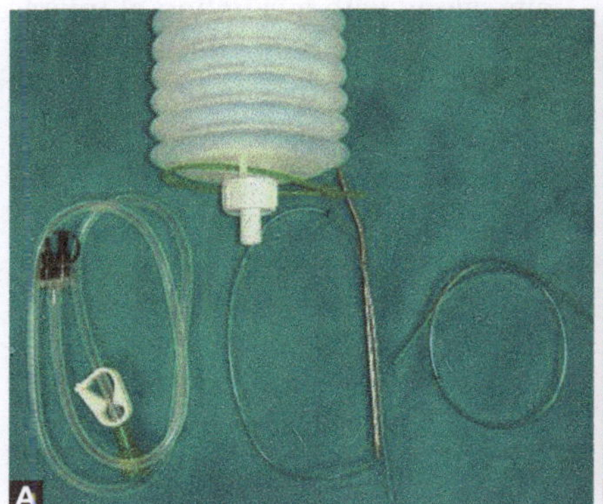

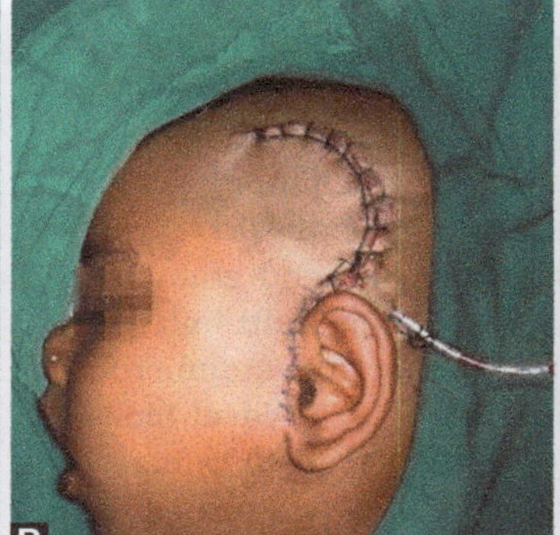

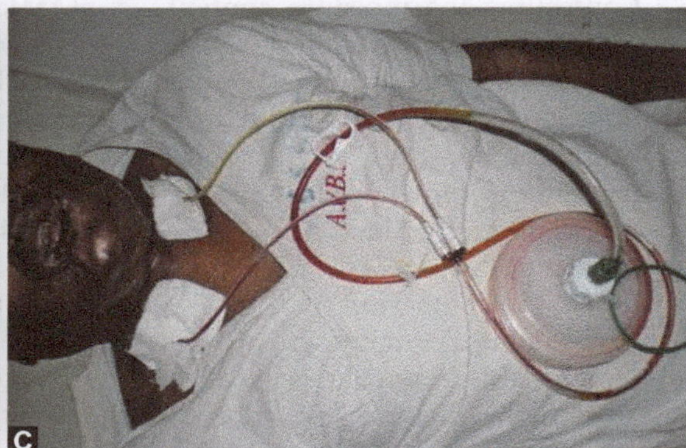

Figs 1.46A to C: Romo-vac drain®

Disadvantage: The continuous negative pressure may induce bleeding.

Dressing

A dressing is an adjunct used by a person for application to a wound to promote healing and/or prevent further harm. A dressing is designed to be indirect contact with the wound, which makes it different from a bandage, which is primarily used to hold a dressing in place. Dressings are frequently used in first aid and nursing.

The ideal wound dressing should have the following characteristics:

- Provide mechanical and bacterial protection.
- Maintain a moist environment at the wound/dressing interface.
- Allow gaseous and fluid exchange.
- Remain nonadherent to the wound.
- Safe in use—nontoxic, non-sensitizing, and non-allergic (both to the patient and the medical personnel).
- Well acceptable to the patient (e.g. providing pain relief and not influencing movement).
- Highly absorbable (for exuding wounds).
- Absorb wound odor.
- Sterile.
- Easy to use (can be applied by medical personnel or the patient).
- Require infrequent changing (if necessary).
- Available in a suitable range of forms and sizes.
- Cost effective and covered by health insurance systems.

Purpose of Dressing

- Controlling the moisture content, so that the wound stays moist or dry, to maintain the optimal wound humidity to prevent wound from becoming dry and forming eschar preventing direct cell migration across the wound bed.
- Protecting the wound from infection.
- Removing slough, and
- Maintaining the optimum pH and temperature to encourage healing. To provide thermal insulation by maintaining a constant temperature of 36 to 37°C to optimize the mitotic activity.

Indications

- Surgical and traumatic wounds.
- Donor site wound dressing.
- Fungating growth.
- On abrasions.

Types of Dressing

- **Glycerine magsulf dressing:** It is the saturated solution of magnesium sulphate ($MgSO_4$) crystals and glycerine, since magnesium sulphate is hygroscopic, it is used to reduce edema in the cases of cellulitis, excessive postsurgical edema.
- **Vaseline gauze dressing:** The vaseline gauze dressing is used to accelerate wound healing. It is nonadhesive and thus ideal for dressing the healthy, raw, granulating wound surfaces. It is also used to cover the raw areas created following the harvesting of split thickness skin grafts.
- **Dry dressing:** Dry dressing is used in wound without granulation, e.g. postoperative sutured, healing incision line.
- **Wet dressing:** Wet dressing is used when ulcer with granulation tissue, i.e. eusol, betadine, saline.
- **Biological dressings:** Such as amniotic membrane dressings, collagen membrane or a skin graft are the best dressings as they prevent wound contamination and promote the healing. The other examples of the biological dressings are aminiotic membrane, collagen membrane, fascia. Amniotic membrane (AM), or amnion, is the innermost layer of the placenta and consists of a thick basement membrane and an avascular stromal matrix. Its properties such as lack of immunogenicity, fluid loss controlling, pain relieving, re-epithelialization and granulation and its stimulating, anti-inflammatory, antifibrotic and antimicrobial properties make it an ideal biological dressing. It has the advantage of ready availability at no extra cost to the patient. It provides secure coverage to the wound site, which reduces exudation from the wound. The AM stimulates epithelialization from the ulcer bed and/or the wound edge, which is considered to be mediated by growth factors and progenitor cells which are released by it. One of the most striking effects is its granulation stimulating effect. This is due to some angiogenic and growth factors which are produced by the membrane. Despite being a human derivative, it is not rejected, because the AM does not express the HLA A, B, C and the DR antigens.

  Collagen materials have been utilized in medicine and dentistry because of their proven biocompatibility and capability of promoting wound healing. Biological dressings like collagen are impermeable to bacteria, and create the most physiological interface between the wound surface and the environment. Collagen dressings have other advantages over conventional dressings in terms of ease of application and being natural, nonimmunogenic, nonpyrogenic, hypoallergenic, and pain-free. Collagen is a biomaterial that encourages wound healing through deposition and organization of freshly formed fibers and granulation tissue in the wound bed thus creating a good environment for wound healing. Collagen sheets, when applied to a wound, not only promote angiogenesis, but also enhance body's repair mechanisms. While acting as a mechanical support these reduce edema and loss of fluids from the wound site, along with facilitation of migration of fibroblasts into the wound and enhancing the metabolic activity of the granulation tissue. Moreover, it is easy to apply and has the additional advantage of stopping bleeding.
- **Occlusive dressing:** An occlusive dressing is an air and water-tight trauma dressing used in first aid.

  These dressings are generally made with a waxy coating so as to provide a total seal, and as a result do not have the absorbent properties of gauze

Table 1.5: Different types of material used for dressing and their examples and properties

Type	Properties
Passive products	Traditional dressings that provide cover over the wound, e.g. gauze and tulle dressings
Interactive products	Polymeric films and forms which are mostly transparent, permeable to water vapor and oxygen, non-permeable to bacteria, e.g. hyaluronic acid, hydrogels, foam dressings
Bioactive products	Dressings which deliver substances active in wound healing, e.g. hydrocolloids, alginates, collagens, chitosan

pads. They are typically used to treat open, or "sucking," chest wounds to alleviate or prevent a tension pneumothorax (a serious complication of a simple pneumothorax). They are also used in conjunction with a moist sterile dressing for intestinal evisceration.

- Occlusive dressings come in various forms, including Vaseline Gauze, which sticks to the skin surrounding the wound using Vaseline.

Classification of Wound Dressings

Synthetic wound dressings would broadly categorized into the following types:

- Passive products
- Interactive products
- Bioactive products

The properties and examples of these products are given in Table 1.5.

Bandage

The bandage is the piece of material used to cover, support, immobilize or exert pressure to the part (Box 1.5).

Bandages commonly used in oral and maxillofacial surgery

- Simple roller bandage—single or double headed.
- Barrel bandage to retain the dressing and support the lower jaw.
- Four-tailed bandage to support the lower jaw (Figs 1.47A and B).
- Mastoid bandage for compression after TMJ surgeries.
- Compression bandage with simple roller bandage, crepe bandage or with elastoplasts. It helps in achieving hemostasis, obliterates tissue dead space and prevents formation of the hematoma.

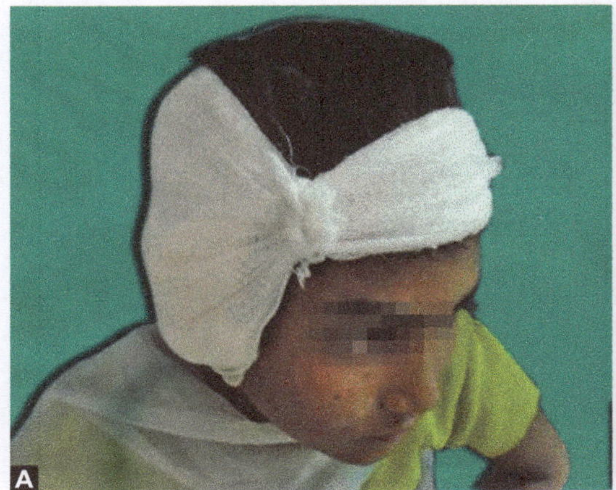

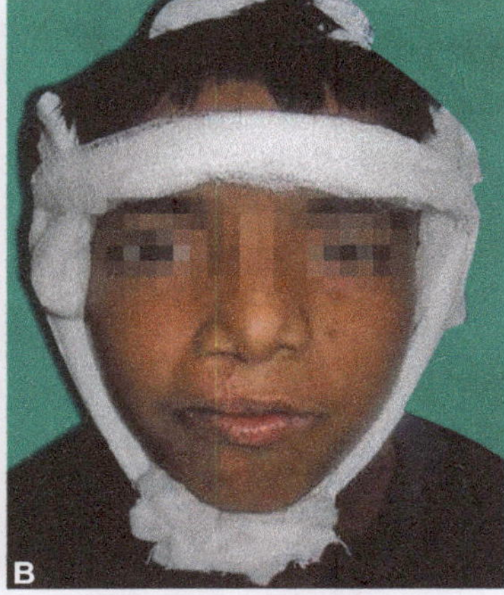

Figs 1.47A and B: Mastoid bandage and 'four tailed' bandage

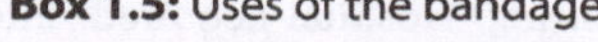

Box 1.5: Uses of the bandage

As a first aid for the injured part, especially to arrest bleeding
To provide rest and support to the part. To retain dressing and to splint the part. To prevent inflammatory edema.

BIBLIOGRAPHY

1. Berger SA, Kramer M, Nagar H, Finklestein A, Frimmerman A, Miller HI. Effect of surgical mask position on bacterial contamination of the operative field. J Hosp Infect. 1993;23:51-4.
2. Dineen P. An evaluation of the duration of the surgical scrub. Surg Obstet. 1969; 129:1181-4.
3. Gupta DS, Borle RM. Operation theater discipline. J Indian Dental Association. 1983;55:437-40.
4. Humphreys H, Russell AJ, Marshall RJ. The effect of surgical theatre headgear on bacterial counts. J Hosp Infect. 1991; 19:175-80.
5. Jordan DM. There is a reason for dress codes. Imprint. 1991;38:46-8.
6. Lippert S, Gutschik E. Bacterial sedimentation during cardiac surgery reduced by disposable clothing. Scand J Thorac Cardiovasc Surg. 1992;26:79-82.
7. Mitchell NJ, Hunt S. Surgical face masks in modern operating rooms—a costly and unnecessary ritual? J Hosp Infect. 1991;18:239-42.
8. Moylan JA, Fitzpatrick KT, Davenport KE. Reducing wound infections.Improved gown and drape barrier performance. Arch Surg. 1987;122:152-7.
9. Nagai I, Kadata M, Takechi M, Kumamoto R, Ucoka M, Matsuoka K. Studies on the mode of bacterial contamination of the operating theater corridor floor. J Hosp Infect. 1984;15:50-5.
10. Orr NW. Is a mask necessary in the operating theatre? Ann R Coll Surg Eng. 1981;63:390-2.
11. O'Hara L. The Operating Theater as a degradation Ritual: A Student Nurse's View, Science as Culture. 1989;6:20-8.
12. Pratt RJ, Pellowe C, Loveday HP. Epic phase 1: The development of National Evidence-based Guidelines for Pre-

venting Hospital-acquired infections in England associated with the use of short-term indwelling urethral catheters in acute care. Different types of material used for dressing and their examples and properties. Technical Report. London: Thames Valley University; 2000.
13. Rehork B, Ruden H. Investigations into the efficacy of different procedures for surgical hand disinfection between consecutive operations. J Hosp Infect. 1991;19:115-27.
14. Tunevall TG. Postoperative wound infections and surgical face masks in a controlled study. World J Surg. 1991;15: 383-8.
15. Verkkala K, Eklund A, Ojajarvi J, Tiittanen L, Hoborn J, Makela P. The conventionally ventilated operating theatre and air contamination control during cardiac surgery—bacteriological and particulate matter control garment options for low level contamination. Eur J Cardiothorac Surg. 1998;14:206-10.

REFERENCES

1. Rubino JR. Overview of Lysol scientific studies. Pediatr Infect Dis J. 2000;19(10 Suppl):S123-4. Review.
2. Ekizoglu MT, Ozalp M, Sultan N. An investigation of the bactericidal effect of certain antiseptics and disinfectants on some hospital isolates of gram-negative bacteria. Infect Control Hosp Epidemiol. 2003;24(3):225-7.
3. Braun A. Survival of skin preserved in weak formalin solutions. Bulletin of Experimental Biology and Medicine. 1996;62(4)1195-966.
4. Dryburgh N, Smith F, Donaldson J, et al. Debridement for surgical wounds. Cochrane Database Syst Rev. 2008; 16(3):CD006214. Review.
5. Joshi HN, Kansagra PJ, Dayal PK. Facial myiasis: report of case. ASDC J Dent Child. 1986;53(1):70-1.
6. Geffen N, Norman G, Kheradiya NS. Chlorhexidine gluconate 0.02 percent as adjunct to primary treatment for corneal bacterial ulcers. Isr Med Assoc J. 2009;11(11):664-8.
7. Topcu O, Kuzu I, Karayalcin K. Effects of peritoneal lavage with scolicidal agents on survival and adhesion formation in rats. World J Surg. 2006;30(1):127-33.
8. Hemani ML, Lepor H. Skin preparation for the prevention of surgical site infection: which agent is best? Rev Urol. 2009 Fall;11(4):190-5.
9. Dias FN, Ishii M, Nogaroto SL, et al. Sterilization of medical devices by ethylene oxide, determination of the dissipation of residues, and use of Green Fluorescent Protein as an indicator of process control. J Biomed Mater Res B Appl Biomater. 2009;91(2): 626-30.
10. Gupta DS, Borle RM. Operation theatre discipline. J Indian Dent Assoc. 1983;55(11):437-40.
11. R. Tomaszewski. Planning a Better Operating Room Suite: Design and Implementation Strategies for Success. Perioperative Nursing Clinics, 2008; 3(1):43-50.

2 Sutures

Borle Rajiv M, Bora Smriti, Rai Anshul

"A suture is a strand of material used to ligate blood vessels and approximate the tissue together[1]."
"To suture is the act of sewing or bringing tissues together and holding them in apposition until healing has taken place."

HISTORICAL ASPECTS[2]

The first description of suture was given by Edwin Smith Papyrus in 16th century BC. Sutures have been used as far back as records go both to hold wounds together and to arrest hemorrhage. The thread and instrument for its application were made from any convenient available method. There is mention in the literature that various material were used for suturing such as gold wires, horses hair, threads plant fibers, etc. and the quest for the ideal material continued.

Primitive men in South America used large black ants to bite the edges of the wound together. Ancient Egyptian Papyri prefer to the use of linen strips, coated with an adhesive mixture of flour and honey for skin closure.

East African tribes ligated blood vessels with tendons and closed wound with strips of vegetation.

Gelen (AD150) comments for the first time on the use of catgut. Although its most important fact that it is absorbed and digested by body enzymes was not discovered until the 18th century. The ancients used it because it was strong and easily available.

In 900 AD Rhazes of Arabia first employed 'kitgut' to suture abdominal wounds.

John Hunter was of opinion that suture were basically undesirable, but if needed they should be interrupted suture. He preferred bandage or sticking plaster across the wound.

In 1867, Hister began to use the catgut treated with an aqueous solution of carbolic acid (sterile suture). Many different materials were tried, viz. linen, cotton, horsehair, tendons, intestinal tissues of various animals, gold, silver wires, etc.

In recent decades, new synthetic filaments such as nylon, polypropylene and polyester have become available. Synthetic absorbable material have also been developed.

With the advancements in suture technology, sterilization techniques also improved. Sterilization with cobalt 60 and ethylene oxide is the new the method of choice.

PROPERTIES OF SUTURES

- **Strength:** It must be strong enough to maintain tissue in apposition for a specified time.
  - *Straight-pull tensile strength:* It is the minimum amount of tension required to break the filaments.
  - *Kno-pull tensile strength:* It is the minimum amount of tension required to break the knot given by the material. It is more important than straight pull tensile strength. It is measured in kilogram during manufacture. The tensile strength increases with increase in diameter of the suture material.
- **Smoothness:** The smoother the suture material, the easier the passage of suture through the tissue with least trauma. For example, monofilament prolene is smooth thus preferred in vascular surgery.
- **Knot security:** Monofilament suture have smooth surface, hence, the knot will slip and open (more knots required). Polyfilament are held more securely (2 to 3 knots are enough). For example, for proline suture the knot stability is poor as compared to the braided silk suture and hence, it is said that the number of knots should be equal to the number of days you want the proline suture to stay, i.e. it requires more knots than the braided material.
- **Infection:** There is relation between the configuration of the suture (multifilament or monofilament) and its propensity to promote infection.
  - Bacterial adherence to the surface of suture

- Ability of the bacteria to gain access.

Braided material can hold bacteria in its interstices where they may be protected from phagocytes. Similarly, the suture having more capillarity tends to attract bacterial colonies and their passage along the suture deep into the wound.

Advantages of monofilament over multifilament are as follows:

- Monofilament provides easy passage through the tissue whereas multifilament tends to provide tissue drag (Fig. 2.1A).
- The smooth surface of monofilament does not support bacterial growth whereas multifilament provides a nidus for infection (Fig. 2.1B).

- **Reactivity:** It is the cellular response to foreign body. It is more for the natural material.
- **Visibility:** Each suture should ideally be distinguishable at a glance from another suture. Similarly the suture material should have good visibility when seen against the bloody surgical field.
- **Handling:** The sutures should run smoothly through the tissue. It should have no memory. Knots should bed down easily and be secure with minimum numbers of throws.
- **Elasticity:** The suture should have degree of elasticity to accommodate the changes of bulk in wound.
- **Memory:** Inherent capability of suture to return or to maintain its original gross shape (related to elasticity, plasticity and diameter).
- **Plasticity:** Measure of the ability to deform without breaking and to maintain a new form after relief of the deforming force.
- **Pliability:** Ease of handling of suture material, ability to adjust knot tension and to secure knots (related to suture material, filament type, and diameter).
- **Capillarity:** Extent to which absorbed fluid is transferred along the suture. The ideal properties of the suture material are summarized in the Box 2.1.

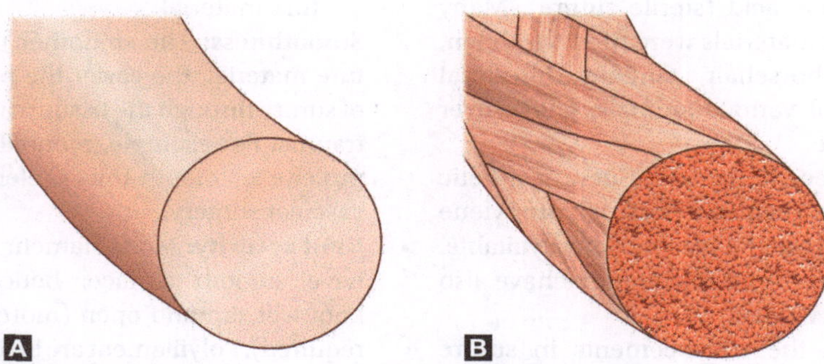

Figs 2.1A and B: (A) Magnified view of monofilament; (B) Magnified view of multifilament

Box 2.1: Ideal properties of suturing material[3]

- It should have a uniform diameter as it avoids breaking points.
- It should maintain its tensile strength until its purpose is over.
- It should have good handling properties.
- It should evoke nil or minimum tissue reaction.
- It should not favor bacterial growth.
- The knot should be stable.
- It should have good tensile strength at a smaller diameter.
- It should not have capillarity, should be non-allergic, non-electrolytic and non-carcinogenic.
- It should be sterilizable without alteration of physiochemical properties.
- It should have good shelf-life.
- It should be economical.

PRINCIPLES OF SUTURE SELECTION[4]

The surgeon has a choice of selecting a suture material suitable for different tissue and the needs of a particular site and surgery. Adequate strength of the suture material will prevent suture breakage. Secure knots will prevent knot slippage. But the surgeon must understand the nature of the suture material, the biologic forces in the healing wound and the interaction of the suture and the tissues. The following principles should guide the surgeon in suture selection.

- When a wound has reached maximal strength, sutures are no longer needed.
  - Tissues that ordinarily heal slowly such as skin, fascia and tendons should usually be closed with non-absorbable sutures.
  - Tissues that heal rapidly such as stomach, colon, oral mucosa and bladder may be closed with absorbable sutures.
- Foreign bodies in potentially contaminated tissues may convert contamination to infection, therefore
  - Avoid multifilament sutures, which may convert a contaminated wound into an infected one.
  - Use monofilament or absorbable sutures in potentially contaminated tissues.
- Where cosmetic results are important close and prolonged apposition of wounds and avoidance of irritants will produce the best result, therefore
  - Use the smallest inert monofilament such as materials such as nylon or polypropylene.
  - Avoid skin sutures and close subcuticularly whenever possible.
  - Under certain circumstances, to secure close apposition of skin edges, skin closure tape may be used.
- Foreign bodies in the presence of fluids containing high concentrations

of crystalloids may act as nidus for precipitation and stone formation.

- Regarding suture size:
  - Use the finest size, commensurate with the natural strength of the tissue.
  - If the postoperative course of the patient may produce sudden strains on the suture line, reinforce it with retention sutures. Remove them as soon as the patient's condition is stabilized.

United States Pharmacopeia Classification

- **Class I:** Silk or synthetic fibers of monofilament, twisted or braided construction.
- **Class II:** Cotton or linen fibers or coated natural or synthetic fibers in which the coating contributes to suture thickness without adding strength.
- **Class III:** Metal wire of monofilament or multifilament construction.

Suture Size

Suture size is based on strength and diameter as decided by the United States Pharmacopeia (USP). This system uses "0" as the baseline, average size suture. As suture diameter decreases, "0"s are added or numbers followed by a "0" (For example, 000 and 3-0 are the same size). As suture diameter increases more "0", numbers are assigned to the suture material.

TYPES OF SUTURE MATERIAL (TABLE 2.1)

Catgut

History: The term 'catgut' is a misnomer. It is derived from the word 'kitgut' which means medieval three stringed violin like instrument (*dancing master's fiddle*), string of which were used by ancient people as suture material.

Lord Baron Joseph Lister (1827–1912) treated it with carbolic acid, hardened this material and reduced the tissue reaction and later treated it with chromic acid.

Manufacture

Prepared from submucosa of sheep's intestine. Sheep submucosa contains rich elastic tissue, which accounts for high tensile strength.

Sterilization

Catgut is sterilized with gamma radiations utilizing 2.5 mega-rads or by ethylene oxide. It is sterilized and preserved in 2.5 percent formaldehyde and denatured absolute alcohol inside spools or foils.

Chromic acid method: Immersed in 20 percent chromic acid and five parts of 8.5 percent glycerin. It sterilizes and secures a longer stay in pack.

Duration of Stay in Tissue

Catgut retains tensile strength for 10 days and chromic catgut for 20 days. Tensile strength is zero after 30 days and completely absorbed in 100 days.

Absorption

Enzymatic digestion by proteolytic enzymes derived from lysosomes from inflammatory cells (polymorphs and macrophages) around catgut. Hence, in the presence of infection catgut is easily absorbed.

Uses

Plain catgut (Figs 2.2A and B)

- Ligation of small blood vessels near the surface of skin.
- Suture subcutaneous tissue, advisable at urinary tract, biliary tract, subcutaneous tissue.

Chromic catgut (Figs 2.3A and B)

- **Size-1-0, 2-0:** Ligation of medium sized blood vessel, peritoneum muscle, rectus sheath, liver and spleen, ligation of pedicle.
- **Size 2-0:** Ligation of cut vessel in vasectomy closure of ureteric and bladder wound and pyelotomy incision.
- **Size-2-0, 3-0:** Intestinal anastomosis.
- **Size-3-0, 4-0:** Muscle layer in cleft lip surgery.
- **Size-5-0, 6-0:** Plastic surgery and circumcision.

Chromic Suture Material

Chromic suture materials have undergone various intensities of tanning with the salt of chromic acid to delay the tissue absorption time. Typical examples of chromic suture and absorption times are:

- **Type A:** Plain—10 days
- **Type B:** Mild chromic—20 days
- **Type C:** Medium chromic—30 days
- **Type D:** Extra chromic—40 days.

ABSORBABLE SYNTHETIC SUTURE

Polyglycolic Acid (Dexon)

Synthetic non-protein suture polyglycolic acid and made by excursion of fine strands are then braided to form uniform size. The filaments are uniform in size.

- **Color:** Green
- **Size:** 8 '0' – 2 '0'
- **Length:** Non-needled length of 150 cm
- **Needle in length:** 45 to 75 mm
- **Tensile strength:** Fourteen days post-implantations about 55 percent of original value and at 21 days 20 percent of original value
- **Packing:** Pre-sterilized form of foil over wrapped without preservative
- **Absorption:** By esterase enzyme
- **Time:** Hundred days.

Advantages

- Minimum tissue reaction
- Less tissue edema
- Uniform absorption
- Can be used in presence of infection (as it is not absorbed by phagocytosis)
- Better knot holding property (braided)
- Less fraying of ends (braided).

Uses

- Intestinal anastamosis
- Ligation of pedicle to ligate superior and inferior thyroid vessel, ligation of splenic and renal pedicle in splenectomy and nephrectomy
- In biliary surgery
- Cosmetic surgery.

Table 2.1: Types of sutures and their properties

Sutures	Classification	Raw material	Absorption rate	Tensile strength	Tissue reaction	Contraindication	Precaution	Use
Catgut Plain Chromic	Natural Monofilament Absorbable	Collagen Derived from sheep or bovine intestine	 70 days 90 days	 Zero after 30 days	 Moderate Moderate	Not to be given when prolonged approximation of the tissue under stress is required	Absorbs faster	Subcutaneous
Linen	Natural, Multifilament, Nonabsorbable	Staple flax fibers Jute fibers	Gradual		Moderate	Cardiovascular surgery	None	Ligation of superficial vessels, mucosal suturing without stress
Surgical silk	Natural, Multifilament, Non-absorbable.	Filament spun by silk worm larva to form its cocoon			Moderate	Cardiovascular surgery	Stich granuloma High infection rate	General, plastic and ophthalmic surgery Ligating body tissues
Surgical cotton	Natural, Multifilament, Nonabsorbable	Staple Egyptian cotton fibers		Low tensile strength	Minimal	None	Frays easily	Most body tissues for ligating and suturing
Surgical steel	Natural, Multifilament, Non-absorbable	Alloy of iron, nickel and chromium	Non-absorbable	Indefinite	Low	Should not be used with a prosthesis of another alloy	Cutaneous dysfunction corrode break at points of bending, twisting and knotting	Abdominal wall and skin closure, sternal closure, retention, tendon repair, orthopedic and neurosurgery
Coated vicryl (polyglactin 410)	Synthetic, Monofilament/ Multifilament, Absorbable	Copolymer of lactide and glycolide coated with polyglactin 370 and calcium stearate	60–90 days	14 days–55% 21 days–20%	Mild	Being absorbable should not be used when prolonged approximation of tissue is required	Safety not proved in neural and cardiovascular tissues	Ligature suture tissues where an absorbable suture is desired

Contd...

Contd...

Sutures	Classification	Raw material	Absorption rate	Tensile strength	Tissue reaction	Contraindication	Precaution	Use
Polydioxanone (PDS)	Synthetic, Monofilament, Absorbable	Polyester polymer	240 days	20 days–70% 40 days–40% 60 days–20%	Minimal	Being absorbable should not be used when prolonged approximation of tissue is required	Absorbs slowly	Abdominal and thoracic closure subcutaneous tissue, rectal and colon surgery, orthopedic and plastic surgery can be used in the presence of sutures
Nylon	Synthetic, Monofilament/ Multifilament, Non-absorbable	Polyamide polymer	Degrades at a rate of 15–20% per year		Extremely low	None	Knot slippery infection due to cervices in braided nylon	Skin closure, Retention, plastic ophthalmic, repair hernia microsurgery
Polypropylene (prolene)	Synthetic, Monofilament, Non-absorbable	Polymer of propylene		2 years	Minimal transient acute inflammatory reaction	None	None	General, plastic, cardiovascular surgery, skin closure, ophthalmology
Collagen	Natural Monofilament Absorbable	Homogenous dispersion of pure collagen fibrils from the flexor tendons of beef	56 days		Minimal	Cannot be used in slow healing tissue		Opthalmic surgery
Polyglycolic acid (Dexon)	Synthetic Absorbable	Nonprotein polymer of glycolic acid	100 days	30 days	Minimal			Intestinal anastomosis Ligation of pedicle

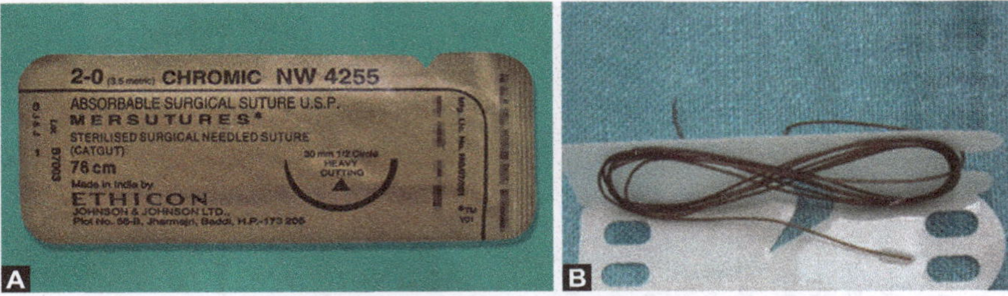

Figs 2.2A and B: Plain catgut

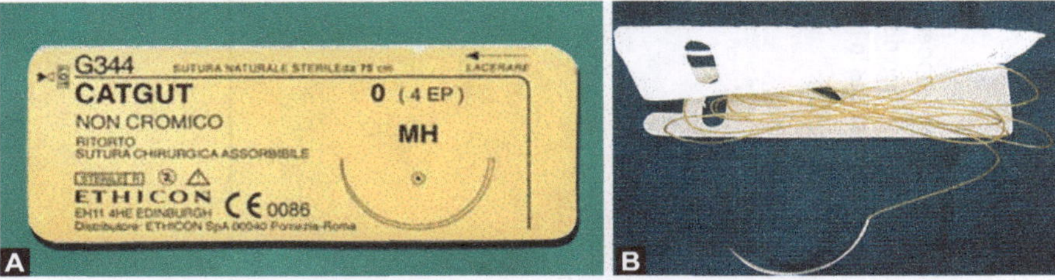

Figs 2.3A and B: Chromic catgut

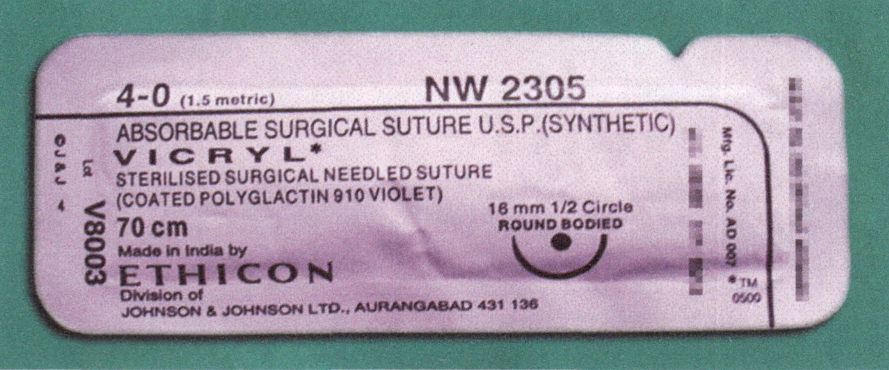

Fig. 2.4: Vicryl suture

Table 2.2: Classification of suture[3]

1. Absorbable			
	a. Synthetic	Monofilament-polydioxanone suture (PDS), polyglyconate	Multifilament—polyglycolic acid (PGA) (DEXON), polyglactin (vicryl)
	b. Natural	Monofilament—catgut	Multifilament—collagen
2. Non-absorbable			
	a. Synthetic	Monofilament—nylon, polyethylene, polypropylene, polybutester,	Multifilament—nylon, polyester
	b. Natural	Monofilament—stainless steel, Tantalum, platinum, silver wire	Multifilament—silk, linen, cotton
Newer		Newer non-absorbable synthetic suture material-Dacron, marlex, polyglyconate	Absorbable synthetic suture material are Poliglecaprone 25 (monocryl), Polydioxanone (PDS), Polyglactin 910 (vicryl coated), Polyglactin 910 (vicryl rapid), Ethibond (polybutylate coated braided polyster

Vicryl (Polyglactin 910)

Vicryl (Fig. 2.4) is a synthetic absorbable suture material. Polyglactin 910 is a co-polymer of glycoline and lactide. It is polyfilament braided suture manufactured by the process of extrusion.

- **Color:** Violet
- **Available size:** 7-0 to 1-0
- **Length:** 70 cm
- **Retention of tensile strength after embedding in the tissue:** 55 percent for 14 days and 20 percent for 21 days
- **Absorption:** Minimal up to 40 percent is completed by 60 to 90 days by slow enzymatic hydrolysis in presence of tissue fluid, then the pieces of fragments are phagocytosed by polymorphs and macrophages. Due to this reason there is least tissue reaction. Its absorption is not affected by infection.

The properties of different suture material are summarized in Table 2.2.

Advantages

- Minimal tissue reaction
- No fraying of edges
- Excellent handling characteristics
- Good knot stability
- Distinct violet color is visible in wound
- The unique molecular structure retains strength during healing period and gets absorbed rapidly after function is served.

Uses

- Intestinal anastomosis
- Ligation of pedicle closure of thoracotomy
- Closure of laparotomy
- Closure of the deeper tissue
- Mucosal suturing especially in transoral surgery
- Cleft palate surgery
- Suturing in pediatric patients
- Deeper layer closure.

Polyglyconate

Monofilament synthetic absorbable suture prepared from a co-polymer of glycolic acid and trimethylene carbonate.

- **Color:** Clear or green

- **Size:** 6-0 to 2-0 (green) and 5-0 to 1-0 (clear)
- **Absorbed:** By nonenzymatic hydrolysis, breaking down into beta-hydroxybutyric acid, glycolic acid and carbonic acid (first two excreted in urine)
- **Retention of tensile strength:** 70 percent up to 2 weeks and 55 percent up to 3 weeks
- **Absorption:** Completed by 6 months
- **Advantage:** Suppleness, flexibility, minimal tissue drag, ease of tying and good knot security.

It is used in most of the soft tissue surgeries.

Polydioxanone

Polydioxanone is a monofilament synthetic absorbable suture prepared from polydioxanone.

- **Color:** Blue, violet or undyed clear form
- **Tensile strength:**
  - 70 percent retained up to 2 weeks
  - 50 percent up to 4 weeks
  - 14 percent up to 8 weeks.
- **Absorption:** Minimal until 90 days and completed by 6 months. It is relatively inert
- **Used:** Where catgut is indicated, but not used due to tissue approximation is under tension.

Poliglecaprone 25 Monocryl (Ethicon)

- **Type:** Monofilament
- **Raw material:** Co-polymer of glycolide and epsilon-caprolactone
- **Retention of tensile strength:** 50 to 60 percent (Violet: 60–70%)—remains at one week. 20 to 30 percent (Violet 30–40%) remains at 2 weeks and lost in 3 weeks (Violet 4 weeks).

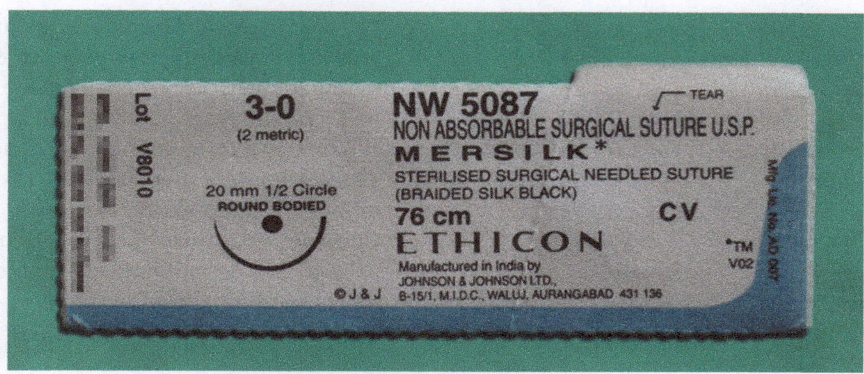

Fig. 2.5: Silk suture

NONABSORBABLE SUTURE MATERIAL

Silk

Silk suture (Fig. 2.5) is also called black, braided silk, due to its black color and the fact that it is multifilament suture prepared by twisting (braiding) these filaments over each other. The black color is for better visibility against the red surgical field. It is natural and nonabsorbable. Although it is categorized under nonabsorbable, it is actually an absorbable material being protein in nature. However, its absorption takes very long time and thus commonly considered to be nonabsorbable (Fig. 2.5). It is the most commonly used suture for the closure of the skin incisions due to its cost effectiveness.

Sizes: The thickness decreases as the size increases 1-0 to 8-0.

Source: Natural silk filament obtained from silk cocoon.

Nature: Consists of protein—70 percent organic protein fibrin, gum—30 percent.

The degumming of silk is done to retain natural body and elasticity; the appropriate number of filaments for each size is tightly braided. The suture is chromicised for noncapillarity.

Tensile strength: Progressive degradation of fibers may result in gradual loss of tensile strength over a period of time. It is not absorbed, but is gradually encapsulated by fibrous connective tissue.

Color: Black for better visibility.

Advantages

- Does not soak-up fluids, it does not limp or become brittle
- Ties down, securely and smoothly and securely
- Economical.

Disadvantages

- Stitch granuloma
- Infection rate is high as compared to synthetic material.

Availability

- Sterile foil over wrap pack as eyeless needled suture
- Sutupac—Precut lengths of sterile sutures in pack of two or six pieces of sutures, without needle
- Non-sterile on reels.

Types

1. According to preparation
   - Perma-hand silk suture
   - Virgin silk suture material prepared from gland of silkworm before pupae stage.

2. According to fibering pattern
   - Braided, twisted, floss
   - Size and length.

Eyeless needled suture

Available size: 9-0 to 3-0
Length: 9-0 to 6-0—36 cm
5-0 to 2-0—76 cm

Reel

Size: 6-0 to 4-0
Length: 25 m

Method of sterilization—autoclaving

- **Tissue reaction:** Acute inflammatory reaction
- **Contraindications:** Known sensitivity or allergies
- **Frequent uses:** Skin sutures.

Uses

- General soft tissue approximation and ligation including neurological, cardiovascular and ophthalmic procedures
- Fixing of skin graft
- To suture nerves and grafts in vascular surgery (atraumatic silk).

Nylon Suture (Ethilon, Dermalon)

Nylon suture (Fig. 2.6) is a synthetic non-absorbable suture. The thickness varies from 1-0 to 8-0.

- **Type:** Monofilament
- **Raw material:** Long chain aliphatic polymers, nylon 6 or nylon 66
- **Tensile strength:** Progressive hydrolysis may result in gradual loss of tensile strength over a period of time
- **Absorption rate:** Gradual encapsulation by fibrous connective tissue
- **Tissue reaction:** Inert, but can evoke minimal inflammatory reaction
- **Contraindications:** Should not be used where permanent retention of tensile strength is required.

Frequent Uses

- General soft tissue approximation and ligation including neurological, cardiovascular procedures.
- Ophthalmic surgery—10-0 and 8-0
- Plastic surgery—6-0 to 3-0.

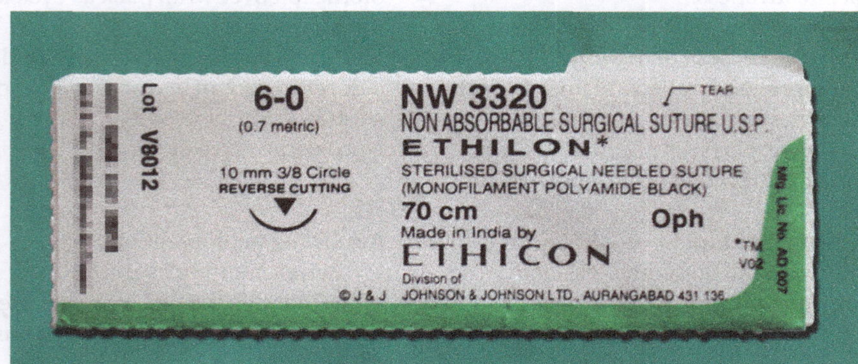

Fig. 2.6: Nylon suture

Polyester Fiber Suture (Mersilene, Dacron)

- **Type:** Braided, monofilament
- **Raw material:** Polyethylene terephthalate
- **Tensile strength:** Not significant change *in vivo*
- **Absorption rate:** Gradual encapsulation by fibrous connective tissue
- **Tissue reaction:** Minimal inflammatory reaction
- **Contraindications:** Not known
- **Frequent uses:** General soft tissue approximation and/or ligation including neurological, cardiovascular and ophthalmic procedures.

Polyproline Suture (Prolene, Surgiline)

- **Type:** Monofilament
- **Raw material:** Isotactic crystalline stereoisomer of polypropylene
- **Tensile strength:** Not subjected to degradation or weakening by action of tissue enzymes
- **Absorption rate:** Non-absorbable
- **Tissue reaction:** Can evoke minimal inflammatory reaction
- **Sterilization:** Available in pre-sterilized state (Fig. 2.7)
- Not known.

Advantages

- Inert as stainless steel and resist breakdown in infection.
- High degree of smoothness so used in plastic and vascular surgery
- Its sky blue (azure) color gives high visibility
- Easy handling
- Knot security—poor
- Least thrombogenic
- Retains tensile strength for years.

Frequent Uses

- Plastic and maxillofacial surgery
- Vascular surgery
- Cardiovascular surgery
- Tendon repair
- Hernia repair.

Surgical Steel

- **Type:** Monofilament
- **Raw material:** An alloy of iron-nickel-chromium
- **Tensile strength:** Indefinite
- **Absorption rate:** Non-absorbable, remain encapsulated in body tissues
- **Tissue reaction:** Minimal
- **Contraindications:** Should not be used when prosthesis of another alloy is implanted as it can cause galvanism.

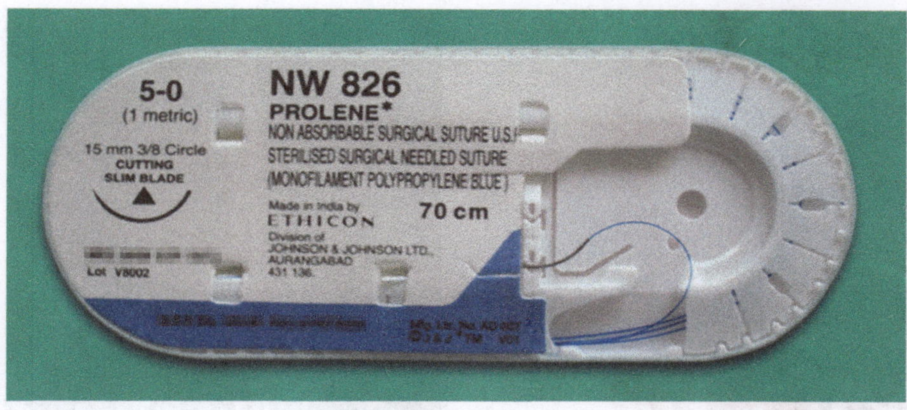

Fig. 2.7: Prolene suture

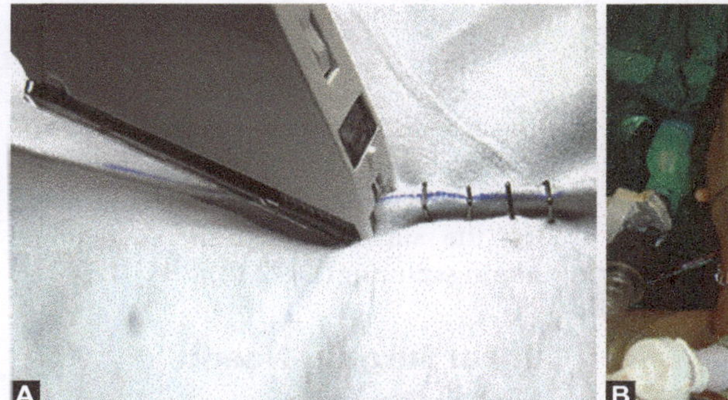

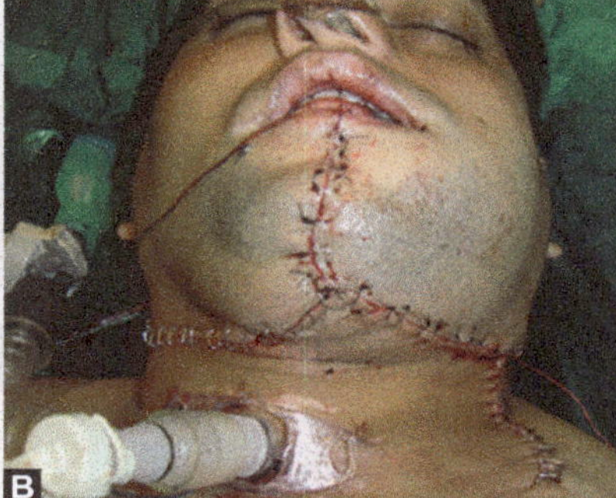

Figs 2.8A and B: Skin staples used for closure of the skin

Frequent Uses

Abdominal wall and skin closure; sternal closure, retention, tendon repair, orthopedic and neurosurgery.

Surgical Cotton

- **Type:** Twisted (braided)
- **Raw material:** Natural long staple cotton fibers (cellulose)
- **Tensile strength:** 50 percent lost in 6 months and 30 to 40 percent lost in 2 years
- **Absorption rate:** Nonabsorbable, remains encapsulated in body tissues
- **Tissue reaction:** Minimal
- **Contraindications:** None
- **Frequent uses:** Most body tissues for ligating and suturing.

Advantages

- It is economical
- Handling properties are good
- Knot stability is good.

Disadvantages

- It has capillarity and can cause wound infection
- Tensile strength is poor and gets degraded by autoclaving
- Not desirable in presence of contamination.

METAL SUTURE AND CLIPS

Humer Hultl[5] in Hungary first used mechanical stapling devise used to close stomach. It gives a strong predictable suture line. It allows access to difficult area.

There are three basic type of gastrointestinal stapling device.

i. Linear stapler—linear everting staple is used for end closure of viscous.
ii. Side-to-side stapler with or without knife blade.
iii. End to end staple—causing everting anastomosis.

Advantages

- Metal clips for skin allow quick closure
- Decreases the operative time
- All clips are easy to remove.

Surgical Staples

It is faster procedures and reduces operating time. The trauma to tissue is reduced because tissue handling is reduced.

Skin Staples

The surgical staples are used for:

- Routine skin closure.
- To secure skin grafts on burn patients.
- For closing the laceration in emergency (Figs 2.8A and B).

Tissue Glues

- **Cyanoacrylate:** It is used for skin closure, but it requires perfect hemostasis, if they are to work well. They are expensive as staple, but quick to use and do not delay healing.
- **Fibrin tissue glue:** Tissue glue involving fibrin works on the conversion of fibrinogen by thrombin to fibrin. The network has good adhesive properties and is used for hemostasis in liver and spleen surgeries. It has been used for neurosurgery in dural tears[6], in ear, nose and throat surgery and ophthalmic surgery to attach implants. It is also used in general surgery for prevention of postoperative adhesion of pericardium to peritonium.

Ligating Clips

Ligating clips offer the surgeon a rapid and secure method of accomplishing hemostasis or ligating arteries, veins, nerves and other small structures. It can be absorbable or non-absorbable. It is of advantage in deep and difficult to reach areas. They are of use particularly in microvascular surgery (Fig. 2.9).

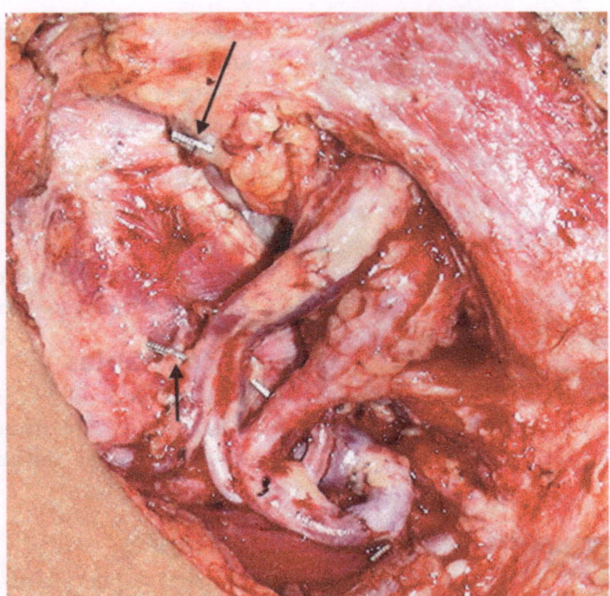

Fig. 2.9: Ligaclips used to clamp the vessels

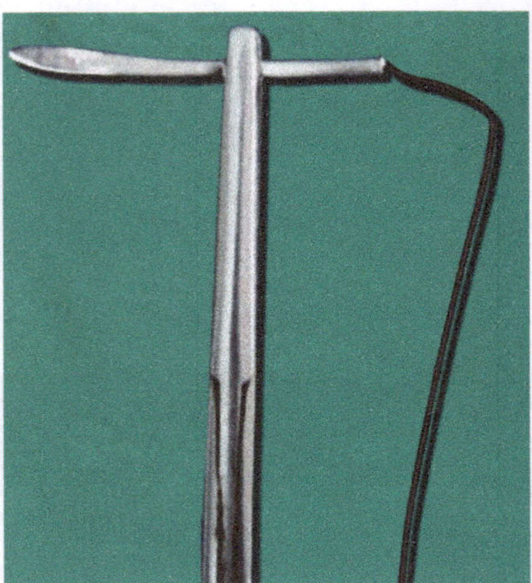

Fig. 2.10: Proper placement of needle holder to hold the needle

Disadvantages

- They do not bring deeper tissue together
- Do not control bleeding from edges
- Fine approximation is difficult.

Clearon

Clearon are a woven polypropylene delnet tape coated with hypoallergenic adhesive mass. It is extremely porous, which ensure adequate wound ventilation. Being transparent progress of wound healing can be checked.

Ethistrips

It is a woven rayon acetate tape coated on one side with a hypoallergenic adhesive mass. It can be used by themselves or to reinforce skin closure. Steristrips are used to buttress the suture and prevent spreading of scar.

Vacum-assisted Closure

It is the vacum assisted closure (VAC) by creating negative pressure within wound. The wounds are closed uniformly by applying controlled localized pressure.

ARMAMENTARIUM

Needle Holder

- Choice of size and type—determined by characteristics of needle and wound or anatomic areas.
- Needle should be grasped at three-fourth distance from tip of needle (Fig. 2.10).
- Always check alignment of jaws of the needle holder. The tip of jaws should meet first.
- Always close needle holder on first or second ratchet.
- Always hold needle holder so that needle point is directed toward surgeons thumb.
- The tripod grip is ideal for holding the needle holder as it provides excellent grip, support and stability (Figs 2.11A and B).
- Always use needle and needle holder as a unit.

Wound closure and healing is affected by the initial tissue injury caused by needle penetration and subsequent suture passage. Needle selection, surface characteristics of the suture (e.g. coefficient of friction) and suture-coating materials selected for wound closure are important factors that must be considered by the surgeon [Instruments required during suturing (Fig. 2.12)].

Ideal Surgical Needle Characteristics

- It should be made up of high-quality stainless steel.
- It should be of smallest possible diameter.
- It should be stable in the grasp of the needle holder.
- It should be capable of implanting suture material through tissue with minimal trauma.
- It should be sharp enough to penetrate tissue with minimal resistance.
- It should be sterile and corrosion-resistant to prevent introduction of microorganisms or foreign materials into the wound.

Needle Performance Characteristics and Definitions

- **Strength:** Resistance to deformation during repeated passes through tissue (Increased needle strength results in decreased tissue trauma).

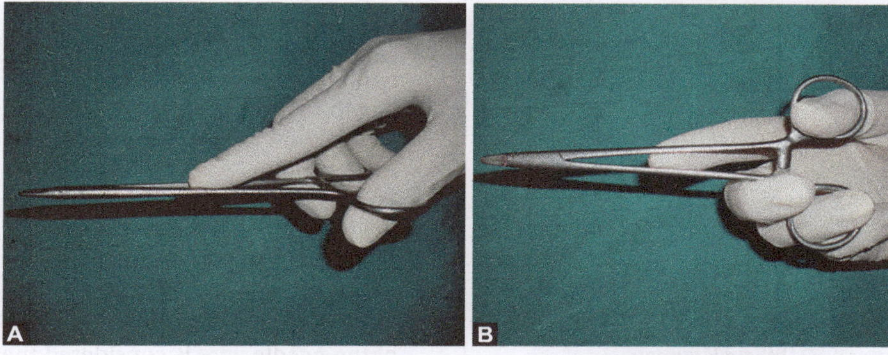

Figs 2.11A and B: Tripod grip of the needle holder

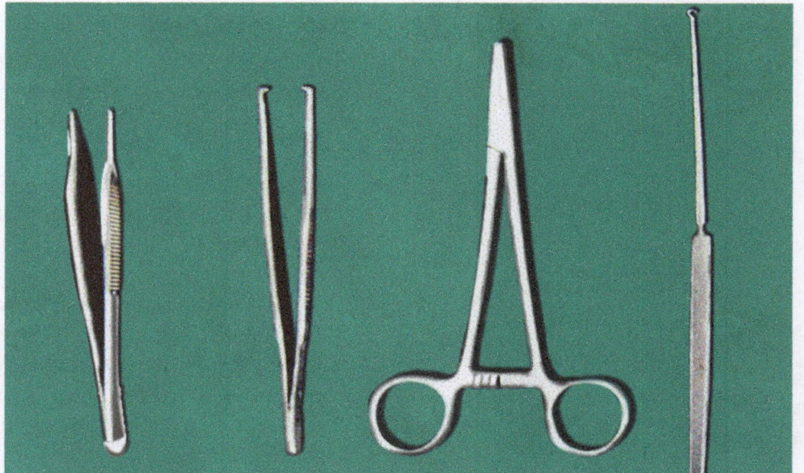

Fig. 2.12: Suturing set tissue holding forceps without and with teeth, needle holder, skin hook

Table 2.3: Point types

Point type	Design	Indication
Conventional cutting	— 3 cutting edges — Triangular cross-section that changes to a flattened body — Third cutting edge is on the inner, concave curvature (surface-seeking).	
Reverse cutting	— Third cutting edge is on the outer convex curvature of the needle (depth-seeking) — Stronger than conventional cutting needles — A reduced risk of cutting out tissue	Skin, tendon sheaths, oral mucosa, cosmetic and ophthalmic surgery
Side-cutting (spatula)	Flat on the top and bottom surfaces to reduce tissue injury	Ophthalmic procedures
Taper-point (round needle)	Sharp tip at the point flattens to an oval/rectangular shape taper ratio (8–12:1) and tip angle (20–35°)	Subcutaneous layers, dura, peritoneum, abdominal viscera
Blunt-point	Dissects friable tissue rather than cuts	Suturing the liver and kidneys

- **Ductility:** Resistance of a needle to breakage under a given amount of deformation/bending.
- **Sharpness:** Measure of the ability of the needle to penetrate tissue.
- **Clamping movement:** Stability of a needle in a needle holder, determined by measuring the interaction of the needle body with the jaws of the needle holder.

Parts of Needle

Point

Point is a portion of the needle extends from the tip to the maximum cross-section of the body (Table 2.3).

Body

Body part of the needle incorporates the majority of the needle length. The body of the needle is important for interaction with the needle holder and the ability to transmit the penetrating force to the point (Table 2.4).

Swage

The suture attachment end creates a single, continuous unit of suture and needle. The swage may be designed to permit easy release of the needle and suture material (*pop-off*).

Types of Swage

- Channel swage
- Drill swage
- Non-swaged.

Figure 2.13 shows suture and their parts.

Needle Coating

The needle may be coated with silicone to permit easier tissue passage. The coating helps reduce the force needed to make initial tissue penetration and the frictional forces as the body of the needle passes through the tissue.

Needle Curvature

The suturing needles are available in various curvatures and sizes of the body. The different curvatures facilitate easy needle manoeuvrability of the needle at different sites. For example, the straight, curved and half circle needles are suitable

Table 2.4: Body types

Body type	Indicated	Use
Straight	Easily assessable tissue that can be manipulated by hand	Microsurgery for nerve and vessel repair
Half-curved-ski	Rarely used in skin closure Difficult to handle.	
Curved	Optimal course for sutures through tissue Even distribution of tension Designed for confined spaces	Intraoral sutures Cleft palate repair
Compound curved	The body has a tight 80° curvature at the tip, which becomes a 45° curvature throughout the remainder of the body	Ophthalmic surgery Microvascular surgery

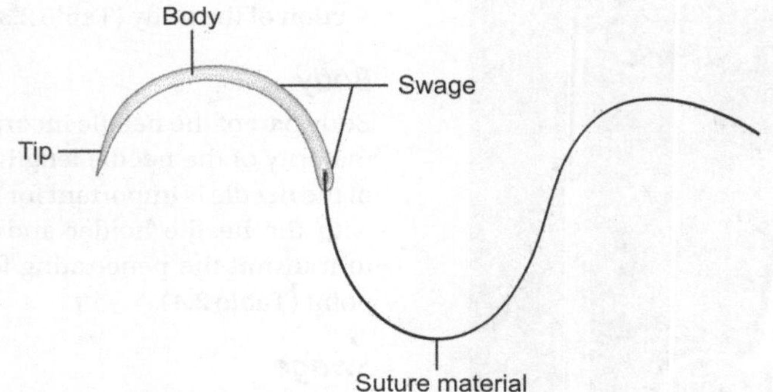

Fig. 2.13: Parts of the suture

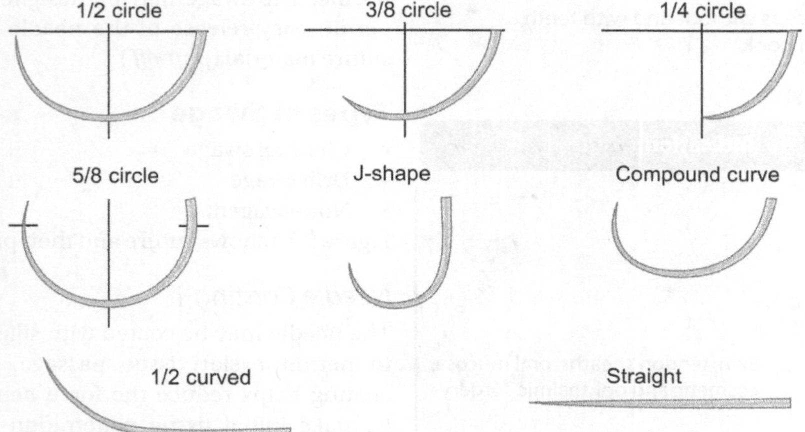

Fig. 2.14: Types of needles according to curvature

for suturing the skin which is on surface while the 'J' curvature is more useful in placing sutures in the depth. The 5/8th circle needle is used for suturing the palatal mucosa (Fig. 2.14). The size of the needle is selected depending upon the toughness of the tissue to be sutured and the place available at the site for easy manoeuvrability of the needle.

Needle Measurements

- **Chord length:** This is the linear distance from the point of the curved needle to the swage (bite width).
- **Needle length:** The distance measured along the needle from the point to the swage is termed needle length. Needle length, not chord length (bite width), is the measurement supplied on suture packages.
- **Radius:** This is the distance from the body of the needle to the center of the circle along which the needle curves (bite depth).
- **Diameter:** The gauge or thickness of the needle wire is considered the diameter.

Suture Principles

- The needle holder should grasp the needle at approximately three-fourth of the distance from the point of the needle.
- The needle should enter the tissue perpendicular to the surface, if the needle pierces obliquely, tear may develop.
- The needle should be passed through the tissue following the curve of needle. The wrists of the surgeon must move as per the curvature of the needle to drive the needle in the tissue smoothly.
- The suture should be placed at equal distance from incision on both sides and at equal depth.
- The needle should be passed from free to fixed end.
- The needle should be passed from thinner to thicker side.
- The needle should be passed from deeper to superficial tissue.
- The distance the needle is passed into the tissue should be greater than the distance from the tissue edge to ensure some degree of eversion in anticipation of some degree of scar contracture.
- The tissue should not be closed under tension to avoid tear or necrosis around the suture, undermining of tissue can be done to avoid it.
- The suture should be tied so that the tissues are merely approximated and not blanched.
- The knot should not be placed on the suture line as it may interfere with the healing/epithelialization.

- Consecutive sutures should be placed at least 3 to 4 mm apart.
- Closer sutures are indicated in areas of underlying muscle activity like tongue.
- Extra tissue on one side of incision can cause *'Dog Ear'*. It can be obliterated by undermining of excess tissue. Incision is made approx 30° to parent incision on the side of undermining. Extra tissue is pulled over incision and the appropriate amount is excised. Incision is the closed in normal pattern.
- Excessively large sutures, which are tightly closed lead to dead space below and epithelialization of the suture tract.

Suture Size

- Use finest permissible size, which commensurate with natural strength of tissues.
- If postoperative course of patient may produce sudden strain on suture line, reinforce it with retention suture. Remove them as soon as patient's condition is stabilized.

Knot Tying

The knot the surgeon prefers to use to secure the suture will vary according to the material used and the location, depth and purpose of the suture. Knots must be tied with a technique appropriate for the tissues to be sutured or ligated and only tight enough to serve their purpose without slipping. Postoperative edema must be anticipated. Generally, synthetic suture materials have very smooth surfaces. They may require a different number of throws to achieve knot security than the natural fibers. Either instrument tie or the one hand or two hand tie is used for tying the knot.

Some general principles govern the tying of all knots, regardless of the suture material to be tied.

- The completed knot must be firmly tied so that slippage will be virtually impossible. The simplest knot is the most desirable.
- The knot must be small and the ends of the suture should be cut as short as possible with a given material to minimize foreign body tissue reaction.
- A seesaw motion or the sawing of one strand down over another, while tying the knot, may materially weaken sutures to the point that they may break when the second throw is made.
- The two ends of the suture are pulled in opposite directions with uniform rate and tension, the knot may be tied securely with less possibility of breakage.
- Clamps and hemostats should never be placed on any portion of the suture, which will remain *in situ.* Avoid the crushing or crimping application of surgical instruments, such as needle holders and artery forceps, to the strand except when grasping the free end of the suture during an instrument tie.
- Sutures for approximation rather than hemostatic purposes should not be tied too tightly as this causes tissue strangulation. While sitting on the knot to prevent its loosening hold the knot firmly but without crushing the thread with plain tissue forceps.
- After the first loop is tied, it is necessary to maintain traction on one end of the strand for control to avoid loosening.
- Extra throws do not add to the strength of a properly tied knot, they only contribute to its bulk.

Types of Knot

- **Square knot:** The suture is thrown around needle holder once and once in the in opposite direction between ties. It is always prudent to provide at least three ties for surface knots. It is indicate in nylon, polypropylene, polyglycolic acid and catgut may require more ties.
- **Surgeon's knot:** Requires two throws of suture around needle holder on first tie and then one throw in opposite direction on the second tie. It has advantage of reducing the slippage, while the second tie is put in the position. The third tie is usually for the security of the previous knot (Fig. 2.15).
- **Granny knot:** First two ties in the same direction followed by third tie squared on the first. The knot involves a tie knot in one direction followed by single tie in the same direction.

Types of Knot Indicated for Different Suture Material

- Square knot is indicated for surgical gut, collagen, surgical silk, virgin silk, surgical cotton, stainless steel,

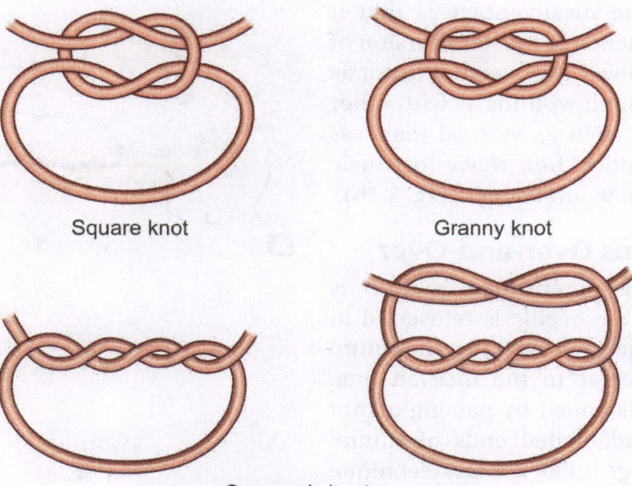

Fig. 2.15: Types of knots

uncoated synthetics, polyester fibers, polyglactin 910. Place first throw in a precise position, for the final knot, using double loop. Tie second throw square. Additional throws advisable in tension.

- For polyster fiber, polyglactin 910, polydioxanone, polypropylene, nylon—a standard technique of flat and square ties with additional throws if indicated by surgical circumstances and experience of surgeon.

SUTURING TECHNIQUES

Simple Interrupted

Simple interrupted is most commonly used technique. The suture is passed through both the ends at equal distance and depth of incision line and knot is tied on one side of the incision line. It is strong and the successive sutures can be placed in a manner to fit the individual requirements of the situation. The loosening of one suture will not cause loosening of other suture. A degree of eversion of the tissue can be produced by ensuring that the depth of the bite is more than the distance from the suture to the wound edge. The advantage of this technique is that it permits good eversion of wound edges and can be rapidly applied. If it gets infected the removal of few sutures would serve the purpose. The disadvantage is that it requires practice to master eversion of edges. However, the eversion is not as good in difficult wounds as with other techniques, such as vertical mattress suture. It does not relive extrinsic tension from wound edges (Fig. 2.16).

Continuous Over-and-Over

First simple interrupted suture is placed and the needle is reinserted in continuous fashion such that the suture is perpendicular to the incision line. The suture is ended by passing a knot over the untightened ends of suture. The advantage is that it is fast technique and there is even distribution of tension over entire suture line. It provides water tight closure, which is important in bone grafting. The apposition and eversion of wound edges is more difficult to achieve and the inclusion cyst may form. If the suture breaks entire suture line opens leading to dehiscence of the wound. It should not be used in the area of existing tension (Figs 2.17A to C).

Continuous Locking Sutures

Continuous locking suture is similar to continuous suture, but locking is provided by withdrawing the suture through its own loop. The suture is passed perpendicular the incision line. The locking prevents excessive tightening of the suture as the wound progresses. Care should be taken not to excessively tighten the individual lock. The locking feature may prevent adjustment of the tensions in the suture line as the tissue swelling occurs. The advantage is that it is applied rapidly; the apposition of wound edges is more complete than with continuous over-and-over suture. There is less epithelialization of tracts. The disadvantage being that the apposition of edges is not as perfect unless procedure is mastered well. If the suture breaks entire suture line opens leading to dehiscence of the wound (Fig. 2.18).

Mattress Suture

The main purpose of the mattress is to provide more tissue eversion. It can be used in the area where wound contracture could cause dehiscence or broad scar formation. Types of mattress are horizontal or vertical.

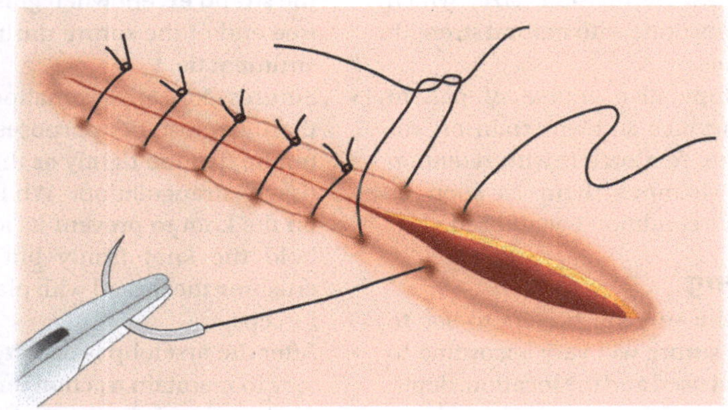

Fig. 2.16: Simple interrupted suture

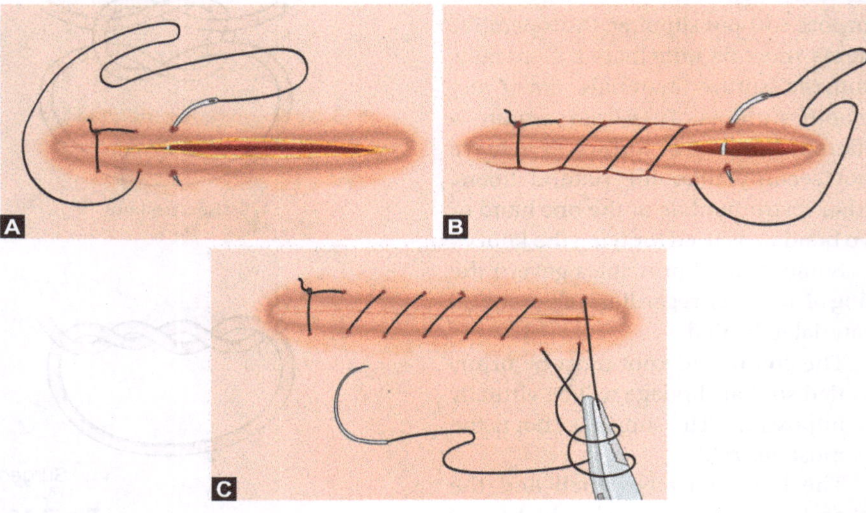

Figs 2.17A to C: Continuous over-and-over

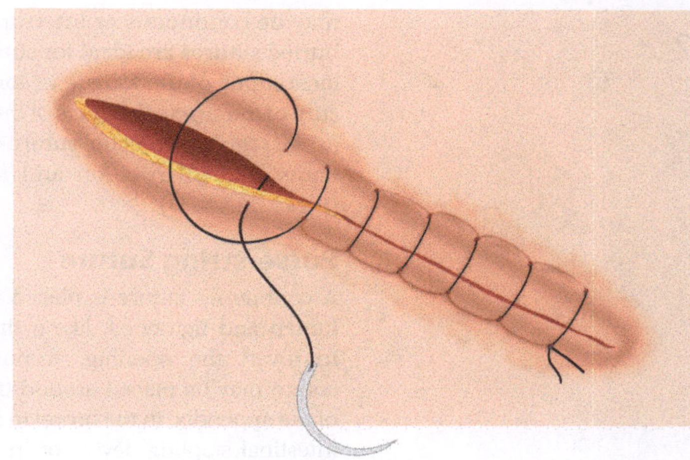

Fig. 2.18: Continuous locking suture

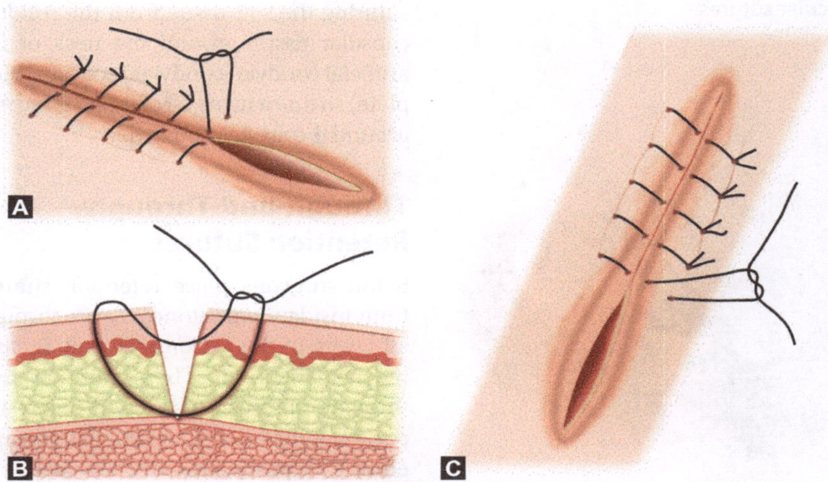

Figs 2.19A to C: Vertical mattress sutures

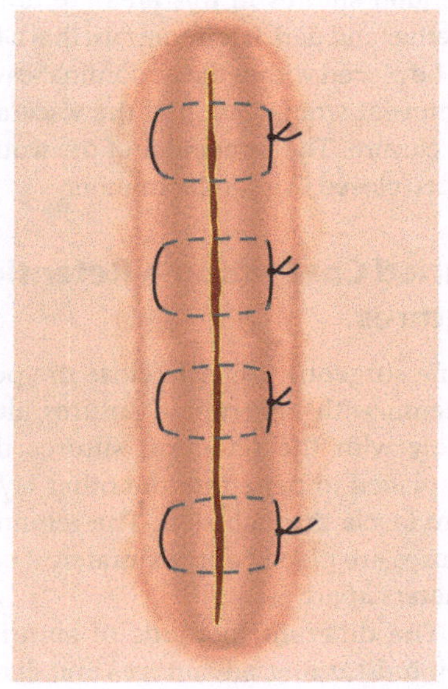

Fig. 2.20: Horizontal mattress

Vertical Mattress

The needle is passed from one edge of the incision to other and again from the latter edge to the first and a knot is tied. When the needle is brought from the second flap to the first the depth of penetration is more superficial. The advantages are that it provides good tissue eversion and there is perfect apposition. It relieves tension from skin edges and runs parallel to blood supply to edge of flap. The disadvantage is that it takes more time to apply and produces more cross-mark (Figs 2.19A to C).

Horizontal Mattress

Similar to vertical mattress, but the depth of penetration from the incision line and the depth of penetration of the needle is same for each entry point. But the horizontal distance of the point of penetration on the same side differs. The advantage is that it produces broad contact of wound margins and reinforces subcutaneous tissue. It relieves extrinsic tension from wound edges. It also helps in hemostasis from the skin edges. It has disadvantage that it constrict the blood supply to the edges of incision casing strangulation and necrosis leading to wound dehiscence if applied too tightly (Fig. 2.20).

Continuous Mattress

Continuous mattress can be rapidly placed in order to approximate large laceration in cosmetically unimportant areas. The disadvantage is that it does not provide good apposition of the wound edge or eversion. If the suture breaks entire suture line opens leading to dehiscence of the wound.

Subcuticular Suture

The subcuticular layer of tough connective tissue if sutured will hold the skin edges in close approximation when cosmetic result is desire. Continuous short lateral stitches are taken beneath the epithelial layer of skin. The ends of suture come at each end of incision and are knotted. This suture gives an excellent cosmetic scar. The advantage is that it is more esthetic and reduces problem associated with suture marking and irritation. The disadvantage is that it does not produce adequate wound approximation, does not evert wound edges and is time consuming (Figs 2.21A and B).

Figure of '8' Suture

Figure of '8' suture is used over extraction site where it provides protection of surgical site and adaptation of gingival papillae around adjacent teeth (Figs 2.22A and B).

Buried Sutures

Sutures placed completely under the epidermal layer of the skin with their knot also in the tissue are considered 'buried' or 'Inverted'. They are not removed postoperatively as only absorbable material is used. Buried sutures

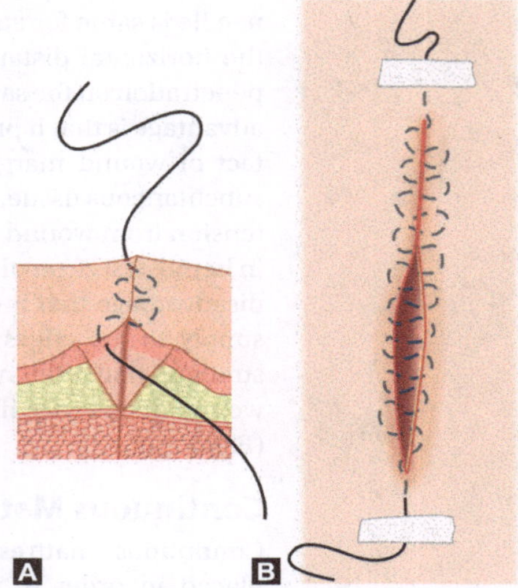

Figs 2.21A and B: Subcuticular sutures

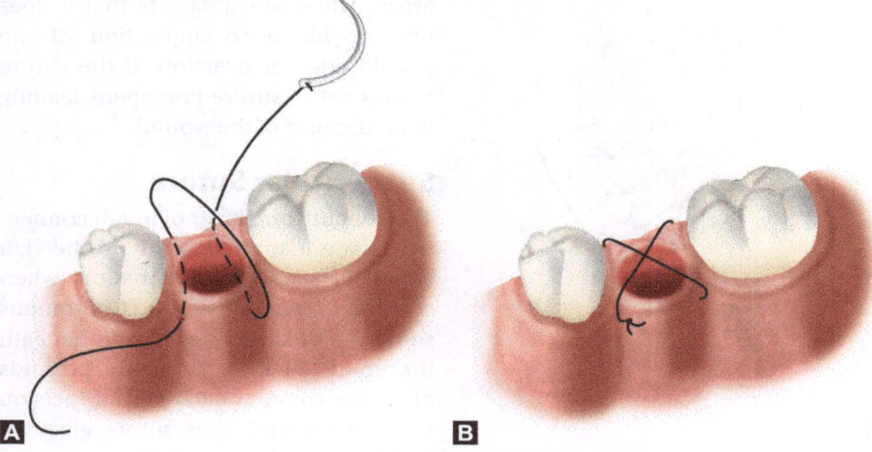

Figs 2.22A and B: Figures of '8' suture

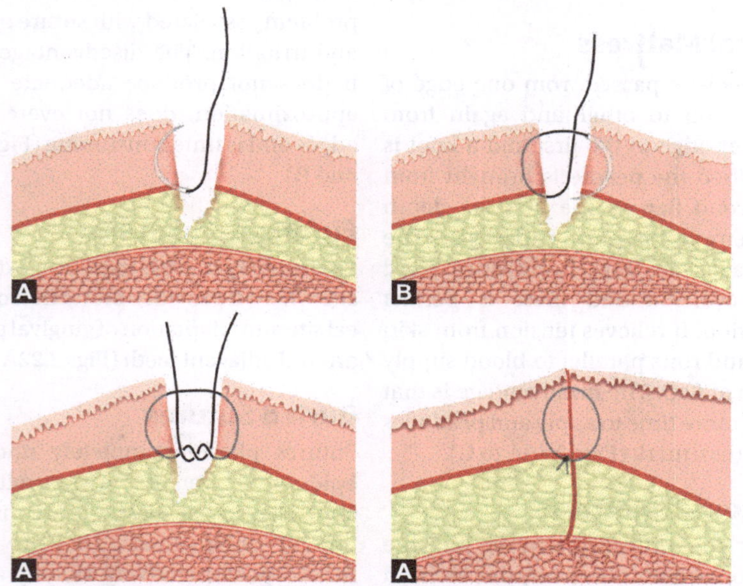

Figs 2.23A to D: Buried sutures

may be continuous or interrupted. The buried sutures are ideal for suturing the lacerations of the tongue or for the closure of the surgical defects of the tongue, as the regular projectile suture ends and knots lead to irritation and salivation (Figs 2.23A to D).

Purse-string Suture

A continuous suture is placed around a lumen and tightened, like a drawstring, to invert the opening. A purse-string suture may be placed around the stump of the appendix, in the bowel to secure an intestinal stapling device or in an organ prior to insertion of a drainage tube. The purse string suture can be used for suturing the soft tissue from the residual capsular tissue around the neck of the artificial condyle (condylar reconstruction plate) so that a nice cuff of tissue is formed around the artificial condyle.

Through-and-Through—Retention Sutures

Some surgeons place retention sutures from inside the peritoneal cavity through all layers of the abdominal wall, including the peritoneum. These "through-and-through" sutures are inserted before the peritoneum is closed. A simple interrupted or a figure-of-eight stitch is used. The wound is then closed in layers for a distance of about three-fourth the length. The retention sutures in this area are drawn together and tied. It is important that a finger be placed within the abdominal cavity to prevent strangulation of the viscera in the closure. The remainder of the wound is then closed in a similar manner.

Buried Coaptation—Retention Sutures

Some surgeons prefer to close the peritoneum with interrupted sutures alternately with the retention sutures that are placed to penetrate the other layers from fascia through skin. The retention sutures are placed approximately 2 centimeters apart.

The different methods of suturing, their indications, advantages and disadvantages are summarized in Table 2.5.

Table 2.5: Methods of suturing along with their advantages, disadvantages and indications

	Suture method	Advantages	Disadvantages	Indications
1.	Interrupted	1. Strong 2. Successive sutures fit individual requirement 3. Individual suture can be removed at the site tension	Require practice to master eversion	1. Area of tension 2. Site of strong closure
2.	Continuous	1. Fast technique 2. Even distribution of tension 3. Provides tight closure	1. Apposition and eversion is difficult to achieve 2. Break in one suture causes dehiscence of entire suture line 3. Not indicated in area of tension	
3.	Locking continuous suture	1. Fast technique 2. Apposition of wound is complete 3. Less epithelialization of tracts	1. Require mastering 2. If one suture breaks entire entire suture line breaks	
4.	Vertical mattress	1. Good tissue eversion 2. Perfect apposition 3. Relieves tension from skin 4. Blood supply parallel to edge	1. Time taking 2. More cross-marks	
5.	Horizontal mattress	1. Broad contact 2. Reinforces subcutaneous 3. Relieves extrinsic tension from wound	Constrict blood supply to edges of incision	
6.	Continuous	Applied over large area	1. Apposition is not good 2. Eversion is not good	Large laceration
7.	Subcutaneous	1. Cosmetically good 2. Less suture marking and irritation	1. Adequate wound approximation 2. Evert wound edges 3. Time consuming	Cosmetic area
8.	Figure of '8'	1. Protection of the surgical site 2. Proper adaptation of the gingival papillae		Extraction socket

LIGATURES

A suture tied around a vessel to occlude the lumen is called a *ligature* or *tie*. It may be used to affect homeostasis or to close off a structure to prevent leakage.

- *Free tie* is a single strand of material handed over to the surgeon or assistant to ligate a vessel. A hemostat is placed on the end of the structure and the suture tied around the vessel under the *tip* of the hemostat. The knot is tightened by the surgeon's fingers or with the aid of forceps, taking care to avoid instrument damage to the suture. As the knot is tightened the assistant gradually releases the clamp to ensure proper seat and tightening if the knot around the open end of the vessel (Figs 2.24A to E).
- *Stick tie,* also referred to as a *suture ligature* or *transfixation suture,* is a strand of suture material attached to a needle. The needle is used to anchor the strand in tissue around the vessel before occluding a deep or large vessel. In other words the vessel is ligated along with the adjacent tissue (Figs 2.25A to E). The strand must be of sufficient length to allow the surgeon to tighten the first knot.

SUTURE REMOVAL

The sutures are removed under aseptic precautions. First the suture site is cleaned. The suture is grasped with an instrument and lifted above the epithelial surface the suture cutting scissor is passed through one loop and transected close to the skin surface. The suture is then pulled out in such a way that the part of the suture, which was inside the tissue will come out and under no circumstances the part of the suture, which was on the surface will pass through the tissue depth as it is contaminated and can carry the infection in deeper tissue planes.

Technique of Suture Removal

Sutures are removed using aseptic and sterile technique. A sterile suture removal tray is prepared for the procedure.

- Cleanse the area with an antiseptic. Hydrogen peroxide can be used to remove dried serum encrusted around the sutures.
- Pick-up one end of the suture with thumb forceps. Cut the suture on one side as close to the skin as possible, where it dips beneath the skin.

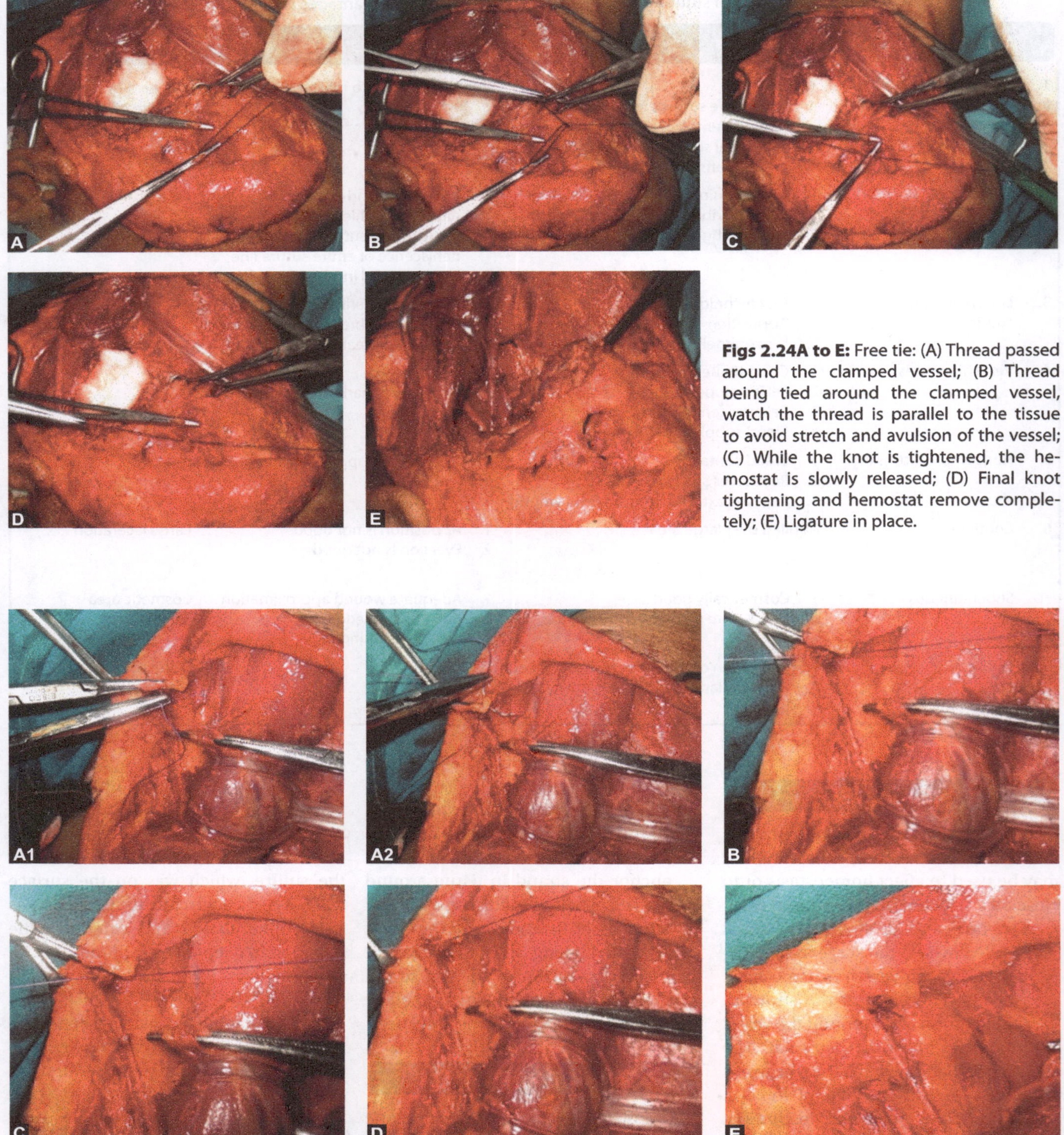

Figs 2.24A to E: Free tie: (A) Thread passed around the clamped vessel; (B) Thread being tied around the clamped vessel, watch the thread is parallel to the tissue to avoid stretch and avulsion of the vessel; (C) While the knot is tightened, the hemostat is slowly released; (D) Final knot tightening and hemostat remove completely; (E) Ligature in place.

Figs 2.25A to E: Transfixing suture: (A) Clamped vessel along with adjoining tissue and the needle takes bite on one side of the clamped vessel; (B) The needle takes bite on the other side; (C) As the knot tightened, the hemostat is slowly released; (D) Final knot tightening after the hemostat is removed; (E) Transfixed vessel with cessation of the blood flow.

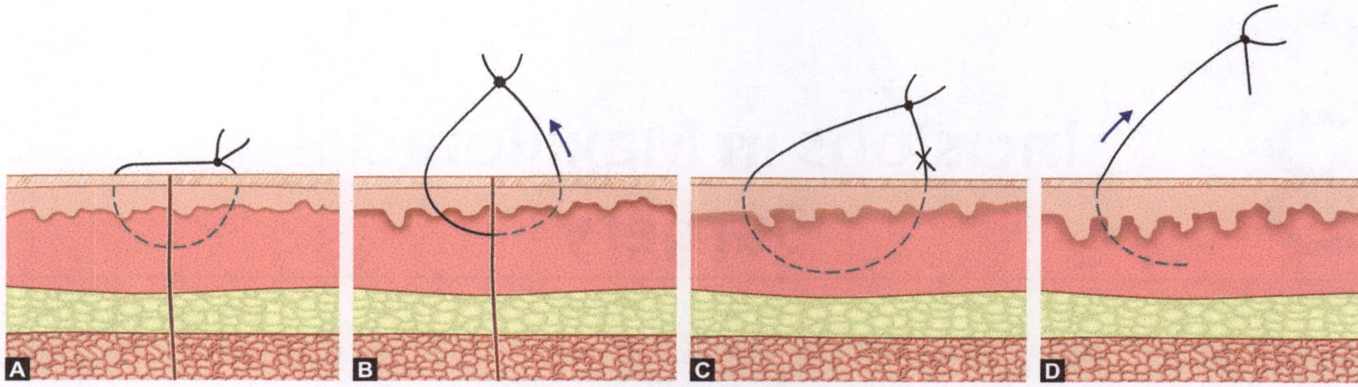

Figs 2.26A to D: Removal of sutures technique

- Gently pull the suture out through the other side while holding the suture with the forceps. The suture should be removed without pulling any portion that has been outside the skin back through the skin (Figs 2.26A to D).

Sutures should be removed "before the epithelium has migrated into deeper parts of the dermis. To prevent widening of the scar, the wound edges may be taped."[7]

Time of Suture Removal

- Skin about face and neck—3 to 5 days
- Other skin sutures—5 to 8 days
- Retention suture—10 to 14 days.

The sutures may not be removed at a time, but alternate sutures are removed from the suture line is done depending on the healing of the surgical site.

REFERENCES

1. Chih-Chang Chu. Wound closure biomaterials and devices. 1st edition, CRC-Press;. 1997.
2. Clifford Snyder. On the history of the suture. Plastic and reconstructive surgery: 1976; 58(4):401-6.
3. Postlethwait RW. Wound healing in surgery, Somerville, NJ: ETHICON, INC., 1971, pp. 8-9.
4. Wound closure manual, ETHICON, INC, 15, 37-8, 50.
5. Hultl H. II Kongress der Ungarischen Gesellschaft fur Chirurgie, Budapest, May 1908. Pester Med Chir Presse 1909; 45:108–10.
6. Toma AG, Fisher EW, Cheesman AD. Autologous fibrin glue in the repair of dural defects in craniofacial resections. J Laryngol Otol. 1992;106(4):356-7.
7. Krizek TJ, Hoopes JE (Eds). Symposium on basic science in plastic surgery, St. Louise: Mosby, 1976;15:87.

3 Incisions in Maxillofacial Surgery

Borle Rajiv M, Rai Anshul

The word '*incision*' is closely associated with surgery. Incisions are placed to drain abscess, excise growths, mobilize tissue and create access to the deeper viscera. Human tissues have an inherent property that makes their response to injury fairly predictable. Depending on this predictability, principles of surgery have evolved, which help to optimize wound healing and formation of an acceptable scar.

While placing the incision, it is imperative to know the regional anatomy, blood supply, nature of tissue and its healing characteristics to achieve the desired results. An incision should not only provide free, passive and unimpeded access to the deeper tissue, but should also be placed in the areas, where the chances of damage to the vital structures is negligible and the tension free closure can be achieved to ensure rapid healing and esthetically viable scar. An incision should ideally be placed in an area, where the ensuing scars are hidden and at the same time do not cause the functional morbidity to the part.

To achieve these objectives certain basic principles of surgery must be adhered to.

A scalpel is used to make an incision. The word scalpel is derived from the *Latin word* '*scalpere*' which means '*to cut*'. A scalpel has two components, a handle and a blade. The blade is usually detachable and is disposable.

BASIC PRINCIPLES OF INCISION MAKING[1]

- A sharp blade of an appropriate size (number) should be used for making an incision. A sharp blade allows incisions to be made cleanly without unnecessary damage to the tissues due to repeated strokes. A number 15 blade is most commonly used for making incisions in oral and maxillofacial surgery. A number 11 blade is used as stab knife for abscess drainage and number 12 blade is used for operculectomy, i.e. excision of pericoronal flaps (Figs 3.1A and B).
- The Bard-Parker blade is mounted on the suitable handle (e.g. number 15 blade and number 3 handle). The surgeon holds the knife with a pen grip, which provides better support to the hand and control over the knife (Fig. 3.2).
- Incision should be given using continuous and controlled pressure and with a single stroke. Multiple soft strokes result in more damage to the incised tissues and increase the amount of bleeding from the surgical site. It also delays healing due to the resultant tissue damage. Hence, long continuous solitary stroke is preferable intermittent strokes to avoid ragged margins. As one approaches towards the end of the incision the direction of the knife should change from oblique to right angle, so that the skin and deeper tissue are incised at the same level.
- An incision should always be deepened layer-wise. A full thickness incision through multiple layers, in a single stroke should be avoided to avoid injury to the deeper vital structures. The reason being the innate variations in the microanatomy

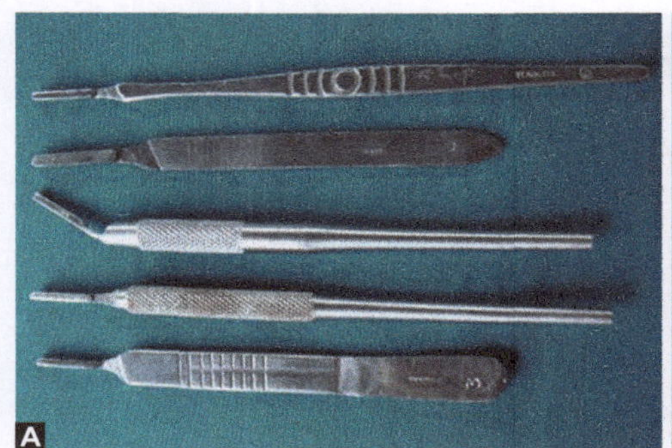

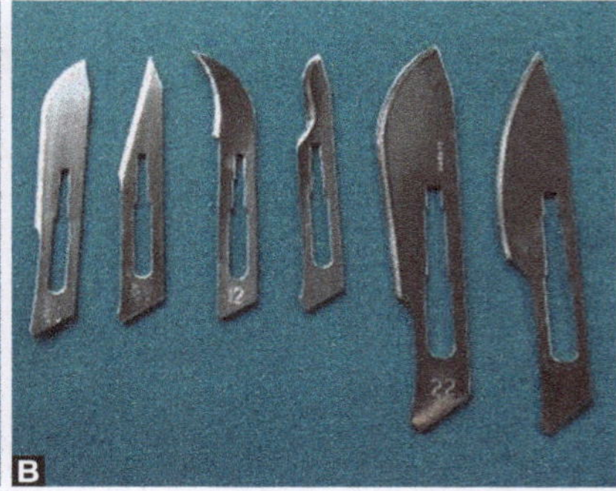

Figs 3.1A and B: Bard-Parker handles and blades

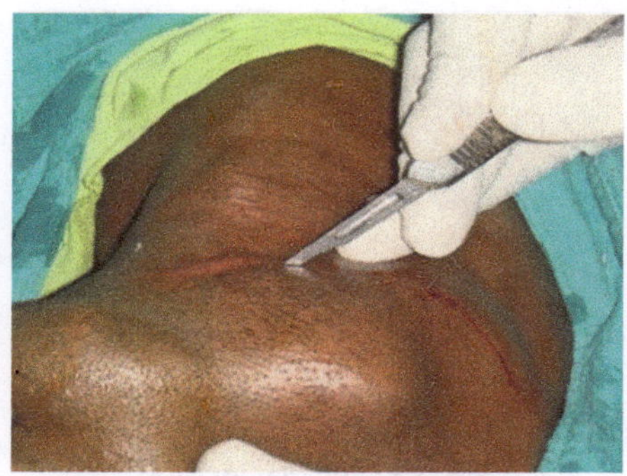

Fig. 3.2: Pen grip for holding knife

and tissue consistency of individuals because of which no two individuals can be treated as similar. It is desirable to incise one layer at a time.

- Incisions on epithelial surfaces should always be made with the blade held perpendicular to the surface. This creates wound edges, which are easier to re-approximate and less susceptible to necrosis.
- While placing incisions on the skin, the skin should be stretched between the thumb and index finger of the other hand to allow a clean incision.
- Mucosal incisions in the oral cavity should always be made resting on healthy bony tissue, so as to provide a healthy base for support of the sutured margins. Also, incision in unhealthy mucosal tissue should be avoided to prevent complication of wound dehiscence. Hence, incisions should preferably be placed on attached gingiva.
- Incisions extending to the marginal and papillary gingiva should be so designed that they do not cut through the papilla or the marginal gingiva. Incision should always cross the free margin of the gingiva at the mesiobuccal or distobuccal line angle of the teeth. If the papilla is cut, it leads to recession of the papillary gingiva and if marginal gingiva is cut, it leads to clefting of the marginal gingiva.
- Extraoral incisions in the head, neck and face region should be given along the existing resting skin tension lines and should not cross them as far as possible. This leads to a better healing and esthetically acceptable scar. If the incisions cannot be placed in the lines of minimal tension, they can be made inconspicuous by placement inside an orifice such as the mouth, nose, or eyelid; within hair-bearing areas or location that can be covered by hair or at the junction of two anatomic landmarks such as the esthetic units of the face.
- Use as long incisions as needed. This provides better exposure and less handling of the tissue. The healing of both long and short incisions takes the same time and longer incisions do not have any disadvantages as far as healing is concerned.

Relaxed Skin Tension Lines

The lines of minimal tension, also called relaxed or resting skin tension lines, are as a result of the skin's adaptation to function and are also related to the elastic nature of the underlying dermis (Fig. 3.3). The intermittent and chronic contraction of the muscles of facial expression create depressed creases on the skin of the face. These creases become more conspicuous with aging. Incisions should be made within these lines of minimal tension. Incision made in or parallel to such a line or crease will become inconspicuous if careful closure is done. Any incision or portion of an incision that crosses such a crease often produces conspicuous and unaesthetic scar.

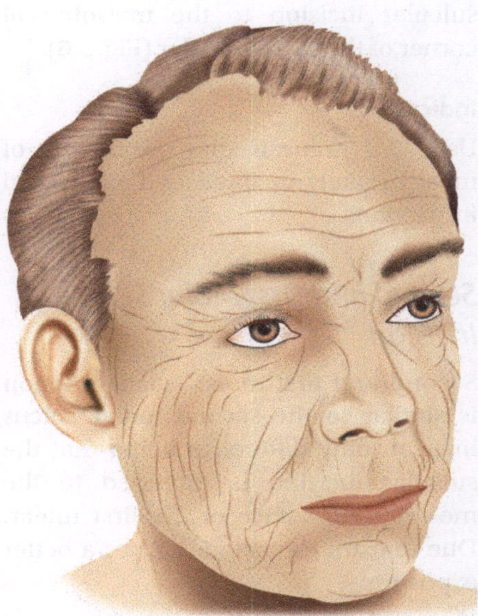

Fig. 3.3: Langerhans lines

On the face and in the neck these lines of minimum tension are known as Langer's lines or tension lines of skin or cleavage lines (Fig. 3.3). They run transversely in the neck and are seen as flexion creases. Incisions taken parallel to these lines heal without the formation of the unsightly scars produced by incisions across them. When tension lines are cut across, they result in undue retraction of the lips of the wound.

INCISIONS USED IN ORAL AND MAXILLOFACIAL SURGERY

Intraoral as well as extraoral incisions are used in the management of the various pathologies in the field of Oral and Maxillofacial surgery. Each incision used is designed based on the basic principles of surgery and is indicated for management of specific conditions.

COMMONLY USED INTRAORAL INCISIONS

Ward I[2]

It consists of mesial release, crevicular and distal incisions. Mesial release incision begins from approximately 5 to 6 mm below marginal gingiva of lower second molar at the mesial root and runs upwards obliquely at an angle of 45° to the distobuccal line angle of the second molar and extends posteriorly cutting the distal papilla and then into the crevice of the third molar, if it is partially erupted and then distally it extends on the anterior border of the ramus of the mandible for a distance of 10 mm. While taking mesial release incision, care should be taken not to allow the knife to slip in the gingivobuccal vestibule as it can lead to damage to the facial artery. It is therefore advisable for the beginners to take this incision from the vestibular depth to free gingiva (bottom to top) to prevent the accidental damage to facial artery (Figs 3.4A and B).

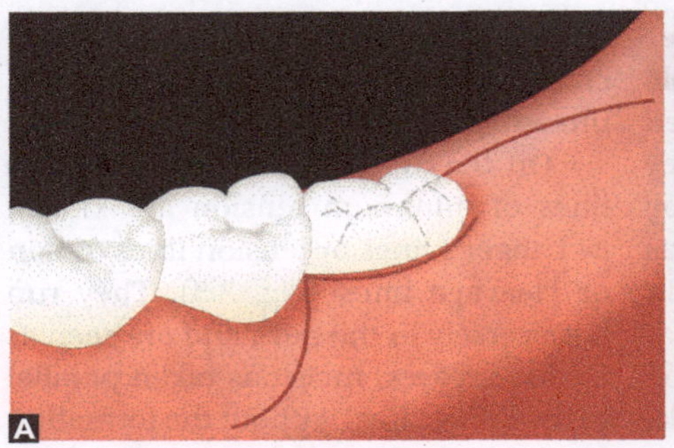

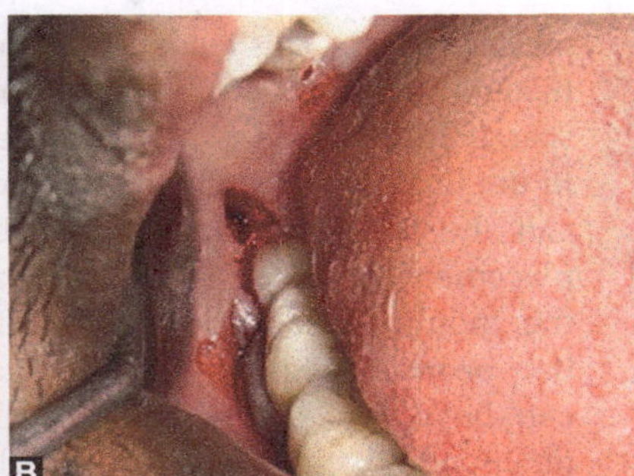

Figs 3.4A and B: Ward I incision

Indications

Transalveolar extractions of the lower third molar, which are partially erupted with adequate depth of buccal vestibule.

Precautions

- Mesial release should not extend too inferiorly to avoid cutting the facial artery.
- Distal release should not be lingually oriented to avoid damaging the lingual nerve or minor bleeding encountered due to presence of nutrient vessels.
- Distal release should be 10 mm long to avoid cutting through tendinous insertion of temporalis or the fibers of the masseter muscle or herniation of buccal fat pad in the oral cavity.

Ward II

It consists of mesial release, crevicular and distal release incisions. Mesial release incision begins from approximately 5 to 6 mm below marginal gingiva of lower first molar at the distal root and runs upwards obliquely at an angle of 45° to the mesiobuccal line angle of the second molar and extends distally into the crevice of the second molar up to its posterior surface and then distally it extends on the anterior border of the ramus of the mandible for a distance of 10 mm (Fig. 3.5).

Indications

Transalveolar extractions of the lower third molar, which are completely unerupted and inadequate depth of buccal vestibule.

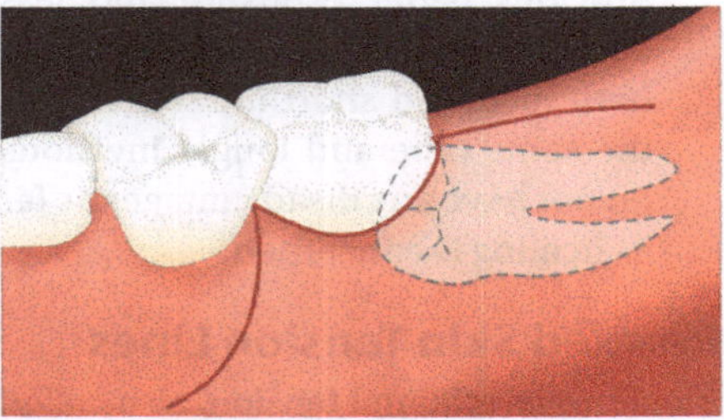

Fig. 3.5: Ward II incision

Precautions

Similar precautions are warranted as mentioned for the ward I incision.

Sulcular Incision

Second Molar Sulcus Incision

Incision starts on the ascending ramus following the center of the third molar shelf to the distobuccal surface of the second molar and then extends as a sulcular incision to the mesiobuccal corner of the second molar (Fig. 3.6).

Indications

Used for transalveolar extraction of most mesially inclined and superficial impactions.

Second and First Molar Sulcus Incision

Second and first molar sulcus incision is similar to the second molar sulcus incision only difference being that the sulcular incision is extended to the mesiobuccal suface of the first molar. Due to extra extension, it gives a better exposure.

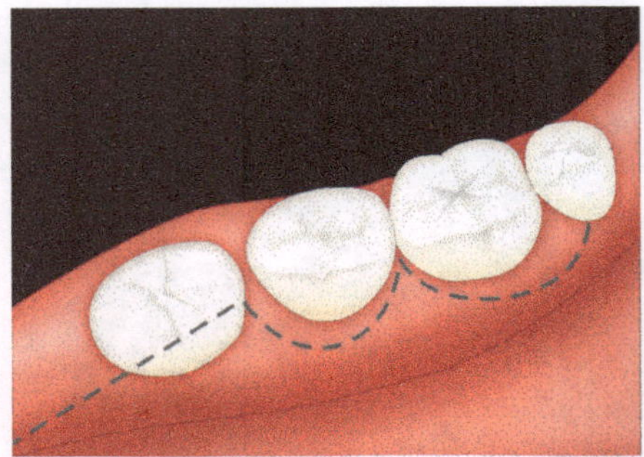

Fig. 3.6: Sulcular incision

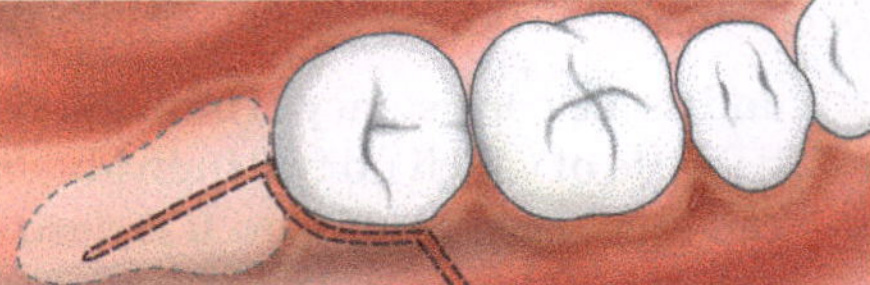

Fig. 3.7: Bayonet flap

Indications

It is used in third molar surgeries when the molar is more lingually situated.

Second Molar Sulcus Incision with Vestibular Extension (Bayonet Flap)

The incision is similar to the second molar sulcus incision with the addition of an oblique vestibular extension in the sulcus area which is angled forward. This gives excellent buccal visibility (Fig. 3.7).

Second Molar Paramarginal Flap with Vestibular Extension (L flap)

L flap is similar to the bayonet flap only difference being that the incision is made a couple of millimeters away from the marginal gingiva. It optimizes marginal attachment healing next to the second molar (Figs 3.8A and B).

Lingual Flap Incision

Lingual flap incision starts on the ascending ramus up to the distobuccal surface of the second molar and follows the distal surface of the second molar as a sulcular incision and then continues lingually to the first molar region.

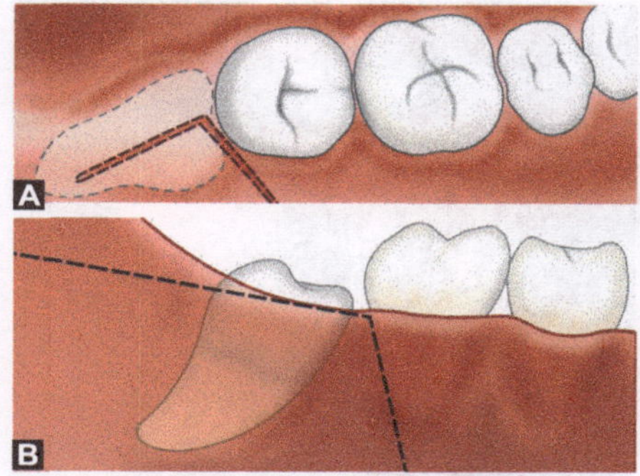

Figs 3.8A and B: Incision for the L flap

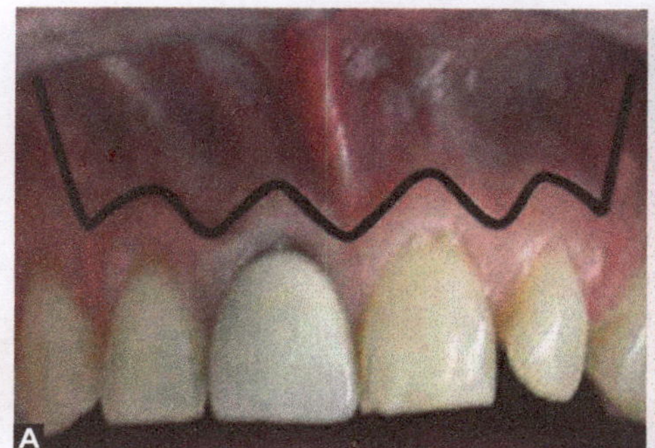

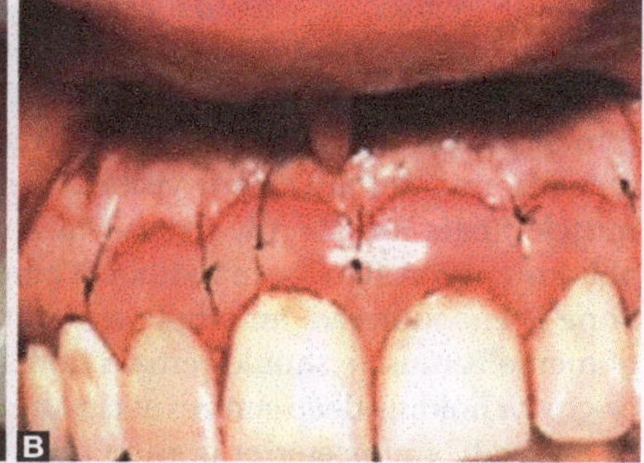

Figs 3.10A and B: Submarginal incision

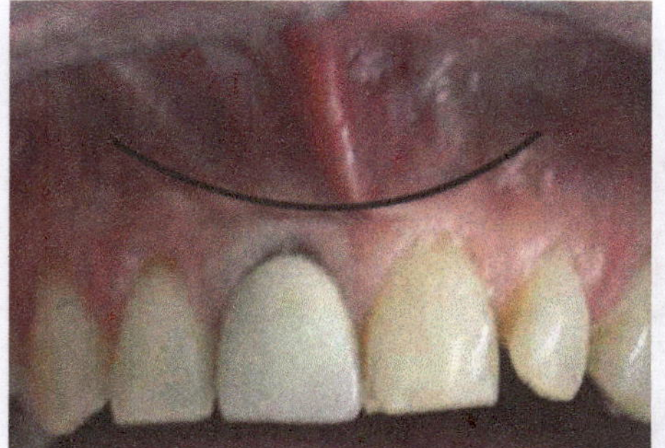

Fig. 3.9: Semilunar incision

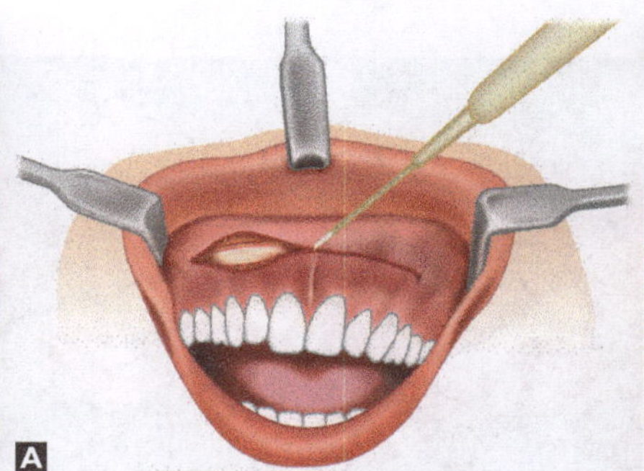

Figs 3.11A and B: Degloving incision (*Source:* Edward Ellis III, Zide MF. Surgical approaches to the facial skeleton. Dallas, Texas)

Indications

It is used for lingual split technique of transalveolar extraction of mandibular third molars.

Semilunar Incision

Semilunar incision is a slightly curved half-moon shaped incision in the alveolar mucosa. It prevents incision and reflection of the marginal and papillary gingiva thus avoiding complications thereof. However, it causes more bleeding, delayed healing and scarring of mucosa. So also, access to the periradicular tissues is restricted. It also carries a risk of flap margins lying over a bony defect thus violating the basic principles of surgery at times (Fig. 3.9).

Indications

It is used for apicectomy of teeth and apical curettage. It can be used for transalveolar removal of retained fractured apical portion of tooth roots.

Submarginal Incision[3]

Submarginal incision has its horizontal component in the attached gingiva with accompanying vertical release incisions. The horizontal incision can be scalloped to conform to the shape of the marginal gingiva. It requires at least 4 mm of attached gingiva. It also results in bleeding into the surgical site (Figs 3.10A and B).

Indications

It is used most commonly in cosmetically important areas such as maxillary anterior teeth for access to the periapical areas of the tooth.

Degloving Incision

The incision is usually placed approximately 3 to 5 mm superior to the mucogingival junction. Leaving unattached mucosa on the alveolus facilitating the closure. Palpation of the inferior extent of the pyriform aperture and/or anterior nasal spine ensures incision placement inferior to these structures in the maxillary anterior region.

Indications

It is used to access the pyriform aperture region anteriorly and zygomatic buttress posteriorly. This incision is used for various surgical procedures performed in the maxilla such as infraorbital nerve neurectomy, Caldwell-Luc operation, Le-Fort osteotomy, low level maxillectomy, fixing of Le-Fort I, II fractures, zygomatic bone fractures, etc. While closing the degloving incision which crosses the midline, there are chances of alar flaring, which can be avoided by taking alar cinch suture (Figs 3.11A and B). The lip lengthening can also be achieved with this incision by doing V-Y closure in the midline.

Curvilinear Incision

Curvilinear incision is used in the mandibular anterior region in the intermental foramina region. It extends anteriorly out into the lip, leaving 10 to 15 mm of mucosa attached to the gingiva. Once through the mucosa, the underlying mentalis muscles are clearly visible. The muscle fibers are sharply incised in an oblique approach to the mandible. When bone is encountered, an ample amount of mentalis muscle should remain on its origin for holding deep sutures at closure. In the body and posterior portion of the mandible, the incision is placed 3 to 5 mm inferior to the mucogingival junction. Leaving unattached mucosa on the alveolus facilitates closure (Fig. 3.12).

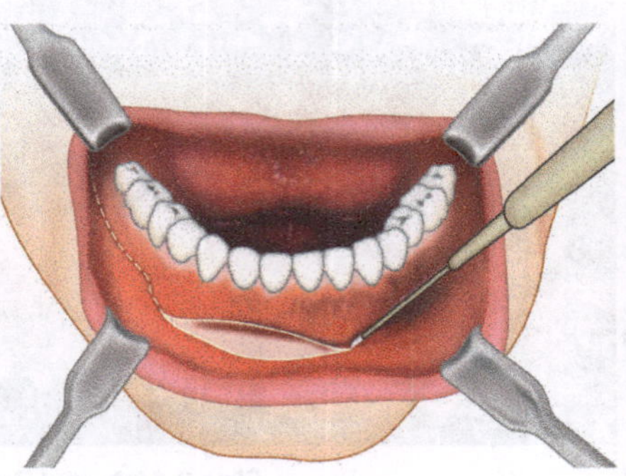

Fig. 3.12: Curvilinear incision

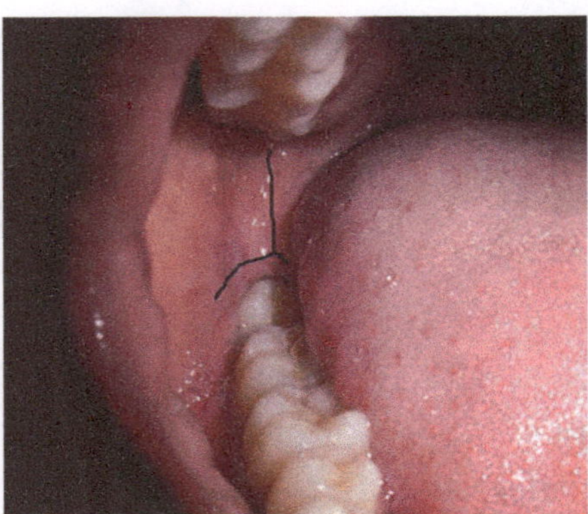

Fig. 3.13: Ginwalla's incision

Indications

For open reduction of mandibular fractures of the symphysis and parasymphysis. For harvesting corticocancellous graft from symphysis region.

Precautions

- In the anterior region, adequate tissue should be left back on the bone for suturing to avoid gaping.
- In the canine area the incision should not be placed lower than 3 to 5 cm to safeguard the mental neurovascular bundle.

Ginwalla's Incision[4]

Ginwalla's incision is placed on the anterior border of the ascending ramus of the mandible and extends both lingually and buccally to end in a 'Y'. It provides better exposure of the inferior alveolar nerve for its avulsion (Fig. 3.13).

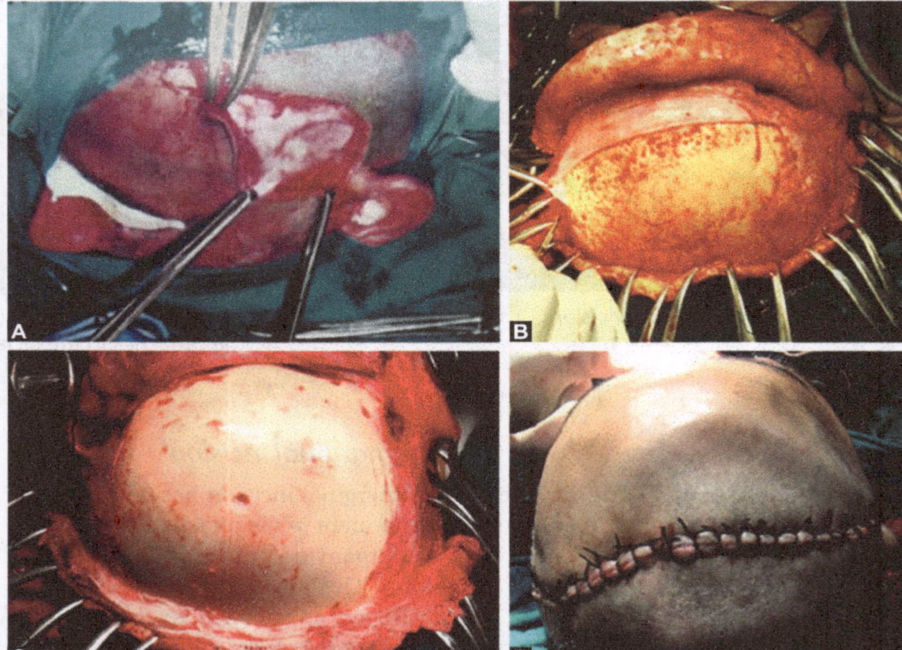

Figs 3.14A to D: Uni and bicoronal incisions

Indications

Ginwalla's incision is used for the inferior alveolar nerve neurectomy for management of trigeminal neuralgia.

EXTRAORAL INCISIONS

Coronal Approach[5]

Uni/Hemicoronal Approach

Two factors are considered, while designing the line of coronal incision. The first is the hairline of the patient. The second factor is the amount of inferior access required for the procedure. The coronal incision can be extended inferiorly, to the level of the lobule of the ear as a preauricular incision to allow exposure of the zygomatic bone and arch, frontozygomatic suture, temporomandibular joint (TMJ). The hemicoronal incision begins in the preauricular area on the desired side of the incision and curves forward at the midline, ending just posterior to the hairline. Curving the hemicoronal incision anteriorly provides the relaxation necessary for retraction of the flap. The incision is made through skin, subcutaneous tissue, and galea revealing the subgaleal plane of loose areolar connective tissue overlying the pericranium (Figs 3.14A to D).

Indications

- Used for exposure of frontozygomatic suture, superior orbital rim, lateral orbital wall, zygomatic arch, for management of unilateral midface fractures.
- For exposure of TMJ in management of ankylosis, trauma.

Precautions

- During finger dissection at the forehead region, there are chances of tearing the pericranium due to its adherence to the frontalis muscle, where sharp dissection is advised.
- During placement of preauricular incision it is essential to mind the superficial temporal artery, which runs in anterior to the tragus.

Bicoronal Approach[6]

Same considerations for location of the incision as above. In the males the hair line recession is not predictable and thus incision line on the cranial side is curved in a zigzag manner, anticipating the future hair loss. The incision begins at one superior temporal line to the other temporal line other temporal line (hair band incision). The incision is made through the skin, subcutaneous tissue, and galea revealing the subgaleal plane of loose areolar connective tissue overlying the pericranium. At the temporal line the incision is carried in the temporalis fascia to maintain the subgaleal plane and extended in the preauricular crease up to the lobule of the ear on both sides (*see* Figs 3.14A to D).

Indications

- Used for exposure of frontozygomatic suture, superior orbital rim, lateral orbital wall, nasoethmoidal area, zygomatic arch, for management of bilateral midface fractures.
- For exposure of TMJ bilaterally, in management of ankylosis, trauma.

Transfacial Approaches to the Mandible

Standard Submandibular Approach[7]

The incision is placed approximately 2 finger breadths or 1.5 to 2 cm below the inferior border of the mandible to avoid injury to the marginal mandibular nerve, which lies within the above mentioned distance from the inferior border of the mandible. The skin creases below the mandible do not parallel the inferior border of the mandible, but run obliquely, posterosuperiorly to antero-inferiorly.

Risdon's Submandibular Approach[8]

Like the standard submandibular incision placed approximately 2 finger-breadths or 1.5 to 2 cm below the inferior border of the mandible to avoid injury to the marginal mandibular nerve and it curls around the angle of the mandible[9] (Figs 3.15A and B).

Indications

- Extraoral approach to mandibular angle and ramus region.
- In management of cysts and tumors of the mandible not amenable to transoral approach.
- In management of low condylar fractures (provides poor access).

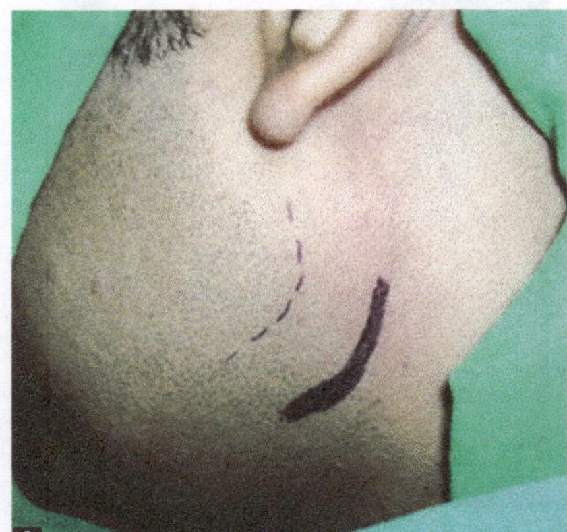

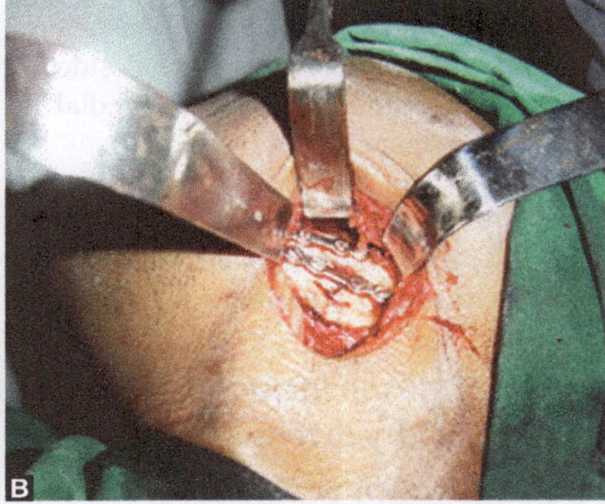

Figs 3.15A and B: Risdon's submandibular incision

Precautions

- Incision should be 1.5 to 2 cm below inferior border to avoid injury to marginal mandibular branch of the facial nerve.
- Facial artery should be palpated before hand to avoid accidental injury.
- Preferably, incision should be placed in the neck crease to avoid ugly perceptible scar.

Retromandibular Incision[10]

The incision for the retromandibular approach begins 0.5 cm below the lobule of the ear and continues inferiorly 3 to 3.5 cm. It is placed just behind the posterior border of the mandible and may or may not extend below the level of the mandibular angle, depending on the amount of exposure needed. A modification[11] to this incision was given by Hind's, where in the incision is placed at the posterior ramus, just below the earlobule; the advantage being direct access to the posterior border of the ramus (Figs 3.16A to C).

Indications

Surgeries of the condylar neck and ramus.

Precautions

- Injury to the main trunk of facial nerve should be avoided.
- Injury to the retromandibular vein should be avoided.

Transfacial Approach to Mid-Face

Lateral Rhinotomy[12]

Lateral rhinotomy was first described by Michaux in 1848, but was popularized by Moure in 1902. The classical lateral rhinotomy described by Moure lies halfway between the medial canthus and the nasal dorsum extending from the inner margin of the eyebrow down along the nasomaxillary groove curving around the ala to enter into the nose. The incision begins from the columella laterally along the vestibule of the nose and then follows the ala of the nostril

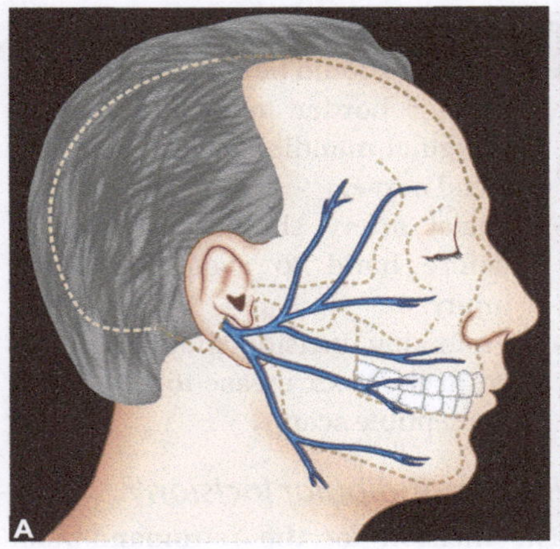

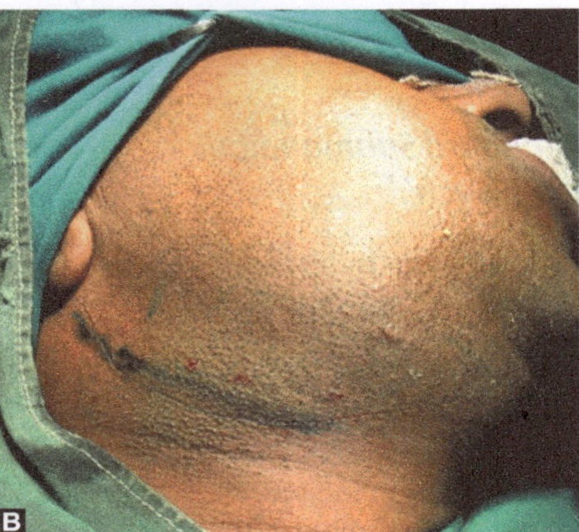

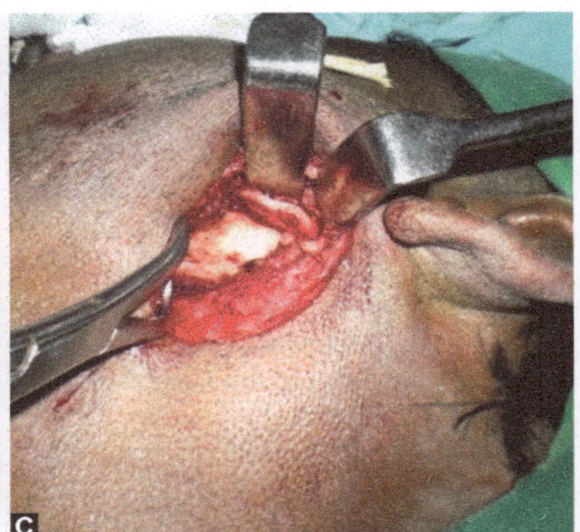

Figs 3.16A to C: Retromandibular incision

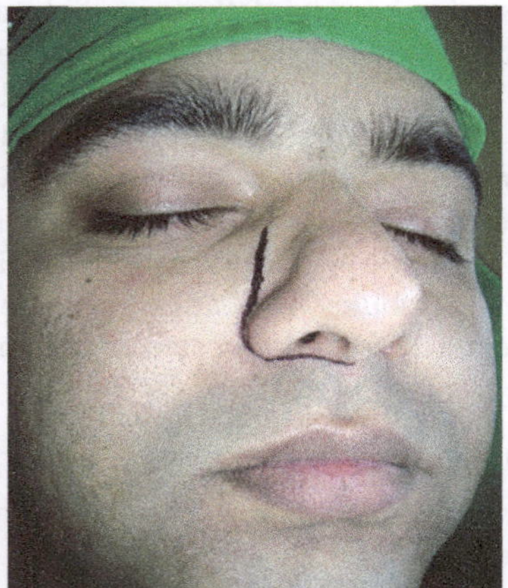

Fig. 3.17: Lateral rhinotomy incision

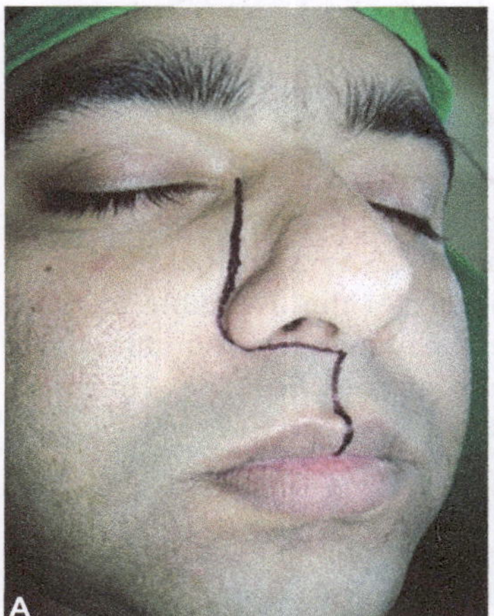

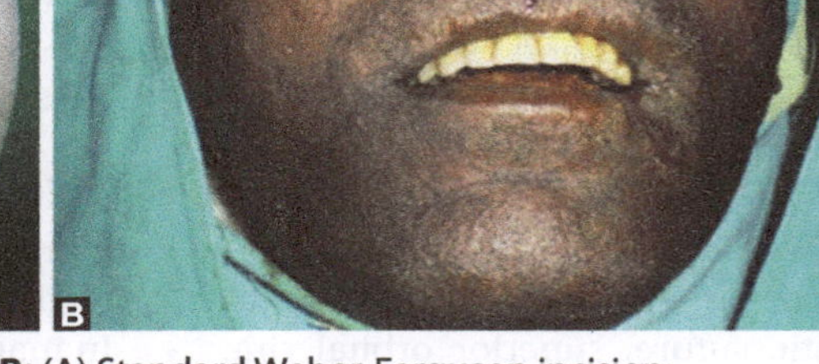

Figs 3.18A and B: (A) Standard Weber-Ferguson incision; (B) Weber-Ferguson incision with subciliary extension

and extends along the lateral aspect of the nose to end a centimeter below the inner canthus of the eye (Fig. 3.17).

Indications

Access to the nasal cavity, for open rhinoplasties and maxillary antrum.

Weber-Ferguson Diffenbach Incision[13]

The basic advantage of Dieffenbach's extension is that it is used for low level subtotal maxillectomy, wedge maxillectomy. It is similar to the lateral rhinotomy incision with the difference being that in this incision the upper lip is split in the area of philtrum (Figs 3.18A and B).

Weber-Ferguson Incision with Lynch Extension

Lynch extension[14]

It is an extension on the medial side from the medial canthus to the medial end of the upper eyebrow (Fig. 3.19).

Indications

It is used for extended maxillectomy and access to the medial orbital wall.

Weber-Ferguson Incision with Subciliary Extension

It is an extension of the lateral rhinotomy incision, wherein inferiorly it

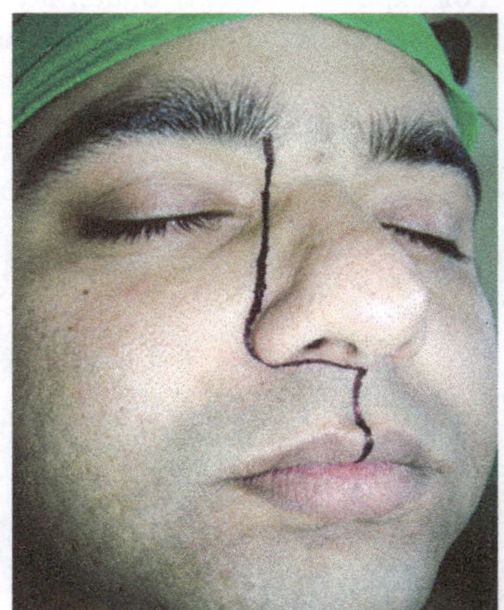

Fig. 3.19: Weber-Ferguson incision with lynch extension

extends from the columella to divide the upper lip in the midline. Superiorly it is 6 to 8 mm medial to the medial canthus, the incision extends laterally, not creating a sharp angle, but forming a rounded curve to avoid necrosis of the tip of the flap and causing a button like dehiscence. The infraorbital extension runs in the crease below the inferior palpebra upto the lateral canthus. A modification for esthetic reasons is that the incision extends into the floor of the nasal cavity from the columella leaving a 60° notch in the nasal floor, where the triangular portion of the upper lip is inserted during closure (Figs 3.20A to C).

Indications

Used for access to the maxilla for partial, subtotal or total maxillectomy.

Precautions

The angle at the junction of the infraorbital and lateral nasal incision should be obtuse to avoid necrosis of the triangular portion of the flap.

Approaches to the Temporomandibular Joint

Preauricular Incision[15]

Preauricular incision is given in the preauricular crease at the junction of facial skin and helix of the ear for the entire length of the attached portion of the pinna. Modifications were suggested to this standard incision such as Blair and Ivy's[16] 'inverted hockey stick incision' and Thoma's[17] 'vertical angulated incision' (Figs 3.21A and B).

Indications

For exposure of the condyle and condylar neck of the TM joint.

Precautions

- Care should be taken to avoid damage to the auriculotemporal nerve.
- Care should be taken to avoid damage to the superficial temporal artery.

Disadvantages

- The access is inadequate.
- The chances of damage to the zygomaticotemporal branch of the facial nerve are very high.
- The horizontal extension of the hockey stick incision lies on the zygomatic arch, producing unsightly scar.

Al-Kayat Bramley's Incision[18]

Al-Kayat Bramley's incision is an inverted question mark incision. It is an extension of the standard preauricular incision, wherein the preauricular incision is extended superiorly and posteriorly around the attachment of the temporalis muscle in an inverted question mark fashion. It provides increased exposure

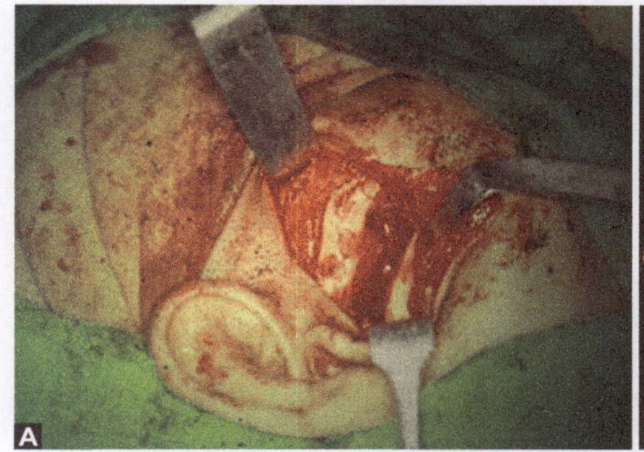
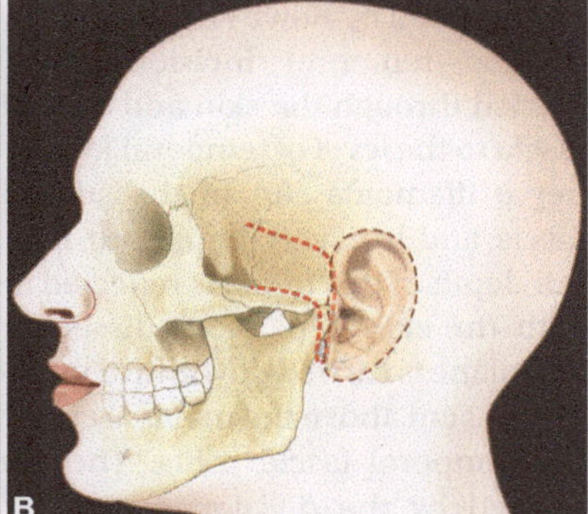

Figs 3.21A and B: Thoma's angulated vertical incision and hockey stick incision

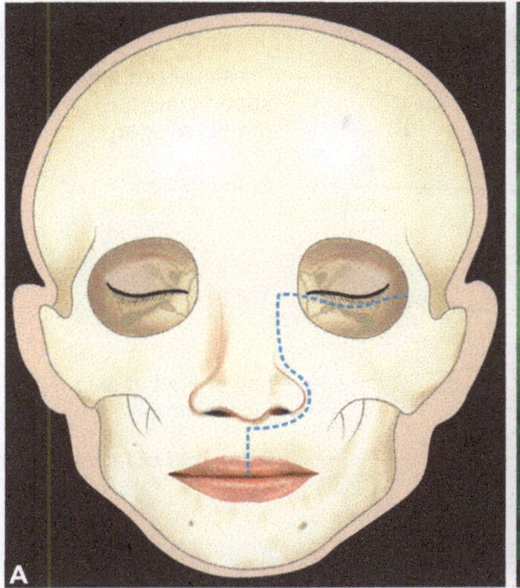
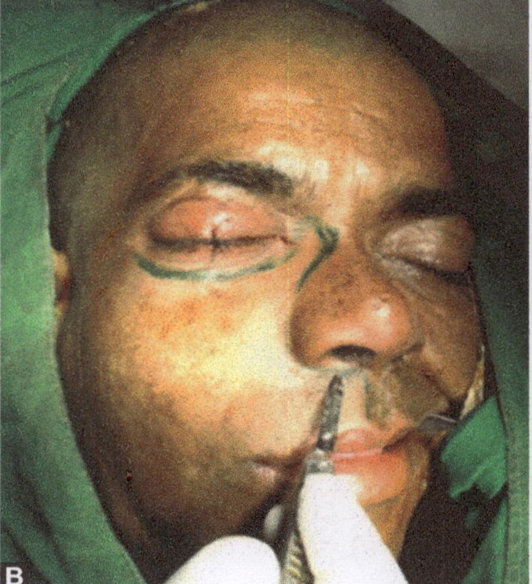
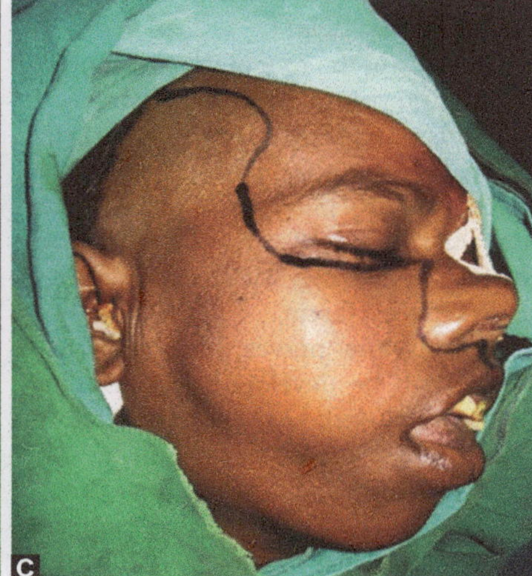

Figs 3.20A to C: (A) Weber-Ferguson incision with subciliary extension; (B) Infraorbital extension; (C) Infraorbital and Borle's temporal extension, used when temporalis muscle flap is planned for the reconstruction (Anshul Rai, et al. modified Weber-Ferguson incision with Borle's extension (Br J Oral and Maxfac Surg. 2010;45(5):e23-4.)

of the TMJ (Figs 3.22A to G). It is the most popular and commonly practiced incision for the TMJ ankylosis surgery.

It is the approach to the malar arch and joint, which gives excellent visibility with safety, but at the price of longer incision and wider exposure than is conventional. It differs from Rowe's description in the positioning of the skin incision and that through the temporal fascia.

The skin incision is question mark shaped and begins about a pinna's length away from the ear, anterosuperiorly just within the hair line and curves backwards and downwards well posterior of the main branches of the temporal vessels, till it meets the upper attachment of the ear. The incision then follows the attachment of the ear and just endaurally as described by Rowe (1972).

The temporal incision must be carried through the skin and superficial fascia to the level of temporal fascia. The nerve filaments run in the superficial fascia and it is very important that the full depth of this fascia is reflected along with the skin flap. Blunt dissection in this plane is carried downward to a point about 2 cm above the malar arch, where the temporal fascia splits. The pocket formed by the division contains fatty tissue, which is easily visible through the thin lateral layer. Beyond this point, there should be no attempt at further dissection of the superficial fascia from the temporal fascia.

Starting at the root of the malar arch, an incision running at 45° upwards and forwards is made through the superficial layer of the temporal fascia. Once inside this pocket, the periosteum of the malar arch can be safely incised and turned forward as one flap with the outer layer of temporal fascia, superficial fascia containing the nerves and skin. The pocket can be developed anteriorly as far as the posterior border of the frontal process of the malar bone and posteriorly joined to the preauricular dissection, which follows closely the cartilaginous external auditory canal beneath the glenoid lobe of the parotid gland and

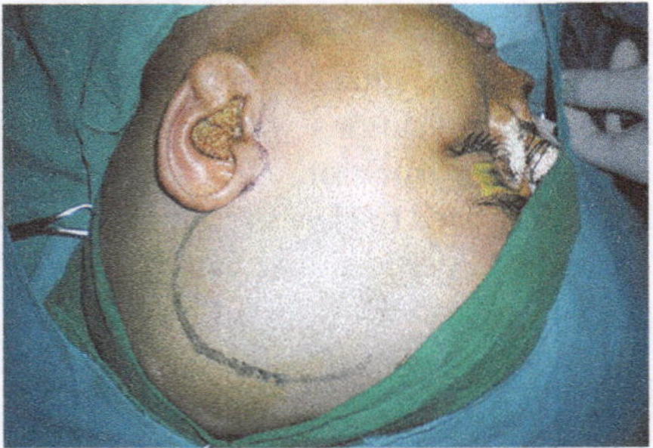

Fig. 3.22A: Al-Kayat Bramley's incision marking

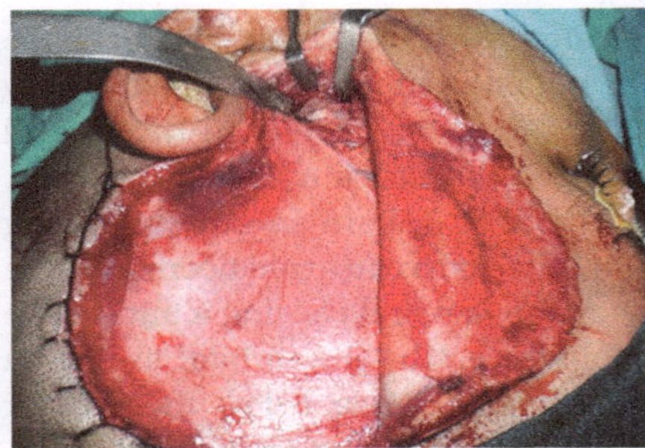

Fig. 3.22B: Temporal fascia

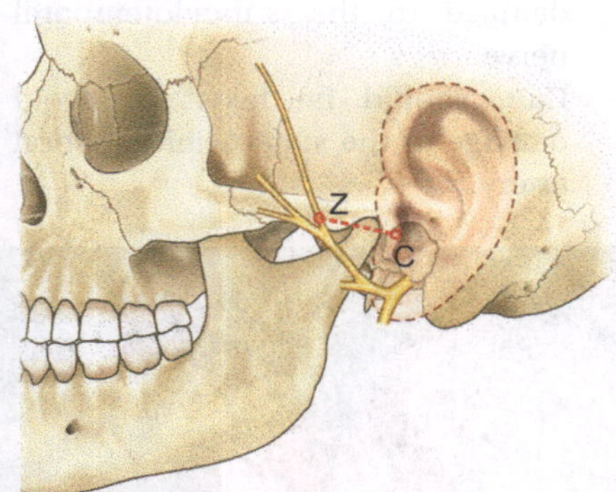

Fig. 3.22C: Point C is the most anterior concavity of the bony external auditory canal. Point Z is the point of the lateral surface of the malar arch midway between the upper and lower border, where the most posterior significant twig of the temporal ramus of the facial nerve crosses the arch

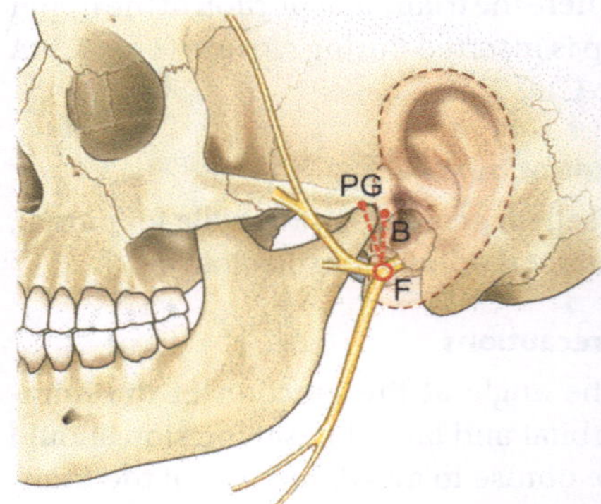

Fig. 3.22D: Point B is the lowest concavity of the bony external auditory canal. Point F is the bifurcation of the main trunk of the facial nerve. Point PG is the lowest point of the postglenoid tubercle

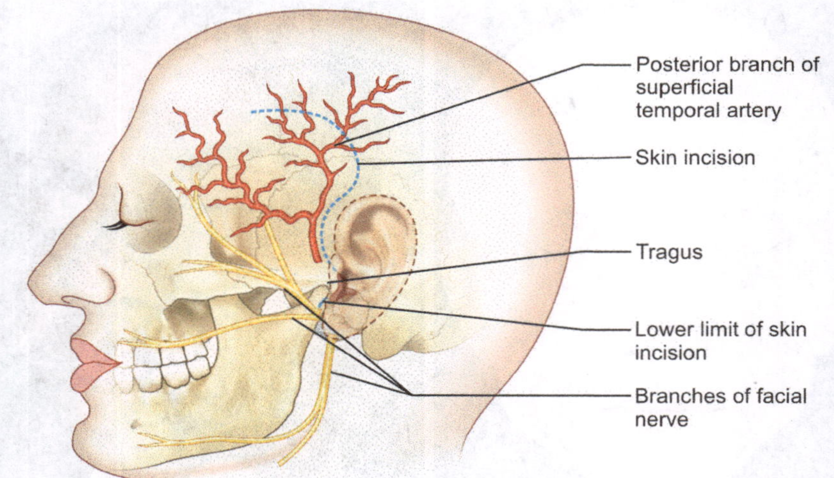

Fig. 3.22E: Skin incision in relation to the underlying structures

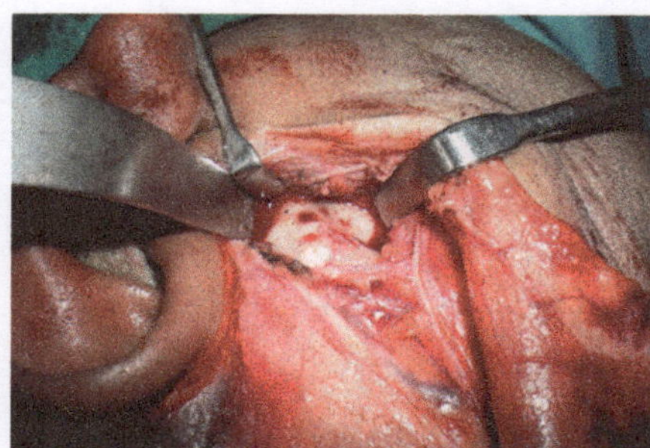

Fig. 3.22F: Incision running at 45° upwards and forwards in made through the superficial layer of the temporal fascia, protecting the vessels and branches of facial nerve, at the same time giving excellent exposure of the joint

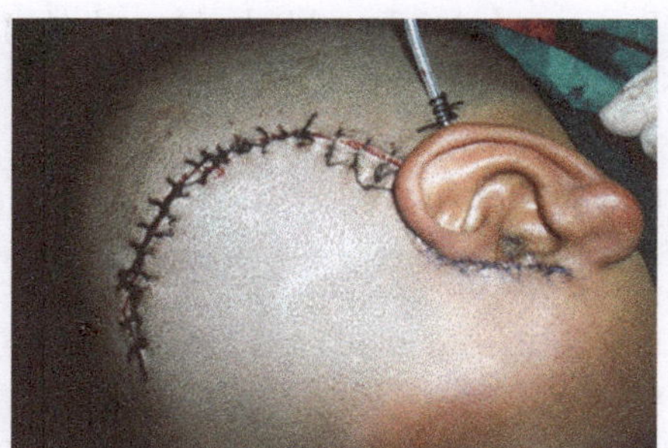

Fig. 3.22G: Closure of Al-Kayat Bramley's incision

superficial temporal vessels. A small torturous branch, the auricular artery, runs backwards from the superficial temporal artery to the ear. The middle temporal artery which comes off the superficial temporal artery perforates the temporal fascia to supply the temporalis muscle. This should be divided and ligated (Fig. 3.23).

Proceeding downwards from the lower border of the arch and articular fossa, the tissues lateral to the joint capsule are dissected and retracted. The base of the neck of the condyle can be exposed. The bifurcation of the facial nerve is not nearer than 2.4 cm in an anterior-posterior direction from the postglenoid tubercle. Care is needed not to extend deep dissection below the lower attachment of the ear.

Repair of the layers presents no problem. The incised outer layer of the temporal fascia can be repaired entirely

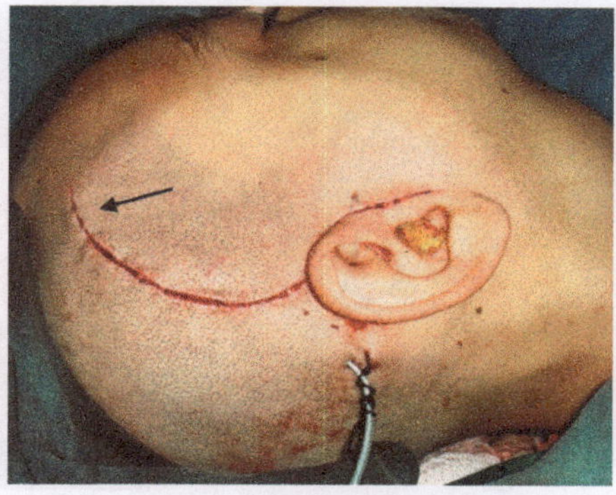

Fig. 3.23: Modified Al-Kayat Bramley's incision. Note that the incision is not curling downwards anteriorly, as it is the area of future hair loss and the scar may become visible

without tension. This is in marked contrast to the near impossibility of approximating the temporal fascia, if it is incised at a higher level, where it is a single layer of tissue.

Advantages of Al-Kayat Bramley's incision are:

- There is minimal bleeding and less sensory loss. The posterior placement of the skin incision and its wide backwards and upwards sweep spares the major branches of the vessels and nerves.
- Facial plane can be easily identified.
- There is excellent visibility. This is partly due to large flap and partly because the unyielding temporal fascia is not reflected with the skin as in the approach described by Rowe and Killey (1968).
- The potential complications of muscle herniation and fibrosis are avoided. The muscle is never exposed and the superficial layer of the temporal fascia can be closed without tension.
- There is remarkably little postoperative discomfort or swelling.
- A good cosmetic result is achieved except in patients with receding hair line.
- The technique is easily teachable and speedily executed.

Indications

- Exposure of the condyle for surgeries of the TMJ.

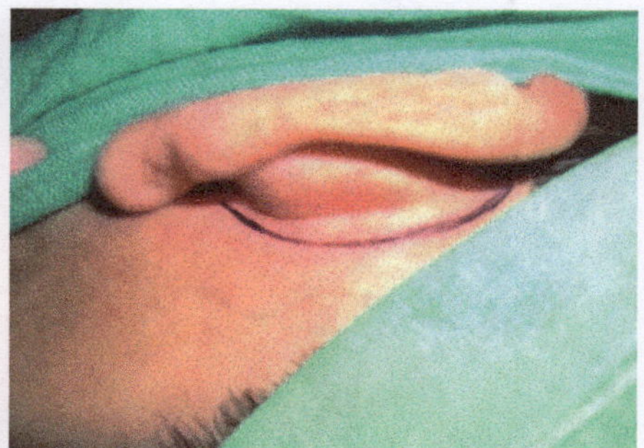

Fig. 3.24: Postauricular approach

- Might also provide exposure of the coronoid process.
- Allows harvesting of the temporalis flap in gap arthroplasty.
- Provides exposure to the zygomatic arch.

Postauricular Approach[19,20]

The incision is placed posterior to the pinna in the retroauricular crease. It is cosmetically viable incision (Fig. 3.24).

Indications

Exposure of the condyle for surgeries of the TMJ.

Disadvantages

- Poor exposure
- Risk of external auditory canal infection.
- Risk of external auditory canal stenosis.
- Temporary or permanent paresthesia of the pinna.

Endaural Approach[21]

The incision begins above the level of the zygomatic arch and extends downward and backward into the intercartilagenous cleft between the tragus and the helix and then extends inwards along the roof of the auditory meatus for approximately 1 cm (Fig. 3.25).

Indications

Used for exposure of the condyle for surgeries of the TMJ.

Disadvantages

- Poor exposure.
- Chances of chondritis.

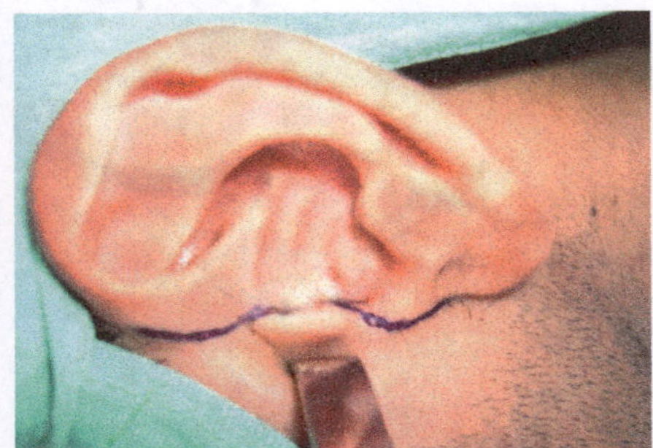

Fig. 3.25: Endaural approach

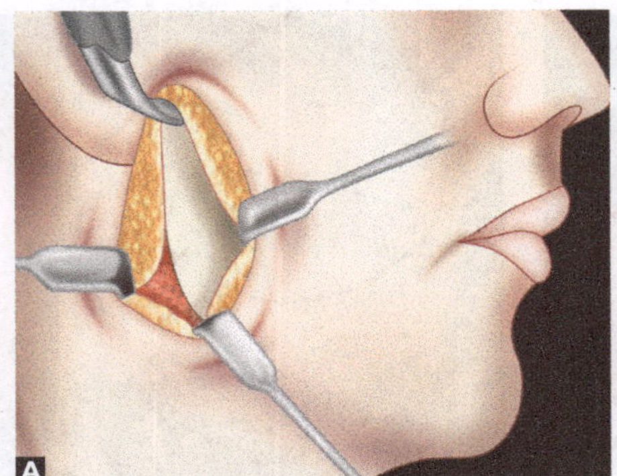

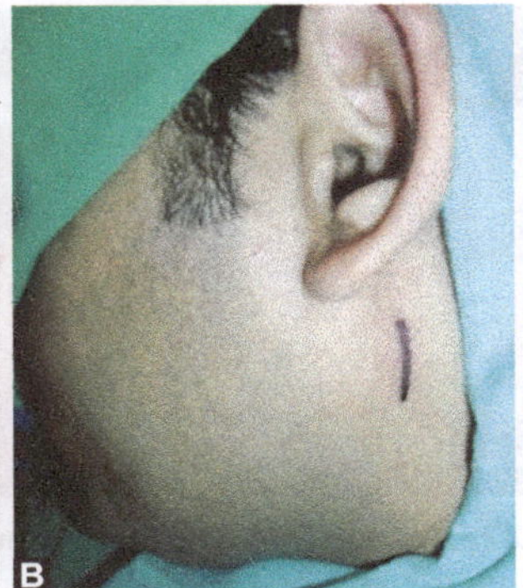

Figs 3.26A and B: Hind's postramal approach (*Source:* Edward Ellis III, Zide MF. Surgical approaches to the facial skeleton. Dallas, Texas)

Postramal (Hind's)[22] Approach

The Hind's Postramal approach is indicated for the surgeries involving the condylar neck and ramal area, e.g. management of the subcondylar or ramal fractures of the mandible. It not only gives excellent exposure but also has very good and acceptable cosmetic results. The incision runs 1 cm behind the posterior border of the ramus, starting a centimeter below the lobule of the ear and extends to the angle of the mandible. After the skin incision the parotidomasseteric fascia is carefully dissected, avoiding damage to the facial nerve and the retromandibular vein (can be identified and ligated if necessary). After exposing the posterior border of the ramus the pterygomasseteric sling is incised and the masseter and the overlying superficial lobe of the parotid gland are reflected superiorly and laterally to expose the condylar neck. After the surgery the pterygomasseteric sling should be repositioned by suturing. Undue force while retracting the parotid and unnecessary dissection through the parenchyma should be avoided to prevent damage to the branches of the facial nerve (Figs 3.26A and B).

Incisions Around the Orbit[23] (Periorbital Approaches)

Infraorbital Incision[24]

Infraorbital incision is placed on the skin. In the skin crease along the infra-orbital ridge from the medial canthus to the lateral canthus. If an extension is required in the lateral side it should be along the line of minimal skin tension along the zygomatic bone (Figs 3.27 and 3.28).

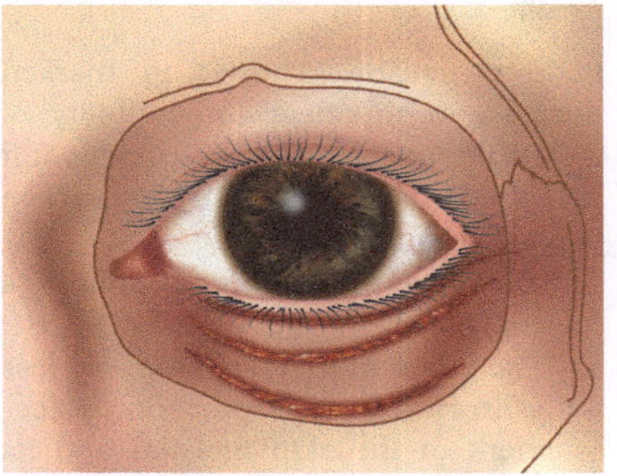

Fig. 3.27: Infraorbital, subtarsal and subciliary incisions (*Source:* Peterson's Principle of oral and maxillofacial surgery. Elsevier)

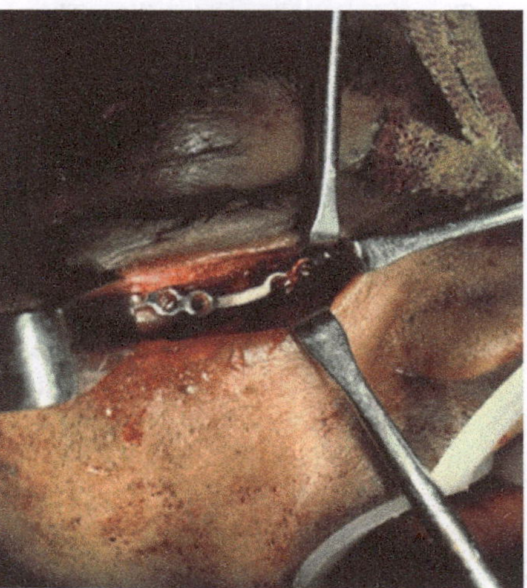

Fig. 3.28: Infraorbital incision

Indications

Exposure of infraorbital ridge during fixing the zygomatic bone and Le-Fort II fractures. Exposure of the orbital floor.

Precautions

It should not cross the lateral canthus to avoid cutting the lymphatic channels that will lead to excess postoperative edema.

Subtarsal Incision[25,26]

Subtarsal incision is placed between the subciliary and infraorbital incision. It is placed in the lower palpebra along the tarsal plate (Figs 3.29A to D).

Indications

Exposure of the infraorbital rim and the orbital floor.

Precautions

It should not cross the lateral canthus to avoid cutting the lymphatic channels that will lead to excess postoperative edema.

Subciliary Incision[27,28]

The incision is made approximately 2 mm inferior to the eyelashes, along the entire length of the lid. The incision may be extended laterally approximately 1 to 1.5 cm in a natural crease, if more exposure is necessary. If no natural skin crease extends laterally from the lateral palpebral fissure, the extension can usually be made straight laterally or slightly inferolaterally. The depth of the

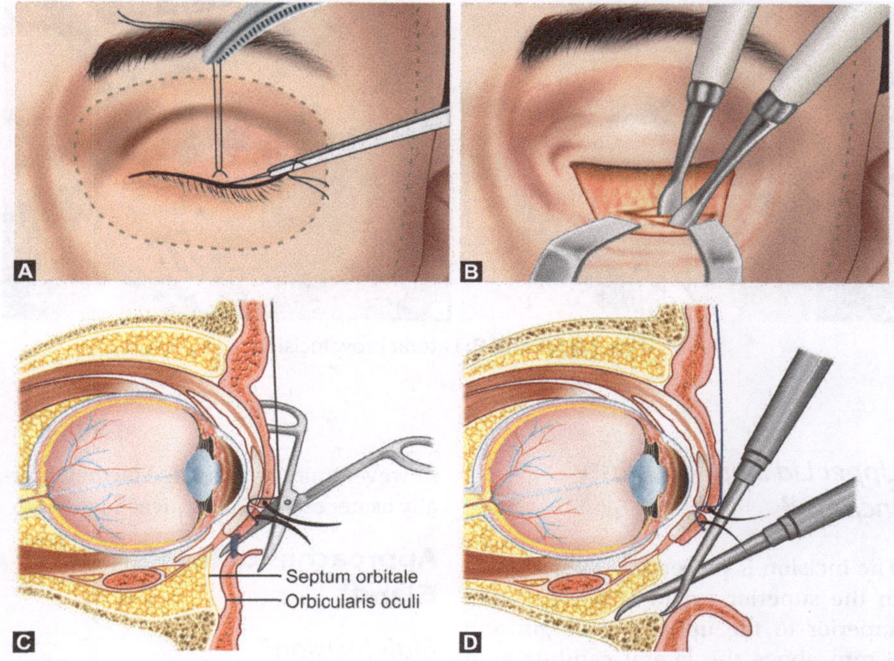

Figs 3.29A to D: Subtarsal incision (*Source:* Edward Ellis III, Zide MF. Surgical approaches to the facial skeleton. Dallas, Texas)

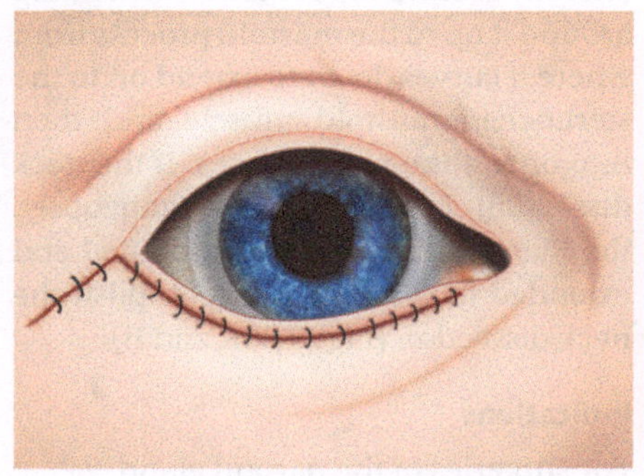

Fig. 3.30: Subciliary incision

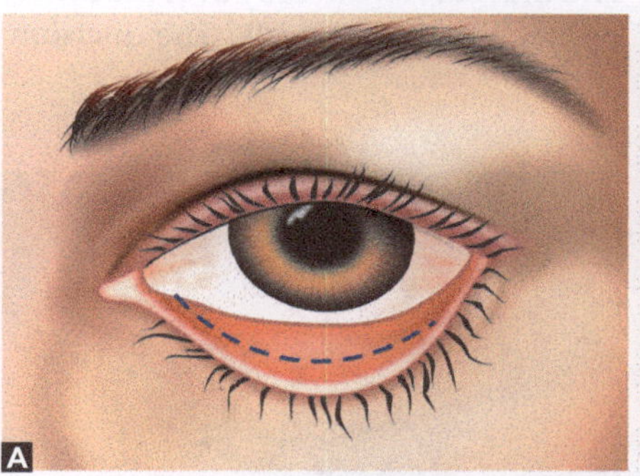

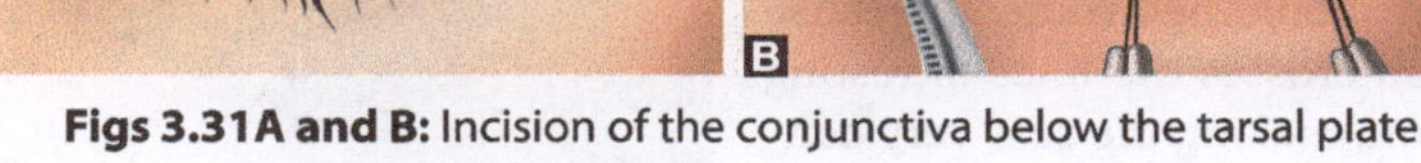

Figs 3.31A and B: Incision of the conjunctiva below the tarsal plate

initial incision is through the skin only such that the underlying muscle is seen when the skin in incised completely (Fig. 3.30).

Indications

For exposure of the infraorbital rim for fixation of fracture passing through the infraorbital rim.

Precautions

Care should be taken not to extend the incision laterally in a superior direction to avoid crossing the minimal tension lines.

The subciliary incision may sometimes cause ectropion due to contracture during healing.

Transconjunctival Incision[29,30]

The lower eyelid is everted with fine forceps and two or three traction sutures are placed through the eyelid approximately 4 to 5 mm below the lid margin to include the tarsal plate in the suture. A lateral canthotomy might be performed if needed (Figs 3.31A and B). Incision is placed on the lower palpebral conjunctiva midway between the inferior margin of the tarsal plate and inferior conjunctival fornix. Medially, incision should not extend beyond the lacrimal punctum (Figs 3.32A and B, 3.33).

Indications

For exposure of the infraorbital rim for fixation of fracture passing through the infraorbital rim.

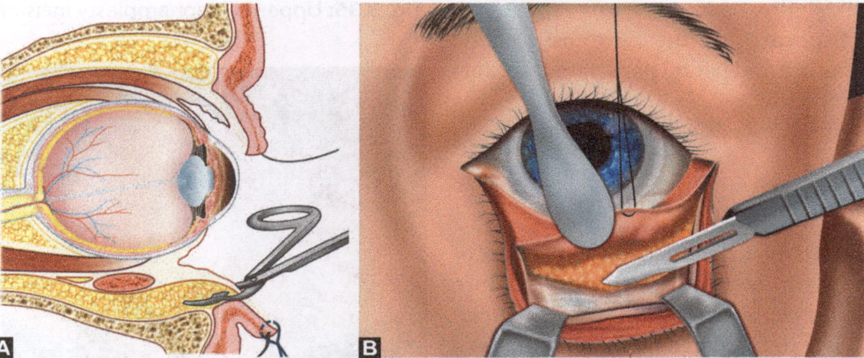

Figs 3.32A and B: Transconjunctival incision (*Source:* Edward Ellis III, Zide MF. Surgical approaches to the facial skeleton. Dallas, Texas)

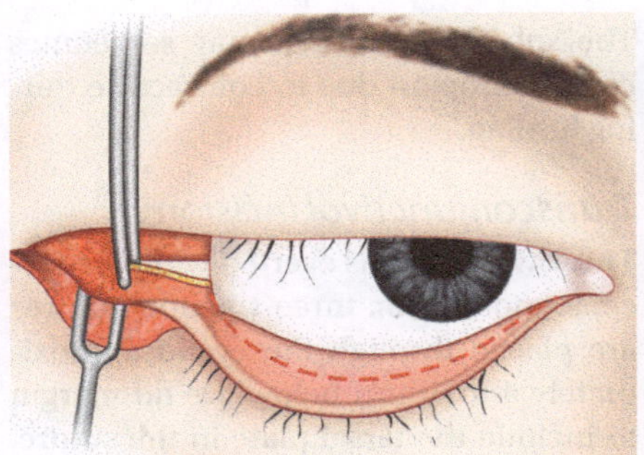

Fig. 3.33: Transconjunctival incision with lateral canthotomy[31]

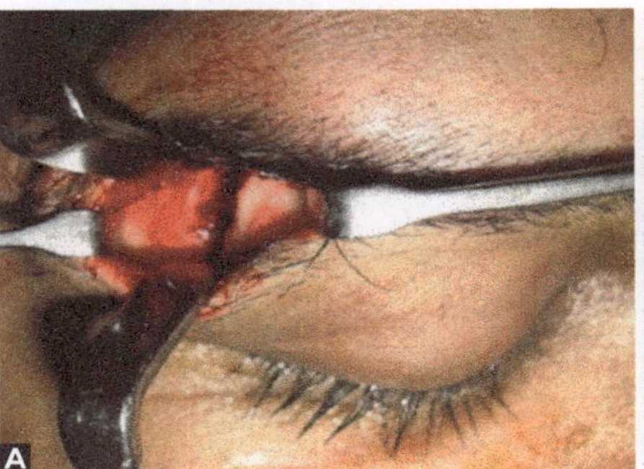

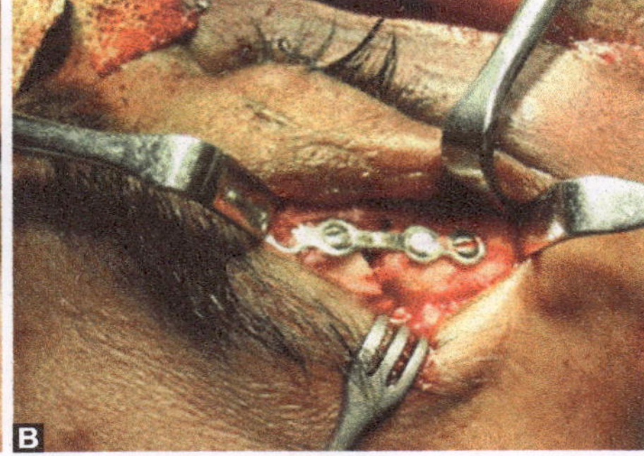

Figs 3.34A and B: Lateral brow incision

Precautions

Care should be taken to protect the globe of the eye from any trauma. Corneal shield can be used for this purpose. Damage to the lacrimal punctum should be avoided by restricting the medial extension of the incision.

Lateral Brow Incision

The eyebrow is not shaved. The skin is stretched over the orbital rim using two fingers and a 2 cm incision is made. The incision should be parallel to the hair follicles of the eyebrow to avoid cutting hair follicles or shafts, which might retard growth of the eyebrow hair. The incision may be made to the depth of the periosteum in one stroke. Extending the incision inferiorly along the orbital rim should be avoided, because the incision crosses the lines of resting skin tension, making the scar very conspicuous (Figs 3.34A and B).

Indications

a. Exposure of the Frontozygomatic suture and lateral part of the supraorbital rim.
b. Exposure of the lateral orbital rim.

Crow's Feet Incision

Crow's feet incision is an extension of the lateral brow incision given if more inferior exposure is required. The incision is extended laterally into a crow's foot wrinkle at least 6 mm above the level of the lateral canthus.

Upper Lid Blepharoplasty Incision[32]

The incision is placed in a skin wrinkle in the superior eyelid at least 10 mm superior to the upper lid margin and 6 mm above the lateral canthus as it extends laterally (Fig. 3.35). If a lid crease is not readily detectable, a curvilinear incision along the area of the supratarsal fold that tails off laterally over the lateral orbital rim works well. The incision, however, may be extended farther laterally as necessary for surgical access.

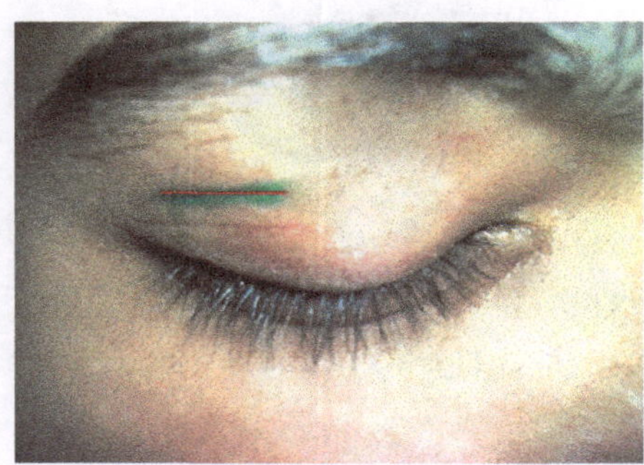

Fig. 3.35: Upperlid blepharoplasty incision

Approaches to the Parotid Gland

Blair Incision[33]

Incision begins in the preauricular crease extending superiorly up to the level of the root of the helix. Inferiorly it turns laterally around the ear lobule extending around it up to the mastoid process from where it curves down to extend on to the sternocleidomastoid muscle and then into one of the neck creases. If the neck dissection is planned simultaneously, the Blair's incision can be modified and extended in the neck to accomplish the neck dissection (Figs 3.36A and B).

Indications

For surgeries of the parotid gland.

Precautions

Care should be taken to avoid damage to the superficial temporal artery, the

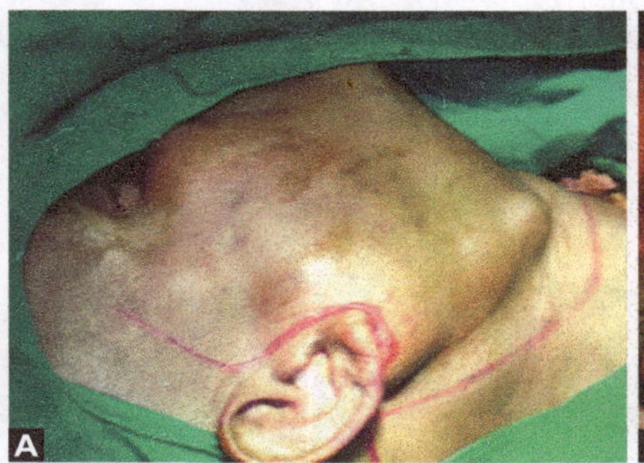

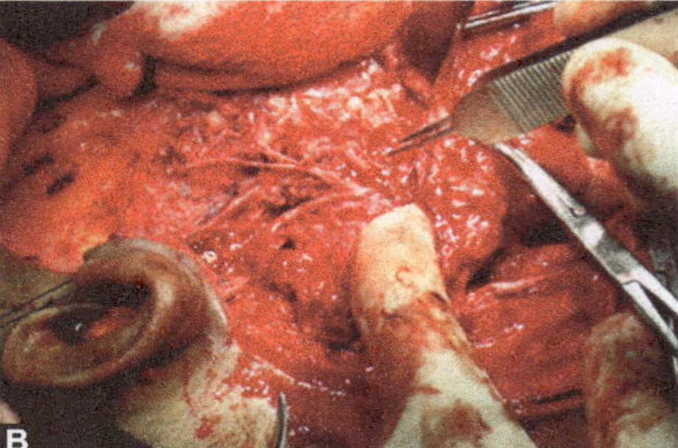

Figs 3.36A and B: (A) Blair incision; (B) Modified Blair incision

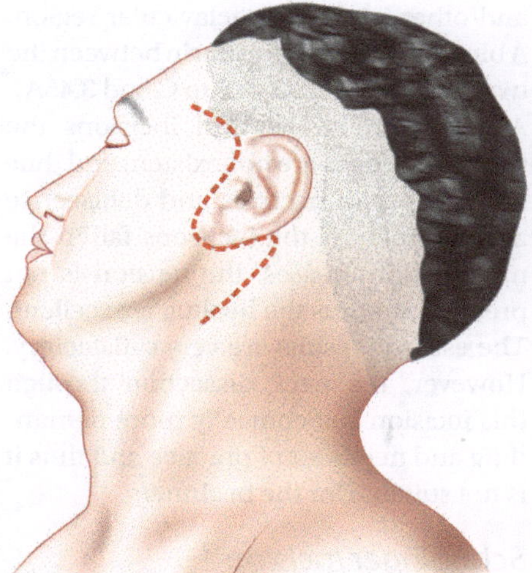
Fig. 3.37: Gutierrez incision

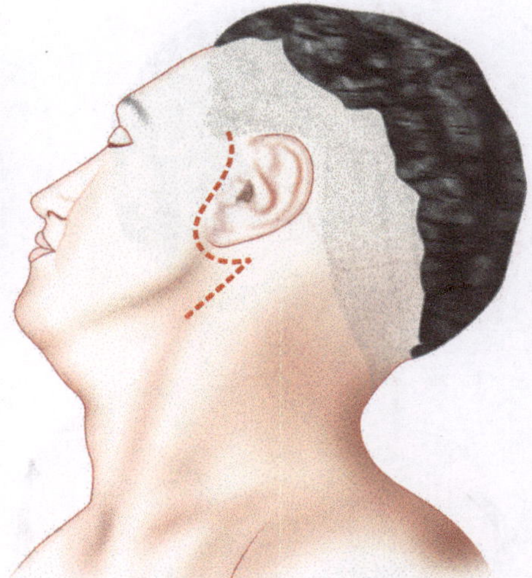
Fig. 3.38: Redon and Vaillant incision

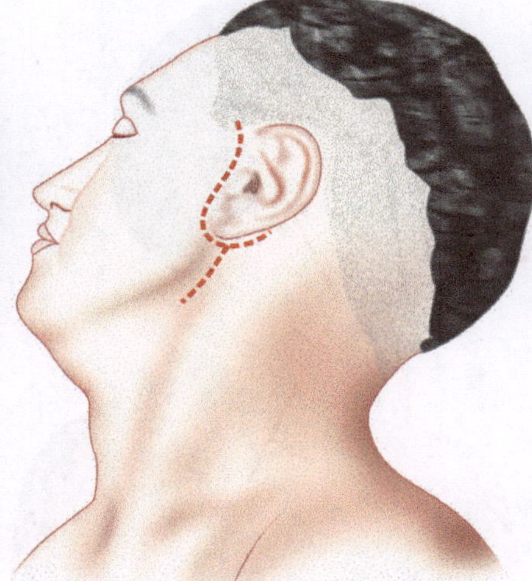
Fig. 3.39: Adson and Ott incision

auriculotemporal nerve, the marginal mandibular nerve while placement of incision in the neck.

Gutierrez Incision[34]

The incision has a temporal extension, a preauricular component and a limb extending on to the neck in one of the skin creases. This was described by Gutierrez in 1903 (Fig. 3.37).

Redon and Vaillant Incision

Their incision was similar to that proposed by Adson. It has a preauricular sector, which curls around the ear lobule and then curls again downwards to extend in one of the neck crease (Fig. 3.38).

Adson and Ott Incision[35]

Adson and Ott incision is a 'Y' shaped incision with a preauricular sector, a postauricular sector and a cervical incision line, that splits off from the site of union of the first two branches. The advantage of this incision is improved esthetics because it lacks a temporal incision line (Fig. 3.39).

Samengo Incision[36]

The incision is similar to the one described above having a preauricular, a postauricular and a neck extension in the incision line (Fig. 3.40).

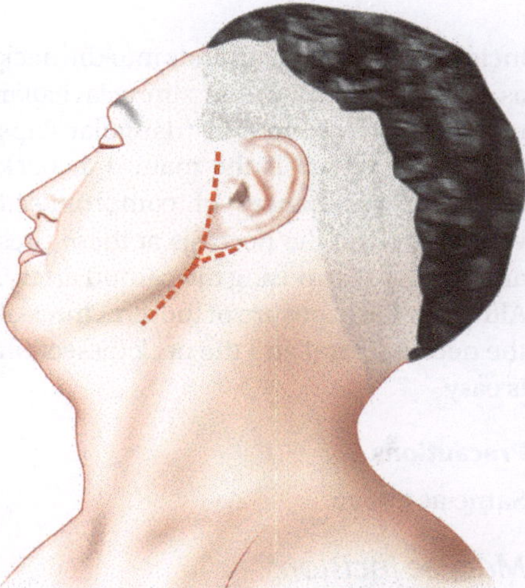
Fig. 3.40: Samengo incision

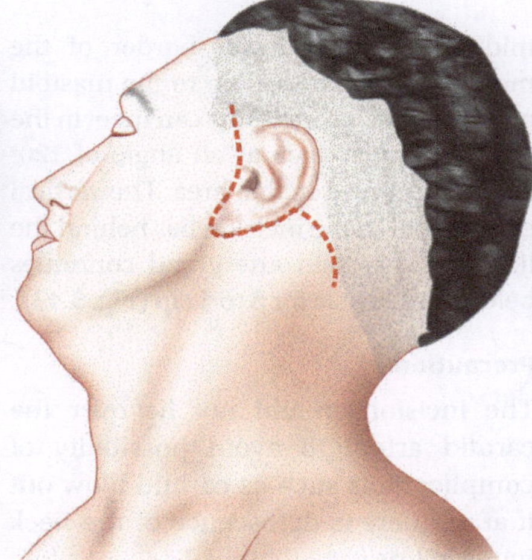
Fig. 3.41: Appiani's incision

Appiani's Incision, 1984[37]

The incision lies within the lower portion of the scalp and is hidden by the hair instead of the vertical incision line. The temporal extension of the incision being short restricts access. To overcome this pitfall, Ferreira JL[38] extended the temporal limb of the incision, but kept it within the hairline (Fig. 3.41).

Approaches for Neck Dissection

Each of the incision advocated for neck dissection represents a compromise between free accesses to the surgical site and need to provide safe skin cover for vital structures left in the neck after the dissection. For the purpose of radical neck dissection, three major incision types were popularized. However, with changing trends in management of neck in various cancers of the oropharyngeal area and management of levels 1 to 3 of the neck nodes, various other incisions have been introduced.

Crile's 'Y' Incision or Triradiate Incision[39]

The submandibular part of the incision begins anteriorly a little beyond the

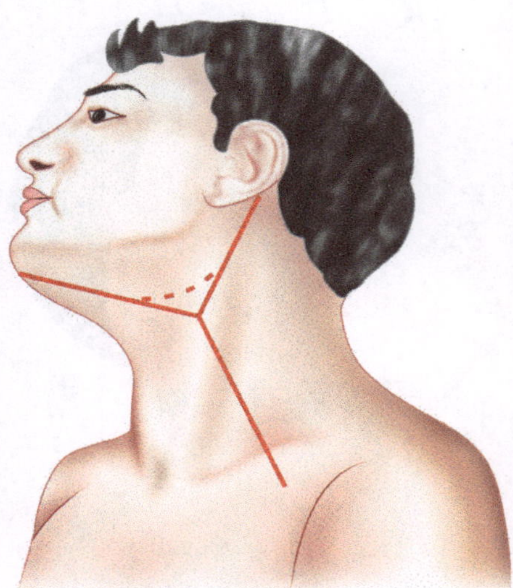

Fig. 3.42: Crile's 'Y' incision or triradiate incision

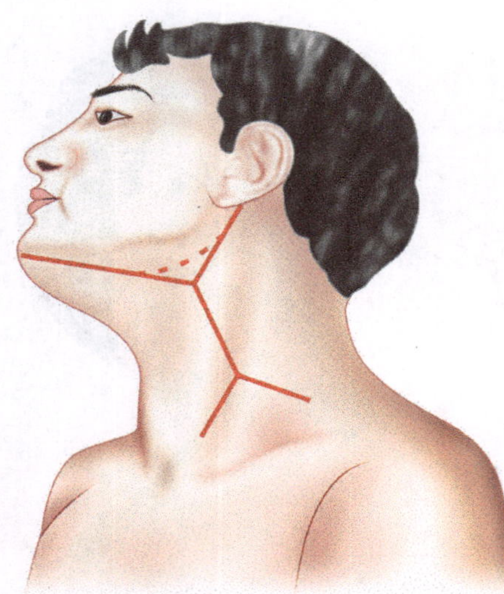

Fig. 3.43: Hayes Martin incision

midline near the lower border of the mandible and extends up to the mastoid process. The two incisions can meet in the submandibular area at an angle of 120° or can be curved in that area. The vertical component of the incision lies behind the line of the carotid artery and continues below the clavicle for 3 to 4 cm (Fig. 3.42).

Precautions

The incision should not lie over the carotid artery to avoid possibility of complications such as carotid blow out if at all there is dehiscence of the neck incision line.

Hayes Martin Incision[40]

Hayes Martin incision has a similar submandibular component like the triradiate incision. However, it extends into the neck as an inverted 'Y' in the supraclavicular region thus creating four triangular flaps (Fig. 3.43). Which is the main drawback as there are chances of compromised vascularity and the necrosis at these sites and danger of exposing the carotid artery. Although the exposure of the structures of the neck is liberal and the neck dissection is easy.

Precautions

Same as above.

MacFee Incision[41]

MacFee incision differs from the above two incisions in that it does not have a vertical limb. It consists of two horizontal incisions, one in the submandibular area and other in the supraclavicular region. A bipedicled flap is present in between the two incisions (Figs 3.44B to C and 3.45A). As there are no vertical incisions the triangular edges are nonexistent and thus the chances of necrosis and dehiscence are minimal. As the incisions fall in the natural skin creases, the tension is not present and thus the healing is excellent. The esthetic results are very satisfactory. However, the neck dissection through this incision is technically more demanding and needs lot of practice and thus it is not suitable for the beginners.

Schobinger Incision[42]

Schobinger incision is a modification of the triradiate incision. In this incision the vertical limb of the incision is curved posteriorly instead of running straight. This modification avoids placement of the vertical component of the incision on the carotid artery (Figs 3.44A and 3.45B). The formation of a sharp triangular area still remains the basic disadvantage of this incision.

Apron like incision of Freund and Latyshevsky[43]: Apron incision is used in management of level 1 to 3 cervical lymph nodes in the neck. It begins at the mastoid process and curves below the lower border of mandible approximately crossing the SCM, where it is crossed by the omohyoid muscle and extends up to the chin (Figs 3.46A to C). This is very effective incision for the supraomohyoid neck dissections. The main advantage being that there are no triangular areas or sharp angles and thus the healing is excellent.

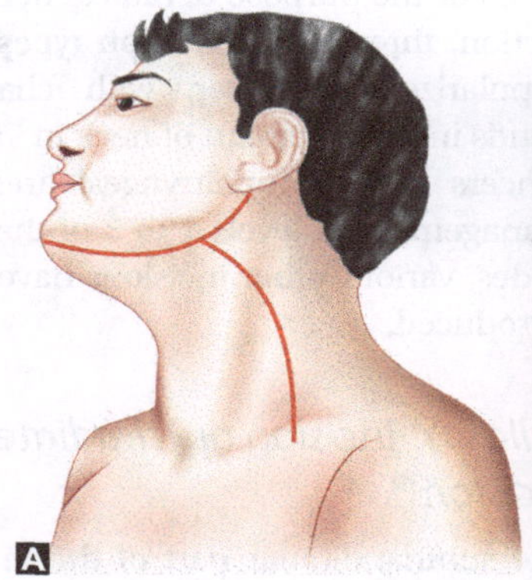

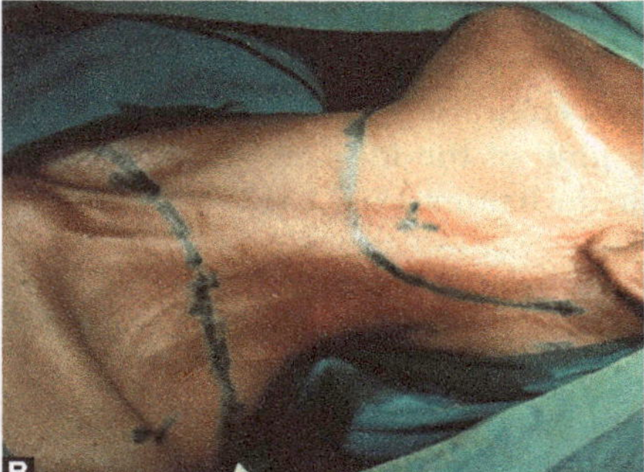

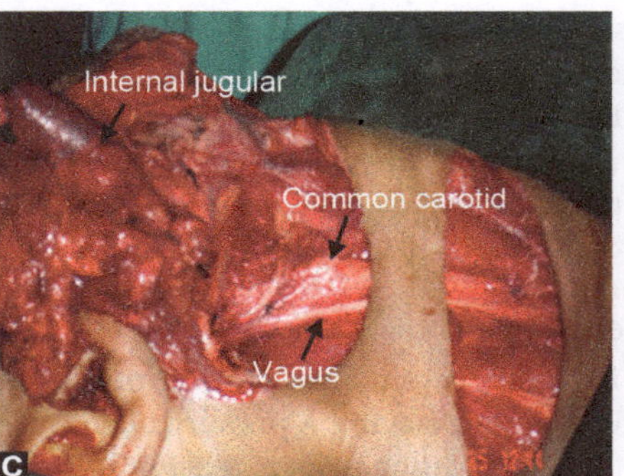

Figs 3.44A to C: (A) Schobinger incision; (B and C) MacFee's ladder incision

Apron Like Incision of Freund[44]

Apron incision of Freund is used in management of malignancies of the larynx. It extends from one mastoid process to the other after crossing the deep neck fold (Figs 3.47A and B). This incision with suitable minor modifications can be used for bilateral supraomohyoid neck dissections for the midline malignancies of the oral cavity.

Conley Incision[45]

Conley incision is a modification of the triradiate incision wherein the anterior limb of the submandibular incision and the posteriorly curved vertical incision are modified to run as a single incision, which begins in the submental region and curves posteriorly at the anterior border of the trapezius muscle up to the clavicle. The posterior part of the submandibular incision is given at a right angle approximately below the ear lobule.

The Conley incision was modified by Lasaridis et al.[46] (1994), which is shown in the figure as dotted line (Fig. 3.48).

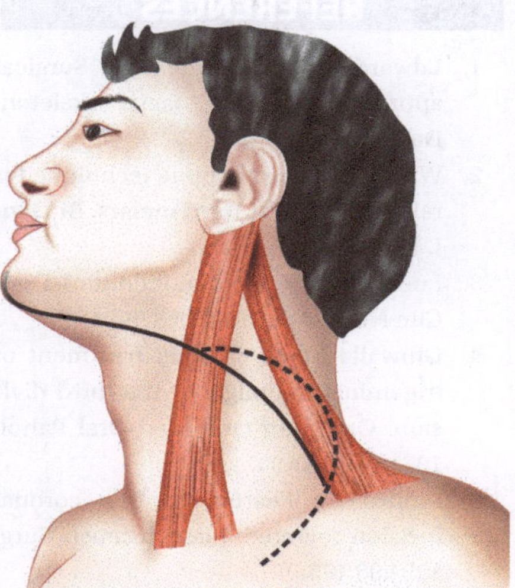

Fig. 3.48: Conley incision

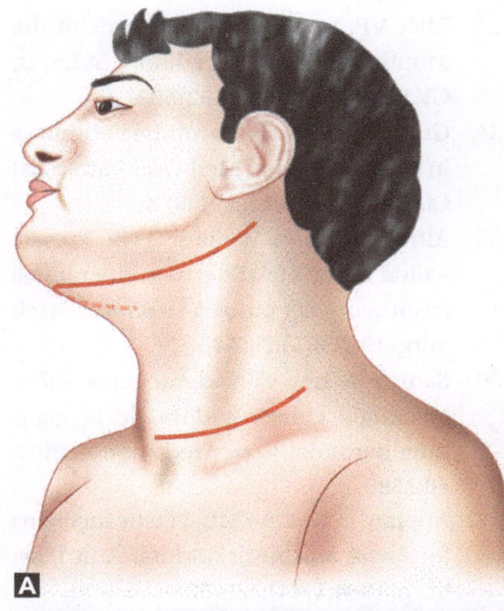

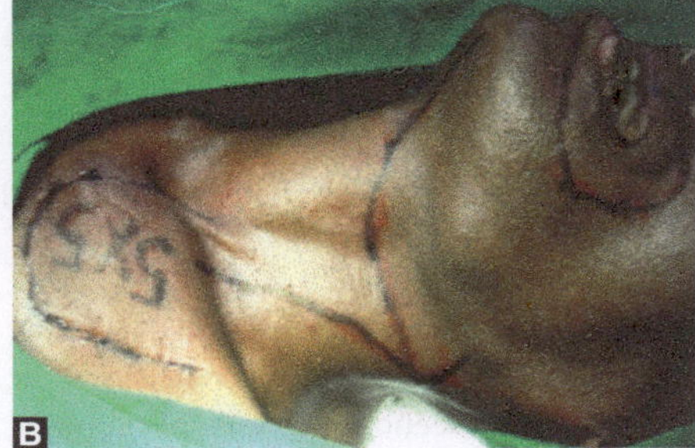

Figs 3.45A and B: (A) MacFee's incision; (B) Shobinger's incision

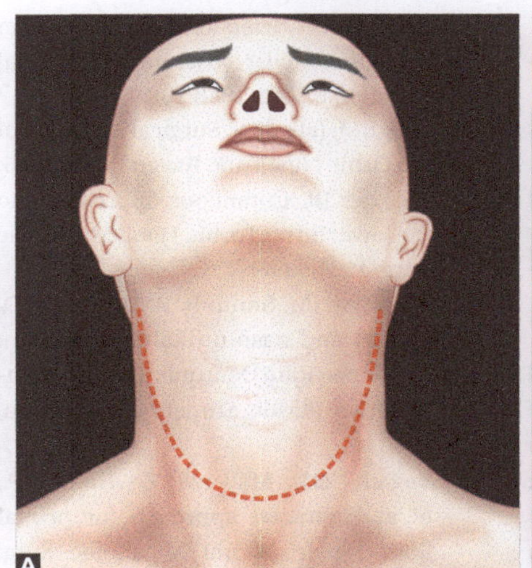

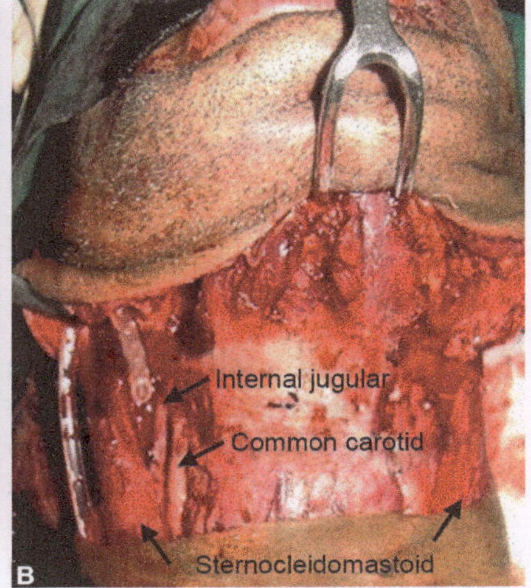

Figs 3.47A and B: Apron like incision of Freund

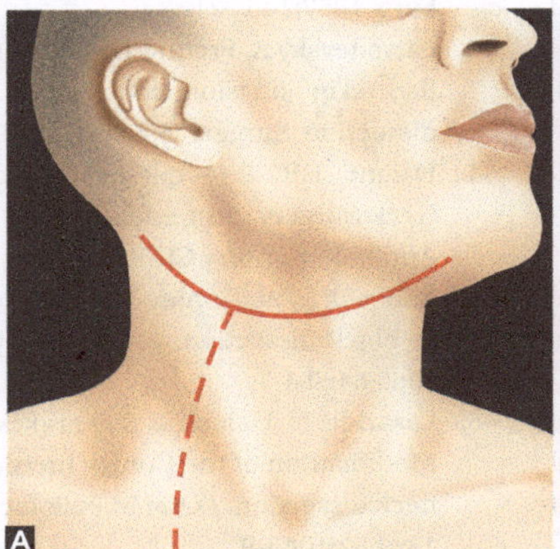

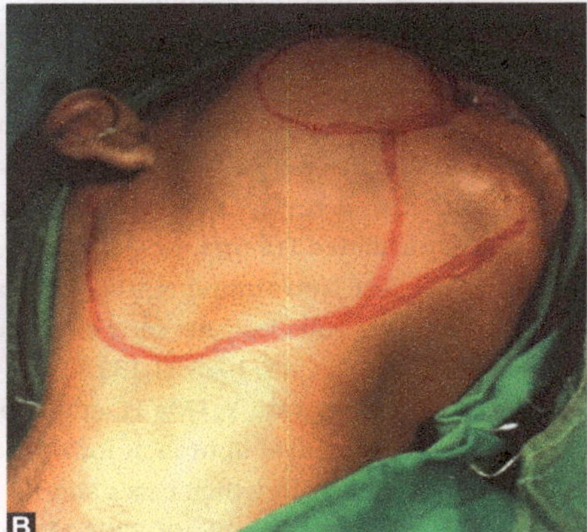

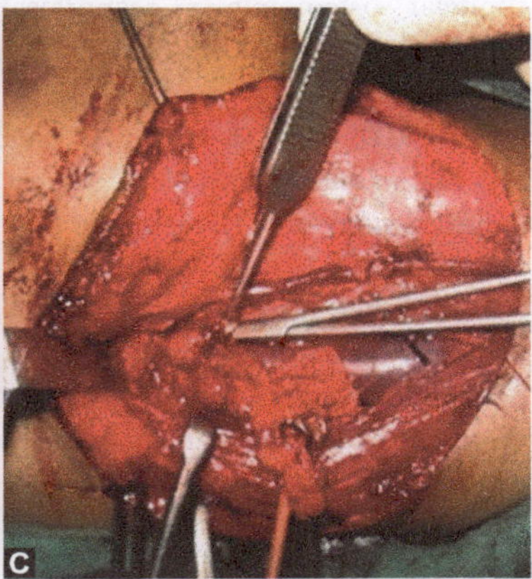

Figs 3.46A to C: Apron like incision of Freund and Latyshevsky

REFERENCES

1. Edward Ellis III, Zide MF. Surgical approaches to the facial skeleton. Dallas, Texas.
2. Ward TG. The split bone technique for removal of lower third molars. Br Dent J. 1956;101:297-304.
3. Luebke RG. Surgical endodontics. Dent Clin North Am. 1974;18:379-91.
4. Ginwalla MSN. Surgical treatment of trigeminal neuralgia of the third division. Oral Surg Oral Med Oral Pahol. 1961;14:1300-04.
5. Munro IR, Fearon JA. The coronal incision revisited. Plast Reconstr Surg. 1994;93:185.
6. Shepherd DE, Ward-Booth RP, Moos KF. The morbidity of bicoronal flaps in maxillofacial surgery. Br J Oral Maxillofac Surg. 1985;23:1-8.
7. Ellis E, Zide MF. Transfacial approaches to the mandible. In: Ellis E, Zide MF III (Eds). Surgical Approaches to the Facial Skeleton, 2nd edition. Philadelphia: Lippincott Williams and Wilkins; 2005. Section 5. pp.151-89.
8. Risdon F. Ankylosis of the temporomandibular joint. J Am Dent Assoc. 1934; 21:1933.
9. Dingman RO, Grabb WC. Surgical anatomy of the mandibular ramus of the facial nerve based on the dissection of 100 facial halves. Plast Reconstr Surg Transplant Bull. 1962;29:266-72.
10. Hind EC. Correction of prognathism by subcondylar osteotomy. J Oral Surg (Chic). 1958;16(3):209-14.
11. Hinds EC, Girotti WJ. Vertical subcondylar osteotomy: a reappraisal. Oral Surg Oral Med Oral Pathol. 1967; 24(2):164-70.
12. Maran AGD, Gaze M, Wilson JA. Stell and Maran's Head and Neck Surgery. Oxford: Butterworth-Heinemann; 1994. pp.176-92.
13. Dieffenbach JF. Die Operative Chirurgie, Vol I. FA Brockhaus, Leipzig. 1845.
14. Bennett JE, Lynch JB, Lewis SR, Blocker TG Jr. The operative treatment of cancer of the lip. Am Surgeon. 1962;28: 537.
15. Rowe WC. Surgery of temporomandibular joint. Proc R Soc Med. 1972;65:383.
16. Blair VP, Ivy RH. Brown JBs Essentials of Oral Surgery, 2nd edition. St Louis: CV Mosby; 1937.
17. Thoma KH. Tumors of the condyle and temporomandibular joint. Oral Surg. 1954;7:1091.
18. Al-Kayat A, Bramley P. A modified preauricular approach to the temporomandibular joint and malar arch. Br J Oral Maxillofac Surg. 1979;17:91.
19. Posnick JC, Goldstein J, Clokie C. Advantages of the postauricular coronal incision. Ann Plast Surg. 1992; 29:114.
20. Alexander RW, James RB, Postauricular approach for surgery of the temporomandibular articulation. J Oral Surg. 1975;33:346.
21. Davidson AS. Endaural condylectomy. Br J Plast Surg. 1956;8:64-7.
22. Hinds EC. Correction of prognathism by subcondylar osteotomy. J Oral Maxillofac Surg. 1958;16:209.
23. Zide BM, Jelks Gw. Surgical Anatomy of the Orbit. New York, Raven Press, 1985.
24. Werther JR. Cutaneous approaches to the lower lid and orbit. J Oral Maxillofac Surg. 1998;56:60.
25. Converse JM, Smith B, Wood-Smith D. Orbital and naso-orbital fractures. In: Converse John Marquis (Ed). Reconstructive Plastic Surgery 2nd edition, 1972.
26. Bagain ZH, Malkawi Z, Hadidi A, et al. Subtarsal approach for orbital floor repair. J Oral Maxillofac Surg. 2008;66:45-50.
27. Wray RC, Holtmann B, Ribaudo JM, et al. A comparison of conjunctival and subciliary incisions for orbital fractures. Br J Plast Surg. 1977;30:142.
28. Patel PC, Sobota BT, Patel NM, et al. Comparison of transconjunctival versus subciliary approaches for orbital fractures: A review of 60 cases. J Craniomaxillofac Trauma. 1998;4:17.
29. Bourguet J. Notre traitement chirurgical de poches sous les yeux sans cicatrice. Arch Fr Bell; Chir. 1928;31:133.
30. Suga H, Sugawara Y, Uda H, et al. The transconjunctival approach for orbital bony surgery: In which cases should it be used? J Craniofac Surg. 2004;15:454.
31. Zide BM, McCarthy JG. The medial canthus revised. An anatomical basis for canthopexy. Ann Plast Surg. 1983;11:1-9.
32. Pospisil et al. Review of the lower blepharoplasty incision as a surgical approach to zygomatic-orbital fractures. Br J Oral Maxillofac Surg. 1984; 22:261-8.
33. Blair VP. Surgery and Diseases of the Mouth and Jaws, 3rd edition, St Louis; CV Mosby; 1920.pp.492-523.
34. Gutierrez-Perez JL. Parotid sialolithiasis in Stensen's duct. Med Oral Patol Oral Cir Bucal. 2006;11(1):E80-4.
35. Alfred W Adson, William O Ott. Preservation of the facial nerve in the radical treatment of parotid tumors. Arch Surg. 1923;6(3):739-46.
36. Samengo LA. Consideraciones sobre la cirugia conserva dora de la glandula parotida. Pren Med Argent 1961; 48:1586.
37. Appiani E, Delfino MC. Plastic incisions for facial and neck tumors. Ann Plast Surg. 1984;13(4):335-52.
38. Ferreira JL, Maurino N, Michael E, et al. Surgery of the parotid region. J Oral Maxillofac Surgery. 1990;48:803-7.
39. Crile GW. Excision of cancer of the head and neck. JAMA. 1906;47:1780-86.
40. Martin H, del Valle B, Ehrlich J, et al. Neck dissection. Cancer 1951;4:441-99.
41. MacFee WF. Transverse incisions for neck dissection. Annals of Surgery. 1960;151:279-84.
42. Schobinger R. The use of a long anterior skin flap in radical neck resection. Ann Surg. 1957;146:221.
43. Latyshevsky A, Freund HR. Long upper flap skin incision for radical neck dissection. Surgery. 1960;47:206-9.
44. Freund HR. Principles of Head and Neck Surgery, 2nd edition. New York: Appleton Century Croft.1979.
45. Babcock WW, Conley J. Neck incision in block dissection. Arch Otolaryngol. 1966;84:554-7.
46. Lasaridis N, Dalabiras S , Karakassis D. Modification of the Conley incision for neck dissection. J Oral Maxillofac Surg. 1994;52:1046-9.

4 Fluid, Electrolyte Balance and Acid-base Equilibrium

Borle Rajiv M, Agrawal Poonam

INTRODUCTION

About a billion years ago, life began in the sea. The sea possessed unique properties for the maintenance of life. The water that surrounds the cells of vertebrates and of humans, i.e. the extracellular water has an electrolyte composition similar to what the sea had in prerecorded times, inspite of all the countless changes in evolution that have occurred.[1]

The total body water (TBW) is usually divided into two main compartments:

1. The extracellular compartment (ECC) and
2. The intracellular compartment (ICC).

The average water content of men is approximately 60 percent of total body weight and of women is 50 percent of total body weight, as the men have more muscle mass, which has higher water content, while females have more fat and less water content. The total body water (TBW) is about 80 percent of total body weight in newborn, which is gradually lost. The young individuals have TBW of about 70 percent which is gradually reduced at old age to 60 percent due to loss of lean muscle mass due to muscle wasting.[2,3]

The water is freely diffusible from one compartment to another, but electrolytes do not as they require an active mechanism. This is of utmost importance in deciding, which intravenous fluids be used during surgery. The volumes of fluid compartments depend highly on sodium and plasma proteins. Sodium is the primary determinant of osmolality and tonicity. It distributes predominantly in the extracellular fluid compartment with nearly equal concentrations in the interstitial fluid and plasma. Intracellular fluid contains only trace amounts of sodium. This is maintained by an active sodium pump in the cells. Any change in sodium concentration in any of the fluid compartments causes a compensatory shift in free water.

The normal adult takes in 2 to 3 liters of water per day in various forms. When normal oral intake (enteral) is impossible or impractical, intravenous fluid replacement (parenteral) is indicated. Among the electrolytes, sodium and potassium are the electrolytes of main concern and their disturbances will lead to varied clinical signs and symptoms. A wide variety of intravenous fluids are available for the replacement of fluid loss and electrolytes. It can be delivered by crystalloid or colloid solutions. Colloid solutions have the advantage of expanding intravascular volume with minimum fluid loss.

The adequacy of fluid and electrolyte replacement must be monitored. Key parameters are weight loss or gain, urine output and electrolyte analysis. Perioperative fluid management is of utmost importance in maintaining homeostasis in the surgical patient. Perioperative hydration improves the recovery process and results in fewer postoperative complications.[2-4]

ACID-BASE BALANCE

The pH of body fluids is maintained within a narrow range despite the ability of the kidneys to generate large amounts of bicarbonate and the normal large acid load produced as byproducts of metabolism.

Compensation for acid-base derangements is either respiratory (for metabolic derangements) or metabolic (for respiratory derangements). Normal acid-base homeostasis prevents metabolic acidosis and alkalosis. Under normal circumstances blood PCO_2 is tightly maintained by alveolar ventilation, controlled by the respiratory centers in the pons and medulla oblongata. If it gets disturbed it will result in respiratory acidosis or alkalosis.[3,4]

A safe and effective parenteral nutrition became feasible in the 1960s as a consequence of the development of inert materials for intravascular feeding catheter, together with pharmaceutical advances in the formulation of feeding solutions. It is the intravenous provision of all nutritional requirements without the use of the gastrointestinal tract (GIT). The primary indication of total parenteral nutrition is for those patients whose gut is not functioning to allow for the delivery of enteral nutrition such as patients with severe inflammatory bowel disease, enterocutaneous fistulae, pancreatitis or short bowel syndrome. Peripheral parenteral nutrition is administered through a peripheral intravenous line with an osmolarity below 900 milliosmoles/L, to prevent venous phlebitis. Nutritional support plays an integral role in the healing and recovery of the trauma patient. It has been shown clearly that the enteral route of feeding is preferable if possible to maintain gut mucosal integrity, enhance immunocompetence and decrease the incidence of septic complications.[5]

In Homeostasis

Water is the most important constituent of the body present in all the tissues (Table 4.1). It accounts for about 55 percent of our weight (range 45%–60%, up to 75% in newborns).

Water is distributed between intracellular and extracellular compartments (Box 4.1). Intracellular water accounts for about two-thirds (80%) of TBW and 40 percent of total body weight. Extracellular water (20% of total body weight) can further be divided into interstitial (three-fourths of extracellular or about 15% of total body weight) and intravascular (one-fourth of extracellular, or 5% of total body weight). Water movement between the spaces is regulated by ionic and colloid osmotic pressure gradients across semipermeable membranes. The normal adult takes in 2 to 3 liters of water per day in various forms. The body easily adjusts to the variations, primarily through renal regulation, conservation or excretion. About 200 mL water is generated as metabolic end product.

Fluid loss has been categorized as sensible and insensible. The sensible loss includes urine, blood loss, gastrointestinal suction and massive diarrhea. Insensible water is lost through vaporization (lungs and skin) and ranges between 500 and 1,000 mL per day, depending on the factors like environmental conditions, presence of fever, etc. This is through the lungs (200–400 mL) and skin (300–600 mL). Normal sensible loss is through the urine (800–1,500) and stool (150–250 mL). These losses depend directly on water intake and diet consistency. The goal of fluid therapy is to balance intake with loss, creating neither deprivation nor extreme excess.[1-3,6]

Table 4.1: Fluid distribution in various compartments

For a 70 kg man	
Plasma	3,500 cc
Interstitial fluid	10,500 cc
Intracellular fluid	28,000 cc

Box 4.1: Percentage wise fluid distribution in various compartments

Total extracellular
Volume—20% of body weight
Plasma—5% of body weight
Interstitial fluid—15% of body weight
Total intracellular
Volume—40% of body weight

Composition of Solutes in Extracellular and Intracellular Water

The composition of solutes in extracellular (EC) water differs from that of solutes in intracellular (IC) water. The principal EC electrolytes are cationic sodium and anionic chloride. Total body sodium includes 30 percent in structural tissue like bone.

The principal electrolytes in the IC compartment are cationic potassium and organic phosphates (Table 4.2). The three electrolytes sodium, potassium and chloride are tightly regulated by renal function. A major mechanism of electrolyte control is regulation of glomerular filtration rate (GFR). The tubular cells reabsorb more than 95 percent of the water and electrolytes filtered and are subjected to paracrine and hormonal influences. Control over the electrolyte composition of EC compartment is affected through selective reabsorption of electrolytes from plasma filtrate generated at the glomerulus.[1-3,6]

Regulation of Osmolality

Sodium in EC compartment and potassium in IC compartment largely determine osmolality and the adjustments in the active transport of these solutes across the cell membrane influence the regulation of body fluid osmolality. However, fluctuations in the volume of TBW principally influence tonicity.

The principal mechanisms for control of tonicity are regulation of antidiuretic hormone released into the blood by the hypothalamus. Osmolality of body water is tightly maintained in the range of 285 to 295 mOsm per liter despite wide variations in salt and water intakes.[1-3,6]

Table 4.2: Ionic concentration of different fluid compartments

Plasma (mEq/L)		Interstitial fluid (mEq/L)		Intracellular (mEq/L)	
Cations (154)	Anions (154)	Cations (153)	Anions (153)	Cations (200)	Anions (200)
Na^+ 142	Cl^- 103	Na^+ 144	Cl^- 114	K^+ 150	SO_4^{--}, HPO_4^{--} 150
K^+ 4	HCO_3^- 27	K^+ 4	HCO_3^- 30	Mg^{++} 40	
Ca^{++} 5	SO_4^{--}, PO_4^{--} 3	Ca^{++} 3	SO_4^{--}, PO_4^{--} 3	Na^+ 10	HCO_3^- 10
Mg^{++} 3		Mg^{++} 2			Proteins 40
	Organic acids 5		Organic acids 5		
	Proteins 16		Proteins 1		

Colloid Osmotic Pressure

Colloid is a term used to collectively describe the large molecular weight (nominally MW > 30,000) particles present in a solution. In normal plasma, the plasma proteins are the major colloids present. As the colloids are solutes they contribute to the total osmotic pressure of the solution. This component due to the colloids is typically quite a small percentage of the total osmotic pressure. It is referred to as colloid osmotic pressure (or sometimes as the oncotic pressure).

Oncotic pressure or colloid osmotic pressure is a form of osmotic pressure exerted by proteins in blood plasma that usually tends to pull water into the circulatory system from the EC compartment.

Throughout the body, dissolved compounds have an osmotic pressure. Because large plasma proteins cannot easily cross through the capillary walls, their effect on the osmotic pressure of the capillary interiors will, to some extent, balance out the tendency for fluid to leak out of the capillaries. In other words, the oncotic pressure tends to pull fluid into the capillaries. In conditions where plasma proteins are reduced, e.g. from being lost in the urine (proteinuria) or from malnutrition, the result of low oncotic pressure can be excess fluid buildup in the tissues (edema). Plasma colloid osmotic pressure (COP) is an important determinant in the appearance of edema especially pulmonary edema.

The normal human plasma COP averages 25.4 mm Hg. The COP is 15 percent less in patients on bed rest than in the ambulatory patients (increase in ambulatory patients is secondary to reduction in plasma volume associated with exercise). There is gradual, but progressive and significant decrease in COP with age. COP is also less in females as compared to males.

FLUID AND ELECTROLYTE IMBALANCE

The disorders in fluid balance are classified into three general categories:

Disturbances of
- Volume,
- Concentration, and
- Composition.[3,7-9]

Disorders of Fluid Volume

Hypovolemia

The term 'hypovolemia' refers to decreased intravascular volume and not decreased EC volume and this disorder results from insufficient function of the normal mechanisms of intravascular volume maintenance.

Pathophysiology

Decreased effective intravascular volume can occur in the presence of decreased, normal or increased EC volume. Decreased EC volume leads to depletion of intravascular volume, which is most common and can arise from increased loss of EC fluid, failure to replete normal losses or a combination of both. Bleeding, diarrhea, vomiting and excessive skin loss of fluid (sweating, burns) can quickly deplete EC and intravascular volumes.[10] Hypovolemia with normal EC volume occurs as a result of any disorder that alters the balance between intravascular and extravascular fluid compartments. Sepsis (peritonitis, septicemia), acute respiratory distress syndrome (ARDS), shock and other critical illnesses alter this balance by increasing permeability of vasculature. The result is an increase in the nonintravascular fluid volume (interstitial compartment, pleural effusions, ascites) at the acute expense of the intravascular volume.

Volume depletion causing inadequate systemic perfusion can lead to altered mental status, confusion, lethargy and coma; cold skin and extremities from vasoconstriction; cardiac ischemia and dysfunction; liver and kidney failure. Reduced skin turgor has been claimed to be the most characteristic finding in the physical examination of dehydrated patient.[10] Cellular dehydration, interstitial space dehydration and poor perfusion are presumably responsible for many of the other classic signs of hypovolemia such as longitudinal tongue furrows, dry mucous membrane, dry axillae and sunken eyes.[6,11-13]

Treatment

- Estimate magnitude of hypovolemia.
- Determine rate of correction of hypovolemia without increasing the preload on the heart.
- Determine appropriate type of fluid to be used.

The replacement fluid should predominantly fill and remain in intravascular space because hypovolemia is depletion of the volume of the intravascular space. Replacement fluids given intravenously consist of crystalloid solution, made of water and small solutes and crystalloid solutions, consisting of water, electrolytes and higher-molecular-weight proteins or polymers.[1,3,7,8,14,15]

Fluid Excess/Hypervolemia

The term 'hypervolemia' denotes increased EC volume with or without increased intravascular volume. Hypervolemia is an increase of EC volume with peripheral edema, ascitis or other fluid collection. The intravascular volume may be low, normal or high.

- **Hypervolemia with decreased intravascular volume:** Sodium along with anions is the predominant solute in the EC space; increased EC volume indicates an abnormally increased quantity of sodium and water. Excessive sodium retention or hypervolemia may occur appropriately in states of inadequate effective circulation, such as heart failure or suboptimal filling of vascular space resulting from loss of fluids in other compartments, as occurs with hypoalbuminemia, portal hypertension or increased vascular permeability to solute and water. The evidence of inadequate circulation may be found, including tachycardia, peripheral cyanosis and altered mental status. If EC volume is high, rales and wheezes consistent with pulmonary edema may be present.

Patients with hypervolemia due to endocrine disorders or renal failure may have findings specific to underlying cause.

Diagnosis

It is diagnosed as follows:

- Edema, ascites or any other evidence of increased EC volume.
- Intravascular volume may be judged to be normal, low (hypovolemia) or high.
- Potential causes of increased EC volume such as renal insufficiency, congestive heart failure, liver disease or some other mechanism of sodium retention, or excessive sodium administration, may be present.

Treatment: The need for treatment and the treatment approach depends on the mechanism of hypervolemia. Hypervolemia associated with severely decreased or markedly increased intravascular volume requires rapid and aggressive treatment.

- **Hypervolemia with primary increased sodium retention:** The other major mechanism of hypervolemia is primary excessive function of the normal mechanisms that ensure sodium and water balance. Normal EC volume is maintained by a complex interactive system that includes renin, angiotensin, aldosterone, glomerular filteration, renal tubular handling of sodium and water, atrial natriuretic factor and antidiuretic hormone along with the intake of sodium and water in the diet. Hyperfunction of some of these mechanisms, such as hyperaldosteronism or excessive intake of sodium or dysfunction of others, such as renal dysfunction or decreased glomerular filteration, cause net positive sodium balance with inevitable expansion of the EC volume. Edema is often a major feature of increased EC volume. Edema always indicates increased EC volume except when there is localized mechanism of fluid transudation or exudation, e.g. local venous insufficiency, cellulites, lymphatic obstruction or trauma. The presence of edema may or may not signify that the intravascular volume is increased.

Hypervolemic hypernatremia (i.e. hypertonic sodium gain) results from an increase in total body sodium and water, where the net increase in total body sodium is greater than that of water (i.e. sodium gain > water gain) and is associated with intravascular and extracellular fluid volume expansion. There is increase in total exchangeable Na^+ and K^+ in excess of the increment in total body water (TBW), resulting in a relative free water deficit.

The causes for hypervolemia with primary increased sodium retention (hypernatremia) are:

- Excessive intravenous sodium administration
  - Hypertonic saline administration (3% saline)
  - Increased sodium bicarbonate administration during management of lactic acidosis
  - Replacing hypotonic insensible loss with 0.9% saline
- Mineralocorticoid excess
  - Hyperaldosteronism
  - Congenital adrenal hyperplasia.
- **Excessive salt intake:** Drinking sea water.
- Chronic orthostatic hypotension

The clinical features of hypernatremia resulting from CNS dysfunction due to brain cell shrinkage are

- Confusion
- Neuromuscular excitability
- Hyper-reflexia
- Seizures
- Coma
- Cerebro-vascular damage with subcortical or subarachnoid hemorrhage
- Venous thrombosis
- Urine sodium is typically greater than 20 mEq/L and urine osmolarity is greater than 300 mOsm/L.

Treatment of these patients should be targeted at both the correction of the hypernatremia and the attainment of a negative H_2O balance.

- Discontinue any sodium sources or offending agents, then induce natriuresis to remove excess sodium.
- Treatment with 5% dextrose in water and/or enteral water will reduce hyperosmolality.
- Loop diuretics like furosemide can be used to induce natriuresis and counteract volume expansion so long as kidney function is preserved.
- Patients with severe renal insufficiency and volume overload may require hemodialysis.
- **Hypervolemia with increased intravascular volume:** In these patients, severely increased intravascular volume will be manifested by pulmonary edema, hypoxemia and respiratory distress. If intravenous fluids are being administered, these should be discontinued unless blood transfusions are necessary for severe anemia. Intravenous furosemide (Lasix, 10–80 mg) is given, with repeated doses every 30 minutes depending on the diuretic response. Supportive care includes oxygen, changes in the patient's position and mechanical ventilation if necessary. The patient need to be monitored critically for the detection of congestive cardiac failure due to increased preload and also signs of pulmonary edema, which require appropriate interventions like oxygen therapy and monitoring of electrolytes especially when potassium wasting diuretics (loop diuretics) are prescribed in high doses for the longer duration.
- **Increased extracellular volume without change in intravascular volume (Table 4.3):** These are usually chronic conditions. Edema and ascites do not by themselves cause immediate problems, but edema may impair skin care and lead to immobility, while ascites may become uncomfortable, may cause respiratory distress and hypoxemia and may become infected (spontaneous bacterial peritonitis).[3,7-9]

Electrolyte Imbalance

Hyponatremia

Hyponatremia denotes decrease in sodium ion concentration.

Table 4.3: Extracellular fluid volume imbalance

Type of sign	Deficit		Excess	
	Moderate	Severe	Moderate	Severe
Central nervous system	Sleepiness, apathy, slow responses, anorexia, cessation of visual activity	Decreased tendon reflexes. Anesthesia distal extremities, stupor, coma.	None	None
Gastrointestinal	Progressive decrease in food consumption	Nausea, vomiting, refusal to eat, silent ileus and distension	At surgery : Edema of stomach, colon, lesser and greater omenta and small bowel mesentery	
Cardiovascular	Orthostatic hypotension, tachycardia, collapsed veins, collapsing pulse	Cutaneous lividity, hypotension, distant heart sounds, cold extremities, absent peripheral pulses	Elevated venous pressure, distension of peripheral veins, increased cardiac output, loud heart sounds, functional murmur Bounding pulse, high pulse pressure, increased pulmonary, 2d sound, gallop	
Tissue	Soft, small tongue with longitudinal wrinkling, decreased skin turgor	Atonic muscles, sunken eyes	Subcutaneous pitting edema, basilar rales	Anasarca, moist rales, vomiting, diarrhea
Metabolic	Mild decrease temperature 97°F–99°F (per rectal).	Marked decrease temperature, 95°F–98°F (per rectal)	None	None

Essentials of diagnosis

Sodium less than 135 mEq/L.

- Altered mental status or new onset of seizure disorder.
- Most cases discovered by review of routinely obtained serum electrolytes.

1. **Hyponatremia with decreased extracellular volume:** Decreased EC volume leads to vigorous water conservation, primarily mediated by increased ADH release stimulated by atrial receptors and increased thirst leading to increased water intake. Hyponatremia is facilitated in adrenal insufficiency because lack of cortisol causes collecting ducts to be excessively permeable to water movement, leading to impaired maximum water excretion. Furthermore, ADH levels in adrenal insufficiency may remain elevated despite hyponatremia, suggesting that there is an abnormal ADH response to decreased serum osmolality.
2. **Hyponatremia with increased extracellular volume:** Hyponatremia in the presence of increased EC volume is seen in congestive heart failure, nephrotic syndrome, cirrhosis, protein-losing enteropathy and pregnancy. These disorders have in common edema, ascites, pulmonary edema or other evidence of increased EC volume. However, these patients appear to have inability to maintain normal effective intravascular volume because of forces generating excessive venous and extravascular volume. Hyponatremia is a consequence of ADH release in response to decreased intravascular volume, even though total EC volume is increased and total body water is high.
3. **Hyponatremia with normal extracellular volume:** Hyponatremia in association with normal EC volume is seen with psychogenic water ingestion, decreased solute intake, and most commonly, the syndrome of inappropriate secretion of ADH (SIADH).
4. **Hyponatremia without hypotonicity:** Hyponatremia without hypotonicity was commonly seen in patients with severe hypertriglyceridemia or hyperproteinemia (> 10 g/dL) when serum sodium was measured by flame photometry. This is no longer a problem with the use of ion-specific sodium electrodes.
5. **Hyponatremia with hyperglycemia (Hypertonic hyponatremia):** Hyperglycemia with hyponatremia is associated with decreased TBW rather than with increased TBW relative to total solute. Hyponatremia in the presence of hyperglycemia can be addressed in several ways. First, laboratory measurement of serum osmolality will give a correct assessment of water balance; serum osmolality will be higher than estimated from serum sodium. Another way is to correct the serum sodium for the degree of hyperglycemia.One empiric correction is to add to the measured serum sodium 1 mEq/L for every 60 mg/dL the serum glucose is increased above 100 mg/dL. Hyponatremia associated with decreased osmolality is often asymptomatic until serum sodium falls below 125 mEq/L, but the rate of change is

clearly important. Severe symptoms-including altered mental status, seizures, nausea, vomiting, stupor and coma occur when serum sodium is less than 115 mEq/L when hyponatremia develops acutely or when it is less than 105 to 110 mEq/L during chronic hyponatremia.

Laboratory findings

Serum electrolytes, glucose, creatinine and urea nitrogen, serum osmolality, urine osmolality, urine Na^+, and urine creatinine (to calculate fractional excretion of Na^+) should be measured. Low serum osmolality 280 mOsm/kg confirms hyponatremia due to increased water relative to solute.

An association has been found between hyponatremia with hypokalemia and severe body potassium depletion. Hypokalemia may also predispose patients with hyponatremia to osmotic demyelination syndromes and encephalopathy.

Treatment

Severity of hyponatremia ($[Na^+] < 120$ mEq/L), acuteness of onset and the presence of neurologic symptoms (confusion, stupor, coma or seizures) determine how quickly treatment should be instituted.

Of the underlying problems leading to hyponatremia, the most straight forward and easily corrected is hypovolemia. Administration of normal saline repletes the intravascular volume and inhibits ADH release by reducing the hypovolemic stimulus. Water excretion is enhanced by the increased GFR, and urine should become quickly and near maximally dilute, facilitating water excretion.

Hypokalemia should be corrected, as this has been associated with complications of hyponatremia and its treatment.

Hypernatremia

Essentials of diagnosis

a. Serum sodium greater than 145 mEq/L.
b. Serum osmolality greater than 300 mOsm/kg.
c. Evidence of increased solute administration.
d. Polyuria with dilute urine (diabetes insipidus).
e. Inadequate water intake.
f. Altered mental status.

Clinical features

Hypernatremia and hyperosmolality should be suspected in patients with decreased access to water, especially with altered mental status or those with a history of polyuria. The elderly patients living in a chronic care facility are especially susceptible. However, many patients are identified through routine electrolyte determinations. The severity of water deficit is estimated from the serum electrolytes and body weight.

Signs and symptoms

As with hyponatremia, hypernatremia and hypertonicity affect primarily the brain. Acute decrease in the size of brain cells can lead to altered mental status, impaired thinking and loss of consciousness is an association of cerebral hemorrhage and hypertonicity and hypernatremia, thought to be due to tearing of blood vessels due to brain shrinkage.

Treatment

1. **Calculation of water deficit:** All patients with hypernatremia have increased serum osmolality and the amount of water needed to correct this state can be calculated from the following equation:

   TBW(L) = Normal TBW(L) × (140/$[Na^+]$).

2. **Rate of correction of hypernatremia:** Just as with hyponatremia, too rapid correction of hypernatremia may be harmful. Cerebral edema with neurologic complications may occur during correction as a result of a compensatory mechanism intended to maintain normal brain cell volume. In response to development of hypertonicity, brain cells fairly rapidly increase the amount of inorganic ions; this restores cell volume to near-normal, but at the expense of disrupted cellular function. With persistence of hypertonicity, brain cells generate and take up idiogenic osmoles, sometimes called 'organic osmolytes'. As cell volume is determined from the amount of solute contained within the cell, organic osmolytes resist the movement of water out of the cells and maintain brain volume close to normal. Many of the organic osmolytes are taken up from the EC space by the formation of specific membrane channels. These channels do not quickly disappear or reverse function when hypernatremia is corrected. Therefore, rapid restoration of water to the body may theoretically cause overexpansion of these cells, resulting in cerebral edema. The following formula is very helpful in calculating the anticipated changes in serum $[Na^+]$ in the hypernatremic patient given intravenous fluids. The rate of correction of serum $[Na^+]$ can be estimated. This formula estimates the amount of change in serum $[Na^+]$ when 1 L of any fluid is administered:

   Serum Na^+ = Fluid $[Na^+]$
   Serum$[Na^+]$ /TBW+ 1

   This formula demonstrates how little the serum $[Na^+]$ changes when normal saline ($[Na^+]$= 154 mEq/L) is given to a hypernatremic patient.[3, 7-9]

Potassium Abnormalities

The normal dietary intake of potassium is approximately 50 to 100 mEq daily and in the absence of hypokalemia, the majority of this is excreted in the urine. Ninety-eight percent of the potassium in the body is located within the IC compartment at a concentration of approximately 150 mEq/L and it is the major cation of IC water. Although the total EC potassium in a 70 kg male would amount approximately to only 63 mEq (4.5 mEq/L × 14 L), this small amount is critical to cardiac and neuromuscular function. In addition, the turnover rate in the EC fluid compartment, may be extremely rapid.

Hyperkalemia

The signs of a significant hyperkalemia are limited to the cardiovascular and gastrointestinal systems. The gastrointestinal symptoms include nausea, vomiting, intermittent intestinal colic and diarrhea. The cardiovascular signs are apparent on the electrocardiogram (ECG) initially, with high, peaked T waves, widened QRS complex and depressed ST segments. Disappearance of T waves, heart block and diastolic cardiac arrest may develop with increasing levels of potassium. Treatment of hyperkalemia consists of immediate measures to reduce the serum potassium level, withholding of exogenous potassium and correction of the underlying cause if possible. Temporary suppression of the myocardial effects of a sudden rapid rise of potassium level can be accomplished by the intravenous administration of 1 g of 10 percent calcium gluconate under ECG monitoring. Serum potassium levels may be transiently decreased by administration of bicarbonate and glucose with insulin (45 mEq $NaHCO_3$ in 1,000 mL/D10% with 20 units regular insulin), which promote cellular uptake of potassium. However, the definitive treatment of hyperkalemia requires the enteral administration of cation exchange resins (Kayexalate) or dialysis.

Hypokalemia

The more common problem in the surgical patient is hypokalemia, which may occur as a result of:

- Excessive renal excretion.
- Movement of potassium into cells.
- Prolonged administration of potassium-free parenteral fluids with continued obligatory renal loss of potassium (20 mEq/day or more).
- Total parenteral hyperalimentation with inadequate potassium replacement.
- Loss in gastrointestinal secretions (persistent vomiting, diarrhea).

Hypokalemia is best dealt by prevention. In the replacement of gastrointestinal fluids, it is safe to replace the upper limits of loss, because an excess is readily handled by the patient with normal renal function. Not more than 40 mEq should be added to a liter of intravenous fluid and the rate of administration should not exceed 40 mEq/h unless the ECG is being monitored. In the absence of specific indications, potassium should not be given to the oliguric patient or to patients during the first 24 hours after severe surgical stress or trauma.[3, 7-9]

Calcium Abnormalities

The majority of the 1,000 to 1,200 g of body calcium in the average-sized adult is found in the bone in the form of phosphate and carbonate. Normal daily intake of calcium is 1 to 3 g. Most of this is excreted via the GIT and 200 mg or less is excreted in the urine daily. The normal serum level is 8.5 to 10.5 mg/dL, about half of which is non-ionized and bound to plasma protein. An additional non-ionized fraction (5%) is bound to other substances in the plasma and interstitial fluid and the remaining 45 percent is the ionized portion that is responsible for neuromuscular stability. Determination of the plasma protein level, therefore, is essential for proper analysis of the serum calcium level.

Hypocalcemia

The symptoms of hypocalcemia, which may be seen when serum levels are below 8 mg/dL, include numbness and tingling of the circumoral region and the tips of the fingers and toes. The signs are of neuromuscular origin and include hyperactive tendon reflexes, positive Chvostek's sign, muscle and abdominal cramps, tetany with carpopedal spasm, convulsions (with severe deficit) and prolongation of the Q-T interval on the ECG. The common causes include acute pancreatitis, massive soft-tissue infections (necrotizing fasciitis), acute and chronic renal failure, pancreatic and small-bowel fistulas. The treatment is directed toward correction of the underlying cause and repletion of the deficit. Acute symptoms may be relieved, by the intravenous administration of calcium gluconate or calcium chloride. Calcium lactate may be given orally, with or without supplemental vitamin D, in the patient requiring prolonged replacement.

Hypercalcemia

The symptoms of hypercalcemia are vague and of gastrointestinal, renal, musculoskeletal and central nervous system origin. The early manifestations of hypercalcemia include easy fatigue, lassitude, weakness of varying degree, anorexia, nausea, vomiting and weight loss. With higher serum calcium levels, lassitude gives way to somnambulism, stupor, and finally, coma. Other symptoms include severe headaches, pain in the back and extremities, thirst, polydipsia and polyuria. The critical level for serum calcium is 15 mg/dL or higher and unless treatment is instituted promptly, the symptoms may rapidly progress to death. The two major causes of hypercalcemia are hyperparathyroidism and cancer with bony metastasis.

A serum calcium concentration of 15 mg/dL or higher requires emergency treatment. Oral or intravenous inorganic phosphates effectively lower serum calcium by inhibiting bone resorption and forming calcium-phosphate complexes that are deposited in soft tissues and bone. If intravenous phosphorus is used, it should be given slowly over a period of approximately 12 hours, once daily for no more than 2 or 3 days. Inorganic phosphates are contraindicated in patients with hyperphosphatemia or renal failure. Intravenous sodium sulfate also lowers serum calcium by increasing urinary excretion of calcium. It is less effective than phosphate salts, however and probably is no more effective than normal saline.[3, 7-9]

ACID-BASE HOMEOSTASIS AND DISORDERS[1,3,7,8]

Pathophysiology

Arterial pH is largely determined by the relative concentrations of bicarbonate HCO_3 and carbon dioxide (CO_2) in the blood. The former is controlled principally by renal conservation or excretion of bicarbonate and hydrogen ion, the latter largely by pulmonary ventilation. Decreased arterial pH is called 'acidemia' and increased arterial pH alkalemia'. The disturbances responsible for these changes are acidosis and alkalosis, respectively and these changes are described as 'metabolic' (not due to an increase or decrease in CO_2) or 'respiratory' (due to primary increase or decrease in CO_2).

Acid-base Buffering Systems

The major acid-base buffering system in the blood involves CO_2 and HCO_3 anion. CO_2, HCO_3 and carbonic acid (H_2CO_3) are interconverted according to the following reaction:

$$H^+ + HCO_3^- \leftrightarrow H_2CO_3 \leftrightarrow CO_2 + H_2O$$

The relationship between the species that define pH is known as the Henderson-Hasselbalch equation:

$$pH = 6.1 + \log \frac{HCO_3^-}{0.0301 \times PaCO_2}$$

Under normal conditions, the balance between these components is tightly controlled. Within 95 percent of confidence limits, the pH of the arterial blood is between 7.35 and 7.43. For $PaCO_2$, the limits are 37 mm Hg and 45 mm Hg. Bicarbonate concentration normally varies between 22 mEq/L and 26 mEq/L. If hydrogen ions are added to the blood, the reaction shifts rightward, with production of CO_2 and water. Normally, the CO_2 so produced is rapidly eliminated by the lungs. The HCO_3 - CO_2 buffering system is the major EC buffer. Other minor EC buffer systems also contribute to stabilization of the pH. After EC buffering occurs, a second IC phase takes place over the next several hours. The main IC buffer systems include hemoglobin, protein, dibasic phosphate and carbonate in bone. The ratio of EC to IC buffering is approximately 1:1 unless the acid load is very large or continues over a long period of time. Contribution by both the EC and IC buffers means that an exogenous acid load (or deficit) has a volume of distribution approximately equal to that of the total body water (50%-60% of ideal body weight). Finally, both HCO_3 and CO_2 act as a 'dynamic' buffering system. For usual buffers, the addition or removal of hydrogen ion, e.g. is countered by corresponding opposite effects of the buffer components. This minimizes pH change at the expense of consumption of some of the buffer components, limiting the maximum buffering capacity. For the HCO_3-CO_2 system, however, physiologic mechanisms greatly increase the buffer capacity. For example, metabolic acidosis can be countered by decreased arterial $PaCO_2$ whereas a respiratory acidosis is countered by increased serum HCO_3. Because the lungs can eliminate a vast amount of CO_2 per day, this serves as a very powerful buffering system. Similarly, the kidneys can eliminate HCO_3 if necessary or can regenerate HCO_3.

Classification of Acid-base Disorders

Acid-base disorders are classified according to whether there is a primary abnormality in plasma HCO_3 concentration, plasma $PaCO_2$ or both (Table 4.4). Abnormal pH due to altered HCO_3 concentration with $PaCO_2$ changes in response to the primary disorder is referred to as either metabolic acidosis or metabolic alkalosis. When the defect in pH is due primarily to altered $PaCO_2$ the condition is referred to as either respiratory acidosis or respiratory alkalosis. A change in HCO_3^- brings about a compensatory change in $PaCO_2$ and a primary change in $PaCO_2$ stimulates a compensatory adjustment in serum HCO_3^-. The compensatory changes may take minutes ($PaCO_2$) or hours to days (HCO_3^-) to reach a steady state.

Metabolic Acidosis

Essentials of diagnosis—as follows:

- Decreased serum HCO_3^- with approximately decreased $PaCO_2$ (simple metabolic acidosis).
- Evidence that low serum HCO_3^- is primary problem (and not due to compensation for hypocapnia).
- May present with peripheral vasodilation; depressed cardiac contractility in severe acidosis; fatigue, weakness, stupor, coma.

It results from an increased intake of acids, an increased generation of acids or an increased loss of HCO_3. The body responds by producing buffers, increasing ventilation (Kussmaul respirations), increasing renal reabsorption and generation of bicarbonate. The kidney will also increase secretion of hydrogen and thus increase urinary excretion of ammonium ions. One of the most common causes of severe metabolic acidosis in surgical patients is lactic acidosis. With shock, lactate is produced as a byproduct of inadequate tissue perfusion. The treatment is to restore perfusion with volume resuscitation rather than to attempt to correct the abnormality with exogenous HCO_3.

Metabolic Alkalosis

Essentials of diagnosis—as follows:

Alkalemia with increased serum (HCO_3).

- Lethargy and confusion progressing to seizures in severe cases.
- Ventricular and supraventricular arrhythmias.
- Altered oxyhemoglobin binding increases $PaCO_2$ and decreases PaO_2.

Metabolic alkalosis consists of the triad of increased [HCO_3^-], increased pH and decreased serum chloride concentration. Because the decline in chloride does not equal the rise in HCO_3, the anion gap always increases.

The principal causes of metabolic alkalosis include:

- Addition of HCO_3 to the plasma
- Loss of hydrogen ion
- Volume depletion
- Chronic use of chloruretic diuretics
- Potassium depletion.

Treatment includes replacement of the volume deficit with isotonic saline and potassium once adequate urine output is ensured.

Respiratory Acidosis

Respiratory acidosis is associated with the retention of CO_2 secondary to decreased alveolar ventilation. The principal causes are narcotics, CNS injury, pleural effusion, pneumonia, mucus plug, pain from abdominal or

Table 4.4: Acidosis – alkalosis

Type of acid-base disorder	Defect	Common causes	$BHCO_3/H_2CO_3 = 20/1$	Compensation
Respiratory acidosis	Retention of CO_2 (decreased alveolar ventilation)	Depression of respiratory center morphine, CNS injury. Pulmonary diseases emphysema, pneumonia	Increase denominator. Ratio less than 20 : 1	
Respiratory alkalosis	Excessive loss of CO_2 (Increased alveolar ventilation)	*Hyperventilation:* Emotional severe pain, assisted ventilation, encephalitis	Decreased denominator. Ratio greater than 20 : 1.	Renal; excretion of bicarbonate, retention of acid salts, decreased ammonia formation
Metabolic acidosis	Retention of fixed acids or loss of base bicarbonate	Diabetes, azotemia, lactic acid accumulation, starvation. Diarrhea, small bowel fistulae.	Decreased numerator. Ratio less than 20 : 1	Pulmonary (rapid); increase rate and depth of breathing; renal (slow); as in respiratory acidosis
Metabolic alkalosis	Loss of fixed acids; Gain of base bicarbonate; Potassium depletion	Vomiting or gastric suction with pyloric obstruction; Excessive intake of bicarbonate; Diuretics	Increased numerator. Ratio greater than 20 : 1	Pulmonary (rapid); Decrease rate and depth of breathing; Rena (slow) as in respiratory alkalosis

thoracic injuries, abdominal distention and ascites. As compensation is primarily renal, it is a delayed response. Treatment is directed at the correction of the underlying cause and at measures to ensure adequate ventilation.

Respiratory Alkalosis

Most cases are acute in nature and secondary to alveolar hyperventilation. Etiologies include pain or anxiety, neurologic disorders, drugs such as salicylates, fever or gram-negative bacteremia, thyrotoxicosis or hypoxemia. Acute hypocapnia can cause an uptake of potassium and phosphate into cells and increased binding of calcium to albumin, leading to symptomatic hypokalemia, hypophosphatemia and hypocalcemia, with subsequent arrhythmias, paresthesias, muscle cramps and seizures. Treatment is directed at the underlying cause, but may also require direct treatment of hyperventilation.

GENERAL PRINCIPLES OF WATER AND ELECTROLYTE THERAPY

Objectives of Therapy

The aims of water and electrolyte therapy are:

- To treat shock.
- To replace electrolyte and water deficits.
- To provide water, electrolytes and nutrients for maintaining the daily needs of the patient.
- To avoid creating new disturbances as a result of the therapy.[1]

Route of Administration

Food and fluids should be given by the oral route (either by mouth or by nasogastric tube). The enteral feeding is the best for the patient and should be started as early as possible. The enteral feeding activates the physiological systems, it facilitates selective absorption of fluid and electrolytes thus the chances of imbalance are less, the fluid is absorbed slowly and excreted and thus the chances of acute increase in preload on the heart and chances of CCF are reduced. The last advantage is more relevant in patients with compromised renal and cardiac function. If this is not possible, intravenous therapy, rather than subcutaneous therapy (hypodermoclysis), should be used.[1]

Rate of Administration

The rate of administration of fluids intravenously can be determined from the following rule.

Drops per minute × drop factor = mL per hour

The drop factor is obtained by dividing 60 by the number of drops that are needed to deliver 1 mL. For example, if 15 drops from an infusion set deliver 1 mL, the drop factor is 60/15 = 4.[1]

Fluid and Electrolyte Therapy[16]

Four general categories of fluid are available for parenteral administration (Table 4.5):

- Red blood cells (RBCs).
- Coagulation replacement products.
- Colloid solutions.
- Crystalloid solutions.

RBCs and coagulation products have excellent volume-expanding capacity.

Colloid Solutions

Colloid solutions are generally administered in a volume equivalent to the volume of blood lost. They are also called plasma expanders as they increase the colloidal osmotic pressure, pull water from interstitial compartment into the intravascular compartment.

Clinically, there are two types of fluids that are used for intravenous drips; crystalloids and colloids. Crystalloids are aqueous solutions of mineral salts or other water-soluble molecules. Colloids

Table 4.5: Solutions used for fluid therapy

Solution	Composition (per 100 mL)	Indications
Lactated Ringer's (Hartman's solution)	Lactic acid 0.24 mL Sodium hydroxide 0.115 g Dilute hydrochloric acid a sufficient quantity Sodium chloride 0.6 g Potassium chloride 0.04 g Calcium chloride 0.027 g Water for injection qs	- To replace body fluids - To buffer acidosis - Shock and other hypoperfusion states
Dextrose and normal saline (DNS)	Dextrose anhydrous 5% w/v Sodium chloride 0.9% w/v Water for injection qs	- To raise total fluid volume - To correct hypoglycemia - Used as a vehicle for administration of drugs
Isotonic saline (normal saline)	Sodium chloride 0.9 g Water for injection qs	- To raise plasma volume, when RBC mass is adequate - To replace body fluid
Isolyte M (maintenance solution with 5% dextrose injection)	Dextrose anhydrous 5.0 g Sodium chloride 91.00 mg Potassium chloride 0.15 g Sodium acetate 0.28 g Sodium metabisulfite 21.0 mg Dibasic potassium phosphate 0.13 g Water for injection qs.	- For IV maintenance therapy
Isolyte G (gastric replacement solution with 5% dextrose injection)	Dextrose anhydrous 5.0 g Sodium chloride 0.37 g Potassium chloride 0.13 g Ammonium chloride 0.37 g Sodium sulfite 15 mg Water for injection qs	- Gastrointestinal/osses (hyperemesis, diarrhea resulting in hypovolemic shock).
Isolyte E (extracellular replacement solution with 5% dextrose injection)	Dextrose amhydrous 5.0 g Sodium a Getate 0.64 g Sodium chloride 0.50 g Potassium chloride 0.075 g Calcium chloride 0.052 g Sodium metabisulfite 0.020 g Magnesium chloride 0.031 g Water for injection qs	- Burns - Fasciitis - Peritonitis
Dextrose 5%	Dextrose anhydrous 5% w/v Water for injection qs	- To raise total volume - To reverse dehydration - To prevent hyperosmolar state - To maintain adequate renal tubular flow (to facilitate water secretion)
Dextrose 10%	Dextrose anhydrous 10% w/v Water for injection qs	- Prevention and correction of hypoglycemia
Dextrose 25%	Dextrose anhydrous 25% w/v Water for injection qs	- Prevention and correction of hypoglycemia
Dextrose 50%	Dextrose anhydrous 50% w/v Water for injection qs	
Mannitol (solution of mannitol in water or normal saline)	Mannitol (inert form of sugar mannose) 20%	- To raise intravascular volume - To reduce interstitial and intracellular edema - To promote osmotic diuresis.
Haemaccel (3.5% infusion solution)	Polymer of gelatin derived Polypeptides 3.5 g Water for injection	- To expand plasma volume (1.5 L blood loss can be replaced with haemaccel)

contain larger insoluble molecules, such as gelatin. The blood itself is a colloid.

Colloids preserve a high colloid osmotic pressure in the blood, while, on the other hand, this parameter is decreased by crystalloids due to hemodilution. However, there is still controversy to the actual difference in efficacy by this difference. Another difference is that crystalloids generally are much cheaper than colloids.

In plasma, the oncotic pressure is only about 0.5 percent of the total osmotic pressure. This may be a small percent but because colloids cannot cross the capillary membrane easily, oncotic pressure is extremely important in transcapillary fluid dynamics.

- **Albumin (5%):** These solutions are chosen when crystalloids fail to sustain plasma volume for more than few minutes due to a low colloidal osmotic pressure. This will be most appropriate when there is an abnormal loss of protein from vascular space, e.g. peritonitis, extensive burns.
- **Albumin (25%):** A colloid solution of 25 percent or 'salt-poor' albumin contains purified albumin at five times the normal concentration. When administered it has the potential to expand the plasma volume by up to 5 times the volume provided. It is selected when the current plasma volume is diminished, but blood pressure is acceptable and the total extra cellular fluid volume is expanded.
- **Dextran 70 (6%):** A colloid solution of 6 percent dextran 70 in normal saline is administered for the same indications as 5 percent albumin.
- **Hetastarch:** Hetastarch (6 G/dL of normal saline) is an alternative to 5 percent albumin for intravascular volume support.

Crystalloid Solutions

Crystalloid solutions are used both to provide maintenance water and electrolytes and for intravascular volume expansion.

- **Normal saline (Isotonic saline):** Osmotic to plasma water sodium concentration, but contains an excess of chloride. It is preferred over lactated Ringer's solution (which contains a hypotonic concentration.

  Normal saline, 0.9 percent NaCl is isotonic and is used when brain injury, hypochloremic metabolic alkalosis or hyponatremia is present.
- **Balanced salt solutions:** Balanced salt solutions (Lactated Ringer's solution/Hartman's solution) are intended to mimic the composition of ECFV. However, the amount of other electrolytes is far less than normal requirements, hence should not be used as a metabolic maintenance fluid.
- **Hypertonic saline:** The rationale for their use is that small volumes will expand plasma volume by osmotic translocation of extracellular and intracellular water. This could minimize storage space requirements at remote sites. However, the very high osmolality (some are more than 900 mOsm/kg H_2O) causes hemolysis at the point of injection.
- **Dextrose (5%):** Five percent dextrose functions as free water, because the dextrose is metabolized. It is iso-osmotic and thus, does not cause hemolysis, which would occur if pure water was injected intravenously, because of rapid movement of water into the RBC interior.

FLUID MANAGEMENT IN VARIOUS SYSTEMIC CONDITION[16-18]

Pediatric Patients

There are a few special considerations relevant to pediatric fluid management in addition to those for the adult. The neonate has limited ability to dilute or concentrate urine and has a high fluid requirement. Thus, neonates should not be without fluid for more than 3 to 4 hours; otherwise, significant dehydration may result.

The pediatric patients are very susceptible to fluid discrepancies and electrolytic imbalance. Whenever possible the enteral route should be used for fluids in pediatric patients. The safe use of IV fluid therapy in children requires accurate prescribing of fluid and careful monitoring.

A calculated dose of desired IV fluid should be administered using pediatric fluid infusion pump to avoid complications.

The fluid requirement for the dehydrated pediatric patients is calculated by Holiday and Segar's formula given as under:

Total fluid replacement per day = Maintenance + Deficit fluids

Deficit is calculated as follows:

- No dehydration = 50 mL/kg
- Some dehydration = 100 mL/kg
- Severe dehydration = 150 mL/kg

Presume the value for the replacement of fluid deficit is 'X'

The Maintenance dose of fluids per day as per the Holiday and Segar's Formula is as under:

- For the first 10 kg of weight of the patient = 100 mL/kg
- Plus the quantity for additional weight from 11 to 20 kg of the patient = 50 mL/kg
- Plus the quantity for additional weight of the patient above 20 kg = 20 mL/kg

For example the maintenance fluids for a patient weighing 24 kg,

- For first 10 kg 100 mL/kg - 1000 mL
- For next 10 kg 50 mL/kg - 500 mL
- For next 4 kg 20 mL/kg - 80 mL

Thus, a patient who weighs 24 kg shall require 1580 mL/24 hours as maintenance fluids, to which the deficit fluids are added to get the whole day's fluid requirement.

Presume the value for the maintenance fluid is 'Y'

Then X + Y = Z becomes the total fluid requirement, per day, for the patient.

Patient with Compromised Cardiac Status

Fluid management of the heart failure patient is directed to maintain the optimal cardiac preload, avoid over administration of sodium, diminish edema and correct common electrolyte abnormalities. Patients with a history of cardiac failure scheduled for major or prolonged surgery should have monitoring instituted preoperatively and an intravascular fluid challenge (i.e. 500–1000 mL of crystalloid/70 kg) performed to identify the optimal preload. Avoid exacerbating tissue edema by frequent monitoring of preload and arterial blood pressure coupled with support of contractility and control of vascular resistance.

These patients have impaired ability to excrete fluids during the fluid mobilization, which occurs postoperatively. The objective in managing fluid postoperatively should be to give as little crystalloid as is consistent with maintaining adequate overall cardiovascular performance. Thus, fluid should be maintained at a low maintenance rate and should include flushing fluid and sodium in that consideration.

Patient with Cerebral Edema

Fluid management of patients with cerebral edema is directed at maintaining cerebral perfusion pressure, avoiding elevations of cerebral venous pressure and hypertension, preventing large changes in plasma osmolality (particularly depression of plasma osmolality) and avoiding hyperglycemia.

Cerebral edema formation is related to capillary pressure, COP, and permeability.

The capillary pressure is between the arterial and venous pressures. Thus, systemic arterial or venous hypertension needs to be prevented. The normal brain capillary bed is essentially impermeable to sodium, mannitol and protein, although water freely crosses. The damaged capillary bed becomes excessively permeable with greatest conductivity to the smallest molecules, thus favoring use of colloid.

Anuric Renal Failure Patient Undergoing Nontransplant Surgery

Fluid management of the anuric renal failure patient for nontransplant surgery should avoid excessive intravascular fluid administration, ECFV expansion and correct (at least not worsen) electrolyte and acid base problems. Attempts should be made to prevent precipitating conditions that would require dialysis during the immediate postoperative period (hyperkalemia, pulmonary edema, metabolic acidosis). Hemodynamics should be closely monitored. If hypovolemia develops, colloid should be used early, one that should avoid producing vascular overexpansion. Likewise, one must avoid interstitial fluid overload, which would require acute postoperative dialysis. Crystalloid replacement of third-space losses should be limited to 1 to 2 mL/kg/h, while blood loss should be replaced with colloid or RBCs. Correction of sodium, potassium and acidosis can be achieved by the use of isotonic fluid without potassium and with reduced amounts of chloride and increased amount of buffer. Initially, an infusion of 30 percent of calculated maintenance fluid rate is important because approximately 70 percent of normal fluid requirements are used in excreting solute via the kidney, a route no longer available. Na, K, pH, HNO_3^-, and glucose should be monitored at regular intervals.

Patient with Adult Respiratory Distress Syndrome

Fluid management of the patient with adult respiratory distress syndrome (ARDS) emphasizes keeping the CVP and pulmonary wedge pressure (PWP) or pulmonary artery occlusion pressure (PAOP) as low as possible, consistent with good ventricular function and maintaining colloid osmotic pressure.

Acute Burn Patient

Fluid management of an acutely burnt patient focuses on restoration of plasma volume and a shift of the ECFV into the burnt but viable tissue, accompanied by increased losses caused by loss of the normal barrier function of the skin. Fluid is mobilized from uninjured tissues by reduced filtration due to compensatory arteriolar vasoconstriction and reduced venous pressure, which diminish capillary pressure and by lymphatic return. The net result is a transfer of fluid from normal tissue into the injured tissue and intravascular hypovolemia. The Parkland formula prescribes fluids based on the percentage of the body surface area burned [% body surface area (BSA) burned] (2 mL/kg)/(% BSA-burned) during the first 8 hours and (2 mL/kg)/(% BSA-burned) during the next 16 hours. The formula prescribes ([0.25 mL/kg]/[% BSA-burned])/h for 8 hours, then ([0.125 mL/kg]/[% BSA-burned])/h for 16 hours, then 5 percent dextrose in water, ([0.8 mL/kg]/[% BSA-burned])/h, plus 5 percent albumin, ([0.015 mL/kg]/[% BSA-burned])/h for 24 hours.

Pregnant Pre-eclamptic Patient

Goals of fluid management of the pregnant pre-eclamptic patient are:

- To restore the contracted intravascular volume.
- To avoid excessive intravascular fluid administration because of normal postpartum fluid mobilization.
- To replace increased sensible (sweat) and insensible (respiratory) losses due to labor.
- To be prepared to replace rapid blood loss.
- To avoid hypotension due to anesthetic induced vasodilation in order to preserve uteroplacental flow.
- To maintain normoglycemia.
- To avoid decreasing the COP further.
- To prevent pulmonary and cerebral edema.

Plasma volume is decreased in pre-eclamptic patients due to elevated lower body venous pressure due to uterine compression, the pressure induced natriuresis seen in hypertension, severe vasoconstriction and hypoproteinemia secondary to proteinuria. After parturition, fluid retained during pregnancy is quickly mobilized and excreted in the normal patient.

PARENTERAL AND ENTERAL NUTRITION

The majority of patients are previously healthy and may be returned to an oral, liquid, blenderized, soft or normal diet in a very short period of time. Although amino acid and lipid solutions are readily available, the condition of an oral and maxillofacial surgery patient rarely warrants the expenses and potential complications. For short-term nutrition, feeding tubes can be easily placed. For long-term nutrition, feeding gastrostomies are less risky than total parenteral nutrition. Total parenteral nutrition is reserved for patients with ineffective gastrointestinal function and not for compromised oral function.

Calories come from three sources carbohydrate, protein and lipid. The yields are 4 Kcal/g and 9 Kcal/g, respectively. Carbohydrate is the most efficient source of calories. In normal circumstances, it is metabolized through the citric acid cycle to CO_2 and water. In anaerobic metabolism (shock), lactic acid accumulates. Small amounts of carbohydrates (100–150 g/dL) ameliorate protein catabolism in starvation by about one-third, termed protein sparing. For peripheral parenteral use, carbohydrate is supplied as dextrose, fructose and invert sugar in 2.5 percent, 5 percent and 10 percent solutions with water or electrolytes. Fructose and invert sugar solutions are significantly more expensive than dextrose and offer no apparent advantage. From, the preceding, it appears that 1 L of 5 percent or 10 percent solution should yield 200 and 400 Kcal respectively. The manufacturers prepare their solutions using hydrated sugars and consequently the yield is 170 and 340 calories, respectively. Five percent alcohol solutions with 5 percent dextrose are also a calorie source. Alcohol yields 7 Kcal/g, or 5.6 Kcal/mL as prepared. For a variety of social reasons, alcohol solutions are not popular for supplying calories, but some clinicians do use them for short-term management of alcohol withdrawal.

Protein represents the building blocks of all tissue. However, the body does not store protein; it is present only as functional tissue. Excess protein not needed for tissue anabolism is metabolized as carbohydrate after deamination. The amino group ends up as urea. Protein metabolism is measured as nitrogen, in which 6.25 g of protein equals 1 g nitrogen. In starvation, 12 to 15 g of nitrogen is lost per day. When intake of nitrogen is less than 5 g/d, body protein is catabolized. A number of amino acid solutions are available. These are supplied in 3 percent, 5 percent, 7 percent, 8.5 percent and 10 percent solutions. The 3 percent and 5 percent solutions are generally used for peripheral intravenous administration. All solutions are expensive. In view of the difficulties, expense and questionable usefulness when administered peripherally, their use in oral and maxillofacial surgery patients.

Lipids are the greatest source of calories per gram. Additionally, lipids add palatability to our diets. Lipids yield 9 Kcal/g by beta oxidation to two carbon fragments, which are then metabolized through the citric acid cycle if carbohydrate is present. In the absence of carbohydrate, the fragments are condensed to acetoacetate and beta-hydroxybutyrate, resulting in ketonuria. Fatty acid emulsions prevent or correct essential fatty acid deficiencies when linoleic acid is provided at 3 percent to 5 percent of total calories. When used, no more than 60 percent of the calories should come from lipid. These solutions are quite expensive and their use in oral and maxillofacial surgery patients seems limited.

A variety of vitamin solutions are available for intravenous administration in both supplemental and therapeutic preparations with or without trace minerals. Most of these do not contain vitamin K. Casual use of vitamin supplements is not without potential risks, as toxic effects of all the fat-soluble vitamins and some of the water-soluble vitamins occurs. Unless signs of vitamin deficiency are present there is no real indication for vitamin supplementation for oral and maxillofacial surgery patients who receive peripheral intravenous therapy for only a short time. Feeding tubes are easily placed and are preferred to intravenous therapy in almost all situations. They should be placed as soon as it is determined that oral intake will be compromised or contraindicated for longer than 24 to 36 hours. The goal is to provide 30 to 35 Kcal/kg/d. The flavored products may also be used by mouth as a complete diet or supplement. Although a blender is all that is needed to prepare tube feedings, the commercial preparations ensure nutritional balance as well as convenience. Liquid diets for tube feeding use casein, soybeans or egg albumin for the protein source Additionally, some use lactose as a carbohydrate and a few are even 'high' in fiber. These compositions may be important in certain patients. For example, lactose intolerance is not uncommon. All of these solutions are hypertonic when used in recommended concentration. It is important to start tube feedings diluted at least 50 percent with water and to gradually increase both the concentration and rate of administration, if no, vomiting and diarrhea may result. Most of the preparations yield between 0.5 and 1 cal/mL when used at recommended strength. Lastly, some of the products are high in sodium content, consideration should be given to patients who are on a sodium restricted diet.[2]

REFERENCES

1. Brensilver JM, Goldberger E. Metabolic acidosis syndromes Hyperkalemia. In: A Primer of Water, Electrolyte and Acid-Base Syndromes. 8th edition New Delhi: Jaypee Brothers Medical Publishers. 1996. pp. 239-49.
2. Davis LF. Fluids, electrolytes, and nutrition in the oral and maxillofacial surgery patient. Oral and Maxillofac Surg Clin of NA. 1992;4(3):720-3.
3. Rosemary A Kozar, Friedrick A Moore. Fluid and electrolyte management of the surgical patient, 6th edition. New York: McGraw-Hill Inc;1994. pp. 61-95.
4. Mengoli LR. Excerpts from the history of postoperative fluid therapy The American Journal of Surgery. 1971;121:311-21.
5. Giannakopoulas Helen, Carrasco Lee, Jason Alabakoff, et al. Fluid and electrolyte management and blood product and usage. Oral and Maxillofac Surg Clin N Am. 2006;18:7-17.
6. Abou-Khalil B, Scalea TM, Trooskin SZ, et al. Hemodynamic responses to

shock in young trauma patients: need for invasive monitoring. Crit Care Med. 1994;22:633-9.

7. Bongard FS, Sue DY. Fluids, electrolytes and acid-base. Current critical care, diagnosis and treatment, 2nd edition. Lange Medical Books: McGraw-Hill; 2002. pp. 14-77.
8. Richard M Langford, Monty C Mythen. Acute life support and critical care: fluid, electrolyte, and acid-base balance and blood transfusion. In: Bailey H, Love McN (Eds). Short practice of surgery. 24th edition. London: Arnold Publishers. 2004. pp. 55-77.
9. Jenkins MT, Giesecke AH, Johnson ER. The postoperative patient and his fluid and electrolyte requirements. Br J Anesth. 1975;47(143):141-50.
10. Dorrington KL. Skin turgor: do we understand the clinical sign? Lancet. 1981. pp. 264-5.
11. McGee S, Abernethy WB, Simel DL. Is the patient hypovolemic? JAMA. 1999 17;281(11):1023-9.
12. Sinert R, Spektor M. Clinical assessment of hypovolemia. Ann Emerg Med. 2005;45(3):327-9.
13. Davis JW, Parks SN, Kaups KL, et al. Admision base deficit predicts transfusion requirements and risk of complications. J Trauma. 1996;41:769-74.
14. Sander-Jensen K, Secher NH, Bie p, et al. Vagal slowing of the heart during haemorrhage: observations from 20 consecutive hypotensive patients. Br Med J (Clin Res Ed). 1986;292: 364-6.
15. Grocott MPW, Mythen MG. Fluid therapy. Baillere's Clinical anaesthesiology. 1991;13:363-81.
16. Tonnesen AS. Anesthesia, 3rd edition. New York: Churchill Livingstone Inc; 1990.pp.1595-616.
17. Salmon JB, Mythen MG. Pharmacology and physiology of colloids, Blood Review. 1993;7:114-20.
18. Vincent JL, Sun Q, Dubois MJ. Clinical trials of immunomodulatory therapies in severe sepsis and septic shock. Clinical Infectious Diseases. 2002;34: 1084-93.

5 Shock

Borle Rajiv M

Although shock is an identified clinical entity for more than hundred years its precise definition has emerged slowly. Elder Gross[1] defined shock as "a rude unhinging of the machinery of the body." It is clear from this definition that it is inaccurate and far from precise. The proper definition is "shock is a clinical condition characterized by a state of hypoperfusion of the tissues secondary to discrepancy between the volume of blood available in vascular reservoir and effective circulating blood volume". The shock may also be defined as "inadequate delivery of oxygen and the nutrients to maintain normal tissue and cellular function". The initial cellular injury due to hypoperfusion is usually reversible, but if the hypoperfusion is severe and prolonged enough it becomes irreversible. The clinical manifestations of the shock are as a result of the sympathetic and neuroadrenergic stress responses, inadequate oxygen delivery and end organ dysfunction. Cannon's observations[2] on the battle field during the World War I led to many contributions to the understanding of the shock. He was first to describe the 'fight or flight response', secondary to elevated levels of the catacholamines in the blood, as a compensatory mechanism.

The state of hypoperfusion can be created by either of the following:

- **Failure of the pump (Heart)**—Cardiogenic shock: Causes—tachyarrhythmias, bradyarrhythmias, cardiomyopathy, conduction disorders, valvular pathologies, congestive cardiac failure (CCF), cardiac tamponade, etc.
- **Loss of fluid (vehicle) hypovolemic shock:** Causes—acute blood loss, loss of fluids due to burns, septicemia, peritonitis, vomiting, diarrhea, crush injuries, etc.
- **Failure of reservoir (loss of peripheral vascular resistance/vasodilatation):** Causes—vasogenic shock, neurogenic shock, endotoxin shock.

In this condition due to vasodilatation the capacity of vascular bed increases, peripheral vascular resistance drops, although the blood volume is normal. The neurogenic shock is a type of vasogenic shock in which the spinal cord injury or spinal anesthesia causes vasodilatation due to loss of sympathetic vascular tone.

HYPOVOLEMIC SHOCK (OLIGEMIC SHOCK)

Hypovolemic shock is the most common type of shock, which results from the loss of circulating blood volume. This may result due to depletion of body fluids due to loss of plasma, (burns, crush injuries), fluids and electrolytes (vomiting, diarrhea, peritonitis, septicemia) or whole blood (acute hemorrhage). It results in a state of hypovolemia. When the whole blood is lost it is called hemorrhagic shock, which is of prime importance to the surgeon.

Hemorrhagic shock is a type of hypovolemic shock, but all the hypovolemic shocks are not necessarily hemorrhagic shocks.

Causes

Traumatic injuries, fractures of the long bones, rupture of viscera, chest injuries, polytrauma, rupture of aneurysm, opening of varices, acute blood loss from peptic ulcer, hemorrhoids, postpartum hemorrhage.

Hemorrhagic Shock

Hemorrhage is defined as an accidental extravasation of blood due to injury or disease of the blood vessel. The blood loss can lead to a stage of hypovolemia and if untreated can lead to a hypovolemic shock secondary to the hemorrhage. Thus, hemorrhagic shock is a type of hypovolemic shock, but all the hypovolemic shock need not be secondary to the hemorrhage. The common cause of severe blood loss are accidental injuries, polytrauma, postpartum hemorrhage, fractures of the long bones, intraperitoneal bleeds secondary to the blunt trauma to the abdomen leading to the visceral injuries such as laceration of liver or spleen, severe, gastrointestinal (GI) bleeding secondary to peptic ulcers, through the verices in cases of cirrhosis of liver, etc. The intraperitoneal bleed is occult in nature and about 2 liters of blood can be lost intraperitoneally. The shaft of femur fracture can lead to sequestration of about 750 mL of blood in the muscle compartment in the vicinity. The scalp lacerations may appear small, but bleed sizably as the scalp vessels do not contract due to presence of dense aponeurosis, which prevents their collapse. Normally in a healthy individual the total blood volume is about 5 to 5.5 liters. When the blood is lost acutely following the trauma the clinical signs of the hypovolemia become evident.

Pathophysiology of Hemorrhagic Shock

Immediately following the trauma due to the sight of blood and pain, the anxiety level is optimum, which leads to secretion of catecholamine in the body and causes vasoconstriction, tachycardia, sweating, breathlessness. Normally, with the blood loss of less than 10 percent there are no gross effects on vital signs (Box 5.1).

However, when the blood loss exceeds 10 percent of total blood volume (TBV) more conspicuous clinical signs and symptoms are apparent. There is restlessness, pallor and perspiration. As the blood volume is depleted tachycardia ensues to maintain adequate blood supply to all the organs. Fall in blood pressure within large vessels results in increase adrenosympathetic activity of autonomic nervous system (ANS) and inhibition of vagal tone. Thus, tachycardia increases further, this is called Marey's reflex. The pulse becomes rapid, low volume and the respiratory rate increases. The selective peripheral vasoconstriction is brought about to maintain adequate blood flow to vital organs like brain, heart and kidneys. Due to the cutaneous vasoconstriction the peripheral blood flow decreases and the venous return also decreases, the skin appears pale and the peripheral veins collapse. The extremities become cold. As a result of hypotension the perfusion pressure falls and the renal perfusion decreases which leads to oligouria (urine output < 20 mL/hour). The body tries to compensate this phenomenon by drawing the extracellular fluid into the intravascular compartment in an attempt to maintain the blood volume. This results into hemodilution, which compromises oxygen carrying capacity of the blood. This phenomenon is facilitated by the fact that the vasoconstriction in the peripheral vessels leads to severe drop in the hydrostatic pressure within the vessels and the drop is so severe that the extracellular fluid migrates into the empty vessels. This complex picture of clinical signs and symptoms is called peripheral circulatory failure[3] (PCF) (Box 5.2).

If the bleeding continues further in excess of 30 percent, the patients become drowsy due to cerebral hypoxia and cyanosed due to tissue hypoxia. The consciousness is lost, the BP falls further and the peripheral pulse becomes extremely rapid and thready and may not be palpable in the peripheral arteries. The metabolism turns anaerobic due to severe hypoxia and results in metabolic acidosis. The body temperature is sub normal and the core temperature falls. The patient become severely pale and when this pallor is super added with cyanosis this is called 'ashen gray pallor'. The respiration is rapid, shallow due to air hunger and the patient may show Cheyne-stokes breathing. This is a picture of hemorrhagic shock. If the blood loss is compensated by fluid resuscitation and blood transfusion and further bleeding is arrested the clinical signs are reversible, this is called reversible hemorrhagic shock. However, the patient can slip into irreversible hemorrhagic shock, if the blood loss continues uninterrupted and is more than 40 percent of TBV, which results into death (Table 5.1).

Box 5.1: Clinical features of the mild blood loss (up to 10%)

Blood loss up to 10%, no gross clinical manifestations apart from
- Tachycardia
- Mild pallor
- Mild hypotension
- Anxiety, tremors

Box 5.2: Clinical features of the mild hemorrhagic shock

Mild shock— loss up to 20%
- Adrenergic constriction
  - Pallor and cool extremities
  - Sweat in hand and feet
  - Patient feels cold and thirsty
    - Tachycardia/hypotension
    - Tachypnea
    - Collapsed peripheral veins oliguria
    - Altered sensorium
    - Peripheral circulatory failure

Compensatory Mechanism

The compensatory mechanism, which occurs after the hemorrhage includes:

- **Adrenergic response:** The loss of circulating intravascular volume results in increased vascular tone, which increases peripheral vascular resistance, resulting in a redistribution of blood flow amongst the organs of the body. The blood flow to those organs that are 'auto regulated' is maintained at the expense of cutaneous, splanchnic and renal bed,

Table 5.1: Clinical features of moderate and severe hemorrhagic shock

Moderate shock (reversible)	Severe shock (irreversible)
• 20–40% blood loss	Loss more than 40%
• Adrenergic constriction—pallor and cool extremities	• Coma/hypoxic encephalopathy
– Sweat in hand and feet	• Severe hypotension
– Patient feels cold and thirsty	• Pulse nonpalpable
• Severe tachycardia/hypotension, peripheral pulse may not be palpable	• Cheyne-Stokes respiration
• Tachypnea	• Deep cyanosis
• Collapsed peripheral veins	• Metabolic acidosis
– Severe oliguria	• Anuria
• Altered sensorium	• Hypothermia
	• Death

which depend upon sympathetic tone for blood flow.

- The increased sympathetic activity increases myocardial contractility, enhances venous return, improves stroke volume and induces tachycardia. The cardiac output increases, the pulmonary circulation improves and so does the myocardial oxygen consumption. The blood pressure is maintained by increase in total peripheral resistance and cardiac output.
- Loss of the circulating intravascular volume decreases capillary hydrostatic pressure. This leads to transcapillary influx of exracellular fluid into the blood vessel as a result of the alteration in sterling forces. This causes expansion of intravascular values and diminished blood viscosity.
- The hemodilution decreases oxygen carrying capacity of the blood. This decreases delivery of oxygen to the tissue, which leads to increased anaerobic metabolism and accumulation of lactic acid. The resultant tissue acidosis produces a rightward shift of oxyhemoglobin dissociation curve, decreasing the affinity of hemoglobin for oxygen, thereby making more oxygen available to tissue. Hypoxia also stimulates respiratory centers leading to hyperventilation and respiratory alkalosis.
- Arteriolar constrictions and loss of circulating volume diminishes renal blood flow. The urinary output decreases as water and sodium are retained. The clearance of urea and acid, as well as buffering capacity are diminished leading to loss of control of acid base balance.
- The change in blood volume leads to marked release of epinephrine and norepinephrine from the adrenal glands early in the course of hemorrhagic shocks. It induces vasoconstriction and tachycardia, resulting in increased cardiac output and blood pressure. Glycogenolysis, lipolysis and skeletal muscles are stimulated and insulin release is inhibited, promoting glucose mobilization, protein catabolism and negative nitrogen balance. It also results into retention of sodium and water in proximal tubules of nephron.
- Adrenocorticotrophin (ACTH) release is stimulated in hemorrhagic shock by decreased blood volume, decreased arterial pressure, pain, hypoxia and hypothermia. Cortisol released by adrenal cortex does not produce feed back inhibition of ACTH release in acute hemorrhagic shock. But the feed back is restored once the blood volume is reexpanded. Cortisol potentiates the action of epinephrine and glucagon on glucose metabolism. Increased cortisol secretion also results in renal sodium and water retention.
- Antidiuretic hormone (ADH) is secreted in response to hypovolemia, which facilitates reabsorption of water in the distal tubule of nephron. ADH is potent vasoconstrictor.
- Activation of renin-angiotensin system occurs in shock in response to increased sympathetic stimulation of juxtaglomerular cells via a beta-adrenergic mechanism, decrease renal perfusion pressure and compositional changes in tubular fluid. Renin liberates angiotesin I from the renal tubules, which is converted to angiotensin II in lungs, which is potent selective vasoconstrictor. It selectively constricts the vasculature of splanchnic organs, kidney and skin. It also stimulates prostaglandin, production and release of aldosteron and ACTH. The aldosteron increases sodium reabsorption in distal nepheron in exchange of potassium and hydrogen ion and represents the principal mechanism by which the kidney may excrete the accumulated by products of anaerobic metabolism and prevent the cellular damage. Prostaglandin particularly PGE2 and kallikreins produced in kidneys increase renal blood flow. The macrophages produce platelet activating factor and the mast cells produce leukotrienes which are potent vasoconstrictor and cardiac depressants.
- During profound acute hemorrhagic shock the transcellular membrane potential difference in skeletal muscle falls from -90 to -60 mV. This produces increased intracellular water and influx of extracellular sodium and chloride and efflux of intracellular potassium, which produces cellular swelling. The decreased production of adenosine triphosphate (ATP) with anaerobic metabolism results in diminish ability to control sodium pump and produces cellular dysfunction. The inflammatory mediators generated in response to injury and hemorrhage like tumor necrosis factor (TNF-alpha), interleukins, platelet activating factor, leukotrienes, thromboxane A2, and complement activation system have been implicated in cellular and hemodynamic dysfunction.

Therapy of Hemorrhagic Shock

Fluid resuscitation

The Ringer lactate solution (balanced salt solution) is the most preferred crystalloid fluid used in shock. It rapidly restores the lost volume and it is safe and economical. When the patient is admitted in emergency room a wide bore needle is inserted into an appropriate vein by venipuncture. If the veins are collapsed, immediate venesection (cut down) is done and a cannula is inserted into the vein, preferably of arm or leg. A catheter is inserted in subclavian vein or jugular vein to measure central veinous pressure (CVP). The Ringer lactate solution is non-sugar, noncolloidal, crystalloid solution with similar concentration of sodium to that of plasma and is suitable in initial stage of fluid replacement. Simultaneously, efforts are made to arrest the bleeding. The infusion is given at a rapid speed so that in 45 minutes about 1,000 to 2,000 mL fluid is given. It is generally observed that BP will return to normal and become steady after infusion of 1 to 2 liters of such fluid.

But it is a transient elevation of BP in view of continued blood loss, hence a blood sample should be sent for blood grouping and cross matching. During massive amount of transfusion, lactate acidosis is feared by some surgeons, however, it is unwarranted as it is rapidly converted into bicarbonate in the liver. The resuscitation should always be started with crystalloid solution even if the blood is available. If the resuscitation is started with cold, banked blood which has more potassium concentration, ensuing hyperkalemia will adversely jeopardize the myocardial contr-actibility. Some clinicians fear the post-resuscitation fluid overload with use of crystalloid solution as it migrates rapidly in the interstitial space to maintain the equilibrium, leading to pulmonary edema; however, effective lymphatic system takes care of it. The use of colloidal substances that remain in the intravascular compartment is advocated by some in place of crystalloid for resuscitation. Administration of fluid preparation which contains colloidal substances like albumin expands intravascular space volume and reduces the resuscitation fluid need to prevent post-resuscitation fluid over load. However, the colloids are costly, may bind to decrease ionized calcium, decrease circulating levels of immunoglobulin, decrease immune response to tetanus toxoid and decrease the levels of serum albumin.[4] More importantly they compromise the extracellular compartment, further which is already compromised in hemorrhagic shock, rather than restoring it. Hydroxyl starch (Hetastarch) and artificial colloid derived from amylopectin, with colloid properties similar to that of albumin, is less expensive than albumin and has longer half life. It is also used in resuscitation.

Hypertonic saline can be effective initial resuscitation solution as it results in lower water load than equivalent resuscitation with balanced salt solution.[5] However, it requires critical monitoring of electrolytes to prevent hypernatremia and hyperosmolar coma. Dextran in 40 kD and 70 kD solutions, is also a colloid which has similar activity as albumin but shorter half life, is used as plasma expander. When the whole blood is not available, blood substitutes like plasma or dextran should be used.[6] When whole blood is available these substances should not be used, before blood transfusion as they may cause difficulty in cross matching and may inhibit clotting system and exacerbate bleeding. These fluids resuscitate the intravascular and interstitial fluid volume rapidly but only quantitatively. For qualitative replacement transfusion of fresh whole blood is indicated. It is better to withhold the transfusion of whole blood until surgical arrest of hemorrhage or at least until just before induction of anesthesia. In case of severe hemorrhage the blood transfusion is started immediately.

To know how much fluid is to be given, blood pressure, pulse rate, urine output, CVP, hematocrit values [hemoglobin, packed cell volume (PCV)] should be monitored.

Adjuvant Therapy

Drugs

Sedatives and analgesics are commonly used in patients with shock to alleviate pain and anxiety. Morphine is used commonly and should be given intravenously as subcutaneous administration in presence of shock will not produce desired results owing to peripheral vasoconstriction. It should be avoided in patients with head injury and in children. In children, barbiturates are preferred. Relief of pain is not mandatory in shock, but if the patient is in severe pain due to fracture, peritonitis, etc. pain control is necessary. Pethidine can be used intramuscularly, but has slight vasodilator effect.

Vasopressors

The use of vasopressors during the shock may increase blood pressure, but at the cost of further increased peripheral resistance and diminished tissue perfusion. Hence, they are seldom used in shock.

Positioning

Most first aid courses teach that the patient in shock should be kept in head low position to improve venous drainage and to maintain cerebral perfusion. However, this position is good in some types of shocks, particularly in neurogenic shock. Its utility in true hypovolemic shock is not established. The patients with multiple trauma often have chest and abdominal injuries and use of Trendelenburg or head low position may interfere with respiratory exchange than those left in supine position. The beneficial effect can be obtained easily by elevating both the legs, while maintaining the head, trunk and arms in supine position.

Mast garment

The on field anti-shock garment (tight trousers) is called MAST garment.[7] With mild pressure applied to extremities, the garment helps in controlling some veinous bleeding. When applied at high pressure, the resultant increase in total peripheral resistance may elevate the systemic pressure, while reducing cardiac output and peripheral perfusion.

Pulmonary support

In hypovolemic shock, the oxygen saturation is usually found to be normal in blood. However, due to hypovolemia the circulatory efficiency is compromised. The oxygen therapy is indicated, if other complicating factors like pneumothorax, pulmonary contusion, aspiration, airway obstruction is present, which may further compound the existing defect in oxygenation due to shock. The patency of airway must be ensured and where ever indicated ventilatory support must be given.

Steroids

In hypovolemic shock adrenocortical depletion was observed, which was supposed to be contributory factor for shock.[8] But subsequent studies have shown that adrenocortical production is stimulated in hypovolemic shock. The use of steroids is indicated in elderly patients, Addison's disease, patients on corticosteroid therapy and postadrenalectomy patients. In trauma patients with hypovolemic shock administration of steroids is not indicated.

Chronotropic agents

These drugs are selectively used in patients with bradycardia. Atropine is most commonly used drug in this group followed by isoproterenol. The latter has an advantage that it increases heart rate and is also vasodilator for systemic arterial and capillary sphincters. The advantages of administering these drugs must be carefully weighed against its disadvantages.

Inotropic drugs

The patients in severe septic, traumatic and cardiogenic shock may require these drugs. The most commonly used drugs in this group are dopamine and dobutamine. These drugs in low dose increase myocardial contractibility and increase renal blood flow by inducing renal vasodilation. They also increase peripheral vascular resistance and should be used carefully in low doses.

Monitoring

Continuous bed side monitoring of circulatory efficacy, including assessment of heart rate, arterial blood pressure, urinary output and peripheral perfusion remains the corner stone of resuscitation. Adequate resuscitation is indicated when adequate cerebral function and renal output is restored. The measurement of CVP is done by passing a catheter in right internal jugular vein. The catheter end is gradually pushed in superior vena cava and the catheter is connected to saline monometer. By the level of saline one can assess the CVP. If the CVP is low, infusion is indicated and if it is more infusion may not be required. A balloon tipped Shwan-Ganz catheter is rarely required in the initial emergency department treatment for hemorrhagic shock. It measures pulmonary artery and pulmonary wedge pressure, thermodilutional cardiac output and allows sampling of blood from pulmonary artery for accurate measurement of blood gases in mixed venous blood.

Electrocardiogram (ECG) in severe hypovolemic shock: ECG will show signs of myocardial ischemia with depression of ST-T segment.

SEPTIC SHOCK

Sepsis, septic syndrome and septic shock define the condition of human response to infection. Although any agent capable of producing infection, including viruses, bacteria, parasites, fungi may generate septic shock, the most common causative organism in this era of antibiotics are gram-negative bacteria and occasionally gram-positive bacteria. The initial infectious process appears to be only stimulus for a series events that may culminate in death, even in absence of infection at the time of death. The gram-negative organisms supplanted gram-positive organisms as the predominant cause of septic shock after the widespread application of antibiotics for gram-positive infections. Despite increasingly powerful gram-negative antibiotics, the incidence of gram-negative sepsis remains very high. Proposed cause for this increasing incidence include a developing reservoir of resistant and virulent organisms, concentration of patients in critical care settings, more extensive operation in elderly and poor risk patients, initial salvage of severely injured and a growing population of patients immunosuppressed by organ transplant protocols, radiotherapy and chemotherapy. The most common source of gram-negative sepsis is genitourinary tract infections secondary to instrumentation of urinary tract. Second most common cause is respiratory tract infections followed by alimentary tract, including biliary system. Prolonged indwelling catheters are major source of infection.

The common organisms, which are concerned with gram-negative shock are *Escherichia coli*, *Klebsiella*, *Aerobacter*, *Proteus*, *Pseudomonas* and *Bacteroides*. Occasionally the septic shock can be seen secondary to the fulminating gram-positive infections.

Predisposing Factors

Extremes of age

- **Primary diseases:** Liver cirrhosis, alcoholism, diabetes mellitus, cardiopulmonary diseases, solid malignancy, hematologic malignancy.
- Immunosuppression
  - Neutropenia, immunosuppressive therapy, corticosteroid therapy, compliment deficiencies.
  - Major surgery, trauma, burns.
  - Invasive procedures.
  - Catheters, intravascular devices, Prosthetic devices, hemodialysis and peritoneal dialysis catheters, endotracheal tubes.
  - Prior antibiotic treatment.
  - Prolonged hospitalization.
  - Other factors—Childbirth, septic abortion, and malnutrition.

Clinical Manifestations

Gram-negative infections usually start with onset of chills and temperature elevation above 38°C (101°F). Two phases are often described:

1. Early warm shock (Box 5.3).
2. Late cold shock (Box 5.4).

Early Warm Shock

Early warm shock is characterized by the cutaneous vasodilatation. The bacterial endotoxins increase the body temperature. To bring the temperature down cutaneous vasodilatation occurs, which decreases peripheral vascular resistance and BP falls, but the cardiac output increases as the left ventricle has less resistance to pump against. Adrenergic response further increases

Box 5.3: Stages of warm shock

Gram-negative sepsis
↓
Stage of red shock (warm shock)
↓
Hypermetabolic state
↓
Heat production
↓
Peripheral vasodilatation for heat loss
↓
Skin appears red, well purfused, veins distended
↓vascular resistance
↑cardiac output
Adrenergic response-further ↑cardiac output
Rapid pulse
BP ↓

Box 5.4: Stages of white shock or cold shock

Circulating toxins cause an intravascular inflammatory response
↓
Damage to capillaries
↓
Exit of fluid from intravascular to extravascular space
↓
Hypovolemia
- Diminished venous return
- Diminished pulmonary circulation
- Shock lung syndrome
- Diminished filling of left heart
- Diminished output
- Hypotension
- Hypoperfusion
- Hypoxia.

Peripheral vasoconstriction and skin becomes cold, pale.

the cardiac output. At this stage the skin appears pink, warm, dry and well perfused. The cutaneous veins remain full. The pulse rate is high and blood pressure is low. The patient may rapidly progress to evidence of altered organ function, most often renal and pulmonary. Unlike most other shocks, the patient who is normovolemic has hypotension in spite an increased cardiac output and reasonable filling pressure. The high cardiac output is often associated with a decrease in oxygen utilization and a narrowed arteriovenous oxygen difference.

Late Cold Shock

In the late cold shock there is increased vascular permeability due to release of toxic products into the circulation. This leads to hypovolemic state, decreased venous return, decreased right heart filling, reduced blood flow in pulmonary bed, decreased left heart filling and so is the cardiac output and the shock results. Early volume replacement frequently increases cardiac output and produces a hyperdynamic circulation, while the patient later in shock is unresponsive to volume replacement and has low cardiac output with increasing metabolic acidosis. Concomitant laboratory investigations show leukocytosis, but leukopenia in immunesuppressed and debilitated patients. Thrombocytopenia may be early indicator of gram-negative sepsis. Mild hypoxia, compensatory hyperventilation, respiratory alkalosis and altered sensorium are seen early in this shock (Box 5.5).

Box 5.5: Stages to septic shock

First stage
Vasogenic component:
- Pooling of large volume of blood in skin due to dilated A-V shunts, reducing the circulating blood volume.

Second stage
Hypovolemic component:
- Generalized leakage of intravascular fluid into the interstitial tissue through the capillary walls, which suffer widespread damage due to bacterial toxins.
  - Subsequently

Deranged cardiac function due to toxins.

Pathophysiology

Septic shock is the result of numerous complex interactions between exogenous and endogenous mediators and host response to these stimuli. As a response to sepsis and bacterial endotoxins many mediators are released in body like interleukin (IL-1 alpha, beta, IL-6, IL-8, IL-11), Cachectin-TNF alpha, TNF beta (tumor necrosis factor), cytokines from macrophages; neutrophils, endothelial cells, prostaglandins, kinins through arachidonic acid and cyclooxygenase pathways particularly PGE2, kallikreins, throboxane-A2, nitric oxide, hormones, etc. This produces a widespread systemic inflammatory response often referred as systemic inflammatory response syndrome (SIRS).[9] It precipitates a series of complex reactions in the body, which results in cellular dysfunction, organ failure, multiple organ failure and death.

Management

The only effective way of reducing mortality in septic shock is prompt diagnosis and treatment. The control of infection by antibiotics and early surgical drainage and debridement is a definitive treatment. USG/CT guided drainage for deep seated infection is indicated. The use of antibiotics based on specific culture and sensitivity tests is desirable.[10] Antibiotic must be selected on basis of suspected organism prior to the sensitivity test and often a combination of antibiotics is used in the beginning, before the sensitivity test. Antibiotics like cephalothin (6 to 8 g/day IV), Gentamycin (5 mg/kg/day), Clindamycin or Chloromycetin, when infection with *Bacteroides* is suspected are the antibiotics to start with.

Correction of pre-existing fluid deficit is essential in septic patients and should proceed rapidly, though carefully, using pulmonary wedge pressure and cardiac output as a guide to target appropriate replacement volumes, so that the detrimental effects of fluid overload can be avoided. Monitoring is essential because fluid replacement is massive in these patients. Resuscitation requirement in excess of 10 L of lactated Ringers solution are common. The use of corticosteroids in the treatment of septic shock was controversial, but after well controlled prospective clinical trials it has been noticed that the use of high doses of corticosteroids did not confer a survival advantage over nonsteroid treated controls. The only indications of steroid treatment are hypoadrenalism and patients taking steroids for immunosuppression and anti-inflammatory action.

Vasoactive Drugs

The vasoactive drugs with only alpha-adrenergic action are of limited value in the treatment of this type of shock. Use of vasoactive drug with mixed alpha and beta-adrenergic receptors may be indicated. Dopamine is initial inotropic drug used. Dopamine has some vasopressor effect at higher doses and that may be required in volume loaded patients with persistent profound hypotension. Augmentation of impaired myocardial performance in septic shock is a reasonable goal. Dobutamine often increases cardiac output with less tachycardia and arrythmias than dopamine. The beta-adrenergic vasodilatation from dobutamine infusion may not be tolerated by these hypotensive patients. Vasodilator drugs have been shown to improve cardiac output and oxygen delivery in normotensive septic patients. Their use in septic shock is limited due to low systemic pressure or decreased cardiac filling pressure. More potent vasopressors despite their obvious detrimental effect on peripheral perfusion, may be transiently unavoidable in patients who have persistent life-threatening hypotension, despite optimal fluid and dopamine infusion. Noradrenaline is a potent alpha receptor and is effective in raising pressure in patients in whom the measures described above have failed. Its use is sometimes preferred over high dose dopamine because the cardiac effects are less. Epinephrine, a potent alpha and beta adrenergic activity, may support the blood pressure, who fail to respond to noradrenaline.

Treatment with steroids,[11] fibronectines and naloxone have been disappointing. Specific immunotherapy with monoclonal IgM antibodies of core lipopolysaccharides[12] have shown to be effective in small group of patients. Monoclonal antibodies[13] to TNF are also available and appear promising in patients with septic shock.

HYPOGLYCEMIC SHOCK

The body tissues require continuous supply of glucose and oxygen to fulfill their metabolic needs. When there is inadequate supply of either of these the metabolism shifts to anaerobic side, there is catabolism and gluconeogenesis to meet the energy needs of the body and metabolic end products of anaerobic metabolism like lactic acid, accumulate in the body, leading to metabolic acidosis. This alternative metabolic pathway is absent in the brain, which depends only on the oxidative phosphorylation, for its metabolic needs. Hence, the brain is very susceptible to hypoxia and hypoglycemia. The deficiency of either of these results in its dysfunction and the patient looses consciousness. The brain requires about 70 mL of blood flow per minute/100 g of brain matter and about 3 to 5 mL of oxygen/min/100 g of brain matter.[14] The glucose requirement is about 5 to 7 mg/min/100 g of brain matter. Any discrepancy in this will lead to its malfunctioning and if it persists for a long, it may lead to irreversible damage or in very severe conditions may lead to death. The normal blood glucose level in the blood is 80 to 120 mg/dL while fasting, and 120 to 140 mg/dL, postprandially. When the blood sugar level drops to less than 50 mg/dL, hypoglycemia results. The children withstand the hypoglycemia a little better and can sustain the falling blood sugar level up to 40 mg/dL. The hypoglycemia is more serious clinical problem than the hyper glycemia, as it may be fatal if not corrected timely.

Causes

The hypoglycemia can occur not only in the patients of diabetes taking oral hypoglycemic or insulin, but it can also happen in nondiabetics, who are starving and are exposed to stress. The chances of the hypoglycemia are more common in the former group.

- Diabetic patient who has taken dose of insulin or oral hypoglycemics, but has missed breakfast or meal. Such patients may land in hypoglycemia, if exposed to stress.
- Strenuous, long procedures in warm, humid environments can precipitate hypoglycemia.
- Starvation—the oral surgical patients, having inflammatory pathologies of jaws (like fracture, pericoronitis, acute infections) are often unable to take adequate diet and are vulnerable to land in hypoglycemia when exposed to stress.
- Postoperative patients who are not supplemented adequately with parenteral therapy taking into account their energy requirements.

Clinical Features

- Mental confusion, giddiness, lack of fine coordination, feeling of weakness.
- Slurred speech, blurring of vision.
- Sweating.
- Fainting, unconsciousness.
- Due to the release of catecolamines, corticosteroids, glucagon the patient will have tachycardia, marginal rise in blood pressure.
- This condition is very dangerous when the patient is in sleep and alteration in level of consciousness may go unnoticed. This can lead to unconciousness, tongue fall and respiratory obstruction.

Prevention

A clinician must evaluate the patient thoroughly. The patients who are diabetic should have adequate control of blood sugar level. They should be given morning appointments so that they had good rest at night and are fresh. Long waiting in crowded, warm waiting rooms adds to anxiety and tends to exhaust the patient. It is important to know whether the patient has taken breakfast or not than the morning dose of insulin or oral hypoglycemic as skipping of breakfast can lead to hypoglycemia. The patient should always be categorized into:

- IDD-insulin dependent diabetics.
- Patients on oral hypoglycemics.
- Patients controlled by diet and exercise.

The first two varieties suggest severe and moderate disease and patients with such disease require more attention.

The patients who have been starving or have skipped their meals should be supplemented with oral glucose, before the clinical procedure. Long sittings should be avoided. The environments should be cool and pleasant and stress should be managed properly.

Management

Management of Hypoglycemia in a Conscious Patient

As soon as the early signs of the hypoglycemia are detected the procedure should be discontinued and patient should be kept in supine position in well aerated environments. The patient should be given oral glucose powder in the form of hypertonic solution. It must be ensured that the patient is conscious failing to which chances of aspiration are high. An ampule of 25 or 50 percent dextrose may be broken and the patient be administered the solution orally. The diabetics who are susceptible to develop hypoglycemia may be asked to keep glucose biscuits with them and eat 2 to 3 biscuits whenever they get feeling of drowsiness.

Management of Hypoglycemia in an Unconscious Patient

In an unconscious patient administration of oral glucose is dangerous as the patient may aspirate. Such patients are given IV dextrose in the form of 25 or 50 percent solution. It may be repeated after some time, if needed. The patients usually recover fast, however, during the period of unconsciousness critical evaluation and monitoring is necessary. Efforts should be made to prevent tongue fall and basic life support (BLS) should be given wherever necessary. Even after the patient has recovered he should be observed for some time to identify and treat any subsequent episode of hypoglycemia.

ANAPHYLACTIC SHOCK

Anaphylaxis is an acute systemic (multisystem) and severe type I hypersensitivity (allergic) reaction in humans and other mammals. The term comes from the Greek words 'ανα', i.e. ana (against) and 'φύλαξις', i.e. phylaxis (protection). Minute amounts of allergens may cause a life-threatening anaphylactic reaction. Anaphylaxis may occur after ingestion, skin contact, injection of an allergen (anaphylactogen) or in some cases, inhalation.

Anaphylactic shock, the most severe type of anaphylaxis, occurs when an allergic response triggers a quick release of large quantities of immunological mediators (histamines, prostaglandins and leukotrienes) from mast cells, leading to systemic vasodilation (associated with a sudden drop in blood pressure) and edema of bronchial mucosa (resulting in bronchoconstriction and difficulty breathing). Anaphylactic shock can lead to death in a matter of minutes, if left untreated.

Anaphylaxis can be typically divided between 'true anaphylaxis' and 'pseudo-anaphylaxis' or an 'anaphylactoid reaction'. The symptoms, treatment and risk of death are identical, but the anaphylaxis is always caused directly by degranulation of mast cells or basophils, i.e. mediated by immunoglobulin E, (IgE) and pseudoanaphylaxis occurs due to all other causes.[15] The distinction is primarily made by those studying mechanisms of allergic reactions.

Causes

Anaphylaxis is a severe, generalized allergic reaction. After an initial exposure 'sensitizing dose' to a substance like bee sting toxin, the person's immune system becomes sensitized to that allergen. On a subsequent exposure to 'shocking dose', an allergic reaction occurs. This reaction is sudden, severe and involves the whole body.

Hives and angioedema (swelling of the lips, eyelids, throat, or tongue) often occur. Angioedema may be severe enough to block the airway. Prolonged anaphylaxis can cause heart arrhythmia.

Common

- **Insect stings:** Most commonly honeybee, Australian native ants, wasps
- **Foods:** Most commonly peanuts, tree nuts, egg, seafood, cows milk, dairy products, seeds
- **Medications:** Most commonly antibiotics, non-steroidal anti-inflammatory drugs
- Unidentified (no cause found).

Less Common

- Physical triggers (e.g. exercise, cold)
- Biological fluids (e.g. transfusions, immunoglobulin, antivenoms, semen)
- Latex
- Tick bites
- **Hormonal changes:** Breastfeeding, menstrual factors
- Dialysis membranes (hemodialysis-associated anaphylaxis)
- Hydatid cyst rupture
- **Aeroallergens:** Domestic/laboratory animals, pollen
- **Food additives:** Monosodium glutamate, metabisulfite, preservatives, colors, natural food chemicals
- Topical medications (e.g. antiseptics).

Allergic reactions to β-lactam antibiotics represent the most frequent cause of drug reactions mediated by immunological mechanisms.[16] The safety profile of cephalosporins is generally good although a wide range of allergic reactions have been caused by β-lactam antibiotics (Fig. 5.1). It is possible to classify these reactions by the Levines classification system, which is based on the time of the onset of the reactions.[17] Some reactions to penicillin and cephalosporin antibiotics are known to be mediated by IgE antibodies. These include anaphylactic and urticarial reactions, while other reactions to β-lactam antibiotics such as serum sickness, hemolytic anemia, maculopapular rashes and Stevens-Johnson syndrome are not IgE mediated.[18] IgE-mediated (immediate onset) reactions are estimated to occur in less than one in 100,000 patients. The frequency of hypersensitivity reactions to cephalosporins is less than to the penicillins. It has been estimated that nearly 75 percent of fatal anaphylactic reactions result from the administration of penicillin. Of all the injectable cephalosporins, ceftriaxone, cefuroxime and oral cefaclor are the most frequently reported ones in allergic reactions.[19] The major antigenic determinant of benzylpenicillin is benzylpenicilloyl, which is formed by the nucleophilic attack on the penicillin molecule by the amino group of proteins found in the plasma or cell membrane.[20]

In penicillin, because of the fusion of a five-member sulfur ring (the thiazolidine ring) to the β-lactam ring, the high tension within the β-lactam ring results in an increased chemical reactivity, while in cephalosporins a six-member sulfur ring (the dihydrothiazine ring) fuses to the β-lactam ring and there is a lower tension in the β-lactam ring for conjugation to carrier protein (Fig. 5.2).

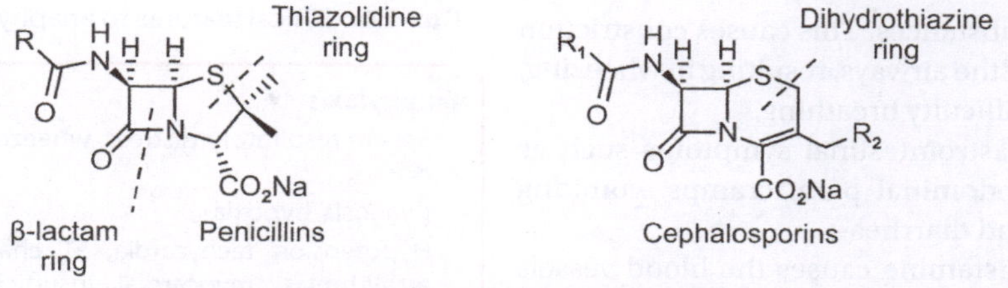

Thiazolidine ring
β-lactam ring
Penicillins
Dihydrothiazine ring
Cephalosporins

Fig. 5.1: Chemical structure of penicillin and cephalosporin

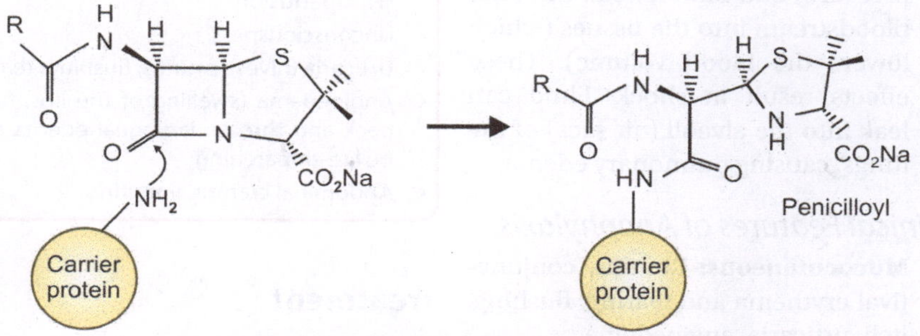

Carrier protein
Penicilloyl

Fig. 5.2: Penicillin conjugation to the carrier protein

Therefore, haptenization of protein by penicillin is quicker and more efficient than by cephalosporin and the conjugate formed by penicillin is more stable.[21]

Some drugs like polymyxin morphine, radiocontrast X-ray dye and others may cause an 'anaphylactoid' reaction (anaphylactic-like reaction). This is usually due to a toxic reaction, rather than the immune system mechanism that occurs with 'true' anaphylaxis. The symptoms, risk for complications without treatment and treatment are the same, however, for both types of reactions. Some vaccinations are also known to cause 'anaphylactoid' reactions. Antitoxins and antivenins may cause similar reactions. In certain individuals, strenuous physical activity can induce anaphylaxis.

Anaphylaxis can occur in response to any allergen (anaphylactogen). Common causes include insect bites or stings, food allergies (peanuts and tree nuts are the most common, (though not the only) and drug allergies. Pollens and other inhaled allergens rarely cause anaphylaxis. In ophthalmology, the dye fluorescein used in some eye exams is a well known trigger. Some people have an anaphylactic reaction with no identifiable cause, in which case the anaphylactic reaction is said to be idiopathic.

Pathophysiology

Classified as a type I hypersensitivity, anaphylaxis is triggered when an antigen binds to IgE antibodies on mast cells based in connective tissue throughout the body, which leads to degranulation of the mast cells (the release of inflammatory mediators).[22]

These immune mediators cause many symptoms, including common symptoms of allergic reactions, such as itching, hives and swelling. Anaphylactic shock is an allergic reaction to an antigen that causes circulatory collapse and suffocation due to bronchial and tracheal swelling.

Different classes of antibodies are produced by B cells to bind and destroy substances that the immune system has identified as potentially dangerous pathogens. Each B cell produces thousands of identical antibodies that can attack a single, small part of a pathogen. In susceptible individuals, antibodies may be produced against innocuous antigens or allergens, such as components of common foods or plants. One class, the IgE antibodies, can trigger anaphylaxis. Production of IgE antibodies may persist for months, even in the complete absence of the allergen. These IgE antibodies associate with a receptor on the surface of mast cells. If the antibody binds to its specific antigen, then the antibody triggers degranulation of the mast cell.

Mast cells become the major effector cells for immediate hypersensitivity and chronic allergic reactions.[23] Mast cells are large cells found in particularly high concentrations in vascularized connective tissues just beneath epithelial surfaces, including the submucosal tissues of the gastrointestinal (GI) and respiratory tracts and the dermis that lies just below the surface of the skin. They contain large granules that store a variety of mediator molecules including the vasoactive amine, histamine. Histamine causes dilation of local blood vessels and smooth-muscle contraction. Other molecules in the mast cell granules include lipid inflammatory mediators such as PG D2 and leukotriene C4 as well as tumor necrosis factor-α (TNF-α), a cytokine. The importance of TNF-α is most noted in the activation of the endothelium. TNF-α, the prototype of the TNF family cytokines, can induce endothelial cells to present E-selectin and ICAM-1, both of which are cell adhesion molecules (CAM) that mediate the 'roll and stick' mechanism of leukocyte extravasation, termed diapedesis. While, this process is essential for the recruit of leukocytes to a localized area during an inflammatory response, it can be catastrophic in cases of systemic infection. Point in case, the presence of said infection in the bloodstream or sepsis, is accompanied by the release of TNF-α by macrophages in liver, spleen and other systemic sites. The systemic release of TNF-α causes vasodilatation, which leads to a loss of blood pressure and increased vascular permeability, leading to a loss of plasma volume and eventually to shock.

TNF-α, along with the other mast cell granule contents become exocytosed upon activation of the mast cell. Activation is achieved only when IgE, bound to the high-affinity Fcε receptors (FcεR1), are cross-linked by multivalent antigen. The FcεR1 is a tetrameric receptor composed of a single α chain, responsible for binding the IgE, associated with a single β chain and a disulfide linked homodimer of γ chains that initiate the cell signal pathway.[24] Cytosolic Ca^{2+} and Phosphokinase C signal the degranulation of the mast cell. Mast cells with bound highly cytokinergic IgE attract other mast cells even in the absence of antigen crosslinking, which explains for the persistence of the allergy to particular allergen.

Pathophysiology of Pseudoanaphylaxis

Pseudoanaphylaxis presents with the same clinical signs and symptoms as true anaphylaxis, but it does not involve IgE antibodies. Instead, mast cell degranulation is triggered either by the activation of the complement system or by a pharmacological reaction on the mast cell's surface.[25] Histamine, which is released in both true IgE-based allergic reactions and in these anaphylactoid reactions, is responsible for the resulting signs and symptoms, which are consequently identical.

The complement system contains three proteins (C3a, C4a, and C5a) that are called anaphylatoxins because of their role in triggering pseudoanaphylaxis. The most common trigger for this mechanism is an intravenous infusion of an iodine-containing radiological contrast medium. The mechanism by which other substances, commonly called histamine liberators, trigger mast cell degranulation, is poorly understood. Some substances are known to be effective liberators in susceptible people, including egg white, strawberries and a variety of medications.

Symptoms

Symptoms of anaphylaxis are related to the action of IgE and other anaphylatoxins, which act to release histamine and other mediator substances from mast cells (degranulation). Histamine induces vasodilation of arterioles and constriction of bronchioles in the lungs, also known as bronchospasm (constriction of the airways).

- Tissues in different parts of the body release histamine and other substances. This causes constriction of the airways, resulting in wheezing, difficulty breathing.
- Gastrointestinal symptoms such as abdominal pain, cramps, vomiting and diarrhea.
- Histamine causes the blood vessels to dilate (which lowers blood pressure) and fluid to leak from the bloodstream into the tissues (which lowers the blood volume). These effects result in shock. Fluid can leak into the alveoli (air sacs) of the lungs, causing pulmonary edema.

Clinical Features of Anaphylaxis

- **Mucocutaneous:** Rhinitis, conjunctival erythema and tearing, flushing, itch, urticaria, angioedema.
- **Abdominal/pelvic:** Nausea, vomiting, abdominal pain, pelvic pain (described as being 'like uterine contractions'), delayed vaginal discharge.
- **Neurological:** Vascular headache (typically described as 'throbbing'), dizziness, collapse (with or without unconsciousness), confusion, incontinence.
- **Respiratory/chest:** Dysphagia and stridor due to upper airway angioedema (laryngeal), throat and/or chest tightness, dyspnea, cough, wheeze, cyanosis.
- **Cardiovascular:** Palpitations, tachycardia, bradycardia (relative or absolute), ECG changes (T and ST changes), hypotension, cardiac arrest (Box 5.6).

Diagnosis

- Diagnosis is based on fulfilling five main clinical criteria
- Sudden onset and rapid progression.
- Life-threatening problem with airway, breathing and circulation.
- Sever-hypoxia and cyanosis.
- Severe hypotension.
- Skin or mucosal changes, for example widespread urticaria/angioedema.

Apart from its clinical features, blood tests for tryptase (released from mast cells) might be useful in diagnosing anaphylaxis.[26]

Box 5.6: Clinical features to anaphylaxis

Anaphylaxis
- Severe respiratory distress, wheeze, stridor
- Cyanosis, hypoxia
- Hypotension tachycardia, ST changes, arrhythmias, myocardial insufficiency, arrest
- Hypoperfusion
- Unconsciousness
- Urticaria (hives), pruritis, flushing, tears
- Angioedema (swelling of the lips, face, neck and throat): laryngeal edema can be life-threatening
- Abdominal cramps, vomiting

Treatment

Box 5.7: Treatment of anaphylactic shock

a. Early identification
b. Basic life support
c. Nasal O_2 8–10 lit/min
d. Inj adrenaline 0.5 to 1 mg (1:10000) SC/IM/IV depending severity
e. Inj hydrocortisone hemisuccinate 100–200 mg IV
f. Inj Soda bicarbonate 1 millimol/kg/min of hypoxia (not to over load)
g. Antihistaminics

Once the patient is reviewed

h. Critical monitoring
i. Maintenance on steroids (dexamethasone)
j. Antihistaminics
k. Nasal O_2 as directed by ABG analysis and clinical condition

Management

Acute Management

Anaphylaxis is a medical emergency that requires immediate treatment. Parenteral epinephrine is the drug of choice, though it is preferred intramuscular or subcutaneous. Intravenous epinephrine (1:10,000 dilution) should be administered only in severe hypotensive shock because of its potential for tachyarrhythmias.

- Place the patient in the supine position (or left lateral position when vomiting is present)

- Resuscitate with intravenous saline (20 mL/kg body weight, repeated up to a total of 50 mL/kg over the first half hour)
- Support the airway and ventilation
- Give supplementary oxygen (8–10 L/min)
- Intramuscular 1:1000 (1 mg/mL) adrenaline at a dose of 0.01 mg/kg (0.01 mL/kg) body weight up to a maximum dose of 0.5 mg (0.5 mL) injected into the lateral thigh (vastus lateralis) has the advantage that it can be given without delay, is absorbed more reliably than injections into other locations or subcutaneously, is anecdotally effective in most cases when given early and avoids the potentially lethal effects of large intravenous bolus injections (Boxes 5.7 and 5.8).

Management of Persistent Airway Tract Obstruction and or Hypotension

If the patient is still unresponsive after the treatments outlined above, there are several further options:

- Persistent bronchospasm may respond to treatment with additional bronchodilators. If intubation is required, continuous puffs of salbutamol through an aerosol port directly into the ventilation circuit may help to 'break' severe bronchospasm.
- Persistent stridor may respond to continuous nebulized adrenaline (5 mg in 5 mL (i.e. five 1 mg ampoules) in addition to parenteral adrenaline. Surgical airway intervention (cricothyrotomy) may be required though not advisable. It serves only purpose of overcoming upper airway obstruction but in view of brochospasm it is not useful.
- Persistent hypotension may be due to either profound vasodilation or cardiac failure. Anecdotally, vasodilation may respond to vasopressors such as metaraminol or vasopressin.[27] In patients who have pre-existing heart failure or are taking β-blockers, a phosphodiesterase inhibitor such as glucagon may be tried.[28]

Box 5.8: Priorities in the management of anaphylactic shock

Emergency management of anaphylaxis
- Stop administration of causative agent (if relevant), assess reaction severity and treat accordingly
- Call for assistance
- Give adrenaline IM (lateral thigh) 0.01 mg/kg (maximum dose 0.5 mg)
- Set-up IV access
- Lay patient flat (elevate legs if tolerated)
- Give high flow oxygen + airway/ventilation support if needed

If hypotensive, also:
- Set-up additional wide-bore IV access (i.e. 14G or 16G in adults) for normal saline infusion
- Give IV normal saline bolus 20 mL/kg over 1–2 mm under pressure
- **If there is inadequate response, an immediate life-threatening situation, or deterioration:**
- Start an IV adrenaline infusion, as per hospital guidelines/protocol

OR

- Repeat IM adrenaline injection every 3–5 mm, as needed

Abbreviations: IM: Intramuscular, IV: Intravenous. Brown SGA. Anaphylaxis: clinical concepts and research priorities. Emerg Med Australias. 2006;18:155-169.

Supportive Therapy

Other supplementary therapy for anaphylaxis includes the use of H_1 and H_2 antihistamines. For example, diphenhydramine, 25 to 50 mg intravenously and ranitidine, 50 mg intravenously or 150 mg orally. Current recommendations are to administer these agents in combination, because H_1 and H_2 blockade is more effective than H_1 blockade alone in preventing symptomatology of anaphylaxis. Inhaled β_2-agonists (e.g. salbutamol) are useful when bronchospasm is present. Corticosteroids (e.g. hydrocortisone in acute emergency and once the patient is stable, methylprednisolone, 125 mg intravenously or prednisone, 50 mg orally; the intravenous route of administration is often used for more severe reactions) may help prevent or minimize second phase reactions. Hypotensive patients should receive intravenous fluid support with crystalloid or colloid and severe cases may require vasopressor agents such as dopamine or high-dilution epinephrine (1:10,000). Individuals who use β-blockers (and possibly angiotensin-converting-enzyme inhibitors, although the evidence is incomplete) may not respond completely to epinephrine, in which case glucagon should be administered at a dose of 5 to 15 μg/min intravenously. Glucagon has inotropic, chronotropic and vasoactive effects that are independent of β-receptors and it also causes endogenous catecholamine release.

Critical Care Monitoring

The time course of anaphylaxis can be classified as 'uniphasic', 'protracted' or 'biphasic'.[29] Although most reactions respond rapidly to treatment and do not recur (uniphasic reactions), an observation period is recommended. This is because, in some patients, symptoms may fail to improve or may worsen as the effect of adrenaline wears off (protracted anaphylaxis) or may return after early resolution (biphasic reaction). No clinical feature consistently identifies patients at risk of a biphasic reaction. Expert consensus is that a reasonable length of observation after symptom resolution is 4 to 6 hours in most patients, with more prolonged observation in those with severe or refractory symptoms and those with reactive airway disease, as most fatalities associated with anaphylaxis occur in these patients.[30]

REFERENCES

1. Gross SG. A System of Surgery: Pathological, Diagnostic, Therapeutic and Operative. Philadelphia, Pa.: Lea and Febiger, 1872..
2. Walter Bradford Cannon. Bodily Changes in Pain, Hunger, Fear and Rage: An Account of Recent Researches into the Function of Emotional Excitement, Appleton, New York, 1915..
3. Dornhorst C. The pathogenesis and management of peripheral circulatory failure. Ann R Coll Surg Engl. 1970; 46(3):172-5..
4. Poole GV, Meredith JW, Pennell T, et al. Comparison of colloids and

crystalloids in resuscitation from hemorrhagic shock. Surg Gynecol Obstet. 1982;154(4):577-86..

5. Chiara O, Segala M. Hypertonic saline solutions in resuscitation in hemorrhagic shock. An experimental study. Minerva Chir. 1997;52(6):753-62..
6. Gruber UF. Volume expansion and flow promotion in shock. Postgrad Med J. 1969;45(526):534-38.
7. Gaffney FA, Thal ER. Hemodynamic effects of medical anti-shock trousers (MAST garment). J Trauma. 1981;21(11): 931-7.
8. Gregory D, Rushing. Effects of Hemorrhagic shock on adrenal response in a rat model. Ann Surg. 2006;243(5):652-6.
9. Alberti C, Brun-Buisson C. Systemic inflammatory response and progression to severe sepsis in critically ill infected patients. Am J Respir Crit Care Med. 2005;171(5):461-8.
10. David Simon. Antibiotic selection for patients with septic shock. Critical Care Clinics-Volume 16, Issue 2 (April 2000), Copyright © 2000 WB Saunders Company.
11. Bone RC, Fisher CJ Jr, Clemmer TP, et al. A controlled clinical trial of high-dose methylprednisolone in the treatment of severe sepsis and septic shock. N Engl J Med. 1987;317:653-8.
12. Fink MP. Adoptive immunotherapy of gram-negative sepsis: use of monoclonal antibodies to lipopolysaccharide. Crit Care Med. 1993;21(2 Suppl):S32-9.
13. Hinds CJ. Monoclonal antibodies in sepsis and septic shock. BMJ. 1992; 304(6820):132-3.
14. Rengachary SS, Ellenbogen RG, Principles of Neurosurgery, (Eds) Edinburgh: Elsevier Mosby, 2005.
15. Limmer D, Mistovich JJ, Krost WS (November 17, 2005). "Anaphylactic and Anaphylactoid Reactions – Prehospital Pathophysiology". EMSResponder.com.
16. Gomez MB, Torres MJ, Mayorga C et al. Immediate allergic reactions to b-lactams: facts and controversies. Curr Opin Allergy Clin Immunol. 2004;4:261-6.
17. Weiss ME, Adkinson NF. β-lactam allergy. In: Mandel GL, Bennett JE, Dolin R (Eds) Principles and Practice of Infectious Diseases. 6th edition Edinburgh:Churchill Livingstone; 2005. pp.318-26.
18. Hoffman DR, Hudson P, Carlyle SJ, et al. Three cases of fatal anaphylaxis to antibiotics in patients with prior histories of allergy to the drug. Ann Allergy. 1989;62:91-3.
19. Romano A, Mayorga C, Torres MJ, et al. Immediate allergic reactions to cephalosporins: cross-reactivity and selective responses. J Allergy Clin Immunol. 2000;106:1177-83.
20. Madaan A, Li JT. Cephalosporin allergy. Immunol Allergy Clin North Am. 2004;24:463-76.
21. Perez-Inestrosa E, Suau R, Montanez MI, et al. Cephalosporin chemical reactivity and its immunological implications. Curr Opin Allergy Clin Immunol. 2005;5:323–30.
22. Murphy, Kenneth (November 27, 2007). Janeway's Immunobiology (7th edition). New York: Garland Science.
23. Kitaura J, Kinoshita T, Matsumoto M, et al. "IgE- and IgE+Ag-mediated mast cell migration in an autocrine/paracrine fashion". Blood. 2005;105(8):3222–9.
24. Paolini R, Jouvin MH, Kinet JP (October 1991). "Phosphorylation and dephosphorylation of the high-affinity receptor for immunoglobulin E immediately after receptor engagement and disengagement". Nature. October 1991;353(6347): 855–8.
25. Joris, Isabelle; Majno, Guido. Cells, tissues, and disease: principles of general pathology. Oxford [Oxfordshire]: Oxford University Press. 2004. pp. 538-9.
26. Schwartz LB. "Diagnostic value of tryptase in anaphylaxis and mastocytosis". Immunology and allergy clinics of North America. 2006;26 (3):451–63.
27. Schummer W, Schummer C, Wippermann J, et al. Anaphylactic shock: is vasopressin the drug of choice? Anesthesiology. 2004;101:1025-7.
28. Zaloga GP, DeLacey W, Holmboe E, et al. Glucagon reversal of hypotension in a case of anaphylactoid shock. Ann Intern Med. 1986;105:65-6.
29. Stark BJ, Sullivan TJ. Biphasic and protracted anaphylaxis. J Allergy Clin Immunol 1986;78(1 Pt 1):76-83.
30. Sampson HA, Munoz-Furlong A, Campbell RL, et al. Second symposium on the definition and management of anaphylaxis: summary report—second National Institute of Allergy and Infectious Disease/Food Allergy and Anaphylaxis Network symposium. J Allergy Clin Immunol. 2006;117:391-7.

6 Medical Emergencies in the Clinical Practice

Borle Rajiv M, Angik Richa

A variety of patients are treated in the clinic for varied ailments and with wide spectrum of procedures with variable degree of invasiveness. All the patients that are treated may not be healthy and may have associated medical conditions which make them prone to develop complications when subjected to stress. No person or no clinic is immune to complications and emergency situations, similarly no clinician can rest assured that an accident will not occur in his clinic or an emergent situation will never crop up with his patient in his carrier. If a clinician says that he/she has never met with complications then there are only two possibilities that either this statement is false or the clinician never treats the patient. The medical emergencies do not occur in the clinic alone, but can occur at any place including home or at any other public place. The patients may have predisposing medical illness or may have a hidden medical disorder which the patient may not be aware of. Such patients have reduced capacity to withstand the increased physical and psychological stress induced by exposure to the surgical procedure. It is therefore imperative to obtain detailed, relevant medical history of the patient to get a forewarning and also perform relevant physical examination to detect the clinical signs of the hidden/unknown medical condition which may predispose the precipitation of the emergent situation. The patients are often ignorant and in the Indian circumstances illiterate also. They do not understand the importance of disclosing the history of medical conditions they suffer from to the surgeon, as they often feel it is irrelevant and unnecessary. Some patients purposefully tend to hide the information about their medical illness for the fear of being advised to undergo some investigations or opinion from the relevant specialist which they feel unnecessary for under going treatment for the present illness. Similarly, some clinicians also tend to be casual towards the history taking and physical examination under the pretex of paucity of time. It has been observed very often in the clinical practice that a patient is asymptomatic and when a blood pressure is recorded or random blood sugar is assessed they turn out to be hypertensive or diabetic. On recollection of the events, they come out with the history of headache, blackouts, giddiness, feeling tiredness after moderate work or feeling of breathlessness, which they kept on ignoring for a long time. They never consult the clinician and remain undiagnosed and untreated for years unless the symptoms are severe or some complication precipitates. Such patients may not have any perceptible problems otherwise, but when an additional stress of surgery is imposed on them the decompensation takes place and complications ensue.

Obtaining history and detecting early clinical signs of underlying medical condition is an art and needs continuous practice. No clinician is immune to these mandatory and important clinical steps at any stage of the carrier and they are required to be carried out religiously as a ritual. The medical history, direct and indirect questions to obtain relevant information, physical examination to know the medical conditions the given patient is having, so that suitable alteration in the surgical/dental treatment plan can be made to minimize the medical complications. In the other words, the famous quotation 'to be forewarned is to be forearmed' is apt and practical.

The average life expectancy has increased due to advancements in the medical science and so has the awareness for health care. Thus, more number of patients from the geriatric age group seek dental treatment. Such patients may have associated illnesses like hypertension, IHD, diabetes as they are more prevalent in the elderly population and as fall out of the modern lifestyle and food habits. The fast lifestyle has created paucity of time and the patient as well as the clinician wants more and more procedures to be done in lesser sittings thus, prolonging the duration of the treatment and increasing the stress associated with long duration of treatment. Certain dental procedures are time consuming and need to be completed in a single sitting. All these factors contribute to increased stress and greater chances of vasovagal episodes and other complications in the dental clinics.

The dental surgeon does not treat a tooth, but he essentially treats a diseased tooth of a living individual. The tooth never walks in the dental clinic, but the person with a diseased tooth seeks the dental treatment. It is therefore imperative to know the individual seeking treatment, thus, 'never treat a stanger'.

PREDISPOSING FACTORS

The medical emergencies can occur more frequently in the patients, who have medical disorders. Usually during the sedentary lifestyle the compensatory mechanisms come into play and due to the physiological compensatory mechanisms the complications do not occur. The stressful conditions such as physical stress, pain, sleepless nights, poor dietary intake and anxiety may impose additional stress and the physiological compensatory mechanisms may not be able to compensate for this additional stress imposed on the body and get exhausted to precipitate a stage of decompensation to produce complications and emergencies which warrant urgent life saving intervention. If not identified in time and left untreated they may lead to life-threatening complications. An average dental clinic may not be well equipped to combat these emergencies nor may the requisite expertise be made available in time. Hence, it is of paramount importance to identify those medical conditions or know the predisposing factors that can lead to catastrophic complications. The preoperative identification of the predisposing condition provides an opportunity to take suitable measures or alteration in the treatment plan to prevent the complications. The medical conditions which can predispose such complications are given in Box 6.1.

Box 6.1: Predisposing factors for medical emergencies

Physiologic conditions
1. Extreme geriatric patients
2. Pregnancy

Pathological conditions
1. CVS disorders
   a. Hypertension
   b. Ischemic heart diseases (angina pectoris, old myocardial infarction)
   c. Patients with previous coronary angioplasty or bypass surgeries
   d. Cardiomyopathies
   e. Disorders of rhythm (sinus bradycardia, ectopic beats, other arrhythmias)
   f. Patients with valvular pathologies and prosthesis
2. Respiratory disorders
   a. Bronchial asthma
   b. Hyper-reactive airway
3. Endocrine disorders
   a. Diabetes
   b. Addison's disease
   c. Thyrotoxicosis and hypothyroidoism
4. Liver disorders
   a. Cirrhosis
   b. Hepatitis
5. Renal disorders—neprotic syndrome, glomerulonephritis, chronic renal failure, azotemia, uremia
6. CNS disorders—epilepsy, cerebrovascular accident
7. Drugs—long-term corticosteroid therapy, antihypertensive, barbiturates, aspirin, oral hypoglycemic, insulin, prolonged therapy with diuretics leading to electrolyte imbalance particularly hypokalemia.
8. Immunosuppressed conditions—HIV, TB, malnourishment, debilitating disorders, cachexia.
9. Psychological disorders—anxiety disorders

CLASSIFICATION OF EMERGENCIES IN CLINIC

The emergencies occurring in the clinic could be mild to severe and life- threatening. They could be further classified as medical emergencies, surgical emergencies and the non-medical emergencies, which could hamper the medical or surgical procedure or complicate the same if no backup mechanism is in place (Box 6.2). The example being power failure and no generator backup in between the surgical procedure. The failure of hand piece or micromotor during the removal of impacted tooth, failure of power saw during the osteotomy could be quiet disturbing if the backup is not available. Explosions due to presence of volatile liquids or gases in the operating room could be of significant concern. The entire medical and dental field has become mechanized and technology dependent and the sophisticated equipment have become a reality in practice thus the aspect of failure of equipment and keeping backup mechanisms has become more significant and relevant.

The common medical emergencies are fainting, bronchospasm, ischemic attack, hypoglycemia to cardiac arrest, etc. which can be fatal if not treated promptly and the surgical emergencies are those which require active surgical intervention failing to which life can be endangered. The example being acute respiratory obstruction secondary to aspiration of foreign body in the larynx or acute laryngeal edema in anaphylactic shock or Ludwig's angina warranting immediate cricothyroidotomy or tracheostomy to maintain patency of airway. Another example being acute hemorrhage requiring surgical intervention to arrest the source of bleeding.

The emergencies can be classified as shown in Box 6.2.

Box 6.2: Classification of medical emergencies

- Medical emergencies
  - Unconciousness
    - Causes—vasodepressor syncope, orthostatic hypotension, Addison's crisis
  - Respiratory distress
    - Causes—bronchospasm, laryngospasm, hyperventilation, anaphylactic shock, Acute pulmonary edema, LVF
  - Altered level of consciousness
    - Causes—hypoglycemic shock, hyperglycemic shock, hypothyroidism, hyperthyroidism, CVA
  - Convulsive disorders
    - Causes—status epilepticus, lidocaine overdose
  - Adverse drug reactions
    - Causes- toxicity, allergic reactions, anaphylactic shock
  - Chest discomfort/pain
- Surgical emergencies
  - Acute bleeding, e.g. rupture of viscera, PPH
  - Aspiration of foreign body in the stomach, larynx, trachea, bronchus
  - Ludwigs angina (laryngeal edema)
  - Acute appendicitis, perforation peritonitis, acute, fulminating cellulitis of limbs)
- Non-medical emergencies
  - Electricity failure
  - Failure of equipment
  - Explosions due to volitile liquids and gases

Table 6.1: Stages of suncope, pathophysiology and clinical signs of syncope

Stage	Causes	Pathophysiological events	Clinical signs
Presyncopal stage or prodroma	Psychogenic stress—fear, anxiety, emotional out break, extreme pain. Physical stress—long upright posture, warm, humid environments	Release of catecholamines and cortisol from adrenal cortex and sympathetic nerves as a result of compensatory mechanism for stress (Fright or flight phenomenon)	• Tachycardia, • Palpitations • Tremors • Flushing • Raised BP, sweating • Palmar sweating • Increased rate of respiration
Syncope	Stimulation of mechanoreceptors (c type afferent vagal fibers in the heart)	• Sympathetic withdrawl • Vagal stimulation • Release of acetyl choline • Slowing of heart • Peripheral vasodilatation • Pooling of blood in veins of extremities and the splanchnic area • Cerebral hypoxia	• Giddiness • Feeling of not well • Nausea, vomiting • Rolling of eyeballs • Fainting • Unconciousness • Bradycardia • Hypotension • Feeble, low volume pulse • Cold clammy skin • Cold sweating

VASOVAGAL SHOCK/ SYNCOPE/VASODEPRESSOR SYNCOPE

Syncope or fainting are the terms which are interchangeably used to designate this benign clinical condition (Table 6.1). It is defined as 'the reversible loss of consciousness secondary to transient cerebral ischemia'.

This is the commonly encountered clinical entity and usually benign and gets reversed fast. The hallmark of this condition is the vagal stimulation leading to vasodilatation, bradycardia and pooling of the blood in the peripheral veins. Diminished venous return, diminished cardiac output and further loss of perfusion pressure lead to diminished blood supply to the brain, cerebral hypoxia and fainting.

The brain is the vital organ which works through out the life even when the person is sleeping the brain functions. Thus, it requires the uninterrupted supply of energy. The brain has only one metabolic pathway, i.e. oxidative phosphorylation.

It means that the brain requires uninterrupted supply of oxygen and glucose for its metabolic activity and without it the functioning of the brain is hampered. If the blood perfusion to the brain is hampered, the brain malfunctions and unconsciousness is precipitated. The brain requires about 70 mL of blood flow per minute/100 g of brain matter and about 3 to 5 mL of oxygen/ min/100 g of brain matter. The glucose requirement is about 5 to 7 mg/min/ 100 g of brain matter. Any discrepancy in this will lead to its malfunctioning and if it persists for a long may lead to irreversible damage or in very severe conditions procedure may lead to death.

The patients seeking dental treatment are often apprehensive and nervous. There is a rampant belief in the population that the dental treatment, especially the extraction of the tooth is very painful. Some people are very apprehensive and some have a phobia of surgical lights, environments of the hospital, sight of blood, needles or surgical equipment and even the smell of the medicaments. On exposure to these things, stress is built up and subsequently vasovagal attack precipitates. Such persons are nervous and to hide their fear, they are often extra talkative or curiously look at the procedures carried out on other patients. Their palms are wet due to palmar sweating when handshake is done with them, such patients need to be identified and counseled before the procedure is started to reduce their anxiety.

Anxiety reduction protocols and premedication with tranquilizers and atropine sulfate (vagolytic) is often beneficial in averting the syncopal episode.

It is usually observed that the children are least prone to have a vasovagal attack as they cry and give way to their emotions. The females also give way to their emotions readily by screaming and thus they have relatively less incidence of the vasovagal attack as compared to the young adult males. The latter group tries to hide their emotions and do not want to express their anxiety and fear due to dominant ego. It builds an emotional stress within them which in turn precipitates a 'fight or flight phenomenon' (release of adrenaline and cortisol) to combat the stress and the reflex vagal stimulation takes place to precipitate the vasovagal attack.[1] The elderly males are matured and have had the experience thus they do not succumb to the stress commonly.

Etiology

Etiology can be divided in two varieties.

1. **Psycogenic:** Fear, anxiety, sight of surgical light, smell of medicaments, sight of blood, sight of surgical instruments, emotional outbreak due to unpleasant news/event, pain, etc.
2. **Non-psycogenic:** Long upright posture, stress, starvation, secondary to acute adrenal insufficiency, etc.

Pathophysiology[2]

Due to any kind of stress on the body there is release of catecholamines and corticosteroids in the body which is manifested clinically as tachycardia, increased myocardial contractibiliy, increased cardiac output, palpitations, flushing, stimulation of sweat glands resulting in sweating, rise in BP, as a compensatory mechanism to combat the stress. This is called 'fight or flight' phenomenon or presyncopal stage. As a result of this stimulation, the vagal afferent C type fibers (mehanoreceptors) situated in the heart are stimulated, which brings about the vagal stimulation (*see* Table 6.1).

Due to the vagal stimulation there is a discharge of acetyl choline in the body which leads to bradycardia, reduced force of contraction, diminished cardiac output and peripheral vasodilatation. Thus, there is expansion in the size of vascular bed and the blood is pooled in dilated peripheral veins, especially that of the leg and splanchnic area. This reduces the venous return, reduces filling of heart chambers during diastole and subsequently the cardiac output also diminishes.

The BP falls due to vasodilatation (loss of peripheral vascular resistance), reduced cardiac output and reduced force of contraction. All these events lead to a discrepancy between effective circulating blood volume and blood available in the vascular reservoir. There is hypotension, fall in perfusion pressure, leading to inadequate tissue perfusion and hypoxia.

The brain is very susceptible to hypoxia and thus patient faints and falls. The flat posture brings the feet and head to same level which improves venous return and improves cerebral blood flow. This brings about improvement in cerebral perfusion, filling of heart chambers and the cardiac output. At the same time the baroreceptors are also stimulated due to hypotension, which leads to abolition of vagal tone, sympathetic stimulation and gradual recovery takes place. The blood pressure improves, bradycardia gets corrected, the perfusion pressure improves and tissue perfusion is restored.

Clinical Presenation

Presyncopal Stage (Aura)[3]

It is characterized restlessness, anxiety, tremors, palpitations, tachycardia, marginal rise in BP, feeling of warmth due to the release of catecholamines in response to stress (fight or flight phenomenon). This is called aura or presyncopal stage.

Syncopal Phase

The stimulation of vagus takes place and the clinical sequence changes. The patient complains of not being well, nausea, and sometimes actually vomits. There is cold sweating, rolling of eyeballs, clenching, jerking and fainting.[4]

There is severe bradycardia, and the pulse volume is very low, that sometimes it is not palpable in peripheral arteries. There is hypotension and the patient looses consciousness due to cerebral hypoxia. The extremities are cold clammy and the patient appears pale. The patient falls down and the pulse improves and gradual recovery takes place.[5]

Management[6]

The vasovagal shock is relatively benign clinical condition. However, may sometimes lead to life-threatening complications like asystole and cardiac arrest. Generally the proper positioning of the patient leads to recovery and no active management may be required. The treatment will ensure a speedy, uneventful recovery. Management of vasovagal syncope is given in Box 6.3.

Box 6.3: Management of vasovagal syncope

a. Stop the procedure
b. Remove instruments—rubber dam, gauze, cotton from oral cavity
c. Position in head-low, feet-up position
d. Lossen tight clothing
e. Aromatic fumes inhalation, mist stimulant or sprinkle cold water on face for reflex stimulation

If no recovery

f. Injection Atropine 0.6 mgIM/IV

If no recovery

g. Look of other causes like hypoglycemia, Addison's crisis (hydrocortisone, dextrose 25%)
h. Start BLS
i. Summon medical help

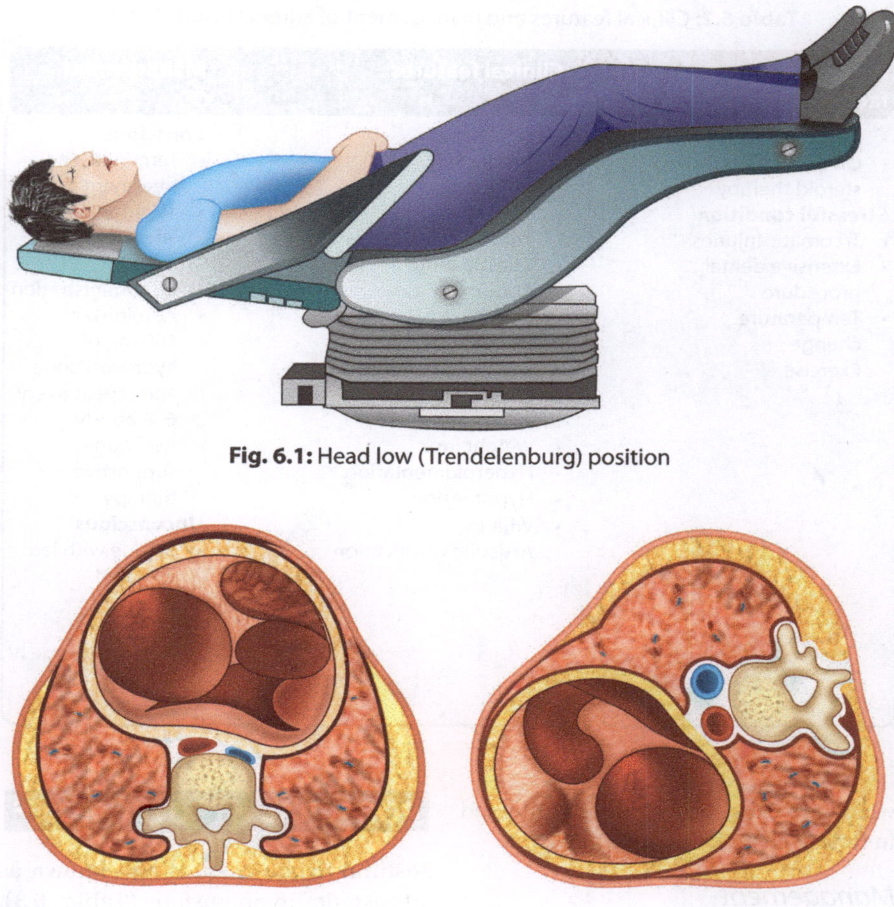

Fig. 6.1: Head low (Trendelenburg) position

Figs 6.2A and B: Compression of the inferior vena cava in supine position: (A) Supine; (B) Lateral

The patient is kept in a head low position, to facilitate venous return to the heart and to ensure gravity assisted blood flow to the brain to correct the cerebral hypoxia. The disadvantage with the head low (Trendelenbrg) position (Fig. 6.1) is that the abdominal viscera presses upon the diaphragm and hampers the respiration by restricting the chest expansion. Hence, rather than putting the patient in a head low position it is desirable to give semirecumbent position (head, chest and abdomen are in one plane as the patient lies in supine position, while the feet are raised to 30° to facilitate the veinous return).

The supine position is not desirable in a pregnant female patient as the gravid uterus will compress the inferior vena cava and obstruct the venous return (Figs 6.2A and B).

Thus, the pregnant females who land into a vasovagal shock are kept in left lateral position with elevation of feet. The reflex medullary stimulation is induced by inhalation of aromatic fumes, asking the patient to swallow liquor of ammonia (mist stimulant), which irritate the nasal and pharyngeal free nerve endings, respectively and induce reflex meduallary stimulation.

Sprinkling of cold water on face stimulates the cutaneous free nerve endings and lead to reflex medullary stimulation. Usually this will help the patient to recover however; if the bradycardia is intense then vagolytic drugs like atropine sulphate (0.6 mg IM or IV) may be injected. Corticosteroids are usually not required but, they are life saving if the vasodepressor syncope is secondary to adrenal insufficiency (*see* Box 6.3). If the patient does not recover with his treatment early then BLS should be started and possibility of other causes should be evaluated.

Vasodepressor Syncope Due to Acute Adrenal Insufficiency[7]

The acute adrenal deficiency or adrenal crisis is a potentially dangerous life-threatening condition. The adrenal glands are the paired glands with two distinctly identifiable structures, a cortex and the medulla. The adrenal cortex secretes about 30 steroid harmones out of which the cortisol, a glucocorticoid is of great importance as it helps the body to adapt to the stressful situations and thus vital for the survival.

Addison[8] (1855) described the clinical signs of adrenal cortical deficiency and it was named after him as Addison's disease, which is an incidious and progressive condition. The incidence of this condition is very low (0.3 to 1, in 100,000) and occurs in both the sexes and at all the sexes including the infants. The clinical features are late to occur and appear only after about 60 to 70 percent of gland is destroyed. During normal life the patient may be asymptomatic, but under the stressful conditions like exposure to the surgery the additional demand of cortisol cannot be met with and the signs and symptoms of acute adrenal deficiency are precipitated. The adrenal gland of a normal adult secretes about 20 mg of cortisol, however in the stressful conditions additional quantities can be secreted. The secretions of the cortex are governed by the hypothalamic-pitutary-adrenocortical axis.[9] In the stressful conditions, this axis is stimulated and the levels of the glucocorticoids are rapidly elevated in the blood.[10]

Predisposing Factors

The patients who can land in an adrenal crisis are:

- Patients with Addison's disease—destruction of the gland due to tumors, infections, hemorrhage, thrombosis

Box 6.4: Rule of TWO

- Patients on 20 mg/day of cortisol therapy
- For two weeks or longer
- Within two years of dental/surgical treatmenta

Box 6.5: Clinical events in adrenal deficiency

- Weakness, fatigue
- Orthostatic hypotension
- Severe hypotension
- Bradycardia
- Loss of conciousness
- Hyperkalemia leading to skeletal muscle paralysis
- Hypoglycemia
- Death occurs due to hypotension and hypoglycemia

Table 6.2: Clinical features and management of adrenal insufficiency

Predisposing factor	Clinical features	Management
• Addison's disease • On exogenous steroid therapy **Stressful condition** • Traumatic injuries • Extensive dental procedure • Temperature change • Exercise	• Weakness • Tiredness • Fatigue • Nausea • Vomiting • Constipating • Abdominal aim • Diarrhea • Salt craving • Postural dizziness • Muscle or joint pain **Sign** • Weight loss • Hyperpigmentation • Hypotension • Vitiligo • Articular calcification	**Conscious** • Terminate the treatment • Position with leg elevated • ABC • O_2 administration • Administer 100 mg of hydrocortisone and repeat every 6–8 hourly • Additional supportive therapy **Unconscious** • Supine with leg elevated • BLS • 100 g hydrocortisone IV or IM • IV access

autoimmune disorders, adrenalectomy for removal of tumors.

- Patients who are on long-term steroid therapy (Rule of TWO—patients on 20 mg/day of cortisol therapy for 2 weeks or longer and within 2 years of dental/surgical treatment) (Box 6.4).
- Sudden withdrawal of the steroid therapy.

The stressful conditions that can precipitate the adrenal crisis in the compromised patients are:

- Surgery
- Anesthesia
- Psychological stress
- Alcohol intoxication
- Hypothermia
- MI
- Acute infarctions
- Hypoglycemia
- Fever
- Asthma

Clinical Features of Adrenal Crisis

The clinical features of the adrenal crisis are similar to that of vasodepressor syncope. The patient becomes dizzy, lethargic, hypotensive and looses consciousness fast. The complications associated with this condition are severe hypotension and severe hypoglycemia, which are usually fatal, if not addressed in time (Box 6.5).

Management

The treatment comprises of (Table 6.2):

- Supine position with feet elevation.
- Basic life support comprising of maintenance of airway, ventilator support, nasal O_2 at the rate of 5 liters/min, establish IV line, circulatory support comprising of inotropic support with dopamine drip (4 mg diluted in 5% dextrose).
- The drug of choice is sodium hydrocortisone hemisuccinate in a dose of 100 to 200 mg IV as it is short acting and the action is prompt. The dose may be repeated if required. Hydrocortisone is a glucocorticoid without any mineralocorticoid action. Dexamethasone in a dose of 8 to 12 mg IV can also be given. It is a long-acting drug and initiation of action is late. Hence, it should not be given in the acute condition, but it can be used for subsequent therapy once the patient has recovered. It has a mineralocorticoid action and thus it is superior in subsequent therapy.[11]

POSTURAL HYPOTENSION[12]

Postural hypotension is also known as orthostatic hypotension (Table 6.3). Postural hypotension is defined as a disorder of autonomic nervous system in which syncope occurs when patient assumes an upright position. It may also be defined as a drop in systolic pressure by 30 mm Hg or greater and 10 mm Hg fall in the diastolic blood pressure. Postural hypotension increases with the age and is relatively uncommon in infants and children. The systolic blood pressure decreases by 2 mm Hg with each inch rise in the level of patients head above heart level and vice versa. There is an immediate drop in 5 to 40 mm Hg of blood pressure when an individual tilts from supine position into upright position. The cardiovascular system brings the pressure to normal in 30 seconds to 1 minute.

Reflex Mechanisms

Various reflex mechanisms are activated to maintain oxygen and glucose supply to brain (Table 6.3).

Table 6.3: Pathophysiology, clinical events and management of postural hypotension

Predisposing factors	Pathophysiology	Clinical manifestation	Management
• Administration or ingestion of drugs • Prolonged convalescence or recumbency • Enadequate postural reflex • Late stage pregnancy • Advanced stage • Venous defects in legs • Recovery from sympathectomy for essential hypertension • Addison's disease • Physical exhaustion or starvation • Chronic postural hypotension (Shy-Drager syndrome)	Failure of the baroreceptor reflex mediated increase in the peripheral vascular resistance in response to postural changes	Prodromal • Pallor • Dizziness • Blurred vision • Nausea • Diaphoresis • Postural hypotension Syncopal • BP low • Heart rate is normal or slightly raised • May exhibit minor convulsions Consiousness return once patient is supine	• Assessment of consciousness • Activation of office emergency system • Supine position • ABC • Administer O_2 • Monitor vitals • Definitive management if delayed recovery • Discharge

Table 6.4: Clinical features and management of hypoglycemia

Predisposing factors	Clinical features	Management
• Diabetics on oral hypoglycemia or insulin who skipping meal or exposed to stress • Starvation • Hot humid stressful conditions	• Feeling of tiredness, fatigue, lethargy • Blurring of vision • Bizarre behavior • Sleepiness • Slurring of speech • Lack of muscle coordination • Sweating—warm, moist skin • Mild tachycardia • Headache • Altered level of consciousness/ unconsciousness • If untreated, coma and death occurs	**Conscious patient** Terminate procedure Hypertonic glucose solution orally Monitor vitals **Unconscious patient** Supine position with elevation of feet Patent airway Nasal O_2 @ 5 lit/min IV dextrose 25% or 50% Monitor vitals Hydrocortisone 100–200 mg IV Injection glucagon 1 mg/kg of body weight

- There is reflex arteriolar contraction mediated by baroreceptors located at carotid sinus and aortic arch increasing the heart rate.
- The arteriolar tone increases and the intrinsic and the sympathetic stimulation causes venous constriction increasing the venous return.
- The reflex increase in respiratory rate and the venous return to right heart via change in intra-abdominal and intrathoracic pressure.
- Release of various neurohormonal substance.

If the cardiovascular system fails to respond to the depressed blood pressure the patient goes into hypotension. Postural hypotension is a result of a failure of the baroreceptor reflex mediated increase in the peripheral vascular resistance in response to positional change. Rapid decrease in blood pressure and no change in the heart rate is pathognomonic for it. The patient does not exhibit any prodromal signs. The patient looses consciousness, when the cerebral blood flow drops below the critical level. Syncope is short lived, once the patient is placed into supine position the blood flow is returned and the conscious regained.

HYPOGLYCEMIA

Glucose is required for the metabolic needs of the body. The energy is derived by oxidation of the glucose in presence of oxygen to meet the metabolic demands. During the homeostasis the excess of glucose is converted in glycogen which is stored in the liver (Table 6.4).

During the stages of starvation this glycogen is mobilized with the help of glucagon and the cortisol. The insulin plays a major role in glucose absorption, its uptake and utilization by the tissue and the conversion into the glycogen. In the conditions of stress and starvation, glucose deficiency is precipitated and the body meets its energy requirements by breakdown of glycogen into glucose (glycogenolysis) or by breakdown of proteins and fats (neoglucogenesis). The process of protein breakdown is referred to as catabolism.[13]

The normal blood glucose level is 80 to 120 mg/dL during fasting and 120 to 140 mg/dL, postprandially. When the blood glucose level falls below 70 mg/dL it is termed as a state of hypoglycemia. The brain is the most susceptible organ to the hypoglycemia as it entirely depends on glucose for its energy requirements for its metabolic functions.[14] The alternative mechanism of energy deriving is not present and thus it gets affected fast and starts malfunctioning. If the blood sugar falls further, the patient faints and becomes unconscious due to the derangement of the functions of the brain. The children tolerate the hypoglycemia better than the adults and the lowered blood sugar levels up to 50 mg/dL are tolerated and hypoglycemia precipitates when the blood sugar level falls below 40 mg/dL.[15]

Predisposing Factors for the Hypoglycemia

Diabetics on Insulin or Oral Hypoglycemic Drug Therapy

If the patient is taking insulin or the drugs like biguanides or sulfonylurea derivatives, it is necessary to keep nice balance between glucose intake and the drugs. As the drugs are important the glucose intake in the controlled manner is equally important. If such patient takes the drugs and misses the breakfast or a meal the chances of precipitating hypoglycemia are high. Similarly during a non-stressful condition the balance between the action of the drug and dietary intake is maintained and the hypoglycemia does not precipitate. But, if such a patient is exposed to the stress and the glucose requirement increases for deriving more energy owing to increased metabolic needs, the increased needs may not be met with and the hypoglycemia precipitates. Secondly, the glucose uptake and the utilization is also defective in the diabetics and thus they are the potent candidates for hypoglycemia in stressful conditions.

Starvation

Even the non-diabetics who are starving fail to comply with the increased stress on the body and are likely to land in hypoglycemia. The inflammatory conditions of the jaws like pericoronitis, fracture, painful ulcers hamper the dietary intake. The patient is also stressed out due to pain and sleepless nights and if such patients are taken for performing dental/surgical procedures without proper evaluation and treatment are most likely to land in hypoglycemic attack. Hence, it is important to understand that not only the diabetics, but also the non-diabetics who are starving are liable to land in hypoglycemia if due care is not taken.[16]

Clinical Features

Hypoglycemia is a more dangerous complication than the hyperglycemia as in the latter case plenty of time is available to treat it and does not result in mortality instantly. Hypoglycemia could be fatal if not treated promptly.[17]

As the patient becomes comatose apart from the damage to the brain the other complications secondary to unconsciousness' such as tongue fall, aspiration may occur which could be fatal (*see* Box 6.5). The hypoglycemia during the sleep is often considered more dangerous the patient is sleeping as when its detection could be very difficult. Thus, while treating the diabetic patients with insulin or oral hypoglycemic the night dose is often less and the patient is counseled for proper dietary regime (Box 6.6).

As the hypoglycemia is more serious complication its timely identification and treatment are of paramount importance. As the prevention is the best treatment the clinician must evaluate the patient properly and identify the subjects who are likely to land in hypoglycemia and take proper precautions to avoid it.

Box 6.6: Clinical features of hypoglycemia

1. Feeling of tiredness, fatigue, lethargy
2. Blurring of vision
3. Bizarre behavior
4. Sleepiness
5. Slurring of speech
6. Lack of muscle coordination
7. Sweating—warm, moist skin
8. Mild tachycardia
9. Headache
10. Altered level of consciousness/unconsciousness
11. If untreated, coma and death occurs.

The detailed medical history, drug history, dietary habits and status, recent episodes of jaw pain which could affect dietary intake, sleepless night, and hot humid environments must be taken into account. In presence of the positive history, suitable alteration in the treatment plan should be done to prevent hypoglycemia.[18]

- Before taking up a patient for dental treatment one must ensure that the patient has had his meal or breakfast. If the patient has missed morning dose of oral hypoglycemic, it would not matter a marginal hyperglycemia is always acceptable than the hypoglycemia.
- If the patient is to be operated under GA and is kept fasting for 5 to 6 hours prior to the surgery, intravenous dextrose should be infused to prevent hypoglycemia.
- The diabetic patients should be given preferably morning appointments so that they had a good sleep in the night and have properly rested and not stressed.
- The long waiting in the waiting room should be avoided.
- The environments should not be hot and humid.

Treatment of Hypoglycemia

Once the hypoglycemic episode is identified it requires a prompt treatment.

Treatment in a Conscious Patient

- Stop the procedure.
- Put the patient in a supine position.
- The environments should not be crowded and poorly ventilated.
- Administer hypertonic glucose solution orally (70–100 g in 50–100 mL water).
- Monitor the level of consciousness and the vital signs.

The patient usually recovers fast. Additional therapy with IV dextrose (25%) infusion or steroid administration is not required in a conscious patient if the hypoglycemia is diagnosed early.[19]

Treatment in an Unconscious Patient

- Place in supine position with feet slightly elevated.
- Maintain patency of airway.
- Establish IV line.
- IV infusion of 1 to 2 ampules of 25 percent dextrose. The first ampule is administered fast. In very severe cases, 50 percent dextrose infusion is administered, which can be repeated depending of recovery of the patient.
- **Glucagon:** It can be given in a dose of 1 mg/kg of body weight, via IM or IV route. The glucagon raises the blood sugar level by breakdown of glycogen in the liver. The response to the glucagon is variable and the onset of action takes place in 10 to 20 minutes with peak action occurring in 45 to 60 minutes.
- Epinephrine can also be given if glucagon or 50 percent dextrose is not available. The epinephrine is given in a dose of 0.5 mg or 1 ampule of 1:1,000 strength and is administered by subcutaneous or IM route. The epinephrine raises the blood glucose levels, but it is not recommended to be used in hypertensive and patients with CVS disorders (*see* Table 6.4).
- Monitor vital parameters.
- Basic life support.
- Prevention of the tongue fall and aspiration.
- IV injection of dexamethasone 4 to 8 mg.

The blood sugar monitoring is done periodically to prevent the recurrence of the condition and the patient is monitored periodically.

HYPERGLYCEMIA

The blood glucose gets elevated after a meal. It remains elevated for 2 to 3 hours later and is slowly reduced by renal excretion or by conversion into the glycogen and uptake by the tissue due to the action of insulin. The blood glucose level remains elevated in the diabetic patients for a longer period either due lack of insulin (type I diabetes) or due to improper uptake of the glucose by the tissue like muscles and adepose tissue (type II diabetes).

The glucose is also produced by glucogenolysis in the liver. The appearance level of the glucose in the urine is called glycosuria. The glycosuria occurs when the blood glucose goes above the renal threshold of 180 mg/dL. The glycosuria could be due to increase in blood sugar level after high carbohydrate meals (alimentary glycosuria), due to renal pathology (renal glycosuria) or sometimes during pregnancy (pregnancy glycosuria). The blood glucose in the diabetics is high and is the cause of persistent glycosuria. The excretion of the glucose in the urine increases osmotic pressure of urine due to its large molecular size and draws water resulting in increased quantity of the urine (polyurea).

The sodium and potassium are also drawn and excreted along with the water. The presence of the ketone bodies promote secretion of the sodium and potassium in urine in the distal tubules to cause further wasting of electrolytes resulting in electrolyte imbalance.

The state of dehydration is produced which results in excessive thirst (polydipsia). The inability of the body tissue to uptake the glucose, mobilization of glycogen and triglycerides, depilation of the muscle mass as the aminoacids are broken down to produce glucose and ketone bodies along with the loss of water contribute to weight loss and increased appetite leading to polyphagia (Box 6.7).

In absence of insulin, the breakdown of glycogen into glucose (glycogenolysis), conversion of proteins into glucose in the liver (gluconeogenesis) takes place. The triglycerides are converted into free fatty acids in the liver which are taken up by the muscle to derive energy and ketone bodies are generated as metabolic end products which provide the breath a typical fruity and sweet odor. This stage is called diabetic ketosis.[20]

Box 6.7: Clinical features of hyperglycemia

- Hyperglycemia (bl glucose > 250 mg/dL)
- Dehydration dry, warm skin, loss of turgor, wrinkling of the tongue
- Fruity, sweet odor to breath
- Kussumaul's respiration
- Tachycardia–thready, weak pulse
- Normal or low blood pressure
- Altered level of consciousness.

If the insulin deficiency is severe the the gluconeogenesis and ketogenosis continue to occur regardless of the blood glucose levels. The utilization of the ketones may not keep pace with its production and the ketones (acetoacetate and beta hydroxybutirate) accumulate in the blood, decreasing its pH and this condition is called diabetic ketoacidosis. The ketones decrease the myocardial contractibility and the response of the arterioles to the catecholamines. The excess of ketone is excreted in the urine (ketonuria).

The ketoacidosis affects the respiration and the respiratory rate increases. The hyperventilation is an attempt by the body to counter the metabolic acidosis with respiratory alkalosis. The typical deep and gasping type of respiration which has variable rate is called kussmaul breathing respiration. The loss of respiratory efficiency leads to loss of consciousness and diabetic coma is precipitated. The very high blood sugar level tend to dehydrate the tissue including the brain.

Etiology of Diabetic Coma

The most common causes for diabetic coma[21] are:

- Severe insulin deficiency.
- Moderate insulin deficiency (hyperglycemic non-ketotic hyperosmolar coma).
- Poor patient adherence to treatment regimen, diet control.
- Alcoholism.
- Severe infections.

Clinical Feature

The Clinical features of hyperglycemia is listed in Box 6.7.

Management

The patient with the presence of clinical signs and symptoms is considered as ASA IV category risk for dental/surgical treatment. Hence, the consultation of the physician is necessary. However, if a patient is detected with hyperglycemia and ketosis in the dental clinic the following treatment may be started:

- Terminate the procedure and remove dental material, instruments from the mouth.
- Put the patient in a supine position with the legs slightly raised.
- BLS to be started.
- Summon medical help.
- Establish IV line and start IV infusion with isotonic saline to keep the IV line patent.
- Administer nasal oxygen through a face mask at the rate of 5 lit/min.
- Shift the patient to medicine emergency.
- Insulin needs to be administered, but has to be administered carefully and only by the competent person where proper monitoring facilities are available. Normally crystalline insulin is administered for rapid action in place of depot insulin. The dose of insulin varies depending on the blood sugar levels. Care must be taken to prevent hypoglycemia as the latter is more dangerous. The hydration of the patients is maintained towards the higher side to flush out the ketone bodies by administrating high quantity of IV fluids taking into account the renal efficiency so as to prevent cardiac overloading and congestive failure. The IV fluids with dextrose are avoided.[22]
- The treatment in a comatose patient is similar except that it should be provided promptly and the life saving support as indicated be provided timely and promptly.

RESPIRATORY TRACT EMERGENCIES

Bronchospasm

The entire tracheobroncheal tree contains smooth muscles which are controlled by the autonomous nervous system. The parasympathetic (vagal) stimulation (release of acetylcholine) brings about the contraction and the adrenergic (release of catecholamines) stimulation produces dilatation. In non-asthamatic patients, the constriction of the smooth muscle protects the lungs by contracting and preventing the aspiration when stimulated by foreign body. However, in an asthamatic patient the response is exaggerated producing the clinical signs of respiratory distress. The bronchoconstriction is more pronounced in small bronchi and bronchioles 0.4 to 0.1 µm in diameter. The inflammation of the airway and edema and the secretions in an asthamatic patient also contribute to narrowing of the bronchial lumen and airway obstruction.

The bronchoconstriction (spasm) can be induced by drugs like aspirin through the activation of cyclo-oxygenase pathway by release of vasoactive amines. Severe allergic reactions to the drugs can also lead to bronchospasm.

The other causes which precipitate the asthamatic (bronchospasm) attack are:

- Allergy to inhaled pollen, fungal spores, drugs like penicillin, vaccines, aspirin, sulfites used as preservative in local anesthetic solution. It is usually a type I hypersensitivity reaction mediated through the IgE antibodies.
- Lower respiratory tract infections.
- Physical exertion.
- Psychological stress.
- Climatic conditions (cold).

Clinical Features

- Feeling of tightness in the chest/ suffocation.
- **Cough:** Dry or productive.
- Dyspnea.
- Audible wheezing on inspiration and expiration.
- Auscultatory rhonchi both inspiratory and expiratory (prolonged).
- Patient prefers to sit or stand up as the breathlessness gets worse in lying position.
- Use of accessory muscle of respiration like intercostals, sternomastoid, abdominal, neck and truncle muscles.
- Supraclavicular, intercostal retraction and nasal flaring.
- Apprehensive and anxious.
- Rapid shallow respiration (40/min).
- Raised BP.
- Tachycardia.
- Diaphoresis.
- Agitation.
- Confusion.
- Cyanosis.

Prevention

- History of asthma, hyper-reactive airway disorders.
- History of allergic tendencies.
- History of drug therapy.
- Avoid local anesthesia solution containing epinephrine (as sulfites are added to prevent oxidation of epinephrine) in susceptible patients.
- Avoid drugs like aspirin, diclofenac sodium, ibuprofen, valdecoxib, mefenamic acid, piroxicam, ketoprofen, rofecoxib, etc. (NSAIDS) in the asthematic patients and patients having allergic tendencies.
- Avoid physical and psychological stress.
- Perform cutaneous sensitivity test before injecting drugs in susceptible patients.

Management

- Terminate dental procedure and remove all materials and instruments from the mouth.
- Keep the patent in the upright position in a well-ventilated environment and loosen all tight clothing.
- Calm down the patient as anxiety can further complicate the things.
- Basic life support
- Administration of O_2 through face mask, nasal hood or nasal catheter at the rate of 5 to 7 L/min. The presence of hypoxia, hypercarbia and cyanosis are indications for oxygen administration. In view of bronchospasm little air enters the zone of pulmonary ventilation, but it must be ensured that whatever small quantity of air is reaching the lungs should be saturated with oxygen.

- Administration of bronchodilator (in case of mild bronchospasm)
  - Through the aerosol inhaler or nebulizers the bronchodilator drugs like β-2 adrenergic agonists (epinephrine, albuterol, isoproterenol drugs) these drugs also have alfa agonistic action and hence should be used judiciously in patients with HT, diabetes, IHD, thyrotoxicosis.
  - In severe bronchospasm apart from the aerosol bronchodilators the drugs are required to be administered intravenously for prompt relief as this is more serious condition.

    The drugs like deriphyllin (theophylline and etofylline) can be given by intravenous or intramuscular routes. It can be given in mild to moderate cases of bronchospasm or as a follow up therapy after the acute phase is managed.

    Injection of aminophylline in a dose of 250 mg, diluted in 20 to 50 mL of 5 percent dextrose by slow intravenous route can be given. Aminophylline has beta agonist action which is not selective and thus it also stimulates the beta receptors in the heart and can produce arrhythmias. To prevent the same, the drug is always given in a diluted form and slowly. Due monitoring of the pulse and heart rhythm is necessary during administration of aminophylline. It can be given as a slow infusion, diluted in one pint of 5 percent dextrose as a follow-up therapy after the acute stage is over to prevent relapse of bronchospasm.

    Epinephrine is the most potent bronchodilator and is the drug of choice in very severe and life threatening bronchospasm. Epinephrine 1:1,000 is administered (0.5 mg), subcutaneously or 1:10,000 (0.5 mg) is administered IV. Epinephrine 1:1,000 should not be administered IV. Due monitoring of BP, heart rate and rhythm is warranted.
  - Other drugs like hydrocortisone sodium succinate can be given in a dose of 100 to 200 mg IV. It helps in reducing the airway edema, suppress antigen antibody reaction and also protects the tissue against the adverse effects of hypoxia to certain extent.
  - Sedatives which can depress the respiration should not be given.
  - The patients should be kept under follow-up to detect and treat any recurrent episode of brochospasm. The follow up therapy with aerosol sprays, oral or parenteral broncodilators like deriphyllin and steroids are prescribed.

Status Asthmaticus

The staus asthmaticus is the most severe clinical form of the asthma and if not treated promptly may be fatal. The patient experiences wheezing, dyspnea, hypoxia and other signs and symptoms which do not respond to the routine 2 to 3 doses of the beta adrenergic drugs. It represents true and severe medical emergency which could be fatal due to severe respiratory distress, hypotension, severe hypoxia, hypercapnea and acidosis.

The management is similar to that of acute, severe bronchospasm, but needs to be given promptly and aggressively.

Hyperventilation

The hyperventilation is defined as the ventilation in excess of that is required to maintain normal PaO_2 (arterial O_2 tension) and PCO_2 (arterial CO_2 tension). It is produced either by increase in frequency or depth of respiration or both.

Majority of the cases of hyperventilation are due to extreme anxiety however organic conditions like pain, metabolic acidosis, cirrhosis, hypercapnia, drug intoxication and central nervous disorders can also cause it.

The hyperventilation secondary to the anxiety is usually seen in the patients who do not give way to their emotions and attempt to tough it out.

Clinical Features

- It is usually precipitated by anxiety and fear at the site of injection, instruments (Table 6.5).
- The patient complains of tightness of chest and suffocation and is unaware that he is overbreathing.
- Palpitations, tachycardia, chest pain. The later could be difficult to differentiate from the angina attack and thus, ECG may be useful.
- Dizziness, light headedness, visual abrasions, numbness or tingling of the finger tips and rarely tetany (carpopedal spasm). These signs are due to the fact that the PCO_2 decreases from normal level of 35 to 40 torr to less than 35 torr and the pH of the blood increases to 7.55 from normal of 7.3 to 7.4, as a result of hyperventilation. The changes are referred to as hypocapnia or hypocarbia and respiratory alkalosis. These changes bring about the cerebral vasoconstriction which could explain the light headedness, dizziness, giddiness and blurring of vision.
- Globus hystericus (feeling of foreign body in the throat), epigastric discomfort.
- Muscle pain/cramps, tremor, stiffness, rarely carpopedal tetany. As the pH of the blood increases to 7.5, the ionic calcium in the blood decreases although the total calcium remains normal. The decrease in the ionic calcium results in the neuromuscular irritability and excitability resulting into tingling, spasm, cramps, numbness of hands and perioral region, carpopedal spasm.

Management

- Prevention by identifying the anxious patients and alleviating the anxiety by counseling and premedication.
- Terminate dental procedure and remove all the material from the mouth.
- BLS
- Calm down the patient by reassurance or drugs like diazepam 5 to 10 mg or midazolam 3 to 5 mg by IM or IV route.

Table 6.5: Clinical features, precipitating factors and management of hyperventilation

Etiology	Clinical features	Pathophysiology	Management
• Extreme anxiety • Pain • Metabolic acidosis • Drug intoxication • Hypercapnea • Cirrhosis • Central nervous system disorder	*CVS* • Palpitation. Tachycardia • Precordial pain *Neurologic* • Dizziness • Light headedness • Disturbance of consciousness • Disturbance of alteration • Numbness and tingling of extremeties • Tetany (rare) *Respiratory* • Shortness of breath • Dryness of mouth *Git* • Globus hystericus • Epigastric pain *Musculoskeletal pain* • Muscle pain • Cramps • Tremor • Stiffness • Carpopedal tetany *Psychological* • Tension • Anxiety • Nightmare	• Increased rate and depth of respiration decreases the CO_2 level leading to respiratory alkalosis causing vasoconstriction of the cerebral vessels and thus ischemia • Catecholamine release due to stress • Alkalosis resulting in decreased ionic calcium ions	• Terminate procedure • Position—comfortable in sitting position • ABC • Remove foreign body and tight bindings • Calm the patient • Correct alkalosis Gaseous mixture of 7% CO_2 and 93% O_2. Patient asked to breathe in full face mask to breathe in and out CO_2 enriched exhaled reservoir • Drug management if necessary Diazepam (10–15 mg orally), midazolam • Subsequent dental treatment • Discharge

- Ask the patient to hold hands in front of nose and mouth like a mask and breathe the exhaled CO_2 rich exhaled air in and out. The face mask or hood can be used to cover the nose and mouth to recirculate the exhaled air in and out during breathing.
- The patient usually recovers with time, calming down and rest.

HYPOTHYROIDISM

The thyroid gland secretes the hormones, thyroxine (T4), triiodothyronine (T3) and calcitonin, which are vital for the regulation of most of the biochemical activities in the body. The thyroid dysfunction could be due to overproduction (thyrotoxicosis) or under production (hypothyroidism) of these hormones. The dysfunction in either form may be subclinical to an acute life-threatening situation.

The clinical features of hypothyroidism vary as per the age of its precipitation and vary in duration and the severity as per the degree of deficiency (Box 6.8). If it precipitates at early fetal life it results in Cretinism and if it precipitates at the adulthood it is called as Myxedema. The hypothyroidism could be primary, (thyroid gland dysfunction), secondary (pituitary dysfunction) or tertiary (due to dysfunction of hypothalamus) the myxedema is 3 to 10 times more common in females. The basal metabolic rate is severly retarded in these patients and their capacity to withstand stress is severely compromised. The patients who are not adequately treated for thyroid deficiency are unusually sensitive to CNS depressant drugs including the sedatives and opioids which are commonly used in dentistry and oral surgery for controlling anxiety and pain. The healing potential is also compromised in such patients.

Box 6.8: Clinical features of myxedema

- Large thick tongue
- Intolerance to the cold
- Muscle weakness
- Dry edematous skin with puffy hands and face
- Lack of sweating
- Bradycardia, BP near normal
- Loss of hair from the brows, alopecia
- Lethargy, slow to speak and react
- Hoarseness of voice
- Altered menstrual pattern in females
- Goiter

The patient when exposed to stress or drugs can land into a myxedema coma characterized by severe hypothermia, hypotension, hypoventilation, hypoxia and hypocapnia.

Prevention of Complications During Dental Procedures

Proper identification of the patients having hypothyroidism is necessary by obtaining detailed medical history, drug history and the clinical manifestations present, if any, before taking such patients for the surgery, medical consultation and proper treatment of hypothyroidism is mandatory.

The patients might be sensitive to sedatives, opioids, antihistaminics, which may be avoided, as even with the normal dose the moderate to severe overdose reactions may be precipitated.

Management of Complications

The patient may loose consciousness in the dental office because of two possibilities

1. Due to fear—in this case the consciousness is regained after the routine steps are undertaken.
2. An undiagnosed, untreated patient having hypothyroidism looses the consciousness and fails to respond to the resuscitative measures.

In both the situations:

- Stop the dental procedure.
- Supine position with elevation of feet.
- Prevent tongue fall.
- Periodic monitoring of vital signs.
- BLS.
- Establish IV line.
- Nasal O_2 through hood or mask.
- Warming blankets to protect against hypothermia.
- Summon medical help.
- Pharmacological support symptomatically, sodium hydrocortisone succinate 100 to 2000 mg, inotropic support raises BP, atropine to correct bradycardia, IV dextrose 25 percent to correct hypoglycemia.
- Definitive treatment comprises of administration of massive doses of T3 and T4, which need to be continued for a long period even after the recovery.

The mortality rate after myxedema coma is very high, i.e. 40 to 50 percent and thus it needs to be identified to prevent it and precautionary measures to be taken rather than facing such severe complications.

HYPERTHYROIDISM—THYROTOXICOSIS

The thyrotoxicosis begins insidiously to produce a more severe crisis the thyroid storm. Although this is a rare emergency it can be seen in the patients with untreated or inadequately treated patients of hyperthyroidism. The patients who have thyrotoxicosis are unusually sensitive to epinephrine and it can precipitate shooting of blood pressure to the dangerous proportions, severe tachycardia and tachyarrhythmias. Such patients should be sedated before the dental therapy, but the sedation could be ineffective if the anxiety is not psychological and is hormonally mediated. The thyrotoxicosis is usually associated with cardiovascular disorders. The patients who are under treatment and are euthyroid (normal levels of thyroid hormone) do not pose increased risk during the dental treatment. Hence, it is necessary to evaluate the patients with positive thyroid dysfunction history and take corrective steps to avoid the serious complications (Box 6.9).

Clinical Features

The patients should be ideally euthyroid before starting the dental therapy. Marginal cases can be treated with due care, with slightly increased risk. The use of vasoconstrictors in local anesthetic solution should be avoided. The epinephrine induces dysrhythmias, angina attacks and precipitate the thyroid storm in hyperthyroid patients whose cardiovascular system is already sensitized (Box 6.9). Similarly drugs like atropine, which is vagolytic should also be avoided. The use of atropine which increases the heart rate by suppressing vagus can initiate the thyroid storm.

Box 6.9: Clinical features of hyperthyroidism

- Anxious, nervous patients
- Warm, wet, sweaty palms
- Tremors
- Elevated BP
- Tachycardia with raised sleeping pulse
- Hyperdynamic circulation and functional cardiac murmurs
- Exophthalmos
- Raised body and core temperature due to increased BMR
- Thyroid nodules.

Box 6.10: Clinical features of thyroid storm

- Hyperpyrexia (105°C)
- Cardiac arrhythmias
- Acute pulmonary edema
- Profound delirium
- Vomiting
- Diarrhea
- Dehydration
- Electrolyte imbalance
- May be fatal if untreated.

The '*thyroid storm*' differs from the severe thyrotoxicosis by the presence of hyperpyrexia (105°F) and may reach lethal level within 24 hours (Box 6.10). This is a severe stage of hypermetabolism and the increased body demand of energy puts additional load on the CVS producing clinical signs and symptoms of cardiac dysrhythmias, cardiac failure and acute pulmonary edema. Thyroid storm also produces profound delirium, vomiting, diarrhea and vomiting leading to a stage of dehydration and electrolyte imbalance.

Management

The untreated and undiagnosed patient of thyrotoxicosis is likely to become unconscious due to vasodepressor syncope and needs to be treated on lines of treating any unconscious patient and basic life support needs to be provided.

- Terminate the dental procedure
- Supine position with elevation of the feet
- Start BLS
- Summon medical help
- Establish IV line
- Nasal O_2
- Transfer the patient to medical emergency department
- Definitive treatment with antithyroid drugs (propylthiouracil)
- Additional measures comprise of administration of propranolol to block the adrenergic mediated effects of thyroid hormone, high doses of glucocorticoid to prevent acute adrenal insufficiency, O_2 administration, cold packs to reduce body temperature, IV fluids to maintain proper electrolyte balance and the hydration.

Anginal Attack in the Dental Office

The chest pain secondary to coronary insufficiency is a common manifestation of ischemic heart disease. The precise description of this condition is "a characteristic thoracic pain, which is usually substernal and usually precipitated by stress, exercise, emotions, heavy meal and is characteristically reduced by vasodilator drugs and rest".

The pain is often described as tightness, stiffness, squeezing, suffocating, strangling rather than a sharp pain and is often radiates to the left arm, lower jaw.

Predisposing Factors

The patients who have coronary insufficiency may not have clinical symptoms at rest or during the sedentary life; however the coronary insufficiency manifests as an angina attack due to the precipitating factors (Box 6.11).

The dental therapy is often stressful and the patient is apprehensive and anxious. Thus, prevention of angina episodes in the dental office, its early detection and management are necessary to prevent life-threatening complications.

Box 6.11: Precipitating factors for angina attack

- Physical activity
- Hot, humid environment
- Cold weather
- Heavy meals
- Emotional stress (argument, anxiety, sexual excitement)
- Caffine
- Cigarette smoking
- High altitude

The steps in identification of the high-risk individuals are:

- History of chest pain, tightness, suffocation (dyspnea) on exertion
- Any previous medical treatment the patient is undergoing (sorbitrate, antihypertensive, aspirin)
- Known cases, cardiac arrhythmias or hypertension
- Thyroid disorders
- Diabetics.

If the patient has a positive history of angina pectoris, a consultation from the physician should be sought to know his coronary status and the severity of the condition. Suitable alterations in the treatment plan and necessary precautions should be taken. The patients with stable angina represent ASA-III risk while as the patients with an unstable angina (daily episodes of angina pain) represent ASA- IV risk.

Management of Anginal Attack in Dental Office

- Stress reduction protocol with proper counselling use of sedatives. The known cases of angina are often prescribed anti-platelet drugs like aspirin. The aspirin therapy prolongs the bleeding due to loss of platelet aggregation. Aspirin irreversibly acetylates platelet cyclo-oxygenase for their life span of 8 to 10 days. Aspirin therefore inhibits the production of proaggregatory thromboxane A2 and is also an indirect antithrombic agent. The aspirin therapy should be discontinued 48 to 72 hours prior to the dental extraction to facilitate new crop of platelets in the circulation and to prevent postsurgical bleeding episode. The decision to stop the antiplatelet therapy should be taken in consultation with the physician.
- Reducing the length of the appointment—the appointments should be preferably in the morning. It is desirable to prescribe sedatives a night before to ensure the patient had a good sleep and rest and is fresh and relaxed. The environments should be cool and comfortable. The appointments should be shorter so that the patient is not over stressed. If the patient shows the signs of fatigue, anxiety or lethargy, the vital signs should be monitored. The BP and pulse may be elevated. The patient should be allowed to rest and then discharged.
- The angina patients are the best candidates to be given O_2 supplements through the nasal catheter or hood during the dental procedure at a flow rate of 3 to 5 liters, to minimize the chances of myocardial ischemia.
- Pain control during the procedure—the acute pain is extremely stressful and efforts must be made to avoid the pain in the angina patients. The pain of a dental procedure is prevented by appropriate local anesthesia. The use of vasoconstrictor should be avoided. Instead of using vasoconstrictor in local anesthetic solution the long acting agents like bupivacaine should be used.
- Premedication with nitroglycerine—the nitroglycerine tablets (0.3–0.6 mg) can be administered 5 minutes prior to the treatment by sublingual route or 30 minutes prior to the treatment by the oral route to prevent angina attack. The nitroglycerine tablets should be available chairside in case the patient develops attack during the treatment.

Ischemic Attack in Dental Office

Management of the Ischemic Attack in the Dental Office

- Terminate the dental procedure.
- The patient does not prefer to be in supine position and wants to sit. Place the patient in the comfortable position.
- BLS.
- Nasal O_2 therapy.
- Administration of vasodilators—the nitroglycerine can be given as sublingual tablets (0.3–0.6 mg) and can be repeated after 5 minutes if needed not to exceed 3 tablets in 15 minutes. The nitroglycerine eliminates the angina pain in 2 to 4 minutes dramatically. The action of the the nitroglycerine is to relax the vascular smooth muscles and produce vasodilatation of the coronary arteries, diminishing the vascular resistance and improving the coronary blood flow. It also causes decrease in peripheral vascular resistance through arterial and more specifically venous dilatation. It leads to diminished venous return, decrease cardiac output and decrease in cardiac workload leading to less O_2 requirement by the myocardium.

  The side effects of nitroglycerine therapy include fullness and throbbing headache, flushing, tachycardia and hypotension. The nitroglycerine therapy is contraindicated in the patients who are in hypotension.

  The patients with coronary artery spasm are known to respond to calcium channel blockers, nifedepine (10–20 mg), when given sublingually. The other examples of calcium channel blockers are veripamil and diltiazem. The veripamil blocks the influx of calcium ions and its supply to the myocardial contractile mechanism and depresses the inotropic state and reduce the myocardial O_2 consumption. It also induces the coronary and peripheral vasodilatation and helps in reducing the systemic vascular resistance. The calcium channel blockers have an additional advantage in its antiarrhythmic action.

  The opioids help only in reducing the angina pain, but are not useful as they do not treat the cause, but are only symptomatic in nature.
- Summon medical assistance and shift the patient to medical emergency for the further management.

MYOCARDIAL INFARCTION

Myocardial infarction[23] (MI) is a clinical syndrome caused by a deficient coronary arterial blood supply to a region of myocardium that results in cellular death and necrosis (Table 6.6).

Predisposing Factors

The predisposing factor for MI is the decreased blood supply to the coronary arteries as occurs with the coronary thrombosis or increased in the level of cardiac workload without increase in the oxygen supply as occurs in the stressed condition. The situation of decreased perfusion is called myocardial ischemia. The anterior descending artery is the most common site for clinically significant atherosclerosis with the occlusion of the vessel and due to the lack of collateral circulation, infarction occurs with myocardial necrosis through the distribution of the occluded artery. The patient with myocardial infarction should be identified and thorough medical history should be taken along with the prescribed medication for the patient.

Management

Post MI patients are on anticoagulants, beta blockers, ACE inhibitors, nitrates or calcium channel blocker. Elective procedures should be avoided at least 6 months after MI. Acute problems should be managed pharmacologically first by antibiotic and analgesics. The extraction should be done under more controlled environment. Stress reduction protocol should be followed and sedation is recommended. Although the endogenous catecholamine released is potentially more dangerous than 0.01 mg/mL of exogenous vasoconstrictor administered in the tissue, the use of vasoconstrictors are a relative contraindication in patients on beta blockers. Elective dental procedure is performed in patients with international normalized ratio (INR) 2 to 3 without the development of bleeding problems. The 80 percent of the patients presents with angina like pain (Table 6.6). The pain is described like 'there is heavy rock or someone sitting on the chest'. A Levine sign (clench at the chest with fist) is present. MI is suspected when the first episode of chest pain is experienced on rest or during dental treatment. The patient may present with previous stable pattern of angina with either increased intensity or frequency.

CARDIAC ARREST

Cardiac arrest is the most serious complication faced by a medical personnel. A prompt diagnosis and immediate CPR can prevent many deaths.[24]

Definition: Cardiac arrest is defined as the abrupt cessation of cardiac pump function that results in death, which may be averted if prompt intervention is instituted.

Etiology

- Hypovolemia
- Hypoxia
- Acidosis
- Hypokalemia/Hyperkalemia
- Hypoglycemia/hyperglycemia
- Hypothermia
- Drugs—tricyclic antidepressants, phenothiazines, beta blockers, Aspirin, acetaminophen
- Cardiac temponade
- Tension pneumothorax
- Thrombosis
- Thromboembolism
- Trauma

Clinical Features

Clinical features of cardiac arrest is given in Box 6.12.

Table 6.6: Precipitating factors, clinical features and management of angina attack

Predisposing factors	Precaution	Clinical manifestation	Pathophysiology	Management
A 90%—Coronary artery disease B Obesity–Male in 5th and 6th decade C Stress	• Stress reduction • Oxygen flow at 3–4 L/min • Sedation $N_2O + O_2$ • Pain control • Less duration of treatment • 6 months after MI	*Symptoms* • Pain—severe intolerable prolonged, 30 min chocking, crushing, retrosternal pain, radiating to left arm, hand, epigastrium, shoulder, neck, jaw. • Nausea • Vomiting • Dizziness • Palpitations • Cold • Perspiration • Sense of impending doom *Signs* • Restlessness • Acute distress • Skin pale and moist • Heart rate—bradycardia to tachycardia	Sudden occlusion of the major coronary artery due to acute thrombosis, subintimal hemorrhage, or rupture atheromatous plaque leading to myocardial ischemia, hypoxia, acidosis and eventually infarction. Infarction causes alteration in the contractility of the heart leading to loss of function to the extent to left ventricular damage	• Terminate procedure • Diagnose—differentiate anginal pain with non-anginal pain. • Position—usually upright is comfortable to the patient • ABC • Summon medical assistance • Administer nitroglycerine (contraindicated in hypotensive patients) • Antiplatelet therapy—aspirin—325 mg orally • Manage pain—parenteral opioid, $N_2O + O_2$ • Monitor vitals • Prepare and manage complication (cardiac arrest) • Transfer to hospital emergency

Box 6.12: Identification of cardiac arrest

- Sudden and abrupt loss of consciousness.
- Absence of respiration (if preceded or intervened by respiratory arrest).
- Loss of central and peripheral pulses.
- Heart sound not audible (blank precardium).

Presentations of Cardiac Arrest

- Asystole
- Pulseless electrical activity (including electromechanical dissociation)
- Ventricular fibrillation
- Pulseless ventricular tachycardia.

The cardiac arrest can also be secondary to:

- Ventricular fibrillation.
- Ventricular asystole.

The time elapsed from the event of arrest is not known in the unwitnessed cardiac arrest. Time available at disposal is very important. As the cardiac arrest takes place profound cerebral hypoxia results. More the time lapse in giving the CPR, more severe is likely to be the ischemic encephalopathy. The brain does not stand hypoxia for more than 3 minutes and if the patient is not resuscitated immediately, irreversible cerebral damage can occur.

Management

Management of cardiac arrest is divided into two protocols.

1. Basic life support (BLS).
2. Advanced cardiac life support (ACLS).

Basic Life Support

Cardiopulmonary resuscitation[25]

Cardiopulmonary resuscitation consists of three main parts, the ABC:

1. A—Airway
2. B—Breathing
3. C—Circulation

Steps:

- Establish unresponsiveness
- Check for breathing
- Maintain patency of airway-neck extension, chin lift, oropharynegeal airway, intubation, suction
- If no breathing give 2 breaths mouth by mouth, mouth to endotracheal tube, ambu bag, etc.
- Look for signs of a pulse in peripheral as well as major arteries (carotid, femoral)

Chest compressions

The chest compressinons are done by keeping the patient on a hard surface. The operator kneels down by the side of the patient if the patient is kept on the floor or stands by the side of the bed. The heels of the hand are kept over each other and on the xiphoid sternum without flexing at elbows, and not on the ribs as ribs can fracture with compression. The sternum is depressed by generating force through the muscles of the trunk and compress 1 ½ to 2 inch.

- Give 15 compressions
- Continue with 4 cycles of 2 breaths to 15 compressions.

Chest compression techniques

- Position yourself at victim's side
- Make sure the victim is lying on his back on a firm, flat surface if the victim is laying facedown; carefully roll him into his back.
- Loosen or remove all cloth covering the victim's chest. You need to be able to see the skin.
- Put the heel of one hand on the center of the victim's bare chest between the nipples.
- Straighten your arms and position your shoulder directly over your hands.
- Push hard and fast. Press down 1½ to 2 inch with each compression. For each chest compression, make sure you push straight down on the victim's breastbone.
- At the end of each compression, make sure you allow the chest to recoil or re-expand completely. Full chest recoil allows more blood to refill the heart between chest compressions. Incomplete chest recoil will reduce the blood flow created by chest compressions.
- A smart blow on the chest can also stimulate the heart, but the chances of fibrillations are high.
- Deliver compression in smooth fashion at a rate of 100 compressions per minute (Fig. 6.3).

Opening the airway and giving the Breaths

- Perform the head tilt-chin lift or jaw-thrust maneuver in case of cervical spine injuries.
- Give mouth-to-mouth breaths to the victim.
- Give mouth to mask breath to the victim.

Performing the head-tilt chin lift:

- Place one hand on victim's forehead and push with your palm to tilt the head back.
- Place the fingers of the other hand under the bony part of the lower jaw near the chin.
- Lift the jaw to bring the chin forward.
- The head tilt-chin lift relieves airway obstruction in the unresponsive victim.
- When a victim is unresponsive, the tongue can block the upper airway, the head tilt-chin lift maneuver lifts the tongue, reliving the airway obstruction.

Things to avoid with head tilt chin lift:

- Do not press deeply into the soft tissue under the chin because this might obstruct the airway.
- Do not use the thumb to lift the chin.
- Do not close the victim's mouth completely (*unless mouth to nose breathing is the technique of choice for the victim*).

Mouth-to-mouth breathing

Mouth-to-mouth breathing is a quick, effective way to provide oxygen to the victim. The rescuer's exhaled air contains approximately 17 percent oxygen and 4 percent carbon dioxide. This is enough oxygen to supply the victim's need.

- Hold the victim's airway open with a head tilt-chin lift.
- Pinch the nose closed with your thumb and index finger.

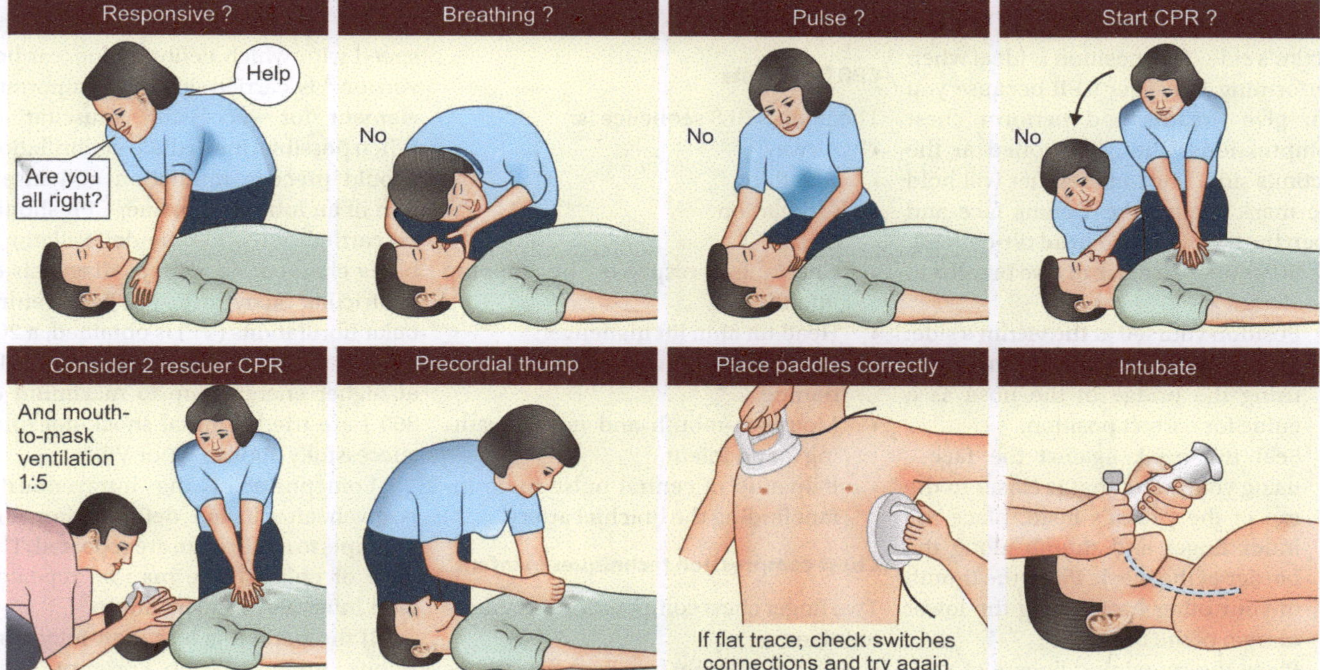

Fig. 6.3: Steps in basic life support

- Take a regular (not deep) breath and seal your lip around the victim's mouth creating an airtight seal.
- Give 1 breath (blow for 1 second) watch for the chest to rise as you give the breath.
- If the chest does not rise, repeat the head tilt-chin lift give a second breath (blow for 1 second). Watch for the chest to rise.

Prevention of risk of gastric inflation

- Giving breaths too quickly or with too much force, air is likely to enter the stomach rather than the lungs. This can cause gastric inflation.
- Gastric inflation frequently develops during mouth-to-mouth, mouth to mask or band to mask ventilation. Gastric inflation can result in serious complications, such as vomiting, aspiration or pneumonia. Reduce the risk of gastric inflation by avoiding giving breaths too rapidly or too forcefully.
  To prevent gastric inflation:
- Taken 1 second to deliver each breath.
- Deliver enough air to make the victim's chest rise.

Mouth to mask technique

To use a mask, the lone rescuer is at the victim's side. This position is ideal when performing 1-rescuer CPR because you can give breaths and perform chest compressions when positioned at the victim's side. The lone rescuer will hold the mask against the victims face and open the airway with a head tilt-chin lift.

Steps to use a mask to give breaths to the victim:

- Position yourself at the victim's side.
- Place the mask on the victim's face, using the bridge of the nose as a guide for correct position.
- Seal the mask against the face—using your hand that is closer to the top of the victim's head, place the index finger and thumb along the border of the mask. Place the thumb of your other hand along the lower margin of the mask.
- Place the remaining fingers of your hand closer to the victim's neck along the bony margin of the jaw and lift the jaw. Perform a head tilt-chin lift to open the airway.
- While you lift the jaw, press firmly and completely around the outside margin of the mask to seal the mask against the face.
- Deliver air over 1 second to make the victim's chest rise.

Cardiopulmonary resuscitation for children (1 year of age to puberty)[26]

Infants and children who develop cardiac arrest often do not have enough oxygen delivery to the brain and heart and other vital organs even before the heart stops pumping blood. It is very important to give effective breaths (breaths that make the chest rise) for infants and children during CPR.

Difference in depth of chest compressions

- **Child age 1 to puberty:** Press down 1/3 to ½ the depth of the chest with each compression.
- **Adult:** Press down 1½ to 2 inches with each compression.

For very small children you may use either one or two hands for chest compressions. Make sure you compress the chest 1/3 to 1/2 the depth of the chest with each compression.

CPR for infants

The infants BLS sequence is:

- Airway
- Breathing
- Circulation.
  Steps:
- Check for response by tapping infant's feet.
- Head tilt chin lift maneuver.
- Relief of airway obstruction by positioning.
- Mouth-to-mouth and nose breathing for an infant.
- Palpation of central pulse in an infant finding the brachial artery.

Chest compression techniques in infant

Two finger chest compression technique in infant:

- Place the infant on a firm, flat surface
- Move or remove clothing from the infant's chest
- Draw an imaginary line between the nipples. Place two fingers on the breastbone just below this line. This will allow you to compress on the lower half of the breastbone. Do not press on the xiphoid process.
- To give chest compressions, press the infant's breastbone down, but 1/3 to 1/2 the depth of the chest.
- After each compression completely release the pressure on the breastbone to allow the chest to recoil or re-expand completely.
- Deliver compressions in a smooth fashion at a rate of 100 compressions per minute (*see* Fig. 6.3).

Advanced Cardiac Life Support[27]

Advanced cardiac life support (ACLS) is intended to achieve adequate ventilation, control cardiac arrythmias, stabilize blood pressure and cardiac output and restores organ perfusion. The activities carried out to achieve these goals include:

- Intubation with endotracheal tube.
- Defibrillation/cardioversion and/or pacing.
- Insertion of an intravenous line.

Ventilation with O_2 (room air, if is not immediately available) may promptly reverse hypoxemia and acidosis. The speed with which defibrillation/cardioversion[28] is carried out is an important element for successful resuscitation. When possible, immediate defibrillation should precede intubation and insertion of an intravenous line; CPR should be carried out while the defibrillator is being charged. As soon as diagnosis of ventricular tachycardia (VT) and ventricular fibrillations (VF) is obtained, a 200 J shock is delivered. Additional shocks at higher energies, up to maximum of 360 J are tried if initial shock does not successfully abolish VT or VF.

Epinephrine 1 mg intravenously, is given after failed defibrillation and attempts to defibrillate are repeated. The dose of epinephrine may be repeated after intervals of 3 to 5 minute.

If the patient is less than fully conscious upon revision, prompt intubation, ventilation and arterial blood gas analysis should be carried out.

Intravenous $NaHCO_3$, is no longer considered routinely necessary and may be dangerous in large quantities, as it abolishes the hypoxic drive of respiration. The patient who is persistently acidotic after successful defibrillation and intubation should be given 1 mEq/kg $NaHCO_3$ initially and additional 50 percent of dose repeated every 10 to 15 minutes.

After initial unsuccessful defibrillation attempts, with persistent electrical instability, bolus of 1 mg/kg lidocaine is given intravaneously and dose is repeated in 2 minutes in those patients who have persistent ventricular arrhythmias or remain in VF. This is followed by a continuous infusion at a rate of 1 to 4 mg/min if lidocaine fails to provide control, other antiarrhythmic therapies should be tried. For persistent hemodynamically unstable ventricular arrhythmia as, intravenous amiodarone, has emerged as the treatment of choice (150 mg over 10 min, followed by 1 mg/min for up to 6 hours and 0.5 mg/min thereafter) intravenous procainamide (loading dose of 100 mg/5 min to a total dose of 500 to 800 mg, followed by continous infusion at 2 to 5 mg/min) may be tried for persisting, hemodynamically stable arrythmias; or bretylium tosylate (loading dose 5 to 10 mg/kg in 5 min; maintenance dose 0.5 to 2 mg/min) may be tried as an alternative for unstable arrythmias. Intravenous calcium gluconate is no longer considered safe for routine administration. It is only used in patients in whom acute hyperkalemia is known to be triggering event for resistant VF, in the presence of known hypocalcemia or in patients who have received toxic doses of calcium channel antagonists.

Cardiac arrest secondary to bradyarrythmias or asystole is managed differently, patient is promptly intubated, CPR is continued, attempt is made to control hypoxemia and acidosis. Epinephrine and/or atropine are given intravenously or by intracardiac route. The prognosis is generally very poor in this form of cardiac arrest even with successful electrical pacing.

DRUG RELATED EMERGENCIES[29]

Local anesthetics are an integral part of the dental treatment plan. Whenever potentially painful procedures are considered, analgesics are prescribed for relief of pre-existing pain or alleviation of potential postoperative pain, antibiotics are used in management of infection and central nervous system depressant are prescribed for all phases of dental treatment for prevention and management of dentistry related fears. These four drug categories constitute the overwhelming majority of all drugs used in the practice of dentistry.

Classifying adverse drug reactions—Pallasch[30] proposed the following classification:

- Overdose—direct extension of the pharmacological action of the drugs.
- Deleterious effects on chemically, genetically, metabolically or morphologically altered recipient.
- Initiation of immune or allergic reaction.

Overdose

A toxic reaction is a condition that results from exposure to toxic amounts of a substance that does not cause adverse effects when administration in smaller amount. It refers to those clinical signs and symptoms resulting absolute or relative over administration of its target organs or tissues. Clinical signs and symptoms of overdose are related to direct extension of the normal pharmacological actions of the drug. Local anesthetic overdose reaction.

Predisposing Factors

Patient factors

- **Age:** Drug absorption, metabolism and excretion may be imperfectly developed in young age group or diminished in older age groups. Underdeveloped or decreased liver function may result in higher blood level of the drugs because the individual cannot transform the local anesthetic into biologically inactive substance.
- **Body weight:** The greater the lean weight, the larger the dose of the drug the individual can tolerate before an overdose develops. This relationship does not apply to obese person since blood flow to adipose tissue is sparse as compared with that supplying muscle. The usual blood level of lidocaine in the brain required to induce seizure activity is 7.5 μgm/mL of blood. Hyporesponsive patients may not exhibit seizure until the brains blood level attains a significantly higher level of lidocaine whereas hyperresponsive patients may exhibit seizures at brains blood level below 7.5 μgm/mL of blood.
- **Pathological process:**[31] The presence of pre-existing disease may alter the bloods ability to transform a drug into a biologically inactive substance. Most amide local anesthetics undergo biotransformation in the liver, with a small percentage of drug unchanged in the kidney. Any disease state that reduces or increases hepatic blood flow is likely to alter various pharmacokinetic parameters of amide local anesthetic. Patients with cardiovascular disease especially CCF demonstrate blood level of local anesthetics almost twice of those found in healthy individual receiving the same doses. This difference results from several factors including a reduced blood volume from drug distribution and diminished hepatic blood flow secondary to low cardiac output.
- **Genetics:** It has been reported that with increasing frequency that certain individual possess genetic deficiency in the enzyme serum cholinesterases reduced in the liver circulates in the blood and is responsible for biotransformation of two important drugs, i.e. succinylcholine and ester type of local anesthetic.
- **Attitude and environment:** The psychological attitude of the patient greatly influences the ultimate effect

of the drug. This is considerably important with sedative hypnotics and opioid analgesics.

- **Sex:** The only instance of sexual difference in the human occurs in females during pregnancy at which time renal function may be altered leading to impaired excretion of certain drugs and their accumulation in the blood, potentially increasing the risk of overdose.
- **Drug factors:** The drugs vasoactivity, dose and root of administration, speed of administration, vascularity of the injection site and the presence of vasoconstrictor influences the risk of overdose.
- **Prevention:** Careful evaluation of the patient before the start of treatment along with careful drug administration can minimize the risk of overdose in almost all situations.

Clinical Manifestation

Onset, intensity and duration—rapid IV injection produces signs and symptoms of overdose rapidly, with seizure or unconsciousness may develop within seconds. These signs and symptoms develop approximately 5 to 10 minutes after drug administration if plain anesthetic solution is administered and 30 minutes if vasopressor is included. The severity of reaction is great, the reaction is self-limiting because of continued redistribution and biotransformation.

Signs and symptoms of local anesthetic toxicity are given in Table 6.7.

Table 6.7: Clinical features of local anesthetic toxicity

Signs	Symptoms
Low to moderate overdose levels • Confusion • Talkativeness • Apprehension • Excitedness • Slurred speech • Generalized stutter • Muscular twitching and tremor of the facer and extremities • Nystagmus • Elevated blood pressure • Elevated heart rate • Generalized tonic clonic seizure followed by CNS depression, depressed blood pressure, heart rate and respiration	• Headache • Lightheadedness • Dizziness • Blurred vision, inability to focus • Ringing in ears • Numbness of tongue feeling • Drowsiness • Disorientation

Local anesthetics depress excitable membranes. The cardiovascular system and CNS are especially sensitive and are considered target organs for local anesthetic drugs. The usual clinical expression of local anesthetic overdose is one of apparent stimulation followed by a period of depression.

Minimal to moderate blood levels—the initial clinical signs of overdose in the CNS are usually excitatory. At low over dose blood levels, the patient usually becomes confused, talkative, apprehensive and excited; speech may be slurred. A generalized stuttering follows, which may progress to muscular twitching and tremor, commonly noted in the muscles of the face and the distal parts of the extremities. The patient may also exhibit nystagmus (involuntary eye movement). The blood pressure, heart rate and respiratory rate increase.

Headache may also be a symptom of overdose (secondary to local anesthetic induced dilatation of cerebral blood vessels). In addition, many patients initially report of having a generalized feeling of lightheadedness and dizziness, i.e. different from that associated with alcohol. These symptoms then progress to visual and auditory disturbances (e.g. difficulty in focusing, blurred vision and ringing in the ears [tinnitus]). Numbness of the tongue and perioral tissues commonly develop, as does a feeling of being either flushed or chilled. As the reaction progresses and if the anesthetic blood level rises, the patient experiences drowsiness and disorientation and may eventually cause unconsciousness. Signs and symptoms of mild local anesthetic overdose may resemble psychomotor or temporal epilepsy.

Moderate to High Blood Levels

As the local anesthetic blood level continues to rise, clinical manifestations of overdose progress to a generalized convulsive state with tonic-clonic seizures. After this "stimulatory" or "excitatory" phase, a period of generalized CNS depression ensues; characteristically of a degree of severity related to the degree of stimulation preceding it. Therefore, if the patient suffers intensive tonic clonic seizures, postseizure depression is more profound, probably characterized by unconsciousness and respiratory depression or respiratory arrest. If the stimulatory phase was mild (e.g. talkativeness or agitations), the depressant phase will also be mild, perhaps consisting of only a period of disorientation and lethargy. Blood pressure, heart rate and respiratory rate are usually depressed during this phase, again to a degree proportionate to the degree of previous stimulation.

Although the sequence just described represents the usual clinical expression of local anesthetic overdose, the excitatory phase of the reaction may be extremely brief or even absent. This is especially true with lidocaine and mepivacaine, in which overdose may appear.

Pathophysiology

CVS effect

On intraoral injection the drug slowly enters the circulation. As the blood level rises, the systemic actions are noted depending on the blood level.

Zero to 1.8 µg/mL—normal blood level after intraoral injection.

No cardiovascular effect 1.8 µg/mL is the minimal effective dose of lignocaine for antidysrhythmic action.

1.8 to 6 μg/mL—antidysrhythmic action. Can be used in the management of ventricular dysarthymia, especially in ventricular extrasystole and ventricular tachycardia.

5 to 10 μg/mL—ECG alteration. There is increase in the P-R interval QRS duration and sinus bradycardia, myocardial depression and peripheral vasodialation.

10 μg/mL and above—it leads to accentuation of the electrophysiological and hemodynamic effects resulting in massive peripheral vasodilation and intensive myocardial depression. The heart rate decreases ultimately cardiac arrest may result.

Central nervous system effect

Central nervous system (CNS) is extremely sensitive to the level of local anesthetic. LA readily crosses the blood brain barrier (BBB) progressively depresses the CNS function. Till the level of less than 5 μg there is no adverse reaction. At cerebral blood levels between 0.5 and 4.0 jig/mL, lidocaine can terminate various forms of seizure. Most clinically useful local anesthetics possess this anticonvulsant property (both procaine and lidocaine having been used to terminate or decrease the duration of grand mal or petit mal seizures). This anticonvulsant action may be related to a depression of hyperexcitable cortical neurons present in epileptic patients.

As the blood level of lidocaine rises above 4.5 jig/mL, early signs and symptoms of CNS alteration appear. These are usually related to increased cortical irritability (e.g. agitation, talkativeness, and tremor). Numbness of the tongue and perioral tissues may result from the rich blood supply to these tissues, allowing the drugs to produce a blockade of the nerve endings.

With further increase in cerebral blood level to 7.5 jig/mL or greater (lidocaine), generalized tonic-clonic seizures develop. Following this period of CNS stimulation, a further increase in cerebral blood level of the local anesthetic results in termination of seizure activity and an electroencephalographic pattern consistent with generalized CNS depression. Respiratory depression and arrest are also noted.

The fact that local anesthetics are CNS depressants on the one hand, but that CNS stimulation is the first clinical manifestation of this depression may seem contradictory. The stimulation and subsequent depression produced by high blood levels of local anesthetics result solely from depression of neuronal activity. The cerebral cortex receives inhibitory and facilitatory (stimulatory) impulses. If it is considered that these two groups of neurons are depressed selectively by different blood levels of local anesthetics, this seeming contradiction is explained. At anesthetic blood levels capable of producing seizures, the inhibitory pathways in the cerebral cortex are depressed, not title stimulatory pathways. This depression of inhibitory pathways allows facilitatory neurons to function unopposed, leading to increased excitation of the CNS and ultimately to seizures. As the local anesthetic blood level increases still further, stimulatory neurons are depressed along with inhibitory neurons, producing a state of generalized CNS depression.

The duration of the seizure, although primarily dependent on the local anesthetic blood level, can be further modified by the acid-base status of the patient. The higher the $PaCO_2$, the lower the local anesthetic blood level required to precipitate generalized seizures. In contrast, the lower the $PaCO_2$ the greater the drug blood level required for producing seizures. Lowering a patient's $PaCO_2$ through hyperventilation raises the cortical seizure threshold to local anesthetics and lessens the chance that a drug may cause seizures.

Drug-induced seizures, in and of themselves, are not necessarily fatal. However, the mortality rate in untreated animals is more than 60 percent. The duration of the seizure appears to be a critical factor in determining the degree of morbidity. The convulsing brain requires greatly elevated oxygen and glucose levels to continue functioning. To a degree, the body's own mechanisms can compensate for this; however, respiratory and circulatory support can enhance the chances of survival significantly. If blood levels of the local anesthetic rise even further, cardiovascular depression is produced and respiration is increasingly impaired by uncoordinated muscle spasm during the seizure. Brain function is affected even more through reduced cerebral blood flow and hypoxia.

Phentolamine mesylate[32] accelerates recovery from oral soft tissue anesthesia in patients who have received local anesthetic injections containing a vasoconstrictor. The proposed mechanism is that phentolamine, an alpha-adrenergic antagonist, blocks the vasoconstriction associated with the epinephrine used in dental anesthetic formulations, thus enhancing the systemic absorption of the local anesthetic from the injection site.

Allergy

Allergy is defined as a hypersensitive response to an allergen to which the individual has been previously exposed and to which that individual has developed antibodies. It manifests itself as drug fever, angioedema, urticaria and dermatitis, depression of blood forming organs, photosensitivity and anaphylaxis. In marked contrast to overdose in which clinical manifestation related directly to the normal pharmacology of the drug, the observed clinical picture in allergy is always a result of an exaggerated response by immune system.

It is desirable that the patient who has history of drug allergies the cutaneous sensitivity must be checked by giving intradermal test dose. If the patient is allergic to penicillin all the drugs falling in the catagory of beta-lactam antibiotics should be avoided. Although the local anesthetics seldom evoke allergic reactions it must be remembered that the preservatives used in the local anesthetic solution are capable of producing allergic reaction.

The milder allergic reactions can be treated with withdrawal of the drug evoking the allergy reaction and administration of antihistaminics and steroids. The major or immediate type of reactions such as bronchospasm to frank anaphylaxis warrant aggressive and prompt treatment to prevent life-threatening episodes. The details of the management of the anaphylactic reaction is discussed in the Chapter 5, on Shock.

Idiosyncrasy

Idiosyncrasy may be defined as an individual's unique hypersensitivity to a particular drug, food or other substance. CNS stimulation after the insertion of known CNS depressant drugs such as barbiturates or histamine blockers. Idiosyncratic reaction covers an extremely wide range of clinical expression any type of expression including depression following administration of a stimulant, stimulation following administration of depressant. Hyperpyrexia following administration of muscle relaxant, such as succinylcholine.

Management

Because of the unpredictable nature of idiosyncratic reaction their management is of necessity symptomatic. The essentials of basic life support—P- A- B- C (position, airway, breathing and circulation) are vital. If idiosyncracy represents as seizure the treatment protocol for seizure is followed.

Dentistry Drug-related Emergencies

The various drugs used in the dentistry are local anesthetics antibiotics and analgesics.

Local Anesthetics

The ester group of local anesthetics carry a risk of allergic reaction, which being the potential reason for the development of the amide group of LA. Although allergic reaction is rare, the common reactions to amide group of LA are psychogenic response (vasodepressor syncope and hyperventilation). Topically applied local anesthetic may also adverse drug reaction. Psychogenic responses rarely occurs. Allergic reaction such as erythema or angioedema of the mucous membrane and lips, are not uncomman after topical application of these drugs. The reason of high level of toxicity is that it is absorbed rapidly and the blood level rises rapidly. Safer use of topical anesthetics may be achieved through either amide type topical anesthetics or benzocaine combined with their judicious application.

Antibiotics

Are given either prophylatically to prevent infection or in special circumstances such as to prevent infective endocarditis. To avoid development of resistance to bacterial strains and allergy antibiotic should be used only when therapeutic indication exists. The dose and the sequence of antibiotic administration should be monitored. The major advantage of oral administration of the drug is the decreased likelihood of adverse drug reaction. If parenteral administration of antibiotic, particularly penicillin, is required the drug should be given only after the sensitivity test and in controlled circumstances where the facilities for managing severe allergic reactions and emergency management are in place. And the patient should be observed for about 1 hour.

Analgesics

The two major categories of analgesics are considered nonopoids and opoids. The NSAIDs such as ibuprofen and naproxen are extremely popular and safe. Most adverse reactions are gastritis, nausea and constipation. Other effects are like headache, dizziness and pruritis. Major side with aspirin and other NSAIDs, includes mild urticaria, renal tubular necrosis to bronchospasm and fatal anaphylaxis. While prescribing the NSAIDs care should be taken to avoid prescribing them to the patients with APD and asthma. Similarly, the patients should be instructed to take the drugs after meals and H_2 blockers or antacids may be prescribed.

SURGICAL EMERGENCIES

The surgical emergencies encountered in the dental office are hemorrhage, aspiration of the foreign body in the larynx, bronchus or the stomach.

Hemorrhage

Hemorrhage is defined as extravasation of the blood from the blood vessels. The commonly encountered hemorrhage is the postdental extraction hemorrhage, however, other causes like accidental injuries to larger blood vessels due to slipping of knife or high speed rotary instruments can also lead to hemorrhage.

Etiology

The common causes of postdental extraction hemorrhage are:

- *Local causes:*
  - Inflammation/granulation tissue.
  - Damage to neurovascular bundle.
  - Excessive soft tissue laceration.
  - Malignant growth.
  - Vascular lesions.
- *Systemic causes:*
  - Coagulopathies—hemophilia A, B, deficiency of other clotting factors, afibrogenemia
  - Bleeding disorders—(ITP), thrombocytopenia, thrombasthenia, von Willibrand's disease
  - Hypertension
  - Liver disorders
  - Renal disorders—uremia
  - Drugs—aspirin, anticoagulants.

Management

The management of the hemorrhage should be undertaken promptly. One should not just rely on the local measures to arrest the hemorrhage as they may not be effective alone if the patient has systemic pathology like a coagulopathy. Similarly, one should not delay the local measures for the want of investigations as by the time the report of the investigations are available, by that time sizable blood loss can occur. Thus, the local measures should be started and simultaneously

Table 6.8: Investigations for the unknown bleeder and their interpretation

BT Normal- 3–5 minute by Duke's or Ivy methods	Platelet count	APTT	APTT	Hemostatic defect	Causes
I	N	N	N	Platelet function, Vascular disorder	von Willebrand's disease (vWD), aspirin therapy, uremia, storage pool defect
I	D	N	N	Thrombocytopenia	Secondary causes, Idiopathic Thrombocytopenic Purpura
N	N	I	N	Extrinsic pathway	Oral anticoagulants, Vitamin K deficiency, deficiency of Factor VII (shortest half life)
N	N	N	I	Intrinsic pathway	Heparin, hemophilia A/B, von Willebrand's disease (vWD)
N	N	I	I	Common pathways	Heparin therapy, liver disease, vitamin K deficiency, Oral anticoagulant therapy, Factor V, X, II, I deficiency
I	D	I	I	Multiple pathways	DIC, Liver disease
N	N	N	N		Mild von Willebrand's disease (vWD), vascular disorder, platelet function defect, Factor XIII deficiency

Abbreviations: I : Increased; N : Normal; D: Decreased

history should be obtained and if necessary samples should be drawn for appropriate investigations to diagnose the systemic pathology.

Local measures

The local site of bleeding should be properly cleaned of blood clots to facilitate proper inspection of the bleeding site to identify the source of bleeding, type of bleeding (arterial, veinous, capillary), presence of granulation tissue, etc. to facilitate selection of proper modality to arrest the bleeding.

- *Mechanical:*
  - Curettage of the granulation tissue.
  - Pressure packs.
  - Suturing.
  - Ligation of the damaged blood vessels.
  - Application of the gel foam, oxidized cellulose.
  - Application of bone wax.
- *Thermal*
  - Hot packs.
  - Cold compressions.
  - Electrocautery.
- *Chemical*
  - Local application of thrombin.
  - Adrenaline packs.

Systemic measures

- History
  - History of bleeding disorders/episodes. Family history for coagulopathy or bleeding disorders.
  - History of drug therapy like aspirin, anticoagulants. Sometimes the patient may not be aware of names of the drug in such cases history of IHD, HT, coronary bypass surgery, angioplasty may be suggestive as such patients are commonly prescribed the drugs like antiplatelet (Aspirin) or anticoagulants (Coumarin derivatives).
  - History of liver and renal disorders.
- Investigations
  - Screening investigations like BT, CT.
  - INR.
  - Platelet count.
  - PT.
  - PPT.
  - Individual factor assay (Table 6.8).

Investigations

- **Bleeding time:** Normal—3 to 5 minutes by Duke's or Ivy methods
- The clotting time (Normal Lee-White 9–14 min)—prolongation of CT is suggestive of coagulopathy, liver disorders, renal disorder (uremia), anticoagulant therapy. It is usually prolonged in Factor VIII, IX, XI, XII and rarely factor X deficiency. However, it is just a gross screening investigation and may not localize the defect accurately. The bleeding time may also be prolonged.
- Torniquet test—positive test is suggestive of capillary fragility and vitamin C deficiency.
- Platelet count (normal 250,000–400,000/cumm) less than 70,000/cumm.
- Prothrombin time (normal 15 seconds by Quick's method)—the prolongation of the prothrombin time is suggestive of deficiency of Factor IV, V, VII, X and fibrinogen deficiency. It is also prolonged in heparinized patients.
- Partial thromboplastin time—the normal time is to be standardized by each laboratory as it depends on the tissue procoagulant used for this test. If it is prolonged it is suggestive of Factor VIII, IX, XI, XII, II, V, VII and X deficiency.
- Combined evaluation of PT and PTT-
  - If PT is Prolonged and PTT is normal.
  - If PT is normal and PTT is prolonged.
- Thromboplastin generation test.
- Individual factor assay—on the basis of the above investigations if the deficiency of a particular factor is determined or suspected then the assay of that factor is to be done for diagnostic and therapeutic purposes.

Systemic Treatment

The systemic treatment comprises of:

- Establish IV line
- Crystalloid infusion to replace the volume
- Injection of vitamin K
- Injection ethambutol
- Transfusion of the whole blood
- Platelet rich plasma
- Fresh frozen plasma
- Platelet concentrates
- Factor VIII concentrate.

ASPIRATION OF THE FOREIGN BODY

The aspiration of the foreign body (FB) during the dental procedure can occur if proper care is not taken during the procedure. It can occur in the anesthetized patients or in conscious patients as well. In the latter case, the foreign body is most likely to be aspirated in the esophagus than the trachea due to the protective reflexes. However, it can be aspirated in the trachea as well. The common types of foreign bodies that can be aspirated are tooth, endodontic instruments, post and core or the rubber dam clamps.

If the foreign body is swallowed accidentally in the esophagus it will not cause any respiratory distress, but does cause discomfort due to abbression of injuries to the lining and gives a persistent feeling of foreign body sensation even after it is removed or has passed in the stomach. The foreign bodies swallowed in the esophagus generally come out on coughing or pass in the stomach and due to peristalsis are passed in the stools. They seldom cause any significant problems, however, sharp foreign bodies may injure the lining of the GI tract and produce clinical manifestations. Periodic radiological examination to know the location of the foreign body and examination of stool is necessary to confirm its safe passage in the stool. If the clinical symptoms develop then the appropriate surgical intervention is required depending upon the site and type of pathology.

If the foreign body is aspirated in the respiratory passage and if it is large it will get lodged in the larynx to produce acute laryngeal obstruction due to mechanical obstruction due to the foreign body and/or acute laryngospasm secondary to it. If the aspirated foreign body is small it will pass through the larynx into the tracheas and subsequently into the main bronchus or small bronchioles, if the aspiration is assisted by the gravity. The foreign body is usually aspirated in the right bronchus as it is vertical and the left bronchus is oblique due to presence of the heart on the left side. The diameter of the trachea and bronchus is small in children the chances of total obstruction are high in them even with the smaller objects.

The aspirated foreign body in the respiratory passage will not produce an immediate life-threatening emergency immediately unless it is lodged in the larynx or the trachea and is of large enough size to cause complete obstruction. The partial obstruction warrants certain important steps to be undertaken to prevent subsequent problems like infection.

Clinical Signs

- Partial obstruction
  - Discomfort and feeling of foreign body.
  - Persistent and vigorous bouts of cough if the FB is in larynx or tracheobroncheal tree.
  - Labored/paradoxical respiration.
  - Wheeze.
  - Tachycardia.
  - Altered voice.
  - Cyanosis may be present.
  - Lethargy, disorientation due to hypoxia.
- Total respiratory obstruction
  - First phase (1–3 minutes)
    a. The patient is conscious
    b. Universal chocking signs, inability to breath
    c. Struggling paradoxical respiration and sounds without air movements
    d. Increased BP
    e. Tachycardia
    f. Inability to speak
    g. Inability to cough
    h. Cyanosis.
  - Second phase (2–5 minutes)
    a. Loss of consciousness,
    b. Decreased respiration
    c. Decreased BP
    d. Bradycardia.
  - Third phase (>4–5 minutes)
    a. Coma
    b. Absent vital signs
    c. Fixed, dilated pupils not responding to the light
    d. Death.

Management

Although not routinely required every dental/oral surgical clinic must have a laryngoscope (working condition) and a Magill's forceps. The identification and prompt action are of vital importance as the airway obstruction is the major cause of sudden cardiac arrest, especially in the children.

- As soon as the condition is recognized, place the patient in the lateral decubitus position.
- Encourage the patient to cough vigorously.
- If the foreign body is retrieved consult the medical specialist before discharging the patient.
- Back blow application and Heimlich maneuver,[33] abdominal thrust, chest thrust.
- Laryngoscope to visualize the FB and if retrievable pick up with a Magill's forceps.
- X-rays to determine the site of FB. This is possible only when the patient has partial obstruction and time is available to do these exercises.
- Bronchoscopy to remove the FB.

In more severe cases where the obstruction is severe and time is more precious efforts are made to establish airway, if the FB is in the larynx then the cricothyroidectomy or tracheostomy should be performed immediately. Once the air-way is established the rest of the treatment for removal of the FB can be undertaken. In the patients who are cyanosed, hypoxic, unconscious appropriate life-saving therapy with oxygen inhalation, pharmacological support to combat hypoxia, acidosis should be started.

The back slaps or blows are applied to remove the foreign body from the airway of the child or the infant. The child is saddled over the rescuer's arm with head lower then the trunk, in a prone position (Fig 6.4). The back blows or slaps are applied between the scapulae.[34]

The manual thrusts are series of exercises applied to the upper abdomen (abdominal or supradiaphramatic thrust) or the lower chest (chest thrust). They increase the intrathoracic pressure suddenly, producing an artificial cough to expel the FB. The abdominal thrust is a soft tissue thrust and does not include pressure on the rib cage or sternum. It can be given in a standing position when the patient is conscious and able to stand. It can also be given in an unconscious patient when the patient kept in a supine position (Figs 6.5A and B). While doing the abdominal thrust, the operator must apply pressure with the heels of the hand just below the rib cage. It is done in such a way that the damage to the rib cage and the intra-abdominal visceral organs like liver and spleen is avoided.

The chest thrust should be given as an alternative to abdominal thrust in special conditions like children below age of 1 year (*see* Fig. 6.4), pregnant females and extremely obese victims, but it is strictly contraindicated in old patients as the ribs are likely to fracture due to osteoporosis.

Prevention

In spite of conscious efforts of preventing the aspiration of the foreign body, the small objects such as burs, endodontic instruments, inlays, debris fall into the oropharynx which can be subsequently swallowed or aspirated by the patient. The concept of sitting dentistry where the patient is kept in a supine or semisupine position in the dental chair enhances the chances of aspiration.[35]

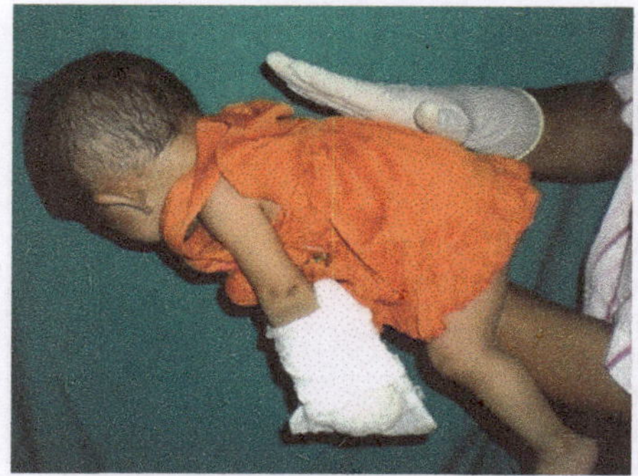

Fig. 6.4: Heimlich maneuver for infants

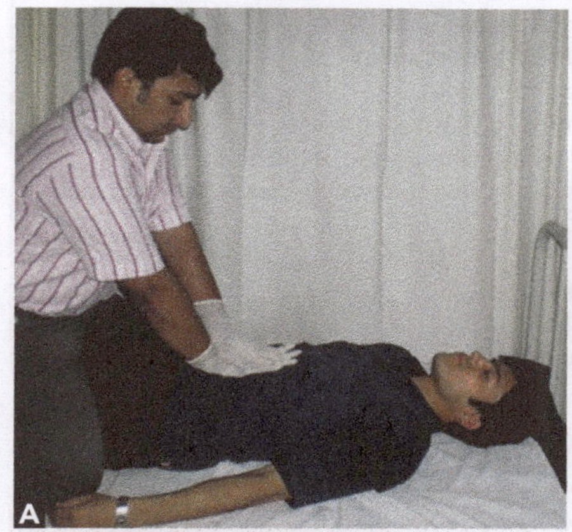

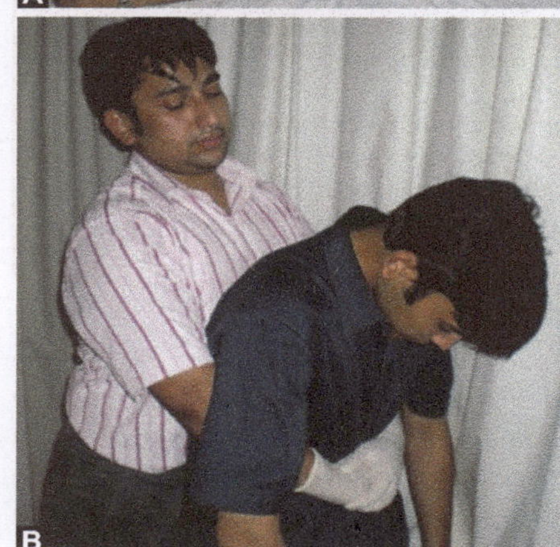

Figs 6.5A and B Abdominal thrust, Heimlich maneuver

Such accidents can be avoided by:

- Application of the rubber dam
- **Oral packing:** A pharyngeal curtain can be created by placing 4 by 4 inch gauze pad in the posterior portion of the oral cavity which effectively prevents the small particles or liquids into the airway. The pharyngeal curtain is especially useful in the patients who are sedated or have been given local anesthesia, where the protective reflexes may be compromised. This cannot be done in the patients who have exaggerated gag reflex. The pharyngeal packing is the most effective way in the patients who are intubated, to prevent the aspiration in the airway.
- **Chair position:** Trendelenburg position (head low) to prevent gravity assisted aspiration of the FB in the airway.
- Suctioning the oral cavity.
- Ligating the dental floss to the endodontic instruments to facilitate easy retrieval.

MAINTENANCE OF EMERGENCY KIT IN THE OFFICE[36] (TABLE 6.9 AND BOX 6.13)

As it has been discussed earlier in this chapter it is quite clear that the dental or minor surgical procedures are not immune to complications. The complications may not be procedure specific and can be related to vital systems of the body because we treat the patient and not the tooth. The patient may have medical compromise or underlying conditions that can precipitate a serious complication. It is necessary that every clinician should have an adequate knowledge of clinical examination; he should be able to asses and identify the clinical signs, interpret the investigations and should be able to at least suspect an abnormality so that proper evaluation and consultation is done prior to the dental therapy and complications are averted. The history taking is an art and needs practice and patience to get relevant information from the patient. This skill can be sharpened by practice only. In the Indian circumstances due to poverty and ignorance, the patients are undiagnosed and untreated for their medical disorders for years together and sometimes they are diagnosed only after a complication is precipitated. Many a times the patients feel that giving

Table 6.9: Composition of the emergency kit[37]

Sl No	Equipment	Drugs
1.	BP apparatus	Adrenaline IP 1:1000
2.	Stethoscope	Atropine sulfate
3.	Percussion hammer	Sodium hydrocortisone succinate
4.	Torch (battery)	Dextrose 25 and 50 percent
5.	Larynoscope	Aminophylline
6.	Magills intubating forcep	Dopamine
7.	Water's oropharyngeal airway	Diazepam, midazaolam
8.	Nasopharyngeal airway	Fortwin
9.	Assorted endotracheal tubes	Sodium bicarbonate
10.	Sterile gloves	Tab nitroglycerin
11.	Artery forceps	Injection nitroglycerin
12.	Needle holder	Phenergan/avil
13.	Scissors	Promethazine (perinorm)
14.	BP handle and blade	Water for injection
15.	Retractors	Furosemide (lasix)
16.	Nebulizer	Aerosol spray epinephrine, salbutamol
17.	O_2 cylinder with flow meter and humidifier	IV fluids dextrose 5 percent Ringer lactate, normal saline
18.	Pulse oxymeter	IV set
19.	AMBU bag	Scalp vein set
20.	Face mask, hood	IV cannula
21.	Tourniquet suction catheters	Disposable syringes with needles 2 mL, 5 mL, and 10 mL

Box 6.13: Norms for maintenance of the kit

- It should be freely accessible
- The place for keeping the emergency kit should be constant and should not be changed. The location should be high lighted by a placard or sign board.
- All the staff working must be oriented towards it.
- It should be periodically checked for the working condition of the equipment, shortfall in the drugs, expiry date of the drugs and prompt rectification should be made. The list of contents should be pasted a chart on the cover of the kit for the convenience of periodic inspection. When ever the drugs are used they should be immediately replaced to maintain proper inventory.

the history of medical disorders to a dental surgeon is unnecessary and if one discloses the history the concerned doctor will advice investigations and medical consultation which as per the patients point of view is unnecessary and will only delay their dental treatment. Hence, it is more important on part of a treating dental surgeon to be meticulous in history taking and in clinical examination.

In spite of due precautions, sometimes the complications occur and it is needless to say that it is the moral duty of the treating doctor to be able to give necessary first aid treatment and BLS to the patient to keep the patient safe until the competent medical help is available or the patient is shifted to the medical emergency department for the definitive treatment. It cannot be done unless the dental office is equipped with necessary life-saving equipment and the drugs. Thus every clinic must have an emergency kit and a place to resuscitate the patient (Box 6.13).

EMERGENCY DRUGS[38]

The injectable (Inj.) drugs are stored in ampules, vials or bulbs. The ampules are single dose, while as the vials or bulbs are multidose (Table 6.10).

Injection Adrenaline IP

Adrenaline tartrate is manufactured under the trademark of adrenaline. Injection of adrenaline is available in 0.5 or 1 mL ampoules, containing 1:1,000 adrenaline in water. It is the life-saving drug in dire emergencies like cardiac arrest, severe bronchospasm.

Dose

- 0.2 to 0.5 mL subcutaneously or intramuscularly.
- 0.25 mL diluted in saline, slow intravenously.
- 0.5 mL intracardiac.

Indications

- Allergic reactions, e.g. analphylactic shock, angioneurotic edema of larynx (Injection is given intramuscularly)
- Acute attack of bronchial asthma (injection is given subcutaneously)
- Cardiac arrest due to drowning, electrocution, during Stokes-Adams syndrome and hypersensitive carotid sinus. The drug is more effective in ventricular standstill. It can be given as an intracardiac injection. 0.2 to 0.3 mL of 1:1,000 adrenaline solution should be injected through a cardiac puncture, most commonly in the 4th or 5th intercostals space, 5 to 7 cm lateral to sternum. Before injecting, make sure that the tip of the needle is in the cardiac chamber by withdrawing the blood, because injection of adrenaline into cardiac muscle precipitates ventricular fibrillation which offers resistance to correction.
- **Hemostasis:** Adrenaline in a concentration of 1:10,000 to 1:20,000 is used topically to control bleeding from arterioles and capillaries, e.g. packs soaked in adrenaline solution are used to control epistaxis, bleeding after tooth extraction, capillary oozing from large raw surface after excision of a tumor, hemorrhage after hemorrhoidectomy, etc.
- **Along with local anesthetic:** To prolong the action of local anesthetic agent because of its vasoconstrictor effect, adrenaline 1:100,000 or 1:200,000 concentration is given along with local anesthetics. Adrenaline should not be used for finger block or ear lobule or for local anesthesia on

Table 6.10: Emergency drugs

Name of the drugs	Dose	Indications/uses
1. Atropine sulfate (anticholinergic)	0.6 mg IM/IV	1. Vasovagal shock 2. Prevention of bradycardia 3. Preanesthetic medication 4. To reduce salivary secretions.
2. Adrenaline tartarate 1:1000	0.5–1.0 mg IV/SC or intracardiac, to be repeated every 5 minute	1. Cardiac arrest 2. Anaphylactic shock 3. Severe laryngobrancheal spasm.
3. Dexamethasone	4–20 mg of base IM or IV 05–50 mg per day orally	1. Cereberal edema 2. Allergic conditions 3. Anti-inflammatory 4. Shock 5. Immunosuppression
4. Sodium hydrocortisone sodium succinate/hemisuccinate (short-acting glucocorticoid). TN-lycortin S.	100 mg IM/IV Stat; may be repeated once or twice	1. Shock 2. Status asthmaticus 3. Acute adrenal insufficiency 4. Anaphylactic reaction 5. Allergic reaction.
5. Pheniramine maleate. TN- avil	Orally—25–50 mg tabs 25 mg 1 tid 50 mg 1 bid ampule—1–2 mL IM 12 hrly Vial 1–2 mL IM 12 hrly	1. Allergic reactions 2. Rigors 3. Sedative 4. Anaphylactic shock 5. Angioneurotic edema.
6. Promethazine hydrochloride. TN-Phenargan	Orally, 10 mg, 2 mg tabs Injection 2 mL	1. Allergy 2. Nausea.
7. Diazepam (benzodiazepine derivative. *Note:* It should not be mixed with other drugs for IV infusion.	Orally 5–40 mg Injection 10 mg, 3–4 times IV	1. Antianxiety 2. In acute muscle spasm 3. Spastic neurological disease 4. Tetanus 5. Electroconsulsive therapy 6. Orthopedic manipulation.
8. Deriphyllin (bronchodialator). Ethophylline 169.4 mg, Theophylline 50.6 mg, per 2 mL injection.	2–4 mL. Up to 2–3 time daily IV. (2 mL in 1 minute IM and SC also; as a combined injection with dextrose).	1. Bronchial asthma 2. Cardiac insufficiency 3. Central respiratory disorder 4. Renal and cardiac edema.
9. Aminophylline (methylxanthine)	250–500 mg diluted in 20–50 mL of 5% dextrose; infuse IV over 20–30 minute repeat as required	1. Status asthmaticus.
10. Mephentermine (adrenergic drug). TN-mephentine	Orally 10–20 mg tabs or IM or IV (to prepare iv drip 2 vials of 30 mg. Each are added to 500 mL of 5% dextrose sol)	1. Shock in myocardial infarction 2. Hypotension due to spinal anesthesia 3. Other hypotensive states.
11. Dopamine(adrenergic alfa and beta agonist)	0.2–1.0 mg per minute	1. Shock cardiogenic 2. Severe congestive heart failure.
12. Frusemide. TN- lasix	Orally, 40 mg tabs. In edema 20–80 mg. Single dose daily	1. Edema in congestive heart failure 2. Hepatic or renal disease 3. Toxemia of pregnancy 4. Mild and moderate hypertension 5. Cereberal edema.
13. Isosorbide dinitrate. TN-sorbitrate	Sublingual 5–10 mg for immediate action, orally 5–10 mg 6 hourly.	1. Angina pectoris.
14. Pentazocin. TN-fortwin	Orally 50–100 mg tabs 30–60 mg IM/SC	1. Moderate to severe pain after surgery 2. Trauma, colic, burns 3. Preanesthetic medications.

Contd...

Contd...

Name of the drugs	Dose	Indications/uses
15. Metoclopramide. TN- perinorm. (more effective if combined with H2 blocker)	25–50 mg IM orally, 5–10 mg thrice daily	1. Premedication 2. Migraine 3. Antiemetic.
16. Ringer lactate	1 pint 2 pint IV	1. Dehydration 2. Burns.
17. Dextrose ampule 25–50%	1–2 amp	Hypoglycemia/Hypoglycemic shock
18. Hemaccel(plasma expander)	1 pint	Hypovolemic shock.
19. Sodium bi carbonate	1 mL mole/kg body weight 50% of dose repeated every 10–15 min IV	Metabolic acidosis.
20. Spirit of ammonia	1 drop in nose	Reflex stimulation in fainting or hysteria.
21. Normal saline	1 pint 2 pint	1. Hypo-osmolality 2. Vehicle for intravenous drug administration.
22. Oxygen	3–5 lit/min	1. Hypoxia 2. Shock 3. Cardiorespiratory failure.
23. Pethidine	50 mg IM	1. Severe pain 2. Preanesthetic medication.

the penis because there are chances of gangrene of these structures are supplied by end arteries.

- **To have bloodless field:** 1:100,000 to 1:200,000 solution is injected subcutaneously before thyroidectomy and palatal surgery.

Adverse Reactions

- Palpitation, tremors, pallor, headache.
- If injected rapidly and intravenously, adrenaline may cause sudden marked increase in blood pressure, precipitating subarachnoid hemorrhage and hamiplegia.
- Ventricular arrhythmias.
- Acute pulmonary edema in patients with cardiac decompensation.
- Anginal pain.

Injection Noradrenaline

Injection noradrenaline is available as 0.2 percent solution in 2 mL (2 mg/mL) ampules. It is inactive in neutral pH. It is a vasopressor.

Dose

2 mL of noradrenaline is added to 1000 mL of 5 percent dextrose solution (acidic) resulting in a concentration of 4 mcg/mL. After judging the response with a test done of 2 to 3 mL, solution is administered at the rate of 0.5 mL per 1 minute, according to the blood pressure response. If noradrenaline is to be used and infused in normal saline, vitamin C (500–1000 mg) should be added to make the solution acidic.

Indications

- Treatment of hypotension of circulatory failure.
- Hypotension following removal of chromaffin cell tumors.

Side Effects

- Same as for adrenaline.
- Extravasation in subcutaneous tissue causes necrosis of the skin.

Injection Dopamine

It is available in 5 mL ampoule, containing 40 mg/mL solution. It is a vasopressor given in cases of hypotension.

Dose

A 5 mL ampoule, containing a total of 200 mg solution, is added to 500 mL of normal saline or 5 percent dextrose. The solution is given by intravenous drip, commencing at the rate of 2 mcg/kg/min (one drop of this solution contains 26.66 mcg or 400 mcg in 15 drops, i.e. 1 mL) to a maximum dose of 50 mcg/kg/min or till central venous pressure (CVP) is 10 to 15 cm of water.

Dopamine drip should not be continued for more than 72 hours otherwise it will lead to tachyphylaxis.

Indications

- Hypotension with inadequate cardiac output, to increase peripheral circulation.
- Open heart surgery.
- Renal failure (renal vasodilator dose is 1–2.5 mcg/kg/min).
- Cardiac failure.
- Shock.

Precautions

- With the rate of 50 mcg/kg/min, ensure adequate urinary output.
- It should be administered via a central vein. Extravasation may cause local ischemia. If any extravasation is noted, the area should be infiltrated immediately with 10 to 15 mL of normal saline containing 5 to 10 mg

of phentolamine as soon as possible to prevent sloughing and necrosis in ischemic areas.

- Over dosage not responding to withdrawal of drip should be treated with phentolamine or other alpha-adrenergic blocking agents.
- Smaller dosage and special care are necessary in patients recently treated with monoamine oxidase (MAO) inhibitors.
- Dopamine should not be added to sodium bicarbonate or other alkaline intravenous agents.
- Dopamine should not be withdrawn spontaneously as due to the development of dopamine dependence, sudden withdrawl leads to severe hypotension.

Contraindications

- Pheochromocytoma.
- Uncorrected cardiac tachyarrhythymias.
- Ventricular fibrillation.

Stop or decrease the dosage, if

- Urine output is diminishing.
- There is increase in tachycardia.
- There is development of new arrhythmias.

Injection Propranolol

It is available in 1 mg/mL ampules. It is nonselective beta blocker.

Indications

- **Thyrotoxic crisis:** Along with other measures, e.g. hydrocortisone, cooling measures, intravenous fluids, etc. Propranolol (intravenous) injection 2 to 10 mg is given slowly with cardiac ECG (electrocardiogram) monitoring and is repeated every 4 hours.
- **Pheochromocytoma:** Alpha-adrenergic blocking agents to reduce blood pressure in pheochromocytoma may lead to severe tachycardia, giving propranolol 1 to 5 mg intravenously controls this complication. However, beta-blockade may lead to severe hypertension in pheochromocytoma.
- Cardiac arrhythmias.
- Acute myocardial infarction (effusion bradycardia).
- Antihypertensive.

Side Effects

- Congestive heart failure (CHF), bradycardia, aggravation of A-V conduction defects.
- Bronchospasm.
- Hypoglycemia unresponsiveness.
- Nausea and vomiting.
- Uterine hypomotility and prolonged labor.
- Thrombocytopenia and leukopenia.

Injection Atropine Sulphate

- **0.65 mg/mL (1 mL) ampules:**
  - As a preanesthetic medication, intramuscularly, 30 minutes before surgery to prevent vasovagal shock and also to dry out the secretions if general anesthesia is to be given.
  - Before pleural taping, ascetic taping, intercostals tube insertion, etc.
  - In treatment of colics and dysmenorrhea, along with morphine
  - Bradyarrhythmias.
  - Parkinsonism—to relieve tremors and rigidity.
- **6 mg/mL (1 mL) ampules:** In the treatment of organophosphorus poisoning, 2 to 4 mg atropine sulphate is injected by slow intravenous injection. More atropine is given depending upon the severity of intoxication and response to first dose to maintain full atropinization. In severe cases the dose is repeated at 5 to 10 minute intervals. The patient's respiration, blood pressure, pulse and salivation should be observed to prevent over-atropinization. The pulse rate should not be allowed to exceed 120/min.
- As a preanesthetic medication to prevent bradycardia and reduce secretions.

Side Effects

- Reduction in salivation, leading to dry mouth and dysphagia.
- Retention of urine.
- Blurring of vision and precipitation of glaucoma in elderly patients.
- Skin rash and local dermatitis.

Precautions

- In the elderly, the drug precipitates glaucoma and causes retention of urine
- In chronic lung diseases it dries up secretions.

Injection Hydrocortisone

Hydrocortisone hemisuccinate powder is available in a bulb containing 100 mg hydrocortisone, reconstituted with 2 mL of water for injection. It is a short-acting glucocorticoid usually preferred for immediate action in emergencies. It lacks mineralocorticoid action.

Indications

- Life-threatening emergencies, e.g. anaphylactic shock, status asthmaticus, hypoglycemia, thyrotoxic crisis, Addision's crisis, hypercalcemia, etc.
- Intra-articularly in osteoarthritis, painful fascial nodules, etc.
- Topically injected in the treatment of keloids.
- As retention enema, 100 mg hydrocortisone dissolved in 120 mL of normal saline is given each night in the treatment of ulcerative colitis.
- Delays wound healing.

Injection Aminophylline

This drug is available in a 10 mL ampule (250 mg/10 mL). It is potent bronchodilator.

Dose

250 mg diluted in 20 mL of 10 percent glucose is injected intravenously and very slowly or given in 5 percent dextrose drip. It is not given undiluted and fast as it can produce severe cardiac arrhythmias. The monitoring of pulse during the administration is very important.

Indications

- Bronchial asthma.
- Cardiac asthma.

- Cheyne-Stokes respiration. Injection may be followed by an intravenous infusion at the rate of 1 mg/kg/h to maintain therapeutic level or injection can be repeated after every 4 hours.

Side Effects

- Nausea, vomiting.
- Epileptiform fits, preceded by twitching of mouth or severe hyperventilation.
- Can precipitate cardiac arrhythmias by virtue of its beta agonist action.
- Collapse and death.

Injection Morphine

It is available in a 1 mL ampule, containing the solution with a concentration of 15 mg/mL. It is natural, potent opioid analgesic.

Dose

5 to 20 mg subcutaneously or intramuscularly. It raises pain threshold and also causes peripheral vasodilation, causing shifting of blood from pulmonary to peripheral vasculature reducing cardiac work and pulmonary pressure.

Indications

- As an analgesic, e.g. in colic (given along with atropine) and myocardial infarction.
- As a preanesthetic medications
- In acute left ventricular failure.

Side Effects

- Hypotension.
- Respiratory depression.
- Drug dependence.
- Urinary retention.
- Tolerance.
- It causes miosis and bradycardia and thus not indicated in head injury.

Injection Pethidine (Meperidine)

It is available in a 2 mL ampule containing the solution with concentration of 50 mg/mL. It is synthetic opioid analgesic.

Dose

50 to 100 mg intramuscularly or intravenously, but slowly.

Indications

Same as morphine except acute left ventricular failure (IVF).

Side Effects

Same as morphine.

Injection Diazepam

Injection diazepam is available in a 1 mL ampule containing 5 mg/mL solution; also available as 10 mL bulp (5 mg/mL). it is anxiolytic, sedative and muscle relaxant.

Dose

5 to 10 mg intravenously or intramuscularly.

Action

- As muscle relaxant in tetanus.
- As preanesthetic medication.
- **In the treatment of convulsions:** Psychomotor epilepsy and status epilepticus.
- As tranquilizers.

Injection Diphenylhydantoin

The 2 mL ampule containing 5 mg/mL solution available for intravenous use only.

Dose

Intravenous dose should not exceed 50 mg/min. It should not be given intramuscularly and should not be given in 5 percent dextrose (acidic solution). Drug precipitates in acidic pH.

Action

It inhibits spread of seizure discharge in brain by decreasing intraneuronal sodium. It restores the balance between excitatory glutamate pathway and inhibitory gamma aminobutyric acid (GABA) pathway. It does not sedate the patient.

Indications

- Convulsions of grand mal epilepsy and status epilepticus.
- Focal seizures in head injury.
- Cardiac arrhythmias, espically digitalis induced cardiac arrhythmias.
- Chorea.
- Trigeminal neuralgia.

Side Effects

- Intolerance.
- Cerebellar ataxia.
- Nausea, vomiting.
- Gum hypertrophy on prolonged use.
- Megaloblastic anemia, lymphadenopathy, osteoporosis.

Injecton Avil (Pheniramine Maleate)

It is an antihistaminic. It is available in 1 mL ampoule containing 22.75 mg/mL solution.

Action

It inhibits the action of histamine release on gastrointestinal tract, uterus and blood vessels, but no effect on bronchospasm, hypotension and gastric secretion.

Indications

- Allergic reaction, e.g. drip rigor, blood transfusion rigors, drug reactions like urticaria, etc.
- Pruritus.
- Hypnotic.

Side Effects

- Sedation, lassitude, fatigue.
- Dryness of mouth, blurring of vision.
- Nausea, vomiting, epigastric distress.
- Blood dyscrasias.

Injection Promethazine Hydrochloride (Phenergan)

It is an antihistaminic and tranquilizer. Ampules of 2.5 percent solution containing 30 mg/mL.

Indications

- Same as for avil.
- As hypnotic.
- As a preanesthetic medication.
- Lytic cocktail to produce hypothermia. The cocktail is prepared from the following drugs and mixture is

injected intravenously in fractional doses:

Promethazine	50 mg
Chlorpromazine	50 mg
Pethidine (meperidine)	100 mg

Injection Insulin

Plain insulin is available in a concentration of 40 units per mL in 10 mL bulb.

Dose

For diabetic ketoacidotic coma, 10 to 15 units intravenous bolus, followed by 5 to 6 units/h or add 100 to 120 units of insulin to 1000 mL of isotionic saline. The solution is given at the rate of 10 drops/min (40–50 mL/h). Reduce the rate by 50 percent once blood glucose comes down to 250 mg percent.

Indications

- Diabetic ketoacidotic coma.
- Glucose insulin drip in hyperkalemia
- Positive Hollander's test-following vagotomy, to test for achlorhydria (completeness of vagotomy). Insulin should be given in a dose of 0.2 unit/kg body weight.
- Other Indications
  - Treatment of diabetes, IDDM, NIDDM with secondary failure, pregnancy with diabetes, surgery of diabetes and complication of diabetes mellitus.
  - Insulin shock for the treatment of schizophrenia.

Side Effect

Hypoglycemia.

Injection Sodium Bicarbonate

Injection sodium bicarbonate is available in 10 mL ampule containing 7.5 percent solution (1 mL contains 1 mmol of sodium bicarbonate). It is buffering agent given in cases of metabolic acidosis.

Dose

To calculate the amount of bicarbonate to correct a base deficit/acidosis; it is assumed that the normal bicarbonate concentration in blood is 26 mmol/L and that the extracellular fluid volume is 20 percent of mean body weight.

Sodium bicarbonate dose in mEq/L = 0.5 × wt in kg × (Desired HCO_3 – Actual HCO_3)

Arbitrarily it can be given in a dose of 1 mEq/kg of body weight/min of hypoxia. Over correction of the acidosis is not recommended as it suppresses the hypoxic drive of respiration.

This drug is used in the treatment of metabolic acidosis.

- Lactic acidosis following D-C shock during cardioversion
- Respiratory acidosis (severe)
- Hyperkalemia.

Side Effects

- Metabolic alkalosis.
- Edema due to sodium retention.

Injection Lasix (Furosemide)

This drug is prepared from furosemide which is also called furosemide or fursemide. Its concentration is 10 mg/mL and 2 mL ampules are available containing 20 mg solution. It acts on the loop of Henley and prolonged use may result in potassium deplition and hypokalemia.

Dose

20 to 40 mg intravenously or intramuscularly.

Indications

- In the treatment of pulmonary edema (given intravenously).
- To induce forced diuresis in the treatment of barbiturate poisoning.
- In the treatment of mannitol-resistant acute oliguria.
- Advanced renal failure.
- In prostatectomy, while closing the urinary bladder and postoperatively, after 4 hours to induce diuresis and thus to prevent clot retention.

Side Effects

- When used unintelligently, Lasix can precipitate serious water and electrolyte disturbances due to excessive loss of sodium (Na), potassium (K), Chloride (Cl) and water, leading to weakness, fatigue, dizziness and cramps.
- Orthostatic hypotension.
- Rapid diuresis in elderly patients may precipitate into retention of urine.
- It can cause hepatic coma in the presence of liver disease.
- Cardiac arrest can occur after intravenous injection.
- Hearing loss, if large doses of furosomide are used in a patient with severe renal failure.

Injection Mannitol

Injection mannitol is a sugar (polyhydroxyaliphatic alcohol) and is available as 20 percent solution in a 350 mL glass bottle. It is an osmotic diuretic.

Dose

10 to 20 percent solution should be infused rapidly in 15 to 20 minutes in a dose of 0.5 to 1 g/kg body weight, but infusion rate should not be more than 3 g/min.

Action

When injected intravenously, mannitol is not metabolized, but rapidly filtered by the glomeruli. Being nonabsorbable, it exerts considerable activity which interferes with the back diffusion of water and reabsorption of sodium in the tubules, causing osmotic diuresis. To be effective, mannitol has to be administered rapidly in sufficiently large doses.

Indications

- To induce diuresis in case of barbiturate poisoning, to increase the urinary elimination of barbiturate.
- Any condition of threatened acute oliguric renal failure from prerenal causes (severe gastroenteritis). In such cases, prior correction of hypovolemia with adequate amount of fluids is necessary. If urine flow rate increases to 100 mL/h more mannitol is given to maintain the high urine flow rate. If no diuresis occurs after the initial mannitol infusion. Patient should be treated for acute renal failure and no more mannitol should be given.
- Preoperatively at the time of certain operations (e.g. aortic surgery, surgery in deeply jaundiced patient) to prevent acute renal failure.

- After severe traumatic injuries and in hemolytic transfusion reactions to prevent renal failure.
- To reduce intracranial tension and to treat cerebral edema, e.g. after cerebrovascular accident (CVA), head injury, hepatic encephalopathy.

Precautions

- Mannitol should be used with caution in a patient with decompensated heart.
- It should not be used in a patient with head injury before confirming or ruling out the subdural or intracerebral hematoma by CAT (Computerized axial tomography) scan, etc. but can be used in rapidly deteriorating patient, to buy time for transfer of the patient to neurosurgical hospital or for special investigations even when diagnosis is not confirmed.
- Potassium chloride, 10 to 20 mEq and sodium bicarbonate may be added to mannitol depending upon blood chemistry report.
- There should not be extravascular leakage.
- Intravenous (IV) set should either be flushed with isotonic saline or changed when mannitol is followed by blood.
- Mannitol infusion should be monitored with serum osmolality and it should not be given if serum osmolality is more than or equal to 320 mOsmol/L.

Adverse Reactions

- Precipitates CHF in a patient with decompensated heart.
- When used repeatedly fluid overload occurs in a patient with established acute renal failure. Maximum dose should not exceed 20 g/h. Infusion can be repeated after 6 hours, provided proper fluid and electrolyte balance is maintained.

Contraindication

Mannitol should not be used in a patient with shock, cardiac failure and established renal impairment.

Injection Mephentine

It is prepared from mephentermine sulfate, 1 mL ampule contains 15 mg/mL solution and 10 mL vial contains 30 mg/mL solution. It is a vasopressor.

Indications

- Hypotension secondary to spinal anesthesia (SA), e.g. in a patient undergoing cesarean section.

  Dose: 15 to 45 mg intravenously in a single injection. The dose is repeated if necessary; or intravenous infusion of 0.1 percent mephentine in 5 percent dextrose. Rate and duration of drip should be regulated by the patient's response.
- Prevention of hypotension attendant to SA or surgical procedures and hypotension that occurs or occurring in recovery room.

  Dose: 30 to 45 mg, intramuscularly or intravenous infusion of 0.1 percent mephentine in 5 percent.

Precautions

- Should be used cautiously in patients taking MAO inhibitors or hypertensive patients.
- When shock is primarily due to loss of blood or fluid, circulating blood volume replacement is done first.

Contraindication

Hypotension caused by phenothiazines.

Injection Potassium chloride

Available in 10 mL Ampule containing 150 mg/mL of KCl.

Dose

Simplest method is to add 1 g of KCl to 500 mL of fluid being infused. Each gram of KCl is equivalent to 13.4 mmol of K^+; 4 g of KCl per day is sufficient to prevent depletion. Not more than 20 mmol should usually be given in 2 hours and each 500 mL fluid infused should never have more than 1.5 g of KCl (40 mmol/liters added to it).

Indication

Hypokalemia.

Side Effect

Cardic arrest, if excessive dose is given rapidly. Cardiac rhythm monitoring is indicated during the administration.

Injection Lignocaine

Injection lignocaine is prepared under the trademark of Xylocard 2 percent. The 2 percent lignocaine HCl, 5 mL vial for dilution in drip infusion. Each milliliter of solution contains lignocaine anhydrous 20 mg.

Dose

- In cardiac arrhythmia, 50 to 100 mg administered as 2.5 to 5 mL of 20 percent lignocaine over a period of 2 minutes, followed by intravenous infusion at the rate of 1 to 2 mg/min, according to the need to the patient (add one 50 mL vial of 2% lignocaine to 500 mL of infusion solution).
- In congestive cardiac failure, shock or renal insufficiency, dose should be reduced to 0.5 to 1 mg/min.
- Intravenous drip should be given for 2 or 3 days or at least for 24 hours.
- If overdose occurs (as shown by prolongation of PQ or widening of QRS and QT complex), the drip rate should be reduced.

Indications

Ventricular arrhythmia (not supraventricular arrhythmia), multiple extrasystoles and tachycardia in connection with:

- Myocardial infarction
- During cardiac surgery
- Diagnostic procedures, e.g. cardiac catheterization and angiocardiography.

Contraindications

- Atrioventricular (AV) block of all degrees.
- Bradycardia
- Patient with a known history of hypersensitivity to local anesthetic or amide group of drugs.

Precautions

- Lower doses are used in cases of severe liver damage and effect is watched carefully.

- Care must be taken in cases of pronounced renal insufficiency.
- Treatment with lignocaine should not be performed without ECG control.
- Too rapid infusion may be lethal.

Injection Calcium Gluconate

Available in 10 mL ampules containing 10 percent w/v calcium gluconate (1 g).

Dose

- In tetany, 2 g intravenous injection is given slowly and repeated if necessary.
- After each 1000 mL of blood transfusion, 1 g is injected intravenously.
- In epididymo-orchitis, 1 g is given intravenously and slowly at 8 hours intervals. The role is yet controversial. Cardiac arrhythmias can be precipitated during the administration of this drug and thus critical monitoring is warrented.

Indications

- Tetany.
- After 1000 mL of blood transfusion.
- As an inotropic drug in cardiac arrest.
- Hypoparathyroidism.
- As a coagulant (Factor V).

Bupivacaine (Sensorcaine)

It is a new local analgesic drug. It is 4 times more potent than lignocaine. It has longer duration of action of about 5 to 6 hours.

Dose

2 mg/kg.

Preparations—Inj bupivacaine 0.5 percent.

Calculation of Dose of Drug for Children

Child dose = Age/(age + 12) × Adult dose (Young's formula).

Child dose = Age/20 × Adult dose (Dilling's formula).

REFERENCES

1. Glick G, Y U PN. Haemodynamic changes during spontaneous Vasovagal reactions. Am J Med. 1963;34:42.
2. Leonard M. An approach to some dilemmas and complications of office oral surgery. Aust Dent J. 1995;40(3).
3. Martin GJ, et al. Prospective evaluation of syncope Ann Emerg Med. 1984;13: 499.
4. Cutino SR. Vasovagal Syncope associated with seizure activity Gen Dent. 1994;42(4).
5. Fried berg CK. Syncope: Pathological physiology, differential diagnosis and treatment. Mod concepts Cardiovasc Dis. 1971;40:55.
6. Leonard M. Syncope: treating fainting in the dental office. Dent Today. 1996;15(1).
7. Webb WR et al. Cardiovascular responses in acute adrenal insufficiency Surgery. 1965;58:273.
8. Addison T. On the constitution and the local effects of diseases of the suprarenal capsules. London: Samuel Highly, 1855.
9. Zaloga GP, Marik P. Hypothalamic-pituitary-adrenal insufficiency. Crit Care Clin. 2001;17:25-41.
10. Guyton AC. The adrenocortical hormones. In human physiology and mechanism of disease, 5th edition. Philadelphia, WB Saunders, 1992.
11. Streeten DHP. Corticosteroid therapy. II. Complications and therapeautic indications. JAMA. 1975;232:1046.
12. Hickler RB. Ortostatic hypotension and syncope, N Engl J Med. 1977;296:336.
13. Olefsky JM. Diabetes mellitus. In: Bennett JC, Plum F (Eds). Cecil Textbook of medicine, 4th edition. Philadelphia: WB Sanders; 1996.
14. University group diabetes programe. Effects of hypoglycaemic agents on vascular complications in patients with adult onset diabetes II. Mortality results Diabetes. 1970;19:785.
15. Barkin RM, Rosen P. Hypoglycemia. Editors: Emergency Paediatrics: A Guide to ambulatory care, 4th edition. St Louis: Mosby; 1994.
16. Owen OE, et al. Pathogenesis and diagnosis of Diabetes mellitus. In: Rose LF, Kaye D (Eds). Internal medicine for dentistry, 2nd edition, St Louis, 1992.
17. Patel JC, Despande PS. Diabetes mellitus. The cause of death: its ranking. Indian J Med Sci. 1977;31:150.
18. Skyler JS. Complications of Diabetes mellitus: Relationship to metabolic dysfunctions, Diabetes care. 1979;2: 499.
19. Little JW, Fallace DA. Diabetes. In: Little JW, Fallace DA (Eds). Dental management of medically compromised patients, 4th edn. St Louis: Mosby; 1994.
20. Kitabchi AE, Wall BM. Diabetic ketoacidosis, Med Clin North Am. 1995;79:9.
21. Nabarro JD. Diabetes in UNITED KINGDOM: A personal series, Diabetic med. 1991;8(1).
22. Raskin P. Treatment of Insulin dependent Diabetes mellitus with portable insulin infusion devices, Med Clin North Am. 1982;66:1269.
23. American heart association: Coronary heart disease and Angina pectoris, Dallas, 1998, American heart association.
24. AHA Scientific position: Sudden cardiac death, Dallas, 1998, American heart association.
25. Cummins RO, Eisenberg MS:Prehospital cardiopulmonary resuscitation: is it effective? JAMA. 1985;253:2408.
26. Orlowski JP. Optimal position for external cardiac massage in infants and children, Crit Care Med. 1984;12:224.
27. Eisenberg MS, Hallstrom A, Bergner L. The ACLS score predicting survival from out of hospital cardiac arrest, JAMA. 1981;246:50.
28. Eisenberg MS and others. Defibrillation by emergency medical technicians, Crit Care Med. 1985;13:921.

29. Caranasos GJ. Drug reactions in Schwartz GR and others, Editors: Principles and practice of emergency medicines Philadelphia, WB Saunders;1978.
30. Pallasch TJ. Principles of pharmacotherapy. V. Toxicology and adverse drug reactions. Anesth Prog. 1989; 36(2):41–45.
31. Arthur GR. Pharmacokinetics of local anaesthetics. In Stri chartz GR, (Ed): Lpcal anaesthetics, Handbook of experimental pharmacology, Vol 81, Berlin, 1987, Springer - Verlag 1987;81.
32. Paul A Moore. Pharmacokinetics of Lidocaine With Epinephrine Following Local Anesthesia Reversal With Phentolamine Mesylate. Anesth Prog. 2008;55(2):40–48.
33. Heimlich HJ. A Life saving maneuver to prevent food choking. JAMA. 1975;234: 398.
34. American heart association and national academy of sciences, National research council: standards and guidelines for CPR and emergency cardiac care. JAMA. 1980;244:453.
35. American heart association and national academy of sciences, National research council: standards and guidelines for CPR and emergency cardiac care. JAMA. 1992;268(16).
36. Malamed SF. Managing medical emergencies. J Am Dent Assoc. 1993;1240.
37. American Dental association: ADA guide to dental therapeutics, Chicago. The association, 1998.
38. Goodman, Gillman's the pharmacological basis of therapeutics, 9th edition. New York. Mcgraw Hill; 1996.

7 Management of Airway in Maxillofacial Surgery

Borle Rajiv M

The oral cavity constitutes the upper part of the aerodigestive tract. The pathologies and the surgeries performed in this area have direct bearing on the airway. A specialized care of the patient is required, while managing the pathologies of the orofacial region to maintain patency of the airway and to prevent airway complications. The chances of aspiration of secretions or blood or foreign bodies in the airway are enhanced during the transoral procedures or the procedures carried out in the nasal or pharyngeal areas. Similarly the handling of this area can enhance the chances of airway obstruction due to edema secondary to surgical handling. There are certain conditions in which there is pronounced trismus and the laryngoscopy is not possible and an alternative access is required to be created to the airway for maintaining its patency, like an endotracheal intubation for administration of the anesthesia and for subsequent airway care. A sound knowledge of the respiratory passage, its anatomy and physiology and the thorough understanding of causes and management of respiratory obstructive conditions are of paramount importance to a maxillofacial surgeon.

The most common cause of respiratory obstruction in an unconscious patient, irrespective of the cause of unconsciousness, is the tongue fall. Hence, even after minor surgical procedures of short duration under general anesthesia the patency of airway is required to be maintained by preventing the tongue fall. The tongue fall is more common in an unconscious patient, who has bilateral parasymphysis fracture of the mandible or who has undergone mandibular resection across the midline.

During severe trauma to the facial skeleton, the fracture segments get displaced posteriorly and cause impingement and narrowing of the airway. Severe bleeding from the fracture sites, presence of clots in the nasal cavity, oral cavity and pharynx and the foreign bodies like avulsed teeth are likely to be aspirated in the tracheobronchial tree, if the airway is not properly guarded. As the inflammatory edema sets in, the airway is further compromised leading to airway obstruction. The facial fractures are usually associated with head injury and the patients are often semiconscious/unconscious and the relative risk of aspiration, acute respiratory obstruction, bronchospasm or pneumonitis are enhanced. The traumatized brain has reduced tolerance to hypoxia and thus any hypoxic environment secondary to airway obstruction can worsen the head injury by inducing irreversible hypoxic brain injury.

The routine endotracheal intubation is not possible in cases of cervical spine fractures. So, to maintain the patency of airway, sometimes an alternative access to the airway is created (cricothyroidectomy or tracheostomy).

The airway complications are also known to happen in the patients with severe maxillofacial infections like Ludwig's angina or sublingual space infection. The laryngeal edema is the common complication secondary to these conditions. Similarly the conditions like cervical necrotizing fasciitis can also cause airway edema. When the cervicofacial infections extend to the mediastinum by either the anterior or posterior facial planes, can cause severe respiratory complications due to sepsis.

The conditions like temporomandibular joint (TMJ) ankylosis, oral submucous fibrosis, etc. are characterized by severe trismus. While performing surgeries on such a patient it is a challenging task to intubate these patients for administration of the general anesthesia and for guarding the airway, as laryngoscopy is also not possible. In such patients either blind nasal intubation, retrograde intubation or fiberoptic bronchoscope guided endotracheal intubation is required. If such facilities are not available or fail then alternative procedures like tracheostomy are required for securing the airway.

After ablative surgical procedures like major head and neck cancer resection the patient requires prolonged anesthesia and prolonged intubation postoperatively. Such patients might also require ventilatory assistance for some time. As the patients are nonambulatory the lower airway care is also imperative, hence to facilitate the maintenance of patency of respiratory passage, to alleviate the respiratory dead space and to facilitate the tracheobronchial suctions to clear the secretions, tracheostomy is preferred over the conventional endotracheal intubation.

In short the knowledge of airway anatomy, physiology and modalities to maintain its patency is of great importance to the clinician in general and a maxillofacial surgeon, in particular. Airway management happens to be the first and the foremost life saving priority in the management of any emergency.

MAINTENANCE OF AIRWAY[1]

Jaw Thrust Chin Lift Maneuver

Jaw thrust chin lift maneuver is an important procedure to prevent the airway obstruction due to tongue fall in an unconscious patient or a patient recovering from general anesthesia. First the upper airway is cleared of saliva, mucous, blood, foreign bodies like fragments, teeth, denture, etc. The neck is then extended, mandibular angles pushed anteriorly and the chin lifted up. This procedure shifts the posterior one-third of the tongue and soft palate away from the posterior pharyngeal wall. The head may be turned on one side, so that the secretions accumulate on the dependent area and the airway is patent (Figs 7.1 and 7.2). To prevent aspiration of the secretions, vomitus or blood into the lower airway, patient may be put into head low position.

Insertion of Airway

Insertion of oropharyngeal or nasopharyngeal airway prevents tongue fall (Figs 7.3A to C). The Water's oropharyngeal airway is inserted transorally. The airway occupies the space between the tongue and the posterior pharyngeal wall and through the lumen of the airway the patient can breathe. The airway has multiple holes. This is to ensure that, if some holes are blocked due to contact with the mucosa or due to mucoid secretions, the patient can still breathe through the remaining patent holes. There is a stellate in the airway which ends short of the length of the airway and does not extend to the other open end (pharyngeal end) of the airway. It is basically meant for administering oxygen to the patient by attaching a catheter to it. As it is short, the stellate cannot be used for sucking out the secretions in the airway. If the airway is blocked due to secretions, a thin rubber catheter is passed through the main opening in the body of the airway to carry out suction.

The nasopharyngeal airway is smaller in diameter than the oropharyngeal airway and it is much smaller in length than the endotracheal tube, as it reaches only up to the hypopharynx. It serves the same purpose as the oropharyngeal airway. It is more suitable, if the airway is required to be maintained in place for longer time and can be secured with adhesive tapes. It is better tolerated by the patients than the oropharyngeal airway. The only disadvantage is that being smaller in diameter it can get blocked due to secretions and needs periodic suctioning to prevent

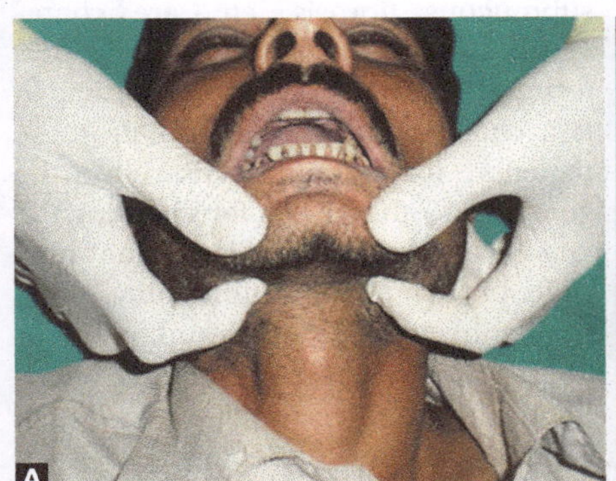

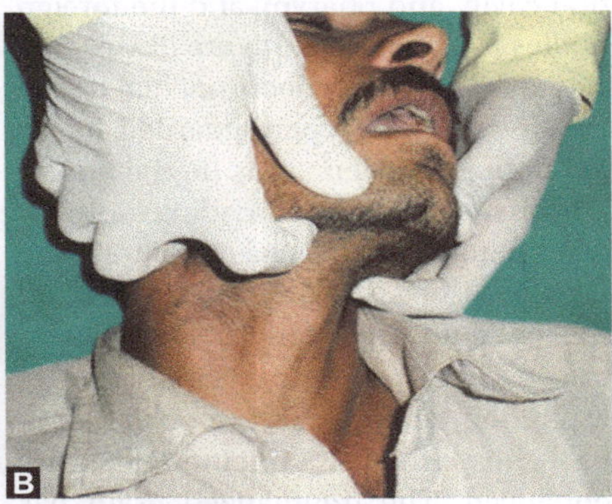

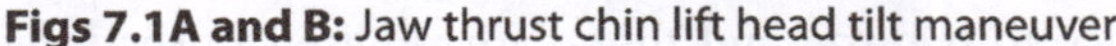
Figs 7.1A and B: Jaw thrust chin lift head tilt maneuver

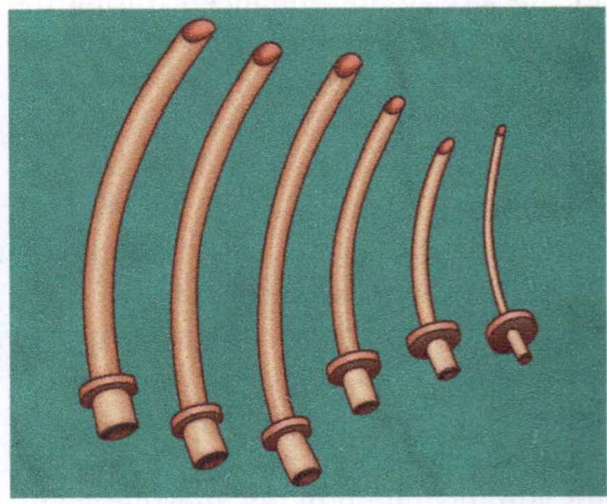
Fig. 7.2: Nasopharyngeal airway

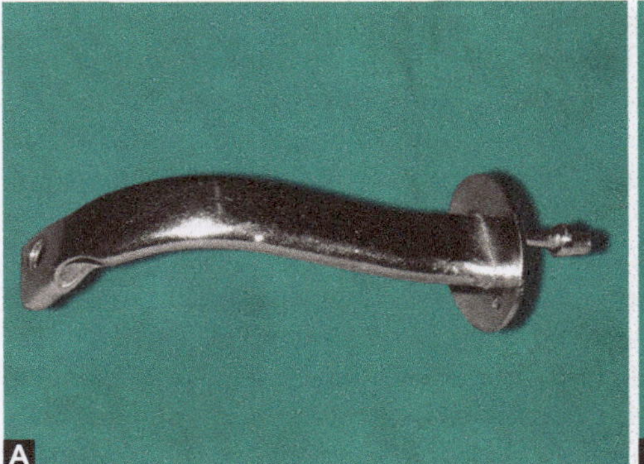

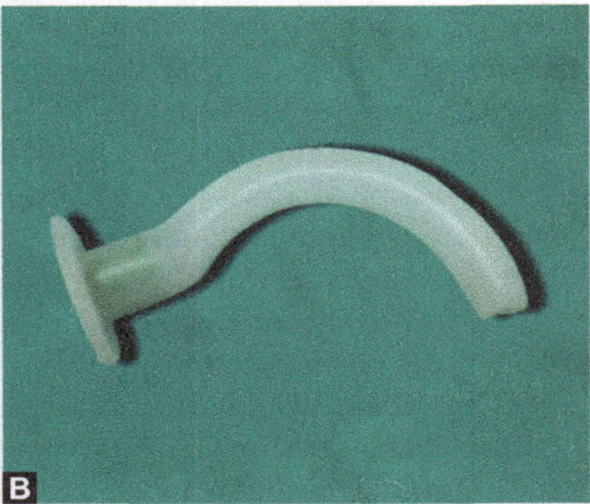

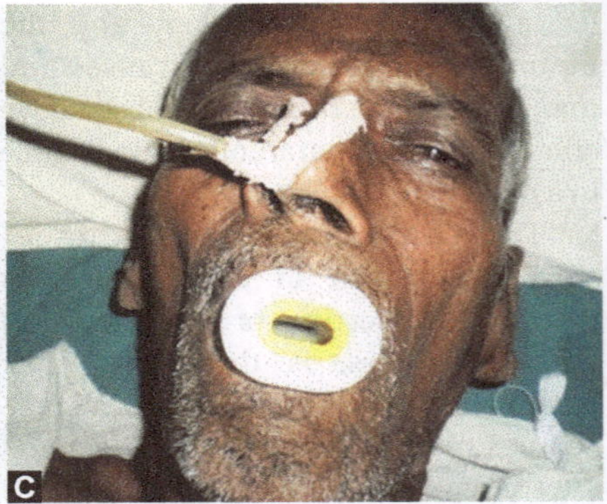

Figs 7.3A to C: (A) Metallic oropharyngeal airway; (B) PVC oropharyngeal airway; (C) Oropharyngeal airway in place

its blockade. Sometimes after the procedure under general anesthesia the endotracheal tube can be partially withdrawn, so that its tip is out of larynx in the hypopharynx and the same can be left in place as a nasopharyngeal airway till the patients recovers completely from the anesthesia.

Application of the Tongue Stitch

Application of tongue stitch horizontally through the tongue substance and drawing the tongue out also prevents tongue fall (Fig. 7.4). The tongue stitch should be given using a large round body needle and a silk thread of 1-0 size should be used. The tongue stitch is never placed vertically in the tongue as during the drawing out of tongue, the tongue may get split in midline due to tear. Both the ends of the thread are held with an artery forceps and clamped to the shirt of the patient, so that the tongue is retained in the protruding state.

Cricothyroidectomy[2]

It is the easiest and the fastest emergency procedure for maintaining the airway patency temporarily. Cricothyroid membrane is punctured with a 16 to 18 gauge hypodermic needle and maintained in position till definitive measures like tracheostomy is performed. The cricothyroidectomy is the procedure, which can be done rapidly and takes lesser time than the tracheostomy. It does not require neck extension (which is contraindicated in case of cervical spine fractures) and can be done with only a stab knife and the handle of the knife can be introduced in the slit incision and rotated to 90° to dilate the incision. A small diameter endotracheal tube is inserted to maintain the airway temporarily. The cricothyroid membrane being superficial is less prone for complications.

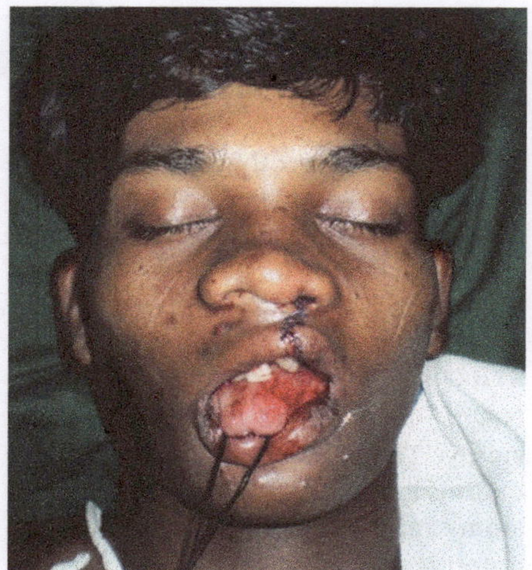

Fig. 7.4: Tongue stitch

The procedure was first described in 1805 by Vicq d'Azyr, a French surgeon and anatomist. A cricothyrotomy (also called thyrocricotomy, cricothyroidotomy, inferior laryngotomy, intercricothyrotomy, coniotomy or emergency airway puncture) is an emergency incision through the skin and cricothyroid membrane to secure a patient's airway during certain emergency situations such as an airway obstructed by a foreign object or laryngeal edema, a patient who is not able to breathe adequately on their own or in cases of major facial trauma, which prevent the insertion of an endotracheal tube through the mouth. A cricothyrotomy is usually performed as a last resort, when control of the airway by usual means (an endotracheal intubation) has failed or is not feasible. This technique is considered easier and faster than a tracheostomy and hence preferred over the tracheostomy in dire emergency. This procedure does not require manipulation of the cervical spine. Cricothyrotomy is only a temporary airway for life-saving situations. It is not suitable for prolonged ventilation due to its small size. A definitive airway (tracheostomy or endotracheal intubation) must be performed later in hospital.

Indications

- Severe facial or nasal injuries (that do not allow oral or nasal intubation).
- Massive midfacial trauma.
- Possible cervical spine trauma preventing adequate neck extension.
- Anaphylaxis.
- Chemical inhalation injuries.

Contraindications

- Inability to identify landmarks (cricothyroid membrane).
- Underlying anatomical abnormality (tumor).
- Tracheal transection.
- Acute laryngeal disease due to infection or trauma.
- Small children under 10 years of age (a 12–14 gauge catheter over the needle may be safer).

Anatomy

The cricothyroid membrane lies between the thyroid cartilage superiorly and the cricoid cartilage inferiorly. It can be felt by palpating the neck anteriorly and finding first the thyroid cartilage that is the most prominent cartilage in the neck. After that you need scroll down your index finger until you can fell the space between the thyroid and cricoid cartilages. This space is the place of the cricothyroid membrane (Fig. 7.5).

Material

- Material required for sterile technique (gloves, mask, cap and gown).
- Povidone-iodine solution for sterilizing the skin.
- Sponges.
- Drapes and rolled bath towel.
- Number 11 scalpel blade mounted on number 3 or 5 handle.
- 1 percent lidocaine without epinephrine in a 10-cc syringe with a 25-gauge needle.
- Two mosquito artery forceps or two Kelly clamps.
- Low pressure cuffed tracheostomy tube.
- A 10-cc syringe to inflate the balloon on the tracheostomy tube.
- Bag-valve-mask (*Ambu bag-airway maintenance breathing unit*) connected to a oxygen source.
- Adhesive tape.

Technique

- Arrange all the necessary equipment/instruments and test the tracheostomy tube by inflating the tube with air from 10-cc syringe. Place the material on a sterile towel placed on a Mayo stand or bedside table.

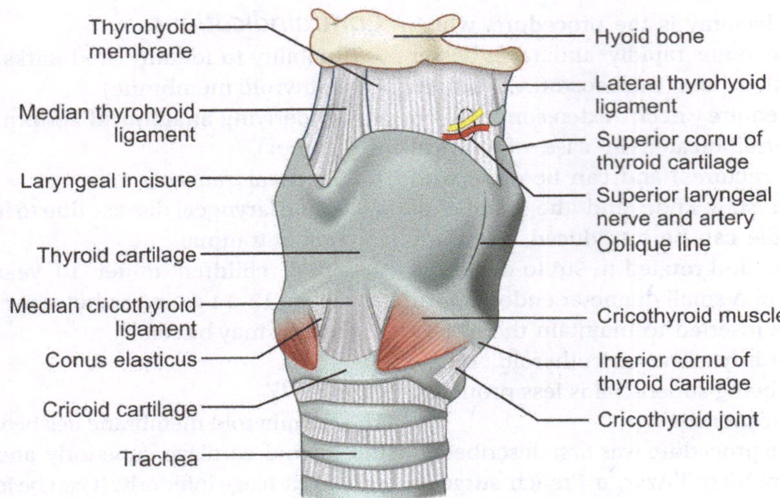

Fig. 7.5: Anatomy of laryngotracheal area

- One of the most important aspect is to position the patient. He or she should be supine, ideally a rolled towel or sand bag under the shoulders and with the neck in hyperextension. The extension of the neck is strictly contraindicated in presence of cervical spine fractures. However, in such situation, it can be performed safely without giving the neck extension or mobilization of the neck.
- Disinfect the skin from the sternal notch to chin and laterally to the base of the neck.
- Observe sterile technique.
- Identify the cricothyroid membrane as described above.
- Anesthetize the skin over the membrane using a syringe with 25-gauge needle with the 2 percent lidocaine.
- Make a transverse incision of the skin over the cricothyroid membrane using the number 11 blade (Figs 7.6A and B).
- Identify the membrane and then continue the incision through it approximately 1 cm on each side of the midline. In dire emergency, the skin and the cricothyroid membrane are incised together with a stab incision and the incision is dilated by inserting the handle of the BP knife and rotating it by 90 degrees. Or by simply introducing a wide bore (no 16) needle through the cricothyroid membrane in the trachea as an interim measure.
- With the mosquito or Kellys clamp in the left hand, insert the clamp into the incision and spread it. This is sufficient to provide an airway for a patient with supraglottic airway obstruction.
- With the right hand insert the small diameter tracheostomy tube or the orotracheal tube through the incision into the trachea, directing it caudally.
- Connect the bag-valve unit to the tube and ventilate the patient with 100 percent oxygen.
- Observe respiratory movements of the chest and auscultate for breathe sounds, which should be bilaterally equal.
- Inflate the tube balloon if cuffed tube is used to prevent aspiration of blood or secretions in the lower respiratory passage.
- Cut a sponge halfway down the middle and wrap it around the tube if an orotracheal tube is being used and then fashion a necklace to place the tube in place. If the tracheostomy tube is used, secure the wings of the tube by tying the tapes around the patient's neck. In both cases do not use the tape to tie tightly because it can cause erosion of the skin.
- Do the suction of the secretions/ blood in the trachea.
- The chest X-ray may be ordered to check the position of the tube.
- It is only an emergency procedure and if the tube is required to be maintained *in situ* for longer period tracheostomy should be performed and the cricothyroid membrane opening should be decanulated. The tracheostomy is more practical and logical option for better airway management for longer duration.

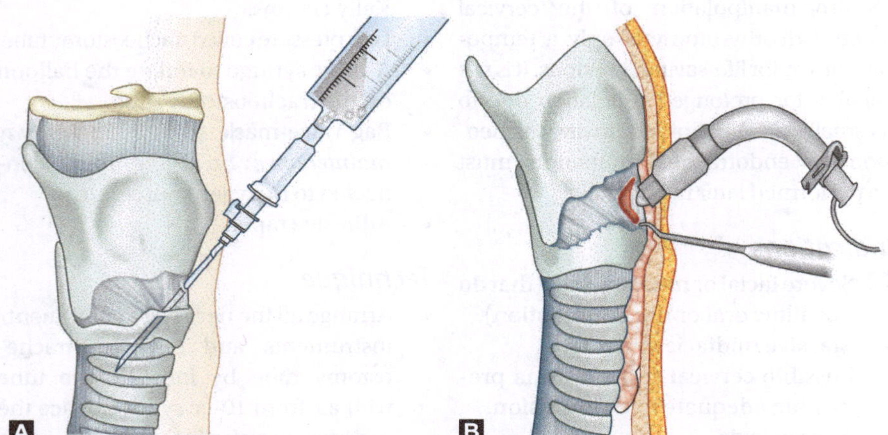

Figs 7.6A and B: Cricothyroidectomy procedure

Tracheostomy[3]

Negus[4] 1938 coined the term tracheostomy. Tracheotomy is an incision or cutting into the trachea while tracheostomy refers to a window made in the anterior wall of trachea just below the larynx. It provides an alternative airway, bypassing the upper passages. It is a lifesaving procedure and every clinician must be competent enough to perform it in emergency.

Surgical Anatomy

The trachea is membranous posteriorly and is formed of semicircular cartilaginous rings anteriorly and laterally. The spaces between the rings are membranous. The cricoid cartilage is present below the thyroid cartilage and is the only complete ring. The trachea has 16 to 20 rings. The upper tracheal rings are covered by the isthmus of the thyroid gland. The trachea extends inferiorly and posteriorly below the manubrium of the sternum and divides into two main bronchi. The point of the bifurcation is called carina. The trachea runs inferiorly and posteriorly. To make it prominent and to draw out the portion of the trachea which goes behind the sternum, the neck is needed to be extended during the tracheostomy. The esophagus is present deep to the trachea. On either side, lateral to the trachea, the carotid sheaths are present which contain the internal carotid artery, internal jugular vein and the vagus nerve. The tributaries of the internal jugular vein may cross the anterior wall of the trachea and need to be ligated during the tracheostomy. The carotid sheath is also required to be retracted laterally, during the tracheostomy to prevent damage to its contents. The strap muscles of the neck such as sternothyroid run parallel to the trachea and if vertical incision is taken for tracheostomy they are easy to retract laterally.

Applied Surgical Anatomy of Trachea

The trachea is a cartilaginous and membranous tube, extending from the lower part of the larynx, on a level with the sixth cervical vertebra, to the upper border of the fifth thoracic vertebra, where it divides into the two bronchi, one for each lung. The trachea is nearly but not quite cylindrical, being flattened posteriorly; it measures about 11 cm in length; its diameter from side-to-side is from 2 to 2.5 cm, being always greater in the males than the females. In a child the trachea is smaller, more deeply placed, and more movable than in the adults. The adult trachea measures 10 to 13 cm from cricoid cartilage to the carina (bifurcation of trachea). If the neck is extended roughly about half, this length is within the confines of the neck making surgery easy. Hence, tracheostomy is performed with the neck hyperextended. This is achieved by placing a sandbag or towel roll under the shoulder blade of the patient.

Relations

The anterior surface of the trachea is convex and covered, in the neck, from above downward, by the isthmus of the thyroid gland, the inferior thyroid veins, the arteria thyroidea ima (when that vessel exists), the sternothyroideus and sternohyoideus muscles, the cervical fascia and more superficially, by the anastomosing branches between the anterior jugular veins. In the thorax, it is covered from before backward by the manubrium sterni, the remains of the thymus, the left innominate vein, the aortic arch, the innominate and left common carotid arteries and the deep cardiac plexus. Posteriorly it is in contact with the esophagus. Laterally, in the neck, it is in relation with the common carotid arteries, the right and left lobes of the thyroid gland, the inferior thyroid arteries, and the recurrent laryngeal nerves. In the thorax, it lies in the superior mediastinum and is in relation on the right side with the pleura and right vagus and near the root of the neck with the innominate artery. On its left side is the left recurrent laryngeal nerve, the aortic arch and the left common carotid and subclavian arteries (Figs 7.7A to C). On either side, lateral to the trachea, the carotid sheaths are present which contain the internal carotid artery, internal jugular vein and the vagus nerve (Fig. 7.8).

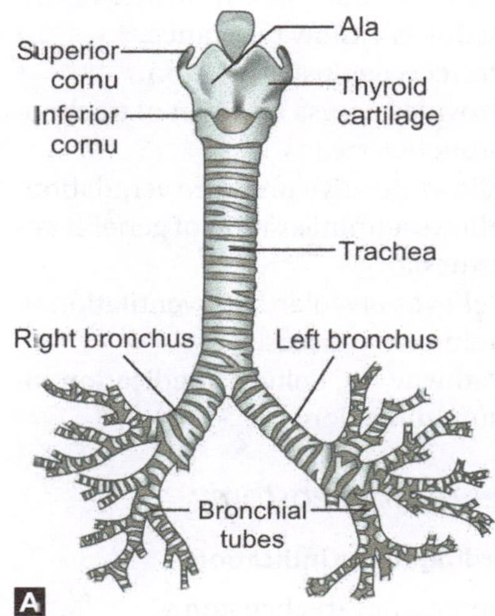

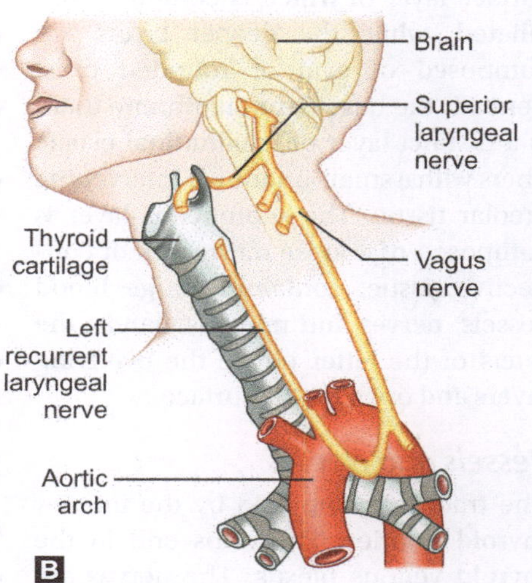

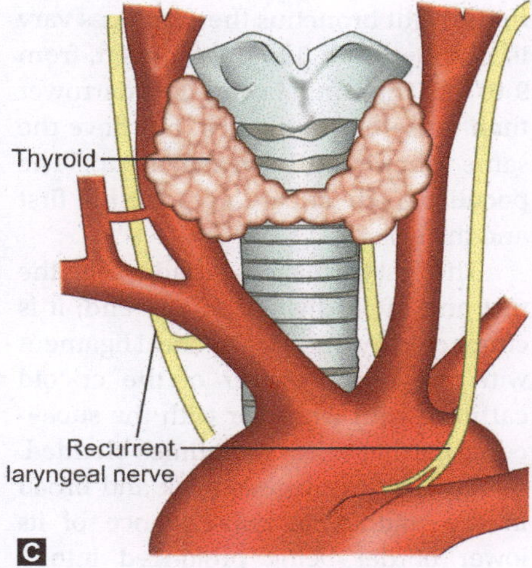

Figs 7.7A to C: Anatomy and relations of trachea

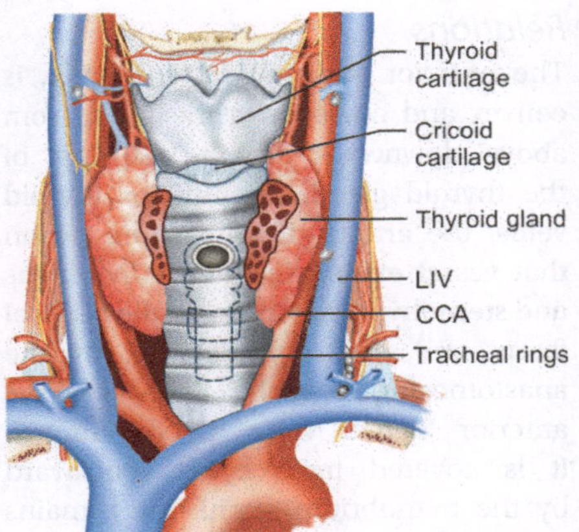

Fig. 7.8: Anatomical structures in relation to trachea

The cartilages of the trachea vary from 16 to 20 in number: each forms an imperfect ring, which occupies the anterior two-thirds or so of the circumference of the trachea, being deficient behind, where the tube is completed by fibrous tissue and unstriped muscle fibers. The cartilages are placed horizontally above each other, separated by narrow intervals. They measure about 4 mm in depth and 1 mm in thickness. Their outer surfaces are flattened in a vertical direction, but the inner surfaces are convex, the cartilages being thicker in the middle than at the margins. Two or more of the cartilages often unite, partially or completely and they are sometimes bifurcated at their extremities. They are highly elastic, but may become calcified in advanced life. In the right bronchus the cartilages vary in number from 6 to 8; in the left, from 9 to 12. They are shorter and narrower than those of the trachea, but have the same shape and arrangement. The peculiar tracheal cartilages are the first and the last.

The first cartilage is broader than the rest and often divided at one end; it is connected by the cricotracheal ligament with the lower border of the cricoid cartilage with which or with the succeeding cartilage, it is sometimes blended.

The last cartilage is thick and broad in the middle, in consequence of its lower border being prolonged into a triangular hook-shaped process, which curves downward and backward between the two bronchi. It ends on each side in an imperfect ring, which encloses the commencement of the bronchus. The cartilage above the last is somewhat broader than the others at its center.

The Fibrous Membrane

The cartilages are enclosed in an elastic fibrous membrane, which consists of two layers; one, the thicker, passing over the outer surface of the ring, the other over the inner surface: at the upper and lower margins of the cartilages the two layers blend together to form a single membrane, which connects the rings with one another. They are thus invested by the membrane. In the space behind, between the ends of the rings, the membrane forms a single layer.

The muscular tissue consists of two layers of nonstriated muscle, longitudinal and transverse. The longitudinal fibers are external and consist of a few scattered bundles. The transverse fibers (Trachealis muscle) are internal and form a thin layer which extends transversely between the ends of the cartilages.

Mucous Membrane

The mucous membrane is continuous above with that of the larynx and below with that of the bronchi. It consists of areolar and lymphoid tissue and presents a well-marked basement membrane, supporting a stratified epithelium, the surface layer of which is columnar and ciliated, while the deeper layers are composed of oval or rounded cells. Beneath the basement membrane there is a distinct layer of longitudinal elastic fibers with a small amount of intervening areolar tissue. The submucous layer is composed of a loose meshwork of connective tissue, containing large blood vessels, nerves and mucous glands; the ducts of the latter pierce the overlying layers and open on the surface.

Vessels and Nerves

The trachea is supplied by the inferior thyroid arteries. The veins end in the thyroid venous plexus. The nerves are derived from the vagus, the recurrent nerves and from the sympathetic; they are distributed to the trachealis muscles and between the epithelial cells.

At the level of thoracic inlet the trachea dives anteroposteriorly behind thymus, innominate vein and innominate artery thus complicating tracheostomy procedure in elderly.

Indications for Tracheostomy

- **Emergency:**
  - Severe laryngeal trauma.
  - Foreign body in larynx.
  - Head injury with unconsciousness is one of the most common indication.
- **Elective:**
  - Elimination of upper respiratory dead space.
  - Inflammation of larynx.
  - Laryngeal malignancy or laryngopharyngeal growth.
  - Laryngeal edema due to allergy, infection, trauma.
  - Laryngeal stenosis secondary to trauma or infection.
  - Sleep apnea.
  - Orofacial injuries.
  - Comatose patient who is put on ventilator.
  - Respiratory failure in adult and children.
- **Others:**
  - Congenital airway anomalies.

Uses of Tracheostomy

- Relieves upper airway obstruction.
- Reduces airflow resistance.
- Protects against aspiration.
- Provides access for toilet of tracheobronchial tree.
- Allows positive pressure ventilation.
- Allows administration of general anesthesia.
- Relieves alveolar hypoventilation in pulmonary disease.
- Pathway to deliver medication or humidification.

Types of Tracheostomy

According to the indication

- Emergency tracheostomy.
- Elective tracheostomy.

According to the level

- **High level tracheostomy:** It is performed above the isthmus of thyroid gland. (1st and 2nd rings).
- **Mid level tracheostomy:** At the level of isthmus (2nd and 3rd).
- **Low level tracheostomy:** Performed below the isthmus (4th to 6th).

Sizes of Tracheostomy Tube

- **Neonates to 3 months:** 4.5 to 5 mm.
- **3 to 12 months:** 5 to 5.5 mm.
- **1 to 3 years:** 5.5 to 6 mm.
- **Adults:** 8 mm.

It is being said that the size of the tracheostomy tube needed for the particular patient is roughly equal to the size of the patient's little finger.

Types of Tracheostomy Tubes

The tracheostomy tubes are available as, PVC tubes and metallic tubes (Figs 7.9 and 7.10). The PVC tubes are with or without cuff. The plain tube is used to maintain the patency of airway. Apart from the maintenance of airway, the cuffed PVC tube serves variety of other purposes like the cuff makes the tube self-retaining, seals the trachea when inflated and prevents aspiration in lower respiratory passage and general anesthesia can be administered through it. However, the basic disadvantage with the PVC tube is that it can get blocked due to thick secretions, if proper care is not taken during the postoperative phase. It is not ideal to be used if the tracheostomy is to be maintained for a long period of time (for months).

The metallic tracheostomy tube has an inner and outer tube and a stellate. It is used, when the tracheostomy is intended to be kept patent for longer period in patients of laryngectomy, head injury; comatose patients or if permanent tracheostomy is planned. The basic advantage is that as there are two tubes, the inner and the outer, the inner tube can be removed and cleaned intermittently, during such periods the outer tube is left indwelling to maintain the patency of airway and thus the chances of blockade are less. The patients can be educated and can do the cleaning themselves at home.

Technique

Keep ready the sterilized standard tracheostomy tray/set, which should be present in every ward (Fig. 7.11). The neck should be extended by placing the sandbags below the shoulder to make the trachea prominent (Figs 7.12A and B). In emergency tracheostomy, a vertical incision is placed in the midline below the thyroid cartilage (Fig. 7.13). As all strap muscles of the neck are placed vertically, it is easy to retract them if vertical incision is taken. In the emergency situations, as the tracheostomy is to be performed in the shortest possible time it is not desirable to do layer-by-layer dissection, but with one or two strokes of the knife the trachea is exposed. In dire emergency cricothyroidectomy is a faster and safer alternative to open the airway and after the airway is secured, the tracheostomy be done.

In the elective tracheostomy the incision is taken horizontally to hide the scar in neck creases for cosmetic reasons (Figs 7.14A and B). After infiltrating the area with 2 percent lidocaine with adrenaline, skin incision is made. The deeper dissection is done by incising the deeper layers one-by-one and retracting them using atraumatic Langenbeck retractors. Care must be taken to avoid damage to the common carotid artery or internal jugular veins, the vagus and the

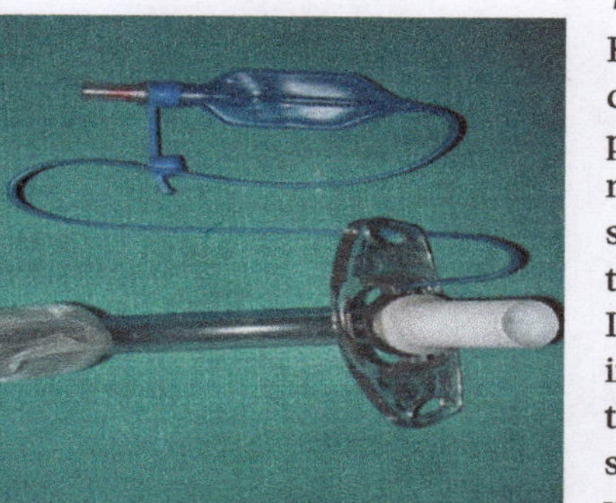

Figs 7.9A and B: PVC tracheostomy tubes: (A) Noncuffed; (B) Cuffed

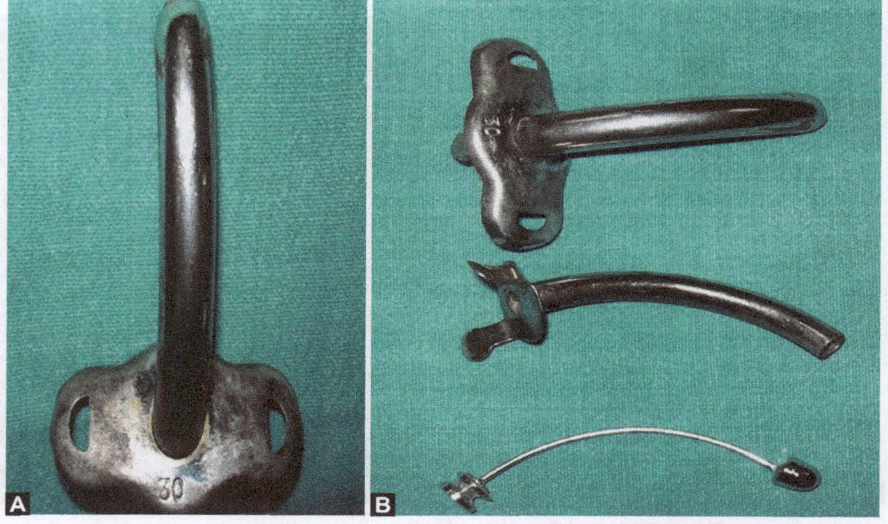

Figs 7.10A and B: (A) Metallic tracheostomy tube; (B) Outer and inner tubes with stellate

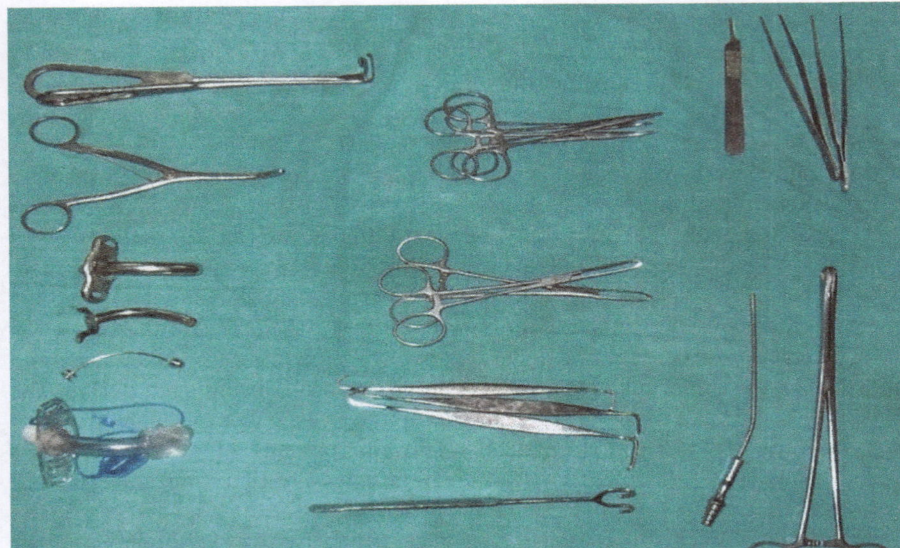

Fig. 7.11: Tracheostomy set

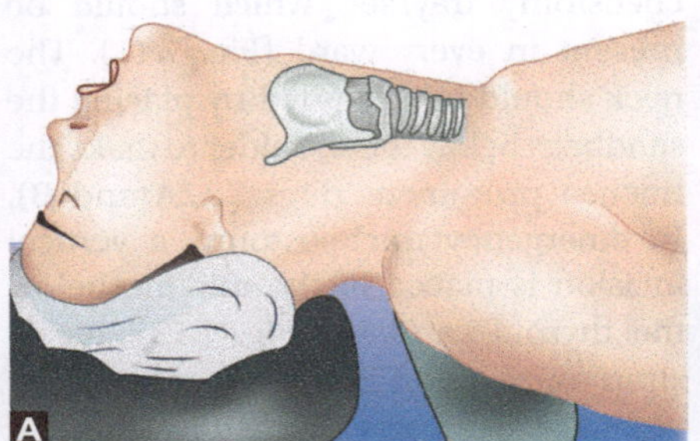

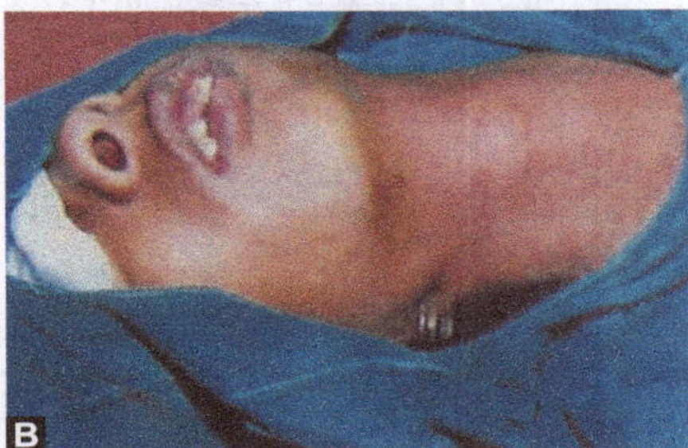

Figs 7.12A and B: Position of the patient for tracheostomy, the neck is extended by placing sandbag below the shoulder and head is supported with a ring pillow

recurrent laryngeal nerve which is the branch of the vagus. The upper rings of the trachea lie deep to the isthmus of the thyroid and by retracting the isthmus the rings are made visible (Fig. 7.15). If the isthmus is bulky and comes in the way of surgery it can be clamped and divided. The trachea can be felt by finger as a cartilaginous, ringed (hoist *pipe-like*) structure. To confirm the presence of trachea, a syringe filled with normal sterile saline is taken and the needle is inserted in the structure and aspiration is done. Aspiration of air in the syringe confirms that it is the trachea. A cricoid hook (Fig. 7.16) is inserted around the trachea to stabilize it and a vertical incision is taken in the anterior wall of trachea over the 3rd, 4th, and 5th tracheal rings. Handling of tracheal lining will result into a bout of cough and after it has subsided the incision is dilated with the tracheal dilator (Fig. 7.17) and tracheostomy tube is inserted into the trachea (Fig. 7.18). In place of the vertical incision a Bjork flap can also be taken to create the opening in the trachea (Figs 7.19A to C). The Bjork flap can be inferiorly or superiorly pedicled. The basic disadvantage with the inferiorly pedicled Bjork flap is that if the flap is not stitched outside, it may fall in the tracheal lumen and block it.

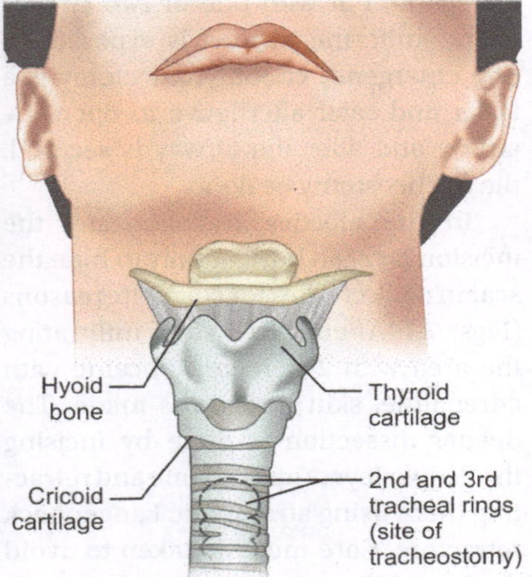

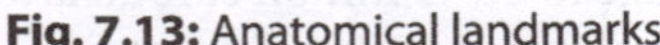

Fig. 7.13: Anatomical landmarks

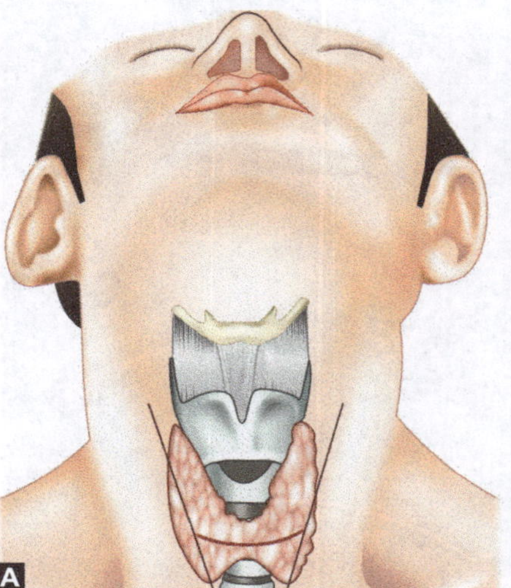

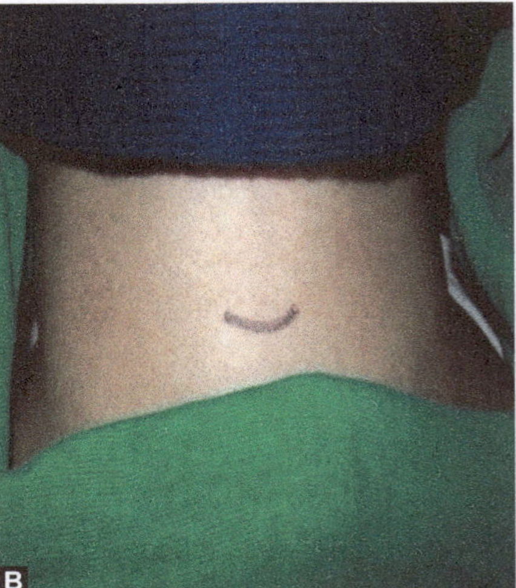

Figs 7.14A and B: Incision for the elective tracheostomy

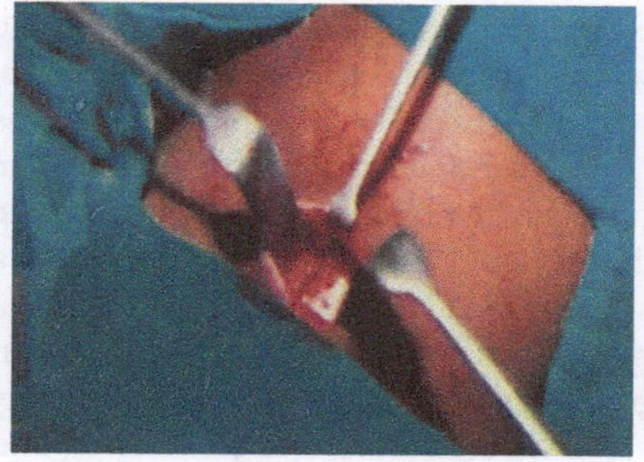
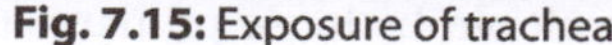

Fig. 7.15: Exposure of trachea

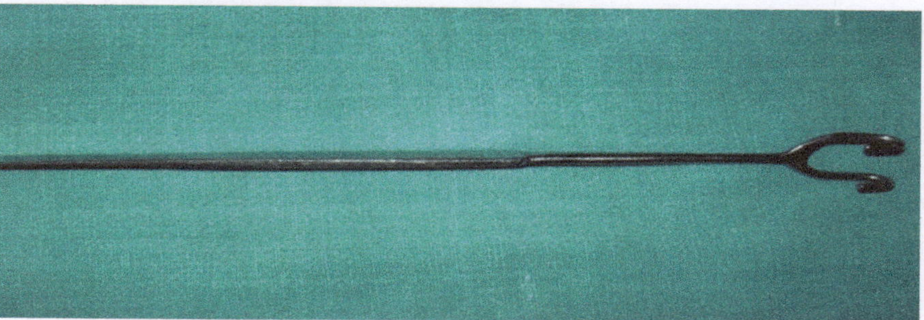

Fig. 7.16: Cricoid hook

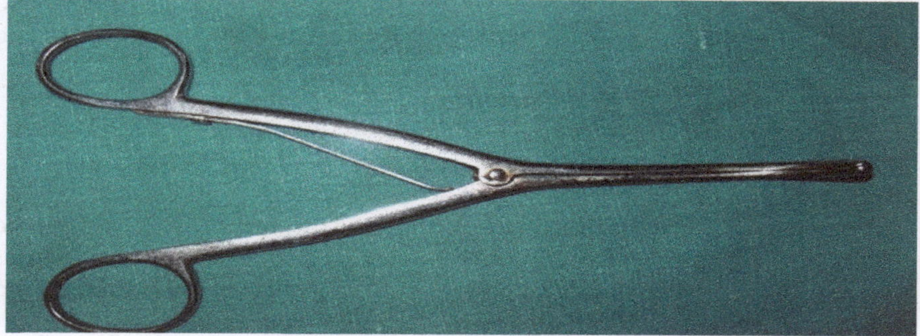

Fig. 7.17: Tracheal dilator

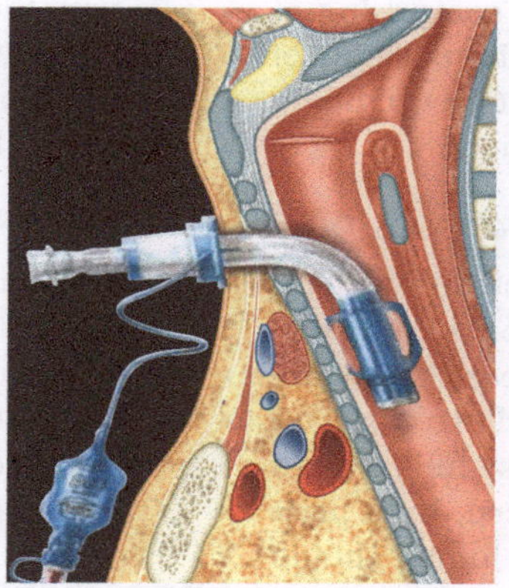

Fig 7.18: Final tube placement

The tube is secured in place by either suturing to the skin or by tying the straps around the neck to prevent accidental decanulation (Figs 7.20A and B).

Subsequent Care of Tracheostomy Tube

- Handle the tracheostomy tube with sterile gloved hands.
- Maintain proper hygiene and asepsis around the tracheostomy site.
- Watch for the signs of surgical emphysema in immediate post-tracheostomy period to detect false passage, if any. Similarly observe for the signs of respiratory distress, intermittently. The air blast should be checked to detect the blockade of the tube due to thick secretions. The air blast is checked by holding the cotton wool fibers over the tube opening and observing its deflection during the expiration.
- Cover the tracheostomy tube with a single layer of moist gauge to humidify the inhaled air.

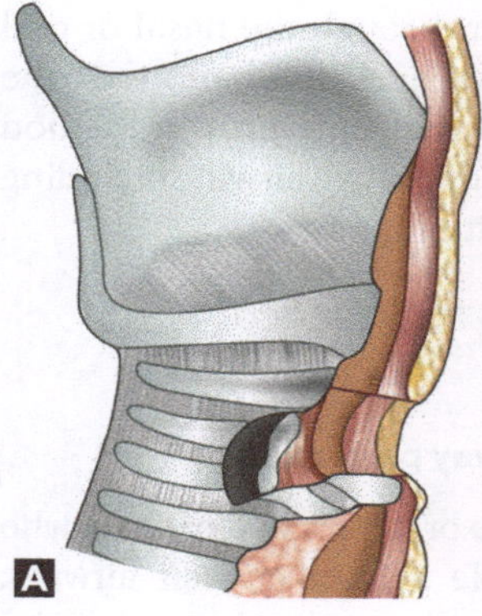

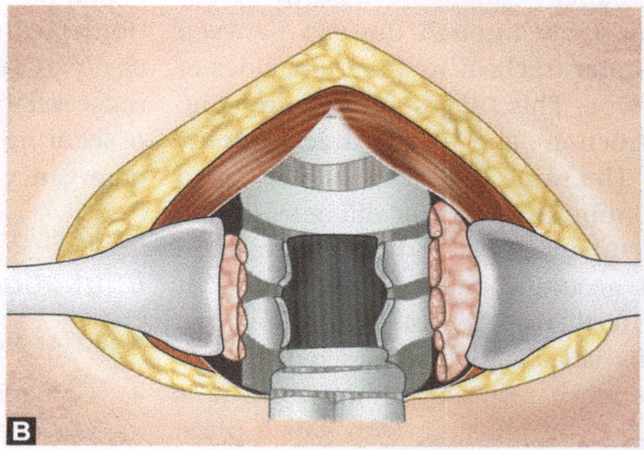

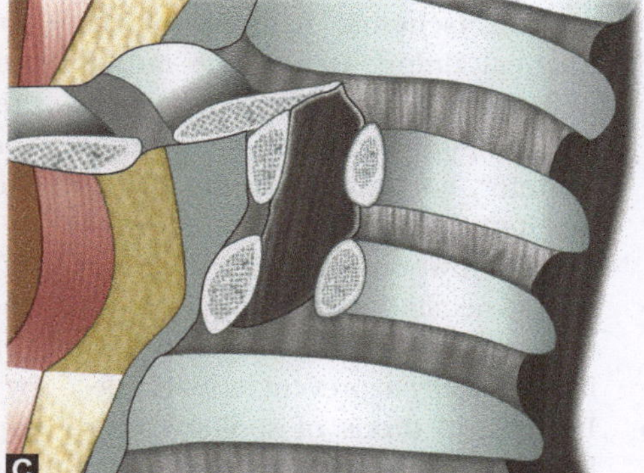

Figs 7.19A to C: Inferiorly and superiorly pedicled Bjork flaps

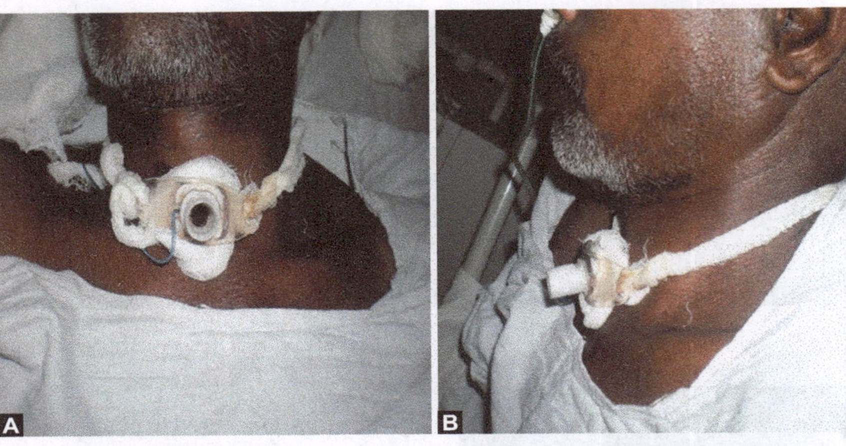

Figs 7.20A and B: Securing the tube with tape straps around the neck

- Perform suctions intermittently to prevent blockage of the tube due to secretion. However, deep tracheal suction should be done judiciously and when needed as it stimulates the vigorous coughing.
- Handle the suction catheters aseptically and do not use open ended catheters at tip, as they may suck the fragile tracheal lining and induce bleeding. Dip the suction catheter in a bottle containing sterile normal saline to flush out the thick secretions present in it to prevent its clogging and after switching off the suction keep the catheter submerged in a dilute, sterile antiseptic solution in a bottle.
- Keep the environment humid by keeping a kettle of boiling water in the room, as dry air tends to irritate the tracheal lining and tends to dry out the secretions, thus blocking the tube.
- If a cuffed tube is used, inflate and deflate the cuff every half hourly to prevent ischemic necrosis of the tracheal lining. Before the cuff is deflated suck the secretions present in the upper airway using separate catheter, so that when the cuff is deflated the secretions are not aspirated in lower respiratory passage.
- If the metallic tracheostomy tube is used, remove the inner tube and clean it periodically to prevent its blockade.
- Put 2 to 3 drops of sodium bicarbonate (soda bicarb) or normal saline through the tracheostomy tube to liquify the secretions.
- Give steam nebulization to the patients every 6 hourly to liquify the secretions (Mucolytic *action*) and reduce congestion of the tracheal and lower airway lining which can be induced due to the tracheal handling, irritation due to nonhumidified air inhalation and subclinical infection.
- Chest physiotherapy comprising of frequent change in the position of the patient, chest exercises, tapping etc. is given to the patient.

Decanulation of the Tracheostomy

Once the purpose is over the tracheostomy tube should be decanulated (removed) as early as possible. More the time it is kept indwelling more are the chances of the chest infection. If the metallic tube is placed, then prior to the removal the tube lumen should be plugged with a gauze piece and the patient should be observed for breathing. The patient should be able to breath comfortably through the gap between the inner tracheal wall and the sides of the tube. This suggests that there is no obstruction above the tracheostomy site. The same is not possible in cuffed PVC tube as the outer diameter of the PVC tube is larger and the deflated cuff also occupies lot of space and does not facilitate the free air circulation by its sides and thus the patient will experience respiratory distress, if it is blocked by plugging with gauze piece unlike the metallic tube. When the PVC tube is decanulated the metallic tube is kept as stand by and the edges of the wound are kept retracted with retractors, so that, in case of any respiratory distress after decanulation of the tube, a metallic tube can be reinserted. The tube must be decanulated under aseptic care. It is a safe practice to observe the patient for a period of atleast 1 hour after decanulation of the tracheostomy tube to detect any signs of respiratory distress. The wound can be closed by loose primary sutures or can just be covered with sterile gauze piece soaked in povidone iodine and taped with adhesive tape, and allowed to heal by secondary intention.

Complications

Perioperative complications of tracheostomy

- **Hemorrhage:** Due to damage to internal jugular vein or its tributaries or as a result of damage to the thyroid isthmus
- False passage
- Surgical emphysema
- Pneumothorax
- Air embolism
- Cricoid cartilage damage
- Recurrent laryngeal nerve damage.

Late postoperative complications

- Complications due to difficult decannulation
- Tracheocutaneous fistula
- Tracheoesophageal fistula
- Tracheal stenosis
- Tracheoinnominate artery fistula.

Endotracheal Intubation

A 'definitive airway' is defined as a cuffed tube passed below the vocal cord (folds), either through the nasal or oral cavity. Orotracheal intubation is the most reliable and time-proven method of securing a definitive airway, including emergency situations.

Indications for Tracheal Intubation

Need for airway protection

- Comatose or intoxicated patients who are unable to protect their airways. In such patients, the throat muscles may lose their tone so that the upper airway obstructs or collapses and air cannot easily enter into the lungs. Furthermore, protective airway reflexes such as coughing and swallowing, which serve to protect the airway against aspiration of secretions and foreign bodies, may be absent. With tracheal intubation, airway patency is restored and the lower airways can be protected from aspiration.

- Risk for aspiration.
- Upper airway bleeding—to prevent aspiration.
- Vomiting—to prevent aspiration.
- Risk for obstruction.
- Severe maxillofacial fractures.
- Neck hematoma.
- Stridor—due to laryngospasm.
- Laryngeal, tracheal injury/fractures.

Where the need for assisted ventilation is felt

- Apnea.
- Inadequate respiratory effort:
  - Hypoxia.
  - Cyanosis.
  - Tachyapnea.
  - Hypercarbia.
- Diagnostic manipulations of the airway such as bronchoscopy.
- Endoscopic operative procedures to the airway such as laser therapy or stenting of the bronchi.
- Patients, who require respiratory support including cardiopulmonary resuscitation.

Contraindications for Tracheal Intubation

Absolute

- The possibility to adequately secure and maintain airway by less invasive means.
- Cervical spine fractures.

Relative

- Severe midface fractures.
- Severe laryngeal trauma with tracheal separation.
- Blind techniques are contraindicated in the setting of major upper airway or neck injuries.

(*Evaluation of the airway before intubation is discussed in this chapter*).

Endotracheal Tubes

The endotracheal tubes may be flexible or preformed and relatively stiff. They are usually made of red rubber, flexible plastic or silicone, though they may be armored with metallic rings to prevent kinking (Figs 7.21A and B). Adult tubes have an inflatable cuff to seal the lower airways against air leakage and gross aspiration and the cuff also makes the tube self-retaining (Figs 7.22A and B). The cuff must be maintained diligently in order to avoid complications from overinflation, which can include rupture of the trachea, tracheomalacia or tracheoesophageal fistula. Many of the complications of overinflated cuffs can be traced to cuff pressure against the tracheal wall causing ischemia of the mucosa underneath.

Smaller pediatric tubes generally are uncuffed, as the cricoid cartilage, the narrowest portion of the pediatric airway, often provides an adequate seal for mechanical ventilation. An excessive leak can sometimes be corrected through the placement of a larger (0.5 mm larger in internal diameter) endotracheal tube, although in difficult-to-ventilate patients even children may need to use cuffed tubes to allow for high pressure ventilation, if the leak is too great to overcome with the ventilator.

The south pole tubes are directed towards the leg end of the patients and are especially suitable for the maxillary surgeries and the cleft lip and palate surgeries (Fig. 7.23). The north pole tubes are directed towards the head and are useful for the surgeries in the lower jaw and face (Fig. 7.24).

Route for Intubation

For infants and young children, oral intubation is easier than nasal. Nasal route carries risk of dislodgement

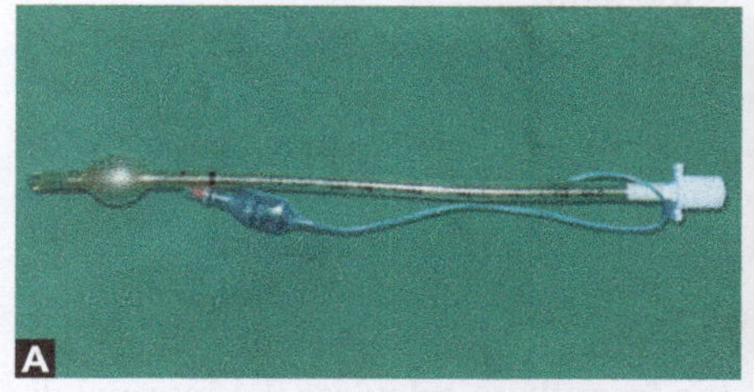
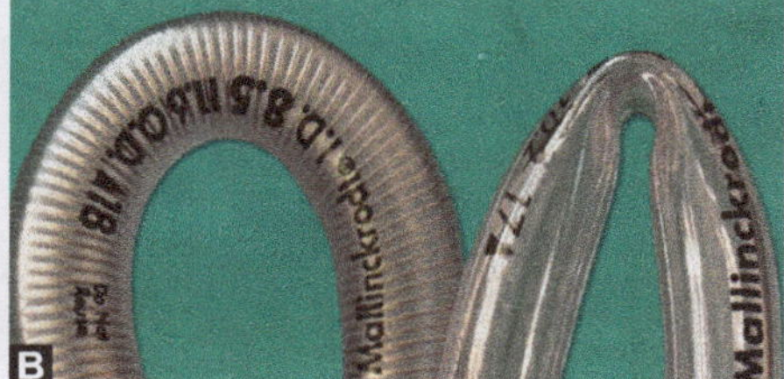

Figs 7.21A and B: (A) Armoured ETT; (B) No kinking in the armoured tube even after acute bending

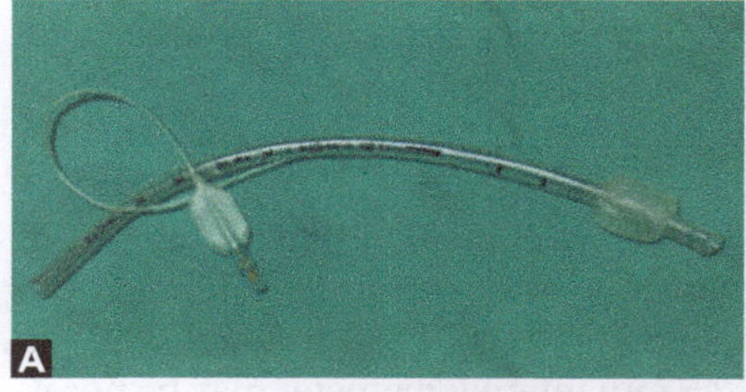
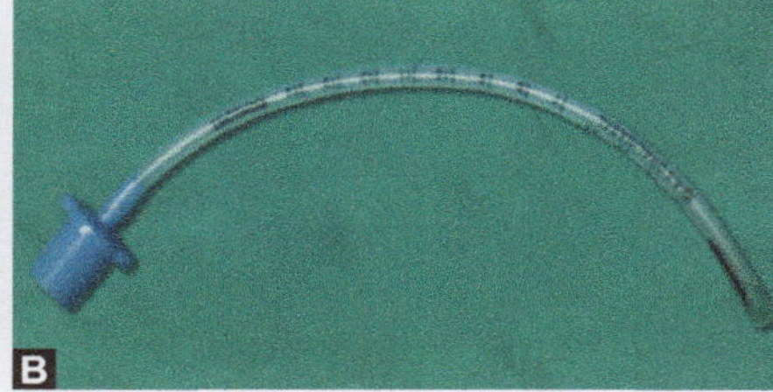

Figs 7.22A and B: (A) ETT with cuff; (B) ETT without cuff

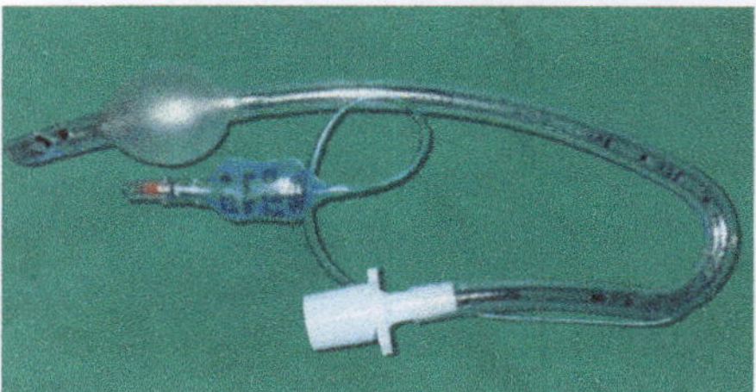

Fig. 7.23: South pole tube

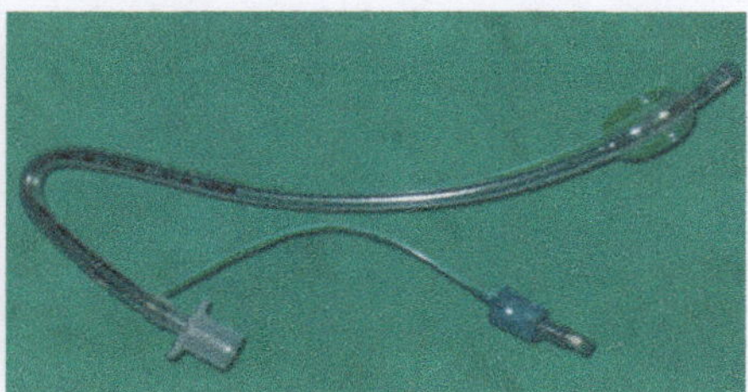

Fig. 7.24: North pole tube

of adenoid tissue and epistaxis, but advantages include good fixation of tube. Because of good fixation, nasal route is preferable to oral route in children undergoing intensive care and requiring prolonged intubation. The nasal intubation is of great help during the transoral surgeries as the oral tube comes in the way of the surgical field. The nasal route is indicated in most of the maxillofacial procedures. Nasal tubes can be left *in situ* after major head neck procedures, where the tube is required to be left *in situ* postoperatively for maintaining the patency of the airway. In the cases of the multiple facial fractures, where nasal intubation is contraindicated and the oral tube is likely to interfere with surgical field and prevent intermaxillary fixation (IMF) during the fracture reduction, the oral intubation is done and the outer end of the tube is drawn out through the floor of the mouth, below the chin. It is called submental or transmylohyoid intubation (discussed under trauma).

Position of Tube

The tip of tube should be at midtrachea (between the clavicles on an AP chest X-ray). The position of the tube is checked by auscultation (equal air entry on each side and by chest X-ray). If the tube is passed too deep it will cross the carina and enter the right bronchus as it has a straight course unlike the left bronchus, which is oblique. In such cases the left lung remains unperfused and air entry will be diminished or absent on the left side. In this case the tube should be withdrawn, so that its tip is above the carina and finally the tube is secured after verification of equal air entry on both the sides.

Type of Tubes

- *Noncuffed tubes (plain tubes)* are commonly used in prepubescent children. In cross section the airway in children is circular, which makes plain tracheal tube fits better than cuffed tube (*see* Fig. 7.23).
- *Cuffed tubes* less than 6.0 mm and not inflated are accepted for use in pediatrics but generally in children less than 10 years old cuffed tubes are avoided to minimize subglottic swelling and ulceration. Inflation of the cuff with air makes the tube self-retaining and prevents aspiration of the secretions and blood in the tracheobronchial tree.
- North pole tube—used for lower face surgeries.
- South pole tube—used for maxillary surgeries such as cleft palate.
- Armoured or flexomettalic tubes—It is flexible and at the same time reinforced with metallic rings and does not kink. It is suitable for head and neck surgeries which require manipulation of the neck (*see* Fig. 7.22).

Size of Tube

Because the airway of a child is narrow, a small amount of edema can produce severe obstruction. Edema can easily be caused by forcing in a tracheal tube that is too tight.

The correct diameter of the tube is that, which results in a small leak at a pressure of about 25 cm of water (the tip should be at midtrachea, between the clavicles on an AP chest X-ray).

For normally nourished children more than about 2 years old, the following formula to calculate the internal diameter of the tube is likely to be of the correct size:

Internal diameter of tube (mm) = (age in years ÷ 4) + 4

Roughly correct tube size can be indicated by:

Inner diameter: It can be estimated by the size of the child's little finger. (For neonates, 3 mm internal diameter is accepted while for premature infants 2.5 mm internal diameter may be necessary).

Length: It can be estimated by doubling the distance from the corner of the child's mouth to the ear canal.

Technique

- A small ring pillow should usually be placed under the occiput to flex the neck and extend the atlanto-occipital joint. This straightens the path from the upper incisors to the larynx. Loose, filled or capped teeth, especially upper incisors, may be protected from the laryngoscope blade by a guard.
- General anesthesia (GA) is induced by an intravenous or inhalational agent along with muscle relaxant. The intravenous agents like thiopental sodium or propofol are commonly used. These agents are pushed slowly and during the same the pulse and respiration are monitored. The short-acting muscle relaxants like succinylcholine is injected quickly, after the patient is administered intravenous anesthesia. The succinylcholine is never mixed with thiopental sodium as they are inpalatable and can lead to precipitation. Similarly, while injecting the thiopental sodium, care must be taken to ensure that the intravenous cannula is indwelling and patent as the extravasation of this drug can produce severe tissue reaction and necrosis.
- Absence of reflexes (pharyngeal, laryngeal and corneal reflex) and adequate muscular relaxation are necessary for laryngoscopy.
- Relaxation must be good and can be monitored by stimulation on the facial nerve.
- The laryngoscope blade is inserted from the right side of the patient's mouth to prevent the tongue blocking the view of the larynx, while watching the blade tip as it is advanced alongside the tongue towards the midline.
- When the epiglottis is seen, the tip is inserted firmly, but not forcibly into the vallecula and is used to lift the base of epiglottis forward to reveal the cords.
- Backward pressure on the thyroid cartilage by an assistant may help to bring the cords into view.
- A gum-elastic bougie may be very helpful for intubations with its tip curved anteriorly, passed into the trachea and used as an introducer.
- The tube, passed over the bougie may be helped by keeping the laryngos cope in the mouth and by rotating the

tube 90 degrees anticlockwise as the bevel reaches the larynx (Fig. 7.25).

- Tube is introduced to the final position using Magill's forceps (Fig. 7.26) and secured using a suture or an elastic tape (Fig. 7.27).

The other modalities for intubation are retrograde intubation, blind nasal intubation, fiberoptic laryngoscope or bronchoscope assisted intubation or laryngeal mask ventilation (Fig. 7.28).

Observational Methods to Confirm Correct Tube Placement

- Direct visualization of the tube passing through the vocal cords.
- Clear and equal bilateral breath sounds on auscultation of the chest.
- Absent sounds on auscultation of the epigastrium.
- Equal bilateral chest movements with ventilation.
- Fogging of the tube due to passage of humid air coming from lungs.
- An absence of stomach contents in the tube.

Concious Sedation[5]

The field of dentistry requires many clinical procedures to be performed in the clinics in the dental chairs. The patients are often apprehensive and anxious. The patient needs to be properly prepared psychologically for effective management. The dental chair is not a place, where general anesthesia can be administered and the patients are set-ups for doing the minor procedures, which was time consuming and costly. In the past there were only two categories of the patients, one those who were not given any medication and only regional (local) anesthesia was given. The other class had those treated under GA. The clinicians felt it necessary to find other modalities, where the patients could be treated in the dental office only without the necessity of GA. The patients compliance, mood, pain perception, pain threshold may be altered in such a way that his/her level of apprehension goes down, pain threshold increases without loosing patient compliance.

In between the stage, where the patient is given only regional anesthesia and the extreme end of the spectrum, where the patient is fully anesthetized by giving GA there is a lot of gray area, which can be used to treat the patients effectively on the OPD basis. If we understand the pain physiology it is seen that the spectrum of pain control is as follows:

- Patient given only regional anesthesia and no medication.
- Regional anesthesia with sedation.
- N_2O + sedation.
- Neuroleptanalgesia.
- Neuroleptanesthesia.
- Dissociative anesthesia.
- General anesthesia.

The width of this spectrum is utilized for the management of the patients.

The conscious sedation does not mean the stage of analgesia of the GA. To understand the conscious sedation the definition of the consciousness should be understood.

It means the patient favorably responds to command, the patient is able

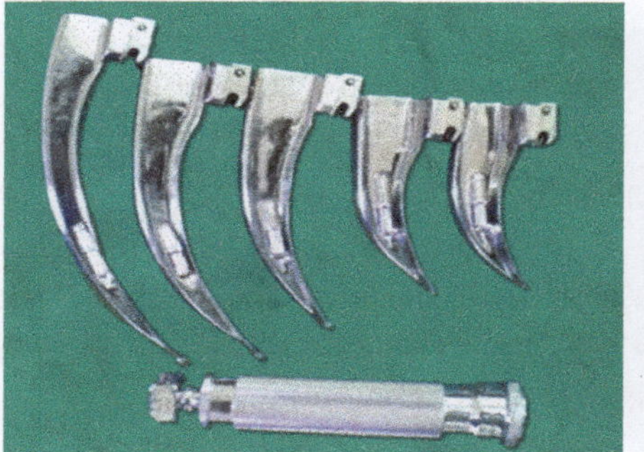

Fig. 7.25: Laryngoscope with blades of different sizes

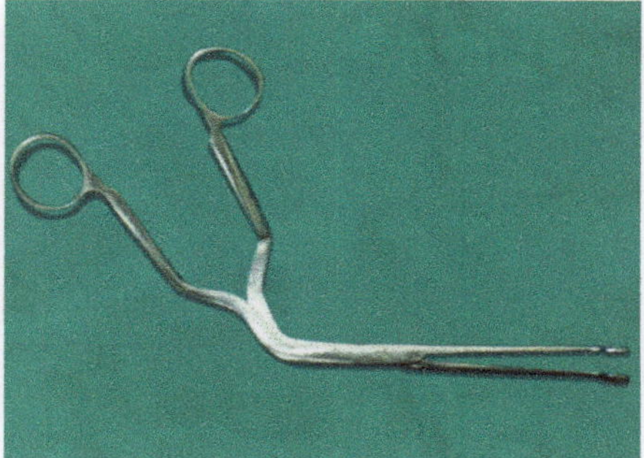

Fig. 7.26: Magill's forceps

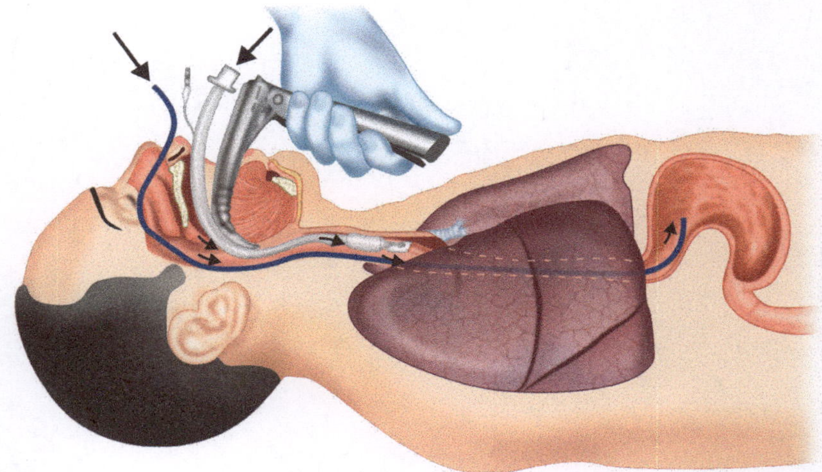

Fig. 7.27: Laryngoscopy and insertion of ETT

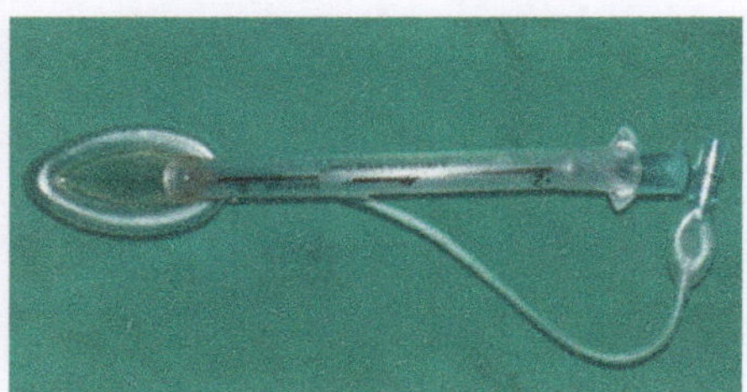

Fig. 7.28: Laryngeal mask airway

to clear his airway as all the protective reflexes are well preserved (Box 7.1).

These goals can be achieved by giving many medications, like benzodiazepines, barbiturates, nitrous oxide, opioids, ketamine and GA. The route of administration could be oral, parenteral or inhalation. There is a thin dividing line between the sedation and anesthesia while using certain drugs like nitrous oxide, thiopental sodium, secobarbital, hexobarbital, etc. as this phenomenon is dose related. If more does are used it can have anesthetic effect and in lower doses analgesic, sedative or tranquilizing effect. The past literature mentions the use of lytic cocktails comprising of pentazocine lactate, diazepam and phenergan to be given preoperatively along with the regional anesthesia. The more refined version is conscious sedation.

In precise, the commonly practiced modalities of conscious sedation are premedication to the patient with pentazocine lactate and or diazepam in a dose 15 to 30 mg and 2.5 to 5 mg, respectively. In children, instead of diazepam, Phenergan (promethazine) is used. Regional anesthesia combined with nitrous oxide is commonly practiced modality for minor oral surgical procedures. The most commonly practiced form of outdoor anesthetics is dissociative anesthesia with ketamine.

Box 7.1: Aims of conscious sedation

1. To alter the mood of the patient, so that the acceptability of the procedure increases the anxiety is alleviated.
2. To alter the pain perception and pain threshold.
3. To alter the physiological parameters minimally.
4. To preserve all the protective reflexes to that the patient is able to clear his own airway.
5. To have patient under command during the procedure.

Box 7.2: Indications for conscious sedation

1. Pediatric patients where compliance is not present.
2. Apprehensive patients.
   a. The procedures where adequate anesthesia/analgesia cannot be obtained by regional anesthesia and GA is not necessary.
   b. Where profound analgesic effect is required.

The conscious sedation is mostly indicated for minor pediatric procedures (Box 7.2).

The procedures that are performed are dental extraction of pediatric patients, removal of sutures of pediatric patients especially after cleft lip surgery, I and D, debridement of facial wounds, burn dressing, reduction of fractures or dislocations, etc. (Box 7.2).

REFERENCES

1. Adams AP, Hevitt PV, Grand CN (Eds): Emergency Anesthesia 2nd edn. Oxford University Press, 1998.
2. Walls RM. Cricothyroidotomy, Emerge Med Clin North Am. 1988;6:725.
3. Benett JD. High Tracheostomy and other errors – Revisited. J Laryngol Otol 1996;110(11):1003-7.
4. Negus VE. Explanation of Respiratory Failure Sometimes Occurring After Successful. Tracheotomy Ann OtoL Bhin and Laryng (Sept). 1938;47:608.
5. Benett CR. Conscious Sedation as an alternative to General anesthesia. NY State dent J. 1976;42:351.

8 Biomedical Waste Management

Borle Rajiv M, Sachdeva Sachin Dev

In accordance with the rules framed by the Ministry of Environment and Forests and notified as the Biomedical Waste (management and handling) Rules, July 1998: every hospital generating biomedical waste (BMW) needs to set-up requisite BMW treatment facilities on site or ensure requisite treatment of waste at common treatment facility. No untreated BMW can be stored beyond a period of 48 hours.

The cost of construction, operation and maintenance of system for managing BMW represents a significant part of overall budget of a hospital, if the BMW rules have to be implemented in their true spirit. Two types of costs are required to be incurred by hospitals for BMW management, internal and external. Internal cost is the cost for segregation, mutilation, disinfection, internal storage and transportation including hidden cost of protective equipment. External costs are offsite transportation, treatment and final disposal.

Hospital is one of the complex institutions, which are frequented by people from every walk of life in the society without any distinction between age, sex, race and religion. This is over and above the normal inhabitants of hospital, i.e. patients and staff. All of them produce waste, which is increasing in its amount and type due to advances in scientific knowledge and is creating its impact. The hospital waste, in addition to the risk for patients and personnel who handle these wastes pose a threat to public health and environment.

Keeping in view inappropriate biomedical waste management, the Ministry of Environment and Forests notified the '*Biomedical Waste (Management and Handling) Rules, 1998*' in July 1998. In accordance with these Rules (Rule 4), it is the duty of every 'occupier', i.e. a person who has the control over the institution and, or its premises, to take all steps to ensure that waste generated is handled without any adverse effect to human health and environment. The hospitals, nursing homes, clinics, dispensaries, animal house, pathological laboratories, blood banks, etc. are therefore required to set in place the biological waste treatment facilities. It is however not mandatory that every institution has to have its own waste treatment facility. The rules also envisage that common facility or any other facilities can be used for waste treatment by entering into a memorandum of understanding with the service provider. However, it is obligatory on part of the occupier to ensure that the waste is treated within a period of 48 hours.[1]

DEFINITION[2]

'Biomedical waste' means any solid and/or liquid waste, including its container and any intermediate product, which is generated during the diagnosis, treatment or immunization of human beings or animals or in research pertaining there to or in the production or testing there of. The physicochemical and biological nature of these components, their toxicity and potential hazard are different, necessitating different methods/options for their treatment/disposal. In *Schedule I* of the Biomedical Waste (management and handling) Rules, 1998, therefore, the waste originating from different kinds of such establishments, have been categorized into 10 different categories (Table 8.1) and their treatment and disposal options have been indicated.

COMPONENTS OF BIOMEDICAL WASTE (BOX 8.1)

- Human anatomical waste (tissues, organs, body parts, etc.).
- Animal waste (as above, generated during research/experimentation, from veterinary hospitals, etc.)
- Microbiology and biotechnology waste such as, laboratory cultures, microorganisms, human and animal cell cultures, toxins, etc.
- Waste sharps, such as hypodermic needles, syringes, scalpels, broken glass, etc.
- Discarded medicines and cytotoxic drugs.
- Soiled waste, such as dressing, bandages, plaster casts, material contaminated with blood, etc.
- Solid waste (disposable items like tubes, catheters, etc. excluding sharps).
- Liquid waste generated from any of the infected areas.
- Incineration ash.
- Chemical waste.

Table 8.1: Color coding for different waste containers

Option	Waste category	Color coding
Category No. 1	Human anatomical	Yellow
Category No. 2	Animal waste	Yellow
Category No. 3	Microbiology and biotechnology	Yellow, Red
Category No. 4	Waste sharps	Blue/White translucent puncture proof
Category No. 5	Discarded medicines and cytotoxic	Black
Category No. 6	Solid	Yellow, Red
Category No. 7	Solid	Red, Blue/White translucent
Category No. 8	Liquid waste	Drained after treatment
Category No. 9	Incineration ash	Black
Category No. 10	Chemical waste	Black

Box 8.1: WHO classification of biomedical waste[3]

Infectious: Waste from surgery and autopsies on patients with infectious diseases.
Sharp: Disposable needles, syringes, saws, blades, broken glasses, nails or any other item that could cause a cut.
Pathological: Tissues, organs, body parts, human flesh, fetuses, blood and body fluids.
Pharmaceutical: Drugs and chemicals that are returned from wards, spilled, outdated, contaminated, or are no longer required.
Radioactive: Waste contaminated with radioactive substances.

Universal symbol of hazardous biomedical waste is shown in Figure 8.1.

INFECTIOUS WASTE

The infectious waste is the material containing pathogens in sufficient concentration or quantity that, if exposed can cause diseases. For example, waste from surgery, autopsy, patients with infectious diseases.

Types of Infectious Waste[4]

- **Isolation waste**: Generated by patients who are isolated.
- **Cultures and stocks** of infectious agents and associated biologicals, e.g. wastes from the production of biologicals, discarded live and attenuated vaccines and culture dishes and devices.
- **Biological wastes:** Blood as well as serum, plasma and other blood products.

Fig. 8.1: Universal symbol of hazardous biomedical waste

- **Pathological wastes:** Tissues, organs, body parts and body fluids.
- **Contaminated sharps:** Needles syringes, pasteur pipettes, broken glass and scalpel blades.
- **Contaminated carcasses:** Body parts and bedding.
- **Miscellaneous contaminated wastes:** Include those from surgery and autopsies, contaminated laboratory wastes, dialysis unit wastes and contaminated equipment.

Color coding of waste disposal containers are given in Table 8.1.

Health Hazards Associated with Poor Management of Biomedical Waste[5]

- Injury from sharps to staff and waste handlers associated with the health care establishment.
- Hospital acquired infection (HAI) (Nosocomial) to the patients due to spread of infection.
- Risk of infection outside the hospital for waste handlers/scavengers and eventually general public.
- Occupational risk associated with hazardous chemicals, drugs, etc.
- Unauthorized repackaging and sale of disposable items and unused/ date expired drugs.

Environmental Concerns

The following are the main environmental concerns with respect to improper disposal of biomedical waste management:

- Spread of infection and disease through vectors (fly, mosquito, insects, etc.), which affect the in-house as well as surrounding population.
- Spread of infection through contact/ injury among medical/non-medical personnel and sweepers/rag pickers, especially from the sharps (needles, blades, etc.).
- Spread of infection through unauthorized recycling of disposable items such as hypodermic needles, tubes, blades, bottles, etc.
- Reaction due to use of discarded medicines.
- Toxic emissions from defective/inefficient incinerators.
- Indiscriminate disposal of incinerator ash/residues.

Infectious Waste Management Plan[6]

The vital steps for safe and scientific management of biomedical waste in any establishment are:

- Handling
- Segregation
- Mutilation
- Disinfection[7]
- Storage
- Transportation
- Final disposal

The key to minimization and effective management of biomedical waste is segregation (separation) and identification of the waste. The most appropriate way of identifying the categories of biomedical waste is by sorting the waste into universally color coded plastic bags or containers. Biomedical waste should be segregated into containers/bags at the point of generation in accordance with *Schedule II* of Biomedical Waste (management and handling) Rules 1998 as given in Table 8.1. The BMW should be segregated at the point of its generation as it is not possible to segregate it later without undue risk. Only 15 to 20 percent of BMW is hazardous, but if it is not segregated then it is 100 percent hazardous. The contaminated sharps are the most dangerous.

- **Designation:** The waste needs to be designated as per the WHO classification.
- **Segregation:** The waste generated in a hospital needs to be segregated and stored in the different containers as per the color coding mentioned in the Table 8.1.
- **Packaging:** The packaging of the waste needs to be done properly to avoid accidental spillage, handling by the children or lay men as it is highly contagious and can lead to hazardous spread of the infection.

Packaging of Infectious Waste[8]

- Liquid infectious wastes can be placed in capped or tightly stoppered bottles or flasks. Large quantities may be placed in containment tanks.
- Solid or semisolid wastes may be placed in plastic bags.
- Select tear-resistant bags. Plastic bags are judged by their thickness or durability as evaluated by the ASTM dart test (ASTM 1975).
- Do not place sharp items or items with sharp corners in the bags (Place sharps in impervious rigid, puncture-resistant containers made of glass, metal, rigid plastic or wood).
- Do not load a bag beyond its weight or volume capacity.
- Keep bags away from coming into contact with sharp external objects.
- Consider double bagging.
- Some treatment techniques required special packaging characteristics. For example, incineration required combustible containers and steam sterilization requires packaging materials such as low-density plastics that allow steam penetration and evacuation of air.
- Carts and recyclable containers that are used repeatedly for transport and treatment of bagged waste should be disinfected after each use. Single-use containers should be destroyed as part of the treatment process.
- Infectious waste should not be compacted before treatment. This process could damage the packaging and disperse the contents or it could interfere with the effectiveness of treatment.
- Outside the hospital, infectious waste should be transported in closed, leak-proof dumpsters or trucks.
- The waste should be placed in rigid or semirigid, leak-proof containers before being loaded onto trucks.

Storage

The BMW must not be stored in the hospital premises for more than 48 hours. It is ideal to do the BMW on daily basis. However, if it is to be stored for its final disposal it must be stored securely ensuring that:

- The area of the storage is in the secluded, remote corner.
- The area is well cordoned by proper fencing and locked.
- The BMW must be stored in rigid or semi-rigid, leak proof containers to prevent spillage and spread of infection through the vectors (flies).
- The universal symbol of hazardous BMW must be prominently displayed and warning notice in the vernacular language must be prominently displayed.

Treatment and Disposal Methods[9]

The following methods are practiced to render the biomedical waste inert and safe for its final disposal so that the risk of infection transmission is minimized to the community as a whole.

- Steam sterilization
- Incineration
- Thermal inactivation
- Chemical disinfection
- Irradiation

After treatment, the wastes or their ashes can be disposed off by discharge into sanitary sewer systems (for liquid or ground-up waste) or buried in sanitary landfills.

Steam/Autoclaving Treatment

- Containers that can be used effectively in steam sterilization are plastic bags, metal pans, bottles and flasks. High-density polyethylene and polypropylene plastic should not be used in this process, because they do not facilitate steam penetration to the waste load. Heat-labile plastic bags allow steam penetration of the waste, but they may crumble and melt. If heat-labile plastic bags are used, they should be placed in another heat-stable container that allows steam penetration such as a strong paper bag or they should be treated with gas/vapor sterilization.
- Waste that contains antineoplastic drugs, toxic chemicals or chemicals that would be volatilized by steam should not be steam-sterilized.

Gas/Vapor Treatment

Gas/vapor sterilization uses gaseous or vaporized chemicals as the sterilizing agents. Ethylene oxide is the most commonly used agent, but should be used with caution since it is a suspected human carcinogen. Because ethylene oxide may be adsorbed on the surface of treated materials, the potential exists for worker exposure when sterilized materials are handled.

Standards for Incinerators

Incineration is a high-temperature dry oxidation process that reduces organic and combustible waste to inorganic, incombustible matter and safe management of wastes from health care activities (Box 8.2).

Waste types not to be incinerated

- Pressurized gas containers.
- Large amounts of reactive chemical waste.

Box 8.2: Standards for incinerators

- Combustion efficiency (CE) shall be at least 99 percent
- The temperature of the primary chamber shall be 800 ± 50°C
- Height of the chimney 80 feet as per environment pollution prevention norms.
- Suitably designed pollution control devices should be installed/retrofitted with the incinerator to achieve the above emission limits, if necessary
- Wastes to be incinerated shall not be chemically treated with any chlorinated disinfectants
- Chlorinated plastics shall not be incinerated

- Silver salts and photographic or radiographic wastes.
- Halogenated plastics such as polyvinyl chloride (PVC).
- Waste with high mercury or cadmium content, such as broken thermometers, used batteries, and lead-lined wooden panels.
- Sealed ampoules or ampoules containing heavy metals.

Standards for Liquid Waste

The liquid waste generated in the hospital should never be passed in the municipal sewerage lines without proper treatment. The liquid waste should be collected in a reservoir, disinfected and treated before releasing it into the sewerage lines. The treated liquid waste must meet the following criteria before it is released in the sewerage:

- pH 6.5 to 9.0.
- Suspended solids 100 mg/L
- Oil and grease 10 mg/L
- Bioassay test 90 percent survival of fish after 96 hours in 100 percent effluent.

Standards for Microwaving

- The microwave should completely and consistently kill the bacteria and other pathogenic organisms that are ensured by approved biological indicator at the maximum design capacity of each microwave unit. Biological indicators for the microwave shall be *Bacillus subtilis* spores using vials or spore strips with at least 1 × 10 to the power of four spores per milliliter.
- Shall not be used for cytotoxic, hazardous or radioactive wastes, contaminated animal carcasses, body parts and large metal items.

Standards for Deep Burial

- A pit or trench should be dug about 2 meters deep. It should be half-filled with waste then covered with lime within 50 cm of the surface, before filling the rest of the pit with soil.
- It must be ensured that animals do not have any access to burial sites. Covers of galvanized iron/wire meshes may be used. The site should be well cordoned off by fencing and the signal of hazardous biomedical waste should be displayed prominently.
- The deep burial site should be relatively impermeable and no shallow well should be close to the site.
- The site should be in an area, which is not flood prone.

Contingency Measures

Contingency measures should be developed to deal with emergencies that occur during the handling, transportation or disposal of infectious waste. Emergencies include spills of liquid infectious waste, ruptures of plastic bags or other containers holding infectious waste and equipment failures.

Staff Training

To practice the healthy methods of the biomedical waste management it is empirical that all the personnel including doctors, nurses, paramedics, lab assistants need to be oriented and trained in the practices of biomedical management. All the practices are ineffective unless every member is oriented and understands the importance of these methods and his/her role in the team.

The personnel protection measures include cap, masks, gloves, gumboots and aprons. Those who handle the BMW need to wear heavy duty gloves to prevent accidental needle pricks or injuries due to sharps. The personnel need to be immunized actively against tetanus and hepatitis B.

LEGAL ASPECTS AND ENVIRONMENTAL CONCERNS[10]

Indiscriminate disposal of infected and hazardous waste from hospitals, nursing homes and pathological laboratories has led to significant degradation of the environment, leading to spread of diseases and putting the people to great risk from certain highly contagious and transmission prone disease vectors. This has given rise to considerable environmental concerns. The first standard on the subject to be brought out in India was by the Bureau of Indian Standards (BIS), IS 12625:1989, entitled 'Solid Wastes-Hospitals-Guidelines for Management', but it was unable to bring any improvement in the situation. In this scenario, the notification of the 'Biomedical waste' (Management and Handling) Rules, 1998 assumes great significance. The Central Govt. has notified these rules on 20th July, 1998 in exercise of section 6, 8 and 25 of the Environment (Protection) Act, 1986. Prior to that, the draft rules were gazetted on 16th October, 1997 and Public suggestion/comments were invited within 60 days. These suggestions were considered before finalizing the rules.

Scope and Application of the Rules

These rules apply to all those who generate, collect, receive, store, transport, treat, dispose or handle biomedical waste in any form. According to these rules, it shall be the duty of every occupier of an institution generating biomedical waste, which includes hospitals, nursing homes, clinics, dispensaries, veterinary institution, animal houses, pathology laboratories, blood banks, etc. to take all steps to ensure that such wastes are handled without any adverse effect to human health and the environment. They have to either set-up their own facility within the time frame or ensure requisite treatment at a common waste treatment facility or any other waste treatment facility. Every occupier of an institution, which is generating, collecting, receiving, storing, transporting, treating, disposing and/or handling biomedical waste in any other manner, except such occupier of clinics, dispensaries, pathology laboratories, blood banks, etc. which provide treatment/service to less than 1,000 patients per month shall make an application in prescribed form to the prescribed authority for grant of authorization to carry on the work. Whenever an accident occurs concerning biomedical waste, it has to be reported to this authority. Each State and Union Territory (UT) Government shall be required to establish a prescribed authority for this purpose. The respective governments would also constitute advisory committees to advise the Governments with respect to implementation of these rules. The occupier or operator can also appeal against any order of the authority, if they feel aggrieved to such other authority as the Government of the State/UT may think fit to constitute.

REFERENCES

1. Garner JS. Hospital Infection control practices advisory committee. Guideline for isolation precautions in hospitals. Infect control Hosp Epi-demio. 1996;17: 54-80.
2. Reinhardt PA, Gordon JG. Infectious and medical waste management. Chelsea, MI: Lewis Publishers. 1991.
3. Tikhomirov E. WHO Programme for control of hospital infections. Chemiotherapia. 1987;3:148-51.
4. Ayliffe GAJ, Fraise AP, Geddes AM, Mitchell. Control of Hospital Infection, 4th edition. London, Arnold. 2000. p. 101.
5. Pratt, et al. The development of national evidence-based guidelines for preventing hospital acquired infections in England associated with the use of short-term indwelling urethral catheters in acute care: Technical report. London: Thames valley university; 2000.
6. Rutala WA, May Hall CG. The society of hospital epidemiology of America. Position paper: medical waste. Infection Control Hosp Epidemiol. 1992;13: 38-48.
7. Johan, et al. Role of disinfectants in infection control. Dent Clin North Am. 1991;35(2).
8. Recommended practice: Selection and use of packaging systems. AORN J. 1992;56(6):1096-100.
9. AAMI: Good hospital practice: Flash sterilization-steam sterilization of patient care items for immediate use, Arlington Va, 1992, American national standards institute.
10. Statutory instrument no 3246. The control of substances hazardous to health regulations. London. HMSO, 1994.

Section 2

Neurological Disorders of Face and General Anesthesia

- Neurological Disorders of the Face
- General Anesthesia

9 Neurological Disorders of the Face

Borle Rajiv M, Rai Anshul

Apart from the motor and sensory innervation, the face has autonomic innervation from the sympathetic chain and the parasympathetic innervation from the mid-brain outflow. The major sensory nerve of the face is the trigeminal nerve (Vth cranial nerve). The muscles of mastication are supplied by the motor division of the trigeminal nerve while muscles of facial expression are supplied by the facial nerve (VIIth cranial nerve). The parasympathetic supply to the orbit comes from the Edinger-Westphal nucleus and is relayed through the occulomotor (IIIrd cranial) nerve. The secretomotor fibers to the parotid and submandibular salivary gland are derived through the inferior and superior salivary nucleus, respectively.[1]

The face is commonly involved in the neurological disorders such as, facial nerve paralysis, trigeminal neuralgia, glossopharyngeal neuralgia, vascular headaches, migraine, Frey's syndrome, neuroparalytic occular conditions such as diplopia, etc. Some of the common neurological disorders involving the face have been discussed in this chapter.

TRIGEMINAL NEURALGIA (TIC DOULOUREUX, IDIOPATHIC TRIGEMINAL NEURALGIA)

The trigeminal neuralgia (TN) is defined as *"An intermittent, paroxysmal, sharp shooting, stabbing, lancinating pain in the distribution of trigeminal nerve"*. It can involve any division of trigeminal nerve, but it commonly involves the mandibular, maxillary divisions than the ophthalmic division. First complete description of TN was given by John Locke in 1677. Nicolas Andre[2] in 1756 coined the term 'Tic Douloureux'. In 1773, John Fothergill gave full and accurate description, henceforth known as Fothergill disease.[3]

Various Other Descriptions of Trigeminal Neuralgia

Trigeminal neuralgia is a sudden, usually unilateral, severe, brief, stabbing, recurrent pain in the distribution of one or more branches of Vth cranial nerve.[4]

Peterson[5] defined it as "It usually presents with sharp, electric shock-like pain in the face or mouth. Pain is intense, lasting for brief period of seconds to 1 min. After which there is refractory period during which pain cannot be re-initiated for a period of time".

IHS definition (*International Headache Society*): Painful unilateral affection of the face, characterized by brief electric shock-like pain limited to the distribution of one or more divisions of trigeminal nerve. Pain is commonly evoked by trivial stimuli including washing, shaving, smoking, talking and brushing the teeth, but may also occur spontaneously. The pain is abrupt in onset; terminations may remit for varying periods.

British Journal of Anesthesia[6] (2001): Paroxysmal episodes of sudden, usually unilateral, severe recurrent pain of shearing, stabbing or lancinating type, in the distribution of one or more branches of the 5th cranial nerve, accompanied by spasmodic contractions of facial muscles, often initiated by a '*trigger zone*'.

Etiology

Although the etiology is not always established, certain etiological factors are proposed. When the etiology is not established it is termed idiopathic.

The proposed etiological factors are divided into the following:

- **Peripheral causes:**
  - Nerve compression.
  - Nerve trauma.
  - Nerve back talk.
  - Aneurysm around the nerve.
  - Demyelination of the nerve.
  - Herpes zoster infection.
- **Central causes:**
  - Microaneurysm around the nerve root.
  - Cerebro-Pontine (CP) angle tumors.
  - Multiple sclerosis.
  - Demyelination of the nerve.
  - Nerve back talk.
  - Pulsations of basilar artery (Fig. 9.1).
  - High petrous ridge.

Clinical Features

- The incidence of trigeminal neuralgia is 4 in 1,00,000 and thus, it is relatively rare.
- The patients are usually in the 5th – 6th decade of life.
- It has a female predilection (Sex: F > M).

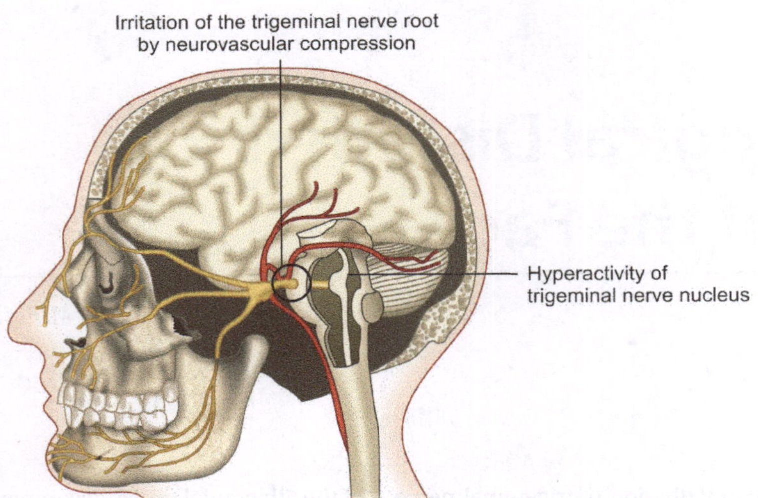

Fig. 9.1: Relation of basilar artery with the sensory root of TN

- It is more commonly seen on the right side (side predilection: right side).
- The mandibular division is most commonly involved followed by the maxillary and the ophthalmic divisions (Division predilection: V3 > V2 > V1).
- The pain is often described as sharp, shooting, stabbing and lancinating.
- It comes in paroxysms, lasts for a few seconds and disappears only to reappear after some time.
- The pain is precipitated by touching certain cutaneous areas in the distribution of the nerve. These areas are described as '*trigger zones*'.
- The pain is invariably unilateral in distribution. It can cross over to other side after the pain on the side has ceased.
- Between the two attacks of pain there is a short period during which the nerve cannot be excited and pain does not occur, this period is called '*refractory period*'. During this period the nerve is hyposthetic. This can be explained due to depolarization of the nerve and the fatigue of the sodium pump, due to repeated stimulation.
- The patient refrains from shaving, cleaning the teeth due to the fear of precipitation of attack of pain.
- During the pain the patient vigorously rubs the cheek to get the relief from the pain. This induces hyperkeratosis of the skin of the face on the involved side.
- During the attack the patient's facial expressions are peculiar and give a significant clue towards the diagnosis. As the pain is precipitated on facial movements the patient tends to guard the facial movements producing a '*mask face*' appearance.
- The pain is present when the patient is awake, it may prevent him from going to sleep but will seldom disturb the sleep.
- The pain responds to the treatment with anticonvulsants.
- The patient may have undergone multiple dental extractions on the involved side due to improper diagnosis of this condition and mistaking it as an odontogenic pain.

Diagnosis

There are no definitive diagnostic tests. The diagnosis is based purely on the history and clinical findings and hence the clinician must give a 'patient listening' and should not jump to conclusions or work with a prejudiced mind. After listening to the complaints of the patient leading questions may be asked to get full information about the pain, its nature, duration, precipitating, aggravating and relieving factors, variations during the day, origin and referred areas, any previous treatment and its results, etc. *It must be remembered that pain is a symptom and not a sign and the fact that it is experienced by the patient only, hence he/she only can describe it in a best way.* The other common causes like caries, periapical infection pulpitis, etc. must be ruled out. Investigations are required to rule out other causes for pain and in some cases may help in locating the cause of trigeminal neuralgia but the diagnosis of TN is often made on basis of history and clinical examination. The radiographs, computed tomography (CT) scan, magnetic resonance imaging (MRI) and angiography may be able to locate the cause in some cases, but it is invariably inconclusive and thus most of the cases are labeled as idiopathic.

Role of Diagnostic Nerve Block

The diagnostic nerve block is often given to confirm the diagnosis of neuralgia. The local anesthetic solution is injected around the peripheral branch, where the trigger zones are located and not around the main nerve trunk in the distribution of which the actual pain occurs. Because, if the main nerve trunk is blocked, all the sensations are lost and pain due to even an inflammatory pathology will also get abolished and the result will be inconclusive. If the trigger zones are not well circumscribed then a local infilteration in the region of the trigger zone should be given. Effort must be made to block the most peripheral part of the nerve and not the main trunk of the nerve.

The diagnostic block will block the trigger areas and the neuralgic pain is abolished. If the pain is due to the organic pathology such as odontogenic pathology will not get eliminated. Secondly the diagnostic block will not only help in differentiating the neuralgic pain from the other pains due to other inflammatory pathologies, but the patient can be explained how the part would remain anesthetic, if any destructive surgical procedure like peripheral neurectomy or alcohol injection is carried out, to get relief of the pain.

Sweet's Diagnostic Criteria for TN[7] *(White and Sweet)*

- The pain is paroxysmal.
- The pain may be provoked by light touch to the face (trigger zone).
- The pain is confined to trigeminal distribution.
- The pain is unilateral.
- The clinical sensory examination is normal.

If the patients' pain fails to meet any of the 5 forgoing criteria, the diagnosis of idiopathic TN is uncertain and the treatment required may be substantially different.

Treatment

The treatment modalities for trigeminal neuralgia are divided into the following:

- Medicinal treatment (conservative)
- Surgical treatment—which can be further divided into:
  - Peripheral:
    - Destructive.
    - Nondestructive.
  - Central:
    - Destructive.
    - Nondestructive.

Medicinal Treatment

The medicinal treatment comprises of drug therapy. The prescription of anticonvulsants is commonly practiced.

- Carbamazepine, (Tegretol®, Mazetol®) in a dose of 100 to 200 mg three times a day, is usually adequate in controlling the pain effectively. The dose of carbamazepine should not exceed 2 g/day. The usual immediate side effects with carbamazepine are dizziness, loss of fine neuromuscular coordination, drowsiness, tremors, gastrointestinal (GI) disturbances. The side effects of long-term therapy are bone marrow depression leading to agranulocytosis, tolerance to the drug which leads to increased dose requirement and ineffectiveness of the therapy.

  Dilantin sodium/Phenytoin sodium is also used to control the pain; it may be used alone or in combination with carbamazepine. Dilantin is given in a dose of 50 to 100 mg 2 to 3 times a day. The side effects are drowsiness and gingival hypertrophy.

  The patient who is prescribed these drugs must always be instructed to refrain from driving, swimming, working in industries near machinery to avoid mishaps. The side effects associated with phenytoin sodium therapy are:
  - Slurred speech
  - Abnormal movements
  - Gingival hypertrophy
  - Folate deficiency.
- The drug like phenobarbitone, diazepam may be prescribed as an adjuvant therapy.
- Gabapentin is also prescribed in a dose of 100 to 200 mg 2 to 3 times a day.
- Clonazepam 1.5 mg/day. The side effects associated with this therapy are drowsiness, fatigue, lethargy.
- Tab oxcarbazepine, 1200 mg/day, the side effects are hyponatremia, double vision.
- The role of B_1, B_6, B_{12} preparations is not established, but they are often prescribed as 'nerve tonic'.

The medicinal treatment is usually the first line of treatment. Apart from the routine complications associated with the medicinal treatment another complication is the drug tolerance. As the treatment is given over a long period the pain does not respond to the doses of the drugs, which were effective earlier to produce adequate pain relief and the doses of the drugs need to be increased or combination of the drugs are required to be prescribed to certain patients for effective pain relief. The patient sometimes does not respond to the medicinal treatment or may not be able to afford the cost of the therapy where the surgical line of treatment comes into consideration.

Surgical Treatment

The surgical treatment can be described under following heads:

Peripheral Procedures

These procedures are further divided into the following:

- Destructive
  - Peripheral neurectomy
  - Inferior alveolor nerve neurectomy
  - Supraorbital nerve neurectomy
  - Infraorbital nerve neurectomy
  - Supratrochlear nerve neurectomy.
  - Peripheral nerve blocks with alcohol, phenol, glycerol, hot water, etc. (Fig. 9.2).

The inferior alveolar nerve neurectomy is done intraorally through a Ginwalla's incision (inverted 'Y' incision, Fig. 9.3), taken in the retromolar area. The mandibular foramen is located on the medial side of the ramus of the mandible. Using a nerve hook, the inferior alveolar nerve and artery are drawn forward, ligated and the distal end is avulsed by performing the

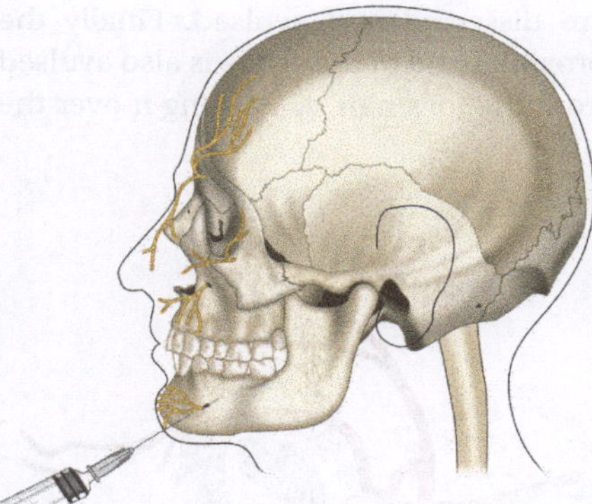

Fig. 9.2: Peripheral branches of the TN where the neurectomies or nerve blocks can be done

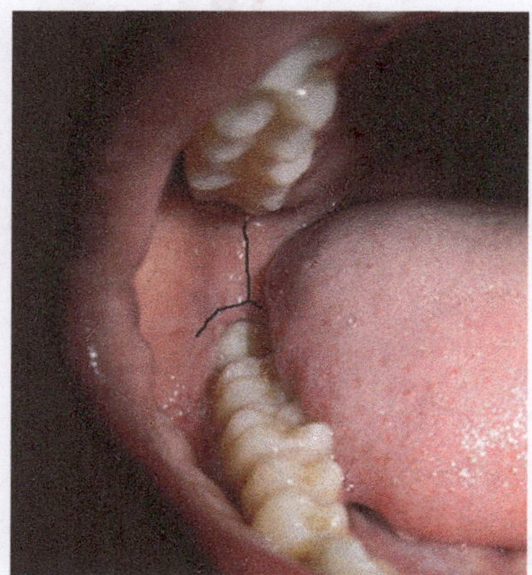

Fig. 9.3: Ginwalla's inverted 'Y' incision

corticotomy in the buccal cortical bone right up to the mental foramen.

The mental nerve neurectomy is done through an intraoral incision taken in the labial vestibule in the lower anterior to premolar area. The mental nerve and its branches are identified and clamped with an artery forcep. The peripheral branches are dissected and avulsed. The proximal end is then avulsed. The mental foramen is decorticated to prevent the nerve regeneration.

The infraorbital nerve neurectomy is also performed intraorally through a degloving incision taken in the upper labial vestibule from the incisor to the second premolar area. A full thickness flap is raised and the infraorbital foramen is located. The infraorbital nerve is grasped with an artery forceps near the foramen; its peripheral branches are dissected and avulsed. Finally the proximal end of the nerve is also avulsed from the foramen by twisting it over the artery forceps. Finally the infraorbital foramen is decorticated, using a bur to prevent the regeneration of the nerve as the decorticated foramen heals completely by bone formation.

Injection of alcohol, phenol, boiling water is given in the vicinity of the nerve, which causes destruction of the nerve by inducing the xanthenes degeneration of the nerve. Proper care must be taken, while giving the injection as these agents can cause sloughing of the soft tissue.

Nondestructive Procedures

The surgical procedures that do not damage the nerve are called nondestructive procedures. These procedures comprise of nerve decompression procedures in cases where the nerve is compressed by bony fragments, impacted tooth, aneurysms, sclerosed and narrowed foramina. Nerve blocks with long-acting local anesthetics (bupivacaine) may be given for temporary pain relief.

Central Procedures

Nondestructive

These procedures are sensory root decompression (Figs 9.4A to D), when aneurysms are present around it. The resection of CP angle tumors or other SOL is the non-destructive procedures. The pulsations of the inferior cerebellar artery are suppose to cause demyelination of nerve and provocation leading to pain. Interpositioning of inert material between the artery and the sensory root causes decompression of the sensory root and relieves the pain.

Destructive Procedures

- Injection of alcohol or glycerol (Glycerol rhizotomy) in the Gasserian ganglion (Fig. 9.5).

  The alcohol or glycerol injection in the Gasserian ganglion results in the destruction of neurons and thus, prevents the conduction of pain and other sensory impulses. It was a popular treatment modality in the past but it lacked specificity. The alcohol diffuses in the adjoining areas and destroys it, resulting into the neurological deficit in the other normal regions of trigeminal nerve. The most catastrophic result was the involvement of ophthalmic division, which resulted in neuroparalytic keratitis, corneal ulcers and in some patients blindness, secondary to it. The other complication was anesthesia dolorosa (phantom pain).

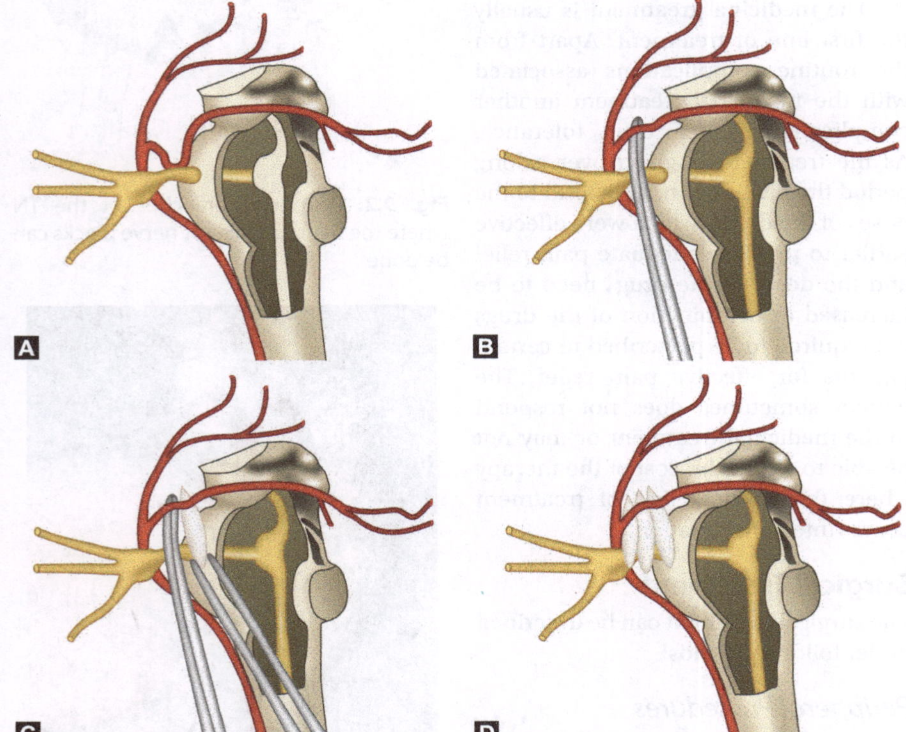

Figs 9.4A to D: Decompression of the sensory root by inserting barrier between the inferior cerebellar artey and the sensory root

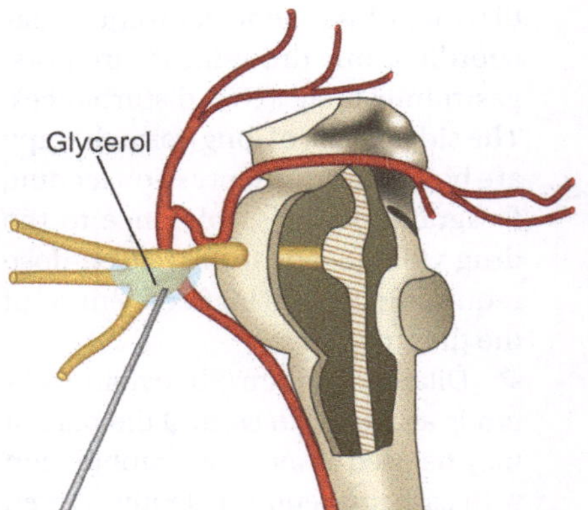

Fig. 9.5: Glycerol injections

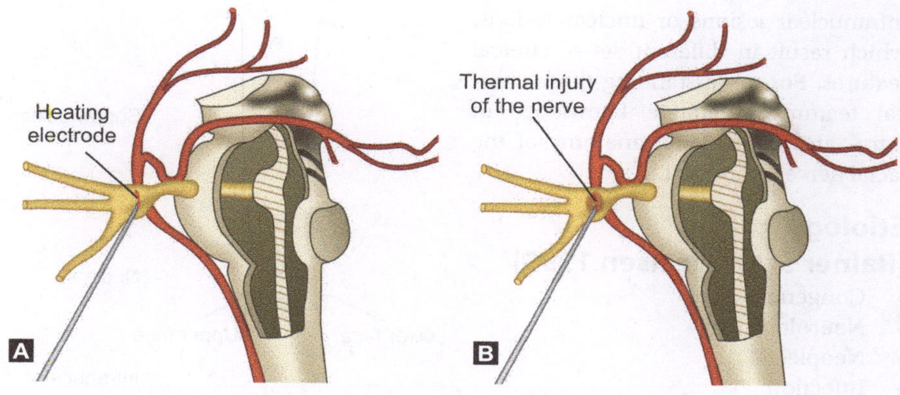

Figs 9.6A and B: Thermocoagulation of the ganglion

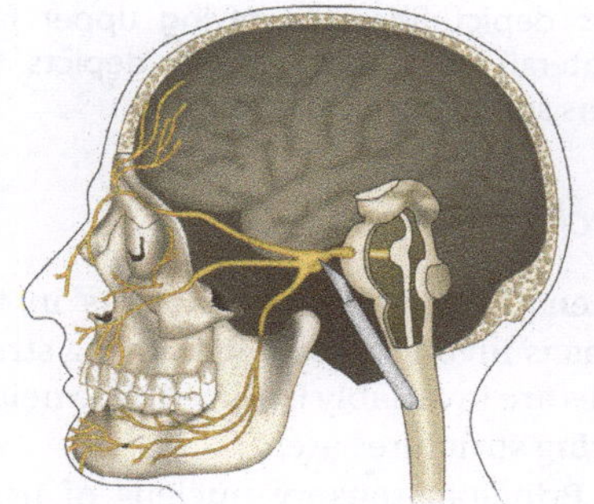

Fig. 9.7: Sectioning to the sensory root (Rhizotomy)

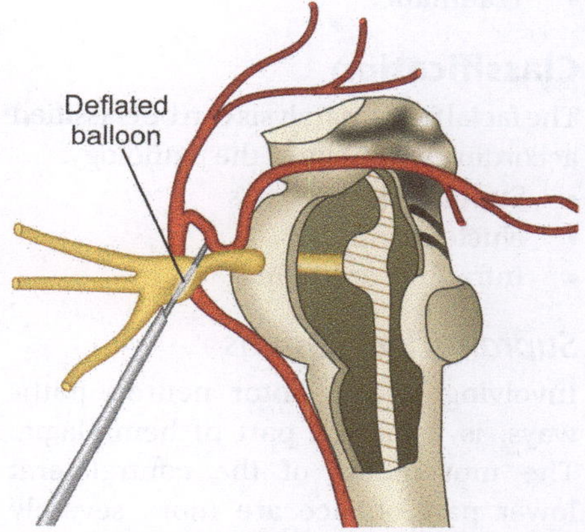

Fig. 9.8: Balloon rhizotomy

- Percutaneous high frequency radio gangliolysis (Thermocoagulation) (Figs 9.6A and B).

  In this procedure an electrode is introduced, percutaneously in the Gasserian ganglion, through the foramen ovale. The patient is not given any anesthesia as per locating the area in which the electrode is present, pain is elicited by applying low-voltage current. The patient gets pain in the corresponding area of trigeminal nerve and that is how the electrode is located in proper area of ganglion. Then a high frequency current is applied, which brings about selective destruction of ganglion, sparing the other uninvolved divisions. The gangliolysis produced by this method results in stereotactic lesions in the gasserion ganglion (*see* Figs 9.6A and B).
- Rhizotomy—division of the sensory root is called rhizotomy (Fig. 9.7).
- Balloon compression rhizotomy (Fig. 9.8).
- Tractectomy—division of spinothalamic tract is the ultimate treatment modality for relief from severe neuralgic pain or pain associated with terminal malignancy.

For these intracranial procedures two common surgical approaches are taken, Dandy's temporal approach and Frazier's posterior fossa approach.

GLOSSOPHARYNGEAL NEURALGIA

Vagoglossopharyngeal neuralgia or glossopharyngeal neuralgia (cranial mononeuropathy IX) is a condition in which there are repeated episodes of severe pain in the tongue, throat, ear and tonsils, which can last from a few seconds to a few minutes. It involves the IX and X cranial nerve in their sensory, motor and autonomic fibers.

Causes

- Etiology of vagoglossopharyngeal neuralgia is unknown. It has been proposed to be due to posterior root demyelination possibly secondary to pressure from intracranial aneurysm or a preceding peritonsillar infection.
- Neuralgia in these areas has been associated with calcified stylohyoid ligament in which chronic pressures on 9th and 10th cranial nerve complex have existed in the region of foramen spinosum.
- Glossopharyngeal neuralgia is believed to be caused by irritation of the 9th and 10th cranial nerve.
- In most cases, the source of irritation is never found. Some possible causes for this type of nerve pain (neuralgia) are:
  - Blood vessels pressing down on the glossopharyngeal nerve.
  - Growths (lesions) at the base of the skull.
  - Tumors or infections of the throat and mouth.

Clinical Features

Symptoms usually begin in people over 40 years of age and there is no predilection for the sex. The left side is involved more than the right side. Symptoms include severe pain in areas connected to the 9th cranial nerve:

- Back of the nose and throat (nasopharynx)
- Back of the tongue
- Ear
- Throat
- Tonsil area
- Larynx.

The pain occurs in episodes and may be severe. It can sometimes be triggered by:

- Chewing
- Coughing
- Laughing
- Speaking
- Swallowing.

The pain is less intense than tic douloureux, but the systemic side effects that accompany an attack are wide-spread and include excessive salivation, lacrimation, vertigo and involuntary movements of the pharynx and larynx. Syncope may occur, with progressive hypotension and bradycardia. In rare cases, asystole and cardiac arrest has been noted.

The attack is usually triggered by swallowing or surface stimulation of the tongue or pharynx or when tasting bitter or spicy foods.

Clinical manifestations are attributed to indiscriminated artificial synpase lesions of the mixed 9th and 10th cranial nerves, of the autonomic areas served by the sensory component of the 9th cranial nerve, the greater petrosal nerve and of the pharngeal plexus of both 9th and 10th cranial nerve and the sinus nerve of Hering.

Investigations

- Computed tomography (CT) scan and MRI of the head to identify tumor or inflammation of the glossopharyngeal nerve.
- Angiography to find out whether a blood vessel is pressing on the nerve.

Treatment

The goal of treatment is to control pain. Over-the-counter pain killers such as aspirin and acetaminophen are not very effective for the relief of neuralgia.

The most effective drugs are anticonvulsant medications, such as carbamazepine, gabapentin and phenytoin. Some antidepressants, such as amitriptyline, may help certain patients.

In severe cases, when pain is difficult to treat, surgery to take pressure off the glossopharyngeal nerve may be needed. This surgery is generally considered effective. If a cause of the neuralgia is found, treatment should control the underlying problem. Intracranial rhizotomy of the posterior root of the 9th and 10th cranial nerves, as well as tractotomies can be attempted for relief.

FACIAL NERVE PARALYSIS

The facial nerve is the 7th cranial nerve. Its paralysis results in paralysis of the muscles of facial expression and certain ocular complications. The paralysis may result from supranuclear lesions, infranuclear lesions or nuclear lesions, which result in different set of clinical features. For understanding these clinical features, adequate knowledge of intra- and extracranial anatomy of the facial nerve is required.

Etiology (Rainer Schmelzeisen 1999)

- Congenital
- Neurological
- Neoplastic
- Infection
- Other causes (idiopathic)
- Iatrogenic
- Traumatic.

Classification

The facial nerve paralysis can be classified according to the site of the pathology:

- Supranuclear lesions
- Nuclear lesions
- Infranuclear lesions.

Supranuclear Lesions

Involving upper motor neuron pathways, is usually a part of hemiplagia. The movements of the contralateral lower part of face are more severely affected than those of upper face and voluntary movements are weak or absent, while the emotional movements are unaffected. This is due to the fact that the corticonuclear fibers going to the upper face are bilateral, while as those going to lower face are unilateral in distribution (Fig. 9.9). The etiological factors for the supranuclear palsy are:

- Infarcts
- Cerebrovascular accident
- Tumors
- Head injury
- Congenital abnormalities and agenesis
- Secondaries.

Clinical Features of Supranuclear Lesions

- Upper motor neuron pool paralysis
- Lower face involved
- Upper face unaffected
- Emotional movements spared
- Voluntary movements affected
- Often associated with hemiplegia.

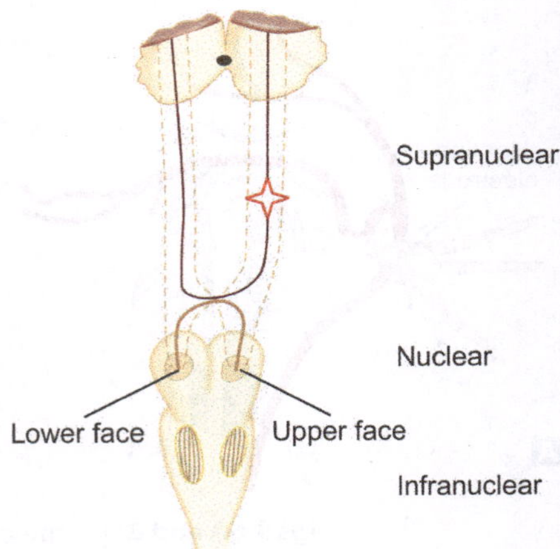

Fig. 9.9: The corticonuclear fibersdotted lines depict fibers supplying upper face (Bilateral) while thick line(✧) depicts the fibers supplying lower face

Nuclear Lesions

When the facial nerve nucleus in the pons is involved the neighboring structures are invariably involved. The neighboring structures are:

- Principal sensory nucleus of trigeminal nerve
- Spinal nucleus of trigeminal nerve
- Nucleus of abducens nerve
- Motor nucleus of trigeminal nerve
- Extrapyramidal tracts
- Vestibulocochlear nerve

The involvement of abducent nerve nucleus results in the paralysis of lateral rectus muscle. Paralysis of muscles of mastication results due to involvement of motor nucleus of trigeminal nerve and sensory loss of face may result due to involvement of principal sensory nucleus or spinal nucleus or spinothalamic tract.

To summarize the clinical features of the nuclear lesions:

- Sensory deficit in distribution of trigeminal nerve.
- Paralysis of muscles of mastication.
- Diplopia due to lateral rectus paralysis.
- Hearing impairment.
  - Lesions at petrous temporal region.
- Lesions in facial canal-chorda tympani involvement—Taste sensation impaired

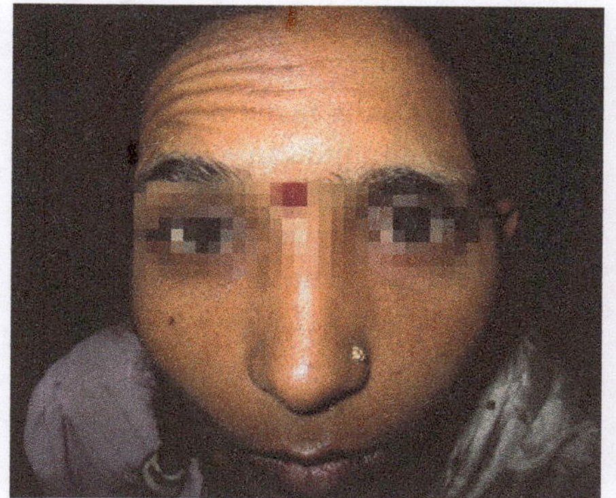

Fig. 9.10: Loss of wrinkling over the forehead (Left) due to paresis of facial nerve

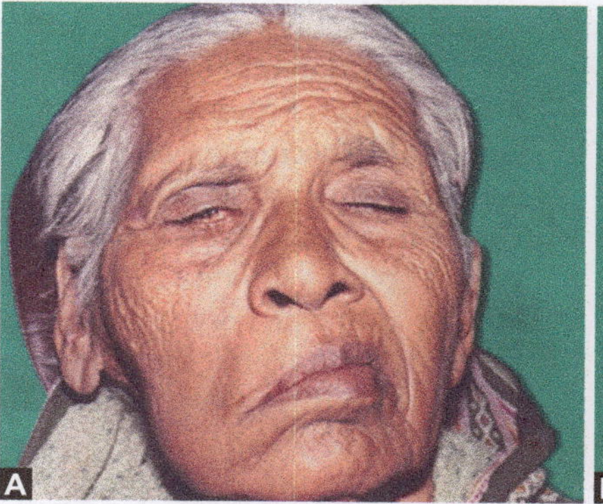

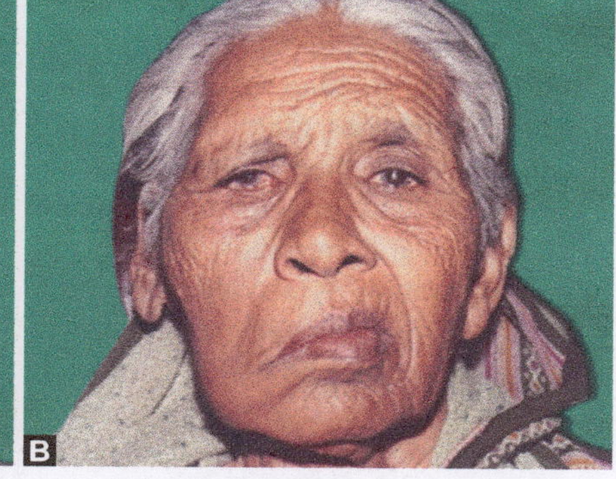

Figs 9.11A and B: Facial nerve paralysis on right side—obliteration of nasolabial fold, drooping of corner of mouth, lagophthalmos, loss of wrinkling on forehead

- Nerve to stepedius damaged—hyperacusis.

Infranuclear Lesions

The lesions that occur at the level of stylomastoid foramen. The etiology is uncertain but results from edema of the nerve and compression of the fibers in the stylomastoid foramen or in the facial canal.

The etiological factors are:
- Exposure to cold.
- Herpes zoster infection.
- Damage or division of the nerve during surgery (parotid surgery, mastoidectomy, middle ear surgery).
- Involvement of the nerve in malignant tumors of the parotid gland.
- Fractures of the base of the skull.

Bell's Palsy

Bell's palsy is defined as an idiopathic paresis or paralysis of facial nerve of sudden onset. The condition was described by Sir Charles Bell (1821), who demonstrated separation of motor and sensory innervation of face. It has female predilection especially pregnant females. It has usually unilateral involvement and can happen at any age.

Clinical Features

The peripheral lesions lead to complete involvement of the face and the voluntary emotional and associated movements are equally involved.
- There is asymmetry of the face.
- Dropping of the corner of mouth.
- Dropping of eyebrow.
- Loss of wrinkling over the forehead (Fig. 9.10).
- Flattening of nasolabial fold (Figs 9.11A and B).
- Inability to blow, whistle.
- The lips remain in contact on the paralyzed side, but cannot be pursed for whistling. When the smile is attempted, the angle of the mouth is drawn up on the normal side but on the affected side the lips remain closed, giving a characteristic '*triangular appearance*'.
- During the mastication the food accumulates in the cheek, due to the paralysis of buccinator and dribbles or is pushed out through the paralyzed lips.
- The tongue appears to deviate to the paralyzed side on protrusion, but if it is seen taking the incisors as guidance it is not so.
- The platysma and the muscle of aurical are paralyzed.
- The ala nasi does not move properly with respiration.
- There is a widening of the palpebral fissure (*lagophthalmos*) due to the unopposed action of levator palpebrae.
- Tears fall down (epiphora) as the lacrimal puncta are not in contact with the conjunctiva and result in the dryness of the conjunctiva.
- Blinking is absent.
- There is loss of corneal reflex and if the patient tries to close the eye, the eyeball rolls up, this is called Bell's sign (Fig. 9.12). Bell's phenomenon or sign is reflex upward, and slightly outward, deviation of the eyes in response to forced closure, or attempted closure, of the eyelids. This is a synkinesis of central origin involving superior rectus and inferior oblique muscles. It is very conspicuous in a patient with Bell's palsy.
- The lagophthalmos (widening of the palpebral fissure) loss of blinking and inability to close the eye results in exposure keratitis, corneal ulceration and may result in blindness.
- The reaction of muscle on electrical stimulation are altered (suggestive of degeneration).
- The involvement of nerve to stapedius results in hyperacusis.

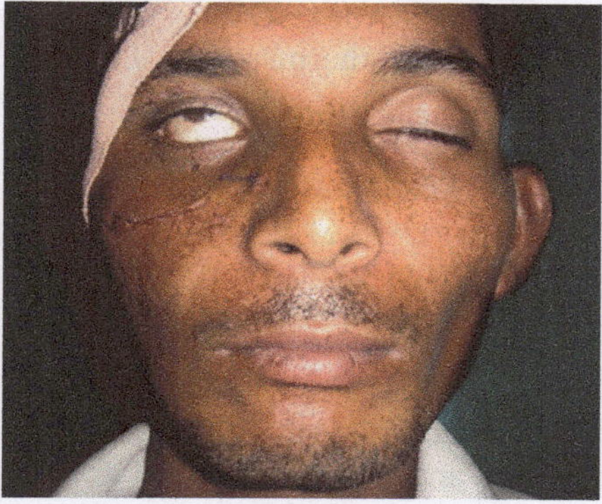

Fig. 9.12: Bell's sign

Management

The management is divided into the following:
- Conservative.
- Surgical.
  - Definitive.
  - Rehabilitative.

Medicinal Treatment

- It comprises of prescription of corticosteroids as they have anti-inflammatory properties. Prednisolone, in a dose of 1 mg/kg/day for 10 days in divided doses, to start with, which is gradually tapered and withdrawn over a period of 2 to 3 weeks. It helps in reducing the nerve edema and inflammation. If the facial nerve paralysis is secondary to the herpes zoster infection, antiviral drugs like acyclovir may be useful. The facial nerve paralysis due to peripheral inflammatory lesions (Bell's palsy) responds well to this treatment and almost complete recovery takes place. However, the lesions causing nerve damage, central lesions may not respond to the treatment. Empirical therapy in form of vitamin B_1, B_6 and B_{12} preparations (Neurontin, Sionneuron® and neurobione, macraberine) are also given.

- Physiotherapy in the form of transcutaneous electrical nerve stimulation (TENS), with galvanic current stimulation is given, which produces satisfactory results. Exercises, massage and hot fomentations are also prescribed.
- Protection of the eye is necessary as the patient has lagophthalmos, lack of blinking, exposure keratitis. Wearing of protective glasses, lubricating eye drops (hydroxy propyl methyl cellulose eye drops, artificial tears) are prescribed, especially when the lacrimal punctum is grossly displaced and the tears do not spread over the eye and fall apart (epiphora). Lubricating eye drops (methylcellulose drops) are prescribed to prevent dryness of the eyes and keratitis.

Surgical Treatment

The surgical treatment can be divided into corrective and rehabilitative. The corrective treatment is done with the intention of restoring the nerve function, before the facial muscles have become flaccid. The essential elements for the successful outcome for surgical treatment are:

- Intact facial nerve
- Healthy muscles (preservation of neuromuscular coordination).

These procedures are as follows:

- Decompression of the nerve trunk
- Anastomosis of the severed nerve ends when it occurs secondary to penetrating injuries, surgical trauma, etc.
- Cross nerve innervations using a cervical plexus C_3 and C_4 (3–12 cm), greater auricular nerve, sural nerve (35 cm) grafts and anastomosing the distal and proximal ends of the severed nerve or to the opposite facial nerve, (Figs 9.13A to D) spinal accessory nerve or hypoglossal nerve, using the microvascular surgical technique. The disadvantage of this procedure is that the facial muscles will contract in unwanted manner with the movements of the part supplied by the nerve anastomosed. Thus, cross innervation from the contralateral facial nerve is most desired. These procedures are useful only when attempted early, before the facial muscles have become flaccid. Even after achieving the anatomical continuity of the nerve by anastomosis the physiological continuity of the nerve is not assured.
- Rehabilitating surgeries like passive fascia lata slings, regional muscle transfers for cosmetic and functional rehabilitation of the patient.

Protocol for Nerve Repair

- The procedures like nerve anastomosis, grafting or cross nerve anastomosis are useful if they are done timely, as the facial nerve paralysis becomes chronic the muscles undergo wasting the muscle atrophy occurs and there is loss of contractile tissue in the muscle and its replacement with collagenous and fatty tissue (Figs 9.13A to D).
- The protocol that needs to be followed for nerve repair or grafting is as follows:
  - Immediate (0–3 weeks)—nerve anastomosis
  - Delayed (3 weeks–2 years)—grafting or nerve cross over
  - Late (over 2 years)—regional muscle transfer or distant microvascular muscle transfer.

Rehabilitating Surgeries

The rehabilitating surgeries are performed to correct the facial deformities for cosmetic rehabilitation of the patient using static fascia lata slings, innervated or denervated muscle slings, which are purely nonfunctional. These surgeries can be described as follows.

Fascia Lata Slings

The fascia lata slings are harvested from the lateral thigh. The slings are nothing but the tendinous insertion of the lateral fascia lata muscle. These slings are used to correct the drooping of the corner of the mouth by suturing the upper end of the sling to zygomatic arch, the lower end of the sling is divided into three and they are sutured to the orbicularis oris, levator labii superioris alaeque nasi and the depressor anguli oris, respectively. These slings lift the corner of the mouth, but it fails to match the movements of the normal side of the face while the patient smiles, as they are passive and the facial deformity becomes obvious. Instead of the fascia lata slings nonabsorbable suture material like prolene can also be used (Figs 9.14A to F). The fascia lata slings can also be used to correct the lagophthalmos by tunneling them in a supratarsal plane below the skin of the eyelids and suturing them on one side to the deep temoral fascia and on the other side to the medial canthal ligament.

Regional Muscle Transfer

Temporal muscle or masseteric muscle slings are used to rehabilitate the patient (Figs 9.15A to D). When these muscles are used they are innervated, during the act of mastication the facial movement takes place, to avoid this undesirable movement the muscle should be denervated. The limitation of this procedure is that it provides only cosmetic correction, when the face is static, but during the movements the deformity is conspicuous and thus, they provide only passive correction.

Correction of lagophthalmos

The complication of lagophthalmos and lack of blinking reflex is exposure

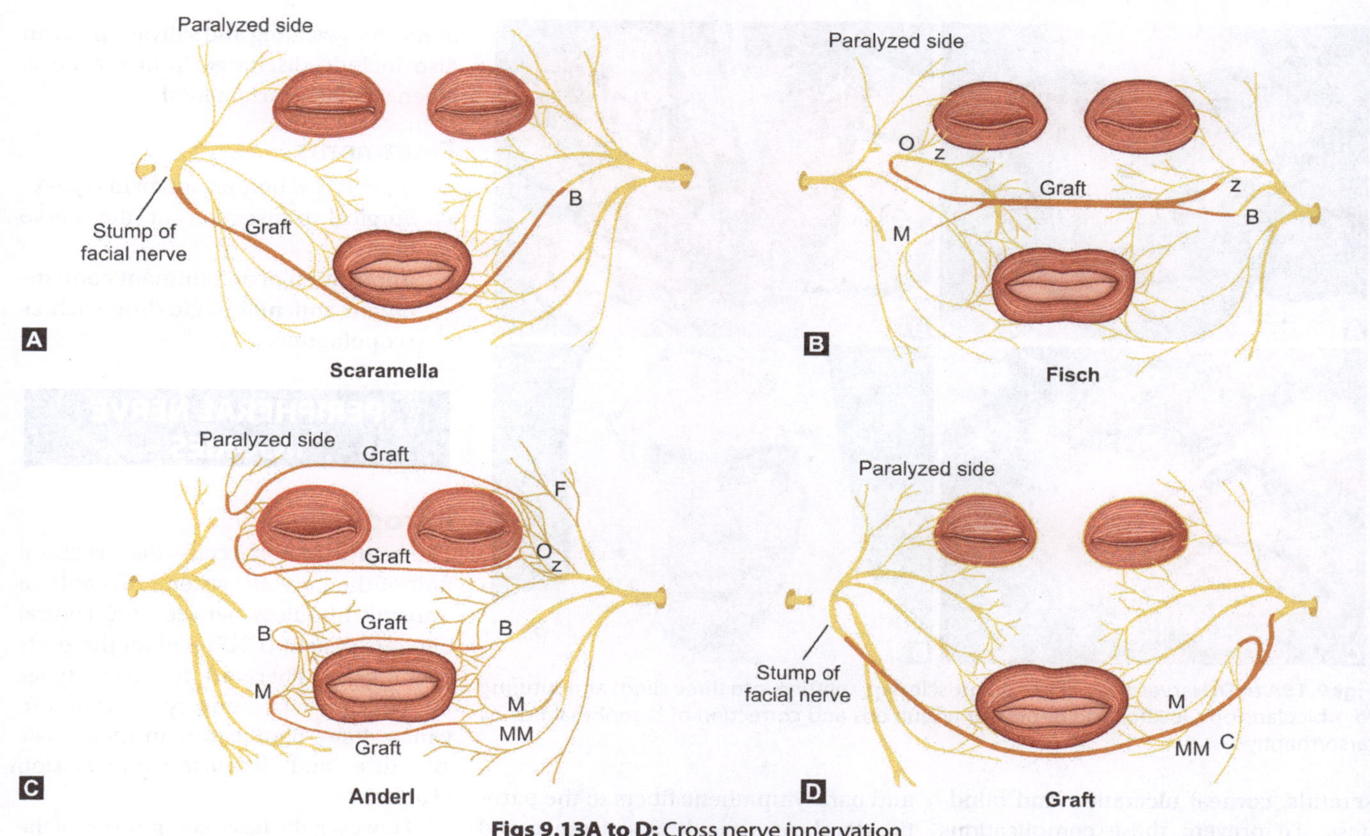

Figs 9.13A to D: Cross nerve innervation

Figs 9.14A to F: Harvesting fascia lata graft, anastomosing with deep temporal fascia and suturing to the corner of mouth and inner canthal ligament after tunneling through the subcutaneous tunnels

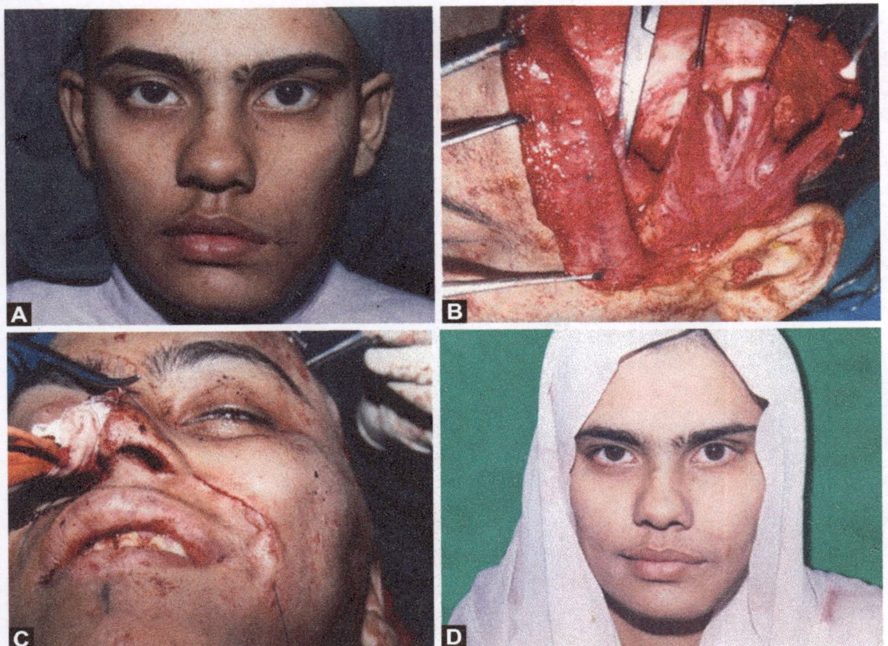

Figs 9.15A to D: Harvesting temporalis muscle flap, splitting into three slings and suturing to orbicularis oris, levator and depressor anguli oris and correction of lagophthalmos by tarsorrhaphy

keratitis, corneal ulceration and blindness. To prevent these complications the lagophthalmos is corrected by either a tarsorrhaphy (Figs 9.15A to D) or by narrowing the wide palpebral fissure using fascia lata slings (*see* Figs 9.14A to F).

FREY'S SYNDROME

Frey's syndrome (also known as Baillarger syndrome, Dupuy syndrome, auriculotemporal syndrome or Frey-Baillarger syndrome) is a food related syndrome, which can be congenital or acquired and can persist for life.

The symptoms of Frey's syndrome are redness and sweating on the cheek area adjacent to the ear. They can appear when the affected person eats, sees, thinks about or talks about certain kinds of food which produce strong salivation. Observing sweating in the region after eating a lemon wedge may be diagnostic.

Frey's syndrome often results as a side effect of parotid gland surgery. The auriculotemporal branch of the trigeminal nerve carries sympathetic fibers to the sweat glands of the scalp and parasympathetic fibers to the parotid gland. As a result of severance and inappropriate regeneration, the fibers may switch courses, resulting in 'gustatory sweating' or sweating in the anticipation of eating, instead of the normal salivatory response. It is often seen with patients who have undergone endoscopic thoracic sympathectomy, wherein part of the sympathetic trunk is cut or clamped to treat sweating of the hands or blushing. The subsequent regeneration or nerve sprouting leads to abnormal sweating and salivation. It can also include discharge from the nose, when smelling certain food.

Treatments

- Injection of botulinum toxin type A
- Surgical transection of the nerve fibers
- Application of an ointment containing an anticholinergic drug such as scopolamine.

PERIPHERAL NERVE INJURIES

Introduction

The neuron or nerve cell is the structural unit of the nervous system. It is able to transmit impulses between the central nervous system (CNS) and all the parts of the body. There are two basic types of neurons, viz. sensory and motor, which differ significantly in their basic structure and impulse transmission (Table 9.1).

However, the basic composition of the axon, dendrite and cell body remain the same, so does the impulse propagation.

Cell body contains nucleus, cytoplasm and various organelles found in other cells. It is located at a distance from the axon or main pathway of impulse transmission in the sensory nerve. Hence, it has no active involvement in nerve conduction and only provides metabolic support for the neuron. The cell body of motor nerve differs from

Table 9.1: Differences between the sensory and motor neurons

Sensory neuron	Motor neuron
Transmit impulses from peripheral organs to the brain	Transmit impulses from brain to peripheral organs
Consists of: 1. Peripheral processes—dendrites, groups of free nerve endings which respond to stimuli 2. Axon which transmits the impulses from the dendrites centrally 3. Centrally located cell body or soma, primarily concerned with vital metabolic functions. Not involved in impulse transmission	1. Cell body of the motor neuron is interposed between the axon and dendrites. 2. Cell body provides vital metabolic support to the neuron in addition to active impulse transmission 3. Axon synapses with muscle cells.

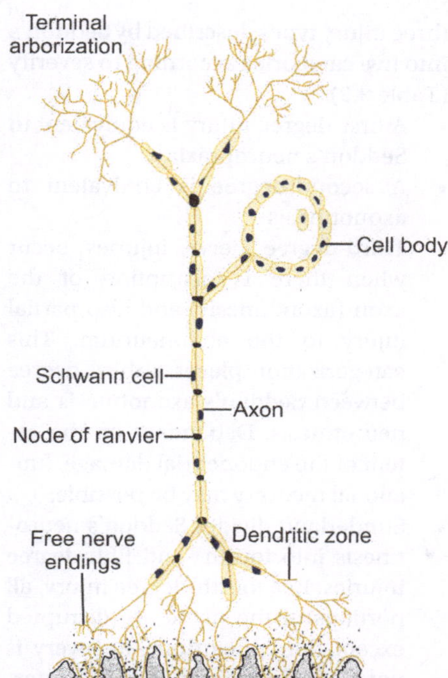

Fig. 9.16: Cell body/soma/perikaryon

sensory nerve cell body, as it is placed between the axon and dendrites. Hence, it has an active role in nerve conduction as well as nutritional support of the nerve (Fig. 9.16).

Axon

It is a single process extending from the cell body and varies in length and diameter. The maximum and minimum length ranges from 1 meter to few millimeters. The diameter of the axon ranges from maximum 20 microns to minimum 1 micron. The diameter is directly proportional to velocity of conduction. The axons conduct impulse away from cell body. Axons terminate in many branched filaments called telodendria and they contain numerous vesicles and mitochondria.

Dendrites

Dendrite means 'tree' in Greek. They are the terminal branches of the multipolar neurons. The distal ends of sensory neurons also called receptors, which are the most distal segment of neuron that carries impulses towards the cell body and is composed of arborization of free nerve endings.

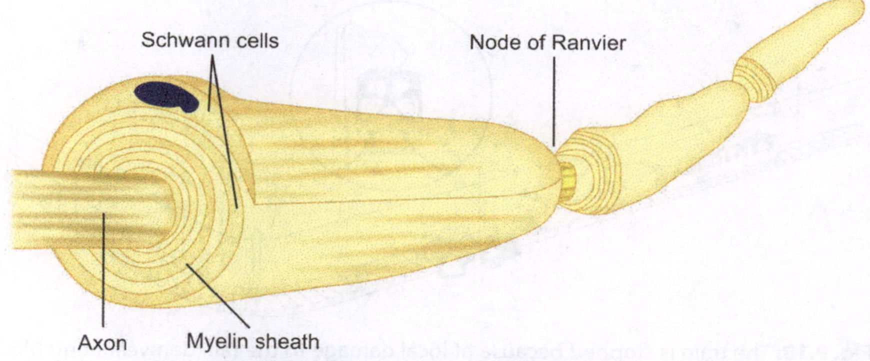

Fig. 9.17: Structure of the myelinated nerve

Myelinated Nerve

It has a central core of axon filled with viscous intracellular fluid—axoplasm, which is surrounded by myelin (lipid sheath) which is specialized secretion form of Schwann cell. The nodes of Ranvier are present at regular intervals of 0.5 to 3 mm (Fig. 9.17).

Nonmyelinated Nerve

It is also surrounded by Schwann cell sheath, but it does not secrete myelin. It has slower rate of conduction as compared to myelinated nerve.

Etiology of Peripheral Nerve Injuries

- Local anesthetic injections
- Impacted third molar removal
- Preprosthetic surgery—mandibular vestibuloplasty
- Endosseous dental implant placement
- Orthognathic surgery—bilateral sagittal split osteotomy
- Facial trauma—fractures
- Gunshot injuries or lacerations
- Endodontic and periradicular surgery
- Salivary gland surgery—parotidectomy
- Treatment of benign and malignant lesions of the head and neck.

Basic Injury Types

It is important to know the basic types of injuries that the neuron is likely to encounter to understand the pathophysiology of nerve injury.

- **Stretch** related injuries are the most common. Peripheral nerves are inherently elastic because of their collagenous endoneurium, but when traction forces exceed the nerve's capacity to stretch, injury occurs. If the force applied is great enough, a complete loss of continuity may occur. More often, however, continuity is retained.
- **Lacerations** such as those created by a knife blade are another common peripheral nerve injury type. Whereas these can be complete transections, more often some nerve element of continuity remains.
- **Compression** is a third common type of peripheral nerve injury. These injuries include the 'Saturday night palsy' due to radial nerve compression as well as entrapment neuropathies and do not involve a severance or tearing of the neural elements. Total loss of both motor and sensory function may occur, but the pathophysiology responsible for these deficits is unclear because complete nerve continuity is maintained. Two pathological mechanisms are believed to be involved in these injuries, mechanical compression and ischemia.

Classification of Nerve Injuries

Seddon divided nerve injuries by severity into three broad categories:

1. Neuropraxia.
2. Axonotmesis.
3. Neurotmesis.

Neuropraxia

The mildest injury type, does not involve loss of nerve continuity and causes functional loss, which is transient. This

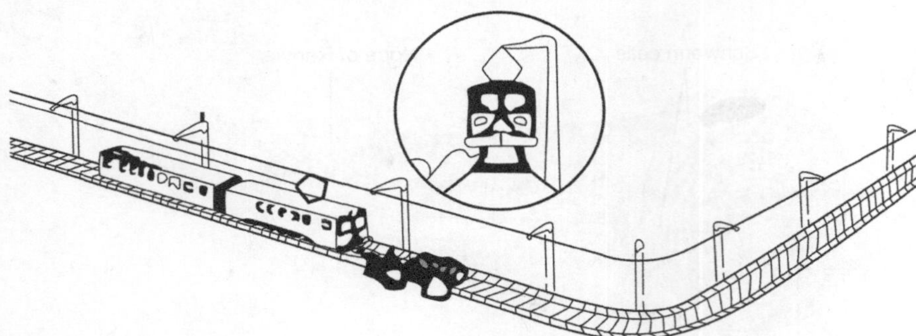

Fig. 9.18: The train is stopped because of local damage to the rail (demyelinating block), more distal parts of the rail as well as energy supply system still being intact. Repair of the local damage might take a considerable time. *Courtesy:* From Lundborg G (Ed): Nerve injury and repair. New York, Churchill Livingstone; 1988. pp. 78-79

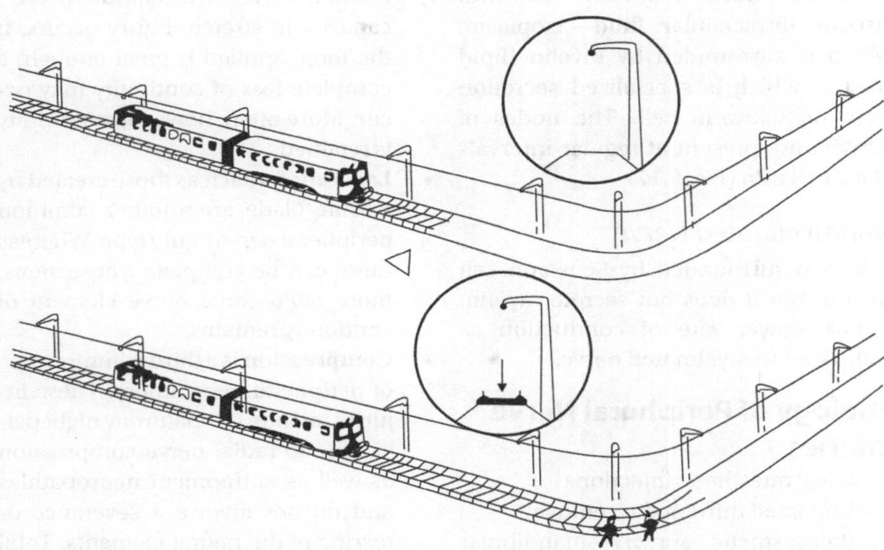

Fig. 9.19: The rail is damaged and has disappeared distal to the level of injury. The track is still intact and new rails can easily be laid down in correct position. *Courtesy:* From Lundborg G (Ed): Nerve injury and repair. New York, Churchill Livingstone; 1988. pp. 78-79

symptom transience is thought to be due to a local ion-induced conduction block at the injury site, although subtle alterations in myelin structure have also been found (Fig. 9.18).

Axonotmesis

Axonotmesis occurs when there is complete interruption of the nerve axon and surrounding myelin, whereas the surrounding mesenchymal structures including the perineurium and epineurium, are preserved. Axon and myelin degeneration occur distal to the point of injury, causing complete denervation. The prospect of recovery is excellent in such injuries because of the remaining uninjured mesenchymal latticework that provides a path for subsequent sprouting axons to reinnervate their target organ (Fig. 9.19).

Neurotmesis

Neurotmesis involves disconnection of a nerve. Functional loss is complete and recovery without surgical intervention does not usually occur, because of scar formation and the loss of the mesenchymal guide that properly directs axonal re-growth (Fig. 9.20).

Sunderland's[8] classification system of nerve injuries further stratifies the three injury types described by Seddon's into five categories according to severity (Table 9.2).

- A first-degree injury is equivalent to Seddon's neuropraxia
- A second-degree is equivalent to axonotmesis
- Third-degree nerve injuries occur when there is disruption of the axon (axonotmesis) and also partial injury to the endoneurium. This categorization places a third-degree between Seddon's axonotmesis and neurotmesis. Dependent on the extent of the endoneurial damage, functional recovery may be possible.
- Sunderland divides Seddon's neurotmesis into fourth- and fifth-degree injuries. In a fourth-degree injury, all portions of the nerve are disrupted except the epineurium. Recovery is not possible without surgical intervention.
- A fifth-degree injury involves complete severance of the nerve.
- A sixth injury pattern was added by Mackinnon and Dellon to describe mixed combination of Sunderland's five degrees of injury. In this some nerve fascicles may exhibit normal function and others have varying degrees of injury.

Physiologic Conduction Block

Type 'A' Conduction Block

Results due to intraneural circulatory arrest/metabolic (ionic) block with no nerve fiber pathology. It is immediately reversible (Fig. 9.21).

Type 'B' Conduction Block

It results from intraneural edema or metabolic block with little or no nerve fiber pathology. It is associated with increased endoneural fluid pressure. It is reversible within days or weeks (Fig. 9.22).

Symptomatic Classification

Anesthesia

It is complete absence of any stimulus detection and stimulus perception, including mechanoreceptive and nociceptive stimuli. It is usually associated with a

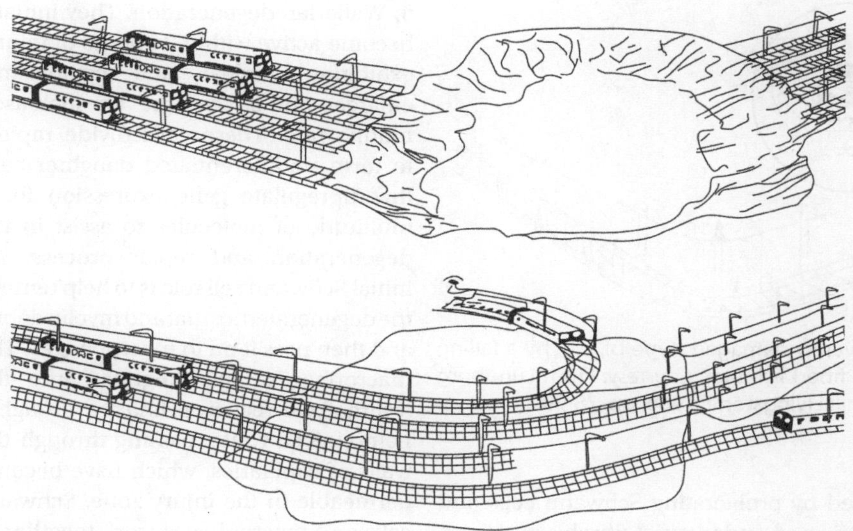

Fig. 9.20: The rails as well as the tracks are destroyed. The result is a great deal of misdirection. *Courtesy:* From Lundborg G (Ed): Nerve injury and repair. New York, Churchill Livingstone; 1988. pp. 78-79

Table 9.2: Comparison between Seddon's and Sunderland's classification

Seddon's classification	Sunderland's classification
Neuropraxia: Stretch injury	First degree
Axonotmesis: Few axons are injured temporary damage, recovery may not be complete	Second degree Third degree Fourth degree
Neurotmesis: Complete severance of nerve—recovery incomplete	Fifth degree

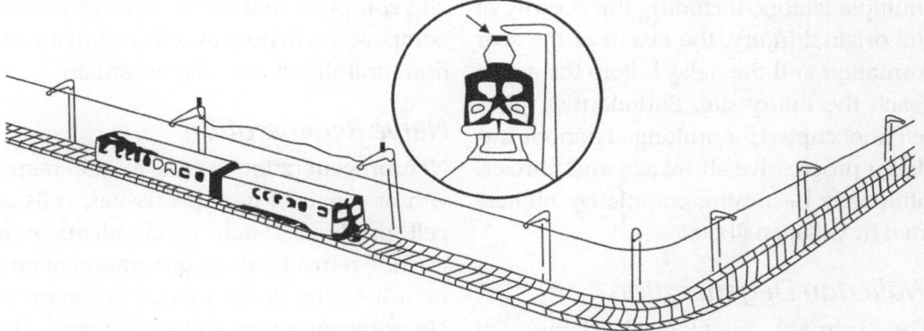

Fig. 9.21: If the local energy supply is interrupted, the train cannot move in spite of intact nerve fiber. The moment the energy supply is restored (electric wire repair) the train can start again. *Courtesy:* From Lundborg G (Ed): Nerve injury and repair. New York, Churchill Livingstone; 1988. pp. 78-79)

severe injury interrupting the integrity of the axons. Sensory recovery is unpredictable and slow.

Paresthesia

It is an alteration in sensibility in which there is abnormal stimulus detection and stimulus perception that may be perceived as unpleasant, but is not painful. Stimulus detection may be decreased or increased and may affect nociception or mechanoreception. Patients may complain of numbness, tingling or itching or swollen sensation. It may be further divided as follows:

- **Hypoesthesia:** Decreased touch and pressure stimuli detection.
- **Hyperesthesia:** Increased touch and pressure stimuli detection.
- **Hypoalgesia:** Decreased nociceptive stimulus detection.
- **Hyperalgesia:** Increased nociceptive stimulus detection.
- **Synesthesia:** Difficulty in quickly and accurately localizing the point of stimulus application.

Dysesthesia

It is an alteration in sensibility in which there is abnormal stimulus detection and stimulus perception that may be perceived as unpleasant and painful. It may be further divided into the following:

- Allodynia—characterized by sharp, first pain perception on light touch.
- Hyperpathia—characterized by dull, second pain on pressure stimulus.

They are associated with neuromas, entrapment, compression and sympathetically maintained pain.

Neural Response to Trauma

Before regeneration of nerve fibers can occur, a series of degenerative processes occur, some of which directly affect regeneration. The success of regeneration depends largely on the severity of the initial injury and resultant degenerative changes.

Pathological changes are mild or absent in first-degree injuries in which the mechanism is conduction block alone and no true degeneration or regeneration occurs.

In second-degree injuries (axonotmesis) there is little histological change at the injury site or proximal to it; however, distal to the injury site, a calcium-mediated process known as Wallerian (or anterograde) degeneration is known to occur.

In third-degree injuries, a more significant trauma-induced local reaction occurs. These intrafascicular injuries involve retraction of the severed nerve fiber ends due to the elastic endoneurium. Local vascular trauma leads to hemorrhage and edema, which results

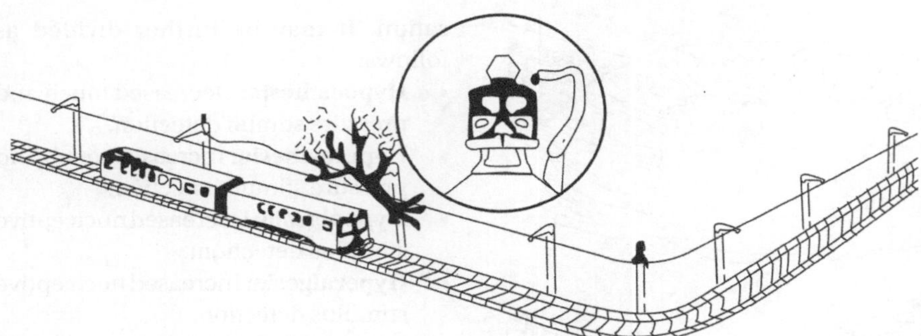

Fig. 9.22: If the electric wire system is more severely damaged (type b), e.g. by a falling tree, the repair takes longer. Still the rail (nerve fiber) is intact. *Courtesy:* From Lundborg G (Ed): Nerve injury and repair. New York, Churchill Livingstone; 1988. pp. 78-79

in a vigorous inflammatory response. Fibroblasts proliferate and a dense fibrous scar causes a fusiform swelling of the injured segment. Interfascicular scar tissue also develops so that the entire nerve trunk, which is left in continuity, is permanently enlarged. Often, it is adherent to perineural scar tissue as well. Distal to the injured segment, Wallerian degeneration follows a sequence very similar to that observed in second-degree injuries. One important difference is that the intrafascicular injury impairs axonal regeneration and therefore, the endoneurial tubes remain denervated for prolonged periods. While denervated, the endoneurial tubes begin to shrink in a process that reaches a maximum at approximately 3 to 4 months postinjury. The endoneurial sheath progressively thickens secondary to collagen deposition along the outer surface of the Schwann cell basement membrane. If the endoneurial tube does not receive a regenerating axon, progressive fibrosis ultimately obliterates it. Stacks of Schwann cell processes representing collapsed endoneurial tubes, known as the bands of Büngner, become important guides for sprouting axons during reinnervation.

In fourth and fifth degree injuries, local reaction to the severe trauma is pronounced. Endoneurial tubes, as well as fasciculi, are disrupted and Schwann cells and axons are no longer confined. The epineurium is also damaged and reactive epineurial fibroblasts are present at the severed ends within 24 hours accompanied by proliferating Schwann cells and peri- and endoneurial fibroblasts. Vigorous cellular proliferation peaks within the 1st week and continues for a prolonged period. The nerve ends become a swollen mass of disorganized Schwann cells, capillaries, fibroblasts, macrophages and collagen fibers. Regenerating axons reach the swollen bulb of the proximal stump and encounter formidable barriers to further growth. Many axons form whorls within the scar tissue or are turned back along the proximal segment or out into the surrounding tissue. Some of the regenerating axons may reach the distal stump, an accomplishment that is dependent on multiple factors, including the severity of the original injury, the extent of the scar formation and the delay before the axons reach the injury site. Endoneurial tubes left unoccupied for prolonged periods undergo progressive shrinkage and fibrosis, ultimately becoming completely obliterated by collagen fibers.

Wallerian Degeneration

The primary histological change in this involves physical fragmentation of axons and myelin, a process that begins within hours of injury. Ultrastructurally, both neurotubules and neurofilaments become disarrayed and axonal contour becomes irregular, due to varicose swellings. By 48 to 96 hours postinjury, axonal continuity is lost and conduction of impulses is no longer possible. Myelin disintegration lags slightly behind that of axons, but is well advanced by 36 to 48 hours. Schwann cells play a key role in Wallerian degeneration. They initially become active within 24 hours of injury, exhibiting nuclear and cytoplasmic enlargement as well as an increased mitotic rate. These cells divide rapidly to form undifferentiated daughter cells that upregulate gene expression for a multitude of molecules to assist in the degeneration and repair process. An initial Schwann cell role is to help remove the degenerated axonal and myelin debris and then pass it on to macrophages. The macrophages have migrated into the traumatized region, primarily through a hemopoietic route, passing through the walls of capillaries, which have become permeable in the injury zone. Schwann cells and macrophages work together to phagocytose and clear the site of injury in a process that requires 1 week to several months.

Endoneural mast cells also play a pivotal role in this process, proliferating markedly within the first 2 weeks post- injury. They release histamine and serotonin, which enhance capillary permeability and facilitate macrophage migration. During the initial stages, the endoneural tubes swell in response to the trauma, but after the first 2 weeks they become smaller in diameter. By 5 to 8 weeks, the degenerative process is usually complete and nerve fiber remnants composed of Schwann cells within an endoneural sheath are all that remain.

Nerve Regeneration

Neuroregeneration refers to the regrowth or repair of nervous tissues, cells or cell products. Such mechanisms may include remyelination, generation of new neurons, glia, axons, myelin or synapses. Neuroregeneration differs between the peripheral nervous system (PNS) and the central nervous system (CNS) by the functional mechanisms and especially, the extent and speed. While the peripheral nervous system has an intrinsic ability for repair and regeneration, the CNS is, for the most part, incapable of self-repair and regeneration. For example the olfactory and the optic nerves are considered as direct extension of the brain matter and once damaged by trauma or inflammation, they fail to regenerate permanently.

There is currently no treatment for recovering human nerve function after injury to the CNS.[9]

Neuroregeneration in the PNS occurs to a significant degree.[10] Axonal sprouts form at the proximal stump and grow until they enter the distal stump. The growth of the sprouts is governed by chemotactic factors secreted from Schwann cells.

Injury to the peripheral nervous system immediately elicits the migration of phagocytic cells, Schwann cells and macrophages to the lesion site in order to clear away debris such as damaged tissue. When a nerve axon is severed, the end still attached to the cell body is labeled the proximal segment, while the other end is called distal segment. After injury, the proximal end swells and experiences some retrograde degeneration, but once the debris is cleared, it begins to sprout axons and the presence of growth cones can be detected. The proximal axons are able to regrow, as long as the cell body is intact and they have made contact with the neurolemmocytes in the endoneurial channel. Human axon growth rates can reach 2 mm/day in small nerves and 5 mm/day in large nerves. The distal segment, however, experiences Wallerian degeneration within hours of the injury; the axons and myelin degenerate, but the endoneurium remains. In the later stages of regeneration the remaining endoneurial tube directs axon growth back to the correct targets. During Wallerian degeneration, Schwann cells grow in ordered columns along the endoneurial tube, creating a band of Büngner (boB) that protects and preserves the endoneurial channel. Also, macrophages and Schwann cells release neurotrophic factors that enhance regrowth. Healing of nerve injuries is unique among tissues, because the process is greatly dependent upon cellular repair rather than tissue repair.

- **Axonal recovery:** Within hours of axotomy, small axoplasmic outgrowths or sprouts protrude from the severed tips. An exaggerated second sprouting occurs after 2 to 3 days. These sprouts advance distally along the Schwann cell tubes on the inside of the basal lamina. The key histologic structures during axonal regeneration appear to be Schwann cell and its basal lamina. Schwann cells multiply in the distal nerve segment and when contacted by an axon sprout undergo a cascade of changes that triggers the production of myelin. Remyelination is a slow process and hence, nonmyelinated axons are likely to regenerate initially.
- **Cellular recovery:** Chromatologic changes are most pronounced between 1 and 3 weeks after axotomy and cells recover from chromatolysis over several weeks to months. The cells are hyperchromatic with predominant Nissl bodies in the mean time. Nissl bodies are stacked endoplasmic reticulum with attached ribosomes indicating massive cellular anabolic response to injury.
- **Receptor recovery:** If regeneration is complete by 6 months following injury, tactile dome receptors are indistinguishable from normal, uninjured receptors.

Neurotrophic Factors

Neurotrophic factors such as nerve growth factor, brain-derived neurotrophic factor, ciliary neurotrophic factor and many others have been identified and are thought to be important in the nerve repair process. Schwann cells also produce neurotrophic factors, including nerve growth factor (NGF), at the site of injury.

Nerve growth factor is involved in nerve cell survival and maintenance in the normal state and appears to be an important component of the nerve repair process as well. It is released from peripheral nerve target organs and transferred to the nerve cell body via retrograde axonal transport. Nerve growth factor receptor concentration on the Schwann cells forming the bands of Büngner increases after injury. The NGF that binds to these receptors on the Schwann cells is presented to the regrowing axon sprouts. This NGF uptaken by the axon is then transferred retrograde from the growth cone to the cell body, providing a continued stimulus for growth as well as a guide for the advancing axon.

Tinel's Sign

Tinel's sign is a way to detect irritated nerves. It is performed by lightly tapping (percussing) over the nerve to elicit a sensation of tingling or "pins and needles" in the distribution of the nerve. It is a sign of regeneration of the nerve.

Central nervous system regeneration

Unlike peripheral nervous system, injury to the central nervous system is not followed by extensive regeneration. It is limited by the inhibitory influences of the glial and extracellular environment. The hostile, nonpermissible growth environment is in part created by the migration of myelin-associated inhibitors, astrocytes, oligodendrocytes, oligodendrocyte precursors and microglia.

The environment within the CNS, especially following trauma, counteracts the repair of myelin and neurons. The growth factors are not expressed or re-expressed, for instance the extracellular matrix is lacking laminins. Glial scars rapidly form and the glia actually produce factors that inhibit remyelination and axon repair. Slower degeneration of the distal segment than that which occurs in the peripheral nervous system also contributes to the inhibitory environment, because inhibitory myelin and axonal debris are not cleared away as quickly. All these factors contribute to the formation of what is known as 'glial scar', which axons cannot grow across. The proximal segment attempts to regenerate after injury, but its growth is hindered by the environment. It is important to note that central nervous system axons have been proven to regrow in permissible environments; therefore, the primary problem to CNS axonal regeneration is crossing or eliminating the inhibitory lesion site.

Management of Peripheral Nerve Injuries

Nonsurgical/Medicinal

- Steroids—reduce the edema around the nerve and is useful in neuropraxia (Prednisolone 5–10 mg TID).

- Nerve tonics—vitamin B_1, B_6, B_{12}—they are supposed to facilitate nerve fiber regeneration and are useful in cases of neuropraxia and axonotmesis.
- In the cases with acute neuralgic pain, drugs like carbamezapine of gabapentine can be prescribed. It is purely symptomatic treatment.
- Physiotherapy—in the form of electrical nerve stimulation (TENS) and in cases of motor nerves exercises and massage therapy can be given.

Surgical

- **Decompression:** It is used if nerve compression occurs resulting into neuropraxia. It is usually done when due to bone deposition in the nerve canal; there is pressure on the nerve leading to neuropraxia. Here, enlargement of the canal boundaries is done to relieve the pressure on the nerve.
- **Anastomosis:** It is microsurgical repair of the severed ends of the nerve. It is useful, when there is no loss of nerve tissue as in accidental clean surgical transection of the nerve.
- **Cross innervation:** It is useful when there is motor nerve deficit due to a lesion in the course of the nerve. In this repair, a nerve is grafted to connect the affected nerve to the normal functional nerve on the other side of the body using microsurgical repair.
- **Nerve grafts:** It is use of a nerve segment from one part of the body to reconstruct and repair an affected nerve in some other part using micrsurgical technique.

Other Painful Conditions

Other painful conditions involving the head, neck and face area such as:

- Myofacial pain dysfunction syndrome
- Eagle's syndrome
- Temporal arteritis
- Migraine
- Cluster neuralgias are discussed in brief.

EAGLE'S SYNDROME

Eagle's syndrome is a rare condition, where an elongated styloid process (> 30 mm) is in conflict with the adjacent anatomical structures. Eagle syndrome was first described by Watt W Eagle in 1937 and is characterized by recurrent pain in the oropharynx and face.

The styloid process is a slender outgrowth at the base of the temporal bone, immediately posterior to the mastoid apex. It lies caudally, medially and anteriorly toward the maxillo-vertebropharyngeal recess (*which contains carotid arteries, internal jugular vein, facial nerve, glossopharyngeal nerve, vagal nerve, and hypoglossal nerve*).

With the stylohyoid ligament and the small horn of the hyoid bone, the styloid process forms the stylohyoid apparatus, which arises embryonically from the Reichert cartilage of the second branchial arch. Eagle defined the length of a normal styloid process at 2.5 to 3.0 cm.

This syndrome was characterized by symptoms typically occurring after pharyngeal trauma or tonsillectomy. It manifests as a nagging dull, long-term ache in the throat, sometimes radiating to the ipsilateral ear and the sensation of a foreign body in the throat. Occasionally, it manifests as odynophagia, dysphonia, increased salivation, and headache.

Frequency

An elongated styloid process occurs in about 4 percent of the general population, while only a small percentage (between 4 and 10.3%) of these patients are symptomatic.[11] So the true incidence is about 0.16 percent, with a female-to-male predominance of 3:1.

Etiology

Eagle (1937–1948) considered surgical trauma (tonsillectomy) or local chronic irritation could cause osteitis, periosteitis or tendonitis of the stylohyoid complex with consequent reactive, ossifying hyperplasia.[12]

Lentini (1975) formulated the hypothesis that persistence of the mesenchymal elements (Reichert cartilage residues) could undergo osseous metaplasia as a consequence of trauma or mechanical stress during the development of the styloid process.[12]

The ossification of muscular tendons leading to irritation of the structures nearby.[13]

The abnormal length associated with abnormal angulation of the styloid process.[14]

Clinical Features

In 1937, Eagle described 2 possible clinical expressions attributable to elongated styloid process, as follows:

The '*classic Eagle syndrome*' is typically seen in patients after pharyngeal trauma or tonsillectomy and it is characterized by ipsilateral dull and persistent pharyngeal pain, centered in the ipsilateral tonsillar fossa, that can be referred to the ear and exacerbated by rotation of the head. A mass or bulge may be palpated in the ipsilateral tonsillar fossa, exacerbating the patient's symptoms. Other symptoms include dysphagia, sensation of foreign body in the throat, tinnitus or cervicofacial pain.

The 'second form' of the syndrome ('*stylocarotid syndrome*') is characterized by the compression of the internal or external carotid artery (*with their perivascular sympathetic fibers*) by a laterally or medially deviated styloid process. It is related to a pain along the distribution of the artery (*carotodinia*), which is provoked and exacerbated by rotation and compression of the neck. It is not correlated with tonsillectomy. In case of impingement of the internal carotid artery, patients often refer supraorbital pain and parietal headache. In case of external carotid artery irritation, the pain radiates to the infraorbital region.

Differential Diagnosis

Temporomandibular disorders, laryngopharyngeal dysesthesia, hyoid bursitis, sluder syndrome, glossopharyngeal neuralgia, esophageal diverticula, trigeminal neuralgia, migraine-type headaches, sphenopalatine neuralgia, cervical arthritis, temporal arteritis, unerupted or impacted molar teeth, faulty dental prostheses, otitis, salivary gland disease, possible tumors.

Treatment

Primary line of management is analgesics and anti-inflammatory medications. Severe cases, which do not respond to analgesics and anti-inflammatory medications, may require partial styloidectomy.

CLUSTER HEADACHE

Cluster headache, nicknamed 'suicide headache', is a neurological disease that involves, as its most prominent feature, an immense degree of pain. 'Cluster' refers to the tendency of these headaches to occur periodically, with active periods interrupted by spontaneous remissions. The cause of the disease is currently unknown. It affects approximately 0.1 percent of the population and men are more commonly affected than women. The condition was originally named Horton's neuralgia after Dr BT Horton, who postulated the first theory as to their pathogenesis.

History

The first complete description of cluster headache was given by the London neurologist Wilfred Harris in 1926. He named the disease migrainous neuralgia.

Cluster headaches have been called by several other names in the past including erythroprosopalgia of Bing, ciliary neuralgia, erythromelagia of the head, Horton's headache (*named after Bayard T Horton, an American Neurologist*), histaminic cephalalgia, petrosal neuralgia, sphenopalatine neuralgia, vidian neuralgia, Sluder's neuralgia and hemicrania angioparalyticia. Sluder's neuralgia (syndrome) and cluster pain can often be temporarily stopped with nasal lidocaine drops.

Pathophysiology

Cluster headaches have been classified as vascular headaches. The intense pain is caused by the dilation of blood vessels, which creates pressure on the trigeminal nerve. While this process is the immediate cause of the pain, the etiology *(underlying cause or causes)* is not fully understood.

Hypothalamus

Among the most widely accepted theories is that cluster headaches are due to an abnormality in the hypothalamus; Dr Goadsby, an Australian specialist in the disease has developed this theory. This can explain, why cluster headaches frequently strike around the same time each day and during a particular season, since one of the functions the hypothalamus performs is regulation of the biological clock. Metabolic abnormalities have also been reported in patients.

The hypothalamus is responsive to light—day length and photoperiod; olfactory stimuli, including pheromones; steroids, including sex steroids and corticosteroids; neurally transmitted information arising in particular from the heart, the stomach and the reproductive system; autonomic inputs; blood-borne stimuli, including leptin, ghrelin, angiotensin, insulin, pituitary hormones, cytokines, blood plasma concentrations of glucose and osmolarity, etc. and the stress. These particular sensitivities may underlay the causes, triggers and methods of treatment of cluster headache.

Triggers

Nitroglycerin (glyceryl trinitrate) can sometimes induce cluster headaches in sufferers in a manner similar to spontaneous attacks. Ingestion of alcohol or chocolate is recognized as a common trigger of cluster headaches, when a person is in cycle or susceptible. Exposure to hydrocarbons (petroleum solvents, perfume) is also recognized as a trigger for cluster headaches. Some patients have a decreased tolerance to heat and becoming overheated may act as a trigger, which may explain the occurrence after aerobic exercise. Napping causes a headache for some sufferers, while for others lack of sleep triggers them. The role of diet and specific foods in triggering cluster headaches is controversial and not well understood.

Smoking

Nicotine may trigger cluster headaches and the affliction is often found in people with a heavy addiction to cigarette smoking.

Signs and Symptoms

Cluster headaches are excruciating unilateral headaches of extreme intensity. The duration of the common attack ranges from, as short as 15 minutes to 3 hours or more. The onset of an attack is rapid and most often without the preliminary signs that are characteristic of a migraine. However, some sufferers report preliminary sensations of pain in the general area of attack, often referred to as 'shadows', that may warn them an attack is imminent. Though the headaches are almost exclusively unilateral, there are many documented cases of 'side-shifting' between cluster periods or even rarer simultaneous (within the same cluster period) bilateral headache. Trigeminal neuralgia can also bring on headaches with similar qualities. However, with trigeminal neuralgia the pain is mostly located around the 'cheek' area and is described as being more lance-like in quality.

Pain

The pain of cluster headaches is markedly greater than in other headache conditions, including severe migraines and experts believe that it may be the most severe pain known to medical science. It has been described by female patients as being more severe than childbirth.

The pain is lancinating or boring in quality and is located behind the eye (periorbital) or in the temple, sometimes radiating to the neck or shoulder. Analogies frequently used to describe the pain are a red-hot poker inserted into the eye or a spike penetrating from the top of the head, behind one eye, radiating down to the neck or sometimes having a leg amputated without any anesthetic.

Other Symptoms

The cardinal symptoms of the cluster headache attack are ptosis, lacrimation, rhinorrhea and less commonly, facial blushing, swelling or sweating. These features are known as the autonomic symptoms. The attack is also associated with restlessness, the sufferer often pacing the room or rocking back and forth. Less frequently, he or she will have an aversion to bright lights and loud noise during the attack. Nausea rarely accompanies a cluster headache. The neck is often stiff or tender in the aftermath of a headache, with jaw or tooth pain sometimes present. Some sufferers report feeling as though their nose is stopped up and that they are unable to breathe out of one of their nostrils.

Cyclical Recurrence and Regular Timing

Cluster headaches are occasionally referred to as *'alarm clock headaches'*, because of its ability to wake a person from sleep and because of the regularity of its timing in that both the individual attacks and the clusters themselves can have a metronomic regularity; attacks striking at a precise time of day each morning or night is typical, even precisely at the same time a week later. This has prompted researchers to speculate an involvement of the brain's 'biological clock' or circadian rhythm.

Episodic or chronic

In episodic cluster headache, these attacks occur once or more daily, often at the same times each day, for a period of several weeks, followed by a headache-free period lasting weeks, months or years. Approximately 10 to 15 percent of cluster headache sufferers are chronic; they can experience multiple headaches everyday for years.

Cluster headaches occurring in two or more cluster periods lasting from 7 to 365 days with a pain-free remission of 1 month or longer between the clusters are considered episodic. If the attacks occur for more than a year without a pain-free remission of at least 1 month, the condition is considered chronic. Chronic clusters run continuously without any 'remission' periods between cycles. The condition may change from chronic to episodic and from episodic to chronic. Remission periods lasting for decades before the resumption of clusters have been known to occur.

Treatment

Cluster headaches often go undiagnosed for many years, being confused with migraine or other causes of headache. Cluster headaches are considered benign, but because of the extreme and often debilitating pain associated with them, a severe attack is nevertheless treated as a medical emergency by doctors, who are familiar with the condition.

Over-the-counter pain medications (such as aspirin, paracetamol and ibuprofen) typically have no effect on the pain from a cluster headache. Unlike other headaches such as migraines and tension headaches, cluster headaches do not respond to biofeedback.

Medications to treat cluster headaches are classified as either abortives or prophylactics. In addition, short-term transitional medications (such as steroids) may be used, while prophylactic treatment is instituted and adjusted. With abortive treatments often only decreasing the duration of the headache and preventing it from reaching its peak rather than eliminating it entirely, preventive treatment is always indicated for cluster headaches, to be started at the first sign of a new cluster cycle.

Abortive Treatment

During the onset of a cluster headache, some patients respond to rapid inhalation of pure oxygen (12–15 liters per minute in a nonrebreathing mask). When used at the onset this can abort the attack in as little as 1 minute or as long as 10 minutes. Once an attack is at its peak, oxygen therapy appears to have little effect, so most people have an oxygen provider close. Alternative first-line treatment is subcutaneous administration of triptan drugs, like sumatriptan and zolmitriptan. Because of the rapid onset of an attack, the triptan drugs are usually taken by subcutaneous injection rather than by mouth. But these drugs are expensive.

Nonnarcotic treatment botox injections along the occipital nerve, as well as sarapin (pitcher plant extract) injections.

Lidocaine and other topical anesthetics sprayed into the nasal cavity may relieve or stop the pain, normally in a few minutes, but long-term use is not suggested due to the side effects and possible damage to the nasal cavities.

Other abortive remedies that work for some include ice, hot showers, cool or lukewarm water sprayed on the face around the sinus, temple and ear areas, breathing cold air, application of White Flower analgesic balm beneath the nostrils, caffeine and drinking large amounts of water in the early stages of an attack. Vigorous exercise has been shown in some cases to be very effective in relieving and aborting an acute attack by increasing the levels of oxygen within the body. This could also be due to an increase in adrenaline and changes in blood pressure.

Hyperbaric oxygen therapy has been used successfully in treating cluster headaches though it was not shown to be more successful than surface oxygen.

Prophylactic Treatment

A wide variety of prophylactic medicines are in use like calcium channel blocker verapamil at a dose of at least 240 mg daily. Steroids, such as prednisolone, are also effective, with a high dose given for the first 5 days or longer before tapering down. Methysergide, lithium and the anticonvulsant topiramate are recommended as alternative treatments. Muscle relaxants and atypical anti-psychotics have also been used.

Magnesium supplements, melatonin, tricyclic antidepressants including amitriptyline and nortriptyline are some of the other drugs used.

Differential Diagnosis

- Chronic paroxysmal hemicrania (CPH) is a condition similar to cluster headache, but CPH responds well to treatment with the anti-inflammatory drug indomethacin and the attacks are much shorter, often lasting only seconds.
- Some people with extreme headaches of this nature (especially if they are not unilateral) may actually have an ictal headache. Anticonvulsant medications can significantly improve this condition.
- It is also possible to have two or more different types of headaches, complicating diagnosis and treatment.

TEMPORAL ARTERITIS

Temporal arteritis or giant cell arteritis is a systemic inflammatory illness that affects people over the age of 50 and is more common in females. It is a primary arterial disorder that manifests as an arteritis with giant cell and chronic inflammatory infiltrate, intimal thickening and thrombosis. It generally starts slowly with the development of fatigue and malaise over several weeks. It may also cause low-grade fevers and weight loss. Patients will also experience muscle and joint aches in their hips and shoulders, but only rarely true joint swelling.

As part of the inflammatory process, major large arteries are inflamed in particular the temporal artery (artery at the side of head near the temples). Since the temporal artery supplies blood to the jaw and top of the head, symptoms include headache, scalp tenderness and soreness of the jaw after chewing or talking. Patient often complains of deep throbbing, unilateral headache over the maxillary, zygomatic, preauricular, temporal and occipital region. The pain is aggravated by lying down or stooping, but can be relieved by carotid compression. There is exquisite tenderness over the course of the superficial temporal, transverse facial and supraorbital arteries, which are torturous, nodular, and often pulseless.

The temporal artery also supplies the optic nerve and one of the most serious and gratefully rare, complications of temporal arteritis is blindness. The treatment of choice for temporal arteritis is prednisone, which is very effective.

The major concern with temporal arteritis is vision loss, although if allowed to progress, it may affect arteries in other areas of the body. This condition is potentially vision threatening, however, if treated promptly, permanent vision loss can be prevented. Vision is threatened, when the inflamed arteries obstruct blood flow to the eyes and optic nerves. If untreated, permanent vision loss can occur from oxygen deprivation to the retina and optic nerve.

The cause of temporal arteritis is unknown, but is assumed to be, at least in part, an effect of the immune response. The disorder has been associated with polymyalgia rheumatica. It has also been associated with severe infections, high doses of antibiotics and chronic disorders such as rheumatoid arteritis and systemic lupus erythematosus. The symptoms occur because of inflammation. The disorder may exist independently or may coexist with or follow polymyalgia rheumatica (a disorder characterized by abrupt development of pain and stiffness in the pelvis and shoulder muscles). About 25 percent of people with giant cell arteritis also experience polymyalgia rheumatica.

Symptoms

- Fever
- Headache
  - On one side of the head or the back of the head.
  - Throbbing.
- Scalp sensitivity, tenderness when touching the scalp
- Jaw pain, intermittent or when chewing
- Vision difficulties
- Blurred vision, double vision
- Reduced vision, blindness in one or both eyes
- Weakness, excessive tiredness
- Loss of appetite
- Weight loss (> 5% of total body weight)
- Muscle aches
- Excessive sweating.

Additional symptoms that may be associated with this disease are:

- Mouth sores
- Joint stiffness
- Joint pain
- Hearing loss
- Bleeding gums
- Facial pain.

Signs and Tests

Palpation of the head shows scalp sensitivity and often shows a tender, thick, palpable artery on one side of the head. The affected artery may have a weakened pulse or no pulse. About 40 percent of people will have other nonspecific symptoms such as respiratory complaints (most frequently dry cough) or mononeuritis multiplex (weakness and/or pain of multiple individual nerve groups). Rarely, ocular palsies (paralysis of eye muscles) may occur. Fever may be the only symptom (the person presents with a persistent fever of unknown origin).

Investigations

Blood tests are nonspecific.

- A sedimentation rate (ESR) is almost always very high.
- A hemoglobin or hematocrit may be normal or low.
- Liver function tests may be abnormal if the disorder is systemic.
- Alkaline phosphatase may be elevated.

A biopsy and analysis of tissue from the affected artery is also done.

Treatment

The goal of treatment is to minimize irreversible tissue damage that may occur, because of lack of blood flow (ischemia).

Corticosteroids such as prednisone are commonly prescribed to reduce inflammation. If symptoms suggest cerebral vasculitis, corticosteroid treatment may be started even before a biopsy confirms the diagnosis (to reduce the risk of complications). Aspirin may be recommended in addition to corticosteroids.

Medications that suppress the immune system (such as cyclophosphamide) are occasionally prescribed.

MIGRAINE

Migraine is a neurological syndrome characterized by altered bodily perceptions, severe headaches and nausea. Physiologically, the migraine headache is a neurological condition more common to women than to men.

The pain associated with migraine is proposed to be vascular in origin. Extra and intracranial vessels like superficial temporal, supraorbital, frontal, internal, external and common carotid, internal maxillary and middle meningeal (extracranial portion) arteries are commonly identified sources.

The onset of this condition is before 16 years of age and disorder affects females twice as often as males.

The typical migraine headache is unilateral and pulsating, lasting from 4 to 72 hours,[15] symptoms include nausea, vomiting, photophobia and phonophobia (*increased sensitivity to sound*).[16] Approximately one-third of people who suffer migraine headache perceive an aura—unusual visual, olfactory or other sensory experiences that are a sign that the migraine will soon occur.[17]

Initial treatment is with analgesics for the headache, an antiemetic for the nausea and the avoidance of triggering conditions. The cause of migraine headache is idiopathic; the accepted theory is a disorder of the serotonergic control system, as PET scan has demonstrated the aura coincides with diffusion of cortical depression consequent to increased blood flow (up to 300% > baseline).

There are migraine headache variants, some originate in the brainstem (featuring intercellular transport dysfunction of calcium and potassium ions) and some are genetically disposed.[18] Studies of twins indicate a 60 to 65 percent genetic influence upon their propensity to develop migraine headache.[19] Moreover, fluctuating hormone levels indicate a migraine relation: 75 percent of adult patients are women, although migraine affects approximately equal numbers of prepubescent boys and girls; propensity to migraine headache is known to disappear during pregnancy, although in some women migraines may become more frequent during pregnancy.

Signs and Symptoms

The signs and symptoms of migraine vary among patients. Therefore, what a patient experiences before, during and after an attack cannot be defined exactly. The four common phases of a migraine attack:

1. The prodrome, which occurs hours or days before the headache.
2. The aura, which immediately precedes the headache.
3. The pain phase, also known as headache phase.
4. The postdrome.

Prodromal Phase

Prodromal symptoms occur in 40 to 60 percent of migraine sufferers. This phase may consist of altered mood, irritability, depression or euphoria, fatigue, yawning, excessive sleepiness, craving for certain food (e.g. chocolate), stiff muscles (especially in the neck), constipation or diarrhea, increased urination and other visceral symptoms.[20] These symptoms usually precede the headache phase of the migraine attack by several hours or days.

Aura Phase

For the 20 to 30 percent[21] of individuals who suffer migraine with aura. This aura comprises focal neurological phenomena that precede or accompany the attack. They appear gradually over 5 to 20 minutes and generally last fewer than 60 minutes. The headache phase of the migraine attack usually begins within 60 minutes of the end of the aura phase, but it is sometimes delayed up to several hours and it can be missing entirely. Symptoms of migraine aura can be visual, sensory or motor in nature.[22]

Visual aura is the most common of the neurological events. There is a disturbance of vision consisting usually of unformed flashes of white and/or black or rarely of multicolored lights (photopsia) or formations of dazzling zigzag lines (*scintillating scotoma*). Scintillating scotoma is the most common visual aura preceding migraine and was first described by 19th century physician Hubert Airy, scintillating scotoma usually begins as a spot of flickering light near or in the center of the visual fields, which prevents vision within the scotoma. The scotoma area flickers, but is not dark. The scotoma then expands into one or more shimmering arcs of white or colored flashing lights. An arc of light may gradually enlarge, become more obvious and may take the form of a definite zigzag pattern, sometimes called fortification spectrum, because of its resemblance to the fortifications of a castle or fort seen from above; often arranged like the battlements of a castle, hence, the alternative terms 'fortification spectra' or 'teichopsia' (*the sensation of a luminous appearance before the eyes, with a zigzag, wall-like outline*). Some patients complain of blurred or shimmering or cloudy vision, as though they were looking through thick or smoked glass or, in some cases, tunnel vision and hemianopsia (*Hemianopsia: the loss of half of a field of vision*). The somatosensory aura of migraine consists of digitolingual or cheiro-oral paresthesias, a feeling of pins-and-needles experienced in the hand and arm as well as in the nose-mouth area on the same side. Paresthesia migrates up the arm and then extends to involve the face, lips and tongue.

Other symptoms of the aura phase can include auditory or olfactory hallucinations, temporary dysphasia, vertigo, tingling or numbness of the face and extremities and hypersensitivity to touch.

Pain Phase

The typical migraine headache is unilateral, throbbing and moderate to severe and can be aggravated by physical activity. Not all these features are necessary. The pain may be bilateral at the onset or start on one side and become generalized and usually it alternates sides from one attack to the next. The onset is usually gradual. The pain peaks and then subsides and usually lasts 4 to 72 hours in adults and 1 to 48 hours in children. The frequency of attacks is extremely variable, from a few in a lifetime to several a week and the average migraineur experiences one to three headaches a month. The headache varies greatly in intensity.

The pain of migraine is invariably accompanied by other features. Nausea occurs in almost 90 percent of patients and vomiting occurs in about one-third of patients. Many patients experience sensory hyperexcitability manifested by photophobia, phonophobia and osmophobia (*Osmophobia or olfactophobia refers to a fear, aversion, or psychological hypersensitivity to smells or odors*) and seek a dark and quiet room. Blurred vision, nasal stuffiness, diarrhea, polyuria, pallor or sweating may be noted during the headache phase. There may be localized edema of the scalp or face, scalp tenderness, prominence of a vein or artery in the temple or stiffness and tenderness of the neck. Impairment of concentration and mood are common. The extremities tend to feel cold and moist. Vertigo may be experienced. Lightheadedness, rather than true vertigo and a feeling of faintness may occur.

Postdromal Phase

The patient may feel tired or 'hungover' and have head pain, cognitive difficulties (*learning difficulties*), gastrointestinal symptoms, mood changes and weakness.[23] Some people feel unusually refreshed or euphoric after an attack, whereas others note depression and malaise. Often, some of the minor headache phase symptoms may continue such as loss of appetite, photophobia and lightheadedness. For some patients, a 5 to 6 hours nap may reduce the pain, but slight headaches may still occur when the patient stands or sits quickly. Normally these symptoms go away after a good night's rest.

Diagnosis

Migraines are underdiagnosed and misdiagnosed. The diagnosis of migraine without aura, according to the International Headache Society, can be made according to the following criteria, the '5, 4, 3, 2, 1 criteria':

- 5 or more attacks.
- 4 hours to 3 days in duration.
- 2 or more of—unilateral location, pulsating quality, moderate to severe pain, aggravation by or avoidance of routine physical activity.
- 1 or more accompanying symptoms—nausea and/or vomiting, photophobia, phonophobia.

For migraine with aura, only two attacks are required to justify the diagnosis.

The pnemonic '*POUNDing*' (Pulsating, duration of 4–72 hours, unilateral, nausea, Disabling) can help diagnose migraine. If 4 of the 5 criteria are met, then the positive is the likelihood ratio for diagnosing migraine.[24]

Migraine should be differentiated from other causes of headaches such as cluster headaches. These are extremely painful, unilateral headaches of a piercing quality. The duration of the common attack is 15 minutes to 3 hours. Onset of an attack is rapid and most often without the preliminary signs that are characteristic of a migraine.

Diagnosis can also be substantiated by exerting digital pressure over the common carotid artery and/or noting the relief of the pain by giving ergotamine tartarate.

Pathophysiology

Migraines were once thought to be initiated exclusively by problems with blood vessels. The vascular theory of migraines is now considered secondary to brain dysfunction[25] and claimed to have been discredited by others.[26] Trigger points can be at least part of the cause, and perpetuate most kinds of headaches.

The effects of migraine may persist for some days after the main headache has ended. Many sufferers report a sore feeling in the area, where the migraine was and some report impaired thinking for a few days after the headache has passed.

Migraine headaches can be a symptom of hypothyroidism.

Depolarization Theory

A phenomenon known as cortical spreading depression can cause migraines.[27] In cortical spreading depression, neurological activity is depressed over an area of the cortex of the brain. This situation results in the release of inflammatory mediators leading to irritation of cranial nerve roots, most particularly the trigeminal nerve, which conveys the sensory information for the face and much of the head.

Vascular Theory

Migraines can begin when blood vessels in the brain contract and expand inappropriately. This may start in the occipital lobe, as arteries spasm. The reduced flow of blood from the occipital lobe triggers the aura that some individuals who have migraines experience because the visual cortex is in the occipital area.[25]

When the constriction stops and the blood vessels dilate, they become too wide. The once solid walls of the blood vessels become permeable and some fluid leaks out. This leakage is recognized by pain receptors in the blood vessels of surrounding tissue. In response, the body supplies the area with chemicals which cause inflammation. With each heart beat, blood passes through this sensitive area causing a throb of pain.[25]

The vascular theory of migraines is now seen as secondary to brain dysfunction.

Serotonin Theory

Serotonin is a type of neurotransmitter, or "communication chemical" which passes messages between nerve cells. It helps to control mood, pain sensation, sexual behavior, sleep, as well as dilation and constriction of the blood vessels among other things. Low serotonin levels in the brain may lead to a process of constriction and dilation of the blood vessels which trigger a migraine.[25] Triptans activate serotonin receptors to stop a migraine attack.

Neural Theory

When certain nerves or an area in the brainstem become irritated, a migraine begins. In response to the irritation, the body releases chemicals which cause inflammation of the blood vessels. These chemicals cause further irritation of the nerves and blood vessels and results in pain. Substance P is one of the substances released with first irritation.[28] Pain then increases because substance P aids in sending pain signals to the brain.

Unifying Theory

Both vascular and neural influences cause migraines.

- Stress triggers changes in the brain.
- These changes cause serotonin to be released.
- Blood vessels constrict and dilate.
- Chemicals including substance P irritate nerves and blood vessels causing pain.

Triggers

A migraine trigger or 'precipitant' is any factor that, on exposure or withdrawal, leads to the development of an acute migraine headache. Triggers may be categorized as behavioral, environmental, infectious, dietary, chemical or hormonal. Migraine attacks may be triggered by:

- Allergic reactions.
- Bright lights, loud noises and certain odors or perfumes.
- Physical or emotional stress.
- Changes in sleep patterns.
- Smoking or exposure to smoke.
- Skipping meals.
- Alcohol.
- Menstrual cycle fluctuations, birth control pills, hormone fluctuations during the menopause transition.
- Tension headaches.
- Foods containing tyramine (red wine, aged cheese, smoked fish, chicken livers, figs and some beans), monosodium glutamate (MSG) or nitrates (like bacon, hot dogs and salami).
- Other foods such as chocolate, nuts, peanut butter, avocado, banana, citrus, onions, dairy products and fermented or pickled foods.

Management

Conventional treatment focuses on three areas:

1. Trigger avoidance.
2. Symptomatic control.
3. Prophylactic pharmocological drugs.

Paracetamol or Nonsteroidal Anti-inflammatory Drugs (NSAIDs)

The first line of treatment is over-the-counter abortive medication.

Simple analgesics combined with caffeine may help. During a migraine attack, emptying of the stomach is slowed, resulting in nausea and a delay in absorbing medication. Caffeine has been shown to partially reverse this effect.

Excedrin migraine: It is a combination of aspirin, acetaminophen and caffeine.

Analgesics combined with antiemetics: Antiemetics by mouth may help relieve symptoms of nausea and help prevent vomiting, which can diminish the effectiveness of orally taken analgesia. In addition some antiemetics such as metoclopramide are prokinetics and help gastric emptying, which is often impaired during episodes of migraine. Combinations available are aspirin with metoclopramide; paracetamol/codeine for analgesia, with buclizine as the antiemetic and paracetamol/metoclopramide. The earlier these drugs are taken in the attack, the better their effect.

Some patients find relief from taking other sedative antihistamines, which have antinausea properties, such as Benadryl (diphenhydramine).

Serotonin Agonists

Sumatriptan and related selective serotonin receptor agonists are excellent for severe migraines or those that do not respond to NSAIDs or other over-the-counter drugs.

Antidepressants

Tricyclic antidepressants have been long established as highly efficacious prophylactic treatments. Nefazodone may also be beneficial in the prophylaxis of migraines due to its antagonistic effects on the 5-HT2A and 5-HT2C receptors.

Ergot Alkaloids

Ergot drugs can be used either as a preventive or abortive therapy. It is a vasoconstrictor, which controls the painful vasodilation thought to be neurhormonally induced. However, ergotamine tartrate tablets (usually with caffeine), though highly effective and long lasting (unlike triptans), have fallen out of favor due to the problem of ergotism.

Steroids

Single dose of IV dexamethasone, when added to standard treatment, is argued to decrease headache recurrence.

Other Agents

If over-the-counter medications do not work or if triptans are unaffordable, the next step for many doctors is to prescribe Fioricet or Fiorinal, which is a combination of butalbital (a barbiturate), paracetamol (in Fioricet) or acetylsalicylic acid (more commonly known as aspirin and present in Fiorinal and caffeine. While the risk of addiction is low, butalbital can be habit-forming if used daily and it can also lead to rebound headaches.

Amidrine®, Duradrin® and Midrin® is a combination of acetaminophen, dichloralphenazone and isometheptene often prescribed for migraine headaches.

Antiemetics may need to be given by suppository or injection where vomiting dominates the symptoms.

Status Migrainosus

Status migrainosus is characterized by migraine lasting more than 72 hours, with not more than four hours of relief during that period. It is generally understood that status migrainosus has been refractory to usual outpatient management upon presentation.

Treatment of status migrainosus consists of managing comorbidities (i.e. correcting fluid and electrolyte abnormalities resulting from anorexia and nausea/vomiting often accompanying status migrainosus) and usually administering parenteral medication to 'break' (abort) the headache. First line therapy consists of IV fluids, metoclopramide and triptans or DHE.

Noninvasive Medical Treatments

Transcranial magnetic stimulation, biofeedback, hyperbaric oxygen therapy are some of the noninvasive techniques employed.

Bruxism, clenching or grinding of teeth, especially at night, is a trigger for many migraineurs. A device called nociceptive trigeminal inhibitor (NTI) takes advantage of a reflex limiting the force of clenching. It can be fitted over the front teeth at night, preventing contact between the back teeth. Massage therapy of the jaw area can also reduce such pain.

REFERENCES

1. Gray's Anatomy: The Anatomical Basis of Clinical Practice, 40th edn (2008), Churchill-Livingstone, Elsevier.
2. Bagheri SC, Farhidvash F, Perciaccante VJ. Diagnosis and treatment of patients with trigeminal neuralgia. J Am Dent Assoc. 2004;135:1713.
3. Wilkins RH. Historical perspectives. In: Rovit RL, Murali R, Jannetta PJ (eds). Trigeminal neuralgia. Baltimore: Williams and Wilkins. 1990;pp. 1–25.
4. International association for study of pain; Clinical Journal of Pain 2002.
5. Peterson AM, Williams RL, Fukui MB, et al. Venous angioma adjacent to the root entry zone of the trigeminal nerve: implications for management of trigeminal neuralgia. Received: 30 March 2001.
6. Trigeminal neuralgia-pathophysiology, diagnosis, and current treatment. British Journal of Anesthesia. 2001;87: 117–32.
7. White JC, Sweet WH. Pain: Its mechanisms and neurosurgical control. Springfield, IL, Charles C Thomas, 1955.
8. Sunderland S (Ed). Nerve injuries and their repair: A critical appraisal. New York, Churchill livingstone; 1991. p. 221.
9. Recknor JB, Mallapragada SK. Nerve Regeneration: Tissue Engineering Strategies, in The Biomedical Engineering Handbook: Tissue Engineering and Artificial Organs, Bronzino JD, (Ed). 2006, Taylor and Francis: New York.
10. Yiu G, Zhigang H. Glial inhibition of CNS axon regeneration. Nature Reviews Neuroscience. 2006;7:617-27.
11. Eagle W. Elongated styloid process: Further observation and a new syndrome. Arch Otolaryngol. 1948;47: 630-40.
12. Lentini A. Gli aspetti clinici e radiologici delle anomalie dell'apparato stilojoideo. Radiol Med. 1975;61:337-3640.
13. Kaufman SM, Elzay RP, Irish EF. Styloid process variation. Radiologic and clinical study. Arch Otolaryngol. 1970; 91(5):460-3.
14. Baddour HM, McAnear JT, Tilson HB. Eagle's syndrome. Report of a case. Oral Surg Oral Med Oral Pathol. 1978; 46(4):486–94.
15. The International Classification of Headache Disorders, 2nd edn. Cephalalgia. 2004;24(suppl 1):1–160.
16. Gallagher RM, Cutrer FM. "Migraine: diagnosis, management, and new treatment options". Am J Manag Care. 2002;8 (3 Suppl): S58–73.
17. 'Guidelines for all healthcare professionals in the diagnosis and management of migraine, tension-type, cluster and medication-overuse headache, January 2007, British Association for the Study of Headache.
18. Ogilvie AD, Russell MB, Dhall P, et al. 'Altered allelic distributions of the serotonin transporter gene in migraine without aura and migraine with aura'. Cephalalgia. 1998;18(1):23-6.
19. Gervil M, Ulrich V, Kaprio J, Olesen J, Russell MB (September 1999). 'The relative role of genetic and environmental factors in migraine without aura'. Neurology. 1999;53(5):995–9. PMID 10496258.
20. Silberstein, Stephen D. Atlas of Migraine And Other Headaches. London: Taylor and Francis Group, 2005.
21. Mathew NT, Evans RW. Handbook of headache. Hagerstown, MD; Lippincott Williams and Wilkins, 2005.
22. Silberstein SD. Headache in Clinical Practice, 2nd edn. London: Taylor and Francis Group, 2002.
23. Kelman L. 'The postdrome of the acute migraine attack'. Cephalalgia. 2006;26(2): 214–20.
24. Detsky ME, McDonald DR, Baerlocher MO, et al. 'Does this patient with headache have a migraine or need neuroimaging?' JAMA. 2006;296(10): 1274–83.
25. Alexander Mauskop; Fox, Barry. What Your Doctor May Not Tell You About (TM): Migraines: The Breakthrough Program That Can Help End Your Pain (What Your Doctor May Not Tell You About...(Paperback). New York: Warner Books; 2001.
26. Cohen AS, Goadsby PJ. "Functional neuroimaging of primary headache disorders". Curr Pain Headache Rep. 2005;9(2):141–6.
27. Lauritzen M. "Pathophysiology of the migraine aura. The spreading depression theory". Brain. 1994;117 (Pt1):199–210.
28. Sheena K Aurora. Pathophysiology of migraine headache. Current Pain and Headache Reports. 2001;5(2):179-82.

10 General Anesthesia

Borle Rajiv M, Angik Richa

HISTORICAL ASPECTS

Surgical procedures were uncommon before 1846. The understanding of the pathophysiology of disease and of the rationale for its treatment by surgery was rudimentary due to lack of satisfactory anesthesia. Limited means of attempting to relieve surgical pain were available such as drugs like alcohol, hashish and opium derivatives taken orally. Unconsciousness induced by a blow to the head or by strangulation did provide relief from pain, although at a high cost. The most common method used to achieve a relatively quiet surgery was simple restraint of the patient by force. Nitrous oxide was synthesized by Priestley in 1776.[1] Diethyl ether and nitrous oxide were first used by Dentists. In 1845, Horace Wells[2] first attempted to demonstrate the use of nitrous oxide for dental extraction at the Massachusetts General Hospital in Boston, but it failed. William TG Morton[3] invented and revealed of the anesthetic inhalation by using ether on the patient, before whom, in all time, surgery was agony.[4]

ANESTHESIA AFTER 1846

Although rarely used today, ether was the first 'ideal' anesthetic agent. Chemically, it is readily made in pure form. It is relatively easy to administer, since it is a liquid at room temperature, but is readily vaporized. Ether is more potent, unlike nitrous oxide and thus, a few volume percent can produce anesthesia without diluting the oxygen in room air to hypoxic levels. It was used to support both respiration and circulation, crucial properties at the time when human physiology was not understood well enough for assisted respiration and circulation to be made possible. Ether is not toxic to vital organs.

In 1847, a Scottish obstetrician James Simpson introduced chloroform.[5] It became quite popular because of its more pleasant odor. The drug is a hepatotoxic and a severe cardiovascular depressant. Despite the relatively high incidence of intraoperative and postoperative deaths associated with the use of chloroform, it was used for 100 years, especially in Great Britain. Nitrous oxide was disused after the apparent failure in Boston in 1845 and was reintroduced in 1863 into American dental and surgical practice, by physician, Gardner Q Colton.[6]

In 1868, the administration of nitrous oxide with oxygen was described by Edmond Andrews,[7] a Chicago surgeon and thereafter the two gases became available in steel cylinders, greatly increasing their practicality.

In 1929, the anesthetic properties of cyclopropane were accidentally discovered by chemists.[8] Cyclopropane was perhaps the most widely used general anesthetic for the next 30 years.

The skeletal muscle relaxants (*neuromuscular blocking agents*) were also discovered. In 1940s, anesthesiologists used curare to provide the muscular relaxation that previously could be obtained only with deep levels of general anesthesia.

INTRODUCTION OF INTRAVENOUS ANESTHETIC AGENTS

In 1935, Lundy[9] demonstrated the clinical usefulness of thiopental, a rapidly acting thiobarbiturate. It was originally considered useful as a sole anesthetic agent, but the doses required resulted in serious depression of the circulatory, respiratory and nervous systems. Thiopental has been accepted as an agent for the rapid induction of general anesthesia. Various combinations of intravenous (IV) drugs from several classes have been used recently as anesthetic agents, usually together with nitrous oxide.[10] The commonly used general anesthetic agents are either inhalational agents or the drugs that can be administered intravenously (Table 10.1).

COMMONLY USED ANESTHETIC AGENTS

Propofol[11]

- It is an alkylphenol sedative-hypnotic.
- Ideal induction agent in many situations except in cases of:
  - Suspected hypotension
  - Patients with preoperative hypovolemia especially in emergency care. It is contraindicated in children < 3 years of age.

Table 10.1: Classification of general anesthetic agents

Inhalational	
Gas	*Volatile liquids*
Nitrous oxide	Ether
	Halothane
	Isoflurane
	Sevoflurane
	Desflurane
	Enflurane
Intravenous	
Inducing agents	*Slower acting drugs*
Thiopentone sodium	Benzodiazepines—Diazepam, Lorazepam, Midazolam
Methohexitone sodium	Dissociative anesthesia—Ketamine
Propofol	Opioid analgesia—Fentanyl
Etomidate	

- **Duration of action:** 5 to 10 minutes—extremely short and desirable.
- It has a very valuable property in examination of the patients with head injury where serial neurological examinations can be performed simply by turning-off the drip and waiting for 10 minutes and assessing neurologic function.
- **Dosage:** Induction dose is 1 to 2.5 mg/kg IV bolus for children and adults. For maintenance the dose is 50 to 200 microgram/kg/min. and for sedation the dose is 25 to 100 microgram/kg/mg.[12]
- Associated desirable side effects—
  - Antiemetic effect
  - Causes amnesia
  - Lowers intra cranial pressure
  - Antiepileptic effect
- Used commonly in oral surgery practice as a day-care anesthetic agent. The patient can be taken under general anesthesia for short procedures, induced on propofol and be discharged on the same day of surgery after regaining consciousness in view of minimal postoperative side effects and hence minimal care is required.
- **Undesirable effects:** It causes significant hypotension especially in cases of hypovolemia.
- **Undesirable side effects after hypovolemia:** The undesirable side effect of long-term infusion is Propofol infusion syndrome.

Ketamine[13,14]

Ketamine is a phencyclidine derivative. Greenfield[15] described the use of ketamine hydrochloride, a drug that alters the patient's awareness for his surroundings, but does not produce the typical state of unconsciousness. Ketamine induces a *'dissociative anesthesia'* characterized by stage of sedation, immobility, amnesia and marked analgesia. Since ketamine acts primarily on thalamus and cortex and not on the reticular activating system, the patient does not appear to be asleep, but rather dissociated from the environment. After the administration the dissociation occurs in 15 seconds and unconsciousness becomes apparent in another 30 seconds. Intense analgesia and amnesia are established rapidly. The state of unconsciousness lasts for about 10 to 15 minutes and the analgesia persists for about 40 to 45 minutes following a single dose administration. Respiration is usually not depressed with proper dosages. The hypoxic and hypercarbic stimulation of the respiration is not seriously affected following usual doses of ketamine. It is associated with increased oral secretions, therefore necessitating premedication with an anticholinergic drug such as an antisialagogue. The important property of ketamine is the preservation of the pharyngeal and the laryngeal reflexes. The airway resistance is decreased and the bronchospasm may be abolished as it has a bronchodilator action. Unlike the routine intravenous anesthetics (thiopental sodium), ketamine does not act upon the reticular activating system of the midbrain, but acts upon the cortex and the limbic system. Thus hallucinations, disagreeable dreams, delirium and excitement are precipitated during the recovery. The unpleasant dreams may persist for several days in adults. It produces postemergence hallucinations and dysphoria, more commonly in adults, but occasionally in children.

Ketamine in an IV dose of 1 to 2 mg/kg of body weight and IM dose of 4 to 5 mg/kg of body weight, has been used as an intramuscular or intravenous injection to sedate combative children in emergency departments at doses of 2 to 5 mg/kg. A revised weight dosage relationship has been established by Greenfield[15] and is based on intramuscular administration.

- Up to 50 Lbs—0.5 to 1.0 mg/Lb,
- 50 to 100 Lbs—1.0 to 1.5 mg/Lb,
- Above 100 Lbs—1.5 mg/Lbs plus $N_2O:O_2$ (50:50).

At these dosage levels, consciousness is generally maintained together with protective reflexes and stable vital signs. The duration of effect varies from 20 to 40 minutes and can be prolonged by the addition of $N_2O:O_2$ in a 50:50 mixture. At higher doses, ketamine is known to produce psychotomimetic effects, including hallucinations, during the recovery period and occasionally there are delayed bizarre disturbances. Precipitation of delirium or violent and irrational response to stimuli is the undesired property during the recovery from ketamine anesthesia.

Ketamine is contraindicated in patients with hypertension, psychiatric disorders and glaucoma. Maintenance of an unobstructed airway is an important property of ketamine anesthesia. Ketamine is found to be a safe anesthetic for minor oral surgical procedures especially in the children.

Isoflurane—2-chloro-2-(difluoromethoxy)-1,1,1-trifluoro-ethane

Isoflurane—2-chloro-2-(difluoromethoxy)-1,1,1-trifluoro-ethane is a halogenated ether used for maintenance of anesthesia. Together with enflurane and halothane, it replaced the flammable ethers used in the pioneer days of surgery. Its use in human medicine is now starting to decline, being replaced by sevoflurane, desflurane and the intravenous anesthetic propofol.

Isoflurane is always administered in conjunction with air and/or pure oxygen. Often nitrous oxide is also used. Although its physical properties mean that anesthesia can be induced more rapidly than with halothane, its pungency can irritate the respiratory system, negating this theoretical advantage conferred by its physical properties. It is usually used to maintain a state of general anesthesia that has been induced with another drug, such as thiopentone or propofol. It vaporizes readily, but is a liquid at room temperature. It is completely non-flammable. Isoflurane, USP, is supplied in 100 mL and 250 mL amber-colored bottles.

Molecular formula of Isoflurane–$C_3H_2ClF_5O$

```
  F  H     F
  |  |     |
F–C–C–O–C–H
  |  |     |
  F  Cl    F
```

Structure of isoflurane

Mechanism of Action

Isoflurane reduces pain sensitivity (analgesia) and relaxes muscles. The mechanism by which general anesthetics produce the anesthetic state is not clearly understood, but likely involves interactions with multiple receptor sites to interfere with synaptic transmission. Isoflurane binds to gamma-amino butyric acid (GABA) receptors, glutamate receptors and glycine receptors and also inhibits conduction in activated potassium channels. Glycine inhibition helps to inhibit motor function, while bonding to glutamate receptors mimics the effects of NMDA (N-methyl-D-aspartate). It activates calcium ATPase through an increase in membrane fluidity and binds to the D subunit of ATP (Adenosine triphosphate) synthase and NADH (Nicotinamide_adenine_dinucleotide dehydrogenase) dehydrogenase. In addition, a number of general anesthetics attenuate gap junction communication, which could contribute to anesthetic action.

Properties

Induction of and recovery from isoflurane anesthesia are rapid. Isoflurane has a mild pungency, which limits the rate of induction, although excessive salivation or tracheobronchial secretions do not appear to be stimulated. Pharyngeal and laryngeal reflexes are readily obtunded. The level of anesthesia may be changed rapidly with isoflurane. Isoflurane is a profound respiratory depressant. Respiration must be monitored closely and supported when necessary. As anesthetic dose is increased, tidal volume decreases and respiratory rate is unchanged. This depression is partially reversed by surgical stimulation, even at deeper levels of anesthesia. Blood pressure decreases with induction of anesthesia, but returns towards normal with surgical stimulation. Progressive increase in depth of anesthesia produces corresponding decrease in blood pressure. Nitrous oxide diminishes the inspiratory concentration of isoflurane required to reach a desired level of anesthesia and may reduce the arterial hypotension seen with isoflurane alone. Heart rhythm is remarkably stable. With controlled ventilation and normal $PaCO_2$, cardiac output is maintained despite increasing depth of anesthesia, primarily through an increase in heart rate which compensates for a reduction in stroke volume. The hypercapnia which attends spontaneous ventilation during isoflurane anesthesia further increases heart rate and raises cardiac output above awake levels. Isoflurane does not sensitize the myocardium to exogenously administered epinephrine.

Muscle relaxation is often adequate for maxillofacial operations at normal levels of anesthesia. Complete muscle paralysis can be attained with small doses of muscle relaxants. All commonly used muscle relaxants are markedly potentiated with Isoflurane, the effect being most profound with the nondepolarizing ones. Neostigmine reverses the effect of non-depolarizing muscle relaxants in the presence of Isoflurane. All commonly used muscle relaxants are compatible with Isoflurane. Isoflurane can produce coronary vasodilation at the arteriolar level.

Side Effects

In susceptible individuals, isoflurane anesthesia may trigger a skeletal muscle hypermetabolic state leading to high oxygen demand and the clinical syndrome known as malignant hyperthermia. The syndrome includes nonspecific features such as muscle rigidity, tachycardia, tachypnea, cyanosis, arrhythmias and unstable blood pressure (It should also be noted that many of these nonspecific signs may appear with light anesthesia, acute hypoxia, etc.). An increase in overall metabolism may be reflected in an elevated temperature (which may rise rapidly early or late in the case, but usually is not the first sign of augmented metabolism) and an increased usage of the CO_2 absorption system (hot canister). PaO_2 and pH may decrease and hyperkalemia and a base deficit may appear. Treatment includes discontinuance of triggering agents (e.g. Isoflurane), administration of intravenous dantrolene sodium and application of supportive therapy. Such therapy includes vigorous efforts to restore body temperature to normal, respiratory and circulatory support as indicated and management of electrolyte-fluid-acid-base derangements.

Nitrous Oxide

Nitrous oxide, commonly known as happy gas, laughing gas and NOX, is a chemical compound with the chemical formula N_2O. At room temperature, it is a colorless, nonflammable gas, with a pleasant, slightly sweet odor and taste.

It is used in surgery and dentistry for its anesthetic and analgesic effects. It is known as *'laughing gas'* due to the euphoric effects of inhaling it. The gas was first synthesized by English chemist and natural philosopher Joseph Priestley[1] in 1775.

Nitrous oxide has been used for anesthesia in dentistry since the 1840s. The most common use is as a 50:50 mix with oxygen, commonly known as Entonox or Nitronox delivered through a demand valve. Nitrous oxide is typically administered by dentists through a demand valve inhaler over the nose that only releases gas when the patient inhales through the nose.

Because nitrous oxide is minimally metabolized, it retains its potency when exhaled into the room by the patient and can pose an intoxicating and prolonged-exposure hazard to the operating staff if the room is poorly ventilated. Where nitrous oxide is administered, a continuous-flow fresh-air ventilation system or nitrous-scavenging system is used to prevent waste gas buildup.

Nitrous oxide is a weak general anesthetic and so is generally not used alone in general anesthesia. It is mainly used as analgesics and not as anesthetic. In general anesthesia it is used as a carrier gas in a 2:1 ratio with oxygen for more powerful general anesthetic agents such as sevoflurane or desflurane.

Nitrous oxide (N_2O) is a dissociative drug that can cause analgesia, depersonalization, derealization, dizziness, euphoria and some sound distortion.

Mechanism of Action

It acts as an NMDA receptor antagonist at partial pressures similar to those used in general anesthesia. The evidence on the effect of N_2O on gamma aminobutyric acid (GABA) receptor currently is mixed, but tends to show a lower potency potentiation by acting as a positive allosteric modulator of the receptor. N_2O, like other volatile anesthetics, activates twin-pore potassium channels, albeit weakly. These channels are largely responsible for keeping neurons at the resting (*unexcited*) potential. Unlike many anesthetics, however, N_2O does not seem to affect calcium channels. Unlike most general anesthetics, N_2O appears to affect the GABA receptor.

Sevoflurane

Sevoflurane is a fluorinated methyl isopropyl ether having properties intermediate between isoflurane and desflurane.

```
  F CF3   H
  |  |    |
F-C--C--O-C-F
  |  |    |
  F  H    H
```

Mechanism of Action

Sevoflurane induces a reduction in junctional conductance by decreasing gap junction channel opening times and increasing gap junction channel closing times. Sevoflurane also activates calcium dependent ATPase in the sarcoplasmic reticulum by increasing the fluidity of the lipid membrane. It also appears to bind the D subunit of ATP synthase and NADH dehydogenase and also binds to the GABA receptor, the large conductance Ca^{2+} activated potassium channel, the glutamate receptor, and the glycine receptor. It is rapidly absorbed into circulation via the lungs, however solubility in the blood is low. The half-life is 15 to 23 hours.

Properties

- The vapor pressure of sevoflurane resembles that of halothane and isoflurane, permitting delivery of this anesthetic via a conventional unheated vaporizer.
- Compared with isoflurane, recovery from sevoflurane anesthesia is 3 to 4 minutes faster and the difference is magnified in longer duration surgical procedures (> 3 hours).
- Sevoflurane is non pungent, has minimal odor, produces bronchodilation similar in degree to isoflurane and causes the least degree of airway irritation among the currently available volatile anesthetics. The acceptability in pediatric patients is good.
- Sevoflurane differs from halothane, enflurane, isoflurane and desflurane, as all these drugs (except sevoflurane) are metabolized to reactive acyl halide intermediates with the potential to produce hepatotoxicity as well as cross sensitivity between drugs.
- Sevoflurane and desflurane because of their lower blood and tissue solubilities permit more precise control over the induction of anesthesia and more rapid recovery when the drug is discontinued.
- Sevoflurane and desflurane, like isoflurane, do not produce evidence of convulsive activity on the EEG either at deep levels of anesthesia or in the presence of hypocapnia or auditory stimulation. Sevoflurane can suppress convulsive activity induced with lidocaine.
- Induction and emergence from the anesthesia are fast and rapid changes in depth can be achieved. It is desirable for use in inpatient and outpatient surgery but its high cost and high open flow system makes it expensive to use.
- It can be used both for induction and maintenance.

Ether

Diethyl ether, also known as ether and ethoxyethane, is a clear, colorless and highly flammable liquid with a low boiling point and a characteristic odor. It is used as a common solvent and has been used as a general anesthetic. Although, it is not commonly used nowadays and sevoflurane is widely used. Alchemist Raymundus Lullus is credited with discovering the compound in 1275 AD, although there is no contemporary evidence of this. It was first synthesized in 1540 by Valerius Cordus, who called it 'oil of sweet vitriol' (oleum dulcis vitrioli), the name given because it was originally discovered by distilling a mixture of ethanol and sulfuric acid. William TG Morton participated the first public demonstration of ether anesthesia on October 16, 1846 at the Ether Dome in Boston, Massachusetts.[16]

Ether was sometimes used in place of chloroform because it had a higher therapeutic index, a larger difference between the recommended dosage and a toxic overdose. Ether is still the preferred anesthetic in some developing nations due to its high therapeutic index (~1.5–2.2).[17] Today, ether is rarely used. The use of flammable ether waned as non-flammable anesthetic agents such as halothane became available. Additionally, ether had many undesirable side effects, such as postanesthetic nausea and vomiting.

Halothane

Halothane vapor (or Fluothane) is an inhalational general anesthetic, supplied in amber colored bottles. Its IUPAC name is 2-bromo-2-chloro-1,1,1-trifluoroethane. It is the only inhalational anesthetic agent containing a bromine atom. It is colorless and pleasant-smelling, but unstable in light. It is available in dark-colored bottles and contains 0.01 percent thymol as a stabilizing agent. Halothane is a core medicine in the World Health Organization's 'Essential Drugs List', which is a list of minimum medical needs for a basic health care system.[18] This halogenated hydrocarbon was first synthesized by CW Suckling[19] of Imperial Chemical Industries (ICI) in 1951 and was first used clinically by M Johnstone[20] in Manchester in 1956. Its properties include cardiac depression at high levels, cardiac sensitization to catecholamines such as norepinephrine and potent bronchial relaxation. Its lack of airway irritation made it a common inhalation induction agent in pediatric anesthesia. Due to its cardiac depressive effect, it was contraindicated in patients with cardiac failure. Halothane was also contraindicated in patients susceptible to cardiac arrythmias or in situations related to high catecholamine levels such as pheochromocytoma.

Repeated exposures to halothane in adults were, noted, in rare cases to result in severe liver injury. This occurred in about 1 in 35,000 exposures.[21] The resulting syndrome was referred to as halothane hepatitis and is thought to result from the metabolism of halothane to trifluoroacetic acid via oxidative reactions in the liver. About 20 percent of inhaled halothane is metabolized by the liver and these products are excreted in the urine. The hepatitis syndrome had a mortality rate of 30 to 70 percent. Concern for hepatitis resulted in a dramatic reduction in the use of halothane for adults. It was replaced in the 1980s by enflurane and isoflurane.

Halothane is clinically the most potent trigger as compared to isoflurane for malignant hyperthermia, due to difference in the calcium releasing potency of individual anesthetics at cellular level, which leads to increased intracellular calcium.

INDICATIONS FOR GENERAL ANESTHESIA

The indications for general anesthesia are as follows:

- The surgical procedures of larger magnitude, which cannot be accomplished under local anesthesia or where the regional anesthesia and or sedation are inadequate to provide satisfactory analgesia.
- When the patients are uncooperative.
- When patient compliance is not required.
- Apprehensive patients where muscle relaxation is required for stabilization.

PREANESTHETIC PREPARATION

For safe administration of the general anesthesia (GA) the patient is thoroughly evaluated and investigated and this procedure is called preanesthetic preparation, which comprises of following steps:

- The patient is hospitalized 2 days prior to the surgery to make him accustomed with environments to reduce the stress.
- Investigations comprising of Hb%, TLC, DLC, BT, CT routine urine tests, assessment of blood sugar levels, are carried out to rule out any associated systemic disease. To evaluate the conditions of the pulmonary parenchyma X-ray chest is done. The renal and hepatic status is evaluated by performing the RFT and LFT respectively. The RFT (also called KFT) comprises of assessment of serum Na^+, K^+, creatinine and urea concentration. The LFT is done by assessing the serum bilirubin SGOT, SGPT levels. The last two investigations (RFT, LFT) are done prior to the administration of GA only when specifically indicated as all the anesthetic agents are metabolized in lever and execrated by the kindeys. Other investigations like PT, platelet, count, hemoglobin electrophoresis, sickling, etc. are done if indicated in a particular case.
- A thorough clinical examination is mandatory in every patient to evaluate the general physical status of the patient and to identify other associated diseases. Cardiovascular status is evaluated by clinical examination and investigations like ECG, echocardiography, Doppler, TMT, etc. when indicated in a particular case. Similarly the pulmonary status is evaluated by clinical examination and posteroanterior (PA) X-ray of chest. Pulmonary diseases like 'chronic obstructive pulmonary disease' (COPD), pulmonary tuberculosis, plural fibrosis, consolidation or even active infection can complicate the administration of GA. The diseases like arrythmias, ischemic heart disease (IHD), hypertension (HT), cardiomyopathies can also make the administration of GA complicated unless controlled satisfactorily before the administration of the anesthesia. The disorders like diabetes, thyroids disorders, Addison's disease, etc. must be adequately controlled before the procedure by giving appropriate treatment. The patients are often referred to physician for such evaluation and management if required.
- The preanesthetic check up is done by the anesthetist, a day prior to the surgery who evaluates the fitness for

the administration of the GA. The anesthetist also evaluates the airway anatomy, degree of mouth opening, nasal patency, pharyngeal and laryngeal anatomy, cervical spine anomalies and neck mobility, which can pose difficulty in intubating the patient.

- The patient is kept nil by mouth/nil per oral (NBM) 5 to 6 hours prior to the surgery to ensure that the stomach is empty and the chances of vomiting and aspirations are minimized. This much time is required as it is the gastric emptying time. If the patient comes for emergency surgery where it is not possible to the patient NBM for 5 hours, the gastric lavage is done to evacuate the contents of the stomach before administration of the GA.[22]
- **Preparation of the bowel:** The patient is prescribed laxatives a night before surgery to ensure that the bowel and rectum are evacuated. The commonly prescribed laxatives are bisacodyl (*Dulcolax*) 5 to 10 mg or liquid paraffin about 5 to 10 mL orally. The former is an irritant cathartic and is not used in patients with APD, ulcerative colitis, etc. The bowel preparation may not be relevant for maxillofacial procedures, but is vital for bowel, anorectal or obstetric and gynecological procedure. In addition to the laxatives the patient is also given enema in the morning with either plain water, warm water or soap water to ensure that the contents are totally evacuated.[23]
- Sedatives are often prescribed to ensure that the patient's anxiety is alleviated and he has good rest and sleep. The anxious patients have raised levels of catacolamines, which make induction of anesthesia difficult. The agitated patient also tends to get exhausted easily.
- The patient is prescribed bland diet to prevent any gastrointestinal (GI) upset.
- Before shifting the patient the loose operation theater (OT) garments are given and tight under garments are removed.
- A written, informed consent of the patient is obtained and wherever necessary, risk consent is also obtained.[24]

PREANESTHETIC MEDICATION

The drugs, which are prescribed prior to the administration of the GA are called preanesthetic medication.[25] The preanesthetic medication (Box 10.1) is given:

- To facilitate smooth administration/induction of general anesthesia.[26]
- To ensure smooth recovery.
- To reduce the dose of general anesthetic.
- To prevent complications.

To achieve the above goals the following drugs are administered intramuscularly (IM) either 30 minutes prior to the administration in the preanesthetic room or IV 5 to 10 minutes before the administration of GA.

- **Sedatives:** The sedatives like diazepam,[27] (5–10 mg), nitrazepam (5–10 mg), phenobarbitone (15–30 mg) are prescribed. These drugs reduce the anxiety and stress and thus the levels of catecholamines.
- **Analgesics:** The analgesics like *Fortwin* (pentazocine lactate) 15 to 30 mg, morphine[28] 10 to 15 mg or pethidine 40 to 60 mg are administered to potentiate the analgesia and to make the induction pain free. The side effect of the narcotic analgesics is emesis, which may not be desirable for oral surgical procedures especially where IMF is required and hence should be avoided.

Box 10.1: Preanesthetic medication

Sedatives—diazepam
Antihistaminics—promethazine hydrochloride (Phenergan), pheniramine maleate (Avil)
Antacids—H_2 blockers (Ranitidine)
Antiemetics—prochlorperazine (Stemetil), metoclopramide (Perionorm)
Vagolytic drugs—atropine sulfate
Steroids—hydrocortisone, dexamethasone
Rationale
To reduce anxiety
To facilitate smooth induction and recovery
To prevent complications

- **Antihistaminics:** The antihistaminics[29] like phenergan (promethazine), Avil (pheniramine maleate), are often prescribed to counter any mild allergic reactions. The IV fluids, IV sets may contain pyrogenes, which may evoke mild allergic reactions like rigors, eruptions, pyrexic reaction, etc. mild to moderate reactions can also occur during blood. The antihistaminics also have tranquilizing effect.
- **Antiemetics:** To prevent the vomiting and thus, its aspiration in the tracheobronchial tree antiemetics are prescribed.[30] The drugs like promethazine or metoclopromide are used in a dose of 25 mg IM or IV.
- **Vagolytic drugs:** Atropine sulfate is vagolytic drug and helps in preventing bradycardia[31] also in reducing the salivary and tracheobronchial secretions thus, keeping the airway patent. It is given in a dose of 0.6 mg IM or IV.
- **Antacids:** The patients are kept NBM and are undergoing stress, both the things can precipitate increased acid secretion and gastritis. To prevent this, drugs like H_2 blockers like Ranitidine[32] are prescribed in a dose of 50 mg IM or IV.
- **Corticosteroids:** They help in inhibiting antigen-antibody reaction, have anti-inflammatory property and help in combating stress. The drugs like sodium hydrocortisone succinate 100 mg or Dexamethasone 4 to 8 mg are prescribed.

PHASES OF GENERAL ANESTHESIA

There are three main phases of general anesthesia:

- Phase of induction

- Phase of maintenance
- Phase of recovery.

STAGES OF GENERAL ANESTHESIA

General anesthesia causes an irregularly descending depression of the central nervous system (CNS) in which the higher functions are lost first and progressively lower areas of the brain are involved,[33] but in the spinal cord lower segments are affected somewhat earlier than the higher segments. The vital centers located in the medulla are paralyzed the last as the depth of anesthesia increases. Guedel[34] in 1920 described four stages with ether anesthesia, dividing the three stage into four planes. These clear-cut stages are not seen now-a-days with the use of faster acting general anesthetics, premedication and employment of many drugs together. The precise sequence of events differs somewhat with anesthetics other than ether.

Stage I—Stage of Analgesia

- Starts from beginning of anesthetic inhalation and lasts up to the loss of consciousness
- Pain is progressively abolished
- Patient remains conscious, can hear and see and feels a dream like state
- Amnesia develops by the end of this stage
- Reflexes and respiration remain normal.

Though some minor operations can be carried out during this stage, it is rather difficult to maintain so the use is limited to short procedures.

Stage II—Stage of Excitement

- Stage starts from loss of consciousness upto gain of rhythmical respiration
- Respiration—Irregular and large in volume
- Heart rate (HR) and BP raises
- Pupils—Large and divergent
- Muscle tone increased—Jaw may be tight
- Patient may shout or struggle
- Involuntary micturation or defecation.

Stage III—Surgical Anesthesia

Extends from onset of regular respiration to cessation of spontaneous breathing. This has been divided into four planes:

Plane 1—Roving eyeballs. This plane ends when eyes become fixed.

Plane 2—Loss of corneal and laryngeal reflexes.

Plane 3—Pupil starts dilating and light reflex is lost.

Plane 4—Intercostal paralysis, shallow abdominal respiration, dilated pupil.

As anesthesia passes to deeper planes, progressively-muscle tone decreases, BP falls, HR increases with weak pulse, respiration decreases in depth and later in frequency also thoracic is lagging behind abdominal.

Stage IV—Stage of Medullary Paralysis

- There is cessation of breathing leading to failure of circulation and death
- Pupils are widely dilated
- Muscles are totally flaccid
- Pulse is thready or imperceptible
- BP is very low or unrecordable.

Many of the above indices have been robbed by the use of atropine (pupillary, heart rate), morphine (respiration, pupillary), muscle relaxants (muscle tone, respiration, eye movements, reflexes), etc. and the modern anesthetist has to depend on several other observations to gauge the depth of anesthesia, such as bispectral index (BIS).

PREANESTHETIC EVALUATION

All the patients who are to be subjected to general anesthesia are needed to be evaluated physically for ascertaining the fitness for anesthesia. The physical evaluation of the patient comprises of LEMON criteria for evaluation of airway which is as under:

L-Look for facial abnormality
E-evaluate 3-3-2
M-Mallampatti grade
O-obstruction
N-neck mobility

- **Evaluation of the nasal cavity:** For presence of polyps, deviated nasal septum and discharge as it may pose problems in nasotracheal intubation.
- **Oral examination:** If the patient has trismus, the laryngoscopy and intubation may become difficult. A large malignant growth over the anterior part of jaws may also make the laryngoscopy difficult and the growth may bleed during laryngoscopy, leading to high chances of aspiration. The loose teeth are likely to be avulsed during larygoscopy and can get aspirated in the air passage. Such teeth should be extracted before hand. The presence of macroglossia, grossly enlarged tonsils and presence of mandibular or maxillary hypoplasia and the other hindering factors.
- **Examination of neck:** The neck should be inspected thoroughly. The short necks are usually considered unfavorable for intubation. Similarly presence of deformities of cervical spine, ankylosing cervical spine conditions preventing the neck movements must be taken into consideration. The injuries to the cervical spine may require special precautions during intubation.
- **The Mallampati score or Mallampati classification:** This score is used to predict the ease of intubation.[35] It is determined by looking at the anatomy of the oral cavity; specifically, it is based on the visibility of the base of uvula, faucial pillars (the arches in front of and behind the tonsils) and soft palate. Scoring may be done with or without phonation. Higher Mallampati score (Class 4) is associated with more difficult intubation as well as a higher incidence of sleep apnea.[36] (Fig. 10.1) and (Box 10.2).

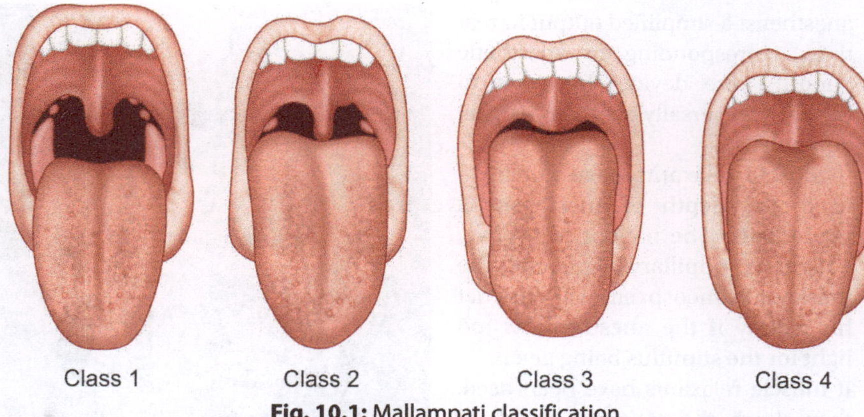

Fig. 10.1: Mallampati classification

Box 10.2: Mallampati classification/score

Class 1: Full visibility of tonsils, uvula and soft palate
Class 2: Visibility of hard and soft palate, upper portion of tonsils and uvula
Class 3: Soft and hard palate and base of the uvula are visible
Class 4: Only hard palate visible

- **Evaluate 3,3,2:** Three of the patient's fingers should be able to fit into his/her mouth when open, three fingers should comfortably fit between the chin and the throat and two fingers in the thyromental distance (distance from thyroid cartilage to chin).
- **Obstructions** (stridorous breath sounds, wheezing, etc.).
- **Cormack-Lehane grading system**[37,38] (according to the percentage of glottic opening on laryngoscopy).

INDUCTION, MAINTENANCE AND REVERSAL OF GA

Induction

Induction is usually the most critical part of the anesthesia process.

- It is the stage of transformation of an awake patient into an anesthetized one.
- This can be achieved by intravenous injection of induction agents (drugs that work rapidly, such as thiopental and propofol), by the slower inhalation of anesthetic vapors from a face mask or a combination of both.
- Adult patients and most children are usually induced with intravenous drugs, this being a rapid and minimally unpleasant experience for the patient. However, the arrival of sevoflurane, a new and well-tolerated anesthetic vapor, has led to something of a renaissance of elective inhalation induction of anesthesia in adults.
- In addition to the induction drug, most patients receive an injection of narcotic analgesic. A wide range of synthetic and naturally occurring narcotics with different properties are available. Induction agents and narcotics work synergistically to induce anesthesia. In addition, anticipation of events that are about to occur, such as endotracheal intubation and incision of the skin, generally raises the blood pressure and heart rate of the patient. Narcotic analgesia helps preempt this undesirable response.
- The next step of the induction process is the securing of the airway. This may be a simple matter of manually holding the patient's jaw such that his or her natural breathing is unimpeded by the tongue or may demand the insertion of a prosthetic airway device such as a laryngeal mask airway or endotracheal tube. A variety of factors are considered when making this decision. The major issue is whether the patient requires an endotracheal tube.
- Indications for endotracheal intubation under general anesthesia include the following:
  - Potential for airway contamination (full stomach, gastroesophageal [GE] reflux, GI or pharyngeal bleeding)
  - Surgical need for muscle relaxation
  - Predictable difficulty with endotracheal intubation or where anesthetist's access to the airway during the case will be difficult (lateral or prone position). For paralysis of vocal cord for intubation a short acting muscle relaxant such as suxamethonium chloride is used.
  - Surgery of the mouth or face
  - Prolonged procedure anticipated.
- Not all surgeries require muscle relaxation.
- If surgery is taking place in muscle groups of the thorax and abdomen areas, then in addition to the induction agent and narcotic, an intermediate or long-acting muscle relaxant drug is administered. This paralyzes muscles indiscriminately, including the muscles of breathing. Therefore, the patient's lungs must be ventilated under pressure, necessitating an endotracheal tube.
- Persons who, for anatomic reasons, are likely to be difficult to intubate are usually intubated electively at the beginning of the when the patient is awake using a fiberoptic bronchoscope or other advanced airway tool. This prevents a situation in which attempts are made to manage the airway with a lesser device, only for the anesthetist to discover that oxygenation and ventilation are inadequate. At that point during a surgical procedure, swift intubation of the patient can be very difficult, if not impossible.

Maintenance Phase

As the effect of the drugs used to initiate the anesthesia begin to wane off, the patient is kept anesthetized with a maintenance agent. According to ASA (American Society of Anesthesiologists) monitoring of oxygenation, ventilation, circulation and temperature should be done by the anesthesiologist throughout the procedures. The $ETCO_2$, SPO_2, pulse rate, blood pressure, ECG and temperature should be monitored.

- For the most part, this refers to the delivery of anesthetic gases/vapors into the patient's lungs. These may be inhaled as the patient breathes himself (spontaneous respiration) or delivered under pressure by each mechanical breath of a ventilator. A continuous infusion of muscle relaxant is also required.
- The maintenance phase is usually the most stable part of the anesthesia. However, understanding that anesthesia is a continuum of different depths is important. A level of anesthesia that is satisfactory for surgery to the skin of an extremity, for example, would be inadequate for manipulation of the bowel.
- Appropriate levels of anesthesia must be chosen both for the planned procedure and for its various stages. In complex plastic surgery, for example, a considerable period of time may elapse between the completion of the induction of anesthetic and the incision of the skin. During the period of skin preparation, urinary catheter insertion and marking incision lines with a pen, the patient is not receiving any noxious stimulus. This requires a very light level of anesthesia, which must be converted rapidly to a deeper level just before the incision is made. When the anesthesia provider and surgeon are not accustomed to working together, good communication (e.g. warning of the start of new stimuli, such as moving the head of an intubated patient or commencing surgery facilitates preemptive deepening of the anesthetic). This maximizes patient safety and ultimately, saves everyone's time.

As the procedure progresses, the level of anesthesia is altered to give the minimum amount necessary to ensure adequate anesthetic depth. Traditionally, this has been a matter of clinical judgment, but new processed electro encephalograph (EEG) machines (BIS monitors) give the anesthetist a simplified output in real time, corresponding to anesthetic depth. These devices have yet to become universally accepted as vital equipment.

- If muscle relaxants have not been used, the depth of anesthesia is inadequate. The patient will move, cough or pupillary signs will be masked. Broncospasm will obstruct his airway if the anesthesia is too light for the stimulus being given.
- If muscle relaxants have been used, then clearly the patient is unable to demonstrate any of these phenomena. In these patients, the anesthesiologist must rely on careful observation of autonomic phenomena such as hypertension, tachycardia, sweating and pupillary dilation to decide that the patient requires a deeper anesthetic.
- This requires experience and judgment. It is from failure to recognize such signs that tragic and highly publicized cases of awareness under anesthesia are caused.
- Excessive anesthetic depth, on the other hand, is associated with decreased heart rate and blood pressure and if carried to extremes, can jeopardize perfusion of vital organs or be fatal. Short of these serious misadventures, excessive depth results in slower awakening and more side effects.

The controlled delivery of inhalant anesthetics and oxygen for maintenance of the proper stage and plane of anesthesia and prevention of hypoxia, are ensured by the use of an anesthetic machine (Boyle's apparatus) is used (Fig. 10.2).

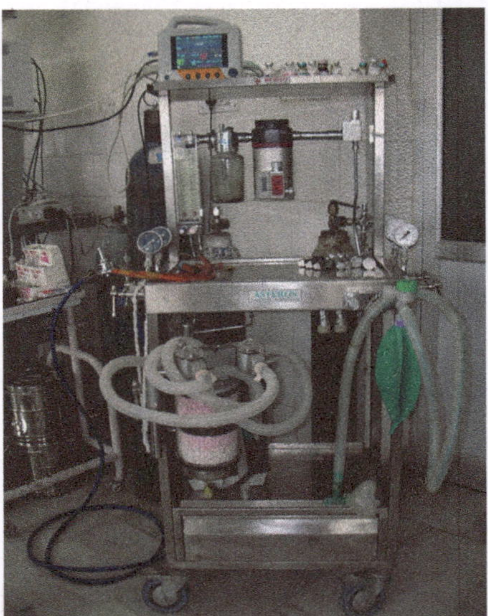

Fig. 10.2: Boyle's machine

Reversal

As the surgical procedure draws to a close, the patient's emergence from anesthesia is planned. Experience and close communication with the surgeon enable the anesthesiologist to predict the time at which the application of dressings and casts will be complete.

- In advance of that time, anesthetic vapors are decreased or even switched off entirely to allow time for them to be excreted by the lungs.
- Excess muscle relaxation is reversed using specific drugs such as neostigmine and adequate long-acting narcotic analgesic to keep the patient comfortable in the recovery room.
- If a ventilator has been used, the patient is restored to breathing by himself (spontaneous) and as anesthetic drugs dissipate, the patient emerges to consciousness.
- Reversal agents—It is a combination of two drugs neostigmine + glycopylorrate in the ratio of 5:1, or Neostigmine + atropine in a ratio of 5:2. Neostigmine is categorized under anticholinesterases group of drugs. Anticholinesterases are agents, which inhibit cholinesterase, protect acetylcholine from hydrolysis. Muscarinic side effects are minimized by concomitant administration of anticholinergic drug (*glycopylorrate*). The effect of neostigmine (0.04 mg/kg) is usually apparent in 5 to 10 minutes, and lasts for more than 1 hour. Pediatric and elderly patients appear to be more sensitive to it's effects, experiencing a more rapid onset and requiring smaller dose. The duration of action is prolonged in geriatric patients. It has been reported that, neostigmine

crosses placental barrier resulting in fetal bradycardia. Thus, atropine is a better choice than glycopyrrolate.

- Emergence is not synonymous with removal of the endotracheal tube or other artificial airway device. This is only performed when the patient has regained sufficient control of his or her airway reflexes.
- The patient must be watched for respiratory distress and should be placed in lateral position and/or an oropharyngeal or nasopharyngeal airway is placed, to prevent tongue fall and prevent aspiration of the secretions even after extubation. In cases of major cancer resections, especially extending across the midline, where the tongue control is doubtful and the chances of tongue fall or aspiration are high, in such cases the patient is not extubated and the naso-tracheal tube is kept indwelling for minimum 24 hours until the patient has fully gained consciousness.

Induction Agents

- For 50 years, the most commonly used induction agents were rapidly acting, water-soluble barbiturates such as thiopental, methohexital and thiamylal.
- These drugs are still commonly in use today, have an enormous record of safety and reliability and are economical.
- More recently, propofol a non-barbiturate intravenous anesthetic, has displaced barbiturates in many anesthesia practices.
- The use of propofol is associated with less postoperative nausea and vomiting and a more rapid, clear-headed recovery.
- In addition to being an excellent induction agent, propofol can be administered by slow intravenous infusion instead of vapor to maintain the anesthesia (total intraveinous anesthesia, TIVA).
- Among its disadvantages are the facts that it often causes pain on injection and it is prepared in a lipid emulsion, which if not handled using meticulous aseptic precautions, can be a medium for rapid bacterial growth.
- Anesthesia can also be induced by inhalation of a vapor. This is how all anesthetics were once given and is a common and useful technique in uncooperative children. It is re-emerging as a choice in adults. Halothane and sevoflurane are the most commonly used drugs for this purpose.

Traditional Narcotic Analgesics

- Morphine, meperidine and hydromorphone are widely used in anesthesia as well as in emergency rooms, surgical wards and obstetric suites.
- In addition, anesthesia providers have at their disposal a range of synthetic narcotics, which in general, cause less fluctuation in blood pressure and are shorter acting. These include fentanyl, sufentanil, alfentanil and remifentanil. Remifentanil is the newest drug in this class and has such a short duration of action that it must be administered as a continuous infusion.

Muscle Relaxants

- Succinylcholine, a rapid-onset, short-acting depolarizing muscle relaxant, is the drug of choice when rapid muscle relaxation is needed.
  - For decades, anesthetists have used it extensively despite a number of predictable and unpredictable adverse effects associated with its use.
  - The search for a drug that replicates its onset and offsets speed without its adverse effects is the holy grail of muscle relaxant research.
- Other relaxants have durations of action ranging from 15 minutes to more than 2 hours.
- Older drugs in this class were often associated with changes in heart rate or blood pressure, but the newer ones are devoid of these adverse properties.
- Muscle relaxants generally are excreted by the kidney, but some preparations are broken down by plasma enzymes and can be used safely in partial or complete renal failure.
- Pancuronium is an established drug that is still in widespread use because of its low cost and familiarity, especially in intensive care units; rocuronium, mivacurium and cisatracurium are more likely to be used by contemporary anesthesiologists.

Anesthetic Vapors

- These are highly potent chlorofluorocarbons, which are delivered from precision vaporizers directly into the patient's inhaled gas stream. They may be mixed with nitrous oxide, a much weaker, but nonetheless useful anesthetic gas.
- The prototype of modern anesthetic vapors is halothane. It has an unparalleled track record of safety and efficacy, though it is associated with rare, but devastating hepatic necrosis to a greater extent than other agents.
- In the 1980s, it was displaced by isoflurane and enflurane, agents that were cleared from the lungs faster and thus were associated with more rapid anesthetic emergences.
- In the late 1990s, two new vapors became very popular, desflurane and sevoflurane. These drugs are much more maneuverable than their predecessors and are associated with much more rapid emergence.
- Sevolurane can be used for volitile induction and maintenance of anesthesia (VIMA).

COMPLICATIONS OF GENERAL ANESTHESIA[39]: INTRA-ANESTHETIC PROBLEMS

Complications of general anesthetia are described in Box 10.3.

Common Problems

- Hypotension—is a significant decrease of arterial pressure less than normal
  - Decreased cardiac contractility
  - Decreased systemic resistance

Box 10.3: Complications of general anesthesia

Common
Hypotension
Hypertension
Dysrhythmias
Hypoxia
Hypercarbia
Oliguria
Hyperthermia
Life-threatening
Laryngospasm
Bronchospasm
Aspiration
Pneumothorax
MI
Air embolism
Malignant hyperthermia
Anaphylactic reaction

- Inadequate venous return
- Dysrrhythmias
- Hypertension—
  - Excess catecholamine release
  - Pre-existing disease
  - Systemic absorption of vasoconstrictors
- Dysrrhythmias
- Hypoxia—occurs when oxygen delivery to the tissue is insufficient to meet the metabolic demands
  - Inadequate oxygen supply
  - Hypoventilation
  - Ventilation perfusion shunt
  - Reduction of oxygen carrying capacity
- Hypercarbia—is either due to inadequate ventilation or increased carbon dioxide production
- Oliguria—defined as urine output of less than 0.5 mL/kg per hour.
- Hyperthermia—is the rise of temperature of 2 degree per hour or 0.5 degree every 15 min.
  - Malignant hyperthermia
  - Inflammation
  - Hypermetabolic state.

Life-threatening Problems

- **Laryngospasm**—is commonly caused by an irritative stimulus to the airway during light plane of anesthesia.
  - The common noxious stimuli to elicit reflex are secretion, vomitus and inhalation of pungent volatile anesthetic agents, oropharyngeal and nasopharyngeal placement.
  - Reflex closure of vocal cords causing partial or total glottic obstruction
  - Hypoxia, hypercarbia and acidosis

  Treatment
  - Deepening of anesthesia level
  - Remove the stimulus
  - Continuous positive pressure ventilation
  - Muscle relaxant—succinylcholine (10–20 mg IV in adults).
- **Bronchospasm**[40]—may be centrally mediated or it may be a local response to the airway.

  May be stimulated by histamine releasing drugs (morphine, atracurium).
  - Detected—Characteristic wheezing, Tachypnea or dypnea in awake patient.

  Treatment
  - Correction of endotracheal tube
  - Deepening anesthetic level—to prevent reverse bronchospam in light anesthesia inhalational or IV agents are used. Ketamine has advantage of causing bronchodilation.
  - Beta-2 adrenergic agonist—IV or inhalational
  - Adequate hydration and humidification of inspired gas.
- **Aspiration**—general anesthesia causes depression of the airway reflexes that predisposes patient to aspirate. Aspiration may cause bronchospasm, hypoxemia, atelectasia, tachypnea, tachycardia and hypotension.
  - Vomiting or regurgitation:
    - Trendelenburg position
    - Head low position
    - Face turned to one side
    - Suctioning and endotracheal tube placement
    - Cricoid pressure used to prevent regurgitation.[41]
  - Bronchoscopy
  - Aspiration of blood
  - Antibiotic, if indicated
  - Close postoperative care.
- **Pneumothorax**—is the accumulation of gas within the pleural space during:
  - Spontaneous rupture of blebs or bullae
  - Accidental surgical entrance
  - Alveolar rupture during excessive positive pressure ventilation.

  Treatment
  - Discontinue nitrous oxide, ventilate with 100 percent oxygen.
  - Introduce wide-bore needle with 10 mL syringe in 2nd or 3rd intercostals space to confirm presence of air and place chest tube in 8th intercostal space in posterior axillary line.
- **Myocardial ischemia**[42]—is the result of imbalance between the oxygen demand and supply.

  Features
  - Chest pain
  - ECG – ST segment elevation

  Treatment
  - Correction of hypoxia and anemia
  - Beta-adrenergic blockers like dobutamine, vasodilators like nitroglycerine.
- **Air embolism**—Venous air embolism (VAE) is a predominantly iatrogenic complication,[43-44] which occurs when atmospheric gas is introduced into the systemic venous system.[45] In the past, this medical condition was mostly associated with neurosurgical procedures conducted in the sitting position.[46-47] More recently, venous air embolism has been associated with central venous catheterization,[48] high-pressure mechanical ventilation, thoracocentesis, hemodialysis, and several other invasive vascular procedures (VAE is detailed below).

VENOUS AIR EMBOLISM

Venous air emboli, pose a risk anytime the surgical wound is elevated more than 5 cm above the right atrium.[2] The presence of numerous, large, noncompressed, venous channels in the surgical field (especially during cervical procedures and craniotomies that breach the dural sinuses) also increase the risk of VAE.

Entrapment of air/gas facilitated by the patient's intraoperative position causing VAE, may result from other surgical procedures. These include, craniofacial surgery, dental implant surgery, vascular procedures (e.g. endarterectomies), liver transplantation, orthopedic procedures (e.g. hip replacement, spine surgery, arthroscopy), lateral decubitus thoracotomy, genitourinary surgeries in the Trendelenburg position and surgeries involving tumors/malformations with high degree of vascularity or compromised vessels, as in the context of trauma.

Venous air embolism may also result from the iatrogenic creation of a pressure gradient for air entry. Procedures causing such a pressure gradient include lumbar puncture, peripheral intravenous lines and central venous catheters.

Venous air embolism is a potentially life-threatening and under-recognized complication of central venous catheterization (CVC), including central lines, pulmonary catheters, hemodialysis catheters and Hickman (long-term) catheters. A number of factors increase the risk of catheter-related VAE, including the following:

- Fracture or detachment of catheter connections (accounts for 60–90%)
- Failure to occlude the needle hub and/or catheter during insertion or removal
- Dysfunction of self-sealing valves in plastic introducer sheaths
- Presence of a persistent catheter tract following the removal of a central venous catheter
- Deep inspiration during insertion or removal, which increases the magnitude of negative pressure
- Hypovolemia, which reduces central venous pressure
- Upright positioning of the patient, which reduces central venous pressure.

Mechanical insufflation or infusion is another cause of venous air emboli.

- Several different procedures involve the use of insufflation, including arthroscopic procedures, CO_2 hysteroscopy, laparoscopy, urethral procedures and orogenital sexual activity during pregnancy (by entering veins of the myometrium during pregnancy and/or after delivery).
- Inadvertent infusion of air can also occur during the injection of IV contrast agents for CT scans. angiography and cardiac catheterization, as well as during cardiac ablation procedures.

Positive pressure ventilation during mechanical ventilation places patients at risk for barotrauma and subsequently, arterial and/or venous air emboli. Entry of gas into the circulation may result if violation of pulmonary vascular integrity occurs at the same time alveoli rupture from overdistension of the airspaces. This complication can occur in the setting of various diagnoses; however, it is most frequently reported in patients with acute respiratory distress syndrome and in premature neonates with hyaline membrane disease.

The occurrence of venous air embolism (VAE) has also been described in the setting of blunt and penetrating chest and abdominal trauma as well as in neck and craniofacial injuries.

Pathophysiology

Two preconditions must exist for venous air embolism to occur:

- A direct communication between a source of air and the vasculature and
- A pressure gradient favoring the passage of air into the circulation.[49]

The key factors determining the degree of morbidity and mortality in venous air emboli are related to the volume of gas entrainment, the rate of accumulation and the patient's position at the time of the event.[50]

Generally, small amounts of air are broken up in the capillary bed and absorbed from the circulation without producing symptoms. Traditionally, it has been estimated that more than 5 mL/kg of air displaced into the intravenous space is required for significant injury (shock or cardiac arrest) to occur. However, complications have been reported with as little as 20 mL of air[51] (the length of an unprimed IV infusion tubing) that was injected intravenously. The injection of 2 or 3 mL of air into the cerebral circulation can be fatal.[52] Furthermore, as little as 0.5 mL of air in the left anterior descending coronary artery has been shown to cause ventricular fibrillation. Basically, the closer the vein is to the right heart, the smaller the lethal volume is.

Rapid entry or large volumes of air entering the systemic venous circulation puts a substantial strain on the right ventricle, especially if this results in a significant rise in pulmonary artery (PA) pressures. This increase in PA pressure can lead to right ventricular outflow obstruction and further compromise pulmonary venous return to the left heart. The diminished pulmonary venous return will lead to decreased left ventricular preload with resultant decreased cardiac output and eventual systemic cardiovascular collapse. With venous air embolism (VAE), resultant tachyarrhythmias are frequent, but bradyarrhythmias can also occur.

The rapid ingress of large volumes of air (> 0.30 mL/kg/min) into the venous circulatory system can overwhelm the air-filtering capacity of the pulmonary vessels, resulting in a myriad of cellular changes. The air embolism effects on the pulmonary vasculature can lead to serious inflammatory changes in the pulmonary vessels; these include direct endothelial damage and accumulation of platelets, fibrin, neutrophils and lipid droplets.

Secondary injury as a result of the activation of complement and the release of mediators and free radicals can lead to capillary leakage and eventual non-cardiogenic pulmonary edema. Alteration in the resistance of the lung vessels and ventilation-perfusion mismatching can lead to intrapulmonary right-to-left shunting and increased alveolar dead space with subsequent arterial hypoxia and hypercapnea.

Arterial embolism as a complication of VAE can occur through direct passage of air into the arterial system via anomalous structures such as an atrial or ventricular septal defect, a patent foramen ovale or pulmonary arterial-venous malformations. This can cause paradoxical embolization into the arterial tree. The risk for a paradoxical embolus seems to be increased during procedures performed in the sitting position.

Air embolism has also been described as a potential cause of the systemic inflammatory response syndrome (SIRS), triggered by the release of endothelium derived cytokines.[49]

Clinical Presentation

History

Most VAE go unrecognized because their presentations are protein and mimic other cardiac, pulmonary and neurologic dysfunctions. Because of the lack of specific signs and symptoms of VAE, a high index of suspicion is necessary to establish the diagnosis and institute the appropriate treatment. The number of procedures that place patients at risk for VAE has increased, and these procedures occur across almost all clinical specialties. This must be considered to aid in the confirmation or ruling out of VAE. If venous air embolism is suspected, inquiry about the following key historical elements should be obtained:

- Invasive therapeutic and/or diagnostic procedures such as central venous catheterization; lumbar puncture; high-pressure infusion of medications, blood products and/or IV contrast agents
- Patients with hemodialysis access catheters or other indwelling central venous catheters
- Patients on positive pressure ventilation.

Physical Examination

Clinical Features

Many cases of VAE are subclinical and do not result in untoward outcomes. However, severe cases are characterized by cardiovascular collapse and/or acute vascular insufficiency of several specific organs, including, but not limited to the brain, spinal cord, heart and skin.

Two additional contributing factors include whether or not the patient is spontaneously breathing (yielding negative thoracic pressure) or is under controlled positive pressure ventilation. These two factors facilitate the entry of air down a pressure gradient. The clinical presentation is also dependent on the patient's body position at the time of the event. Generally, if the patient is in a sitting position, gas will travel retrograde via the internal jugular vein to the cerebral circulation, leading to neurologic symptoms secondary to increased intracranial pressure. In a recumbent position, gas proceeds into the right ventricle and pulmonary circulation, subsequently causing pulmonary hypertension and systemic hypotension.

An arterial air embolism can also form if passage of air occurred through a right-to-left shunt, as in the case of a patent foramen ovale. The arterial air emboli can then lodge in the coronary or cerebral circulation, causing myocardial infarction or stroke.

Symptoms (Awake Patients)

- Acute dyspnea
- Continuous cough
- 'Gasp' reflex (a classic gasp at times reported when a bolus of air enters the pulmonary circulation and causes acute hypoxemia)
- Dizziness/lightheadedness/vertigo
- Nausea
- Substernal chest pain
- Agitation / disorientation / sense of 'impeding doom'

Signs

Cardiovascular

- Dysrhythmias (tachyarrhythmias/bradycardias)
- 'Mill wheel' murmur—A temporary loud, machinery like, churning sound due to blood mixing with air in the right ventricle, best heard over the precordium (a late sign)
- Jugular venous distention
- Hypotension
- Myocardial ischemia
- Non-specific ST-segment and T-wave changes and/or evidence of right heart strain
- Pulmonary artery hypertension
- Increased central venous pressure (CVP)
- Circulatory shock/cardiovascular collapse

Pulmonary

- Adventitious sounds (rales, wheezing)
- Tachypnea
- Hemoptysis
- Cyanosis
- Decreased end-tidal carbon dioxide, arterial oxygen saturation and tension
- Hypercapnia
- Increased pulmonary vascular resistance and airway pressures
- Pulmonary edema
- Apnea

Neurological

- Acute altered mental status
- Seizures
- Transient/permanent focal deficits (weakness, paresthesias, paralysis of extremities)
- Loss of consciousness, collapse
- Coma (secondary to cerebral edema)

Ophthalmologic

Funduscopic examination may reveal air bubbles in the retinal vessels.

Skin

Crepitus over superficial vessels (rarely seen in setting of massive air embolus).

Livedo reticularis (vascular condition characterized by purplish mottling of the skin).

The above hemodynamic, pulmonary, and neurologic complications primarily result from gas gaining entry into the systemic circulation, occluding the microcirculation and causing ischemic damage to these end organs.

Treatment

The best management of this condition is precautions to avoid it and if it has occurred inadvertently then it is treated symptomatically.

Malignant Hyperthermia

It is hypermetabolic syndrome occurring in genetically susceptible patients[53] when exposed to anesthetic triggering agents.

Triggering agents: Halothane, enflurane, isoflurane, desflurane, sevoflurane and succinylcholine.

The syndrome is thought to be due to reduction of reuptake of calcium ions by the sarcoplasmic reticulum leading to sustained muscle contraction. This results in signs of hypermetabolism like tachycardia, acidosis, hypercarbia, hypoxemia, and hyperthermia.

Treatment

- Discontinue all anesthetic agents
- Administer—dantrolene[54] 2.5 mg/kg/IV initially and repeat to a total of 10 mg/kg (it inhibits the release of calcium ions from sarcoplasmic reticulum)
- Sodium bicarbonate administration
- Hyperkalemia may be corrected with insulin and glucose
- Dysrrhythmias can be treated with procainamide
- Treat hyperthermia by cold sponging
- Monitor urine output.

Anaphylactic reaction[55]—is an immediate type of life-threatening allergic/hypersensitivity reaction. Characterized by severe hypotension and larygo-bronchospasms leading to severe hypoperfusion of the tissue secondary to hypoxia. It is initiated by IgE antibodies.

Treatment

- Discontinue anesthetic agents
- Administer 100 percent oxygen
- Epinephrine 5 to 100 μg IV/SC
- Steroids (sodium hydrocortisone hemisuccinate 250 mg - 1 gm IV)
- Prophalactic drug to hypersensitivity-h_1 and h_2 antagonist and corticosteroids.

POSTANESTHETIC CARE[56]

The patient recovering from the GA needs a good care as the patient is yet to regain full consciousness and the protective reflexes. The patient is susceptible to airway obstruction due to tongue fall, aspiration of secretions, blood or vomitus in the tracheobronchial tree, thus requires good care. The care of the respiratory passage and maintaining its patency is of paramount importance in oral and maxillofacial surgery due to its intimate relation with upper aerodigestive tract. Handling of this part leads to bleeding, edema, loss of anchorage of tongue to the mandible in the cases where midline resection has been done; enhance the chances of respiratory obstruction and aspiration.

- The patient is kept nil per orally till he regains full consciousness. Till such time the patient is kept on parenteral therapy to fulfill the nutritional, fluid and electrolyte requirement using appropriate IV fluids.
- The patient is kept in lateral position with head low position to prevent aspiration. The periodic suctioning of oral cavity, pharynx and nasal cavity are done to make them free of secretions. However, vigorous deep suction using a catheter having opening at the tip should be avoided as it provokes gagging and may suck the friable mucosa and bleeding may take place. Therefore recommended to use plain rubber catheter with rounded end and opening at the side, which is less traumatic. In the tracheostomized patients it is desirable to use separate catheters to suck oral cavity and tracheostomy tube to prevent contamination and lower respiratory tract infections.
- The tongue fall is the most common cause of respiratory obstruction in an unconscious patient. It is more common complication in oral and maxillofacial surgery in patients undergoing mandibular resection across the midline. The tongue fall of the tongue is prevented by lateral position of the head, extension of neck, thrusting the angles of the jaw forwards.
- The other modalities for preventing the tongue fall are placing oropharyngeal (*Water's oropharyngeal airway*) or nasopharyngeal airway. Placing a tongue stitch to draw the tongue out and prevent fall is also practiced. The tongue stitch is always placed using a thick silk suture and the needle bite is taken horizontally deep in the tongue, as the vertical bite in the midline can lead to splitting of the tongue when it is drawn out by pulling. The O_2 saturation in the blood can be monitored by pulse oxymetry.
- The vital parameters like pulse, temperature and respiration (TPR) are monitored periodically, initially in the immediate postoperative period the frequency of recoding could be every 1/2 hourly and as the patient gets settled then 2 to 4 hourly recording of vitals could be enough. In very critical patients continuous monitoring is warranted. All the patients are monitored using multipara monitors now-a-days.
- The periodic BP monitoring is done. The continuous monitoring of the blood pressure is also possible using the multipara monitors.
- Renal perfusion is monitored by measuring the urine out put. Urine out put less than 15 to 20 mL/hr is suggestive of oliguria and poor renal perfusion secondary to hypotension or hypovolmia. Appropriate action should be taken to rectify the cause. The input and output chart is maintained.
- Signs of respiratory distress should be checked and auscultation should be done to know air entry, signs of bronchospasm like ronchi/wheeze. In case, the tracheostomy has been

done or the endotracheal tube is kept indewelling, the patency of the tube must be ensured by periodic suctions and observing air blast. Saline nebulization, few drops of soda bicarbonate or plain saline may be put in the tubes to prevent crustation and drying of the secretions to prevent its blockage due to thick, tenacious or dried secretions.

- Other care includes periodic change of position (if permissible) to prevent from a particular area of lung to become dependent for a long-time. Because the secretions stagnate and accumulate in that dependent part by gravity and that part becomes hypoperfused, increasing physiologic dead space of respiration. The chest physiotherapy should be initiated to prevent the same and facilitate drainage of stagnated secretions. The airway, handling and irritation due to inhaled gases leads to mild inflammation and edema of airway and the secretions are enhanced. Steam nebulizations are given to reduce airway congestion and liquefy the secretions for their easy drainage. After a major surgery the patients remain confined to the bed for long time without physical activity. In such cases, the chances of venous stasis occur especially in the lower extremity due to lack of muscle activity and the chances of deep vein thrombosis and risk of pulmonary embolism are increased, especially in elderly patients. In such patients calf physiotherapy should be initiated. Similarly in cases of long-term non-ambulation, the back care is important to prevent pressure sores (bed sores). A frequent change in position, back massage, use of ring air cushions or water beds is indicated.

REFERENCES

1. Priestley, Joseph. Experiments and Observations on Different Kinds of Air. London W. Bowyer and J. Nichols, 1774. Vol. 1 to 6..
2. Wells, Horace. A History of the Discovery of the Application of Nitrous Oxide Gas, Ether, and Other Vapors to Surgical Operations. Hartford: J. Gaylord Wells, 1847..
3. Bigelow HJ. Insensibility during surgical operations produced by inhalation. Boston Med Surg J. 1846;35:309-17..
4. Atkinson RS, Rushman GB. A synopsis of anesthesia 8th edn. London, John Wright and Son, Ltd. 1977..
5. Wawersik J. History of chloroform anesthesia. Klinik fur Anasthesiologie und Operative Intensivmedizin, Klinikum der Christian-Albrechts-Universitat zu Kiel. Allerg Immunol (Paris). 1998;30(5):135-7..
6. Colton, Gardner Q. Anesthesia. New York: AG Sherwood and Company. 1886.
7. Andrews, Edmund. The relative dangers of anaesthesia by chloroform and ether, from statistics of 209893 cases. Chicago, Robert Fergus' Sons, 1870. 12 p.
8. Lucas GHW, Henderson VE. 'A new anaesthetic gas: cyclopropane.' Canad. Med. Assoc. Journ. 1929;xxi, 173.
9. Lundy JS. Intravenous Anesthesia: Preliminary Report of the Use of the Two New Barbiturates, Proc. Staff Meet. Mayo Clin. 1935;10:536-43.
10. Dripps RD, et al. Introduction to anesthesia–The principle's of safe practice, 5th edn. Philadelphia WB: Saunder's Co. 1977.
11. Kay B, Rolly G. ICI 35868, a new intravenous induction agent. Acta Anaesthesiol Belg. 1977;28:303.
12. Irwin MG, Thompson M, Kenny GNC. Anesthesia; 1977;52:525-30.
13. Ngan Kee WD, Khaw KS, Ma ML, et al. Postoperative analgesic requirement after cesarean section: a comparison of anesthetic induction with ketamine or thiopental. Anesth Analg. 1997;85:1294–8.
14. Amiot JF, Bouju P, Palacci JH, et al. Intravenous regional anaesthesia with ketamine. Anaesthesia. 1985;40(9):899-901.
15. Greenfield W. Neuroleptanalgesia and dissociative drugs. Dent Clin North Am. 1973;17(2):263–74.
16. Guy K Tallmadge. The Third Part of the De Extractione of Valerius Cordus. Isis. 1925;7(3):394-411.
17. Calderone, F.A. J. Pharmacology Experimental Therapeutics, 1935;55(1): 24-39.
18. "WHO Model List of Essential Medicines". World Health Organization. 2005.
19. Suckling CW. Some chemical and physical factors in the development of fluothane. Br J Anaesth. 1957;29(10):466-72.
20. Johnstone M. The human cardiovascular response to fluothane anaesthesia. Br J Anaesth. 1956;28(9):392–410.
21. Subcommitee on the National Halothane Study of the Committee on Anesthesia, N. Summary of the national Halothane Study. Possible association between halothane anesthesia and postoperative hepatic necrosis. JAMA. 1966;197(10):775-88.
22. Strunin L. How long should patients fast before surgery? Time for new guidelines. (Editorial). Br. J. Anaesth. 1993;70:1-3.
23. Nimmo WS. Gastric emptying and anaesthesia. Can J Anaesth, 1989;36(3): S45-S47.
24. McDonough JP, McMullen P, Philipsen N. Informed consent: an essential element of safe anesthesia practice. CRNA, 1995;6(2): 64-9.
25. Alexander F, Cullen S. Preanesthetic medication. The American Journal of Surgery. 1936;34(3):428-34.
26. Cetina J. Smooth induction of anaesthesia in children by means of oral or rectal ketamine dehydrobenzperidol application. Anaesthesist. 1982;31(6):277-9.
27. Aono K, Yoshinaga H. Use of intravenous diazepam for preanesthetic medication-with special reference to sedative effects and changes in vital signs. Masui. 1971; 20(6):556-60.
28. Wilson DV, Evans AT, Miller R. Effects of preanesthetic administration of morphine on gastroesophageal reflux and regurgitation during anesthesia in dogs. Am J Vet Res. 2005;66(3):386-90.
29. Alfano G, Manicastri F. Meprobamate-antihistaminic combination as a preanesthetic medication for surgical patients. Minerva Anestesiol. 1959;25:447-9.
30. Saur P, Kazmaier S, Buhre W, et al. Clinical use of antiemetic drugs for prevention and therapy of postoperative nausea and vomiting. Anaesthesiol Reanim. 1996;21(6):153-8.
31. Koichi Maruyama. Can intravenous atropine prevent bradycardia and hypotension during induction of total intravenous anesthesia with propofol and remifentanil? Journal of Anesthesia. 2010: 24:(2):293-96.

32. Kemmotsu O, Mizushima M, Morimoto Y, et al. Effect of preanesthetic intramuscular ranitidine on gastric acidity and volume in children. J Clin Anesth. 1991;3(6): 451-5.
33. Barry Wyke. A neurological analysis of the stages of anaesthesia. Irish Journal of Medical Science (1926-1967). 1960; 35(11).
34. Guedel AE. Third stage ether anesthesia. A subclassification regarding the significance of the position and movements of the eyeball. Am J Surg. 1920; 34:53-6.
35. Mallampati S, Gatt S, Gugino L, et al. "A clinical sign to predict difficult tracheal intubation: a prospective study." Can Anaesth Soc J. 1985;32(4):429–34.
36. Nuckton TJ, Glidden DV, Browner WS. "Physical examination: Mallampati score as an independent predictor of obstructive sleep apnea". Sleep. 2006;29(7):903–8.
37. Cormack RS, Lehane J. Difficult tracheal intubation in obstetrics. Anaesthesia. 1984;39:1105-11.
38. Cormack R, Lehane J. Cormack-Lehane laryngoscopy grades. In Maltby JR (ed) Notable names in anaesthesia. London, Royal Society of Medicine Press, pp. 43-5, 2002.
39. Gravenstein N, ed. Manual of Complications during Anesthesia. Philadelphia. USA: JB Lippincott, 1991.
40. Daniele RP. Pathophysiology of asthma. In: Fishman ap, (Ed.). Pulmonary diseases, Vol 1 New York, Mcgraw-Hill: 1998: 1055-68.
41. Sellick BA, Cricoid pressure to control regurgitation of stomach contents during induction of anaesthesia. Lancet 2 (1961), pp. 404–6.
42. Alpert JS, Francis GS. Handbook of coronary care, 6th edn. Lippincott Williams and Wilkins, London, 2000.
43. Mirski MA, Lele AV, Fitzsimmons L, et al. Diagnosis and treatment of vascular air embolism. Anesthesiology. 2007; 106(1): 164-77.
44. Sviri S, Woods WP, van Heerden PV. Air embolism—a case series and review. Crit Care Resusc. 2004;6(4):271-6.
45. van Hulst RA, Klein J, Lachmann B. Gas embolism: pathophysiology and treatment. Clin Physiol Funct Imaging. 2003;23(5):237-46.
46. Muth CM, Shank ES. Gas embolism. N Engl J Med. 2000;342(7):476-82.
47. Wong AY, Irwin MG. Large venous air embolism in the sitting position despite monitoring with transoesophageal echocardiography. Anaesthesia. 2005;60(8): 811-3.
48. Pronovost PJ, Wu AW, Sexton JB. Acute decompensation after removing a central line: practical approaches to increasing safety in the intensive care unit. Ann Intern Med. 2004;140(12):1025-33.
49. Kapoor T, Gutierrez G. Air embolism as a cause of the systemic inflammatory response syndrome: a case report. Crit Care. 2003;7(5):R98-R100.
50. Sheasgreen J, Terry T, Mackey JR. Large-volume air embolism as a complication of augmented computed tomography: case report. Can Assoc Radiol J. 2002;53(4): 199-201.
51. Moon R. Air or Gas Embolis. Hyperbaric Oxygen Committee Report. 2003;5-10.
52. Ho AM. Is emergency thoracotomy always the most appropriate immediate intervention for systemic air embolism after lung trauma?. Chest. 1999;116(1): 234-7.
53. Denborough MA, Lovell RRH. Anaesthetic deaths in a family, Lancet. 1960;2:45.
54. Harrison GG. "Control of the malignant hyperpyrexic syndrome in MHS swine by dantrolene sodium". British Journal of Anaesthesia. 1975;47(1):62–5.
55. Caranasos GJ. Drug reactions. In: Schwartz Gr (Ed). Principles and Practice of Emergency Medicine. Philadelphia, Lee and Febiger. 1992.
56. Mcgrath B, Chung F. Post operative recovery and discharge. Anesth Clin North Am. 2003;21.

Section 3

Dentoalveolar Surgeries

- Exodontia
- Management of Impacted Teeth
- Preprosthetic Surgeries

11 Exodontia

Borle Rajiv M, Arora Aakash, Magarkar Shashwat D

HISTORY

From the very earliest times, humans have been plagued by dental problems and have sort a variety of means to alleviate them. Egyptians, Greeks, Japanese, Indians and many more are associated with the history of dentistry.

Although the Ebers Papyrus from Egypt makes no mention of surgical intervention for dental ills, the Edwin Smith Papyrus, of the 17th century BC, cites numerous operations of fractures and dislocations of mandible, maxilla. Since forceps are so prominently pictured in various caves and wall carvings, we can assume that extractions were indeed carried out.

Hippocrates (5th century BC) referred dental forceps, made up of iron known as 'odontagra', have been discovered sites of Greece.

Pierre Fauchard, Father of modern dentistry in 16th century coined the term 'Surgeon Dentist'. He devised many forceps for extraction of teeth. He used to call it 'pelican', which had a fixed part and a movable arm, with hooked end. The hooked end was to engage a tooth to be extracted, while the fixed ends presses against the adjacent teeth, acting as a brace and fulcrum.

In Indian history, Sushruta has described two kinds of surgical instruments *'yantra or blunt'* and *'sastra or sharp'*. Among yantra *'dantasanka'*—a special forcep is described for extraction of teeth. However, Sushruta disapproved extracting firmly rooted teeth, preferring to remove only those that were loose.[1]

DEFINITION OF EXODONTIA

Exodontia or tooth extraction is defined as the painless removal of a whole tooth or tooth root, with minimal trauma to the investing tissues, so that the wound heals uneventfully and no postoperative prosthetic problem is created.[2]

APPLIED SURGICAL ANATOMY OF TEETH AND JAW BONES

The teeth are firmly anchored in the alveolar process of the jaw bone in the alveolar sockets with the help of sharpey's fibers of periodontal ligament. The joint between the teeth and the alveolar bone is called a *'gomphosis'*. The bones are more elastic and resilient in the younger individuals and are more amenable to pressure and expand readily thus, the extractions are easier in the younger patients. In the elderly patients, the bones become less vascular, less cellular and become more compact and brittle and do not yield to pressure easily. Similarly, the teeth also become brittle owing to the regressive changes in them. As a result of this the tooth and the alveolar bone can fracture during the extraction making, the extraction more difficult and complicated. The non-vital and the endodontically treated teeth are often more fragile and brittle due to carious undermining and desiccation of the tooth structure due to loss of the pulp and fracture readily during the extraction and thus, require more careful approach. The teeth have varying crown forms and varied root patterns and need to be assessed thoroughly before proceeding for the surgical procedure to prevent fracture of the tooth or its root. The bulbous crowns warrant selection of forceps with heavier beaks, while as the tapering or peg-shaped crowned teeth require lighter beaked forceps. The multirooted teeth offer more resistance and cannot be luxated or extracted with rotational force as the chances of root fracture are high. Similarly if the roots are divergent, the delivery of the tooth becomes difficult and application of excess force may lead to fracture of the root or the alveolar bone. The roots which are dilacerated thin and slender are also liable to fracture during the extraction. While the roots which are fused, tapering and conical offer simple proposition.

Mandible

The mandible is the only mobile bone of the craniofacial skeleton and is the heaviest too. It has thick cortices, less spongy bone and also has less vascular supply as compared to maxilla (Fig. 11.1). Thus, the chances of complications are more and healing is also slower as compared to the maxillary sockets. The mandible is depressed during the jaw

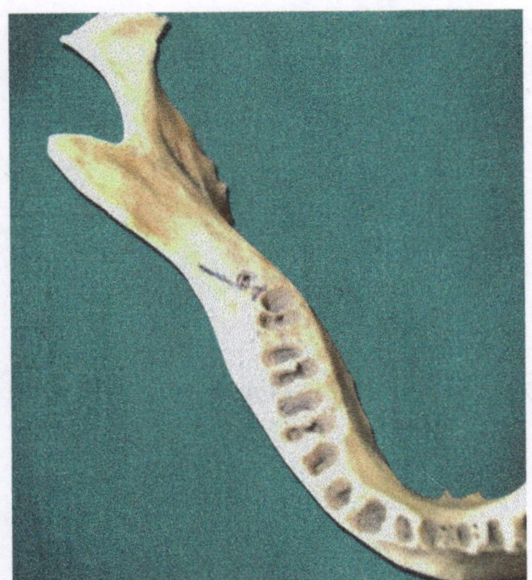

Fig. 11.1: Mandibular alveolar bone showing thick cortices and less spongy bone

opening and if the procedure is long and the mandible is unsupported during the application of the forces during the extraction, the chances of injuries to the temporomandibular joint or its dislocation are very high. The cortical plates in relation to the mandibular incisors are thinner as compared to the cortical plates in the molar and premolar area and hence, local infiltrations with local anesthetic solution, may work in the anterior region but, fails to penetrate the thick cortical plates around the posterior teeth and local anesthetic effect is inadequate and thus, nerve block is the modality of choice for anesthetizing the mandibular teeth. The local infiltrations may work in the anterior area, but it is not a reliable method.

Nerve Supply of Mandibular Teeth

The main nerve supply to the mandibular teeth, the alveolar bone and the periodontal ligament, is derived from the inferior alveolar bone, which enters the inferior alveolar canal through the mandibular foramen present on the lingual cortex of the ascending ramus. The nerve travels in the canal and supplies the mandibular molars and their supporting alveolar bone and periodontal ligament fibers. At the level of the premolar, the inferior alveolar nerve divides into the incisive nerve and the mental nerve. The incisive nerve continues in the bone and supplies the mandibular anterior teeth and their supporting alveolar bone and periodontal ligament fibers, up to the midline and never crosses over to the other side. The mental nerve makes its exit from the mental foramen situated between the premolars and supplies the labial mucoperiosteum and gingiva of the mandibular anterior teeth, as well as the lining of the lower lip.

The gingiva over the mandibular molars is supplied by the long buccal nerve, which also supplies the mucosa of the cheek up to the level of the corner of the mouth.

The lingual gingiva of all the mandibular teeth are supplied by the lingual nerve up to the midline and the lingual nerve also supplies the floor of the mouth and half of the tongue, ipsilaterally.

Maxilla

The maxillary bone has more spongy bone and thin cortical plates and excellent vascularity (Fig. 11.2). Due to the presence of the more spongy bone, it is more amenable to expansion when the pressure is applied during extraction. Owing to its better vascularity as compared to the mandible and thus, the healing is faster and less eventful. However, maxilla being the weaker bone, heavy elevators like cross bar elevators cannot be used for luxating the teeth as the chances of fracture of the alveolar bone and the tuberosity are very high.

The apices of the maxillary molars are in close proximity to the floor of the maxillary sinus. Sometimes due to the anatomical variations, the sinus floor extends deep between the roots of the molars and only thin bone separates the floor of the sinus and the root apices. Any chronic periapical infection may lead to destruction of this thin bone and the periapical infection from the tooth may extend into the sinus causing odontogenic maxillary sinusitis. In the event of fracture of the root and injudicious use of force or injudicious instrumentation may displace the fractured root into the sinus.

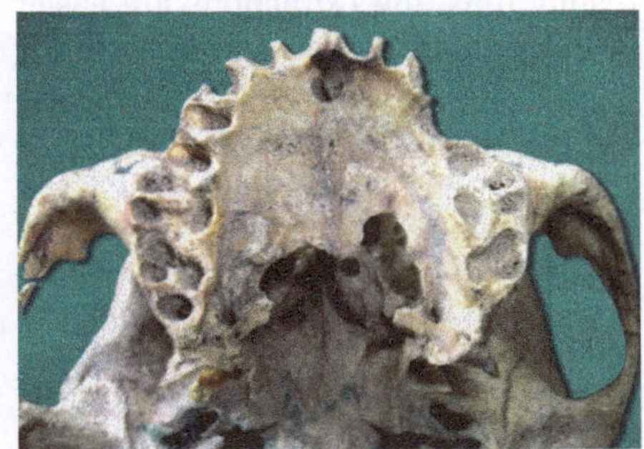

Fig. 11.2: Maxillary alveolar bone showing thin cortices and plenty of spongy bone

The maxillary third molars are last teeth to erupt and are invariably present in the maxillary tuberosity, which is the structure having spongy bone. It has been observed that in majority of cases, the roots of the maxillary third molars are fused, conical and tapered and thus, the extraction of this tooth is a simple procedure. However, when the roots are unfavorable and especially in elderly patients, where the bone becomes more compact and brittle, the extraction of the maxillary third molar may become a difficult task and injudicious use of force or use of heavy elevators for luxation of these teeth may lead to fracture of the tuberosity and the formation of oroantral communication.

As the maxillary alveolar bone has thin cortical plates simple paraperiosteal infiltrations of local anesthetic solution can produce adequate anesthesia for facilitating the exodontias procedures. However, to ensure proper anesthesia, it is desirable to give nerve blocks, where ever feasible.

Nerve Supply of Maxillary Teeth

The maxillary teeth, alveolar bone and the periodontal ligament fibers are supplied by the branches of the maxillary nerve namely the posterior, middle and the anterior superior alveolar branches. The first and the second molars are supplied by the posterior superior alveolar nerve. While the distobuccal and palatal roots of the first molar are supplied by the posterior superior alveolar nerve, its mesiobuccal root is supplied by the middle superior alveolar nerve. Because of this, separate infiltration is required to be given for anesthetizing the middle superior alveolar nerve in addition to the PSA nerve block, while extracting the maxillary first molar. The middle and the anterior superior alveolar nerves are the branches originating from the infraorbital nerve in the infraorbital canal and descend inferiorly in the maxillary bone to reach the teeth supplied by them, i.e. the premolars and the anteriors respectively. The infraorbital nerve block is good enough to block these two nerves. All these three nerves form a plexus in the maxillary alveolar bone called a '*superior dental plexus*'.

As the cortical plates are thin and there is more spongy bone in maxilla, even paraperiosteal infiltrations of local anesthetics work and produce adequate anesthesia. However, in presence of local infections or acute inflammatory reaction the local infiltration may fail and nerve block becomes the ultimate choice of anesthesia. The local infiltrations can also fail in presence of osteosclerotic conditions and thus, nerve blocks are more reliable.

The buccal gingiva up to the molars is supplied by the posterior superior alveolar nerve, in the premolar area by the middle superior alveolar nerve and the labial gingival of the anterior teeth are supplied by the anterior superior alveolar nerve. The palatal gingival of molar and the premolar area are supplied by the branches of the greater palatine nerve, while as the palatal gingival of the anterior teeth is supplied by the nasopalatine nerve.

INDICATIONS FOR EXTRACTION OF TOOTH

The teeth can be extracted for either therapeutic or prophylactic considerations. The indications for extraction of the teeth can be enumerated as follows (Box 11.1):

- Severe caries where the teeth are not restorable.
- Pulpal necrosis.
- Severe periodontal disease leading to severe irreparable periodontal loss and mobility.
- Orthodontic reasons—for creation of space, prevention of arch collapse, serial extractions and removal of malposed teeth, which cannot be corrected orthodontically.

Box 11.1: Indications for exodontia

- Severe caries where the teeth are not restorable
- Pulpal necrosis
- Severe periodontal disease
- Orthodontic reasons
- Malposed teeth which hinder with the designing and fabrication of the prosthesis or cause trauma from occlusion
- Fractured teeth which cannot be conserved
- Preprosthetic extractions
- Teeth in fracture line
- Teeth associated with pathologies
- Teeth in firing line of radiations
- Supernumerary teeth.

- Malposed teeth which hinder with the designing and fabrication of the prosthesis or cause trauma from occlusion causing recurrent ulcers or lead to non-self cleansing areas thus leading to periodontal or carious disease.
- Fractured teeth which cannot be conserved.
- Preprosthetic extractions—total extraction for fabrication of complete dentures or removal of undesirable teeth, which come in the way of fabrication of proper dentures.
- Teeth in fracture line—all the teeth in fracture line need not be removed, however, when the fracture occurs in dentate patient in the denture bearing area the fracture becomes essentially a compound fracture and the chances of infection are very high and thus, the teeth in fracture line may be removed. Similarly the teeth which hinder with the proper reduction of the fracture may also be extracted.
- Teeth associated with pathologies such as cysts, tumors, granulomas or chronic infections.
- Teeth in firing line of radiations the patients undergoing the radiation therapy for the management of malignancies of the head neck area were usually subjected to prophylactic extractions of the teeth in the way of radiations as the effects of radiations on the bone (*avascularity*) and the teeth (*radiation caries*) lead to high chances of complicated osteoradionecrosis. However, due to advent of better technology and care, now-a-days it is not practiced widely.
- Supernumerary teeth.

CONTRAINDICATIONS FOR EXTRACTION

All the patients undergoing the dental extractions need not be healthy and may have associated medical disorders, which can complicate the dental extraction. Proper control of the underlying medical or local pathology minimizes the chances of complications and makes the surgical procedure safe. The identification of the medical disorder, its evaluation, assessment and proper control is mandatory before the dental extraction is undertaken. It requires adequate knowledge of medical condition, proper history taking, short but relevant general clinical examination, appropriate and judicious investigations and timely referral to the specialist for the treatment and advise. In the medically compromised patients, where the chances of developing life-threatening complications are high, it becomes a teamwork for ensuring proper safety of the patients. Similarly, undertaking this procedure under the controlled environments is of paramount importance to provide necessary medical help and care to the patient promptly, if needed. In most of the dental clinics the facilities and infrastructure may not be available to combat the emergency and it is advisable that such high risk patients be operated under controlled environments, where such facilities are available. The dental surgeon must be in position to suitably alter the treatment plan or premedicate the patient during the perioperative phase to take adequate care to avoid complications. Hence, it can be said that the associated medical conditions are only relative contraindications and not the '*absolute contraindication*' for the dental extraction in majority of cases, if due care and control is established. Any medical condition which is uncontrolled, severe or acute may become absolute contraindication at a given time, however the same patient may be fit to undergo dental extraction, once the underlying medical condition is brought under control. One has to assess the severity of the condition, general condition of the patient and his ability to withstand surgical stress as against the advantages of dental extraction. Most of the times there are conservative and less invasive options available for dental extraction, e.g. simple opening of the root canal will decompress the periapical infection and provide temporary pain relief to the patient. One must weigh the advantages of dental extraction as against the chances of severe complications that can occur in a medically compromised patient and should try to defer the procedure by opting for conservative approach for time being. An extraction must be regarded as a minor surgical procedure like any other surgical procedure on human body and thus, the focus should be on the patient as whole rather than only on the local dental pathology.

The contraindications (conditions that warrant proper care) are (Table 11.1).

Physiological Contraindications

Menstruating Females

Menstruation is a stressful condition and adding further surgical stress may not be a good idea. Secondly, owing to high circulating levels of the estrogen in the blood, the tissues tend to bleed more[3] and thus, the elective extractions should be avoided during the menstruation.

Pregnancy

Pregnancy is a major event in any woman's life and is associated with many physiological changes affecting especially the endocrine, cardiovascular and hematological systems. The levels of most of the hormones rise, especially the sex hormones, prolactin and thyroid hormones, but levels of luteinizing hormone and follicle-stimulating hormone fall.

The first and the third trimesters of the pregnancy are more risky. Fetal development during the first 3 months is a complex process of organogenesis and the fetus is at a risk of from developmental defect. The most critical period is the 3rd week to 8th week, during differentiation. All drugs should be avoided unless a potential benefit outweighs potential risk, as during the first trimester the organogenesis is taking place in the fetus and the drugs prescribed may have teratogenic effects. The patient may have severe toxemia and may not tolerate the procedure.

During second and third trimesters, the fetus is growing and maturing, but can still be affected by infections, drugs and possibly other factors.

In the third trimester supine hypotension syndrome[4] may result, if the patient is laid flat. The patient should, therefore, be put on one side to allow venous return to recover. Elective dental care should be avoided in the last month of pregnancy, as it is uncomfortable for the patient. Moreover, premature labor or even abortion may also be ascribed.

The second trimester is supposed to be relatively safe for minor surgeries. However, if the tooth is causing recurrent sepsis and infections and bacteremia/septicemia, its extraction can be undertaken with due care as retaining it is equally hazardous.

Because of the risk of coincidental mishaps, it is wise to try to avoid giving any drugs, possibly even local anesthetics, conscious sedation or general anesthesia. As much treatment as possible should be postponed until after parturition in those with bad obstetric history (the history of abortion). During first trimester the only safe course of action is to protect all patients from infections and avoid the use of drugs and radiographs. Dental treatment is best carried out during the second trimester.

Extreme Geriatric Patients

The physiologic compensatory mechanisms are severely compromised and the stress combating capacity is very poor and such patients may not be able to cope up with minor surgical procedure and thus they need to be avoided.

Table 11.1: Contraindications for exodontia

Local	Systemic
• Acute infection • Tooth in malignant growth • Tooth associated with vascular lesion • Proximity with vital structures • Irradiated jaw	**Physiologic** Menstruation Pregnancy Extremely geriatric patients **Pathological** CVS—HT, IHD, CCF, valvular pathologies, conduction disorders Immunosuppression Hepatic disorders Endocrinal disorders—Addisons disease, hypo- and hyperthyroidism, diabetes Neurological—epilepsy, stroke Hematological—leukemia, agranulocytosis, bleeding disorders, coagulopathies, anticoagulant or antiplatelet therapy Renal disorders RS—asthema, pulmonary tuberculosis, COPD, active chest infections

Pathological Contraindications

Systemic Contraindications

Unstable systemic disease:

- Unstable endocrine disorders like myxedema, thyrotoxicosis, diabetes, Addisons disease and patients on long term steroid therapy.
- Renal disorders, e.g. chronic renal failure, glomerulonephritis, uremia.
- Cardiovascular, e.g. hypertension, ischemic heart diseases, cardiomyopthia, valvular disorders, CCF, conduction disorders.
- Pulmonary—bronchial asthma, COPD, active chest infections such as tuberculosis.
- Hepatic disorders—cirrhosis of liver, acute liver infections.

- Neurological disorders—stroke, epilepsy.
- Hematologic disease—thrombocytopenia, agranulocytosis, leukopenia, leukemia, bleeding and clotting disorders, patients on anticoagulants.
- Immunosuppressed conditions.

Local Conditions

- Irradiated jaws—as the chances of osteoradionecrosis are very high due to severe impairment of the vascularity of the bone.
- Vascular lesions, like AV malformations, hemangiomas, aneurysms may lead to catastrophic bleeding.
- Malignant tumor—a malignant growth in the region of the offending tooth should be taken as an absolute contraindication for the dental extraction as the tooth associated with malignant lesions is mobile due to destruction of investing periodontal tissues. The extraction of such teeth may lead to seeding of malignant cells in the capillaries and may lead to distant metastasis of the tumor to viscera. The patients always tend to insist for the extraction of such teeth, which should not be done.
- Proximity to vital structures—the teeth which are in close proximity of vital structures such as inferior alveolar nerve, maxillary sinus and extraction of such teeth can lead to damage to these structures thus should not be extracted, unless it is absolutely unavoidable.
- Presence of acute infection—the tooth having acute infective pathology should not be extracted as there are chances of local extension of the infection in the deeper tissue planes due to handling and breaking the barriers during the surgery. At the same time with the exposure of the capillaries, the microorganisms may get ingress into the bloodstream and lead to bacteremia and complications associated with it. The most common complication apart from pyrexia associated with bacteremia is bacterial endocarditis. If the tooth is to be extracted in presence of acute infection, suitable antibiotic prophylaxis in the form of Amoxicillin, given intravenously half an hour before extraction in a dose of 500 mg or Ampicillin 500 mg to 1 g IV, is given to prevent bacterial endocarditis. As far as possible, the infection is controlled by antibiotic therapy and local measures for its drainage/decompression (e.g. opening the root canal) are undertaken to control it and relieve pain and discomfort to the patient.

PRESURGICAL ASSESSMENT

Medical Risk Assessment

As already stated earlier a dental surgeon must understand that he is 'not treating a tooth, but he is treating an individual with a diseased tooth'. Therefore, the approach should not be localized and restricted to dental pathology alone and the patient as a whole should be taken into consideration. Every dental extraction should be considered as a minor surgery and should be done with utmost care to prevent complications. All the patients walking in a dental surgery may not be absolutely healthy and may have associated medical conditions, which may lead to severe life-threatening complications and it is also true that the complications do not occur with prior warning, but effort must be made to make the dental extractions safe and uneventful for the patient. The patients are sometimes unaware of their medical ailments and it is the test of skill of history taking, where a dental surgeon should make comprehensive effort to extract the desired information by direct or indirect questioning. It has been observed that even if the patient is aware of his medical illness, he will not reveal it to a dental surgeon as he often considers it unnecessary for undergoing dental extraction due to illiteracy and ignorance. It is therefore, necessary for a dental surgeon to establish a proper rapport with the patient, communicate well and should not resort to shortcuts, while obtaining the history. The drug history can also indirectly suggest the type of pathology he might be suffering from. It is therefore reemphasized that relevant, concise history and brief relevant general clinical examination is key to successful clinical practice. In patients who are above 40 years of age, history of hypertension, diabetes, IHD must be obtained as these diseases are commonly seen due to urbanization and changing lifestyles in this age group. Blood pressure should be recorded in such patients, as they may be undetected hypertensive patients. The past history of dental treatment or extraction may also give useful information and should also be recorded.

Emotional Condition

By and large there are many misconceptions prevailing in the society about the dental extractions, especially in rural area, such as 'weakening eye sight' following the dental extraction. The patients are always very apprehensive to undergo dental extraction, as they often consider it to be a very painful procedure as it is narrated to them by someone. Such patients are very anxious and are liable to go into a syncope or aggravation of their medical problems leading to complications, due to emotional stress. The anxious patients may be unnecessarily talkative, behave in a peculiar way and have palmar sweating. Such anxious patients need to be identified, counseled and premedicated prior to the extraction as a part of anxiety reduction protocol. Normally the counseling is good enough, but in the patients who are extremely anxious premedication with tranquilizers/anxiolytics (*Diazepam*) and atropine sulphate (*vagolytic*) may be beneficial. The former reduces the anxiety and calms down the patient and the latter prevents bradycardia by its vagolytic action, reducing the chances of syncope during the procedure.

Clinical Evaluation

Local clinical evaluation of the patient should be done thoroughly. Any extraoral swelling, presence of cellulitis, abscess, lymphadenopathy and trismus should be noted. The extraoral swelling is suggestive of extension of dental infection to the soft tissue spaces around the jaws and may warrant separate procedures apart from dental extraction such as, incision and drainage or decompression to bring about its resolution. The presence of trismus is associated with inflammatory pathology is suggestive of protective muscle spasm secondary to pain and may obstruct the access to the surgical site. Acuteness of these clinical signs of infection should also be assessed and the procedure should be preferably carried out under antibiotic cover to prevent bacteremia. The bacteremia related complications like bacterial endocarditis are more serious and should be prevented by antibiotic prophylaxis.

Intraoral examination should be carried out to assess proper access to the surgical site, bulky buccal fat of pad, trismus, large tongue, hyperactive gag reflex usually prevent proper access and handling of the intraoral structures. The condition of gingiva, acuteness of inflammation, edema, congestion and pus discharge should be noted as such tissues are friable and bleed during the surgery and their healing may be complicated. It is desirable not to extract the tooth in presence of acute infection as it may and lead to bacteremia and spread of the infection to the deeper tissue planes. Such cases should be treated after proper control of infection with antibiotics and local care.

The dental arches should be evaluated. The periodontal condition of the teeth, mobility, missing teeth, crowding should be noted. If the tooth in question is crowded or malposed, the application of forceps or elevator may be difficult. If the adjacent tooth is missing then the interdental bone cannot be used as fulcrum to luxate the tooth and the extraction may be carried out using forceps only. Presence of generalized periodontal disease associated with pockets and pus discharge render the teeth mobile, which are easy to extract, but the presence of septic focus may cause wound infection and requires antibiotic coverage to prevent it.

The tooth in question should be thoroughly evaluated for its crown size, form, shape, carious undermining, previous endodontic therapy, angulation, malposition, etc. as carious undermining and endodontic therapy may make the tooth structure brittle and the tooth may fracture, while extracting. The adjacent tooth should also be evaluated for mobility, caries and presence of any restoration.

Radiographic Evaluation

The tooth in question should be evaluated radiographically. It is necessary to know the normal radiographic landmarks on a radiograph. The size, shape, form, number of roots, presence of dilacerations, resorption and hypercementosis should be noted. The condition of adjacent tooth should also be evaluated. The condition of the bone should also be evaluated as the chronic infections make the bone sclerotic owing to the periosteal bone apposition and such bone resists expansion during extraction. Presence of periapical pathologies like cyst, granuloma should also be noted and presence of any other bony pathology associated with the tooth should be ruled out. The periapical cyst and granuloma needs to be curetted as failure to do so may lead to residual cyst in the former case and prolonged oozing of the blood in latter case. The proximity of the tooth with vital structure like neurovascular bundle, maxillary sinus also needs to be evaluated radiographically.

Overall Difficulty

When all the findings derived from the history, general examination, local and radiological examination are summed up, the overall difficulty can be determined. Once the difficulty index is determined suitable preoperative evaluation, referral to consultant for control of underlying medical condition, alteration in treatment plan and preparation for surgery can be undertaken to ensure smooth conduct of the procedure and to minimize the complications.

METHODS OF EXODONTIA

Intra-alveolar Extraction

Intra-alveolar extraction is usually practiced to extract an erupted, intact tooth with the help of a forceps, elevator or both. It is also referred to as extraction by closed method.

Indications for intra-alveolar extraction:

- Loose teeth.
- Firm teeth with intact crown.
- Teeth facilitating proper access to forcep and/or elevators.

Transalveolar Extraction

Transalveolar extraction is practiced to remove the teeth, which are impacted or to remove the root pieces or teeth which have unfavorable roots. It is also called a surgical extraction, which is misnomer as irrespective of the technique; the extraction is a surgical procedure. In this technique, the tooth is approached and accessed by removing the alveolar bone over it (*transalveolar*) (Box 11.2).

Box 11.2: Indications for transalveolar extraction

- Root pieces
- Severely undermined crowns
- Fractured teeth
- Brittle teeth (RC treated)
- Unfavorable root form
- Dense bone
- Malposed teeth—crowding, incomplete eruption
- Proximity with vital structures

SEQUENCE OF PROCEDURES TO BE UNDERTAKEN DURING EXTRACTION

Administration of Local Anesthesia

Most of the cases of exodontia are performed effectively and successfully under local anesthesia. Hence, the first step in the extraction of the tooth is administration of local anesthesia through an appropriate agent and technique. One must wait for the local anesthetic to act and verify the same by subjective and objective symptom evaluation.

Position of the Operator and the Patient

Position of the Operator

- Standing or sitting.

- In front or behind patient—for the maxillary teeth and the mandibular teeth on the left side, the operator should stand at 7 to 8° clock position and for the mandibular posterior teeth on the right side, the operator should stand at 11° clock position (Figs 11.3A to C and 11.4A to C).
- Be comfortable. Back straight. Head not bent forward blocking light.
- The operator should not lean over the patient and contaminate the sterile field created by draping and isolation.

Position of the Patient

- Patient should be kept in comfortable position with head nicely supported at the occiputs for maxillary teeth supine position (back 10° to ground) is recommended.
- Patient almost supine or semi-sitting (back 20°–30° to ground) for the mandibular teeth.
- Both the above positions are recommended when the operator is operating in sitting position.
- If the operator is standing then the chair is raised and head of the patient is tilted backwards, so that the mandibular arch is parallel to the floor and the maxillary arch is at 45° angle to the floor.

The level of the head of the patient should be at the level between the shoulder and the elbow of the operator while the level of the head should be at the level of elbow of the operator.

Sequence of Tooth Extraction

To prevent blood from the sockets of extracted teeth obscuring the field of operation, it is usual to remove mandibular teeth before the maxillary. However, this sequence has disadvantage as well, if the maxillary teeth are extracted after the mandibular teeth, the loose fragments of calculus or fractured tooth fragments may fall in the sockets of the extracted mandibular teeth. Such foreign bodies could hamper the healing. Hence, it is recommended by some authors to extract maxillary teeth before the extraction of the mandibular teeth. The posterior teeth are extracted before the anterior teeth as it will not obstruct the access due to placement of the pack. Unnecessary movement to and fro around the chair is avoided by starting multiple extractions with the right mandibular teeth, which are extracted from behind the sitting patient.

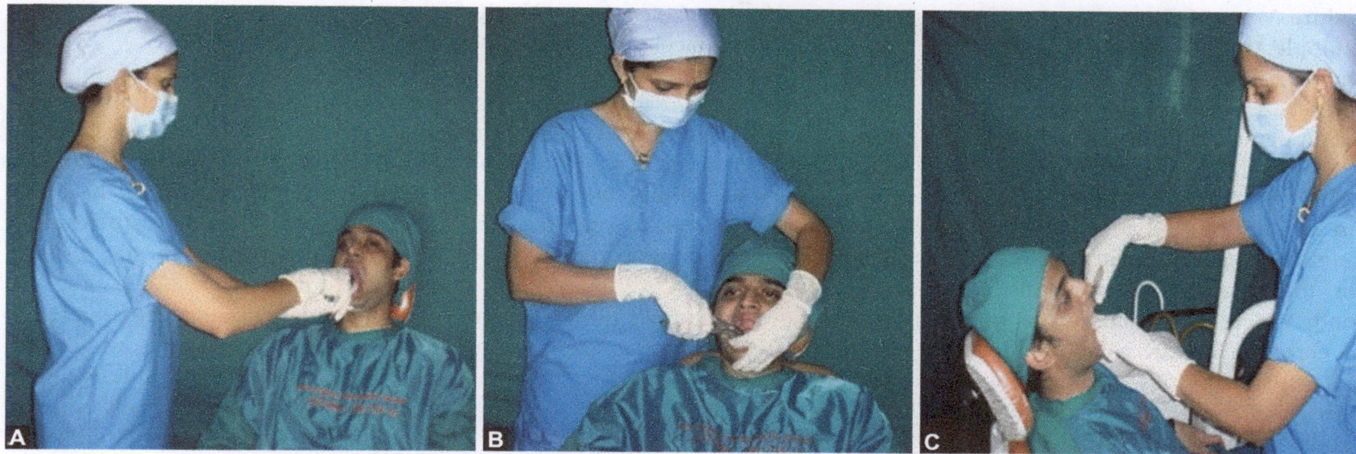

Figs 11.3A to C: Position for mandibular anterior, right posterior, left posterior teeth

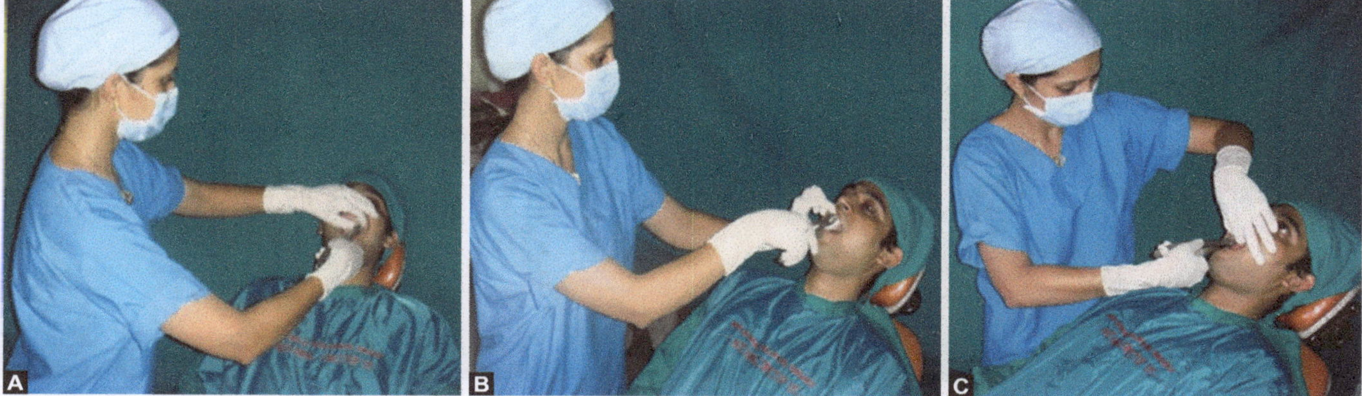

Figs 11.4A to C: Position of the operator for maxillary posteriors on left side, anteriors and right posterior teeth

It is wise to begin with the most painful tooth when undertaking multiple extractions lest any surgical or anesthetic difficulty prevents the completion of the operation. Similarly, when working under local anesthesia only one quadrant of the mouth should be injected at a time. When the surgery in this area has been successfully completed a new quadrant may be injected. It is better to take out teeth from one side of the arch only, at one visit, thereby leaving the other for chewing.

The extraction of many teeth at one outpatient sitting is contraindicated as it may produce significant inflammation and discomfort to the patient and the blood loss can be considerable. It is not possible to standardize as to how many teeth should be extracted at a single sitting as it depends on the surgical difficulty, patient's health, morale and other factors relevant to the surgical procedure. Where it is necessary to extract multiple teeth at one visit, the patient should be kept in the recovery room for at least an hour postoperatively and then accompanied home by an attendant.

Access

An adequate access and visibility of the surgical site are important requirements for the uneventful extraction of the tooth. Never try to apply the forceps of elevators blindly as it may lead to soft tissue injuries, slippage of the instrument and fracture of the tooth. Proper access to the surgical site can be created by gently retracting the lips, cheek and the tongue using Bishops/Austin/Minnesota retractors and Wieder tongue blade, respectively (Fig. 11.5). The mouth needs to be kept open during the procedure to facilitate proper access to the surgical site and prevent accidental biting on the operator's finger, especially while treating children and epileptic patients. Mouth props, bite block, side action mouth prop can be used for this purpose, but they are not usually required in an awake patient. The mouth mirror can also be an effective tool in the retraction of the cheek and the tongue during the extraction.

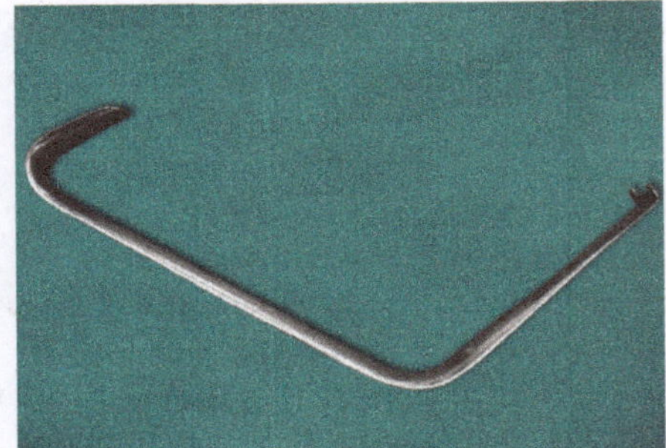

Fig. 11.5: Modified Austin's retractor

The visibility to the surgical site must be good and after retraction proper illumination of the surgical site should be ensured. Any secretions, blood should be readily sucked out to keep the surgical site clear to impart uninterrupted visibility.

The fundamental requirements for the exodontia procedures are summarized in Box 11.3.

Box 11.3: Fundamental requirements

To summarize the fundamental requirements:
- Adequate access
- Good visualization of the field
- Unimpeded pathway of delivery of the tooth
- Controlled forces to retract adjacent structures and remove tooth

Gingival Retraction

Before proceeding for extraction, the gingival attachment on the tooth needs to be detached and retracted to facilitate proper application of the forceps as apically as possible below the CE junction and to prevent laceration of the gingiva, while performing extraction. The gingival retraction should be liberal to facilitate passive retraction (Figs 11.6A to C). The gingival papilla on either side of the tooth should be reflected to expose the entire tooth to be extracted. The gingival retraction can be done using a number 15 BP blade, Moon's probe or a sharp periosteal elevator.

Use of the Elevator[5,6]

Elevators are single-bladed instruments for extracting or luxating the teeth and roots, which they do by moving them out of the sockets along a path determined by the natural curvature of the roots. They are applied on the cementum of any surface, usually the mesial, distal or buccal, at a point.

The dental elevators are used either to elevate/luxate the tooth or to deliver the tooth. The elevators are simple machines designed specially to suit different requirements and to deliver maximum mechanical advantage with minimum efforts. It is not necessary to

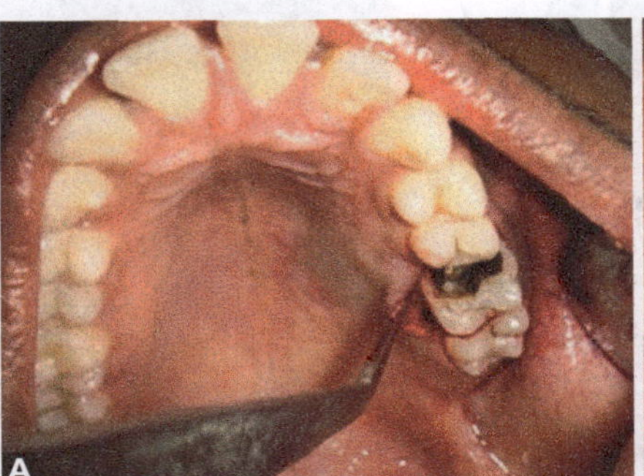

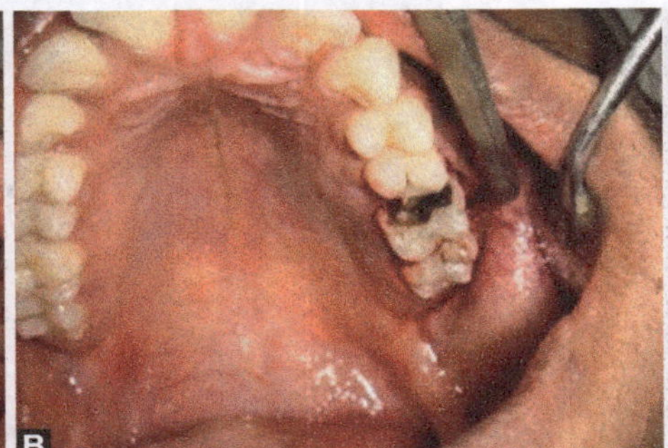

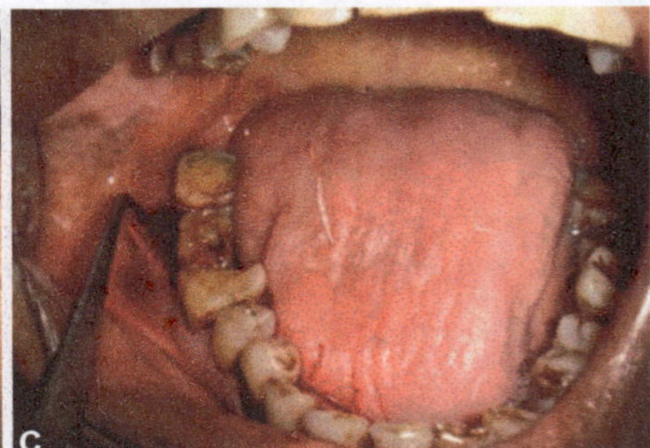

Figs 11.6A to C: Liberal gingival retraction

use elevators always, however, the teeth which are firm and malposed and where the forceps cannot be applied, the tooth is luxated and then either delivered using the elevator or with forceps.

The elevators are to be used judiciously and following rules must be followed, while using the elevators:

- Do not use heavy elevators like cross bar elevators to luxate/deliver the maxillary teeth, as it is a weak bone and can get readily fractured.
- Do not use the adjacent tooth as a fulcrum unless it is also to be extracted.
- Never use the buccal cortical plate at the gingival line as a fulcrum, except where odontectomy is performed, or in the third molar areas.
- Never use the lingual cortical plate at the gingival line as a fulcrum.
- Use controlled guided force and do not use injudicious forces as it may lead to fracture of the tooth, alveolar bone or basal bone.
- Engage the tip of the elevator on a natural undercut area such as below the cervical line (purchase groove) or artificially created point on to the tooth to be extracted (*purchase point*) to prevent slippage.
- Support the jaw and head to prevent slippage of the elevator and dislocation of the mandible, especially while elevating the lower tooth.
- Use finger guard to prevent accidental soft tissue injury due to accidental slippage of the elevator, but make sure that the finger is protected against the injury by the gauze piece as a wrapping (Figs 11.7A and B).
- When cutting through interseptal bone, take care not to engage the root of an adjacent tooth.

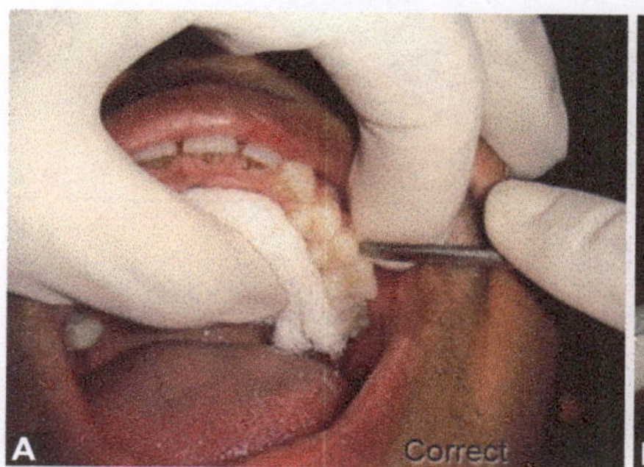

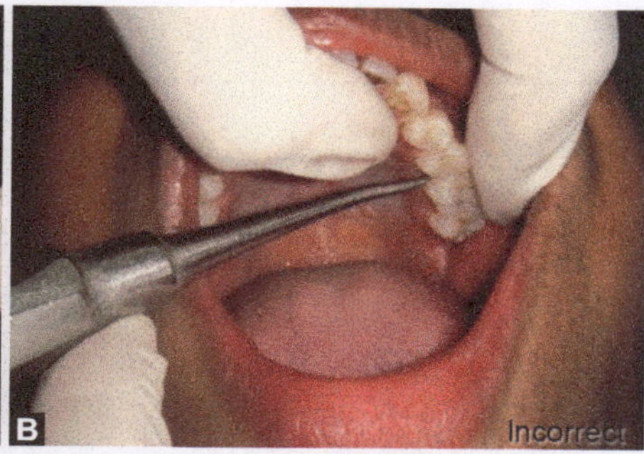

Figs 11.7A and B: (A) Correct; (B) Incorrect method of application of elevator

Indications

Elevator is generally used to luxate or extract those teeth, which cannot be engaged by the beaks of the forceps such as in impactions, malposed teeth, to remove roots, fractured or carious teeth.

Elevator should be used with utmost caution at all times because of the dangers of damaging or even of extracting adjacent teeth, fracturing maxilla or mandible, fracturing the alveolar process, slipping and plunging the point of the instrument into the soft tissue, with the possible perforation of major vessels and nerves, penetrating the maxillary antrum or forcing the root into the antrum, or forcing the apical third of the root of the lower third molar into the mandibular canal or through the lingual plate of the mandible into the submandibular or pterygomandibular space depending upon the position of the third molar.

Parts of the Elevator

- Handle—this may be a continuation of the shank or at a right angle to it.
- Shank.
- Blade—part which engages the crown. The shape of blade differs for each elevator type and each is used as the need dictates.

According to form, elevators can be classified as follows:

- **Straight:** Wedge type.
- **Angular:** Right and left.
- Cross bar (handle at right angle to shank).

According to use, elevators can be classified as:

- Elevators designed to remove the entire tooth.
- Elevators designed to remove roots broken off at the gingival line.
- Elevators designed to remove roots broken off halfway to the apex.
- Elevators designed to remove the apical at the apical third of the root.
- Elevators designed to reflect the mucoperiosteum.

Work Principles in use of Elevators

The work principle as for the use of the elevators may be that of the lever, the wedge, the wheel and axle or the combination of the above mentioned principles (Figs 11.8 to 11.10).

Lever principle: Elevators most frequently make use of this principle. The elevator is the lever of the first class-position of the fulcrum is between the effort and the resistance. In order to gain mechanical advantage in a lever of the first class, the effort arm, on one side of the fulcrum must be longer than the resistance arm on the other side of the fulcrum.

Long arm is ¾ of the total length and short arm is ¼ of the total length, to get the mechanical advantage of 3.

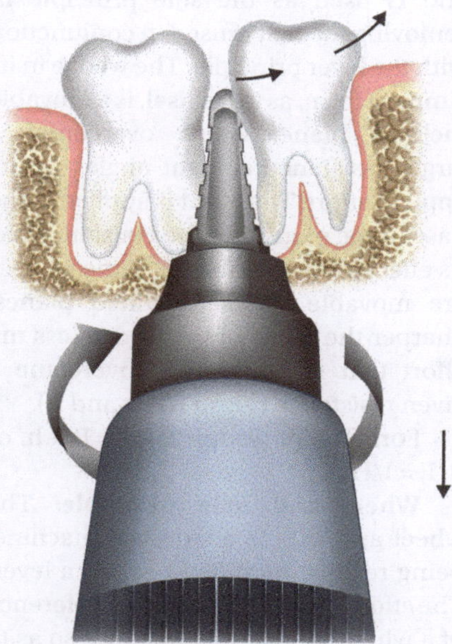

Fig. 11.8: Straight elevator used as a lever

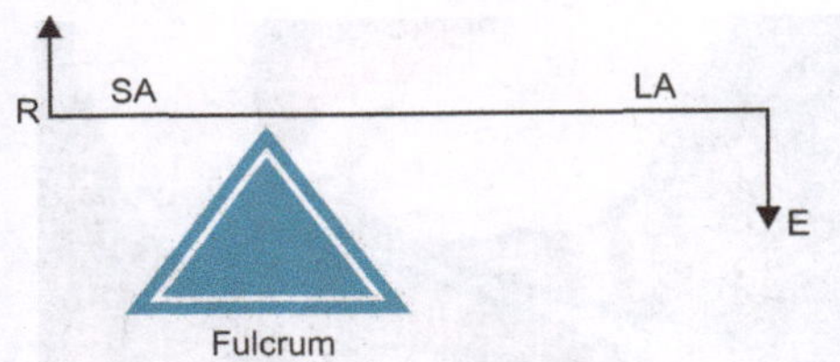

Fig. 11.9: Lever principle (*Abbreviations:* R: Resistance; E: Effort, SA: Short arm; LA: Long arm).

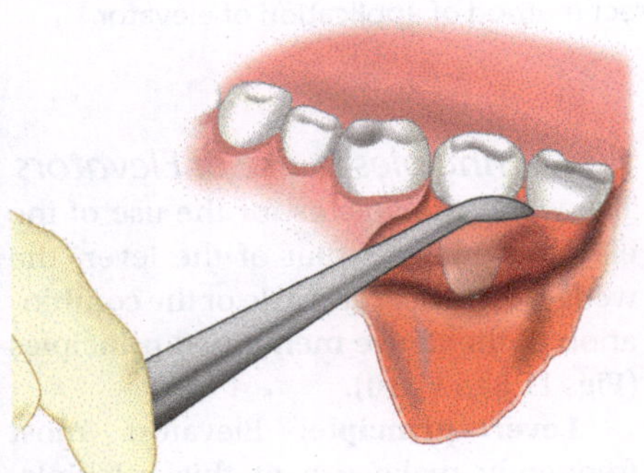

Fig. 11.10: Axo lever elevator

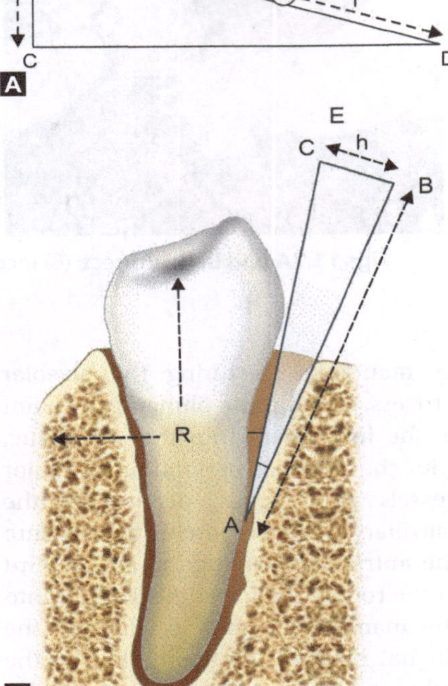

Figs 11.11A and B: Wedge principle—apexo elevator in use (*Abbreviations:* R: Resistance; E: Effort; L: Length; H: Height).

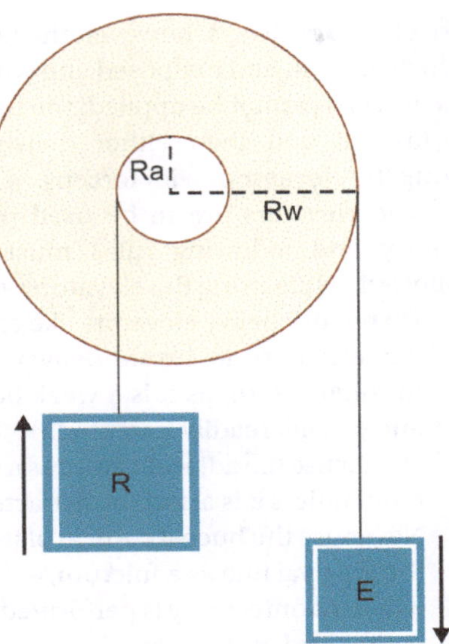

Fig. 11.12: Principle of wheel and axle (*Abbreviations:* R: Resistance; E: Effort; Rw: Radius of wheel; Ra: Radius of axle)

Wedge principle: Some elevators are designed to work on this principle called wedge elevators. The wedge elevator is pushed between the root and the investing bony tissue parallel to long axis of the root, by hand pressure or by mallet force.

While the wedge principle can be and is used as the sole principle in removing teeth, it is used in conjunction with the lever principle. The wedge in its simplest form, as in a chisel, is a movable inclined plane, which overcomes a larger resistance at right angles to the applied effort. The effort is applied at the base of the plane and the resistance has its effect on the slant side. Some wedges are movable double inclined planes. Sharper the angle of the wedge less the effort that is required to overcome a given resistance (Figs 11.11A and B).

Formula for wedge: E × I = R × h, or R/E = I/H

Wheel and axle principle: The wheel and axle is a simplest machine, being really a modified form of a lever. The effort is applied to the circumference of a wheel, which turns the axle so as to raise a weight.

While the wheel and axle principle can be and is used as the sole work principle in removing teeth, it is also used in conjunction with the wedge principle and in some cases with the lever principle (Fig. 11.12).

Effort × Radius of wheel = Resistance × Radius of Axle

Formula for the wheel and axle principle: R/E= Rw/Ra

Specific use of Certain Elevators

Straight apexo elevator no. 81 (Fig. 11.13A) is primarily used on the maxilla, where the upper central, lateral, cuspid or bicuspid has fractured at gingival line.

The straight apexo elevator is used as a wedge. Place this wedge on the mesiolabial in the space occupied by the periodontal membrane. Apply apical pressure and a slight labiolingual movement, then enter the elevator on the distal and repeat; then enter the elevator at the mesial and repeat. Surgical mallet can be used to drive elevator along the route.

Apexo elevator, with concavity always turned towards root, is wedged into space occupied by periodontal membrane. After forcing the tip alongside the root for approximately 5 mm, rotate the handle.

Caution:

- Protect the surrounding tissue.
- On the maxilla grasp the dental arch with the index finger and thumb, so that alveolus containing the root is between them. On the mandible the first and second finger should straddle the alveolus and the thumb is placed beneath the mandible, supporting it, thus offsetting the downward pressure of the elevator, which might otherwise dislocate the mandible. It is far better for the dental surgeon to injure his own finger than to run risk of seriously injuring the patient, with a possible lawsuit ensuing.

Nos. 4 and 5 apexo elevators on the mandible R and L:

In these apexo elevators, (Fig. 11.13B) the blade is at a 45° angle to the handle and the shank is at a angle to the handle 90°. The principle of their use is the same as that for the straight apexo elevator, that

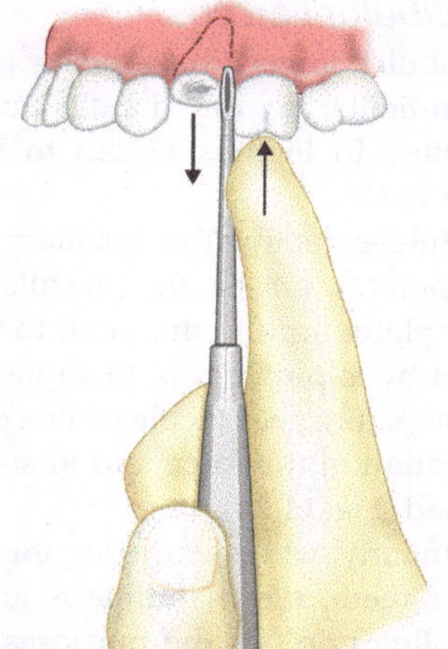
Fig. 11.13A: Straight apexo elevator no. 81

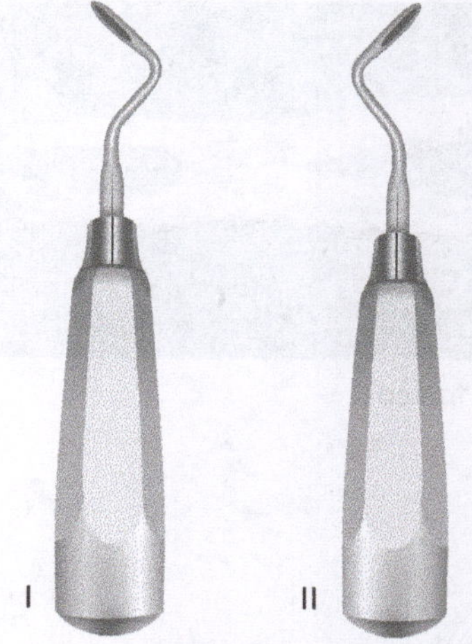

Fig. 11.13B: Apexo elevator no. 4 (I) and no. 5 (II)

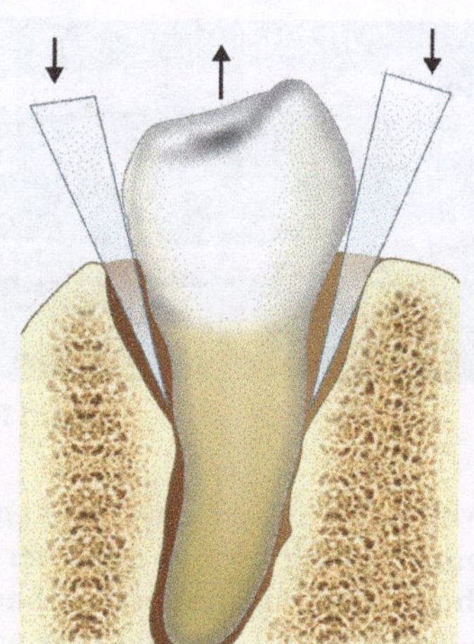
Fig. 11.13C: Double apexo elevator technique

is, they are used as wedge. These elevators may be used in on all lower teeth, where fracture of the root has occurred at the gingival line.

Insert, with a rotary motion and simultaneous apical pressure, the point of the no.4 apexo elevator along the mesial surface of the root, until a depth of 2 to 3 mm.

Next take the no. 5 apexo elevator and repeat the procedure. Next insert the point of the no. 4 apexo elevator on the mesial surface of the root using more and more rotary and apical pressure, until a depth of 6 mm.

Double apexo elevator technique: Place the no. 4 apexo elevator in the left hand and the no. 5 in the right hand. Then place the points of both elevators in against the root on opposite surfaces and using both elevators with lever pressure occlusally, elevate the root to the surface (Fig. 11.13C).

Apical fragment ejectors: Apical fragment ejectors are shaped just like the straight and right and left apexo elevators, the only difference being that the apical fragment ejectors are smaller. Apical fragment ejectors are used to remove roots, or parts of roots, fractured at the apical third of the root (Fig. 11.14).

Use of crossbar elevator on the mandible: Cross bar elevator are used on the mandible for the following purposes (Figs 11.15A to C).

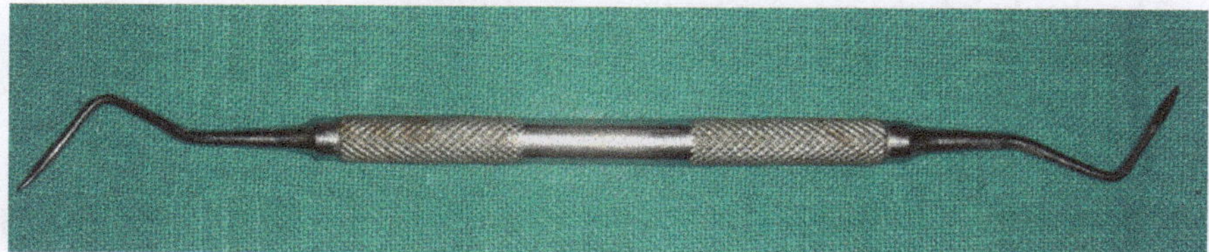
Fig. 11.14: Apical fragment ejector

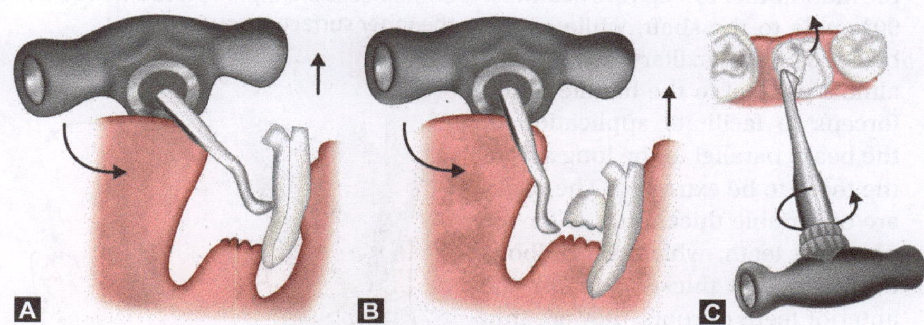

Figs 11.15A to C: Crossbar elevator

- To remove molar roots fractured at or below the gingival line.
- To fracture off crown or split roots after a groove has been cut in with a crosscut fissure bur.
- In cases of impacted teeth.

Forceps

The forceps are based on the principles of simple machine. They are designed in such a way that the access to the tooth in question is unimpeded and the adjoining structures are not damaged, while extracting the tooth with a forceps. The forceps have basically three components (Fig. 11.16):

- **The handle:** It is longer as compare to the beaks, which gives maximum mechanical advantage. The handle or the shaft is designed in such a way that it provides an unimpeded access to the tooth so as to prevent damage to the adjoining or opposing teeth and also prevents injury to the lips and at the same time facilitates the application of the beaks parallel to the long axis of the tooth. The shaft of the forceps have serrations,

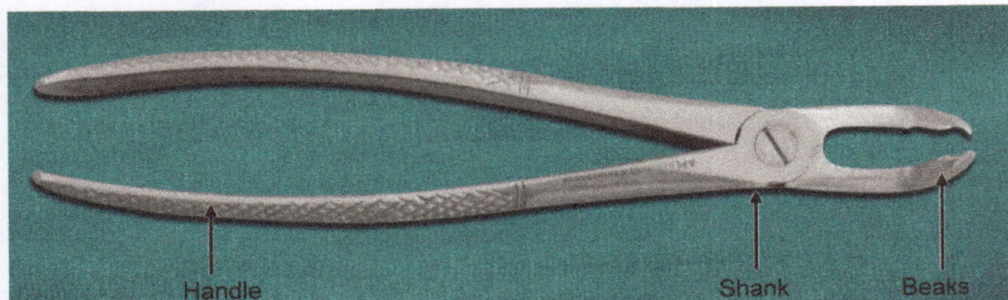

Fig. 11.16: Parts of forcep

which are away from the shank to provide long arm of the lever and thus, offer maximum mechanical advantage and it is the part where the operator holds the forceps with a palm grip. The serrations facilitate firm grip.

- **The shank:** It is the area, where the beaks unite with the handle. It also corresponds to the fulcrum of the lever.
- **The beaks:** These are much shorter as compared to the shaft and provide short arm of the lever for optimum mechanical advantage. The beaks of the mandibular forceps are at almost 90° angle to the shaft, while as the beaks of the maxillary forceps are almost parallel to the handle of the forceps to facilitate application of the beaks parallel to the long axis of the tooth to be extracted. The beaks are of variable thickness, i.e. for the posterior teeth, which are bulbous the beaks are thicker and for the anterior teeth or roots, they are thin and slender. The outer surface of the beaks is smooth and tapering to facilitate wedging of the beaks between the alveolar bone and the root surface in the periodontal ligament space to get an apical seat (beaks are applied apical to the CE junction). The inner surface of the beaks has serration to facilitate firm grip on the tooth. (Figs 11.17A and B). The ideal contact between the tooth to be extracted and the beaks of the forceps is described as 'two point contact' (Figs 11.18A and B).

The design of the forceps is variable for different teeth to achieve the objectives of:

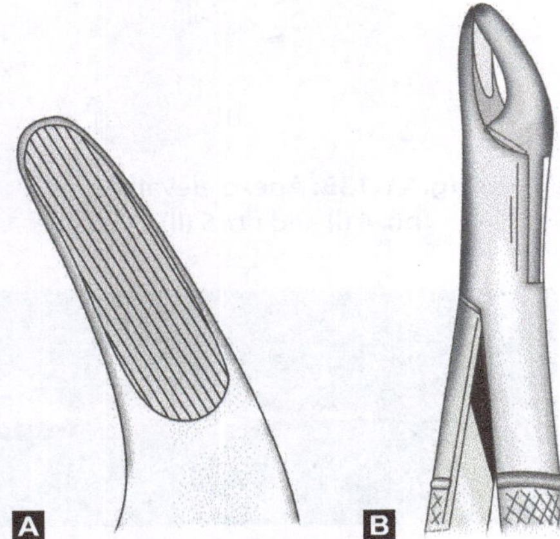

Figs 11.17A and B: Note the outer surface of the beaks are tapered and smooth, while the inner surface is serrated

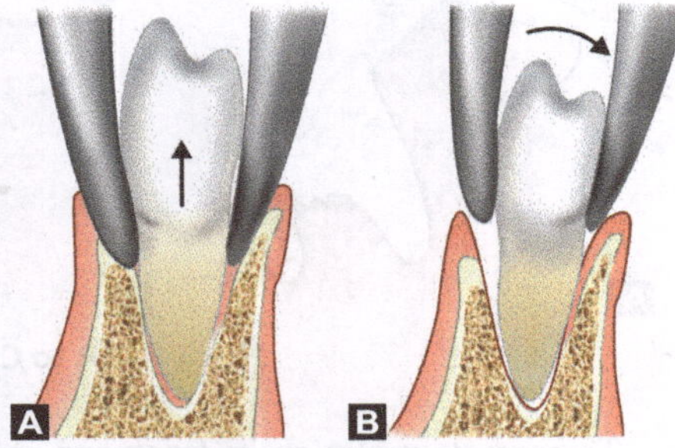

Figs 11.18A and B: (A) Wedge principle; (B) Bone expansion

- Unimpeded access.
- Application of the beaks apically and parallel to the long axis of the tooth, without injuring adjacent structures.
- To get maximum mechanical advantage.
- To get firm grip.

Maxillary Forceps

Maxillary forceps are illustrated in Figures 11.19 to 11.21.

Mandibular Forceps

Mandibular forceps have beaks almost perpendicular to the handle and are illustrated in Figures 11.22A to E and 11.23A to C.

While extracting the maxillary teeth, the operator grasps the maxillary alveolar plates around the tooth to be extracted by a 'pinch grip' to support the cortical plates, get a tactile feeling during application of the force and to stabilize the head (Fig. 11.24).

Similarly, while extracting the mandibular teeth, the mandible is grasped with 'sling grip' for the purposes mentioned above and also for giving support and counter traction to the mandible, while applying forces with the forceps to prevent its dislocation (Figs 11.25A to C).

Forceps Extraction

The forceps help in extraction of the tooth by way of severing the periodontal ligament fibers and expanding the cortical plates. The pressures that are applied with a forceps to achieve the same are (Fig. 11.26):

- **Apical pressure:** For wedging the forceps beaks in the PDL space and to gain an apical seat.
- **Buccal pressure:** It is the major movement as the buccal cortical plate is thin and can be expanded easily. The periodontal ligament fibers on the opposite side get severed.
- **Lingual pressure:** It is the minor movement as the lingual cortical plates are thick and do not expand adequately when subjected to pressure. The periodontal ligament fibers on the opposite side get severed. Moreover, there are chances of fracture of the root, especially in cases of maxillary molar extraction due to thick palatal bone. The fracture of the lingual cortical plate can lead to sublingual hematoma or damage to the lingual nerve in cases of mandibular molar extraction.
- **Rotation:** These forces are applied for breaking the PDL fibers. Rotational forces are not applied to the multirooted teeth and the maxillary lateral incisors as they have distal

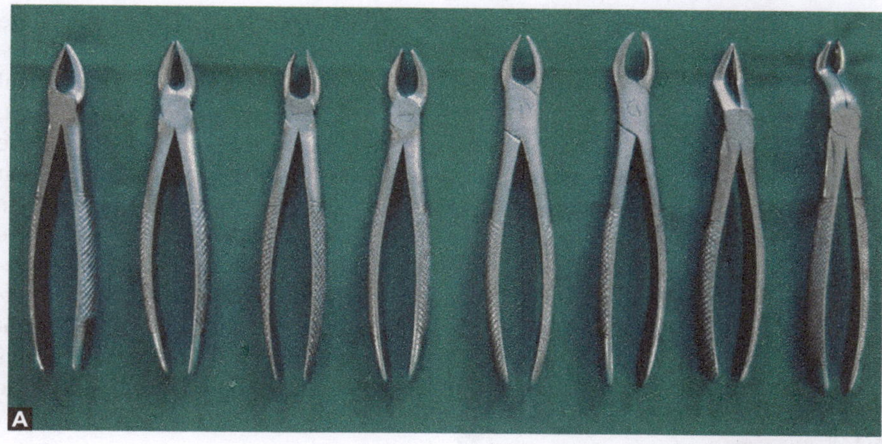

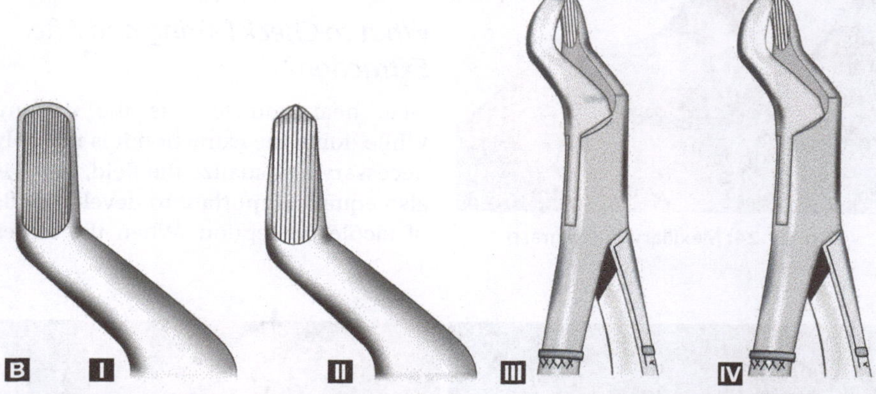

Figs 11.19A and B: Maxillary molar forceps: (I) The rounded tip of the palatal beak; (II) Buccal beak with a triangular projection, which engages the furcation area between two buccal roots; (III) The maxillary molar forceps left side; (IV) The maxillary molar forceps right side

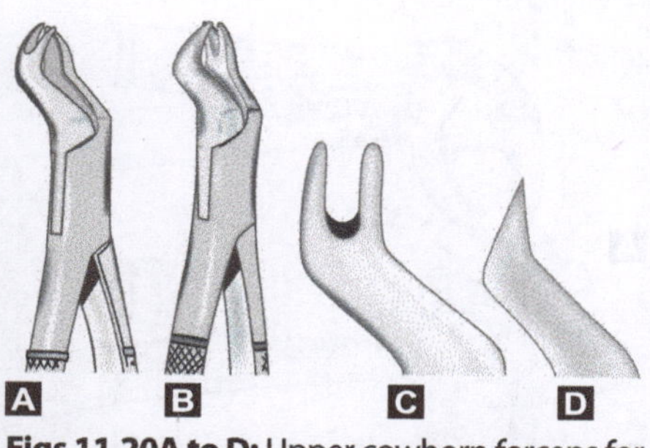

Figs 11.20A to D: Upper cowhorn forceps for molars: (A) Left side; (B) Right side; (C) Bifurcated palatal beak engages single palatal root; (D) Pointed (horn like) buccal beak engages the bifurcation between two buccal roots. The cowhorn forceps are used to extract the teeth with severe carious undermining of the crown

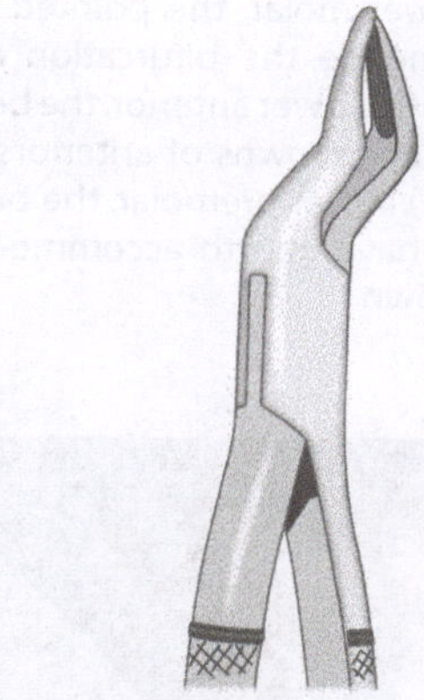

Fig. 11.21: Upper bionet forcep used for the extraction of the root fragments

curvature of the root and there are chances of fracture of the root. The rotational forces are best suited for the teeth having conical roots.

- **Traction:** It is applied to deliver the tooth from the expanded socket and with severed periodontal ligament fibers.

Special Consideration while doing an Orthodontic Extraction

The premolars are often extracted for orthodontic considerations to create space for correcting the crowding of the teeth. When such an extraction is planned, care must be taken to cause minimal trauma to the bone. The expansion of the socket should be minimal and the buccal cortical plate should not be fractured by application of the

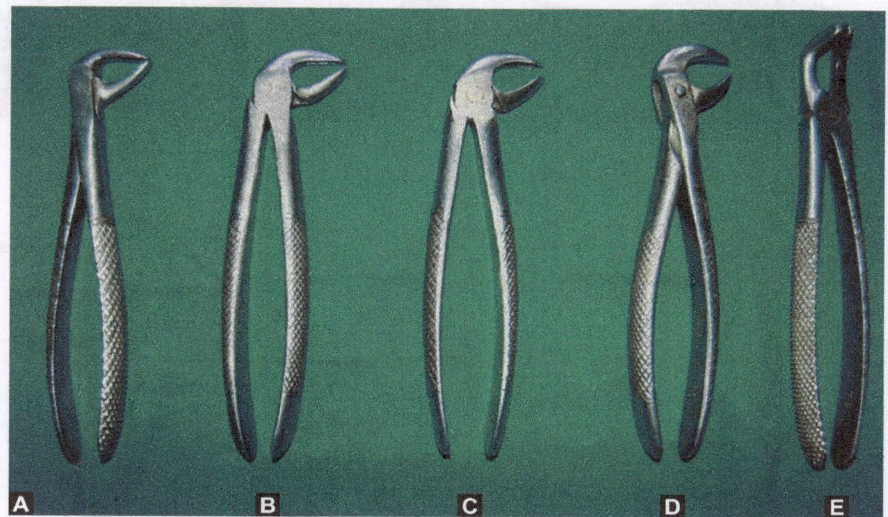

Figs 11.22A to E: Mandibular forceps: (A) Anterior; (B) Premolar; (C) Molar; (D) Cowhorn for molars; (E) Third molar forceps

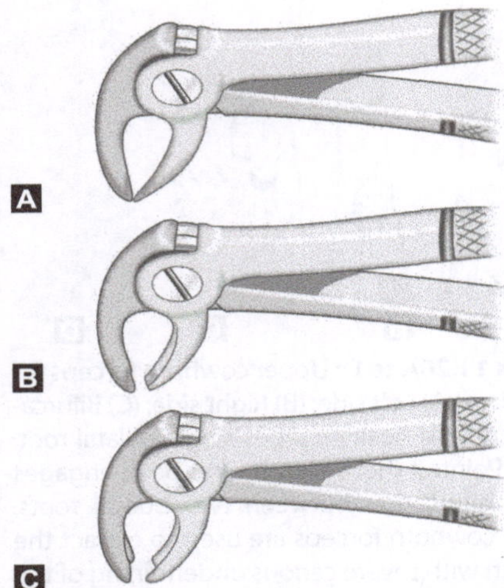

Figs 11.23A to C: Mandibular extraction forceps: (A) Lower molar, the pointed tips if the beaks engage the bifurcation area buccolingually; (B) Lower anterior, the beaks are meeting as the crowns of anteriors are less bulbous; (C) Lower premolar, the beaks are heavy and have gap to accommodate the bulbous crown

excessive force, nor the root should fracture as removal of the residual root fragment may require transalveolar technique resulting into damage to the buccal cortical plate. Fortunately, the patients requiring orthodontic extractions are young and the bones have excellent elasticity and if proper preoperative evaluation is done and adequate care is taken, the tooth is often extracted uneventfully. It is desirable to evaluate the roots of the premolar prior to extraction by obtaining intraoral periapical X-rays to prevent the fracture of the root. The use of elevator is avoided during the extraction for orthodontic reason, as it may create undue stresses in the bone and the indentations produced in the bone used as fulcrum will resist movement of tooth during orthodontic treatment. Secondly, the socket should not be compressed after the extraction as the space is needed for movement of the tooth in the socket.

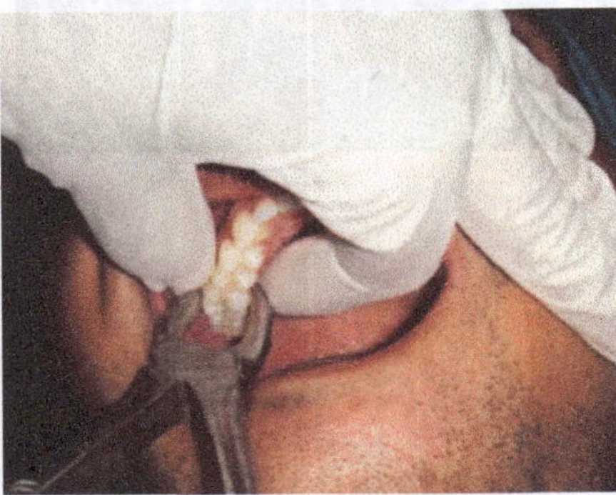

Fig. 11.24: Maxillary pinch grasp

What to Check During and After Extraction?

'See, hear and feel' is the dictum. While doing the extraction it is not only necessary to visualize the field, but it is also equally important to develop skills of tactile perception. When the forces

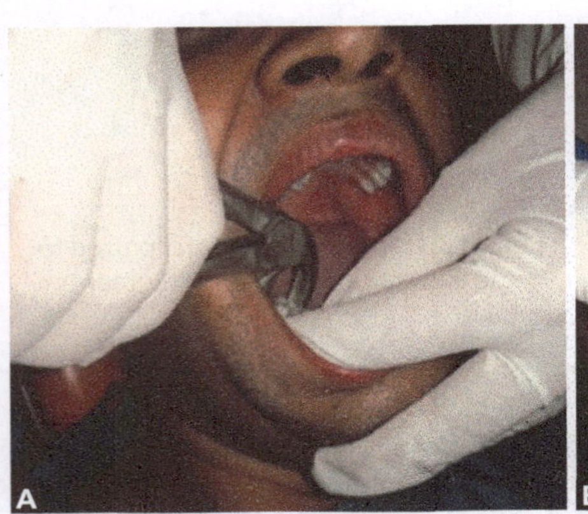

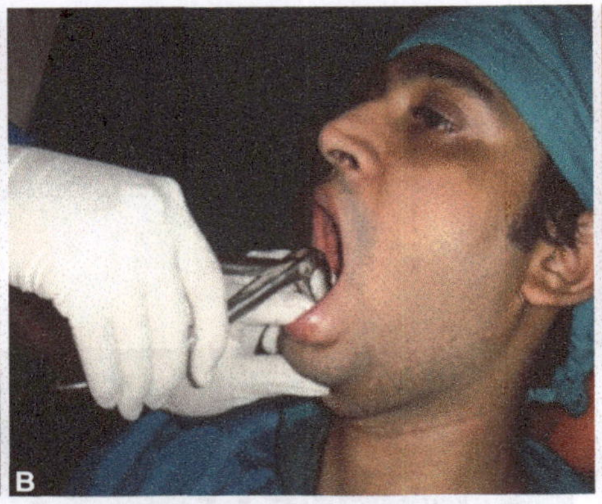

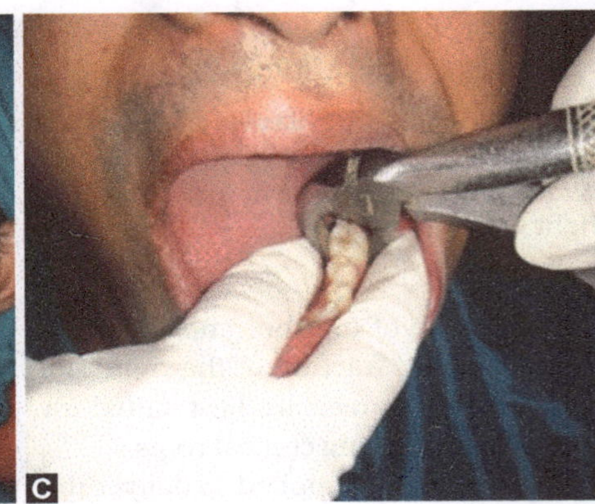

Figs 11.25A to C: Mandibular sling grasp

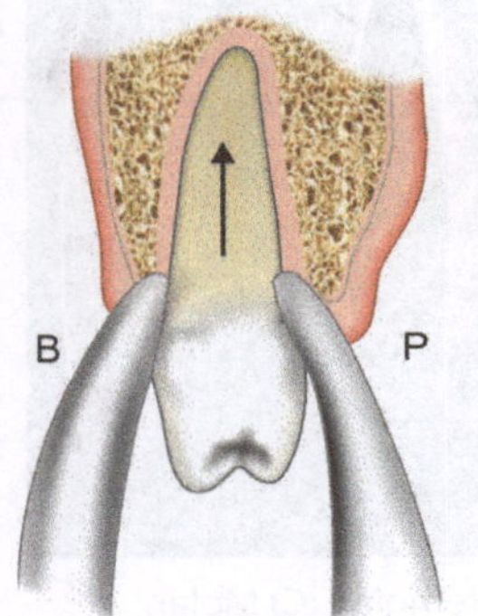

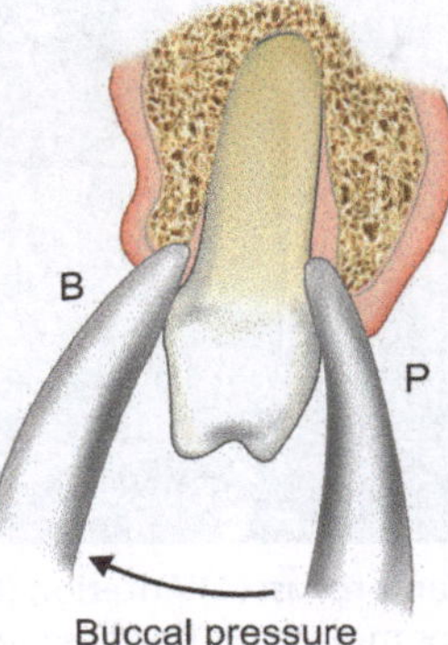

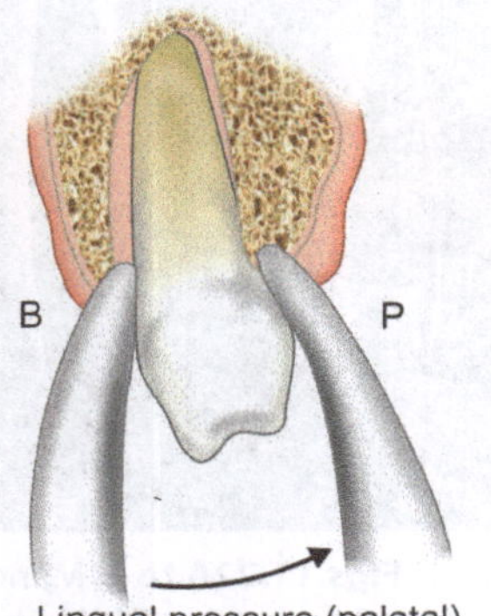

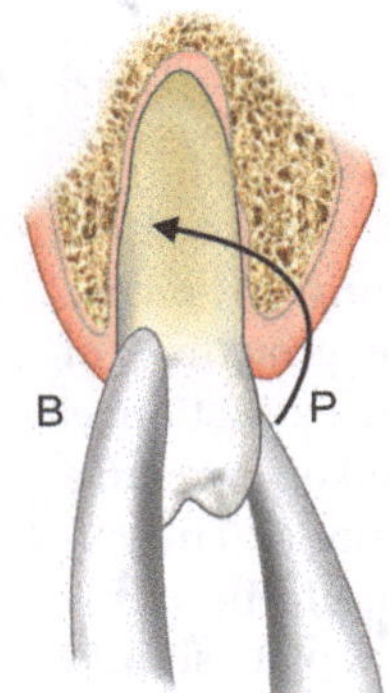

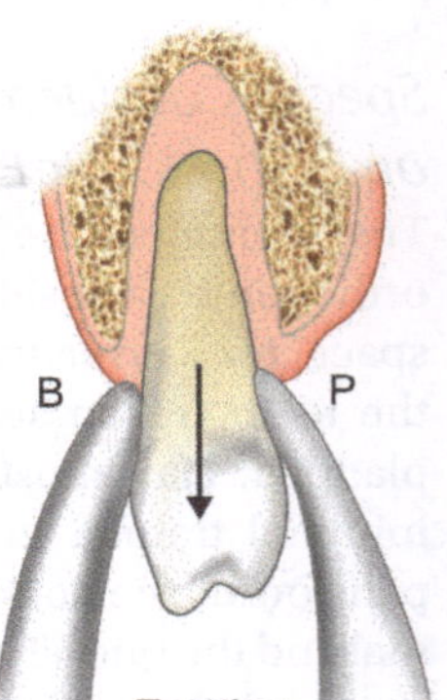

Fig. 11.26: Forcep extraction

are applied with the help of either the elevators or the forceps the movement of the tooth can be seen, but it is equally important to feel the movement through the tactile feeling that is perceived by the hand holding the forceps. This skill needs to be developed purely by practice and cannot be explained in the words. A skilled person will always know, which direction the forces are more effective and can be suitable to extract the tooth. The ears are also required to be kept vigilant to hear the sound, while luxating or extracting the tooth as any clicking sound could be as a result of fracture of the alveolar bone or the root of the tooth.

Once the tooth is delivered, the first thing that is to be done is to inspect the tooth and its root for their completeness. The roots normally taper and are conical any incompleteness would suggest either fracture or resorption of the root. Fracture will always show a sharp line, while as the resorption will show irregular margins. If the evidence of fracture is present determine, which root is fractured and what would be its approximate length. Never discard such tooth until the remaining fragment is also removed.

The next step is to wipe the socket dry and make the field dry by sucking out the saliva or blood in the vicinity to visualize the socket. Inspect the socket thoroughly for any excessive bleeding, foreign bodies like fragments of the tooth, calculus tags, granulation tissue or any sharp or loose bony fragments. If they are present remove them by grasping with a mosquito artery forceps. Any loose bony fragment which is devoid of periosteal attachment is unlikely to survive and must be removed. Excessive bleeding could be due to injury to blood vessels (*inferior alveolar or nutrient vessels*) or presence of the friable granulation tissue in the socket. In the latter case, the blood will well out from in the socket steadily and in the former case, it will flow more forcefully. Pack the socket with gauze and try to curette the socket and remove all the residual granulation tissue. The bleeding will not stop, until all the granulation tissue is curetted out. If the injury to the blood vessel is suspected, pack the socket or use bone wax or gel foam to control the bleeding. The other cause of excessive bleeding is gingival laceration and if it is present, pressure pack or sutures are beneficial to control it.

Palpate the edges of the socket for any sharpness in the bony margins. If the sharp bony margins are present nibble or file them off to make them smooth. Such sharp margins irritate the gingival flap, cause pain and delay healing. The patients always feel them with tongue and complain of incomplete extraction of the tooth.

As the cortical plates are expanded during the extraction, they are gently compressed with digital pressure to reduce the expanded cortical plates to their original position. This procedure is called a 'simple alveoloplasty'. This is done to facilitate fabrication of subsequent prosthesis. Some clinicians do not recommend simple alveoloplasty if an implant is planned.

The next step is application of pressure using pressure pack to achieve hemostasis. The material used for pressure pack is either rolled and moistened sterile gauze or a pressure pad prepared by rolling gauze over the absorbent cotton wool. The cotton wool absorbs the blood and saliva and gauze prevents the sticking of the cotton fibers to the raw surgical area. Never use cotton wool to apply pressure directly over the raw area, as the fibers may stick to the wound surface and may subsequently interfere with the healing. The pressure pack is placed on the top of the socket and the patient is asked to bite on it for minimum 30 minutes to 1 hour to achieve hemostasis. The normal clotting time is 8 to 12 minute, but still the pack is maintained for longer time, because one must remember the following the extraction, the bleeding occurs from the gingival margins, severed periodontal fibers and the apical vessels of the tooth. The gingiva get compressed between the pack and the alveolar bone and the bleeding from the same stops rapidly due to direct pressure what keeps on bleeding is the inside of the socket. As the pack is kept on the top of the socket and not inside the socket, to develop pressure on the inner walls and base of the socket is its filling with clotted blood, which gets compressed and exerts pressure on the bleeders inside the socket thus, it requires more time. Secondly the initial clot is soft, flabby and is unstable and liable to be dislodged readily with routine activities. The clot retraction takes place in 30 to 45 minutes and the serum is expressed out from the clot making it drier and more stable. The pressure pack should thus, be kept for about 60 minutes. The sutures are not always indicated as the healing is by secondary intention, however, the suture help to stop bleeding, prevents food impaction. Generally dehiscence takes place even after placing the sutures as the flaps do not get properly approximated, unless the cortical plates are trimmed significantly and the suture line lies on the defect. The sutures should be loose approximating sutures.

The patient is given following postoperative instructions:

- To maintain pressure pack for 60 minutes—for hemostasis.
- Not to spit and swallow the saliva, as during the act of spitting the jaw moves and the pressure pack may get disturbed.
- Not to do forceful gargles or smoke—as the negative pressure generated, while smoking may dislodge the clot and lead to bleeding.
- Soft diet—as the pain may get aggravated, while making more masticatory effort and the wound/clot does not get disturbed.
- No hot fomentations but to give cold compressions—in the immediate postoperative phase, the vascular phase of inflammation is predominant and is manifested by vasodilatation, hot fomentations may aggravate it and lead to excessive edema and discomfort. Hence, application of cold compressions helps in reducing the edema by inducing vasoconstriction. Once the edema sets in the mounting pressure within

the interstitial compartment blocks the lymphatics and venules, which are the draining channels and help in reabsorbtion of the interstitial fluid to reduce the edema. It leads to stasis of circulation.
- Warm saline gargles after 48 hours: These induce vasodilatation and facilitates the reabsorption of interstitial fluid and edema thus, improving local circulation, which also helps in faster healing and drug delivery.

Policy for Leaving Root Fragments

The roots that are fractured at the time of extraction should ideally be removed as the root fragment may serve as a septic focus or may give rise to pathologies such as cyst. It is therefore imperative to assess the root fragment for its length, presence of any pathology, its proximity with vital structures and the depth of the fragment in the bone. One has to evaluate the advantages of removing the root fragment against the complications that can be encountered, while attempting its removal. It is not advisable to remove a small root fragment of about 2 to 3 mm by removing large quantity of bone, while attempting a transalveolar removal or damaging vital structures such as the neurovascular bundle or maxillary sinus. Large root fragments, i.e. the roots which are fractured at or below the CE junction must be removed. They can be removed either using the intra-alveolar technique by using apexo or cryers elevators or by using the apical ejectors. The prerequisite is thorough evaluation including the radiographs and proper visibility. The procedure must not be attempted blindly as the chances of displacement of the root fragment in the maxillary sinus, sublingual space or trauma to the adjacent vital structures are more. In case of any doubts or difficulty in gaining proper access or visibility, it is better to resort to transalveolar technique. Judicious removal of buccal cortical bone, splitting of the roots in case of multirooted teeth and elevating the root with the help of an elevator creating a purchase point on the root is less traumatic than blindly doing the instrumentation and traumatizing the adjacent tissue.

Smaller root fragments may be retained with due information to the patient. The patient should be advised to report in case the root piece becomes symptomatic. The criteria for retaining the root fragment may be summarized as follows:
- Small (≤ 5 mm in length).
- Root fragment must not be superficial.
- Tooth involved must not be infected or have apical lesion on radiograph.
- If near vital structure, which may be injured.
- If has potential to be displaced into sinus, inferior alveolar canal, or submandibular space or would require excessive destruction of bone.

Transalveolar Extraction

The teeth when extracted by creating surgical access to it through the alveolar bone, fall in the category of transalveolar extraction technique. As it requires reflection of the flap and removal of the cortical bone, it is also called 'extraction by open method'. The teeth which cannot be removed by conventional intra-alveolar method and require more complex procedure for their removal are termed a complicated exodontia.

The indications for the transalveolar extraction are:
- Root pieces.
- Severely undermined crowns.
- Fractured teeth.
- Brittle teeth (endodontically treated teeth, geriatric patients).
- Unfavorable root form.
- Dense bone.
- Malposed teeth—crowding, incomplete eruption.
- Proximity with vital structures.
- Lone standing tooth with grossly carious crown (Fig. 11.27).

The factors that complicate the extraction of the tooth are:

Crown

Destruction of the crown (Fig. 11.28) (e.g. caries, complex restorations, fixed prosthesis) prevents the application of instruments and therefore, the application of forces. Such teeth fracture readily on application of forceps or the elevators.

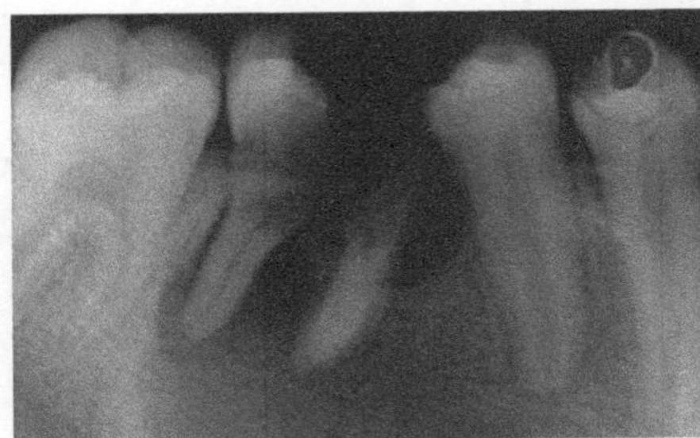

Fig. 11.27: Lone standing tooth with grossly carious crown

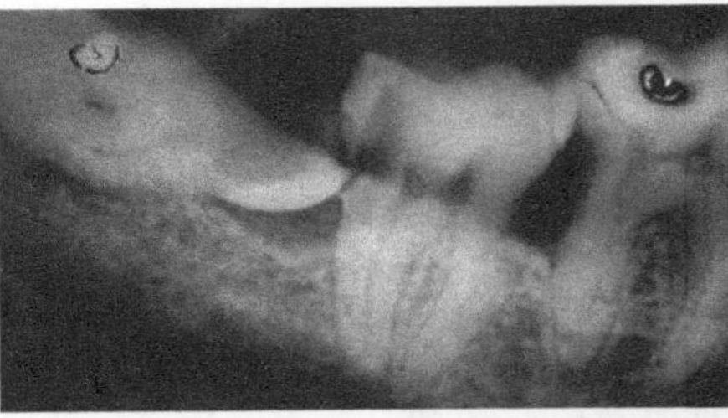

Fig. 11.28: Destruction of crown

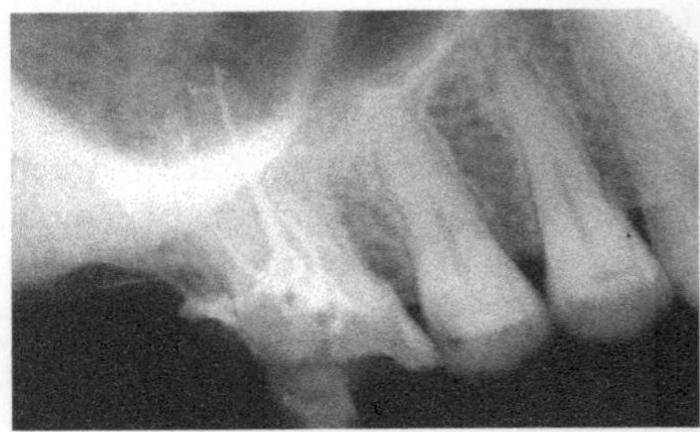

Fig. 11.29: Endodontically treated tooth

Roots

All those factors that result in unfavorable path of removal or increased resistance.
- Multiple roots
- Bulbous roots
- Endodontically treated teeth (Fig. 11.29)
- Hypercementosis (Fig. 11.30)
- Ankylosed teeth (Fig. 11.31)
- Divergent/dilacerated roots (Figs 11.32 and 11.33)

Bone: Increased density of the bone due to chronic periosteal reaction (osteocondensation) and loss of resilience of the

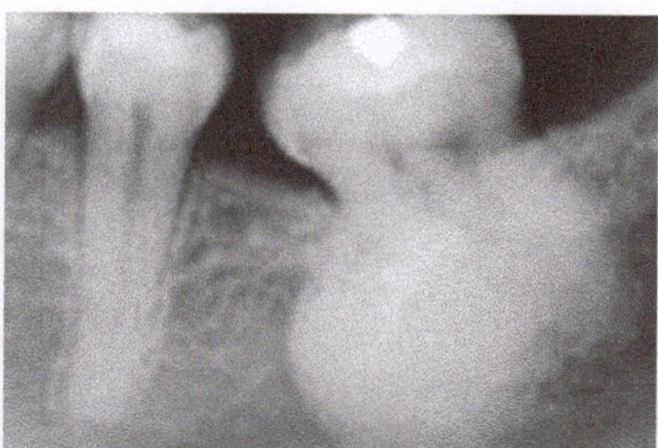

Fig. 11.30: Hypercementosis

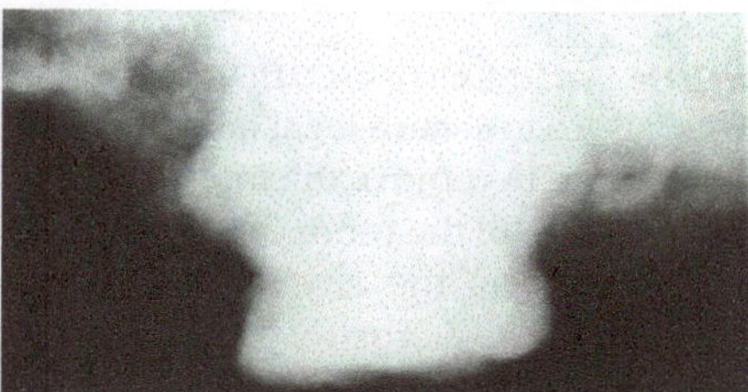

Fig. 11.31: Ankylosis

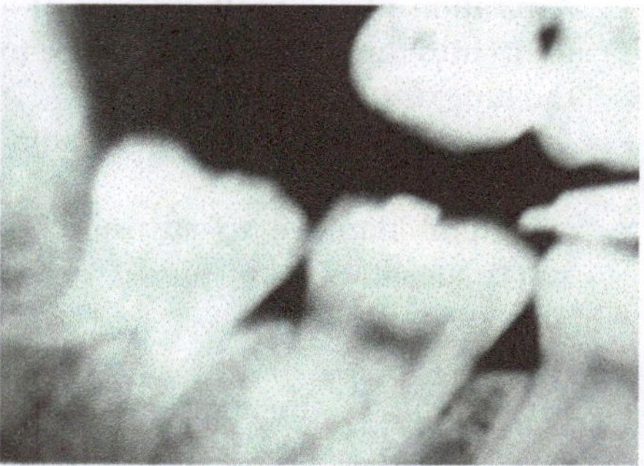

Fig. 11.32: Divergent roots

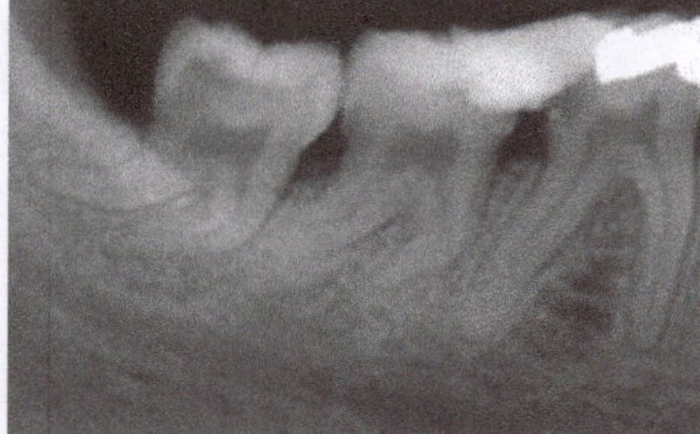

Fig. 11.33: Dilaceration roots

bone in the old age makes the bone less amenable to pressure and the expansion of the socket is in adequate during the extraction, which can lead to fracture of the cortical plates or the roots. During the extraction in some osteodystrophies like Paget's disease and fibrous dysplasia, the bone bulk increases making the extraction more difficult.

Diminished access: The major cause of diminished access is due to trismus and the common causes for the trismus are:

- Oral submucous fibrosis
- Ankylosis
- Muscle spasm
- Scleroderma
- Microstomia
- Interferes with application of instruments due to crowding, supernumerary, malposed teeth, hypertrophied buccal fat pad and macroglossia.

Adjacent/nonadjacent teeth

- Highly carious adjacent teeth.
- Root canal on adjacent teeth.
- Heavily restored adjacent teeth.
- Periodontally involved adjacent teeth.
- Lone maxillary molar or canine.

Malposed teeth: The teeth which are positioned out of arch or are crowded the correct application of forceps may not be possible. Even the creation of the 'purchase point' for correct application of elevators may not be available. The transalveolar extraction may be the only choice in such situations.

Adjacent vital structures: The close proximity with vital anatomical structures may lead to damage to these structures during the extraction, if due care is not exercised. The structures which are likely to be damaged are (Fig. 11.34):

- Inferior alveolar bundle
- Lingual nerve
- Maxillary sinus.

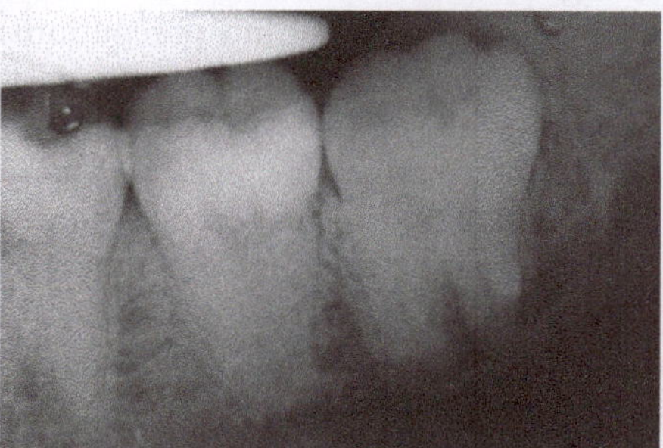

Fig. 11.34: Adjacent to vital structures, i.e. inferior alveolar canal

Prosthetic concerns:

- Preservation of alveolus
- Alveolar contour
- Preservation of attached gingiva.

Technique

After a thorough preoperative evaluation the decision of transalveolar extraction is taken. The patient should be explained the treatment plan and the procedure is performed under local anesthesia.

To create proper access to the tooth or the root fragment, an appropriate mucoperiosteal flap is raised (*details of the basic principles of flap designing are given in Chapter 1*) (Fig. 11.35). The bone is removed from the buccal cortical plate to expose the roots up to cementoenamel junction in an intact tooth or in case of the root fragment, the bone is removed to visualize the root, using burs or chisel (Fig. 11.36). The bone should be removed judiciously.

Once the root fragment is exposed, a hole is drilled in the root fragment, which is used to engage the tip of the elevator. This point is called a 'purchase point'. While creating the purchase

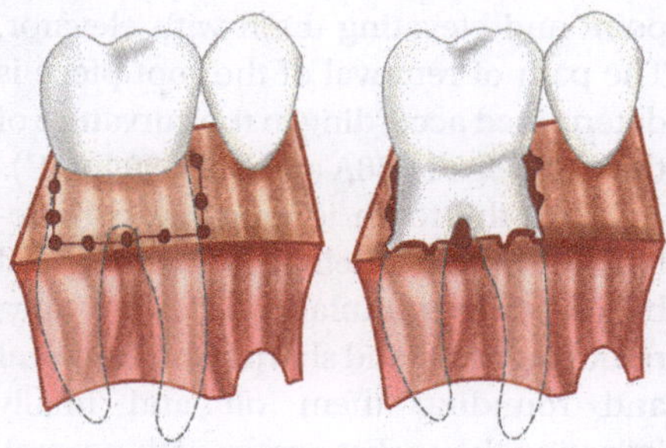

Fig. 11.35: Reflection of the mucoperiosteal flap and removal of the bone to expose the furcation area

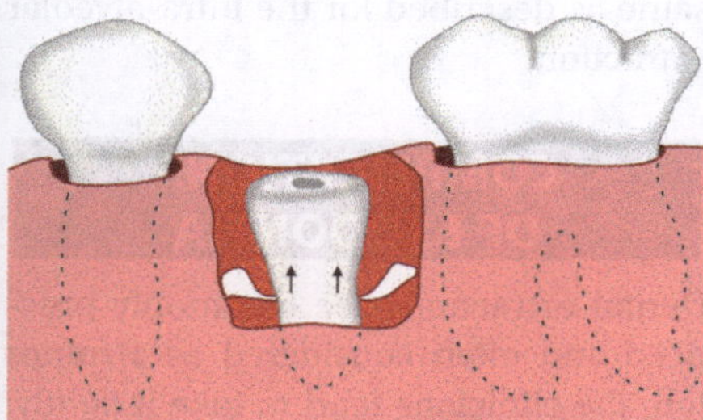

Fig. 11.36: Removal of the bone to expose the root fragment and its removal by elevation

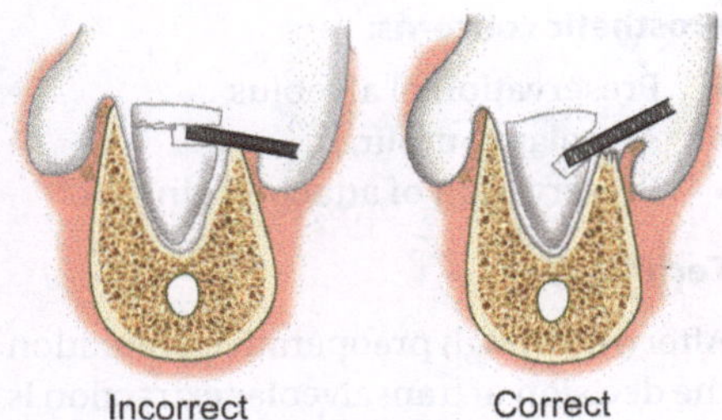

Fig. 11.37: The incorrect and correct way of creating the purchase point

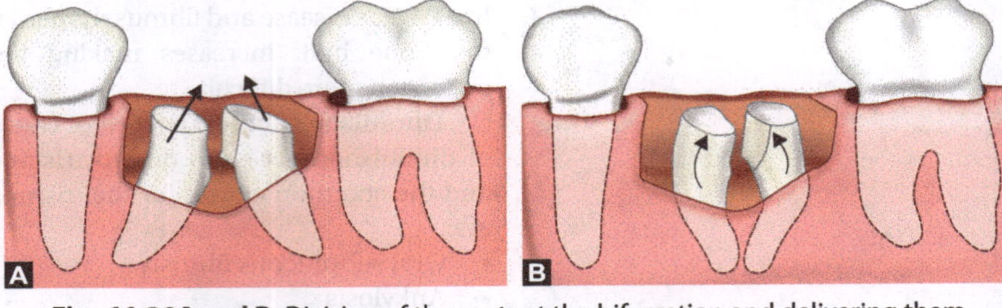

Figs 11.38A and B: Division of the roots at the bifurcation and delivering them separately as per their curvature

point, care should be taken that it is created in healthy root area, so that it has adequate strength to withstand the force applied through the elevator and does not fracture easily. The purchase point should be deep enough to engage the tip of the elevator securely (Fig. 11.37).

In case of an intact tooth, the tooth is sectioned and removed. If the crown is fragile, it can fracture in an unplanned manner, making the removal of remaining roots difficult. Hence, it is desirable to section it (odontectomy) in a planned manner, so that the remaining fragment can be removed easily. The roots are sectioned and removed separately in a multirooted tooth by creating purchase point and elevating them with elevator. The path of removal of the root piece is determined according to the curvature of the root (Figs 11.38A and B, 11.39A to C).

After the tooth is removed completely, the wound is debrided and prepared by curetting granulation tissue if any, removing loose and sharp bone fragment and rounding them off and finally irrigating the socket gently, with normal, sterile saline. The primary closure of the flap is done with sutures.

Postoperative care remains the same as described for the intra-alveolar extraction.

COMPLICATIONS OF EXODONTIA

Dental extractions are commonly practiced and often considered as a minor job, the clinicians tend to take it lightly. No surgical procedure is guaranteed to be free of complications and tooth extraction is no exception.

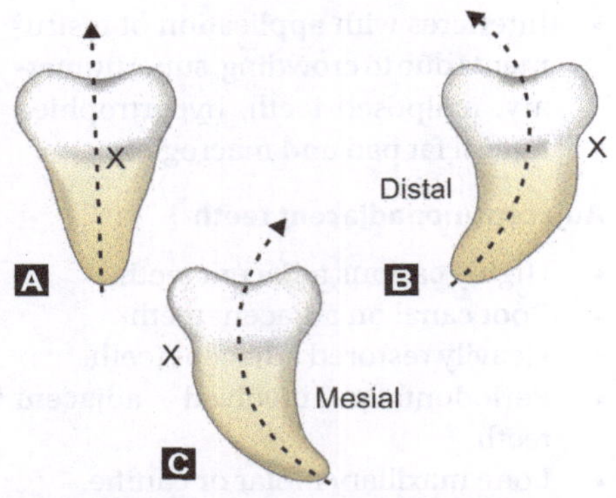

Figs 11.39A to C: Showing the direction of tooth elevation according to curvature of the root. The elevator is applied on the convex side and the tooth is delivered towards the concave side

Exodontia is essentially a surgical procedure and warrants all the judicious precautions and the aseptic care to prevent complications. Whenever the basic principles of the surgery are violated, the relative chances of developing complications are increased significantly. Similarly when the patients are medically compromised and due precautions are not taken; the likely hood of precipitating complications is high. The complications can occur in spite of good care and precautions, but their incidence is minimized. It therefore, necessitates the clinician to take a comprehensive approach and have sound knowledge of complications, their prevention and management. The postdental extraction complications can be classified as:

- Local complications
  - Immediate
  - Delayed.
- Systemic complications.

Local Complications

Immediate Complications

- Failure to secure local anesthesia.
- Failure to remove the tooth.
- Fracture of the tooth.
- Fracture of the alveolus (including maxillary tuberosity).
- Oroantral communication.
- Displacement of the tooth or a root into the adjacent tissues.
- Aspiration of the tooth or part of a tooth into the pharynx and hence to the lung or stomach.
- Fracture or subluxation of an adjacent tooth.
- Collateral damage to surrounding soft tissues.
- Thermal injury.
- Bleeding.
- Dislocation of the temporomandibular joint.
- Fracture of mandible.
- Damage to branches of the trigeminal nerve.

Delayed Complications

- Excessive pain, swelling and trismus.
- Hemorrhage.
- Localized alvelolar osteitis (dry socket).
- Acute osteomyelitis.
- Infection of soft tissues.
- Oroantral fistula.
- Failures of the socket to heal.
- Nerve damage.

Late Complications

- Chronic osteomyelitis.
- Osteoradionecrosis.
- Nerve damage.
- Chronic pain.

Failure to Secure Anesthesia

It is usually due to faulty technique, insufficient dosage of the anesthetic agent, infection at the site of injection or poor quality of local anesthetic solution. A thorough evaluation of the anesthesia by subjective and objective methods is done to assess the effect of local anesthetic. If the anesthesia is not secured properly, additional dose of local anesthetic should be injected.

Failure to Remove the Tooth with Either Forceps or Elevators

If the tooth does not yield to reasonable displacing forces applied with forceps or elevators, this normally indicates that either the bone texture is dense and inelastic, or that the root shape is obstructing its path of withdrawal. Ankylosed teeth, abnormal root anatomy these also yield difficulty, while removing the tooth. In such a situation, the cause of the obstruction should be sought, by taking a radiograph. A mucoperiosteal flap should raise and remove bone and/or divide the tooth and remove the tooth.

Fracture of the Tooth

The causes of crown or root fracture are:

- Improper and excessive force applied to the tooth.
- A tooth weakened by caries or large restorations or endodontically treated teeth.
- Inappropriate application of force resulting from failure to grasp enough of the root mass or using forceps with blades too wide to make two point contacts on the root.
- Unfavorable root anatomy of dense and non-elastic bone.
- Inspection of the fractured tooth shows the likely size and position of the retained root.
- If there is no preoperative radiograph, it should be taken at this stage.
- When only the crown has been removed, it may be possible to reapply root forceps to remove the roots.
- When the root itself has fractured, retrieval of the retained portion normally requires a surgical (transalveolar) approach.

Fracture of the Alveolar Bone

Fracture of the alveolar bone is one of the common complications of tooth extraction. It occurs due to accidental inclusion of alveolar bone within the forceps blades or to the configuration of roots. Examination of extracted teeth reveals alveolar fragments adhering to the teeth. The extraction of canines is frequently complicated by fracture of the labial plate, especially if the alveolar bone has been weakened by extraction of the lateral incisor and/or the first premolar prior to the removal of the canine, hence, the canine should be extracted prior to lateral incisor and canine. It is advisable to remove any loose alveolar fragments, which are devoid of the periosteal attachment as they tend to undergo avascular necrosis.

Fracture of the Maxillary Tuberosity[7]

Fracture of the maxillary tuberosity is a specific type of alveolar bone fracture (Fig. 11.40), which may be predisposed by:

- The presence of a large antrum that weakens the maxillary alveolus.
- A large or splayed root mass of the upper second or third molar.
- Fusion of an unerupted third molar to the root of the second molar.

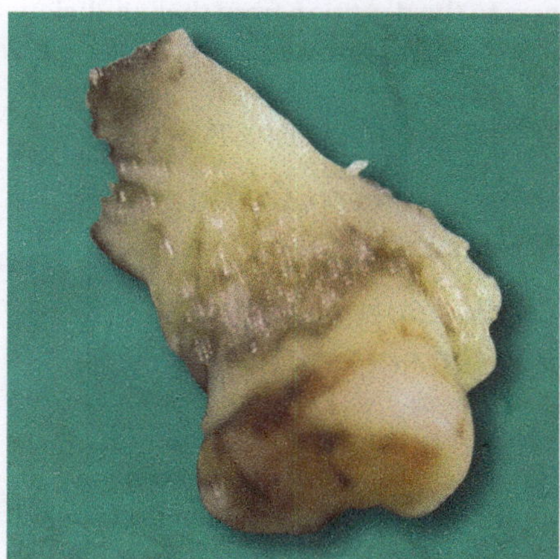

Fig. 11.40: Extracted tooth with fractured tuberosity

When the fracture occurs, the forceps are discarded and a large buccal mucoperiosteal flap is raised. The fractured tuberosity and the tooth is then freed from the palatal soft tissues by blunt subperiosteal dissection and lifted from the wound. If the removal of fractured fragment is tried without detaching its soft tissue attachment, the mucosa may get torn/lacerated and the lacerations might extend up to lateral pharyngeal wall. Once the fragment is removed, the oroantral communication must be ruled out. The soft tissues flaps are then apposed with mattress sutures, which evert the edges and are left *in situ* for at least 10 days. If a large oroantral communication is present, which is unlikely to be closed by suturing the flaps, proper plastic closure of the communication be done using appropriate technique and flap.

Oroantral Communication[8]

Oroantral communication is a pathological communication between oral cavity and the maxillary antrum. An oroantral fistula is an epithelized, pathological, unnatural communication between these two cavities. The root apices of the maxillary cheek teeth are closely related to the antral floor. With increasing age the nasal sinuses slowly enlarge, so that the tooth roots often appear in a two-dimensional radiographic view to be protruding into the antral cavity. In the elderly patient, the bony barrier between tooth and sinus is thin and brittle.

As the tooth is manipulated in the forceps, there is a risk that the bone of the antral floor, which may be adherent to the roots, will fracture and be removed with the tooth, so leaving a defect and creating a communication from the mouth to the antrum via the socket. The detailed description of this condition is given in the Chapter 14 (*Diseases of Maxillary Sinus*).

Dislocation of the Temporomandibular Joint

Dislocation of the temporomandibular joint during forceps extraction is normally the result of failure to support the mandible, while a difficult lower tooth is being loosened. Dislocation may also be caused by the injudicious use of gags. To avoid this complication, the operator's left hand should ideally stabilize the jaw during this maneuver. If dislocation occurs it should be reduced immediately. To reduce the dislocation, the operator stands in front of the patient and places his thumbs intraorally on the external oblique ridges lateral to any mandibular molars, which are present and his fingers extraorally under the lower border of the mandible (Fig. 11.41). This complication of mandibular extractions can usually be prevented if the lower jaw is supported during extraction. An extraoral support to the joint should be applied and worn, until tenderness in the affected joint subsides.

Fracture of the Mandible

Fracture of the mandible is a rare event during dental extraction. It usually signifies that either there is some predisposing weakness of the jaw, which then exhibits a pathological fracture when 'normal' forces are applied to a tooth, or that an excessive force, sufficient enough to break a 'normal' mandible has been used.

Examples of conditions predisposing to pathological fracture include:

- Large cysts
- Tumors (including bone metastases)
- Impacted/buried teeth
- Generalized osteoporosis
- Paget's disease
- Osteogenesis imperfect
- Hyperparathyroidism.

Fracture or Subluxation of an Adjacent Tooth

Fracture or subluxation of an adjacent tooth complication should be avoidable using appropriate techniques with forceps and elevators. The rule is that no force should be applied to teeth other than the one being removed. Careful preoperative examination will reveal, whether a tooth adjacent to that to be extracted is either carious, heavily restored, or in the line of withdrawal.

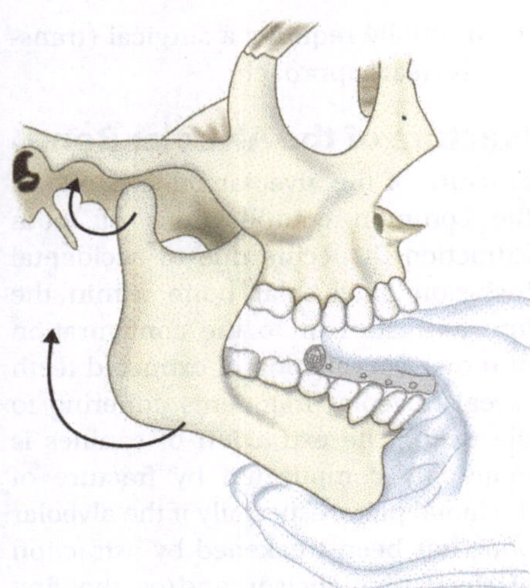

Fig. 11.41: Reduction of dislocated condyle

Certain situations make inadvertent damage to other teeth more likely:

- Overhanging restorations in adjacent teeth.
- Bulbous full crown restorations on adjacent teeth.
- If the tooth for extraction is a bridge abutment, the bridge must either be removed completely, or sectioned to isolate the tooth to be extracted.
- Lack of proper space between two teeth, i.e. crowding.

Caries and loose or overhanging fillings should be removed from an adjacent tooth and a temporary dressing inserted before the extraction. Extractions under general anesthesia pose possible dangers to the dentition from the injudicious use of the mouth gags or props, laryngoscopes, oral endotracheal tubes and airways used during recovery of the patient.

Injury to Surrounding Structures

Displacement of a Root into the Antrum[9]

Displacement of a root into the antrum can occur following fracture of a maxillary molar/premolar and ineffective attempts to retrieve the retained palatal root. Incidence of this complication can be reduced, if the following basic rules are observed.

- Do not apply forceps to a root below the antrum, unless there is sufficient exposure of the root to allow the blades to grasp the root securely under direct vision.
- Be content to leave the apical third of maxillary molar palatal roots, unless there is an overriding indication for their removal.
- Never attempt to retrieve a root below the antrum by passing an instrument up into the tooth socket.

Any root in the antrum should be removed. The patient should be taken for sinus exploration and root retrieval. Raise a buccal flap and remove bone to allow adequate access for the root to be elevated away from the antrum. The remaining defect into the antrum from the socket also should be taken care of.

Displacement of the Tooth or a Root into the Tissues

Displacement of the tooth or a root into the tissues is a rare, but potentially serious complication. The tooth or part of it may be lost under mucoperiosteal flap, into the lingual pouch through the thin lingual cortex of bone in the lower third molar region, or into the infratemporal fossa around the back of the maxillary tuberosity from the upper third molar region.

If a tooth or root is lost from view during the course of an extraction, it may be in one of the following sites:

- Swallowed into the stomach or inhaled into the respiratory passage. If either of these is suspected, the patient should be sent to hospital for abdominal and chest radiographs.
- Pushed into the antrum.
- Displaced into a soft tissue space.
- Collected inadvertently by the suction apparatus (check the filter).
- Still in the socket.

Collateral Damage to Surrounding Soft Tissues

A certain amount of disruption to the gingival tissues around an extracted tooth is to be expected. However, it can be minimized by judicious gingival retraction.

The incidence of the following modes of soft tissue injury can be reduced with care and forethought:

- Gingival tissue lacerated by the forceps blades.
- To avoid this complication, be sure to place the blades inside the gingival crevice after liberal gingival retraction. This is a particular dangerous on the lingual aspect of lower teeth.
- Lower lip crushed against the lower teeth while extracting resistant upper molars: This is due to incorrect angulations of the forceps and is more likely to happen under general anesthesia or when the patient's lower lip is also anesthetized. The best way for prevention of this complication is awareness of the patient.
- Damage to the tongue, floor of mouth or the palate due to elevator: To avoid this complication, elevators should always be held with the index finger down the shank of the handle towards the tip to act as a 'stop' in case the instrument slips. The damage to the soft tissue can also occur due to slippage of the bur if proper tissue retraction is not done and guards are not placed. The poor maintenance of the rotary instruments like handpieces also leads to lot of frictional heat during the use. As the patient is administered the local anesthesia and as the surgeon is wearing gloves, sometimes double gloves, the heating of the handpiece may go unnoticed during the surgery and the patient may report subsequently with thermal injuries especially at the oral commissures.

Self-inflicted Tissue Injury

Self-inflicted tissue injury is common in children and mentally retarded adults. It is seen in the form of self-inflicted trauma to lips, tongue and cheek. During the postoperative phase when the part is still anesthetized such patients tend to bite heavily on the lips, tongue or cheeks producing severe lacerations.

Prevention

- Use minimum effective dose of local anesthetic agent.
- Warn the patient's guardians or parents against biting of lips and tongue.
- Also warn against eating and drinking hot fluids; while the effect of anesthesia is still present.
- Gauze pack can be placed after treatment to prevent lips trauma.

Management

Symptomatic: It comprises of analgesics and if necessary antibiotics.

Topical application of petroleum jelly or local anesthetic or antibiotic cream to relieve the pain and achieve comfort during eating.

Thermal Injury

Thermal injury results from the continued use of a handpiece with worn bearings, so that the instrument overheats. Awareness of the problem and regular maintenance of equipment will reduce the incidence of this unfortunate event.

Hemorrhage

- Primary hemorrhage—the bleeding may be at the time of surgery.
- Reactionary hemorrhage—within a few hours after surgery when the vasoconstriction of damaged blood vessels ceases.
- Secondary hemorrhage—present up to 14 days postoperatively as a result of infection.

Excessive bleeding from the socket occurs not infrequently even in patients who have no pathological hemorrhagic tendency. To avoid this proper history (previous hemorrhagic episode; onset, duration and amount of bleeding) should be taken. The drug history of the patient is also very important to find out, whether the patient is on oral anticoagulants, heparin therapy. Most of the patients having hypertension, valvular pathologies, prosthesis, CVA, neuroparalytic disorders are often prescribed antiplatelet agents most common being acetyl salicylic acid (aspirin) in low doses of 75 to 150 milligrams per day. By virtue of its antiplatelet effect, it prevents the platelet aggregation and such patients are at a risk of prolonged bleeding following surgery. It is therefore desirable to with hold the aspirin therapy in consultation with the physician, at least 72 hours prior to the surgery, to allow new platelets to be produced by the body, which would not be influenced by aspirin and help in the hemostasis. The platelets once influenced by aspirin do not recover.

Precautions to minimize the risk of hemorrhage include:

- Proper medical history.
- Careful handling of the tissues to avoid unnecessary trauma.
- Placing a gauze pack over the socket for at least 10 minutes.
- Avoiding vigorous mouth rinsing or chewing.
- If hemorrhage is systemic then proper case history should be taken, investigations like coagulation profile done.

If there is excessive bleeding at the time of extraction:

- Good suction apparatus should be used.
- Injecting further local anesthetic solution containing a vasoconstrictor.
- Inspecting the socket for the presence of friable granulation tissue and if it is present it should be curetted out.
- Horizontal mattress/figure of 8—suture is placed across the margins of the socket.
- A small pack of resorbable oxidized cellulose (*Surgicel*) or gelatin foam (*Gelfoam*) placed into the superficial part of the socket. The Gelfoam is made wet in saline before packing, while as the Surgicel is used in dry form. They act as an artificial clot and provide scaffold for the clot formation. With the absorption of the blood/fluid, they gain weight and seal the open ends of the capillaries. The Gelfoam can be impregnated with adrenaline or thrombin before packing.
- If a single blood vessel is seen to be the bleeding point then that can be tied off using a suture or coagulated with diathermy.

If there is persistent oozing from the cancellous bone then that can be stopped by using bone wax in the bone marrow. The bone wax mechanically

Box 11.4: Composition of bone wax

- Bees wax IP
- White hard paraffin wax, IP
- Isopropyl palmitate, USP

occludes the blood vessels. Bone wax is made of beeswax containing a softening agent such as paraffin (Box 11.4). Bone wax is used to mechanically stop bone bleeding during surgical procedures. The bone wax is smeared across the bleeding edge of the bone, blocking the holes and causing immediate bone hemostasis through a tamponade effect. Bone wax is supplied in sterile sticks and most often requires softening before it can be applied. Once applied, it essentially never goes away.

It is opaque in color and has a shelf life of 5 years. It can be sterilized with gamma radiations. Although inexpensive, easy to use and immediate, bone wax has a number of adverse reactions associated with it. Bone wax inhibits formation of new bone osteogenesis and acts as a physical barrier preventing bone union.[10,11] Bone wax remains as a foreign body for many years, and can cause a giant cell reaction and local inflammation.[12] In skull base surgery, bone wax has been reported to cause granuloma formation and CSF leak.[13,14] The bone wax is also known to inhibit the osteoblast migration, retard the healing and may increase the chances of infection.

The FDA has recently approved a new water soluble bone hemostasis material called Ostene, which is designed to look and feel like bone wax. This material comprises a sterile mixture of water-soluble alkylene oxide copolymers, derived from ethylene oxide and propylene oxide. These copolymers are considered inert. These compounds are not metabolized, but eliminated from the body unchanged. It is anticipated that with the introduction of these new hemostatic materials, the incidence of surgical bone infections, non-union and inflammatory complications will decrease with time.

If the patient is an unknown bleeder, when the local measures are being carried out for arresting the bleeding, simultaneously the blood samples should be drawn to evaluate the systemic cause of the bleeding if any. The different investigations along with their interpretations are given in Table 11.2.

When it is established that the patient has a coagulopathy along side the local measures mentioned above, the systemic supportive therapy and definitive treatment should be undertaken.

Supportive treatment:

- Monitor vitals for the signs of hypovolemia periodically.
- Intravenous administration of crystalloids (Ringer's lactate)/colloids (hexastarch solution as plasma expander).
- IV calcium gluconate injection (should be given carefully as it can precipitate cardiac arrythmias).
- Administration of vitamin K and vitamin C.

The definitive treatment for the individual coagulopathy is given in the table (Table 11.3).

Table 11.2: Different investigations and their interpretation

S. No	Test	Method	Reagent	Normal value	Causes of abnormality
1.	Bleeding time	Duke's Ivy	—	3.5 minutes 5 minutes	Thrombocytopenia 70,000/mm³ Thrombasthenia, thrombocytopathia—asprin, uremia, cirrhosis of liver
2.	Tourniquet test	Rumple leed	—	3–4 petechiae of 2.5 cm in diameter at 40 mm of Hg	— Capillary fragility — Vitamin C deficiency
3.	Platelet count	Brecher and Cronkite	Phase contrast microscope	160,000–3,5000/mm³	
4.	Euglobulin clot retraction time	—	—	3–4 hours	Platelet deficiency < 1,00,000/mm³
5.	Clotting time	Lee-White	—	9–14 minutes	F VIII, IX, XI, XII rarely factor X deficiency
6.	One stage PT	Quick's	Tissue procoagulant, acetone, dehydrated rabbit brain, Ca⁺⁺, citrated plasma	15 seconds	F IV, V, VII, X, fibrinogen, heparin (antithrombin action) deficiencies
7.	Partial thromboplastin time	—	Tissue procoagulant + blood	Variable as per product used	F VIII, IX, XI, XII and II, V,VII, X deficiencies
8.	PTT + PT	—	—	—	PTT prolonged, PT Normal : PT
9.	Thrombin time	—	Thrombin + plasma	Variable	Fibrinogen < 1,000 mg/dL

Table 11.3: Treatment for the individual coagulopathy

Component	Contents	Indications for use	Approximate volume	Amount of active substance per transfused unit	Risk of hepatitis	Shelf life of product
Platelet concentrate	Platelets, few white blood cells, some plasma	Bleeding resulting from thrombocytopenia	30–50	3–5 × 10^{10}	2	1–5 days depending on the storage and preperation
Whole blood						
Cryprecipitate	Coagulation factors I and VII	Hemophilia, Von-Willebrand disease, fibrinogen deficiency	10–25	80–100 units factor VIII	2	12 Mo frozen, 2 hours thawed
Factor	**Normal level**	**Life span**	**Fate during coagulation**	**Level required for safe hemostasis**	**Stability in ACD hemostasis**	**Ideal agent for replacing deficit**
Factor I	200–400 mg/100 mL	72 hours	Consumed	60–100 mg/100 mL	Very stable	Bank blood concentrate fibrinogen
Factor II	20 mg/100 mL (100%)	72 hours	Consumed	15–20%	Stable	Bank blood, concentrate preparation
Factor V	100%	36 hours	Consumed	5–30%	Labile (40% at 1st week)	Frozen fresh plasma, blood under 7 days
Factor VII	100%	5 hours	Survives	5–30%	Stable	Bank blood, concentrate preparation
Factor VIII concentrate proconvertin serum prothrombin conversion accelerator (SPCA) stable factor	100% (50–150)	6–12 hours	Consumed	30%	Stable	Fresh frozen plasma, bank blood, concentrated preparation
Factor IX [Christmas factor, plasma thromboplastin component (PTC), Hemophilia B factor]	100%	24 hours	Survives	20–30%	Stable	Bank blood, concentrated preparation
Factor X (Stuart Prower factor)	100%	40 hours	Survives	15–20%	Stable	Bank blood, concentrated preparation
Factor XI [plasma thromboplastin antecedent] (PTA)	100%	Probably 40–80	Survives	10%	Probably stable	
Factor XII (Hageman factor)	100%	Unknown	Survives	Deficit produces no bleeding tendency	Stable	Replacement not required

Table 11.4: Postdental extraction hemorrhage

Causes	Management
Local 1. Trauma 2. Laceration 3. Friable granulation tissue 4. Clot dislodgement: Mechanical infection 5. Hemorrhagic lesions	1. *Preventive* • History • Investigations 2. *Local* • Curettage • Mechanical (sutures, ligatures, clamps, pressure packs, bone wax) • Thermal (application of hot and cold packs) • Electrocoagulation • Chemical: – Gel foam – Topical thrombin – Oxidized cellulose - Oxicell - Surgicel - Methyl-2-cyanoacrylate
Systemic 1. Coagulopathies 2. Anticoagulant therapy 3. Antiplatelet drugs 4. Liver dysfunction 5. Chronic liver failure 6. Uremia 7. LE 8. Steroid therapy (prolonged) 9. Multiple myeloma 10. Leukemia 11. HT 12. Thrombocytopenia.	*Systemic* 1. Supportive: Commercially available nonspecific coagulants (Hemlock, Botropase, Pause, etc.) 2. Vitamin K 3. Calcium gluconate 4. Fluids, Hematocrit, monitoring 5. Investigations and definitive adequate substitute.

Postdental Extraction Hemorrhage[15,16]

The causes and management of post dental extraction bleeding are illustrated in Table 11.4.

Excessive Pain, Swelling and Trismus[17]

Swelling and discomfort occurs after any surgical procedure; tooth extraction is no exception. Appropriate postoperative instructions and reassurance, is normally adequate management of these symptoms.

The inflammatory edema can be minimized to a great extent by following the aseptic principles like aseptic care, gentle tissue handling, judicious bone cutting and use of coolent and by placing sutures loosely. Judicious use of physiotherapy in the form of cold compressions, warm saline gargles can also help in reducing the inflammation. Heavy dependence on the drugs can be avoided by following these principles. Suitable pharmacological support using anti-inflammatory and analgesic drugs can be prescribed.

Causes for Trismus

- Muscle spasms.
- Injury to ligament and medial pterygoid muscle.
- Infection in pterygomandibular space and/or submasseteric space.

Trismus is an inability to open the mouth to a normal gap, and is commonly seen following extractions, particularly lower molars. Inflammation and edema may spread from this region to affect the powerful jaw closing muscles, masseter and medial pterygoid, which are then painful when stretched and undergo protective myospasm. Severe and progressive trismus occasionally follows a few days after an inferior dental nerve block as the result of the development of a hematoma in the medical pterygoid muscle. The hematoma may undergo fibrosis. Trismus due to edema normally resolves spontaneously with the inflammation. The needle injury to the sphenomandibular ligament during the pterygomandibular block can also lead to pain and trismus.

The patient can be made more comfortable by the application of heat to the affected area.

Management

Management depends on the cause of trismus and consists of the following:

- Heat therapy (short waive diathermy)
- Warm saline rinses
- Analgesics
- Anti-inflammatory
- Muscle relaxants (role is questionable)
- Application of glycerin magnesium sulfate dressing
- Physiotherapy
- Surgical decompression
- Antibiotics

Nerve Damage

The following branches of the trigeminal nerve may be at risk during tooth extraction.

- The mental nerve—damaged by overextension of relieving incisions in the depth of the buccal sulcus in the lower premolar region.
- The inferior dental nerve—the roots of the third molars are in close proximity of the inferior alveolar nerve thus there are chances of damage to the nerve during extraction. Similarly, injudicious instrumentation can also lead to damage to the nerve.
- The lingual nerve—nerve is at risk of crush injury during periosteal elevation lingual to the lower third molar.

Management

Most paresthesias resulting from the nerve damage, resolve within 8 weeks without treatment.[18] However, if the damage to the nerve is severe, then only the paresthesia may require longer time or can be permanent.[19] The recovery is variable and depends upon the extent of the nerve injury.

- Reassurance to the patient.
- Administer vitamins (vitamins B_1, B_6 and B_{12}), parenteral and oral.
- If dental treatment is to be continued, avoid readministration of the local anesthetic agent into the same region of traumatized nerve.
- Nerve decompression or anastomosis surgeries whenever indicated.

The details of nerve injuries are covered under the Chapter on Neurological Disorders.

Dry Socket (Synonym: Alveolar Osteitis)[20]

Definition

Dry socket clinical entity is a localized osteitis involving either whole or part of the condensed bone lining a tooth socket, the lamina dura.

Causes

The exact etiology of the dry socket cannot be ascertained; however, the following factors are believed to precipitate it:

- Excessive trauma to bone.
- Use of vasoconstrictor along with the local anesthetic solution.
- Menstruating females and the patients on oral contraceptives.
- Infection (*treponema denticola*, fusospirochetes, *Borrelia vincentii*)—although these microorganisms have been isolated from the lesions of the dry socket, they are opportunistic and anaerobic, which might grow in the hypoperfused, sloughy tissue. The other studies have shown that there is a mixed infection and no single organism could be held responsible for the dry socket. Moreover, the clinical picture is not similar to that of the other infective pathologies.
- Abnormal clot retraction.

Pathogenesis

Birn[21,22] suggested that trauma and infection cause inflammation of the bone marrow with the resultant release of tissue activators that convert the plasminogen in the clot to plasmin. This fibrinolytic agent then dissolves the blood clot and at the same time release kinins from the kininogen, which is also in the clot, leading to severe pain. The loss of clot makes the bone bare and leads to alveolitis and neuritis of the free nerve endings in the bone, which is also the cause for the pain (Fig. 11.42).

Clinical Features

The dry socket is characterized by:

- The onset of acute pain and a foul odor 3 to 4 days after the extraction.
- There is loss of blood clot in the socket, exposing vital bone, which is very tender to touch due to neuritis in the exposed nerve endings.
- The socket may have small quantity of grayish slough, but there is no suppuration.
- Similarly, the gingiva around the socket may not show the signs of inflammation and the swelling is usually absent.
- The healing of the socket is delayed process and pain normally continues for at least 10 to 14 days.

Management

- As the pain is severe the patient is given sedative dressings in the form of zinc oxide and oil of cloves on cotton wool or gauze, is loosely tucked into the socket. This dressing is often referred to as 'pom-pom'.
- The curettage of the socket to induce fresh bleeding is recommended, however, it is not advocated as the pain may get aggreviated and there are chances of the infection spreading in the deeper tissue planes.
- Prophylactic use of antimicrobial drugs such as metronidazole and clindamycin has been shown to reduce its incidence though it is not universal finding. The antibiotic therapy with betalactum group of antibiotics with metronidazole is usually adequate. It must be understood that it is not an infective pathology as it is evident from the clinical and microbiological finding. The role of the antibiotics should not be overemphasized.

Osteomyelitis[23]

Osteomyelitis is 'an infection of the bone and the bone marrow, which can be caused by an infection in the body spreading in the blood stream from the point of origin to the bone'.

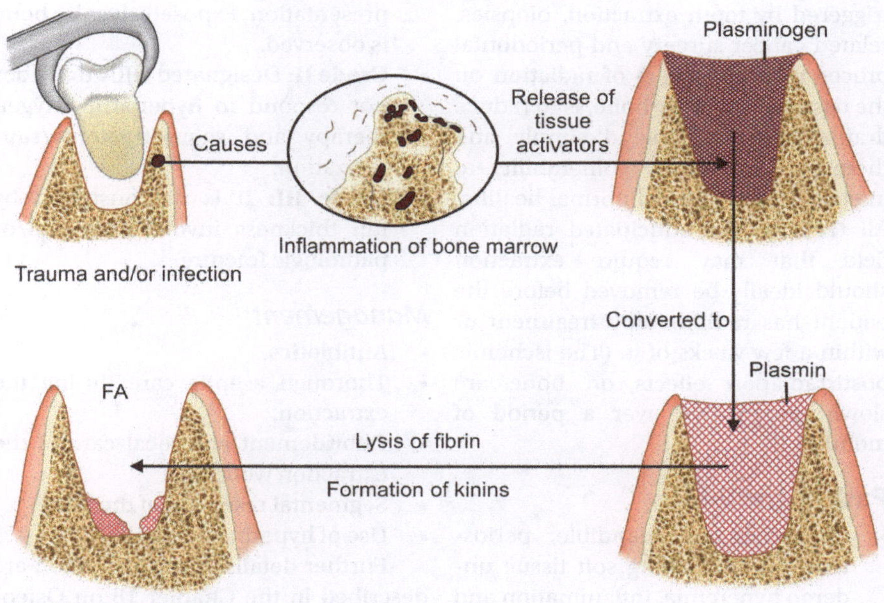

Fig. 11.42: Etiology and pathogenesis of fibrinolytic alveolitis (Birn's hypothesis[22])

Etiology

- Extractions done in presence of acute infections.
- Severe infection.
- Immunocompromised patients, e.g. uncontrolled diabetes.

Symptoms of Osteomyelitis

- Intense penetrating bone pain, prolonged healing of the socket, anesthesia of the lower lip and general malaise.
- Swelling and warmth in the infected area.
- Fever.
- Drainage of pus through the skin.

Treatment

High dose of an appropriate antibiotic for an extended period, normally several weeks. Chronic suppurative osteomyelitis demands surgical debridement of the affected area to remove any sequestra of dead bone. *The details of this condition are described in the Chapter on Osteomyelitis.*

Osteoradionecrosis[24]

Osteoradionecrosis was first described by Marx[25] in 1983 as hypovascularity hypocellularity, and local tissue hypoxia. It is an extremely serious complication of radiotherapy to the jaws that can be triggered by tooth extraction, biopsies, related cancer surgery and periodontal procedures. The effect of radiation on the tissues, especially bone, is to reduce dramatically their blood supply and therefore to increase vulnerability to infection and failure of normal healing. All teeth in the anticipated radiation field that may require extraction should ideally be removed before the patient has radiotherapy treatment or within a few weeks of it. (The ischemic postirradiation effects on bone are slowly progressive over a period of months).

Pathophysiology

- The irradiated mandible, periosteum and overlying soft tissue undergo hyperemia, inflammation and endarteritis.
- These conditions ultimately lead to thrombosis, cellular death, progressive hypovascularity and fibrosis.
- The radiated bed is hypocellular and devoid of fibroblasts and osteoblasts.

Contributing factors to the Development of ORN:

- Dental trauma
- Tumor location
- Radiation dosage
- Elapsed time since radiation
- Nutrition
- Alcohol and tobacco use
- Concomitant surgery and chemotherapy.

Clinically there are three types of ORN[25,26]

- Types I is trauma-induced ORN, which occurs when radiation or surgical wounding are coupled closely together.
- Type II, also trauma-induced ORN, most common which occurs years after radiation therapy.
- Type III or spontaneous ORN can occur anytime after radiotherapy, but commonly occurs 6 months to 2 years following radiotherapy, without any obvious preceding surgical or traumatic event.

Grading

- **Grade I:** ORN is the most common presentation. Exposed alveolar bone is observed.
- **Grade II:** Designated ORN that does not respond to hyperbaric oxygen therapy and sequestrectomy/saucerization.
- **Grade III:** It is demonstrated by full thickness involvement and/or pathologic fracture.

Management

- Antibiotics.
- Thorough aseptic care during the extraction.
- Debridement and local care of the extraction wound.
- Segmental resection of the bone.
- Use of hyperbaric therapy.

Further details of this condition are described in the Chapter 18 on Osteomyelitis of the Facial Bones.

REFERENCES

1. Malvin E King. Dentistry: An Illustrated Histroy. New York: Abradale Press 1993.
2. Geoffrey L. Howe. The Extraction of Teeth. 2nd edition revised. Bristol: J. Wright. 1974.
3. Kemal Findikcioglu. Effect of the menstrual cycle on intraoperative bleeding in rhinoplasty patient. European Journal of Plastic Surgery. 2009;32(2).
4. Beard RW, Gillian M Roberts. Supine hypotension syndrome. Br Med J. 1970; 2(5704):297.
5. William Harry Archer. Oral Surgery: A step-by-step atlas of operative techniques, 4th edn, WB Saunders Company. 1966.
6. Moore US, Principles of Oral and Maxillofacial Surgery, 5th edn. Blackwell Science Ltd, 2001.
7. Norman JE Cannon PD: Fracture of the maxillary tuberosity. Oral Surg. 1967;24:459-67.
8. Ehrl PA. Oroantral communications. Int J Oral Surg.1980;9:351-8.
9. Fickling BW. Oral surgery involving the maxillary sinus. Br Dent J. 1957;103: 199-214. Ann R Coll Surg. 1957;20:13-35.
10. Wang MY, Armstrong JK, Fisher TC, et al. 'A new, pluronic-based, bone hemostatic agent that does not impair osteogenesis'. Neurosurgery. 2001;49: 962-8.
11. Schonauer C, Tessitore E, Barbagallo G, et al. 'The use of local agents: bone wax, gelatin, collagen, oxidized cellulose'. Eur Spine J. 2004;13:S89-96.
12. Allison RT. 'Foreign body reactions and an associated histological artefact due to bone wax'. Br J Biomed Sci. 1994;51:14-7.
13. Patel RB, Kwatler JA, Hodosh RM. 'Bone wax as a cause of foreign body granuloma in the cerebellopontine angle: Case illustration'. J Neurosurg. 2000;92:362.
14. Bolger W, Tadros, M, Ellenbogen R, et al. 'Endoscopic management of cerebrospinal fluid leak associated with the use of bone wax in skull-base surgery'. Otolaryngol Head Neck Surg. 2000;132: 418-20.

15. Milam SB, Cooper RL. Extensive bleeding following extraction in a patients undergoing chronic hemodialysis. Oral Surg. 1983;55:14.
16. Olson RA, Roberts DL, Osbon DB. A comparative study of polylactic acid, Gelfoam, and surgical in healing extraction sites. Oral Surg. 1982;53:441.
17. Young HR. Resolution of postoperative swelling following oral surgery: chymoral. Oral Surg. 1967;23:12-8.
18. Nickel AA, Jr. A retrospective study of paresthesia of the dental alveolar nerves. Anesth Prog. 1990; 37(1):42-5.
19. Haas DA, Lennon D. A 21 year retrospective study reports of paresthesia following local anesthetic administration. J Can Dent Assoc. 1995; 61:961-7.
20. Krogh HW. Incidence of dry socket. J Am Dent. Assoc.1937;24:1829.
21. Birn H. Fibrinolytic activity in dry socket. Acta Odont Scand. 1970;28:37-58.
22. Birn H. Etiology and pathogenesis of fibrinolytic alveolitis ('dry socket'). Int J Oral Surg. 1973;2:211-63.
23. Alling CC. Postextraction osteomyelitis syndrome. Dent Clin North Am. 1959; 621.
24. Epstein J, van der Meij E, McKenzie M, et al. Postradiation Osteonecrosis of the mandible: a long-term follow-up study. Oral Sury Oral Med Oral Pathol Oral Radiol Endod. 1997;83:657-62.
25. Marx RE. Osteoradionecrosis: a new concept of its pathophysiology. J Oral Maxillofac Surg. 1983;41(5):283-8.
26. Marx RE, Johnson RP. Studies in the radiobiology of osteoradionecrosis and their clinical significance. Oral Surg Oral Med Oral Pathol. 1987;64(4):379-90.

12 Management of Impacted Teeth

Borle Rajiv M, Arora Aakash, Magarkar Shashwat D

The tooth, which fails to erupt in the oral cavity due to obstruction to its path of eruption is called 'impacted tooth'. The obstruction could be due to adjacent tooth, thick bone, fibrous tissue, any cyst or tumor. Archer[1] has defined impaction as "The tooth, which fails to erupt in oral cavity in its functional position and which has lost its further potential of eruption."

It should be differentiated from the embedded tooth in which the tooth does not erupt in the oral cavity due to lack of eruptive forces.

The man has evolved from apes to the current civilized state. The food habits have also changed from raw food to the cooked and processed food. The jaws have evolved due to the change in food habit and the need for heavy jaws is no more felt. The size of the jaws has receded, but the number of teeth has remained constant, which resulted in discrepancy between the size of the dentition and the space available to accommodate it in the jaws. Thus, the teeth often get obstructed and fail to erupt in the oral cavity, in the desired position. The third molars are by far the most commonly impacted as they are the last to be formed and erupt in the oral cavity. By the time they start erupting in the oral cavity the other teeth have already occupied the available space in the jaw and thus, the third molars face the space constraints. The second tooth commonly found impacted is maxillary canines and then the mandibular canines, as they also erupt later than their adjacent teeth and face the space problem due to the small size of the jaw which is not fully grown at that age and secondly due to mesial drift phenomenon.

THEORIES OF IMPACTION[2]

- **Phylogenetic theory:** Due to evolution, the human jaw size is becoming smaller and since the third molar tooth is the last to erupt there may not be room for it to emerge in the oral cavity.
- **Mendelian's theory:** Here genetic variation plays a major role, if the individual genetically receives a small jaw from one parent and large teeth from other parent.
- **Nodine theory:** The modern diet (soft diet) does not require a decided effort in mastication and hence, according to Nodine et al.[3]; the growth stimulus of jaw is lost and modern man has impacted teeth.

ETIOLOGY

Apart from the above mentioned factors certain etiological factors have been mentioned for impacted teeth. They are:

Local Factors

The local factors are as follows:

- Micrognathia
- Crowing of teeth
- Condensing osteitis
- Cysts
- Tumors
- Thick fibrous bands under the mucosa.

Systemic Factors

The systemic factors are as follows:

- Prenatal causes—heredity.
- Postnatal—rickets, anemia, tuberculosis, congenital syphilis, malnutrition.
- Endocrinal disorders of thyroid, parathyroid, pituitary glands like hypothyroidism, achondroplasia, etc. Here the primary retention of teeth is seen due to lack of osteoclastic activity, which does not provide resorption of the bone overlying the developing tooth.
- Heredity linked disorders—Down's syndrome, Hurler's syndrome, osteopetrosis, Cleidocranial dysostosis, cleft palate, etc. There is failure of the overlying bone to resorb and development of an eruption pathway is absent.

IMPACTED MANDIBULAR THIRD MOLARS

The mandibular third molars are the most common teeth to be impacted[4] and the most challenging impaction to be treated.

APPLIED SURGICAL ANATOMY

- When the mandible is viewed superoinferiorly it is noticed that the third molars are located in the lingual shelf of the bone and buccally a strong buttressed bony ridge is present.

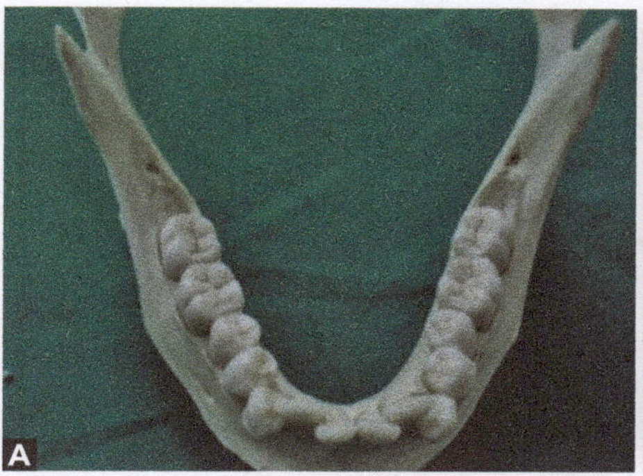
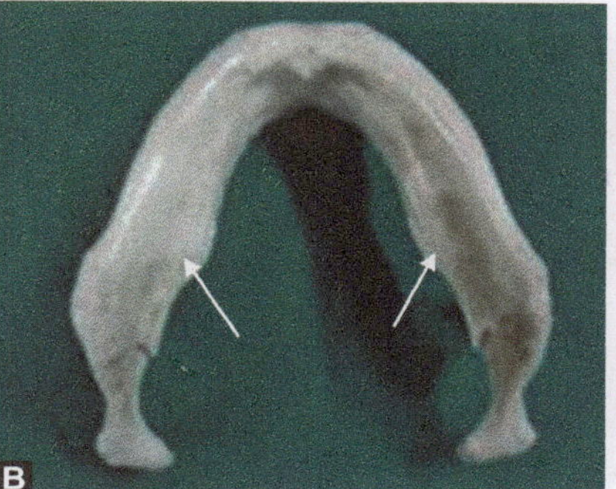

Figs 12.1A and B: Lingual shelf for mandibular third molars

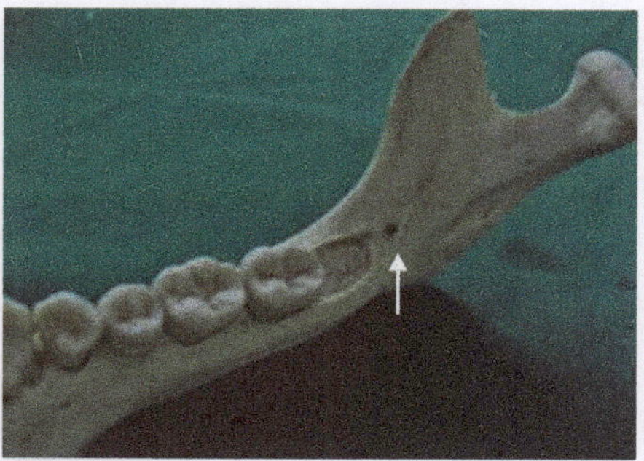

Fig. 12.2: Showing the nutrient foramen in the retromolar area

When viewed from inferior side the lingual shelf is conspicuously seen and it is noticed that the lingual shelf is thin as compared to the buccal bone (Figs 12.1A and B).

- Third molars are situated close to the junction of the thin vertical ramus and thick body of the mandible. The junction between the thick and the thin portions of the bone constitutes a line of weakness. The bone grains also change their course from vertical to the horizontal direction in this area, which also makes the bone weak in this area.[5] When the third molars are impacted and placed deep in the bone, they occupy lot of space in the bone and undermine it making it further weak. The reinforcement is provided to this area by the presence of buttressed external and internal oblique ridges. If bone is removed injudiciously from this area during the surgery or excessive force is applied the bone can fracture readily at the angle of the mandible.
- The lingual nerve lies very close to the lingual cortical plate in the third molar area and can get damaged during the surgery due to following reasons:
  - If vertical incision at the anterior border of the ramus is taken too far lingually.
  - If the soft tissues on the lingual side are not properly guarded by placing a guard then the accidental slippage of the sharp instrument or clogging of the bur in the soft tissue may damage the nerve.
  - The thin lingual cortical plate may fracture readily and the lingual nerve may get damaged.

  The inferior alveolar nerve also lies close to the roots of the deeply placed impacted mandibular third molar.[6] It may be in close proximity of the apices, may pass between the two roots or may groove the surface of the root and pass through it. The relation of the roots with the nerve must be carefully assessed and the treatment plan must be suitably modified to prevent the damage to the nerve.
- The facial artery lies at the anteroinferior angle of the insertion of the masseter muscle and ascends anteriorly and upwards in the cheek. It is close to the buccal vestibule in the molar area. During taking the vertical relieving incision if the knife slips accidentally the vessel can get damaged and lead to profuse hemorrhage. To stop the bleeding, firm digital pressure may be applied at anteroinferior angle of the insertion of the masseter, over the inferior border of the mandible, exrtaorally. The facial artery gets compressed between the finger and the bone and the bleeding can be stopped, until the artery is ligated. To avoid such accident, a beginner, while taking the vertical relieving incision, must direct the knife from the depth of the vestibule to the gingival margin and not the other way round.
- There are small nutrient foramina on the lingual side of the retromolar area in some mandibles. If the vertical incision is taken lingually the nutrient vessels may get traumatized and results into disturbing bleeding during the surgery (Fig. 12.2).
- The Buccal fat pad is present laterally and superiorly to the ramus. If the vertical incision is placed too far laterally to the ramus or taken too long, the fat pad can get exposed and prolapse into the oral cavity. It is difficult to reduce it to its original position and may get necrosed and delay the healing.
- The bone grains in the ramus area are placed vertically. They change their course in the body and become horizontal. While removing the bone with the help of chisel and mallet, first two stop cuts, which are cortex deep, must be marked at the anterior and posterior ends of the proposed bone removal and then only the intervening bone should be removed. If the chisel is directly used parallel to the bone grains, without marking the vertical stop cuts, the whole bone may get split along the bone grains.

CLASSIFICATION OF THE IMPACTED THIRD MOLAR IMPACTIONS[7]

Winter's Classification[8]

The third molars are classified according to the position of its long axis as follows (Figs 12.3A to G):

- Mesioangular

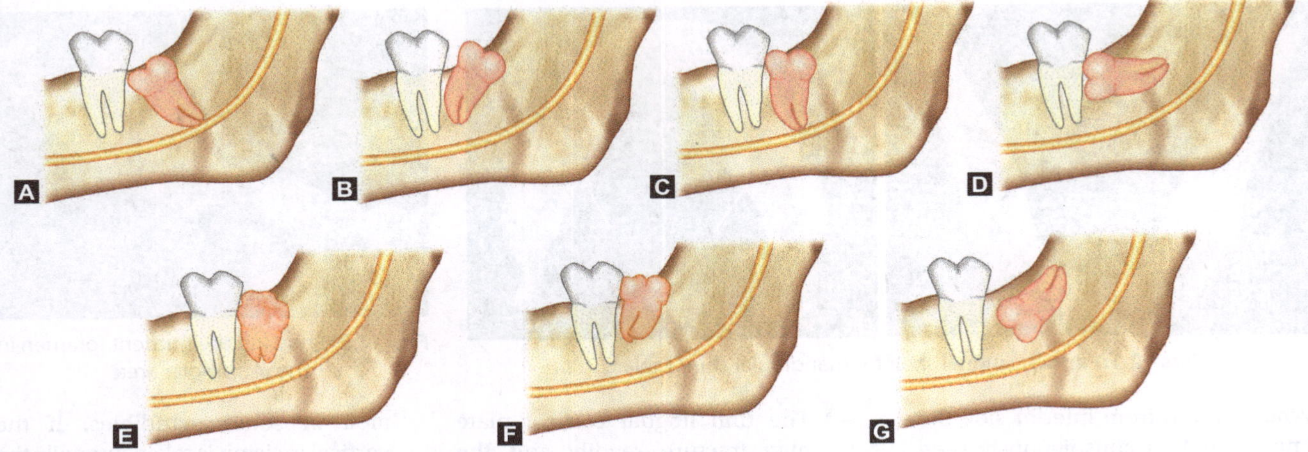

Figs 12.3A to G: Classification according to position: (A) Mesioangular; (B) Distoangular; (C) Vertical; (D) Horizontal; (E) Buccoversion; (F) Linguoversion; (G) Inverted

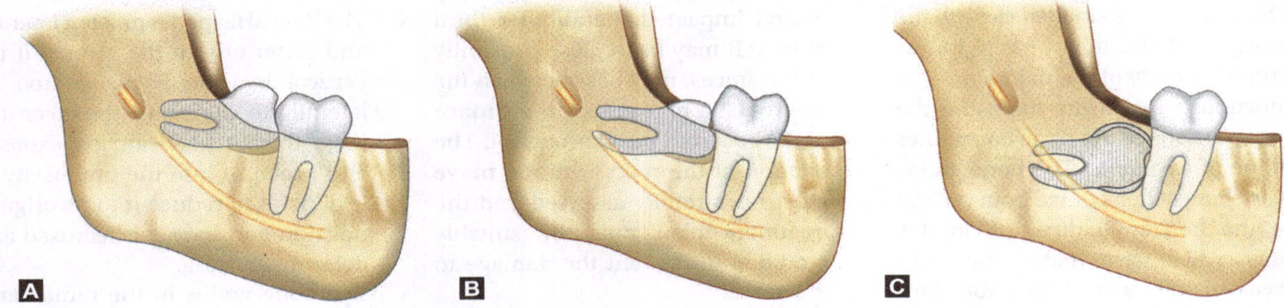

Figs 12.4A to C: Position A, B and C as per Pell and Gregory's classification

- Horizontal
- Vertical
- Distoangular
- Crown in buccoversion
- Crown in the linguoversion
- Inverted

Pell and Gregory's Classification[9]

According to the relative depth of the third molar in the bone in relation to the second molar, the third molars are classified as:

- **Position A:** When the highest portion of the impacted third molar is at or above the occlusal level of the second molar.
- **Position B:** When the highest portion of the impacted third molar is between the occlusal and cervical level of the second molar.
- **Position C:** When the highest portion of the impacted third molar is below the cervical line of the second molar (Figs 12.4A to C).

According to the space available between the distal surface of the second molar and the anterior border of the ramus of the mandible third molars can be classified as:

- **Class I:** When there is sufficient space available between the distal surface of the second molar and the anterior border of the ramus to accommodate the third molar.
- **Class II:** When the space is inadequate and the third molar is partly present in the space between the second molar and the anterior border of the ramus and partly in the ramus.
- **Class III:** When the third molar is totally present in the ramus due to the lack of space (Figs 12.5A to C).

Winter's Lines

White, amber and red (WAR) lines given by George Winter[8]—based on imaginary lines drawn on radiograph to determine position and depth of impaction:

W—White line
A—Amber line
R—Red line

- White line—imaginary line joining enamel cusps of erupted 2nd molar extending posteriorly over 3rd molar
- Amber line—imaginary line joining crest of interdental septum between molars
- Red line—imaginary line perpendicular to amber line to an imaginary point of application of elevator (usually on mesial side except for distoangular molar) (Fig. 12.6).

Why the Classification is Important?

The third molar impactions should be classified for:

- Better understanding and communication.
- To assess the degree of difficulty in its surgical removal.

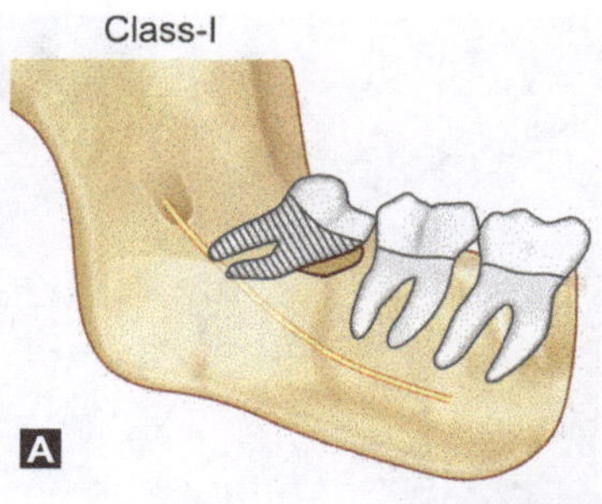

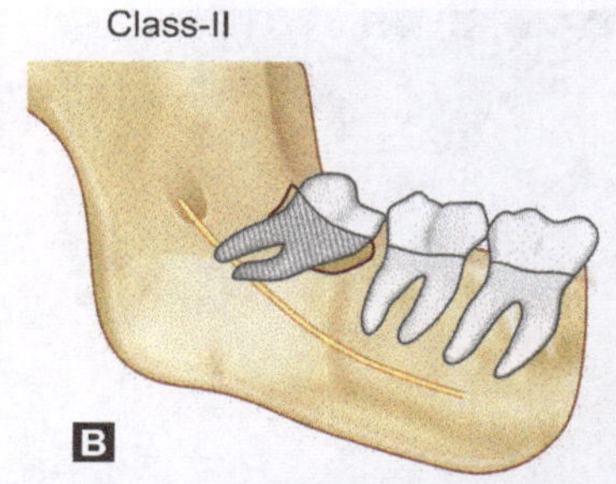

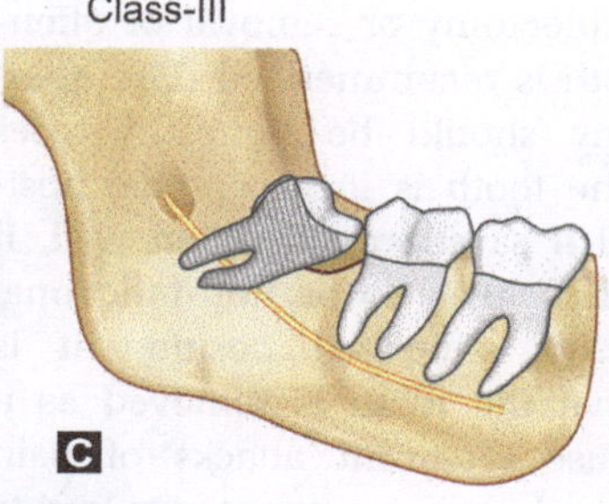

Figs 12.5A to C: Class I, II and III as per Pell and Gregory's classification

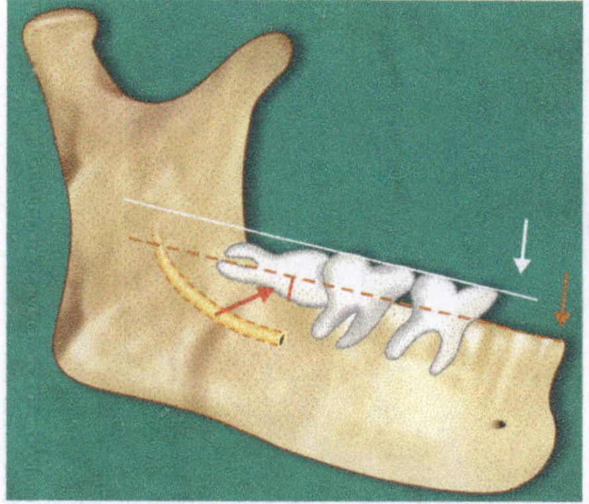

Fig. 12.6: WAR lines

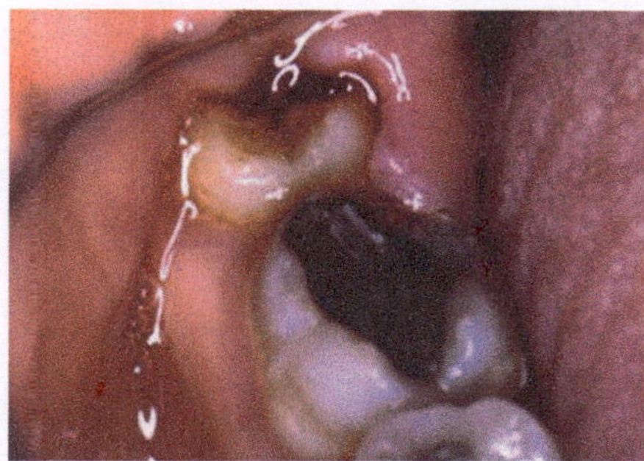

Fig. 12.7: Pericoronitis

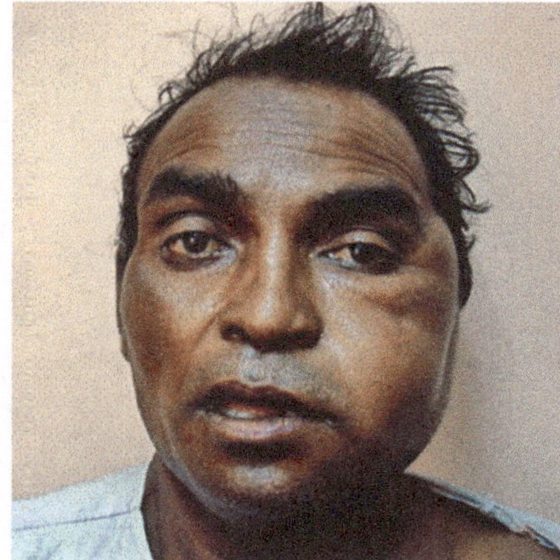

Fig. 12.8: Buccal space infection secondary to pericoronitis

- To assess the bone cover.
- To assess the proximity with the vital structures.

SEQUELAE OF THE IMPACTED THIRD MOLARS

The clinical problems caused by the impacted third molars are the sequel. In other words they are the indications for their removal.[10]

Pericoronitis

Pericoronitis is defined as the inflammation of the soft tissue that covers or surrounds the crown of an unerupted tooth. When the third molars are not fully erupted or when they are abnormally placed, the area does not remain self-cleansing. The food particles tend to accumulate and get degraded. The microorganisms get an opportunity to proliferate. Due to the irritation and infection the soft tissue under goes inflammation and pericoronitis ensues. The covering of the soft tissue on the crown of an unerupted tooth is called 'operculum'. The accumulation of food particles below it or due to recurrent trauma from occlusion, inflammation sets in, resulting in pericoronitis. Secondary infection worsens the condition (Fig. 12.7).

Clinical Features

The clinical features of the pericoronitis are:

- In acute condition there is severe, persistent pain.
- Trismus due to protective myospasm secondary to the pain.
- The pericoronal tissue is inflamed, congested and edematous.
- In acute condition due to surrounding cellulitis, mild extraoral swelling may be present.
- The patient experiences difficulty in mastication and swallowing.
- Due to the edema the tissue swells and the opposing tooth (upper third molar) traumatizes this inflamed tissue. It results in indentations of the cusp on the soft tissue operculum or sometimes traumatic ulceration.
- The acute inflammation localizes to form an abscess (pericoronal abscess), which is characterized by localized swelling, surrounded by inflamed and congested mucosa and pus discharge.
- The acute stage may resolve or progress to a chronic stage, which is characterized by dull pain, fibrous tissue around the crown, which has a tendency to undergo acute exacerbation recurrently, especially when the tooth is impacted and non-self-cleansing. The infection may spread along the soft tissue plane to the buccal space or submasseteric space (Fig. 12.8).

Management

The management of acute pericoronitis is usually conservative, with antibiotics and analgesics, anti-inflammatory drugs and local measures like irrigations with normal saline, warm saline gargles and soft diet, selective cuspal grinding of the opposing tooth causing trauma from occlusion.[11] The only surgical intervention recommended at an acute state is drainage of the pericoronal abscess. After the acute stage is subsided and proper evaluation is completed, definitive surgical treatment comprising of operculectomy or removal of offending tooth is recommended. The operculectomy should be done in cases where the tooth is in acceptable position and if saved can function well. If the tooth is likely to be non-functional because of abnormal position it is better that the tooth is removed as it may cause recurrent attacks of pain and operculectomy may not give lasting relief to the patient.

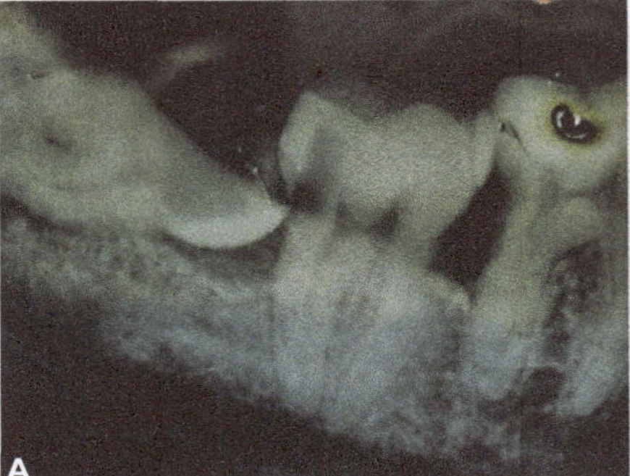

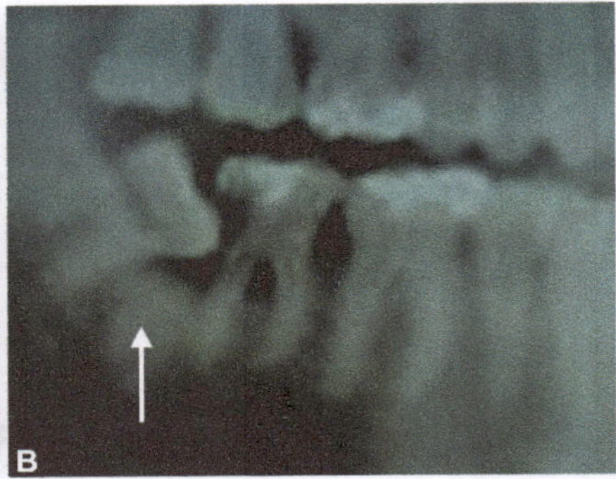

Figs 12.9A and B: Carious involvement of (A) 3rd; (B) 2nd molars

Caries

Caries is generally observed as the tooth, which is impacted and partially erupted in the oral cavity fails to maintain good contact with the adjacent tooth. Due to this, the chronic food impaction results and moreover it is not accessible site for cleaning. This results in caries, not only in the impacted tooth, but also in the adjacent tooth, which like any other carious tooth causes further complications (Figs 12.9A and B).

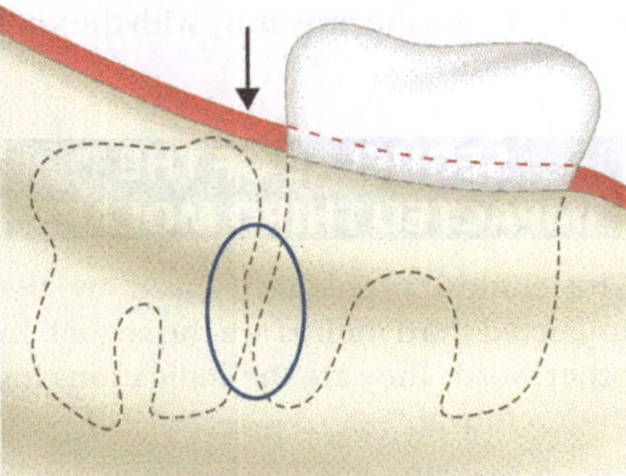

Fig. 12.10: Lack of contact, plunging of food debris and pocket formation

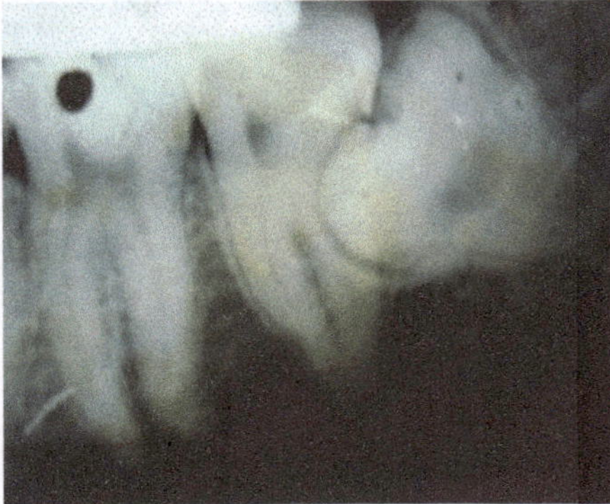

Fig. 12.11: Pressure resorption of the root of second molar

Periodontal Pocket Formation

The food impaction leads to periodontal pocket formation more commonly between the second and the third molars. The food impaction distal to the third molar results in apical migration of the gingival attachment and results in distal pocket formation. The periodontal pockets lead to recurrent attacks of periodontitis and sensitivity to hot and cold and cemental caries (Fig. 12.10).

Pressure Symptoms

The deep seated third molars impinge upon the neurovascular bundle and produce pressure symptoms like dull pain, hypoesthesia and tingling sensation.

Root Resorption of the Second Molar

Due to chronic pressure on the roots of the adjacent tooth (second molar), the roots of the second molar may undergo resorption (Fig. 12.11).

Anchorage Loss

The impacted third molars exert a mesial pressure on the arch, thus the teeth have a tendency to drift mesially. It is very important to note during the orthodontic treatment, as drift can cause anchorage loss and the orthodontic treatment can be complicated. Thus, the elective removal of the impacted third molars is advocated before the orthodontic treatment (Fig. 12.12).

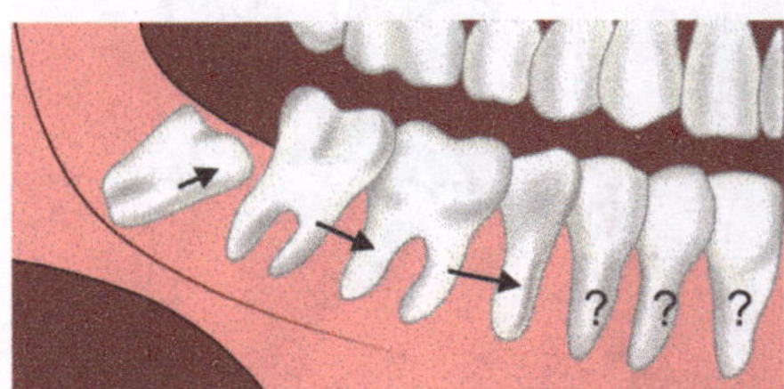

Fig. 12.12: Mesial collapse of the arch due to pressure from the third molar

Cyst and Tumor Formation

The unerupted and impacted third molars are covered with the reduced enamel epithelium, which is the embryonic tissue and has pleuripotentiality. Such embryonic tissues are capable of differentiating in variety of other tissues and can lead to pathological conditions like cyst, ameloblastoma. The dentigerous cysts are commonly seen to be associated with the impacted third molars, in which the Ameloblastic transformations are a common occurrence.[12] To prevent such a development, prophylactic removal of the third molar is recommended. A procedure called lateral trephnization[13] is recommended in the literature in which the developing bud of the third molar is surgically removed to prevent further complications (Fig. 12.13).

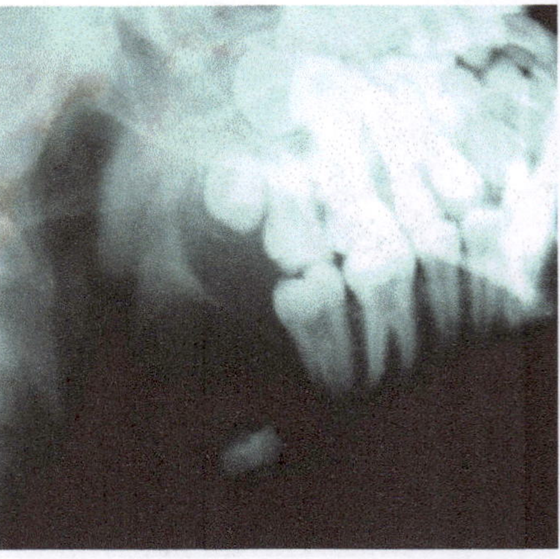

Fig. 12.13: Dentigerous cyst associated with the impacted third molar

Cheek Biting/Trauma from Occlusion

When the third molars are too far posteriorly and buccally placed they impinge upon the soft tissue and traumatize it leading to traumatic ulceration. The upper third molars, which are buccally erupted and supraerupted due to lack of opposing tooth, often traumatize the soft tissue in the retromolar area. The soft tissue is entrapped between the anterior border of the ramus and the cusps of the third molar, it leads to ulceration, pain and trismus. Although the pain is due to the trauma from upper molars, at the sight of impacted mandibular molars the clinician tends to jump to a conclusion that the pain is due impacted mandibular molar and often remove them although they may not be the actual cause of pain. In such cases, both the upper and lower third molars, which are non-functional and cause recurrent TFO are indicated for surgical removal.

Fracture of the Mandible

Impacted teeth occupy lot of space in the bone and undermine the bone, making the bone weak and vulnerable to fracture, in case of trauma (Fig. 12.14). When the mandibular third molars are in normal position or have been removed earlier prophylactically, the bone at the angle region is no more weak and the chances of subcondylar fractures following trauma are increased. The fractures at the angle are easier to treat than the subcondylar fractures and thus, it is recommended by some authors not to remove the third molars prophylactically (Duan D H et al. 2008).

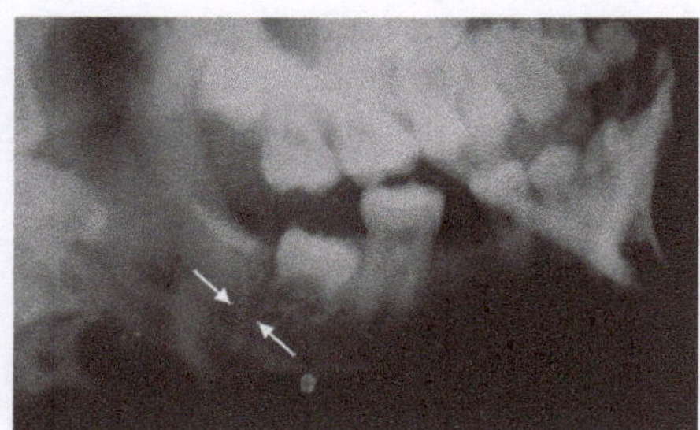

Fig. 12.14: Fracture of mandible at angle. Note the third molar is unerupted occupying space in the bone

EVALUATION OF THE PATIENT FOR THE THIRD MOLAR SURGERY[14]

The patients who are posted for surgery need a careful evaluation to ensure smooth and uneventful procedure. Poor planning is one of the major causes for encountering difficulties during the third molar surgery, increasing the surgical time and postoperative complications. The evaluation is as follows:

History

A short relevant medical history and physical examination is mandatory to rule out any associated medical disorder, which will adversely affect the outcome of the surgery. A thorough local examination is carried out and following points are noted.

- **Age of the patient:** As the age of the patient increases (more than 40 years) the bones tend to become more compact and loose their resilience. Thus, the simple looking impactions are more difficult to remove in an elderly patient due to the compact bone. The removal of impacted teeth in younger individuals is easier to remove as the bones are more resilient and elastic.
- Presence of acute infection.
- Presence of trismus
- Level of eruption of the tooth, i.e. whether it is erupted, partially erupted or unerupted.
- Condition of the soft tissue around the crown as the inflamed and congested tissue oozes during the surgery and the healing in such tissue is retarded.
- The size of the tongue, hypertrophied buccal pad of fat, excessive salivation, exaggerated gag reflex should also be noted as these factors interfere with access and the conduct of the procedure.
- Condition of the crown, the non vitality, carious undermining of the crown tends to make it fragile and lead to unplanned fracture of the crown during the surgery. The size of the crown should also be assessed as bulky crown needs removal by splitting (odontectomy) to prevent damage to the adjacent tooth and to prevent weakening of bone due to its removal during the surgery.
- **Condition of the adjacent tooth:** The second molar should be evaluated for caries, fractures, endodontic treatment and prosthesis. The carious exposure in the second molar or periapical infection may cause pain. Sometimes at the sight of an impacted tooth in the vicinity the clinician tends to jump to a conclusion that the pain is due to impacted tooth and its surgical removal is undertaken. But, the pain persists as the cause lies in adjacent tooth. Similar erroneous planning can occur in the cases of crack tooth syndrome associated with second molar. If the second molar is treated endodontically, it becomes brittle and can readily fracture during elevation of the third molar if the elevator is not used properly. Similarly, the filling or prosthesis on second molar may be damaged during luxation of the third molar.
- Relation with the adjacent tooth—the relation of the third molar with the adjacent tooth must be assessed. The crown of the third molars, which are mesioangularly or horizontally impacted may lie below the height of contour of the second molar and may require odontectomy for its safe removal without damaging the second molar. These teeth are also known to cause resorption of the interdental bone and the roots of the second molar, due to chronic pressure. Removal of the interdental bone during surgery should be avoided as it may lead to pocket formation, cemental sensitivity and caries.
- Associated diseases like oral submucous fibrosis not only restrict the mouth opening, but also render the oral mucosa stiff. The removal of third molars in such patients is difficult as the access is difficult and the forceful retraction may lead to tearing of the stiff buccal mucosa and significant bleeding. This is a common occurrence in the patients from this part of the world.

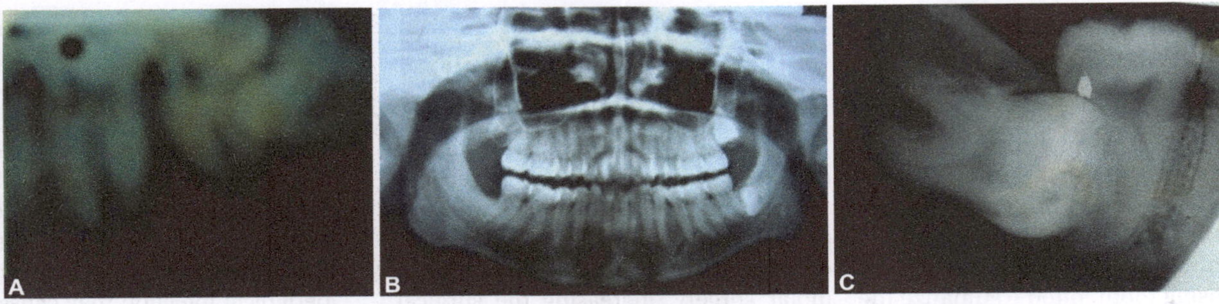

Figs 12.15A to C: (A) Improper; (B and C) Proper radiographs

- Position of the tooth in relation to the external oblique ridge, adjacent tooth, presence of divergent ramus, should also be evaluated to facilitate the decision regarding the incision, bone removal, odontectomy.

Radiological Evaluation

The radiological evaluation is very crucial for the third molar surgery.[15] A good quality periapical X-ray should normally be adequate to evaluate the third molars properly. However, if they are placed very deep or posteriorly their complete visualization on the periapical radiograph is not possible, in such cases an extraoral X-ray like lateral oblique view or panoramic view of mandible should be taken and the complete tooth should be visualized (Figs 12.15A to C). The impacted mandibular third molar will produce a classical 'Bull's eye' image on periapical radiograph when it is in linguoversion (Fig. 12.16).

The findings that should be studied on the X-ray are:

- The size of the crown and roots.
- The number and form of the roots, i.e. fused, conical, divergent, dilacerated, hypercementosed, etc.
- The relation with the adjacent tooth, resorption of the roots of the adjacent tooth.
- Any carious undermining of the crown which can make the tooth structure fragile.
- Presence of any periapical pathology.
- Associated pathologies like cyst or tumor.
- Depth of the tooth in the bone and its angulations.
- Relation of the apices of the root of the third molar with inferior alveolar canal—the inferior alveolar canal starts lingually near the foramen as it goes inferiorly and anteriorly towards the mental foramen; it gradually curls to the buccal side. Normally, the roots of the third molar are present buccal to the canal, however, as the X-rays are two dimensional pictures, due to superimposition it will appear as if the roots are in very close proximity of the canal. In some cases the roots are really in a very close proximity of the canal and if proper care is not taken may lead to damage to the nerve. To avoid such accidents the following points must be critically observed on the X-ray. The relation of the apices with the canal could be as follows as per the JP Rood criteria (Figs 12.17A to E):

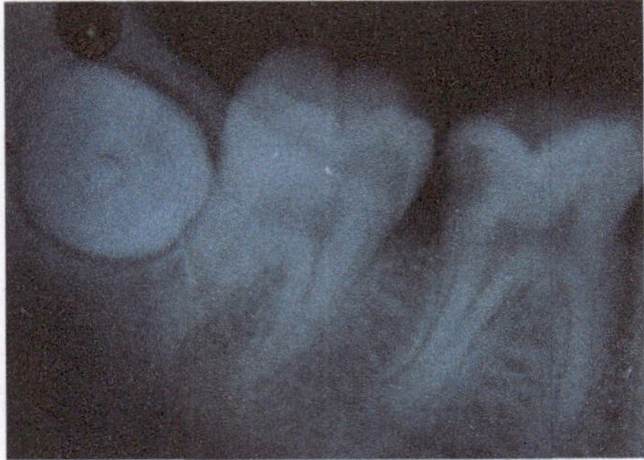

Fig. 12.16: Classical 'Bull's eye' image of impacted mandibular third molar when it is in linguoversion

Related but not Involving the Canal

- Separated
- Adjacent
- Superimposed.

Related to Changes in the Roots

- Darkening of the root (radiolucent)
- Dark and bifid root
- Narrowing of the root
- Deflected root.

Related with Changes in the Canal

- Interruption (loss) of white line
- Converging canal (narrowing)
- Diverted canal

Tube Shift Technique (Clark's Rule;[16] Buccal Object Rule) (Figs 12.18A to F)

The rationale of this procedure is derived from the manner in which the relative positions of radiographic images of two separate objects change when the projection angle at which the images were made is changed.

If the tube is shifted and directed at the reference object (e.g. the apex of a tooth) from a more mesial angulation and the object in question also moves mesially with respect to the reference object, then the object lies lingual to the reference object. Alternatively, if the tube is shifted mesially and the object in question appears to move distally, it lies on the buccal aspect of the reference object. These relations can be easily remembered by the acronym SLOB: same-lingual, opposite-buccal. Thus, if the object in question appears to move in the same direction with respect to the reference structures as the X-ray tube, it is on the lingual aspect of the reference object, if it appears to move in the opposite direction as the X-ray tube, it is on the buccal aspect. If it does not move with respect to the reference object,

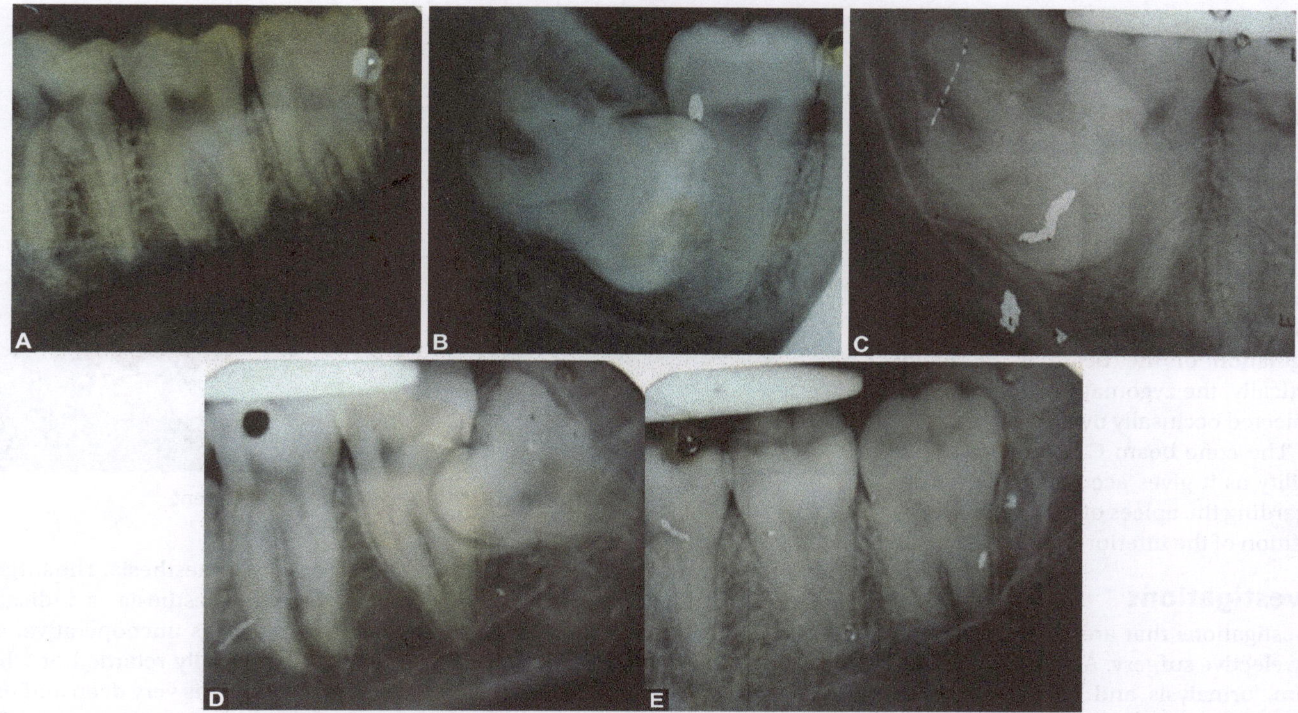

Figs 12.17A to E: (A) Darkening of the roots; (B and E) Loss of cortication of the canal; (C) Deflection of the canal; (D) Narrowing of the roots; (E) Break in continuity of the canal (Rood's JP criteria 1990[6])

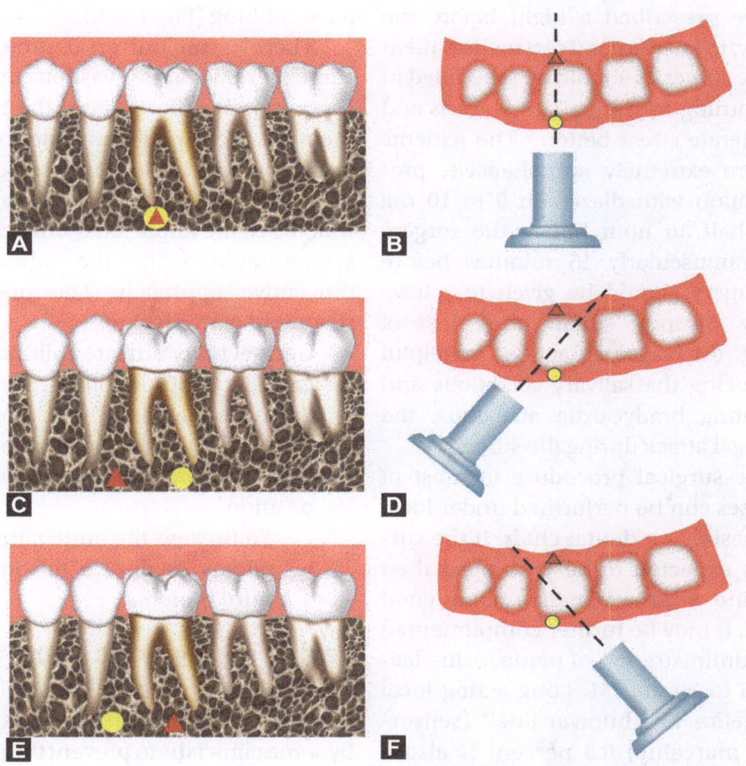

Figs 12.18A to F: Tube shift technique

it lies at the same depth (in the same vertical plane) as the reference object.

Examination of a conventional set of full-mouth films with this rule in mind will demonstrate that the incisive foramen in indeed lingual (palatal) to the roots of the central incisors and the mental foramen is buccal to the roots of the premolars. This procedure will assist in determining the position of impacted teeth, foreign objects or other abnormal conditions. It works just as well as when the X-ray machine is moved in the vertical plane as in the horizontal plane.

As sometimes happens, the surgeon may have two radiographs of a region of the dentition that were made at different angles, but there is no record of the orientation of the X-ray machine. Comparison of the image fields (i.e. the changed positions of the bony anatomy with respect to the teeth) will help distinguish changes in horizontal or vertical angulations. For instance, the image of lateral incisor on an incisor view will be projected from the mesial than it will on a canine view. Similarly, the relative positions of the osseous landmarks—such as the inferior border of the zygomatic process of the maxilla or the anterior border of the mandibular ramus, with respect to the teeth will help identify changes in horizontal or vertical angulations. These two structures lie buccal to the teeth and will appear to move mesially as the beam is oriented more from the distal. Similarly, as the angulation of the beam is increased vertically, the zygomatic process will be projected occlusally over the teeth.

The cone beam CT is a very useful facility as it gives accurate information regarding the apices of the roots and the position of the inferior alveolar canal.

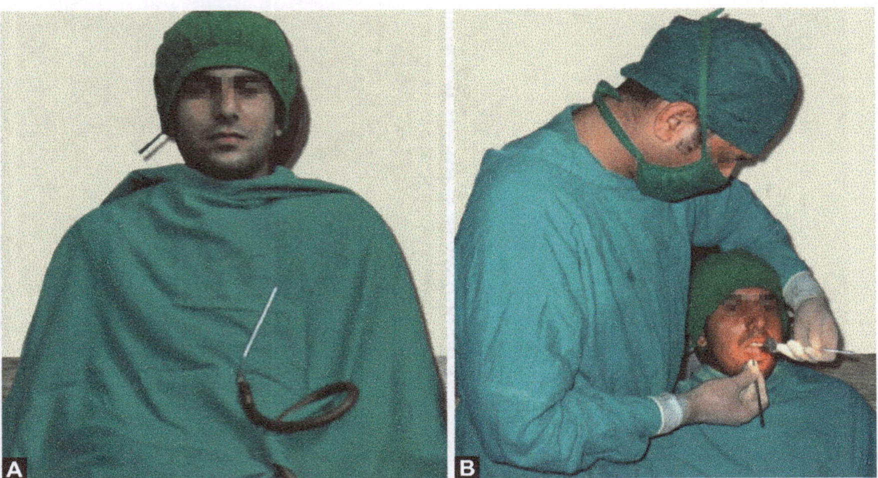

Figs 12.19A and B: Proper draping of the patient

Investigations

Investigations that are desirable before any elective surgery. A complete hemogram, urinalysis and coagulation profile (BT, CT) are the minimum required investigations. Other relevant investigations should be done, whenever indicated in a particular case.

Part Preparation

As the surgery is performed intraorally the mouth preparation should be done to prevent infections. It comprises of scaling, eradicating any active septic focus, preoperatively. The patient is prescribed antiseptic mouth wash like Chlorhexidine or Povidine iodine to reduce the count of microorganisms, at least 24 hours prior to the surgery. The final intraoral and extraoral part preparation is done immediately preceding the surgery. The skin of the perioral area needs to be prepared as the surgeon and assistant touch it during the retraction of the tissue and during supporting the mandible, while the elevators are used. The final preparation can be done using 5 percent povidone iodine solution. After the part is prepared, the surgical field is isolated by draping (Figs 12.19A and B).

Premedication[17]

The patient should be prescribed preoperative prophylactic antibiotics. The Beta-lactam group of antibiotics give good prophylaxis as the organisms causing contamination are gram- positive and come from oral flora. Higher antibiotics are usually not required unless specifically indicated or the patient is immunocompromised. Immunization against the tetanus may be done by giving 0.5 mL tetanus toxoid, intramuscular, for the patients who are previously not immunized. The sedatives may be prescribed a night before the surgery, to ensure good rest to the patient and the surgeries should be scheduled in the morning as the patient is fresh and can tolerate stress better.[18] The patients who are extremely apprehensive, premedication with diazepam 5 to 10 mg orally half an hour before the surgery or intramuscularly 15 minutes before the surgery should be given to relieve anxiety. Atropine sulfate, in a dose of 0.6 mg. IM (vagolytic action) is helpful in reducing the salivary secretions and preventing bradycardia and thus, the vasovagal attack during the surgery.

The surgical procedure in most of the cases can be performed under local anesthesia, in a dental chair. If the surgery is expected to be prolonged then lidocaine with adrenaline is a good choice. It may be further complimented with administration of pentazocine lactate 15 to 30 mg IM. Long acting local anesthetics like bupivacaine[19] (sensorcaine, marcaine) 0.5 percent is also a good anesthetic agent, which gives sufficient duration of anesthesia. The surgery under general anesthesia is indicated when the patient is uncooperative, apprehensive, mentally retarded or when he impacted tooth is very deep and may require long and extensive surgery. The surgical trolley should be thoughtfully arranged and all the required instruments should be properly arranged and checked by the surgeon before he goes for scrubbing (Fig. 12.20).

There is no universal protocol for surgical removal of wisdom tooth as every case is different and the requirement of every patient is variable. The preferences and opinions of the surgeons are also variable. Some dental surgeons wait to see the impacted tooth becoming symptomatic, while the others have preventive approach. The preventive treatment comprises of:

- Germectomy[20] in late childhood
- Lateral trephination and removal during adolescent.
- A curative approach involves exposure of crown if tooth has good position
  - To prevent the anticipated complications due to the impacted third molars.

Early Prophylactic Removal

The early prophylactic removal of the impacted third molar is recommended by some clinicians to prevent the possible complications related to the impacted

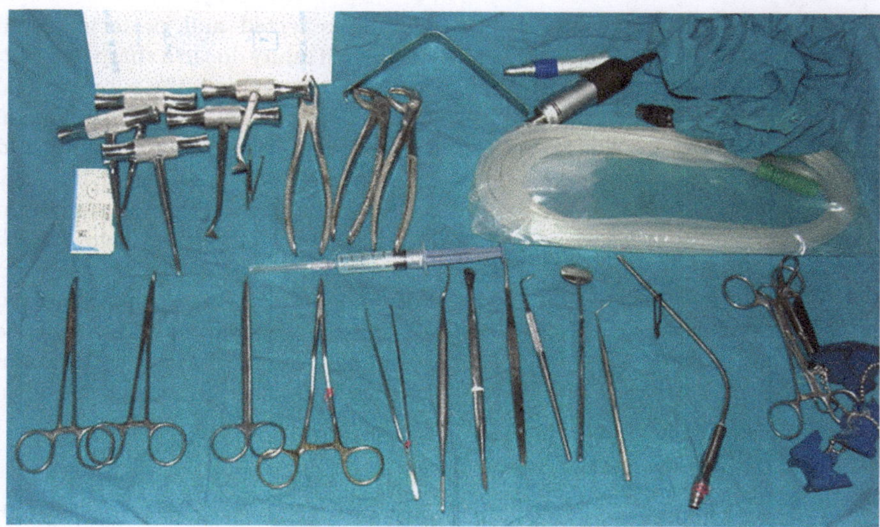

Fig. 12.20: Armamentarium for the third molar surgery

third molar such as pain, recurrent pericoronitis, development of pathologies, etc. It is also argued that if the impacted third molars are removed late the surgery is more difficult and surgical complications can occur. On the other hand removal of developing tooth bud before the root formation is complete, the removal is easy and in the younger age the bones have excellent elasticity and facilitate the surgical procedure. The healing is also faster and uneventful in younger patients.

Advantages

The early prophylactic removal is easy:

- Root formation not complete
- Pericoronal space is wide
- Bone is more elastic in early age
- Operative and postoperative complications are less
- Healing is uneventful
- Morbidity of periodontal tissue is reduced.

Disadvantages

Excellent clinical judgment and motivation for extraction in early age is challenging to clinician.

Late Therapeutic Removal

Disadvantage of Advancing Age

- Unfavorable and bizarre root morphology
- Bone becomes brittle and sclerosed
- Healing is not satisfactory
- More amount bone removal is required
- More discomfort to patient.

Advantages

- Therapeutic removal is done to treat inflammatory component.
- Patient motivation is not a problem. However, it is very difficult to motivate the patients to undergo prophylactic surgical removal of the third molar as they are totally asymptomatic. Most of the third molars are removed only when they become symptomatic.

SURGICAL PROCEDURE

The surgical procedure will be discussed under the following heads:

- Incision, designing and reflection of the flap
- Removal of the bone
- Odontectomy
- Preparation of the wound for closure
- Suturing
- Postoperative care.

Designing of the Flap

While designing the flap all the basic principles of flap designing must be followed. The incisions and flaps recommended for the third molar surgery are:

- Envelope flap (Fig. 12.21A)
- Three cornered flap
  - Ward I incision[21] (Fig. 12.21B)
  - Ward II incision (Fig. 12.21C)
  - Modified ward incision
  - L shaped incision.

The ward I and II incisions are more commonly practiced. The vertical leg of the incision is placed along the anterior border of the ramus. The incision follows the anterior border of the anterior border of ramus and is slightly lateral to it. If the incision is placed lingually there are chances of damage to the lingual nerve and the nutrient vessels in the retromolar area. The length of the incision is decided as per the requirement in a given case. One centimeter length of the incision is

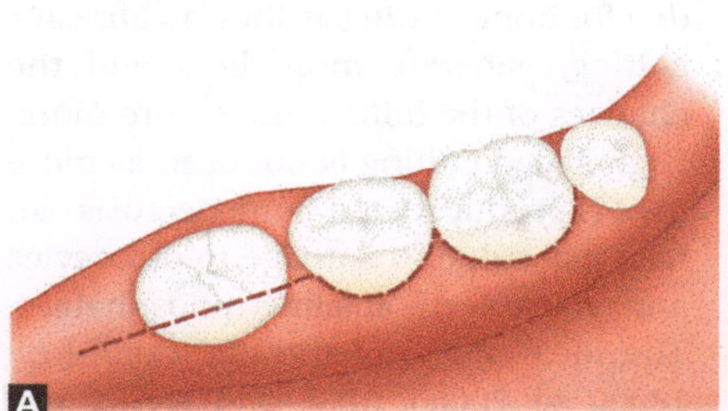

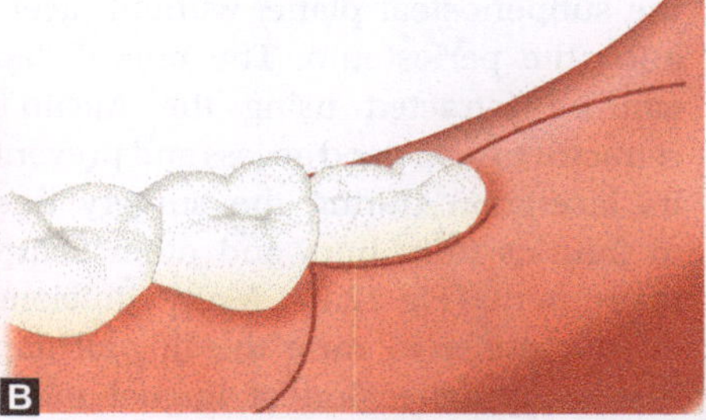

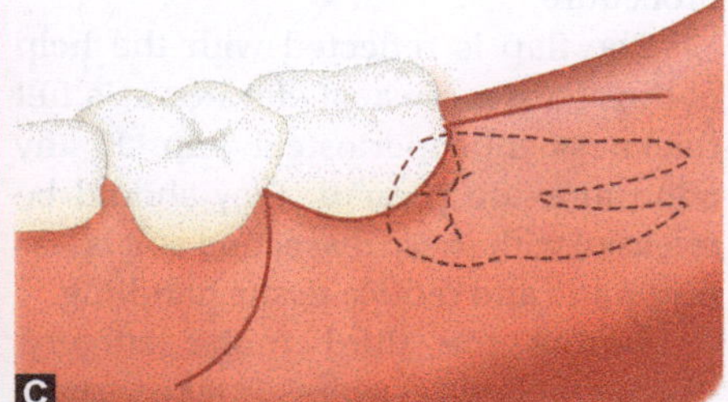

Figs 12.21A to C: (A) Envelope incision; (B) Ward I incision; (C) Ward II incision

usually adequate. If the incision is too long and lateral, there may be exposure of the buccal pad of fat. If the tooth is erupted then the incision extends anteriorly in the gingival crevice of the third molar up to the distal aspect of the second molar. In ward I incision the vertical relieving incision is placed distal to the second molar and in ward II incision it is mesial to the second molar, which inclines over the buccal alveolar bone at an angle of 45 degree to the horizontal incision in the gingival crevice. If the third molar is unerupted then the vertical incision directly starts from distal of the second molar. While taking the vertical relieving incision if the knife slips the facial artery may get injured and profuse bleeding may take place. To avoid such an accident a beginner must direct the knife from the depth of the vestibule to the gingival margin and not the other way round. The incision must be full thickness and the tissues must be incised in one stroke. The flap should be designed in such a way that the access to the surgical site should be direct and passive. The proposed surgical defect must be taken into account and the suture line should rest on the healthy bone and cover and defect adequately. Small incisions do not facilitate free and passive access to the surgical site and forceful retractions of the tissue is required which enhances the tissue handling, tissue trauma and thus, more postoperative edema. It is incorrect to think that the shorter incisions are less traumatic or they heal faster than the long incisions. The healing across the incision is a simultaneous process and is not affected by the length of the incision. The degloving incision is recommended only for the teeth, which are very deep in the bone or for lateral trephnization procedure.[22]

The flap is reflected with the help of the sharp periosteal elevator as a full thickness mucoperiosteal flap. If any adhesions are present, they should be released with sharp dissection as it is less traumatic and reduce tissue handling.

During the third molar surgery, usually the buccal access is taken as the lingual split technique is complicated. The buccal flap is raised, necessarily in the subperiosteal plane, without lacerating the periosteum. The buccal flap can be retracted using the Austin's retractor to gain good access and prevent its laceration during the surgery due to injuries from burs and other sharp instruments (Fig. 12.22). Many clinicians do not prefer to raise the lingual flap due to apprehension of lingual nerve damage. However, it is safe to reflect the lingual flap as well, as the tissue can be reflected and protected from accidental injury due to a sharp object. It is mandatory to be in the subperiosteal plane to avoid damage to the lingual nerve as it lies supraperiosteally and is safely reflected along with the flap. (Figs 12.23A and B). The second reason for reflecting the lingual flap is that the bone on the distolingual aspect (distolingual lock) of the impacted third molar should be removed to facilitate the luxation of the third molar and without raising the lingual flap the bone removal is difficult.

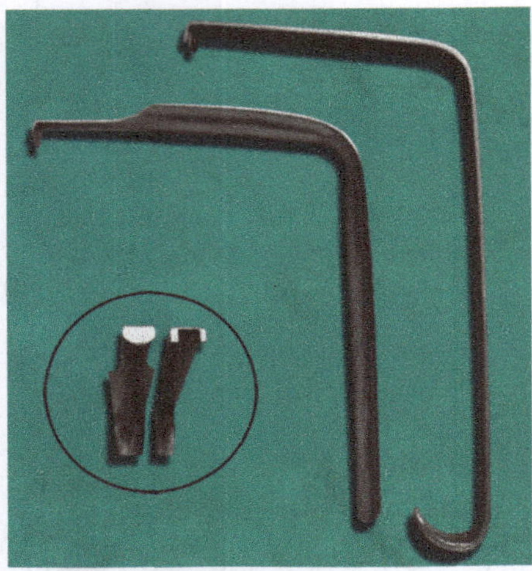

Fig. 12.22: Austin's retractor, traumatic and atraumatic used for retraction of the mucoperiosteal flap

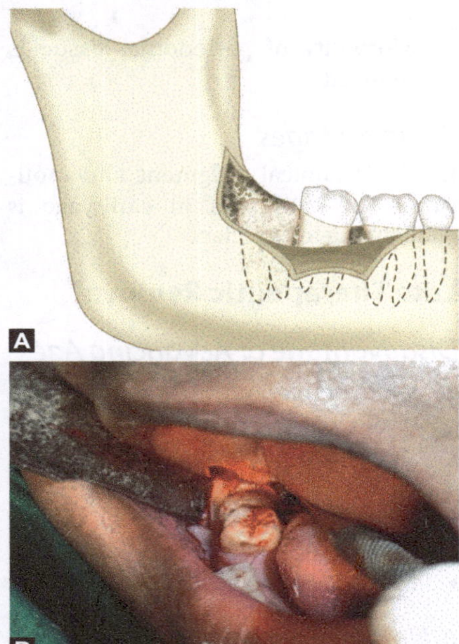

Figs 12.23A and B: Flap reflection—showing reflection of (A) Buccal; (B) Lingual flaps

Removal of Bone

As the third molars are covered with bone, to create the access it is removed. The bone cutting can be done with the help of a bur and dental motor or with the help of a chisel and mallet.[23] The chisel and mallet is not a preferred method as better and more effective rotary instruments are available. The use of the chisel and mallet evokes more anxiety in a patient operated under local anesthesia. If the chisel and mallet is used two vertical stop cuts are first made at the anterior and posterior boundaries of the proposed bony defect and then the intervening bone is removed to prevent the splitting of the bone along the bone grains. The chisel should be sharp and heavy mallet blows should be avoided to prevent fracture of the bone. The chisel must have a good purchase on the bone to prevent its slipping and a guard must be kept to prevent damage to the soft tissue. The mandible must be supported, while applying the mallet blows to prevent dislocation.

The sharp stainless steel or carbide burs should be used for the bone cutting. The diamond burs are not recommended for bone cutting as they do abrasive cutting, generate more heat and the chances of the bone necrosis are more. High speed cutting is not used as more heat is produced and bone necrosis can take place due to damage to osteocytes and release of alkaline phosphatase. The ideal speed of the bur should be 18000 to 20000 RPM and the motor should have good torque to facilitate the bone removal at the lower speed.

Use of air rotors is contraindicated not only for the above reason, but due to the chances of surgical emphysema as air under pressure can enter in the open tissue planes. During the bone cutting with the help of a bur, first round bur is used to mark the incision and then the fissure bur is used. The round bur gets good purchase on the bone and does not slip. The soft tissues are protected by retraction and by placing guard. Copious irrigation with normal saline is done during the bone cutting to dissipate the heat and to flush the bone particles to prevent the clogging of the bur.[24]

The bone is removed judiciously as the bone is to be preserved. The tooth is to be sacrificed and thus, the tooth should be sectioned and removed in pieces to prevent excessive bone cutting. The bone in the area is weak due to the reasons already discussed. It is buttressed by the external oblique ridge and if the excessive bone is removed from this area it is rendered weaker and may fracture during the surgery. The bone removal should be just enough to expose the crown up to the CE junction (Figs 12.24A and B). The bone in the distolingual area usually prevents the elevation of the tooth (distolingual lock) and hence, should be removed carefully. Usually the bone is removed distobucally to expose the crown and facilitates the application of the elevator; it is called preparation of the distobuccal gutter (Moore Gilby's collar technique). The bone must be removed under the direct vision and after carefully observing where the tooth is getting locked during the elevation. The bone removal done blindly will invariably lead to unnecessary and excessive bone removal. When the tooth is placed deep in the bone, horizontally or mesioangularly impacted, the crown is bulbous and lies very close and below the height of contour of the second molar, it is advisable to split the crown in pieces rather than doing excessive bone cutting or damaging the adjacent tooth or bone.

After the removal of the bone a purchase point or groove is prepared on the third molar for engaging the tip of the elevator. The purchase groove should not be very superficial as proper purchase may not be obtained. It should be made with plenty of margin of tooth structure or else the thin tooth structure will fracture when the force is applied with an elevator. The elevator should not be wedged between the second and third molar for creating purchase as the second molar may get damaged. The bone in the younger individuals is elastic and resilient and yields to the pressure easily and thus, the younger individuals the tooth can be easily elevated and removed. The similar kind of tooth will not be easily elevated in the older patient as the bone tends to be more compact and brittle.

ODONTECTOMY

The splitting of the crown of the tooth is called odontectomy. It is done to facilitate removal of the tooth in pieces without excessive bone cutting. The dictum that "*tooth belongs to surgeon and bone belongs to patient*" must be followed. As the tooth is to be discarded it can be cut as per the need but bone is precious and need to be dealt judiciously. If the tooth is sectioned in a planned manner the operator will have good control over the remaining portion of the roots and will be able to remove them with ease than removing the fragments of the tooth, which fractures haphazardly during the forceful elevation. The indications for odontectomy are:

- Large bulbous crown.
- Deep horizontal or mesioangular impactions.
- Disto angular impactions with plenty of bone cover.
- Unfavorable root form like divergent, locking or dilacerated roots.
- Hyper cementosed roots.
- Roots in close proximity of the inferior alveolar canal.
- Badly carious and fragile tooth structure.

The other advantage of the odontectomy is that after the crown is sectioned and removed it creates a space for delivering/removal of the roots. This avoids the rotation of the roots in the bone, while elevating the tooth and prevents the damage to the inferior alveolar nerve (Figs 12.25A to C). The odontectomy may be performed with the help of the burs or sharp chisels. If straight hand piece does not facilitate proper access then contra angled or modified contra angled handpiece may be used. The odontectomy cuts are marked with stainless steel or carbide burs. The use of diamond bur is very convenient for this purpose. It is not necessary to split the tooth by taking a full thickness cuts with the help of bur. The tooth is split up to two third of its thickness with the bur and the remaining portion may be split with a chisel or with the help of an elevator wedged in the cut and giving slight leverage to fracture the remaining portion. The tooth may be split in two, three or four pieces, as shown in the figure, depending upon the requirement in an individual case[7] (Figs 12.26A to E).

Many a times in spite of all precautions the apical third of the root

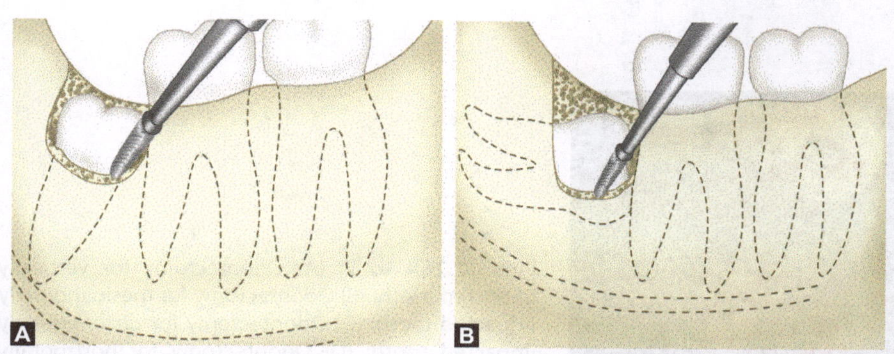

Figs 12.24A and B: (A) Bone removal for vertically impacted tooth; (B) Bone removal for horizontally impacted tooth

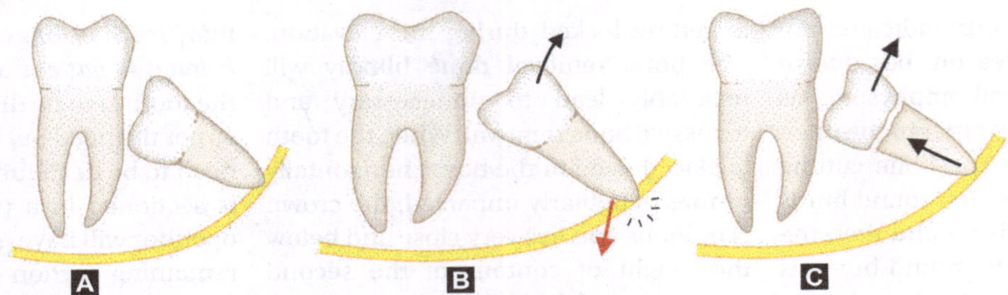

Figs 12.25A to C: Arc of rotation of the third molar while elevation resulting in the damage to the nerve, odontectomy avoids the damage to the nerve

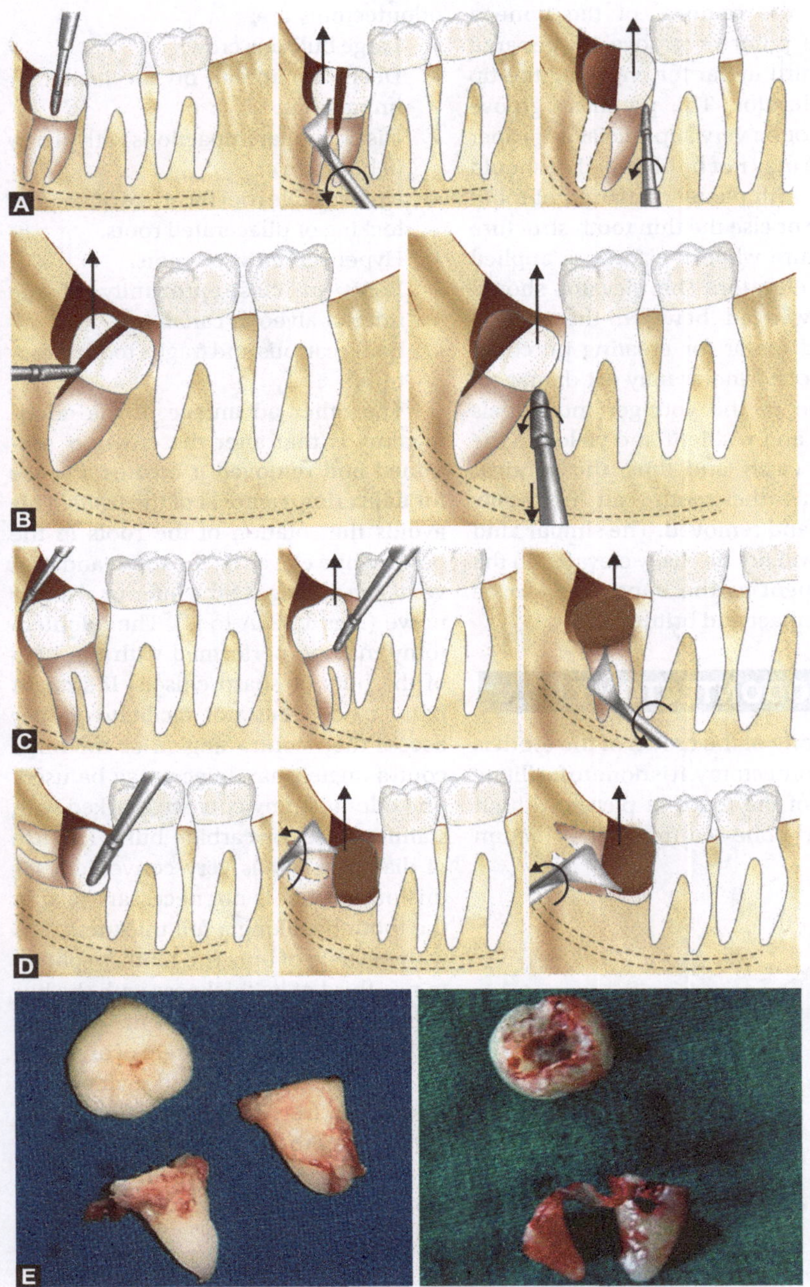

Figs 12.26A to E: (A) Odontectomy for vertically impacted tooth; (B) Odontectomy for mesioangularly impacted tooth; (C) Odontectomy for distoangularly impacted tooth; (D) Odontectomy for horizontally impacted tooth; (E) Odontectomy specimen

fractures, while delivering the roots. Purposefully leaving the root fragment, root tip does not necessarily mean the negligence of surgeon, but it could be deliberate decision and as a part of standard care.[25]

Criteria for Leaving the Root Fragment

- When the root is free of any periapical pathology, which is true in majority of cases of impacted third molars.
- When there is possibility of damage to the vital structures, while attempting the removal of the root fragments.
- If the root is inaccessible to direct vision or reflected vision with the mouth mirror or when the root is likely to be displaced in an inaccessible area where it is going to be very difficult to remove.
- If it is a minor fragment of about 5 mm length.

Usually the root tips remain harmless in and should be observed periodically for detecting any pathological changes in the bone and undergo some degree of resorption. As the alveolar bone recedes following the removal of the tooth the fragments often become superficial and their removal becomes easy subsequently, however this takes a long time. If the root becomes symptomatic due to infection, the root fragment becomes loose due to inflammatory process and its tracking and removal becomes easy. If the root fragment is left it must be informed to the patient.

Debridement and Preparation of the Wound for Closure

The key words to be remembered after the tooth has been extracted are '*see, feel and freshen, close*'. The wound is thoroughly prepared for closure. The area is packed to achieve initial hemostasis and then thoroughly inspected for the presence of any foreign bodies like fragments of the tooth, loose bony fragments, granulation tissue or any periapical pathological tissue like cystic lining. The foreign bodies are picked up and the granulation tissue and the residual cystic lining are curetted. The alveolar bone margins are palpated and any loose bony fragments, devoid of periosteal attachment, which can turn non-vital are removed. The sharp bony margins are filed off and made smooth as they can interfere with the healing by inducing irritation and inflammation of the flap. Any lacerated margins of the flap are carefully trimmed as they can get necrosed and result in the dehiscence of the wound. When the impacted third molar is partially erupted in the oral cavity, the gingival margin around it has reduplicated epithelial edge (*gingival cuff*). It should be freshened up by excising the margin as the epithelium to epithelium contact can prevent healing.

Suturing

The closure of the prepared surgical wound is done with 3'0' silk or vicryl suture. The simple interrupted sutures are placed. The first suture that should be placed is the suture at the distal end of the second molar, because if there is dehiscence in the suture line, distal pocket formation will take place with the second molar and recurrent periodontal complications can occur. The sutures should not be placed too tightly, as it can result in strangulation of the wound edges and avascular necrosis of the wound edges leading dehiscence. The tight closure will prevent decompression of the wound and lead to excessive inflammatory edema. Hence, the sutures should be placed loosely. The purpose of the suture is to approximate the tissue and not to achieve the water tight closure. The sutures should be equidistant and should exert uniform pressure on the wound edge, throughout the length of the incision. The knots should be placed on one side and not on the incision line. The sutures are removed on the seventh postoperative day. Figures 12.27A to J illustrates step-by-step technique for the removal of an impacted mandibular third molar.

Follow-up

The patient is called periodically for the follow-up. The first visit is preferably on subsequent day wherein apart from edema, pain, trismus, wound condition the evaluation of the lingual and inferior alveolar nerves is carried out. The neurological evaluation is planned on first postoperative day because the effect of local anesthesia totally wanes off by then and early detection and explanation to the patient can be done, if the neurological deficit is present. The neurological examination is done by assessing the perception of fine touch, prick and two point discrimination. Similarly the taste sensation on the tongue can also be ascertained.

Postoperative Care

A pressure pack is given postoperatively, which should be maintained for about an hour to achieve adequate hemostasis. In the immediate postoperative phase the vascular phase of the inflammation is predominant which is characterized by vasodilatation and increased capillary permeability. This leads to formation of inflammatory edema. To prevent the excessive edema formation, cold compressions are advised, intermittently for first 24 hours. The application of cold induces vasoconstriction and prevents excessive edema. The edema leads to raised interstitial fluid pressure, compression of lymphatics, capillaries and venules, stasis of circulation and may retard healing. The excessive edema distends the tissue and generates tension across the suture line, which can lead to dehiscence of the wound. To reduce the edema and to correct the stasis of circulation, the patient is prescribed anti-inflammatory drugs. One should not heavily rely on the drugs but, simpler things like warm saline gargles and Glycerin-magnesium sulfate dressings, given extraorally can be very helpful. The warm saline gargles improve the circulation by inducing vasodilatation and facilitate the reabsorption of the interstitial fluid, thus reducing interstitial fluid

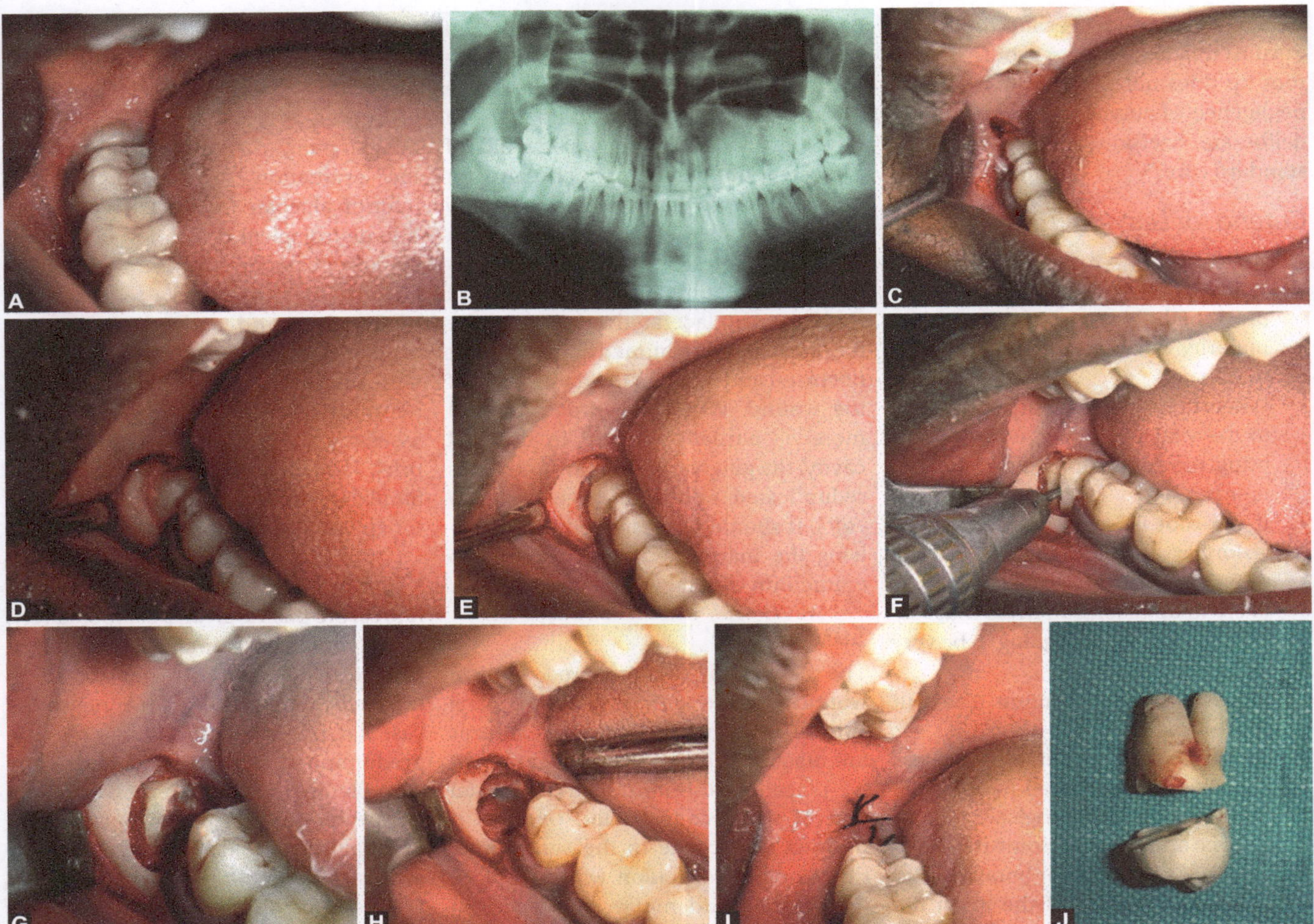

Figs 12.27A to J: Step-by-step procedure for removal of impacted third molar: (A) Preoperative clinical photograph; (B) OPG; (C) Ward I incision; (D) Reflection of the flap; (E) Removal of the bone by Gillby collar technique; (F) Odontectomy; (G) After odontectomy; (H) Removal of the complete tooth; (I) Loose suturing; (J) Odontectomy specimen

pressure. The glycerin magnesium sulfate dressing is hygroscopic in nature and thus draws the fluid across the skin, which acts like a semipermeable membrane. The reaction of glycerin with magnesium sulfate is exothermic and works as hot fermentations and induces vasodilatation and improves the circulation. The warm saline gargles have dual effect the warmth induces vasodilatation and improves the circulation, reduces stasis, mucosal congestion, improves local drug delivery and ensures that humoral factors necessary for promoting healing reach the site. The saline solution has more tonicity than the tissue fluid and thus, draws the fluid from the tissue across the mucosa. This should be done after 24 hours, as by this time the vascular stage of inflammation settles and cellular stage starts which is important to prevent infection and promote healing. The use of steroids as anti-inflammatory drug has been mentioned in the literature and some clinicians do recommend them but, it must be remembered that simpler things like tissue respect (less tissue handling), sound surgical technique, less bone trauma, good wound preparation before closure, loose sutures, aseptic technique help in reducing the changes of generation of excessive edema. The measures mentioned above help in preventing and reducing the edema and should be tried rather than opting for steroid therapy. The patient is prescribed antibiotics and analgesics apart from anti-inflammatory drugs. Normally the edema increases up to first 48 to 72 hours and then gradually starts receding. The oral hygiene and the wound hygiene are maintained by antiseptic gargles using chlorhexidine or povidone iodine solution or by toileting (irrigation) of the wound with normal saline solution. The patient obviously has trismus, edema and pain and discomfort postoperatively. The movements of jaw will further aggravate the pain and discomfort, hence, the patient is prescribed soft and semisolid diet.

Alternative Technique

The above mentioned technique is a standard surgical technique. As the third molar is situated in the lingual shelf of bone, which is thin, William Kelsyfry recommended "Lingual split technique".[26] According to him it is easy, less traumatic to remove the thin lingual bone and deliver the tooth lingually. In this technique a good bucco-lingual flaps are raised. After guarding the lingual soft tissues adequately, the lingual cortical bone is removed and the tooth is delivered lingually. This technique is difficult to master and the chances of lingual nerve damage are more.

Coronectomy

The removal of crown of the impacted tooth and leaving behind the roots is a procedure described as coronectomy. It is indicated in the cases where the third molars are deep (position C) and the roots are in proximity with the inferior alveolar nerve. To prevent the damge to the nerve it is recommended that the crown should be excised and the roots should be left behind. As the tooth becomes non-functional the roots become resorbed and with the resorption of the alveolar bone and its remodeling, they become superficial and are easy to remove and the chances of damage to the inferior alveolar nerve are minimized. It is practiced with variable success by many clinicians. The complications with this technique could be infection and development of pathology with the retained root could be late complication.

COMPLICATIONS OF THIRD MOLAR SURGERY

- **Edema:** Certain amount of inflammatory edema is a normal occurrence after the third molar surgery. The excessive edema is as a result of excessive tissue handling, excessive bone cutting, bone necrosis, tight wound closure preventing the drainage of exudate or as a result of secondary infection.

  The edema can be prevented by ensuring that the tissue is handled judiciously, bone is cooled during removal with copious saline irrigation and the sutures are loosely placed to facilitate the drainage of inflammatory exudates and collected blood. The edema resolves fast in 72 hours and no vigorous treatment is warranted. The other interventions necessary to reduce the inflammatory edema are discussed earlier. The suture line of vertical reliving incision of Ward incision which rests on the alveolar bone may be left open without suturing to ensure decompression and it helps in reducing the edema.
- **Trismus:** The trismus is usually a temporary phenomenon secondary to protective muscle spasm, secondary to pain at the site of surgery and gets relieved within 4 to 5 days. But if it is severe and persists longer it could be due to injury to the tendon of temporalis muscle or injury to the medial pterygoid muscle or ligaments during the administration of the inferior alveolar nerve block. If the surgery is prolonged or if the lower jaw is not adequately supported during elevation of the tooth, the TMJ can get strained and arthritis can result leading to trismus, pain during mandibular movements and the tenderness over the joint. Such cases often require extended medicinal treatment with anti-inflammatory drugs and physiotherapy. The physiotherapy comprises of short wave diathermy, forceful jaw opening using mouth gags after the acute stage has subsided, followed by jaw exercises.
- **Dry socket:** The details of this condition are described under the exodontias.
- **Infection:** The infection could be the exacerbation of the previous pericoronitis, which was not adequately resolved or the infection acquired postoperatively. If the local signs of infection like congestion, purulent discharge are evident in the wound, one suture may be removed to decompress/drain the infective material to prevent its spread. As the tissues are dissected during the surgery and the anatomical barriers are broken the infection rapidly spreads to pterygomandibular or buccal spaces. The incidence of infection following the removal of third molars is very low.[10]
- Osteomyelitis
- Fracture of the alveolar bone, especially the lingual cortical plate
- Fracture of the jaw—due to injudicious application of excessive force with heavy elevators and injudicious bone removal.
- Damage to the lingual nerve—the lingual nerve damage results from injury to the lingual nerve due to fracture of the lingual cortical plate, sharp instruments or slipping of the burs. The taste fibers are relayed in the lingual nerve from chorda tympani nerve and once they are damaged, the taste sensations are very seldom restored.
- Hemorrhage—damage to the facial artery, inferior alveolar artery.
- Dislodgements of the tooth in the sublingual space.
- Damage to the second molar—distal pocket formation, sensitivity due to exposure of the root, luxation fracture.

MAXILLARY CANINE IMPACTIONS

Introduction

The permanent maxillary canines are developed deep within the maxilla, complete their development late and emerge into the oral cavity after the neighboring teeth have erupted. Due to these circumstances, eruption disturbances are more common with maxillary canines than with other teeth, except for third molars.

Mineralization of the primary canine starts at 4 to 12 months of age and is complete by 6 to 7 years of age. Tooth germs are in close contact with apices of primary canine as well as lateral incisor and first premolar. During eruption the canine moves down along the distal aspect of the lateral incisor, not in very close contact with it.

Clinically, palpation of the buccal surface of the alveolar process distal to the lateral incisor may reveal the position of the maxillary canine about 1 to 1/2 years before its emergence. During the active phases of eruption, i.e. 1 to 2 years before oral emergence, the width of the dental follicle increases, whereas the size of the follicle decreases in cases of impacted teeth.

Incidence

The prevalence of non-eruption or ectopic eruption of maxillary canine is reported to a range from 0.8 to 2.3 percent. It is seen with a higher frequency in females as compared to males. Most commonly, it is found unilaterally. The most common position of the impacted canine is palatal to the lateral incisor. In only 15 percent of the cases the direction of impaction is seen buccally.

Etiology[27,28]

- **Space loss:** It can occur in dentition with severe crowding, but most frequently it is seen in dentitions without crowding.
- Ectopic position of tooth germ.
- **Delayed resorption of root of primary canine:** It is most commonly a sequlae of impacted canine rather than being an etiologic factor.
- **Lack of guidance from gubernacular canal:** If the gubernacular canal does not widen normally during development or if there is an obliteration of the canal, impaction may result.
- Root tip deflection.
- **Heredity:** An autosomal recessive trait has been suggested for canine impactions.
- **Space augmentation:** In cases of excessive space availability, the guidance of the root of lateral incisor for eruption of the canine is not available and may result into impaction.
- **Obstruction to eruption pathway:** The eruption may be prevented by presence of supernumerary teeth and odontomas. In addition; increased bone density, narrowed alveolar process and excessive fibrous mucosa may restrict eruption of canine.
- Cleft lip and palate cases.
- Trauma, due to partial destruction of follicle and subsequent development of ankylosis of tooth.

DIAGNOSTIC AIDS

Clinical inspection and palpation of the alveolar process in the canine region should be performed every year from the age of 8 years. Clinical examination should include an evaluation of number of permanent teeth in position and inclination of incisors as well as asymmetries between eruption patterns between both sides and its correlation with age and somatic maturity.

The alveolar process must be palpated from both buccal and palatal sides to feel for the canine bulge. Normally a bulge appears in the buccal sulcus in the canine region 1 to 1/2 years before eruption.[29]

If the canine bulge cannot be palpated between 8 and 10 years, a radiographic investigation is indicated. A normal IOPA and occlusal radiograph must be taken to study the canine form and position.

CLASSIFICATION

- **Class I:** Impacted canine located in the palate:
  - Horizontal
  - Vertical
  - Semi-vertical.
- **Class II:** Impacted canine located in the buccal side:
  - Horizontal
  - Vertical
  - Semi-vertical.
- **Class III:** Impacted canines located in both palatal as well as buccal alveolar bone.
- **Class IV:** Impacted canines located vertically between incisors and premolars.
- **Class V:** Impacted canines located in edentulous maxilla.

Management

Numerous treatment options exist for the ectopically erupting or impacted canines. These include:

- No treatment
- Prophylactic space augmentation
- Extraction of primary canine (guided eruption)
- Surgical exposure and orthodontic repositioning
- Surgical repositioning-not useful
- Removal of canine.

NO TREATMENT

Few cases of initially ectopic positioned canines spontaneously upright and show a normal eruption. The most common complication in absence of this spontaneous correction is development of a follicular cyst. So also, development of odontogenic tumors from the follicle is rarely seen. There is loss of attachment of the neighboring teeth with which the impacted canine is in close approximation.

Prophylactic Space Augmentation

Elimination of crowding in the dental arch to make room for the eruption of the impacted canines in some cases may stimulate eruption.

Extraction of Primary Canine

Extraction of primary canines is carried out to align a palatally erupting maxillary canine wherein there is no resorption of the incisor. This technique shows less favorable results with ectopic permanent canines.

Exposure and Orthodontic Repositioning

This is usually the treatment of choice in cases of ectopic positioning and normally leads to a predictable and successful result. However, the prognosis for orthodontic correction depends on several factors including age, space conditions and sagittal and transverse position of the canine crown and root. Even if there is a dentigerous cyst associated with an impacted canine and the canine is in favorable position and likely to erupt in oral cavity, marsupialization of the cyst is carried to conserve the canine.

Surgical Removal

Surgical technique varies with the position of the canine. Either a labial or palatal approach is used according to the position of the crown. Damage to adjacent tooth roots should be avoided.

Labially positioned canines are accessed by raising a semilunar flap or marginal flap according to the position of the crown. Pericoronal bone is removed with burs/chisel until the widest part of the crown and half of the root has been uncovered. Then the crown can be sectioned and elevated out. A purchase point is created in the root and it is elevated out. Socket is irrigated and flap repositioned (Figs 12.28A to F).

Palatally positioned crown is accessed from palatal side. A palatal flap is raised from premolar to premolar. Palatal gingiva can be spared by giving an incision a few millimeters from the marginal gingiva. Release incision should be avoided on the palatal side to avoid damage to the greater palatine neurovascular bundle. However, a midline palatal relieving incision can be given to manage unilateral impacted canine. Once the palatal flap is raised, bulge of the crown is located and a small access hole is made to visualize the crown and it is enlarged to uncover the entire crown and a part of the root. The crown is sectioned and elevated out. A purchase point is created in the root and it is elevated out. Socket is irrigated and flap repositioned (Figs 12.29 and 12.30). When the tooth is placed in class III position a combined buccal and palatal approach is taken first the buccal flap is raised and through the access created in the bone the root is sectioned from the crown and delivered buccally and then the crown is removed through the palatal access (Figs 12.31A to K).

Complications

- Perforation of maxillary sinus floor forming an oroantral communication.
- Perforation of nasal floor forming an oronasal communication.
- Hemorrhage from greater Palatine artery due to accidental damage, while using palatal approach.
- Damage to adjacent tooth roots from bur/chisel or application of excessive forces with elevator.

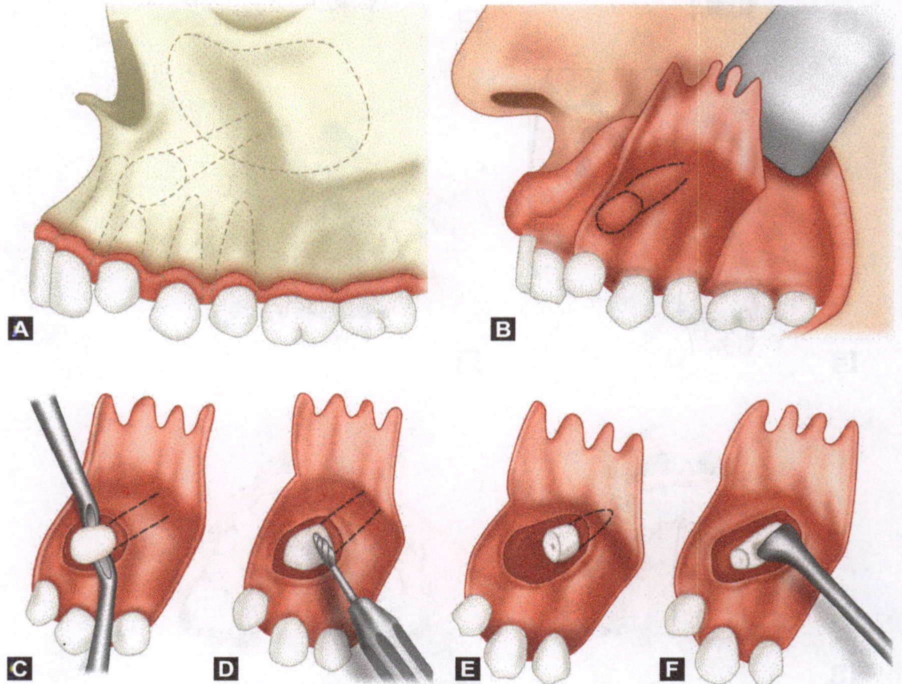

Figs 12.28A to F: Labial approach (*Source:* Archer HW, 1966)

IMPACTED MAXILLARY THIRD MOLAR

Introduction

The maxillary third molar starts its development at the cervical neck of the second molar and with the occlusal surface facing posteriorly. Start of mineralization can be seen radiographically at 8 to 10 years of age. The posteriorly tilted tooth gradually uprights during further crown and root formation and ends up with its axis being almost vertical. Maxillary third molars erupt at approximate age of 20 years, being 6 months late in females than males. However, extraction of any tooth anterior to it, results in advancement of eruption by 1.4 years and 1.3 years in males and females, respectively.

The maxillary third molars are often seen erupted in buccoversion. This position results into impingement of the soft tissue between the cusps of the tooth and the anterior border of coronoid process leading to traumatic ulcers and recurrent pain. The selective cuspal grinding of the third molar relieves the trauma from occlusion temporarily. If the clinician is not alert, it is observed that many a times this condition is labeled as pain due to pericoronitis with mandibular third molars and the lower third molars are subjected to surgical removal. Sometimes the operculum of the impacted mandibular third molar is traumatized by the upper third molar leading to pain. It is therefore recommended that the examination of the third molar should be comprehensive and both the upper and lower third molars should be thoroughly evaluated together. If one of the third molars is in a non-functional position and unlikely to be corrected in normal functional position and if there is no other consideration for their retention the decision needs to be taken for their removal simultaneously because if one tooth is removed the other becomes non-functional and supraerupts to cause trauma from occlusion, abnormal contact with adjacent tooth, food

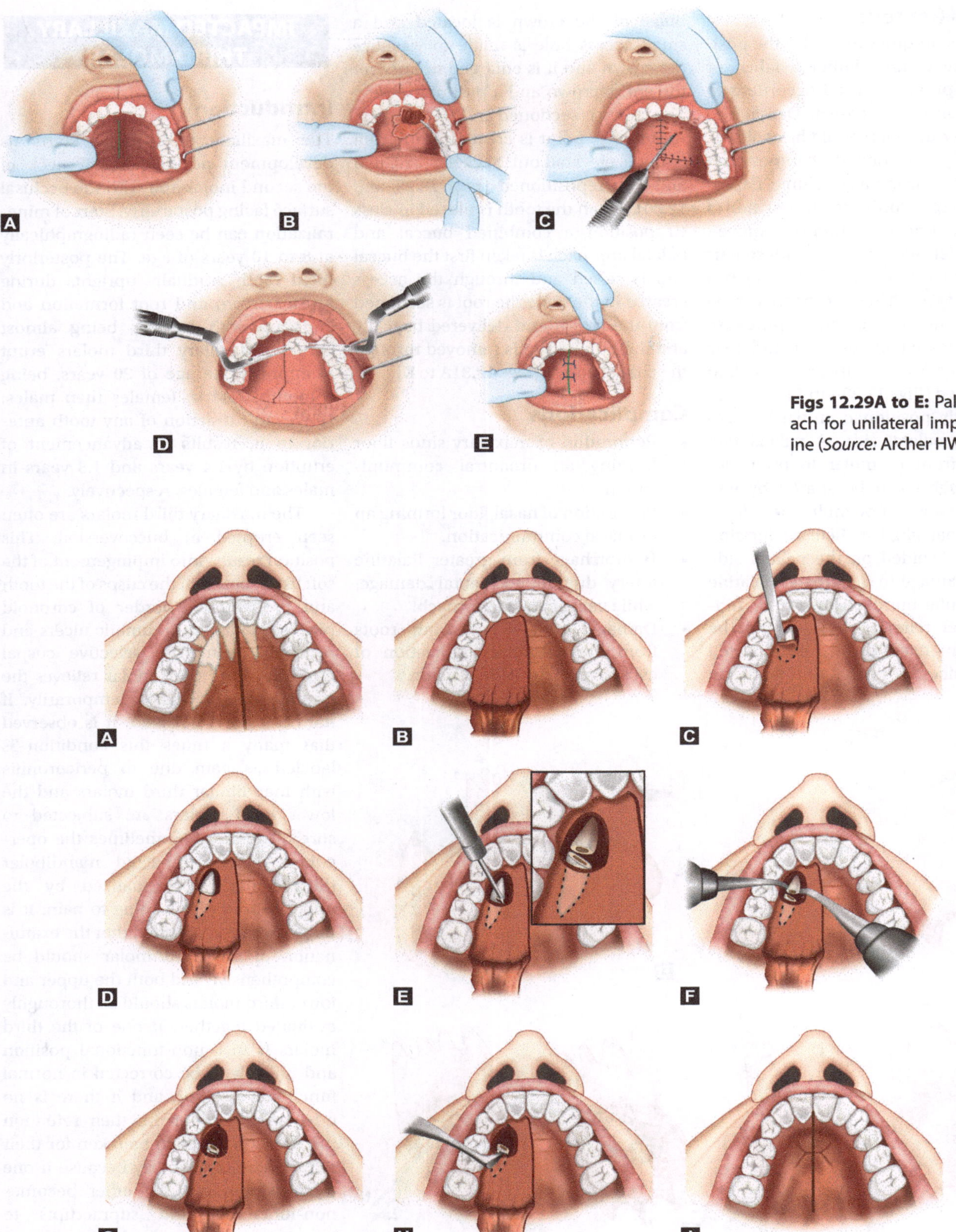

Figs 12.29A to E: Palatal approach for unilateral impacted canine (*Source:* Archer HW, 1966)

Figs 12.30A to I: Palatal approach with tooth sectioning (*Source:* Archer HW, 1966)

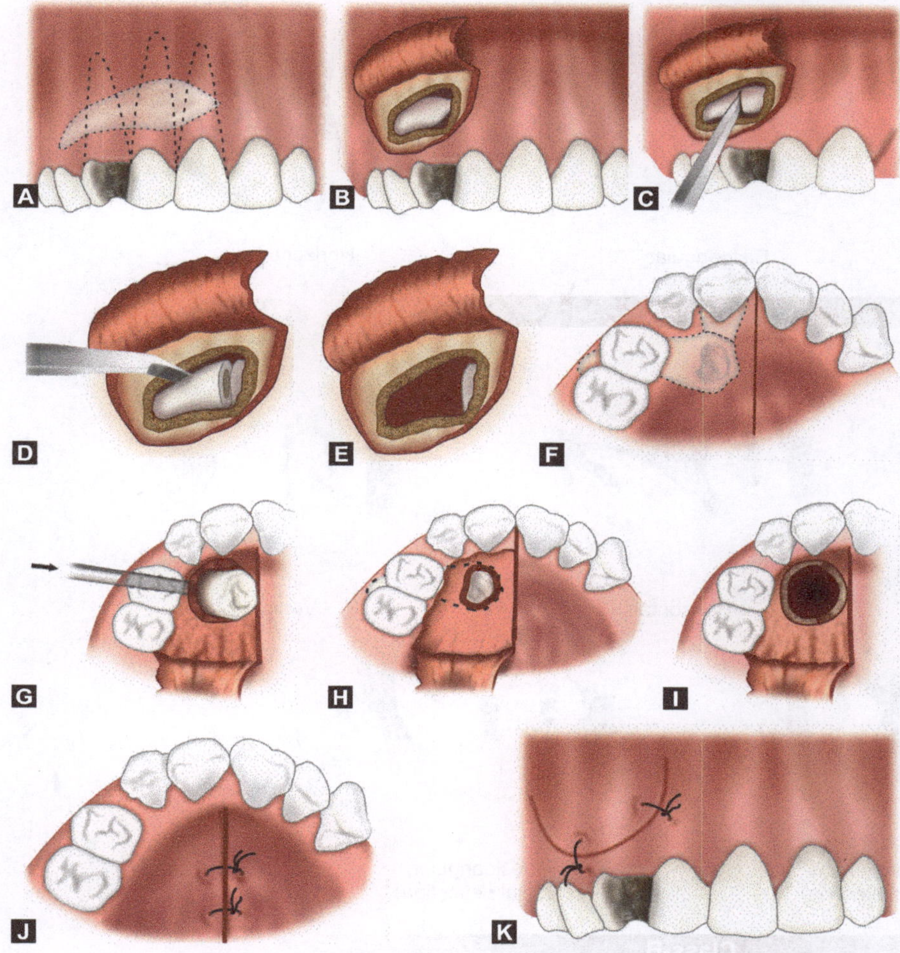

Figs 12.31A to K: Surgical approach for removing Class III impacted canine

impaction, caries or periodontal problems, subsequently.

Classification[1]

- Based on relative depth in bone (Figs 12.32A to C)
  Class A: Lowest portion of the crown is in level with or below the occlusal surface of the maxillary second molar
  Class B: Lowest portion of the crown is in between level of occlusal surface and cervical line of the maxillary second molar
  Class C: Lowest portion of the crown is at or above the cervical line of the maxillary second molar.
- Based on position of long axis with relation to second molar:
  - Vertical
  - Horizontal
  - Mesioangular
  - Distoangular
  - Inverted
  - Linguoangular
  - Buccoangular

  These may also occur in buccoversion, linguoversion and torsoversion.
- Based on relation to Sinus
  - *Sinus approximation (SA):* No bone or a thin partition of bone between impacted maxillary third molar and maxillary sinus.
  - *No-sinus approximation (NSA):* 2 mm or more bone is present between impacted maxillary third molar and maxillary sinus.

DIAGNOSIS

The presence and position of maxillary third molars should be evaluated before the age of 20 years although malposition and its sequelae are less frequent in maxilla than mandible. The panoramic radiograph is used frequently for screening the patient for presence of impacted maxillary third molars. However, IOPA, oblique occlusal views are also used for preoperative assessment of the maxillary third molars. However, no imaging technique can predict the possibility of complications such as tuberosity fracture and perforation into the maxillary sinus.

TREATMENT

The treatment modalities for management of impacted maxillary third molars are:

- No treatment
- Surgical exposure
- Guidance into mesial eruption path
- Surgical removal.

NO TREATMENT

Treatment of a maxillary impacted third molar can be deferred for some time in any of the following two conditions.

Firstly, the tooth is so deeply impacted that progression of marginal periodontal inflammation from adjacent 2nd molar is not likely to occur.

Secondly, it can be left as it is when there is no radiographic sign of pathologic changes such as cyst, tumors arising from the impacted teeth.

Surgical Exposure

It is done very rarely, only if there is a need for functional third molars. In this procedure, the mucosa covering the crown is removed to allow for spontaneous eruption of the molar.

Guidance into a Mesial Eruption Path

It is carried out if the prognosis of the second molar is poor and it is doubtful that the 2nd molar will serve purpose for a long time. In this procedure, the 2nd molar is extracted and the third molar is allowed to erupt normally. It is found that the 3rd molar will drift anteriorly such that it erupts upto the occlusal

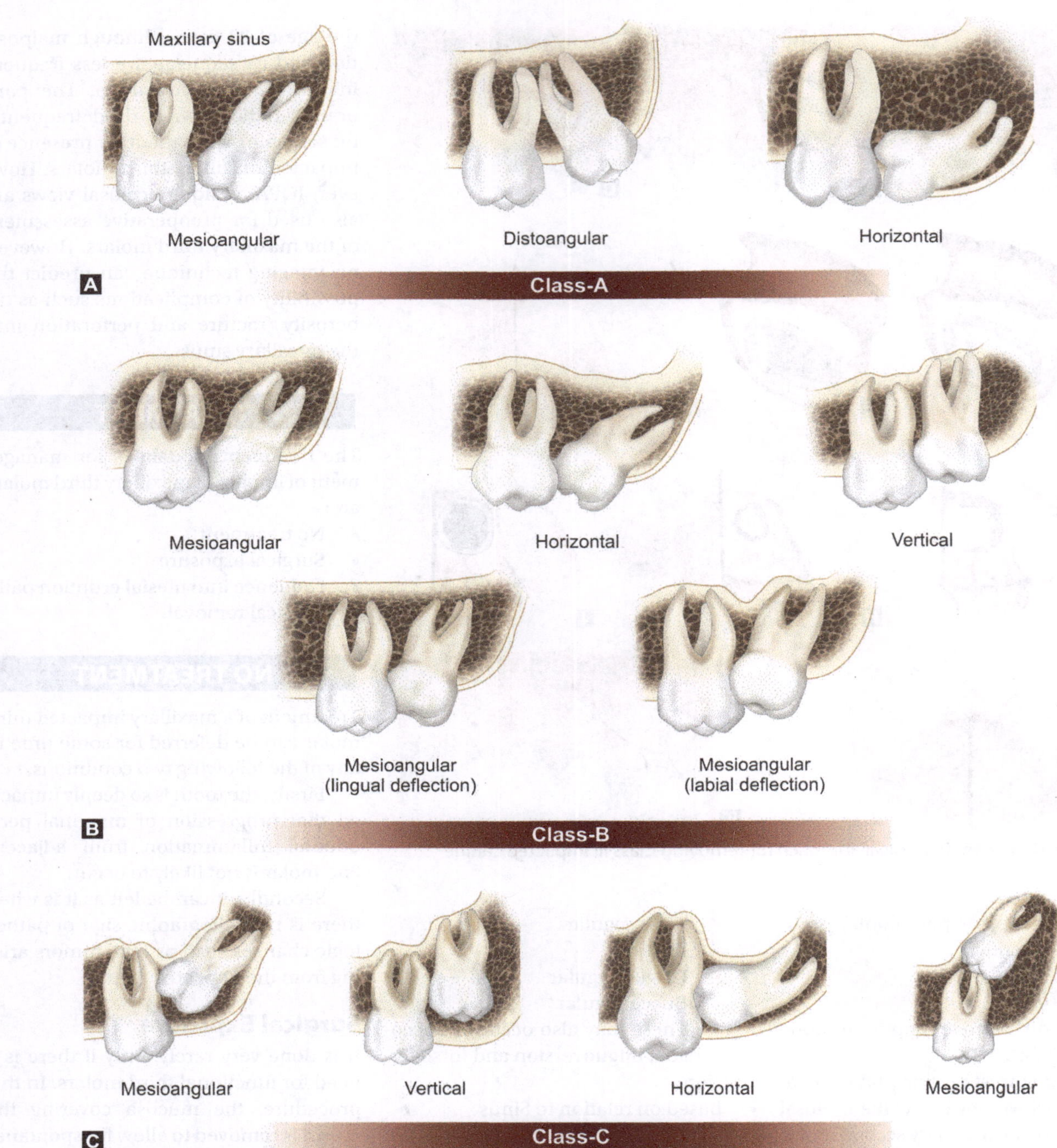

Figs 12.32A to C: Classification of the impacted maxillary third molars.[1] (A) Class-A; (B) Class B; (C) Class C (*Source:* Archer WH. Oral and Maxillofacial Surgery, 5th edn.,1975. WB Saunders Co., Philadelphia).

level and achieves a normal proximal contact with the 1st molar.

Surgical Removal

Several incisions can be used for removal of the impacted 3rd molars based on the whether a buccal or palatal approach is used. They include the following:

- **Buccal sulcular incision:** This incision starts from the distal part of the tuberosity upto the distal surface of the 2nd molar and extends in the gingival sulcus of the 2nd molar and 1st molar if required.
- **Buccal sulcular incision with vestibular extension:** This is similar to the previous flap with the only difference of having an additional

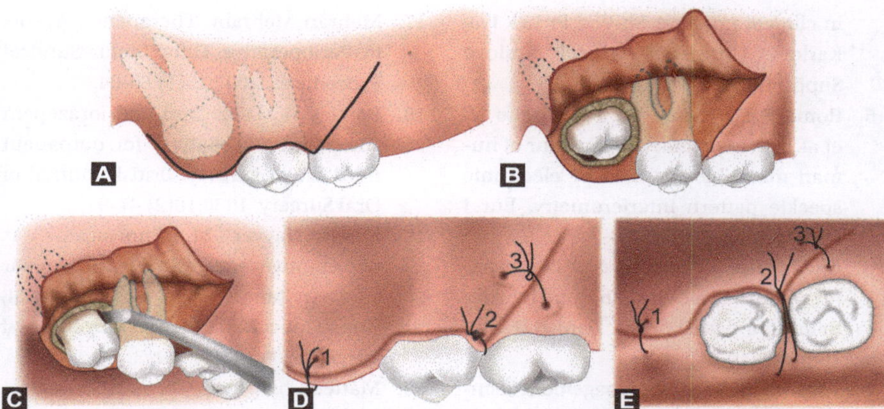

Figs 12.33A to E: Removal of the third molar by Buccal approach[1] (1, 2, 3 depicts the sites for placement of the three sutures)

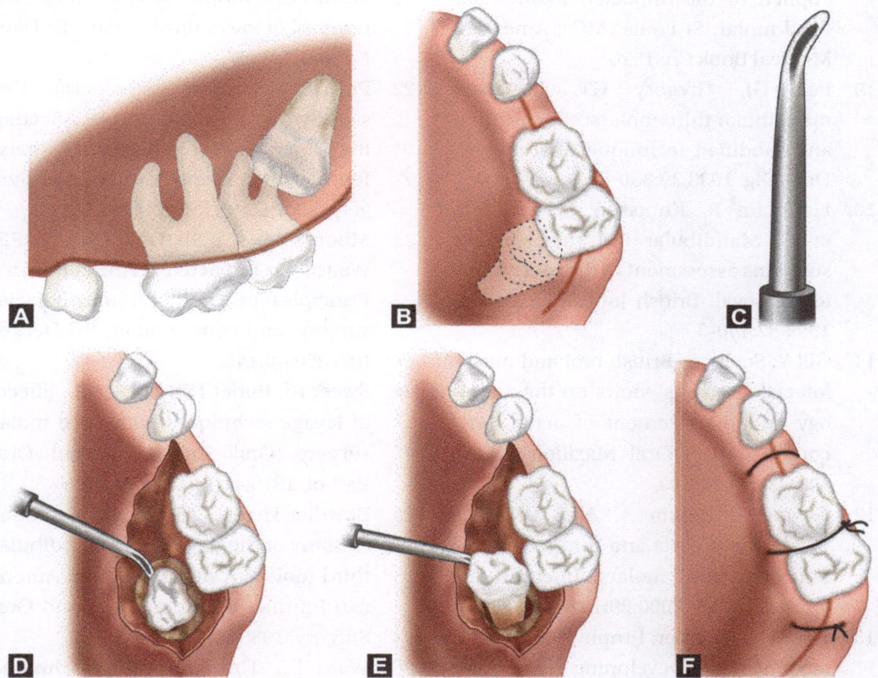

Figs 12.34A to F: Removal of the third molar by Palatal approach[1] (*Source:* Archer WH. Oral and Maxillofacial Surgery, 5th edn., 1975. WB Saunders Co., Philadelphia)

release incision at the anterior end of the sulcular incision at 45° extending onto the attached gingiva on the buccal sulcus (Figs 12.33A to E).

- **Palatal incision:** A palatal sulcular incision is made from the distal of the tuberosity to the mesial of the 1st molar.

A mucoperiosteal flap is raised irrespective of the incision and approach used. The flap is retracted to visualize the tooth and surrounding bone easily. The most common direction of removal of the 3rd molar is distobuccal. Usually only a thin cortical plate covers the impacted maxillary tooth. Hence, most commonly bone covering the buccal and distal surface of the 3rd molar is removed with either with the periosteal elevator, unibeveled chisel or a surgical bur. The bur should be used cautiously as the space available for operating the bur is less and the chances of injuring the flap are more. Instead, a bone fracturing technique using a periosteal elevator or chisel can be employed safely (Figs 12.34A to F).

The tooth is then elevated out of the socket by placing elevators mesiobuccally between the 2nd and 3rd molars. The force is applied in the distal and lateral direction with the retractor placed distally to guard against the tooth slipping into the pterygopalatine fossa.

In cases of divergent roots it might be necessary to section the roots to facilitate the elevation of the roots separately. In case the tuberosity is fractured, it should be repositioned with the fingers and suturing done to maintain the position.

Complications

- **Resistance to removal:** Resistance to distobuccal removal is usually due to a divergent palatal root. This can be avoided by sectioning of the roots.
- **Herniation of buccal fat pad into surgical site:** This complication arises due to damage to the flap by burs or instrument slippage. The extruded fat can be repositioned or excised. However, entire fat pad should not be removed.
- **Displacement of tooth into infratemporal fossa:** It can occur if distal guard is not kept. The incision is enlarged distally, to locate and retrieve the tooth.
- **Displacement into the sinus:** This may occur in sinus approximation impactions due to deficient bone in the floor of the sinus. The tooth can be retrieved by accessing the sinus through the Caldwell Luc's approach.
- **Hemorrhage:** Hemorrhage may occur due to damage to posterior superior alveolar artery or the pterygoid plexus of veins.
- **Fracture of the tuberosity:** It may happen due to enlargement of sinus into the tuberosity or divergent roots of the 3rd molar (Fig. 12.35). Management of this complication can be by three ways:
  1. Immediate excision of the tuberosity results into formation of

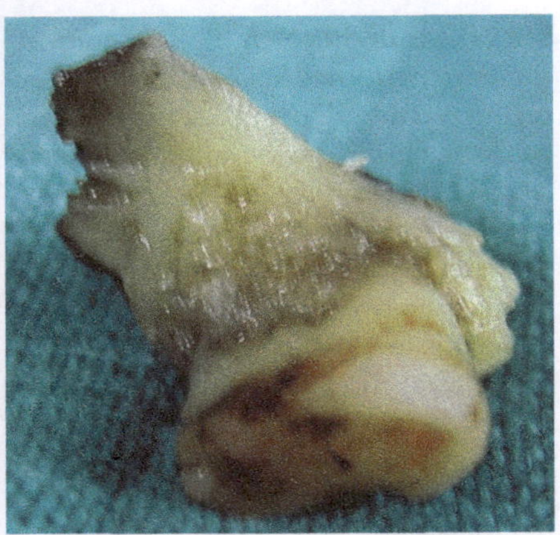

Fig. 12.35: Specimen showing fractured tuberosity during maxillary third molar extraction

oroantral communication and this should be closed primarily.

2. Removal of third molar from mobile tuberosity is performed by sectioning the roots and controlled removal of bone from the tuberosity. The mobile tuberosity is supported with finger pressure and primary suturing is done.
3. Immobilization until bony healing and tooth removal is done when prevention of oroantral fistula may not be possible with the previous two techniques. In this method the surgical procedure is stopped and tuberosity is immobilized and the wound is closed with sutures. Fracture is allowed to heal for 2 to 6 months after which transalveolar extraction is performed. However, it takes a prolonged treatment time.

REFERENCES

1. Archer WH. Oral and Maxillofacial Surgery, 5th edn. WB Saunders Co., Philadelphia. 1975 pp.524-705.
2. Archer WH. Impacted Teeth: Oral Surgery—A Step by step Atlas of Operative Techniques. 4th edn. Philadelphia and London, WB Saunders Comp. 1966;122.
3. Nodine AM. Aberrant teeth, their history, causes and treatment. Dent Items of Interest. 1943;65:440-51.
4. Antalovská Z, Skalská H, György A. The significance of the lower third molar in clinical practice. Sb Ved Pr Lek Fak Karlovy Univerzity Hradci Kralove Suppl. 1974;17(5):451-65.
5. Roman JF, Fernandez P, Moreno V, et al. The mechanical behaviour of human mandibles studied by electronic speckle pattern interferometry. Eur J Orthod 21. 1999;413-21.
6. Rud J. Third molar surgery: relationship of root to mandibular canal and injuries to inferior dental nerve. Danish Dent J. 1983;87:619-31.
7. Fonseca RJ. Surgical management of impacted teeth: oral and maxillofacial surgery, vol-1. 1st edn, Philadelphia, Pennsylvania. Saunders comp, 2000.pp.256-9.
8. Winter GB. Principles of exodontia as applied to the impacted mandibular third molar. St Louis (MO): American Medical Book Co; 1926.
9. Pell GJ, Gregory GT. Impacted mandibular third molars: classification and modified technique for removal. Dent Dig. 1933;39:330-8.
10. Liedholm R, Knutsson K, Lysell L, et al. Mandibular 3rd molars: Oral surgeons assessment of the indications for removal. British journal of OMFS. 1999;37:440-3.
11. Gill Y, Scully C. British oral and maxillofacial surgeons' views on the aetiology and management of acute pericoronitis. Br J Oral Maxillofac Surg. 1991;29(3):180-22.
12. Guven O, Keskin A, Akal UK. The incidence of cysts and tumors around impacted third molars, International journal OMFS. 2000;29:131-5.
13. Henry C. Bowdler, Prophylactic Odontectomy of the Developing Mandibular Third Molar. Am J Orthodontics and Oral Surg. 1938;29:72.
14. Shriniwasan B. Impacted teeth: Text book of oral and Maxillofacial Surgery. 2nd edn. New Delhi, Churchill Livingstone. 1996. p.68.
15. A Öhman. Preoperative radiographic evaluation of lower third molars with computed tomography. Dentomaxillofacial Radiology. 2006;35:30-5.
16. Clark, CA. A method of ascertaining the relative position of unerupted teeth by means of film radiographs. Odont Sec Roy Soc Med Proc. 3:87-90,1909-1910.
17. Mehran Mehrabi. Therapeutic Agents in Perioperative Third Molar Surgical Procedures. 2007;19(1):69-84.
18. Barclay JK. Diazepam and lorazepam compared as sedatives for outpatient third molar surgery. British Journal of Oral Surgery. 1980;18(2):41-9.
19. Sharif Nayyar M, Bupivacaine as pre-emptive analgesia in third molar surgery: Randomised controlled trial. British Journal of Oral and Maxillofacial Surgery. 2006;44(6):501-3.
20. Matteo Chiapasco. Germectomy or delayed removal of mandibular impacted third molars: The relationship between age and incidence of complications. 1995;53(4):418-22.
21. Ward TG. The split bone technique for removal of lower third molars. Br Dent J. 1956;101:297.
22. Peter D. Waite Soft Tissue Incision Design. Symposium on Strategies Affecting the Outcome of Third Molar Surgery. Journal of Oral and Maxillofacial Surgery. 2007;65(9): (Suppl), pp. 1-120.
23. Miloro M, Ghali GE, Larsen PE, Waite PD. Impacted teeth: Peterson's Principles of Oral and maxillofacial surgery. 2nd edn. London, BC Decker Inc. 2004.p.145.
24. Sweet JB, Butler DP, Drager JL. Effects of lavage techniques with third molar surgery. Oral Surg Oral Med Oral Pathol. 1976;41(2):152-68.
25. Bowdler Henry C. Prophylactic odontectomy of the developing mandibular third molar : A new operation. American Journal of Orthodontics and Oral Surgery. 1938 ;24(1):72-84.
26. Ward TG. The Split Bone Technique for Removal of Lower Third Molars. Br Dent J. 1956;101:297-304.
27. Marks SC Jr, Schroeder HE, Andreasen JO. Theories and mechanisms of tooth eruption. In: Andreasen JO, Ko "lsen-Pedersen J, Laskin DM (Eds). Textbook and Color Atlas of Tooth Impactions. Copenhagen, Denmark: Munksgaard; 1997. pp. 19-64.
28. Marks SC Jr, Schroeder HE. Tooth eruption: theories and facts. Anat Rec. 1996;245:374–93.
29. Williams BH. Diagnosis and prevention of maxillary cuspid impaction. Angle Orthod 1981;51(1):30-40.

13 Preprosthetic Surgeries

Borle Rajiv M, Bhoyar Anjali, Garg Ketan

INTRODUCTION

Preprosthetic surgery is a part of oral and maxillofacial surgery that deals with preparation of oral tissues and structures favorable to placement of subsequent prosthesis for their proper placement, retention, stability, function and cosmesis.

The loss of teeth and their replacement by artificial dentures has always been associated with many problems. These may have existed before extraction, but are exaggerated by the edentulous state. An example is the loss of alveolar bone through extensive periodontal disease. Other abnormalities develop after dentures have been worn for some time. Irritation of the soft tissues can occur, if excessive resorption of the jaws occur; as the alveolar process resorb further, the vestibule becomes shallow and makes wearing of dentures difficult or impossible. If excessive atrophy of the entire bone occurs, grafts or implants may be the only solution for this difficult problem. Finally, atrophy can become so severe that a pathological fracture may occur and then the only remedy is a bone graft. Thus, the main functions of preprosthetic surgeries are elimination of pathology in the denture-bearing soft and hard tissue, and making the edentulous ridges and supporting structures favorable for receiving prosthesis.

There may be many unfavorable situations such as high frenal attachments, sharp bony ridges, undercuts, abnormal muscle attachments, flabby soft tissue, hypertrophied maxillary tuberosity, etc. which can come in the way of fabrication of a good prosthesis. The surgical correction of such conditions prior to the prosthesis enhances the result outcome and the quality of the prosthesis and thus the quality of life for the patient.

Willard (1853)[1] was the first person to recommend preprosthetic surgery as an aid in preparation of the patient for complete dentures. Preprosthetic surgery emerged from a ridge trimming service to a truly reconstructive service.

It is essential for every member of the dental profession to possess adequate knowledge of biologic considerations, which will aid in prosthodontic practice.

SCOPE OF PREPROSTHETIC SURGERY

Preprosthetic surgeries includes the following:

- Ridge preservation procedures.
- Corrective recontouring procedures.
  - Soft tissue corrective procedures.
  - Hard tissue corrective procedures.
- Ridge extension procedures.
- Ridge augmentation procedures.
  - Alloplastic bone grafting material.
  - Rib/Iliac crest bone grafting.
    Sinus lift techniques.
  - Implants.
- Correction of abnormal ridge relationships.
- Correction of soft tissue deformities.
- Implant supported restorations and adjuvant procedures.

ANATOMICAL AND PHYSIOLOGICAL CONSIDERATIONS

Bone

In general, a loss of calcified tissue and a concomitant increase in the porosity of bone with age is seen, especially in women. In addition, the bone is often more brittle due to myelofibrosis and decreased vascularity. On the microscopic level, a decreased number of lacunae and osteocytes are seen, along with an associated decrease in the number of viable precursor cells in the bone of elderly persons.[2]

The blood supply is impaired to both the mandible and the maxilla with age. Angiographic studies of the blood supply to the mandible have demonstrated that the inferior alveolar artery is absent or reduced in size in older individuals.[3] This finding may be due to the atherosclerotic changes in the artery itself or to loss of the teeth. Further investigation has demonstrated the presence of a periosteal plexus of vessels along the inferior border of the mandible, which is composed of branches from the buccal, lingual and facial arteries. This plexus is contiguous with the periosteum of the mandible and is thought to contribute to the major part of the blood supply to the mandible as it ages. The maxilla has less age-related vascular compromise than the mandible. The maxillary artery is more prone to atheroma than any other artery,[4] but because of the abundant collateral circulation of the midface, the maxilla remains well perfused.

Bone Loss in the Edentulous Jaw

Approximately 50 percent of the population becomes edentulous by the age of 60. It is generally held that the alveolar bone relies on the presence of dentition for its maintenance. The loss of the teeth leads to lack of functional stresses on the bone and subsequently leads to disuse atrophy of the bone, leading to tooth loss accentuating the normal rate of alveolar bone resorption in the jaws. The physiology of this bone loss remains a mystery. However, biomechanical forces are believed to be the control mechanism for bone remodeling.[5] Any imbalance of forces applied to the bone stimulates both osteoblasts and osteoclasts. Tension forces result in bone deposition and pressure forces result in bone resorption. Remodeling of the bone continues until the forces are balanced and the equilibrium returns.

Once the teeth are extracted and denture wearing commences, a different pattern of force is applied onto the alveolar bone. Certain areas are underloaded and other areas are overloaded, causing bone remodeling. Denture wear accentuates alveolar bone loss and this bone loss is four times greater in the mandible than in the maxilla or basal bone. This may be due to the fact that the stress bearing area of the maxilla is 1.8 times greater than that of the mandible. Therefore, more compressive forces per square centimeter are placed on the mandible than on the maxilla during normal function. Other factors that may modulate the remodeling of alveolar bone include heredity, hormonal factors, local pH, enzymatic agents, local oxygen tensions, bioelectric potentials and local induction phenomena.

Differences are found in the remodeling pattern of alveolar and basilar bones of the jaws. Generalized remodeling activity occurs at a much higher rate in alveolar bone than in the adjacent basal bone in the mandible. This may be because the rate of deposition and resorption in alveolar bone is greater than that for the non-tooth-bearing bone tissues. This is thought to be because alveolar bone is much more vascular and porous than basal bone. Atwood (1986) gave a classification of resorption of residual alveolar ridges (Fig. 13.1).

The edentulous ridges are molded by differential forces delivered onto the bone, determined by the timing and sequence of tooth loss, prosthesis wear and facial morphology (brachycephalic versus dolichocephalic). The usual pattern is resorption of the maxilla on the labial and inferior portions of the alveolar ridge. Consequently, the residual ridge moves posteriorly and superiorly. The palatal vault becomes shallow and the residual ridge approaches the anterior nasal spine anteriorly and the hamulus posteriorly. This is often accompanied by pneumatization of the maxillary sinus into the tuberosity regions of the maxilla. If resorption is allowed to continue, the maxilla may become flat and 'egg shell' thin. In contrast, resorption of the mandible occurs such that the residual ridge is located slightly to the anterior. The mental foramen, genial tubercles and muscle attachments are all located nearer to the crest of the ridge with continued resorption. With severe resorption, the basilar bone of the mandible can get affected, giving a concave shape to the superior surface of the mandible.[6] The differential patterns of resorption of maxilla and mandible, coupled with autorotation of the mandible, place the residual alveolar ridges in a pseudo-Class III relationship.[7]

Facial Changes Associated with Aging

Cutaneous Changes

In addition to the effects of long-term exposure to the physical environment (e.g. sun exposure), the skin has intrinsic age changes that are thought by many to be genetically controlled. These changes begin at about 30 years of age and progress to 80 to 90 years. Facial skin thickness declines sharply at about age of 60 years. As the skin becomes thinner, underlying blood vessels become more noticeable. Wrinkling of the facial skin is progressive, especially on the forehead, near the lateral canthus of the eyes, and in the regions of nasolabial fold and perioral area. These perioral changes

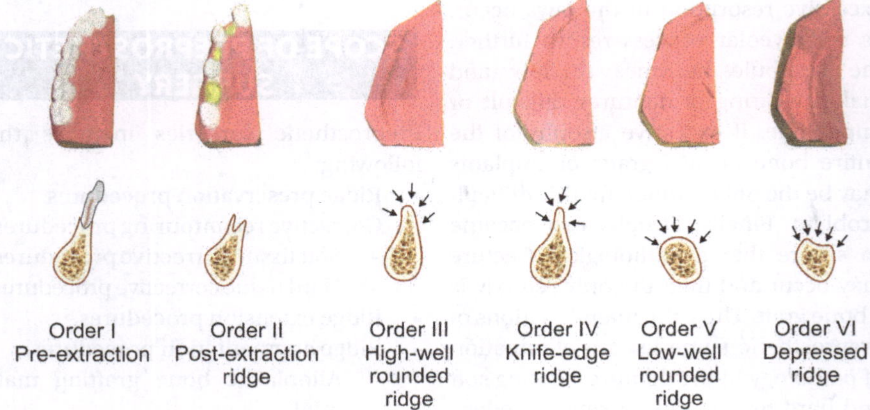

Fig. 13.1: Atwood's classification of ridge resorption. Order I—Pre-extraction; Order II—Post-extraction ridge; Order III—High well rounded ridge; Order IV—Knife edge ridge; Order V—Low-well rounded ridge; Order VI—Depressed ridge (*Courtesy:* Prosthodontics Department Museum, SPDC, Wardha, India)

are magnified with tooth and alveolar bone loss and with the loss of the vertical dimension of occlusion. This wrinkling is due to the loss of elastin fibers in the facial skin and is exacerbated by dermal changes and loss of the subcutaneous fat. There is also decreased function of the skin appendages, thought to be due to a loss of vascularity, causing a fibrosis of the glands of the skin. Collagen synthesis is reduced and fibroblasts are relatively inactive in aged facial skin. A decrease in hyaluronic acid production leads to a dehydration of the facial skin due to a decreased water-binding capacity. Subcutaneous fat is lost and the melanocytes appear to lose the ability to spread their melanin granules evenly throughout the skin. The dermis becomes relatively dehydrated and loses vascularity, strength and elasticity.

In addition to wrinkling of the skin, clinical facial changes associated with aging include a progressive weakening of the orbital septum leading to down-slanting of the lateral canthus of the eye, resorption of adipose and subcutaneous tissues of the cheeks and temporal areas, drooping of the nasal tip, downturning of the commissures of the mouth, and eversion of the lower lip with accentuation of the labiomental fold.

Sensory Changes

A generalized decrease in perception of sensory nerves of the head and neck occurs with age. This is due to senile neuropathy in both, the central and peripheral segments of the nervous system. The peripheral nervous system component is due to accumulated damage to the peripheral nerves and segmental demyelination. The central nervous system element is due mostly to the central neuronal degeneration.

Breakdown in the alveolar ridge can have various causes:

- Disuse atrophy following the removal of teeth.
- An accelerated mucosal and bony pathologic atrophy associated with faulty metabolism.
- Pressures from the prosthesis.
- Overclosures.
- Poor cusp angles of artificial teeth.
- The type of denture tooth materials used.
- Occlusal disharmonies.
- Deformation of the denture bases.

Normally a mean alveolar bone loss of 0.1 mm per year is noted in the anterior maxilla and a 0.4 mm per year loss is found in the mandible.[8]

Alveolar ridge preservation can be achieved through a variety of approaches:

- Supramucosal vital root retention.
- Submucosal vital root retention.
- Root cone implants.
- Transcortical or endosseous implants.

Supramucosal Vital Root Retention

Retained teeth and roots have been used for long periods to support a complete denture. Such prosthesis is called an overdenture, telescopic denture or a sleeve-coping denture.

The advantages of a retained root structure along with an expected decreased ridge resorption include more favorable crown-to-root ratio (through crown root disproportionate length reduction), increased denture retention and stability with intracoronal or intraradicular attachments, increased proprioception, increased masticatory efficiency and psychological benefits to the patient.[9,10] Additionally, since the retained roots are the patients own tissues, there is no risk of rejection as with the implanted materials.

The obvious disadvantages remain those of caries and of periodontal diseases such that patient motivation in the maintenance of a high level of oral health and prosthodontic follow-up care becomes bottom line in this type of denture service.

There are associated technical difficulties in the more commonly retained lower teeth and roots such as the canines, where a buccal undercut is frequently found. This may preclude denture fabrication, but more often can be managed by over-contouring the denture flange to assure relief on the tissue side or by the use of resilient liners.

An additional potential disadvantage is that the retained teeth frequently will require endodontic therapy to achieve appropriate crown-root length ratios, which adds to the cost of therapy along with the frequently required amalgam or gold copings and attachments. In the final analysis the cost of over-dentures compares favorably with alternative treatment methods because of the ease of maintenance and the low percentage of remakes.

Submucosal Vital Root Retention

Studies of human roots unintentionally fractured at surgery and retained in alveolar bone suggest that they generally remain asymptomatic until they break through the overlying mucosa and enter the mouth.[11] Clinical symptoms occur only with root exposure in the oral cavity and periradicular radiolucency.

A series of early animal studies showed that with roots appropriately reduced to a level 2 mm below the alveolar crestal bone and with primary watertight closure of the overlying mucosa, roots would remain vital.[12] The severed root would be covered again with regenerated bone with a structural periodontal ligament and with a layer of cementoblast over cut dentin.

This was confirmed by early human reports, although vitally submerged teeth appear to have a greater potential for healing than those treated with root canal filling prior to submerging.

All teeth are to meet the following criteria for retention as proposed by Garver et al (1978).[13,14]

- No more than 1 mm horizontal mobility.
- No infrabony pockets that could not be reduced at the time of surgery.
- Sufficient healthy mucogingival tissues for watertight closure of the mucosa.
- Remaining supporting tissue atleast one-third of the total root length.
- Should be asymptomatic, test vital, or show only calcific metamorphosis.

Technique of Submucosal Vital Root Retention

A full thickness mucoperiosteal flap is raised using a reverse bevel incision facially and lingually. Crown amputation is done using either a high speed bur or chisel mallet. Following complete removal of crevicular epithelium and granulations, periosteal relaxing incisions are given to allow for tension-free apposition of the flap. This is sutured with a running horizontal mattress suture of nonwicking monofilament to provide eversion closure, which is then oversewn by a continuous running suture to effect a watertight closure.[15]

Denture placement is either at the time of surgery with pressure paste relief and autopolymerizing treatment resin reline inserted or is delayed until 6 weeks after surgery. Conventional denture fabrication techniques are observed, with special emphasis placed on obtaining a balanced occlusion without undue pressure that could cause decubital ulcers and subsequent root exposure in the mouth.

Complications

Immediate complications include tissue dehiscence (due to closure under tension) or pressure dehiscence (due to immediate denture). Immediate postsurgical root exposure requires endodontic therapy and conversion of the root to an overdenture abutment.

Delayed problems usually occur 14 to 20 days postoperatively and are usually related to a small dehiscence into the mouth over individual roots that cannot easily be covered surgically because of their small size, making tissue free grafts or flap closures questionable. The delayed dehiscence is usually not pus production, but if persistent can become fistulous and require root extraction. These complications are related to faulty prosthesis pressures, to alveolar bone resorption allowing sharp root surfaces to penetrate the mucosa, or to the presence of retained epithelium over the root.

Root Cone Implants

Current studies have shown that porous and non-resorbable particulate and block forms of hydroxylapatite can be used clinically as tooth root, bone augmentation and bone replacement materials. Hydroxylapatite induces neither an inflammatory nor immune response when in contact with bone. It forms a nidus for new bone growth. It does not resorb and bonds chemically to bone without an intervening fibrous capsule.[16]

Ridge Extension Procedures

The goal of ridge extension is to uncover existing basal bone of the jaws surgically by repositioning the overlying mucosa, muscle attachments and muscle to a lowered position in the mandible or to a superior position in the maxilla. The resultant advantage is that a larger denture flange can be accommodated, thus contributing to greater denture stability and retention.

All the cases of maxillary or mandibular basal bone atrophy cannot be surgically treated by sulcus extension. There must be an adequate alveolar bone with sufficient height remaining to allow for repositioning of the mental nerves and the buccinator and mylohyoid muscles in the mandible. In the maxilla the anterior nasal spine, the nasal cartilage and the malar buttresses may interfere with repositioning the sulcus superiorly.

Conversely not all cases require a full skin or mucosal graft vestibuloplasty with floor of the mouth lowering. Many cases have success with a vestibular extension anterior to the mental foraminá or a lingual procedure to reduce the genial tubercles or release the mylohyoid muscle posteriorly in the floor of the mouth, which may very well solve the problem of lack of denture stability and retention.

Ashley et al. (1953)[17] gave the following principles of plastic revision of tissues:

- Bare soft tissue should be covered surgically with epithelium to prevent subsequent scars and contracture.
- Whenever the local tissue is not available to obtain the anticipated final result or to cover the defect without tension, distant tissue should be used.
- In creating a new cavity, allowance should be made for contracture whenever the cavity is lined with remote grafted tissues or local flaps. Contracture is usually prevented by overcorrection of the cavity defect without tension on the lining tissue.
- The greater the thickness of split-skin graft the lesser the tendency for contracture.

Sulcoplasty

Following removal of the natural teeth, remodeling of the alveolar process results in a reduction in the height and width of the residual ridge. As the basal seat area becomes smaller, denture stability and retention decrease.

Ideally, it would seem desirable to restore the alveolar ridge to its former size by bone grafting. However, since several methods of sulcoplasty are available to extend the denture foundation, bone grafting is indicated only when these methods of sulcoplasty cannot provide satisfactory results.

If a denture flange is overextended in an attempt to gain added resistance to lateral displacing forces, the mucosa at the fornix of the vestibular or sublingual sulcus becomes traumatized, ulcerated and scarred and the denture gets easily displaced. Ultimately the flange must be shortened to its physiologic limits.

If an incision is made at the fornix of the sulcus to accommodate a longer flange, granulation tissue and scar tissues form around the flange and the flange must be shortened. The incision heals and the sulcus returns to its former position with a scar in the fornix, making it even worse.

For successful extension of the vestibular or sublingual sulcus both the osseous and the soft-tissue sides must be lined with epithelium. If the extended sulcus is to be an aid in denture construction, the mucosa of the sulcus must be free of scar tissue. To prevent relapse of the sulcus to its former condition there must be a minimum of connective tissue between the mucosa and the periosteum on the osseous side of the sulcus and the epithelial lining of the sulcus must be free of tension.

There are three general methods of sulcoplasty, as follows:

1. Mucosa adjacent to the sulcus can be advanced to line both sides of the extended sulcus.
2. Neighboring mucosa can be advanced to line one side of the sulcus, while the other side heals by granulation and secondary epithelization.
3. Epithelium, either skin or mucosa, can be transplanted as a free graft to line one or both sides of the extended sulcus.

VESTIBULOPLASTY PROCEDURES

Mucosal Advancement

When the vestibular sulcus is to be extended, the first choice of procedure should be the one whereby the neighboring mucosa can be advanced to line both sides of the sulcus. The prime criterion for this type of procedure is the presence of an adequate amount of healthy mucosa. Obwegeser[18] used a simple clinical test to determine whether or not there is sufficient mucosa available. With the lips in a relaxed position, a mouth mirror is inserted into the sulcus to the required depth required prosthetically. If the upper lip is not displaced upward or drawn inward by the maneuver, it can be assumed that there is sufficient mucosa for an advancement procedure. A similar test can be used in the lower labial vestibule.

Obwegeser's Submucous Vestibuloplasty[19]

In many cases of a clinically short alveolar ridge there actually is enough bone present. The difficulty lies in the fact that the mucosa and muscles of the sulcus are attached too closely to the crest of the ridge. The objectives in this surgical procedure are to extend the sulcus to provide additional ridge height and to transfer the submucous connective tissue and the adjacent muscles to a position farther from the crest of the ridge.[20] The purpose of the second objective is to prevent relapse of the sulcus to its preoperative condition. This procedure is applicable to the entire maxillary sulcus and to the anterior mandibular sulcus, but better results are obtained in the maxillary vestibule. This procedure is one that can be performed with local anesthesia in the dental office. An important feature of the operation takes place before the incision is made. A copious amount of saline, or a dilute solution of local anesthetic, is injected superficially in the submucosa of the sulcus, lip and cheek to facilitate dissection of the mucosa from the submucosa. A vertical incision is made in the midline of the sulcus through the mucosa only, extending from the mucogingival junction to a level in the lip corresponding to the proposed sulcus extension (Figs 13.2A to D). With the lip everted in the horizontal plane, a scissor is introduced through the incision and by blunt spreading dissection the mucosa is separated from the submucosa on the right and left sides. A tunnel is formed between the mucosa and the submucosa, extending from the mucogingival junction well out into the lip and cheek so that the mucosa is completely undermined. The tunnel is carried posteriorly to the zygomatic buttresses of the maxilla and to the mental foramen areas of the mandible.

When the submucosal tunnels have been created, the vertical incision is deepened to bone at the midline. If the anterior nasal spine is prominent, it can be reduced through the median incision. Supraperiosteal tunnels are made to the right and left with the scissors, separating the connective tissue and muscles from the periosteum. The supraperiosteal dissection should be extended as far as the proposed sulcus extension requires. A wedge-shaped strip of connective tissue remains between the two tunnels. This strip of connective tissue may be cut close to the bone with the scissors. The tissue may be excised, or it may be permitted to retract into the lip and cheek. The freely movable mucosa is adapted into the deepened sulcus with finger pressure and blood is milked out of the surgical field. The vertical incision is sutured. A roll of gauze is placed into each sulcus to temporarily support the mucosa

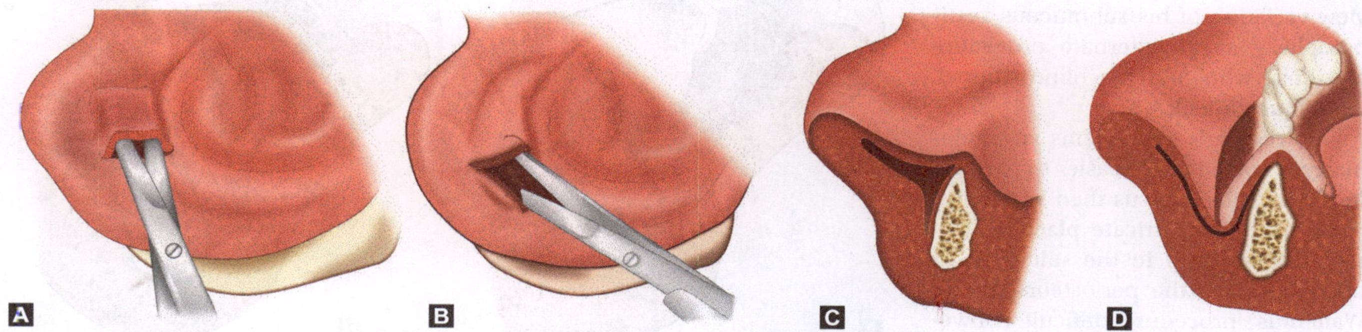

Figs 13.2A to D: Obwegeser's submucous vestibuloplasty: (A) Incison in vestibule; (B) Blunt dissection by scissors; (C) Tunnel formed; (D) Denture/splint with extended flanges secured to alveolar bone (*Courtesy:* Artist Kombe SPDC, Wardha, India)

and prevent hematoma formation, while the denture is being prepared.

A compound impression is made of the new sulcus with use of the patient's denture or a previously prepared splint. The compound is chilled and trimmed. The denture or splint with the extended flanges is secured to the maxilla or mandible for 1 week with peralveolar wires or pins or with circumzygomatic or circummandibular wires.

The postoperative course is accompanied by moderate pain and facial swelling that subside after 4 or 5 days. A new denture can usually be made after 2 or 3 weeks.

Wallenius' (Open-View) Technique

Wallenius[21] (1963) accomplished—the same mucosa-lined sulcus extension as Obwegeser, but he used an 'open view' procedure instead of a 'tunneling' technique. An incision is made along the mucogingival junction through the mucosa only. The supraperiosteal dissection is performed to the extent desired for the proposed sulcus extension. Care must be exercised not to cut or tear the periosteum. The mucosa is dissected from the submucosa far out into the lip so that a large flap of mucosa is mobilized. Stay sutures are placed in the flap to fix it to the periosteum deep in the sulcus. The free margin of the flap is then returned to its original position and sutured.

Wallenius uses stay sutures to fix the mucosa at the fornix of the sulcus to the periosteum rather than use a stent or percutaneous sutures.

Obwegeser also suggested an open-view variation of his submucous vestibuloplasty as an alternate procedure for those who find the blind 'tunnel' technique difficult.

Obwegeser's submucous vestibuloplasty is considerably easier to perform in the maxillary sulcus than Wallenius' technique. The intricate placement of stay sutures deep in the sulcus to fix the mucosa to the periosteum makes Wallenius' procedure difficult. Obwegeser's use of an extended denture flange to hold the fornix of the sulcus in its new position is considerably easier. If the patient's denture is lined with a soft liner, sufficient retention can frequently be obtained so that osseous fixation is unnecessary.

Vestibuloplasty by Secondary Epithelization

The success of Obwegeser's submucous vestibuloplasty and Wallenius' mucosal advancement operation depends on the presence of a sufficient amount of healthy mucosa in the vestibule. When inflammatory hyperplasia and scar tissue are present, these mucosal advancement procedures are contraindicated. Secondary epithelization techniques should be considered as the first alternative.

There are two basic techniques of vestibuloplasty by secondary epithelization with several variations. In one technique (Kazanjian) a mucosal flap is raised in the lip and transferred to line the osseous side of the deepened sulcus. In the other (Clark) a flap of alveolar mucosa is raised and transferred to line the soft tissue side of the sulcus. Variations in the two basic techniques relate to the periosteum.

Kazanjian Technique

Kazanjian[22] (1935) made an incision in the mucosa of the lip and reflected a large flap of labial and vestibular mucosa. He then performed a supraperiosteal dissection to deepen the sulcus (Figs 13.3A and B). The flap of mucosa was turned downward from its attachment on the alveolar ridge and placed directly against the periosteum to which it was sutured. A rubber catheter stent was placed in the deepened sulcus and fixed through the lip to the outer surface with percutaneous sutures. The catheter helped to hold the flap in its new position and to maintain sulcus depth during the first stages of healing. The catheter was removed after 7 days. The labial donor site was coated with tincture of benzoin and was otherwise left raw to granulate and heal by secondary epithelization. The basic disadvantage of this technique is that the raw area is in the soft tissue, which brings about scarring of the vestibule and relapse is common.

Godwin Technique

Godwin[23] (1947) performed a similar procedure to deepen the lower vestibular sulcus. Like Kazanjian, he raised a flap of labial mucosa, but he deepened the sulcus by means of a subperiosteal stripping. The periosteum and the attached connective tissue was either excised or pushed downward. Godwin placed the flap of labial and vestibular mucosa directly against the bone and sutured it to the connective

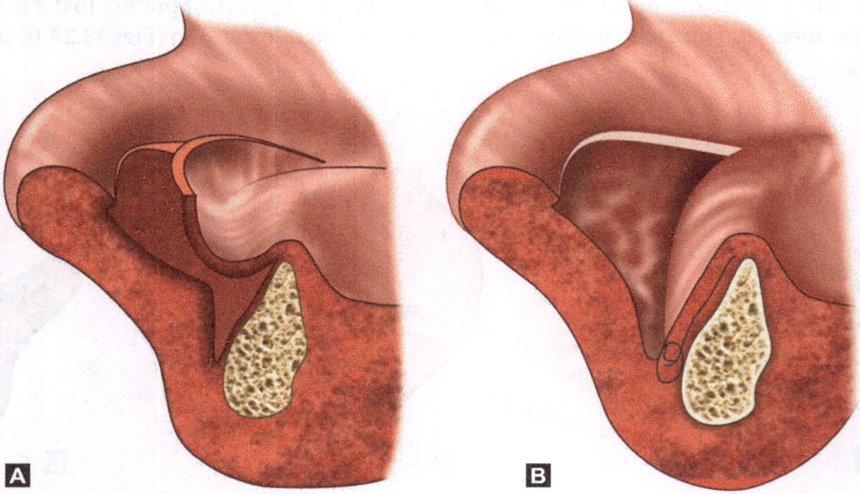

Figs 13.3A and B: Kazanjian's technique: (A) Flap harvested from lip mucosa; (B) Flap sutured to periosteum of bone

tissue beyond the deepened sulcus, using absorbable suture. By stripping the periosteum, Godwin exposed the bone and was able to smoothen the bone with files, before the flap was positioned in the sulcus. The raw tissues healed by granulation and secondary epithelization, with a contracture line on the labial side of the sulcus.

Both Kazanjian's and Godwin's procedures have the disadvantage of scar contracture on the labial side of sulcus, with a loss in sulcus depth. Godwin's technique has the added disadvantage of inviting additional bone resorption by removing the periosteum.

Cooley Technique

Cooley[24] (1952) presented a method for deepening the mandibular and maxillary sulci. With his technique he was also able to smoothen any bony irregularities on the crest of the ridge and reposition the mental nerve. He made an incision on the crest of the mandibular ridge from second molar area on one side to the same position on the opposite side. Short lateral relaxing incisions were given at the posterior ends of the primary incision. A full thickness labiobuccal mucoperiosteal flap was reflected down to the level of the proposed sulcus extension. The mental nerve was repositioned inferiorly on each side. The labial and buccal mucosa was undermined thoroughly. Three drill holes were placed through the alveolar ridge, one in the midline and one in each cuspid area. The gingival margin of the labial flap was sutured through the peralveolar holes to the lingual mucoperiosteum leaving the crest of the ridge bare.

A previously prepared acrylic splint with extended flanges was secured to the mandible for 6 days with circumferential wires. This splint was worn by the patient after the immediate postoperative period until a new denture could be constructed.

Cooley's maxillary sulcoplasty procedure was similar to the mandibular except that the primary incision, instead of being on the crest of the ridge, was made to the palatal side of the crest.

The advantages of Cooley technique are as following:

- Bony irregularities on the crest and labial surface of the ridge can be corrected.
- The crest of the ridge is left raw to granulate and heal by secondary epithelization. Since there can be no scar contracture over bone, this technique is an improvement over Kazanjian and Godwin techniques in which a scar is formed on the labial side of the sulcus.
- The mental nerve can be repositioned bilaterally, if indicated.

Collett Technique

Collett[25] (1954) used a previously prepared denture with overextended flange borders to support full-thickness labiobuccal mucoperiosteal flaps. In his technique the amount of sulcus extension is determined preoperatively on a study cast and a clear surgical template with appropriately extended borders are made from the corrected cast.

An incision is made on the crest of the maxillary ridge from one tuberosity to the other. The external mucoperiosteum and muscles are elevated and a large full-thickness flap is reflected. The transparent template is inserted and used to reposition the flaps higher in the vestibular sulcus. The position of the flaps can be observed through the template. No sutures are placed. The denture is inserted to support the newly deepened sulcus. The bone is protected by the denture until granulation tissue forms and surface epithelization occurs.

In Collett, Cooley, and Godwin procedures the periosteum is stripped from the bone. Godwin covered the bone with the mucosal flap. Cooley repositioned the mucoperiosteal flap with only the ridge crest remaining bare. In Collett procedure the entire external surface of the maxillary ridge is left bare, thus inviting infection and additional bone resorption of a previously resorbed ridge.

Clark's Technique

Clark[26] (1953) described a sulcus extension procedure that can be considered to be the reverse of Kazanjian technique. Clark based his operation on four principles of plastic surgery:

1. Raw surfaces on connective tissue contract, whereas the same surfaces undergo minimal contraction when covered with epithelium.
2. Raw surfaces overlying bone cannot contract.
3. Epithelial flaps must be undermined sufficiently to permit repositioning and fixation without tension.
4. Soft tissues undergoing plastic revision have a tendency to return to their former position so that overcorrection and firm fixation are necessary.

In Clark's operation an incision is made on the alveolar ridge and a supraperiosteal dissection is done to the depth desired. The mucosa of the lip is undermined to the vermilion border (Figs 13.4A and B). Three non-absorbable mattress sutures are placed in the free margin of the mucosal flap and are carried through the skin and tied over a cotton roll. The soft-tissue side of the sulcus is covered with mucosa, whereas, on the osseous side, the raw periosteal surface is left to granulate and epithelize. Clark technique is particularly applicable for the mandibular labial sulcus.

In 1953, Edlan[27] recommended an incision on the lip mucosa with full thickness mucoperiosteal dissection followed by incision of periosteum over the crest of the ridge. The periosteum was then used to cover the mucosal wound over the lip. In 1954, Collett[25] described the procedure of secondary epithelization without suturing, which resulted in scar contracture on the labial aspect and finally there was loss of vestibular depth. In 1955, Caldwell[28] recommended that the incision should be made on the top of the crest and that it should extend from the retromolar pad to the bicuspid region through the periosteum down to the bone. It must be carried sufficiently to the buccal side so as to assure a table of bone to which the lingual periosteal flap can be returned for closure of the wound. After cutting the ridge and severance of all muscle attachment the wound is closed.

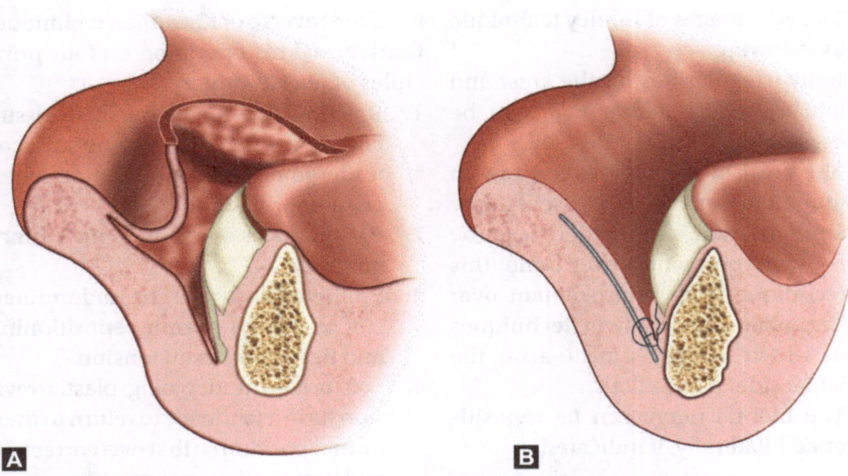

Figs 13.4A and B: Clark's technique: (A) Flap harvested from alveolar mucosa; (B) Flap sutured to labial mucosa

A rubber tube is sutured in position to maintain the sulcus depth.

Obwegeser Secondary Epithelization Vestibuloplasty

Obwegeser[29] technique was published in 1967, coauthored by Macintosh. It is essentially a modification of Clark's technique. Obwegeser used secondary epithelization in cases in which there is enough bone, but insufficient healthy mucosa for his submucous vestibuloplasty technique. He used this procedure primarily to extend the maxillary vestibule. The incision is made at the mucogingival junction and the supraperiosteal dissection is extended quite high, almost to the infraorbital foramen. The labial and buccal mucosa are undermined. The free margin of the mucosal flap is sutured to the periosteum high in the extended sulcus with 000 chromic catgut sutures. Percutaneous sutures are not used in maxillary sulcoplasty operations.

Obwegeser suggested that the denture flange be shortened so there is no contact with the raw periosteal surface. Irritation from the flange that could cause proliferation of an excessive amount of granulation tissue is thereby avoided. 4 to 5 weeks postoperatively a flange is added to the denture. In such cases the denture is lined with a soft acrylic resin that is changed weekly until the tissues have healed, usually in 3 or 4 weeks.

Obwegeser stated that within 3 years 50 percent of the sulcus depth obtained by secondary epithelization was lost by regression. As a result overcorrection is indicated. He stated that he had better results with this procedure in cases of maxillary vestibuloplasty than in mandibular.

Conclusion Regarding Secondary Epithelization Vestibuloplasty

- The Clark procedure, which leaves a raw periosteal surface that cannot contract, is preferred to the Kazanjian procedure, which leaves a raw lip that does contract.
- The mucosal flap must be free of tension and must be fixed for a sufficient period of time to prevent relapse.
- Relapse can be further minimized, if the periosteum is scarified at the base of the sulcus.
- The denture flange should not irritate the granulating periosteal surface.
- A new prosthesis may be made after 4 to 5 weeks. The flange of the denture should be of sufficient length to maintain the new sulcus depth.
- Inspite of all the best efforts to avoid a relapse, a 30 to 50 percent relapse in sulcus depth can occur and so overcorrection of the sulcus should be attempted whenever possible.
- If the bony ridge is too small to permit overcorrection, or if the raw operative defect is large, a free epithelial graft should be placed to cover the wound.

Effects of Vestibuloplasty

Mechanical Resistance to Displacement Forces

The vestibuloplasty with the skin grafting (VSG) and lowering the floor of the mouth (LFM) provides increased sulcus depth, especially in the lingual flange area, which materially helps to control lateral displacement.

Stable Denture Seating Area

The atrophic mandibular ridge has only a small line of attached mucosa forming the crest of the ridge. All the remaining mucosa of the denture seating area can be elevated by the movement of the lips cheek and tongue. The vestibuloplasty with skin grafting and lowering of the floor of the mouth (VSG and LFM) produces a non-displaceable tissue covering the entire denture-bearing area. The skin's firm attachment to the periosteum permits denture stability even in the severely atrophied mandible where no significant ridge height can be created.

Skin as a Load Bearing Tissue

Whereas mucosa tends to ulcerate in response to pressure, skin tends to form a benign hyperkeratosis similar to the callus response on the hand. This hyperkeratosis is rarely painful. The pain threshold of grafted skin is higher than that of mucosa and touch perception is somewhat diminished. Patients are usually more comfortable with skin than mucosa as a load bearing tissue. Both skin and mucosa will rarely exhibit problems like candidiasis.

Probable Slower Mandibular Resorption Beneath Skin

Advantages of use of stents

The stent is more versatile than the suturing method because the skin can be adapted with accuracy to any contour of the labial-buccal area whereas with suturing method, there should be minimal depressions in the labial-buccal contour. With the stent technique the skin can be adapted to the lingual undercut via the Protaform-type adaptation material and poor crestal soft tissue or sharp crestal bone can be dealt with at the time of grafting. With the suturing method, these problems need to be dealt in with a separate procedure.

A graft with voids can be tolerated using the stent method, as it can be manipulated on the stent to give proper coverage. This allows a thinner graft than may be used in the suturing method, thus predisposing to better donor site healing.

Advantages of submucosal suturing

Without the stent the patient is more comfortable for the first week postoperatively. In addition, no stent construction or adaptation materials are required.

Skin Graft

Skin grafts have been used for years to cover wounds of the oral tissues in the plastic repair of trauma and in tumor surgery. In preprosthetic oral surgery when there is an inadequate amount of oral mucosa that can be repositioned to deepen the vestibular sulcus, the addition of a free skin or mucosal graft may make the difference between success and failure.[30]

Obwegeser[31,32] (1963, 1967) used skin grafting almost exclusively in mandibular vestibuloplasty, usually combined with a lowering of the floor of the mouth (lingual sulcoplasty). The initial steps of the operative procedure are the same as those of secondary epithelization vestibuloplasty in which a labiobuccal flap is sutured to the periosteum low in the deepened sulcus (Figs 13.5A to C). When ridge skin-grafting vestibuloplasty is combined with lingual sulcoplasty, the free margin of the labiobuccal flap is sutured, not to the periosteum, but to the free margin of the lingual flap with chromic gut sutures that pass under the inferior border of the mandible. The split-thickness skin graft is placed inside a previously prepared stent and secured with an adhesive. The stent and skin graft are secured to the mandible for 1 week by circumferential wires or heavy nylon sutures. After a week the stent is removed. The graft has healed to the raw periosteum. Excess skin may be removed with a scissor. The stent or temporary denture should be replaced to prevent contracture and loss of the newly deepened sulcus. After 4 to 5 weeks a new denture may be constructed.

Morbidity, complications and side effects of vestibuloplasty

- Dysesthesia is a relatively frequent postoperative complication. Avoidance of surgical error is of importance in reducing dysesthesia, i.e. the avoidance of physical injury to the nerve of the surgical area.
- Soft tissue profile changes of considerable magnitude and uniform pattern have been found, even when the surgical preparation is restricted.

Lingual Sulcoplasty

For the patient with a grossly resorbed mandible, extension of the lingual sulcus, or lowering of the floor of the mouth, can extend the denture foundation and improve the stability and retention of the mandibular denture. The mylohyoid and genioglossus muscles and the mucosa of the floor of the mouth can be repositioned inferiorly without undue impairment of function. Cooley[24] (1952) suggested lingual frenotomy and transplantation of the superficial fibers of the genioglossus muscles to improve the contour of the anterior lingual sulcus.

Trauner Technique

Trauner[33] (1970) stated that lingual sulcus extension was indicated when the mucosa of the floor of the mouth

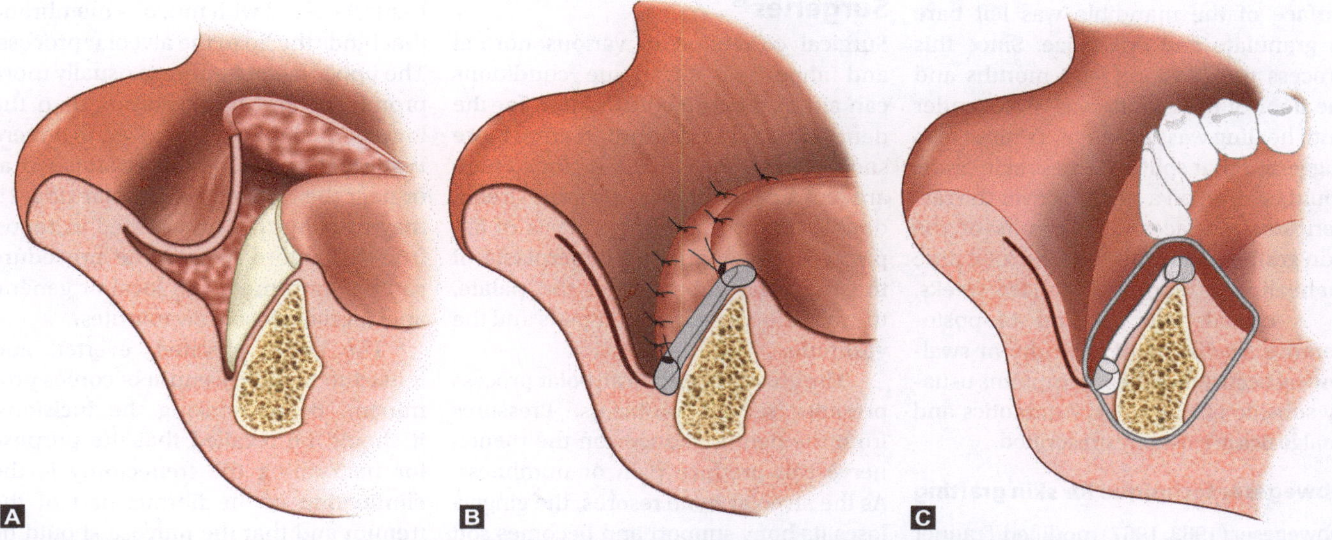

Figs 13.5A to C: Obwegeser's secondary epithelization vestibuloplasty: (A) Flap harvested from alveolar mucosa; (B) Flap sutured to lip and skin graft secured; (C) Temporary denture placed as stent

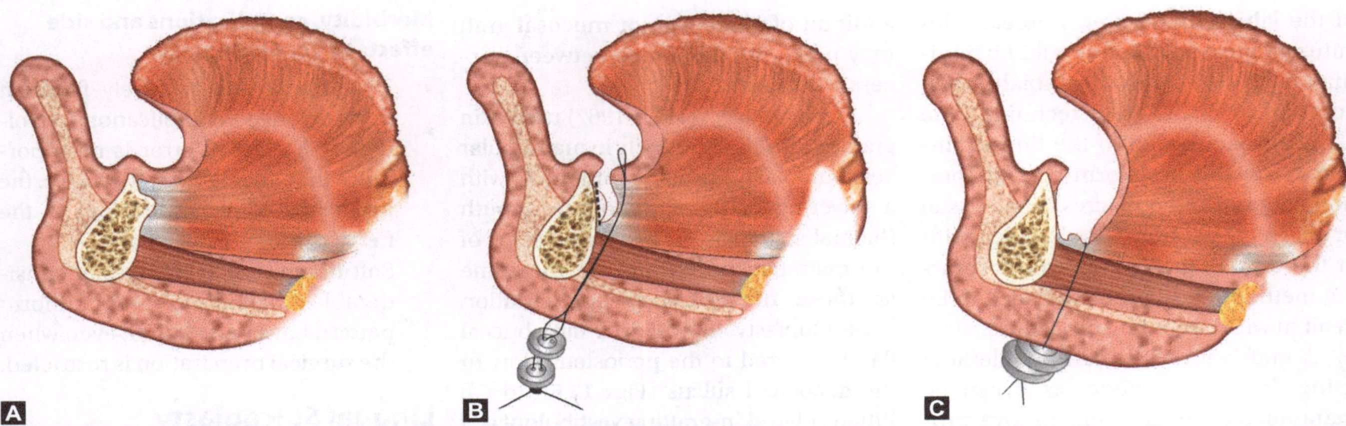

Figs 13.6A to C: Lingual sulcoplasty (Trauner's technique): (A) Incision near lingual crest of ridge; (B) Release of periosteum and genioglossus muscle; (C) Mucosa sutured to skin under the mandible

rose as high as the mandibular ridge when the tongue is elevated and when the mylohyoid muscle is attached at the level of the ridge.

Trauner made an incision in the mucosa of the floor of the mouth close to the mandible from the third molar region on one side to the same location on the opposite side (Figs 13.6A to C). By blunt dissection the connective tissue was separated from the periosteum until the inferior border of the mandible was encountered. The mucosa of the floor of the mouth and the mylohyoid muscle were sutured with heavy nylon mattress sutures through the skin to buttons under the mandible. The medial periosteal surface of the mandible was left bare to granulate and epithelize. Since this process took as long as 2 months and the floor of the mouth was quite tender until healing was complete, Trauner also suggested that split-thickness skin grafts could be used on a stent to cover the raw periosteal surfaces. The results of the skin grafts were favorable. The total time for healing was shortened to a few weeks.

A considerable amount of postoperative swelling and difficulty in swallowing occurs, but these symptoms usually subside after a week. Antibiotics and analgesics are usually prescribed.

Obwegeser technique for skin grafting

Obwegeser (1963, 1967) modified Trauner technique. He combined a ridge skin-grafting vestibuloplasty with a lingual sulcoplasty (Figs 13.7A to D).

Moore[34] (1970) suggested a modification of Obwegeser technique. Moore used a soft silicone lining in the splint. He sutured the mucosal flaps to the stent and fixed the stent to the mandible with Steinman pins. With this modification, Moore was able to avoid making the ten submandibular awl punctures that are part of Obwegeser procedure.

CORRECTIVE SURGICAL PROCEDURES

Soft Tissue Corrective Surgeries[35]

Surgical correction of various normal and abnormal soft tissue conditions can aid in denture construction for the dentist and make denture wearing more successful for the patient. Included here are correction of hypertrophic frenii, double lip, papillary hyperplasia of the palate and submucosal hyperplasia of the maxillary tuberosities, the palate, the mandibular retromolar pads and the vestibule.

The grossly resorbed alveolar process presents several problems. Pressures from the denture flanges on the mental nerve can produce pain or numbness. As the alveolar bone resorbs, the gingiva loses its bony support and becomes soft and mobile and the denture becomes progressively more unstable. As the alveolar ridge resorbs and becomes shorter, the denture flange must be shortened a little amount to prevent the formation of decubiti and hyperplastic folds of vestibular mucosa. As the denture flanges are shortened, both stability and retention decrease. This situation can be partly overcome by certain surgical procedures designed to deepen the vestibule and the sublingual sulcus.

Labial Frenectomy

One of the easiest corrective surgical procedures to perform is the excision of a hypertrophic labial frenum. The labial frenum is a band of fibrous connective tissue, covered with mucous membrane that binds the lip to the alveolar process. The upper labial frenum is usually more prominent and more fibrous than the lower, which often is reduced to a mere vestige. When a frenum is attached at or near the crest of the alveolar ridge, it may be subjected to repeated irritation from a denture flange. The procedure can be performed with local or general anesthesia in just a few minutes.

The lip is elevated, everted and tensed so that the frenum becomes prominent. Before making the incisions, it should be recalled that the purpose for performing the frenectomy is the elimination of the fibrous part of the frenum and that the mucosa should be repositioned to cover the surgical defect.

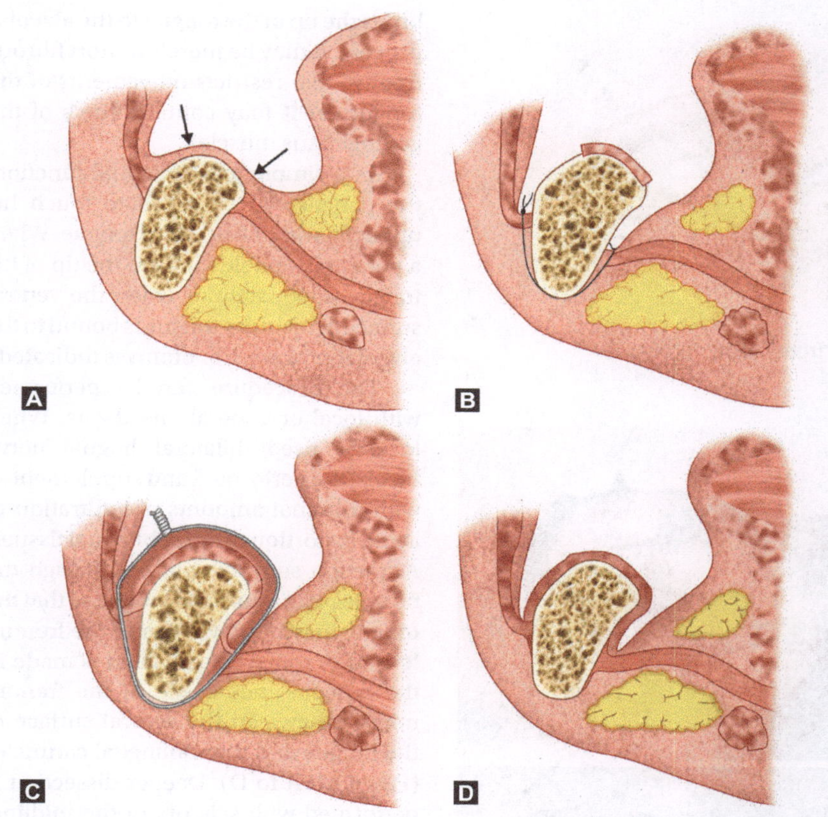

Figs 13.7A to D: Obwegeser's modified linguosulcoplasty: (A) Incision sparing mucosa at crest of ridge; (B) Labial and lingual ridge extensions; (C) Raw bone is skin grafted and covered with surgical stent; (D) Final result

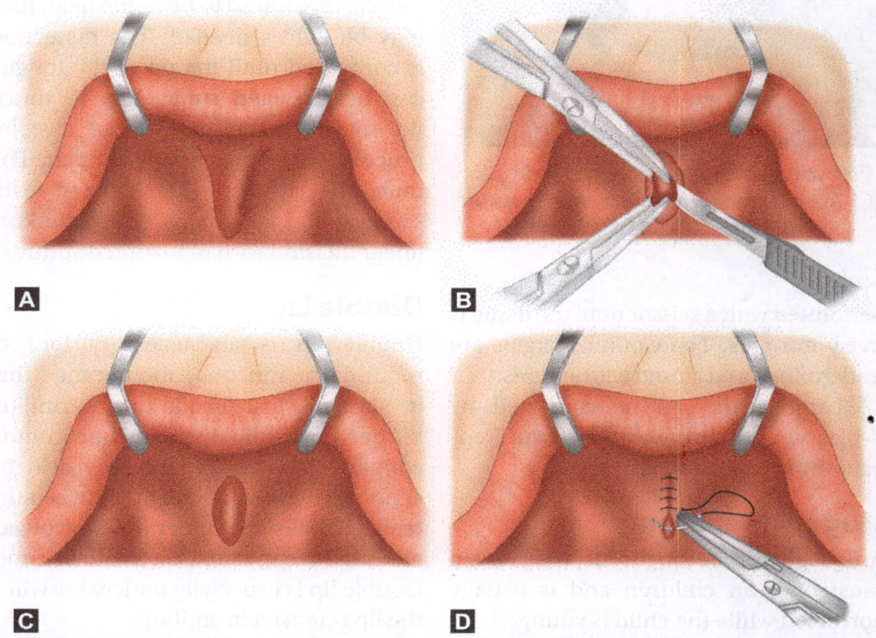

Figs 13.8A to D: Labial frenectomy: (A) V shaped incision; (B) Frenum detached from bone; (C) Diamond shaped defect; (D) Closure

The incisions are given in the mucous membrane around the frenum and are carried down to the bone (Figs 13.8A to D). If the frenectomy is performed to aid the orthodontic closure of a median diastema, the apex of the V should be at or near the incisive papilla on the palate. The two limbs of the V incision should be closely placed and often are nearly parallel. When the frenum is detached from the bone with a periosteal elevator, most of the connective tissue fibers retract upward into the lip. The small tag of labial mucosa and any surplus connective tissue can be removed easily with scissors. The margins of the resulting diamond-shaped defect can be undermined with a scissor and closed with interrupted sutures. The first suture should be placed across the middle of the wound (usually the widest part) and should engage both mucosal margins and the periosteum at the midline. This deeply fixed suture helps to maintain the height of the vestibular sulcus in the midline and to minimize the formation of a hematoma under the alveolar mucosa. Additional sutures are placed to close the wound in a vertical line. Sutures should be removed in 7 days.

Buccal Frenectomy

Buccal frena are composed mainly of folds of mucous membrane with only a thin fibrous stroma. They occur in the first bicuspid regions of the mandible and the maxilla. Their correction can be accomplished by a V-Y plasty or a V-diamond plasty if the frena are large. Since most buccal frena are small, a transverse incision through the frenum with a scalpel or scissors is all that is required to produce a diamond-shaped wound, the margins of which are undermined and closed longitudinally, or perpendicular to the original incision (Figs 13.9A and B). When correcting a lower buccal frenum, the surgeon should remember that the mental neurovascular bundle is often found in the connective tissue and trauma to the mental nerve should be avoided.

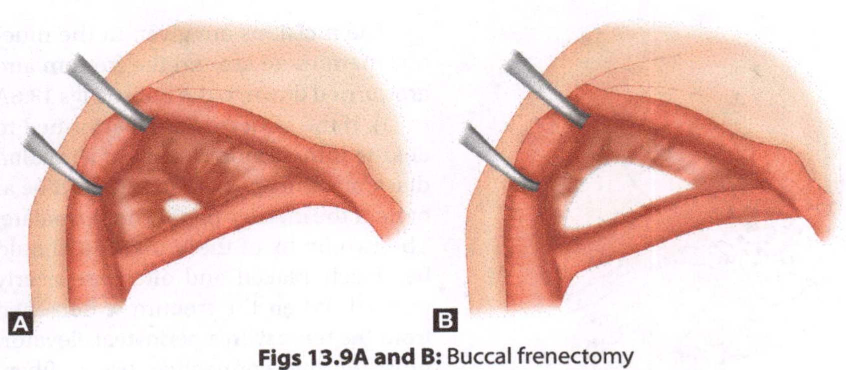

Figs 13.9A and B: Buccal frenectomy

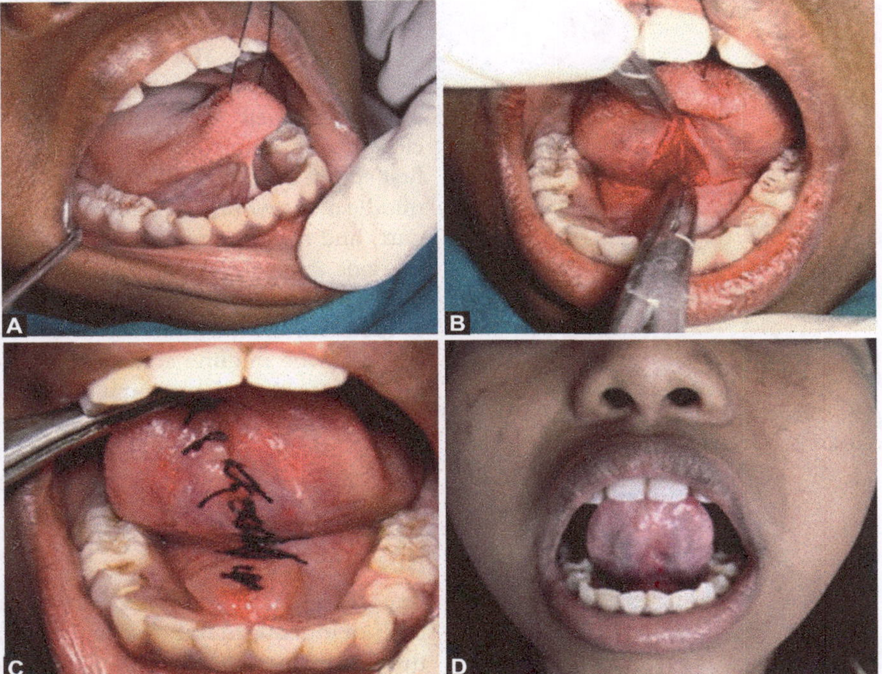

Figs 13.10A to D: Lingual frenectomy: (A) Preoperative limited tongue protrusion; (B) Transverse incision along lingual frenum; (C) Approximation of mucosa and suture; (D) Preoperative free tongue movement

Correction of Scar Contractures of the Lips and Buccal Mucosa

Depending on the size of the scar contracture and its location, a variety of corrective procedures can be performed. Thin scars can be corrected by a simple transverse incision across the scar similar to that made for a buccal frenum. The wound is converted from a transverse incision to a longitudinal diamond-shaped wound by tensing the tissue. Deeper dissection of the fibrous scar band can be performed with a scissor until the tissue is freely movable. The wound margins are undermined and closed with sutures.

Large scars can be corrected by Z-plasty, V-Y plasty or other tissue-repositioning procedures.

Lingual Frenotomy

Ankyloglossia, or tongue-tie, is observed most often in children and is usually corrected while the child is young.

The lingual frenum may consist of a fold of mucous membrane only, or it may contain a dense fibrous septum that binds the tip of the tongue to the alveolar process. It may be merely a short fibrous frenum that restricts movements of the tongue, or it may contain fibers of the genioglossus muscles.

As a simple test of lingual function, the patient can be asked to touch his upper lip with the tip of his tongue. When a patient is unable to move the tip of his tongue adequately or when the ventral surface or tip of the tongue is bound to the alveolar process, frenotomy is indicated.

The procedure can be performed with local or general anesthesia. When local is used, bilateral lingual nerve blocks are performed and supplemented with minimal amounts of infiltration to avoid distortion of the sublingual tissues. A traction suture is placed through the muscles of the tip of the tongue so that the tongue may be elevated and the frenum tensed. A transverse incision is made in the mucous membrane of the frenum midway between the ventral surface of the tongue and the sublingual caruncles (Figs 13.10A to D). Deeper dissection is performed with scissors in the midline, avoiding the ducts of the submandibular salivary glands and the sublingual veins, which are usually found lateral to the surgical field. If fibers of the genioglossus muscles are found to be in the field, they may be cut as needed. The dissection is continued until the tip of the tongue can be retracted sufficiently to touch the maxillary incisor teeth or alveolar process, while the mouth is open. The mucosal flaps are undermined with scissors and closed as a longitudinal linear incision with interrupted sutures.

Double Lip

Double lip is an accessory fold of redundant mucous membrane that is situated just inside the vermilion border of the lip. It is an uncommon congenital anomaly and may also be acquired by sucking the lip between the teeth. Usually the upper lip is involved, although it can occur on the lower one. Double lip is especially noticeable when the lip is tensed in smiling.

The procedure is performed in the dental office with local anesthesia. Bilateral infraorbital nerve blocks are

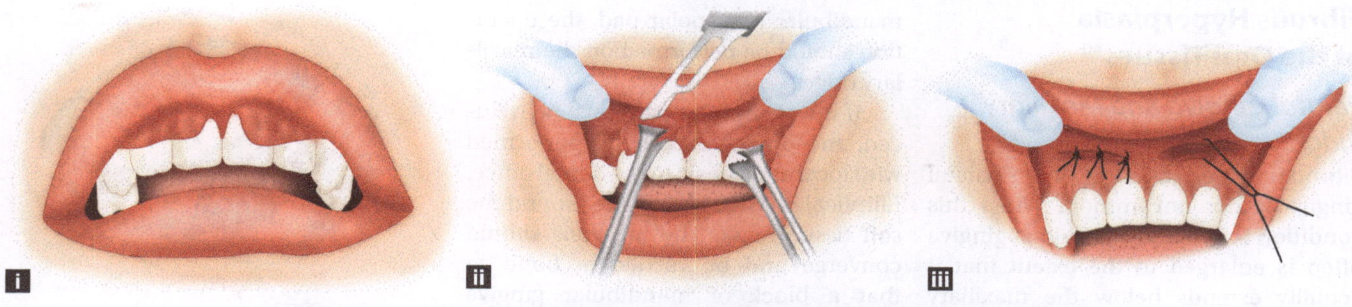

Figs 13.11A: Diagrammatic representation of the double lip surgery: (i) Presurgical; (ii) Intraoperative excision with knife; (iii) Closure

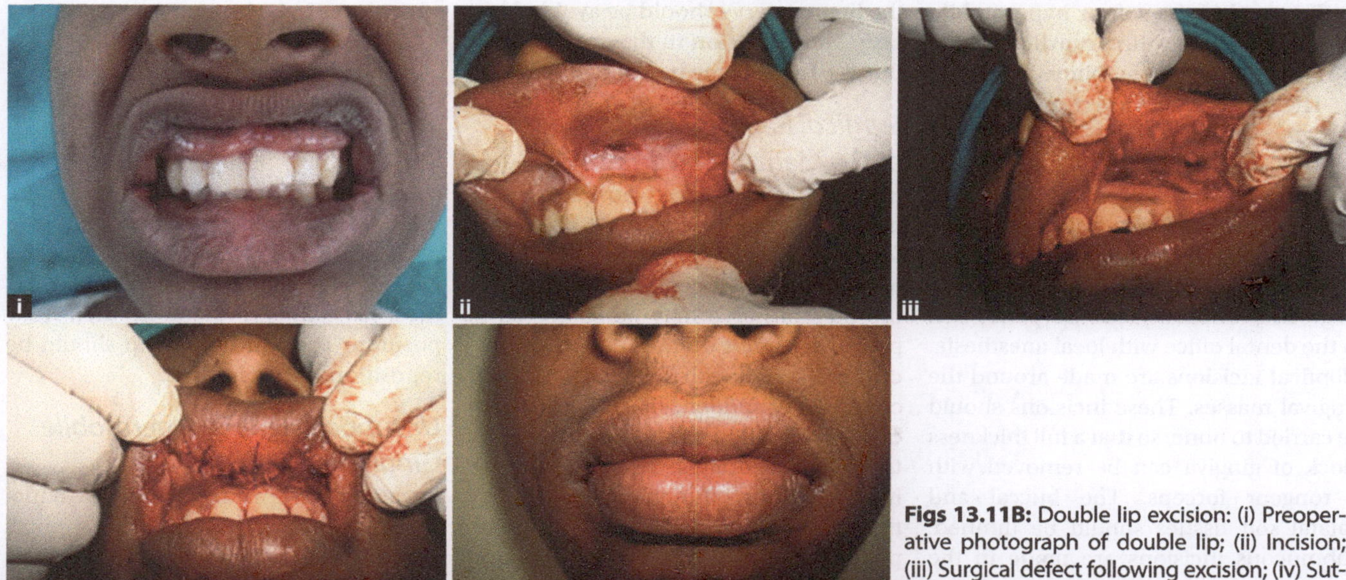

Figs 13.11B: Double lip excision: (i) Preoperative photograph of double lip; (ii) Incision; (iii) Surgical defect following excision; (iv) Suturing of the surgical wound; (v) Postoperative photograph

administered so that infiltration into the lip, producing distortion of the contour, can be avoided. The redundant folds of labial mucosa are grasped gently with Allis forceps and elliptical incisions are made around the masses (Figs 13.11A and B). The incisions are carried deep into the submucosa so that one or two blocks of tissue, wedge-shaped in cross section, are removed. A few small bleeders are ligated/cauterized. The wounds are closed in layers with 4 '0' absorbable sutures.

Inflammatory Papillary Hyperplasia of the Palate

Inflammatory papillary hyperplasia is a painless, irreversible disease of the oral mucous membrane. It occurs most commonly on the hard palate, although it is not restricted to this location. It has been observed primarily, but not exclusively, in patients who wear a complete maxillary denture.[36] It also occurs in patients who wear a maxillary partial denture and in patients with natural teeth and no prosthetic dental appliances.

The etiology is obscure. However, many authors agree, at least in part, on a number of contributing factors:[37]

- Poorly fitting denture.
- Wearing the denture 24 hours a day.
- Poor oral hygiene.
- Use of palatal relief.
- Predisposing factors.

Treatment of this disease can be accomplished in a variety of ways. In every case a biopsy is indicated to verify the benign nature of the disease. Removal of the denture for several days helps to reduce the inflammation, but does not eradicate the lesions.

Split-thickness, supraperiosteal excision is the treatment of choice for most lesions of inflammatory papillary hyperplasia. Small lesions can be removed with sharp curettes or by mucoabrasion with a rotary instrument. Use of electrocautery[38] and cryosurgery[39] by liquid nitrogen have also been reported. They have found that 2 to 4 treatments at weekly intervals are necessary, but the postoperative pain reportedly is less than that occurring after other methods of treatment. In all cases the patient's denture or a specially prepared surgical splint should be used to cover the raw wound.

Fibrous Hyperplasia of the Oral Tissues[40]

Palatal Gingiva and Maxillary Ridge

Fibrous hyperplasia of the palatal gingiva is not uncommon. When this condition is present, the palatal gingiva often is enlarged to the extent that it actually extends below the maxillary occlusal plane. This condition should be corrected for the following reasons:

- Removal of the soft or hypermobile gingiva leaves a firm maxillary ridge for good denture stability.
- The palatal gingiva is recontoured to remove soft-tissue undercuts.
- The crest of the maxillary ridge is shortened, thus providing space for a denture base.

Surgical reduction of the hyperplastic submucosa of the posterior maxillary ridge and tuberosity can be performed in the dental office with local anesthesia. Elliptical incisions are made around the gingival masses. These incisions should be carried to bone, so that a full thickness block of gingiva can be removed with a rongeur forceps. The buccal and palatal soft tissues should be thinned. Submucous incisions are made in the buccal and palatal connective tissue, parallel with the mucosal surface, and are carried to bone. The blocks of submucous connective tissue are removed, leaving buccal and palatal flaps of appropriate thickness, which are repositioned and sutured.

Mandibular Retromolar Pad Reduction

Fibrous hyperplasia of the mandibular retromolar pad occurs infrequently. When it does occur, the retromolar pad may contact the maxillary tuberosity or teeth. The fibrous portion of the retromolar pad supports the posterior border of the mandibular denture. Complete excision of the retromolar pad deprives the mandibular ridge of a valuable protective covering and permits excessive settling of the denture and ridge resorption. If a choice is available between surgical reduction of the maxillary gingiva and the mandibular retromolar pad, the operation should be performed on the maxillary ridge.

If the retromolar pad must be reduced, the operation can be performed with local anesthesia in the dental office. Elliptical incisions are made around the soft tissue mass. The incisions should converge and be carried to bone so that a block of mandibular gingiva can be removed. The gingival flaps are approximated and sutured. Trauma to the lingual nerve should be avoided lost taste and sensation to the anterior two-thirds of the tongue be interrupted.

Surgical Repositioning of the Mental Nerve

In patients with gross atrophy of the mandibular alveolar process the mental foramen may be found at or near the crest of the residual ridge. When this occurs, the mental nerve may be subjected to pressure from a denture during mastication. Patients with this condition often complain of sudden, sharp, severe pain of short duration similar to the pain of trigeminal neuralgia. The pain may be initiated during functional loading of the denture during mastication. Some patients complain of both pain and numbness in the lower lip.

For many patients the symptoms can be eliminated by relieving the denture to avoid pressure on the mental foramen. This method is successful when, there is sufficient support provided by the remaining denture-bearing area. When the denture support is insufficient, the denture should not be relieved, as this would reduce the support even more. Instead, the mental neurovascular bundle should be surgically repositioned.

The surgical procedure can be performed with local anesthesia in the dental office. A long incision is made on the crest of the residual ridge. If the mental foramen has been found by palpation to be located on the crest of the ridge, the incision should be curved lingually to avoid the foramen. The mucoperiosteal flap is carefully reflected to expose the mental foramen and the neurovascular bundle, which should be carefully retracted.

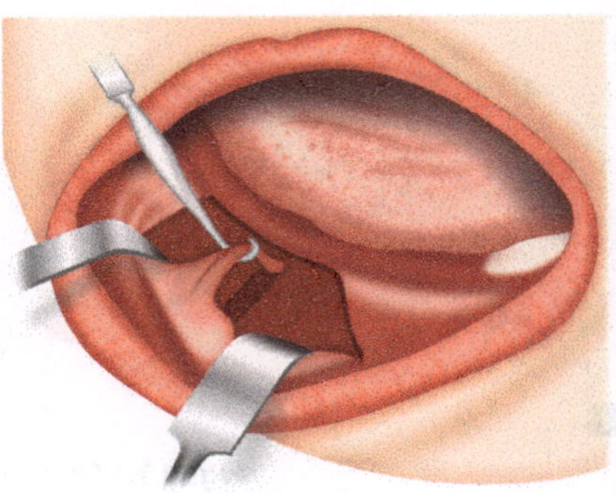

Fig. 13.12: Mental nerve repositioning

A vertical groove should be made in the bone beneath the mental foramen with a dental drill (Fig. 13.12). When the osseous preparation has been completed, the neurovascular bundle may be carefully positioned in the newly formed foramen. Surgicel may be placed over the neurovascular structures to maintain them in their new position. The soft tissue flap should be repositioned and sutured.

Unsupported and Hypermobile Gingiva[41]

In cases of severe atrophy of the residual ridge, the gingiva loses its bony support and becomes freely movable. As a result, the denture becomes increasingly more unstable. Treatment is directed towards providing a firm basal seat area for the denture. The operation may be performed with local anesthesia. Two incisions are made along the crest of the residual maxillary ridge, one to the labial and the other to the palatal side. The two incisions converge at the right and left ends of the surgical field and are carried to bone so that a long strip of gingiva may be removed. The wound margins are approximated and sutured. A soft denture-lining material may be placed inside the denture to compensate for the change in tissue contour.

The excision of hypermobile mandibular gingiva usually is complicated by the presence of a very thin and short residual ridge. Since there is a deficiency of mandibular gingiva, it is desirable not to excise too much when the hypermobile gingival crest is removed. Sutures are rarely necessary. A soft denture-lining material may be placed inside the denture to improve the tissue-denture contact and to protect the tender mandibular ridge, which heals in a week with minimal postoperative pain and swelling.

Excision of hypermobile gingiva, whether maxillary or mandibular, does not consistently produce good results. In some cases of extreme alveolar atrophy, removal of the hypermobile gingiva results in a short ridge with a soft mucosal covering. Sulcus-deepening procedures are necessary to permit construction of a denture with a flange of sufficient length to provide some measure of denture stability.

Recognizing the limitations of surgical reduction of the hypermobile ridge, Laskin (1970) had injected a sclerosing solution into the hypermobile gingiva in an effort to produce fibrosis within the soft tissue and a resultant reduction in the mobility of the ridge. He recommends that the patient should not wear his denture after the injections lest tissue movement interfere with the fibrosis of the ridge. After 4 to 6 weeks, the ridge should be sufficiently rigid that a new denture may be made.

Inflammatory Hyperplasia of the Vestibular Mucosa

Chronic irritation from a poorly fitting denture frequently results in the formation of areas of hyperplastic enlargement of the alveolar mucosa (Fig. 13.13) and the mucous membrane of the vestibular sulcus. The terms '*epulis fissurata*' and '*denture fibroma*' have been used to describe this lesion. These hyperplastic masses are composed of fibrous connective tissue with a mucous membrane covering and occasionally some labial mucous glands in the stroma. Inflammation is a common feature.

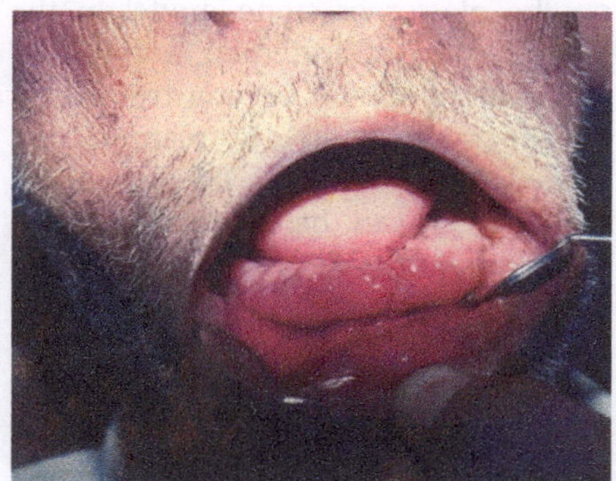

Fig. 13.13: Gingival hyperplasia

These masses should be excised in such a way that minimal scarring of the vestibule occurs and the depth of the sulcus is maintained. Usually the wound margins cannot be sutured together without reducing the depth of the sulcus. As a result, many of these wounds heal by granulation and secondary epithelization.

HARD TISSUE PROCEDURES

Alveoloplasty

Alveolectomy has been defined by Boucher[42] as the excision of a portion of the alveolar process. Only recently 'alveoloplasty' has been adopted to signify recontouring of the alveolar process rather than its removal. Alveoloplasty is generally performed to facilitate the removal of one or more teeth, and to prepare the residual ridge for the reception of artificial dentures.

Willard[1] AT first reported (1853) a case of alveolectomy, where he removed the interdental papilla and alveolar margin, permitting edge-to-edge closure of the soft tissues. Dean[43] (1936) introduced 'Intra-Septal Alveolectomy' a procedure he had been using since 1916. He advocated preservation of labial cortex at the expense of inter radicular medullary bone.

Types of Alveoloplasty

Alveolar compression: The easiest and quickest form of alveoloplasty is the compression of outer and inner cortical plates between the fingers. This procedure should be done for all the extractions in which considerable manipulation of the tooth with expansion of buccal cortex was necessary. Compression reduces the width of the socket and eliminates many otherwise troublesome bony undercuts. Suture may or may not be used to maintain soft tissues.

Simple alveoloplasty: It is used to trim the buccal or palatal cortical margins after extraction of isolated tooth in the oral cavity. Overerupted teeth have elongated alveolar process so that vertical reduction of bony margins of socket often is indicated when such teeth are removed. An envelope flap is generally enough for access to the cortical plates, when indicated a trapezoidal flap can be used with one or two releasing incisions. With a rongeur bone-cutting forceps held parallel to bony margin of alveolar process, just right amount of bone can be removed. Schram suggested that only one-half the desired amount of bone be removed, as this amount would be enough.

Cortical Alveoloplasty

In normal circumstances the residual alveolar ridge is allowed to resorb and mould itself after extraction, without any additional surgical procedures. However, if the denture construction is more urgent, cortical alveoloplasty is indicated. Cortical alveoloplasty may be performed after extraction of a single tooth, multiple teeth and teeth in the entire arch.

A crestal incision is made through the extraction site. The projecting bone is removed with rongeur or surgical bur and smoothed with a bone file. Soft tissue can be removed from the mesial and distal sides of the socket to facilitate linear closure of the wound. The wound is closed with interrupted or mattress sutures.

Dean alveoloplasty: Dean[43] gave this successful technique for preparing the alveolar ridge for dentures. Thoma described this procedure as inter-cortical rather than interseptal to describe the removal of inter-radicular bone.[44] 'Crush technique' is also a common term used for the same procedure. Regardless of the descriptive terminology, Dean technique and its results are based on sound biological principles:

- The prominence of the labial and buccal alveolar margin is reduced to facilitate the reception of dentures.
- The muscle attachments are undisturbed.
- The periosteum remains intact.
- The cortical plate is preserved as a viable onlay bone graft with an intact blood supply.

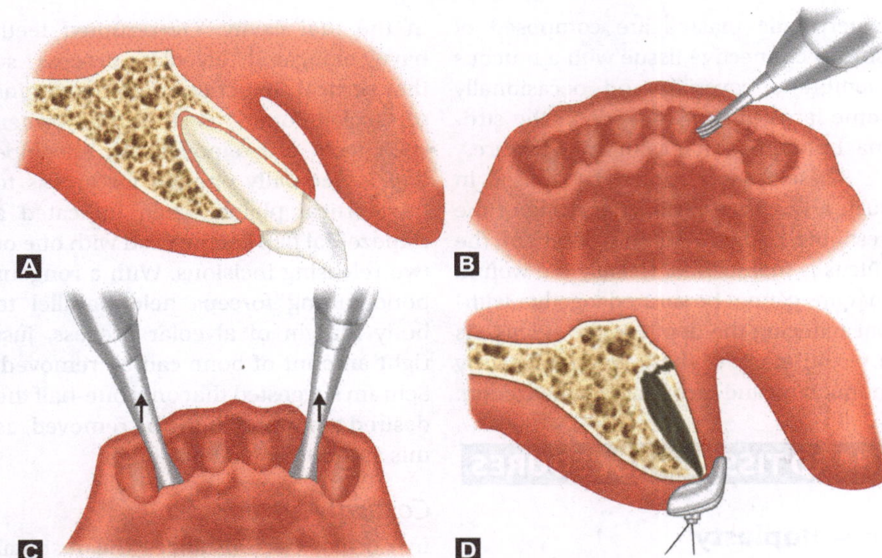

Figs 13.14A to D: Dean's alveoloplasty: (A) Cross-sectional view prior to extraction; (B) Removal of interdental bone; (C) Fracturing of labial cortex; (D) Approximation and suturing of mucosa

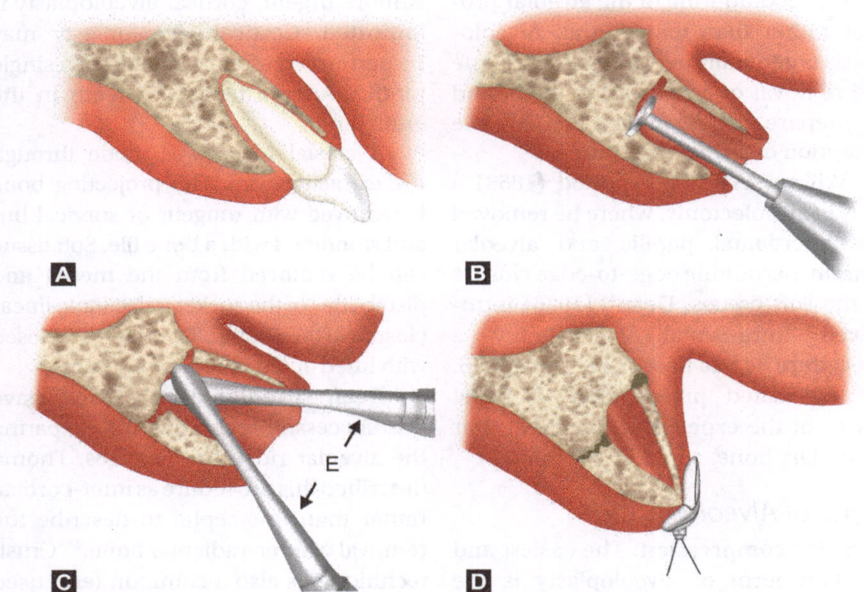

Figs 13.15A to D: Obwegeser's technique: (A) Cross-sectional view of ridge prior to extraction; (B) Scoring of labial and palatal cortex; (C) Both cortical plates fractured; (D) Approximation of cortices and closure

- Because the cortical bone is spared, postoperative resorption is minimized.

After removal of the teeth the interradicular bony septa should be removed with a rongeur forceps (some operators prefer chisels or burs) (Figs 13.14A to D).

To permit the labial cortex to be moved palatally, some relief is necessary to permit the telescoping of the labial cortex, Dean used a chisel to make an inverted V-shaped excision of bone in the labial cortex of the cuspid socket. Thus, three sides of the labial cortical flap were freed. At this point finger pressure usually was sufficient to compress the cortex palatally. Doing so the labial cortex became a freely movable bone graft attached to only the mucoperiosteum from which it received its blood supply. The horizontal fracture line in the apical area was smoothened with a bone file from within the socket to produce a smooth labial surface. Dean used this technique on posterior ridges as well as anterior ridges, making a buccal cortical relief at the most posterior socket.

Obwegeser Technique for Alveoloplasty

Obwegeser[29] suggested further modification of Dean's technique. In cases of extreme premaxillary protrusion, Dean's technique would produce a V-shaped anterior ridge instead of the desired U-shaped ridge. To avoid such a ridge, Obwegeser fractured both the labial and the palatal cortices.

Removal of teeth is done as usual. Sockets are connected using rongeurs or burs to remove the medullary interradicular bone. Both the labial and palatal plates are cut with burs in the cuspid area to weaken the bone and to form the three-sided bone flaps in both cortical plates (Figs 13.15A to D). A small mounted disk is inserted into the sockets and through to score or groove the labial and palatal plates, horizontally weakening them along the proposed fracture lines. Finger pressure is then used to mold the alveolar process into its desired shape. Sutures close the gingiva over the sockets and help to hold the bone in position. A denture on splint is used to stabilize the fractured alveolar process, which heals in 4 to 6 weeks.

The operation should be 'performed' on the plaster or stone model in the laboratory first, and then a splint or the denture should be constructed on the 'operated' model. By planning the procedure on plaster in the laboratory, the surgery can be performed more accurately in the dental office or operating room.

Buccal and Labial Alveoloplasty

Reduction of the outer cortical plates is the oldest and most popular method of alveoloplasty.

An incision is made in gingival and a full thickness muco-periosteal flap that extends at least one tooth on either side of area of bony surgery is elevated. A sharp side cutting ronguer forceps is held with one beak beneath the bony rim of the socket and other on the crest of the ridge. Small pieces of the bone can be nibbled off the ridge. After the bone is removed, a bone file can be used to smooth and perfect the bony contour. This type of alveoloplasty is most suited in cases in which minimal bone reduction is indicated.

Alveolectomy and Alveolotomy[45]

The extraction of isolated posterior teeth commonly leaves prominent cortical bone with superficial buccal undercuts. A single longitudinal crestal or a narrow elliptical subperiosteal incision permits access to these and their removal where indicated.

Troublesome undercuts are frequently found on the labial surfaces of both upper and lower anterior regions, some patient for unknown reason undergo grossly uneven alveolar resorption particularly of the labial or buccal plates, which produces multiple irregular horizontal bony protuberance on which it is impossible to fit satisfactorily denture.

Reduction of the Knife-edged or Saw-tooth Ridge

Extreme alveolar atrophy of the mandibular ridge and occasionally of the maxillary ridge often results in a sharp residual alveolar crest that literally cuts into the mucoperiosteum from the deep surface whenever pressure is brought to bear on the area. Denture wearing becomes extremely painful in this situation. The pain is usually relieved when the denture is removed, but mere finger pressure on the tender area will produce the pain again.

The incision should be made horizontally in the gingiva just apical to the alveolar crest, with a small relaxing incision at each end. The labial and lingual flaps are reflected just far enough to expose the sharp bone at the crest. Any sharp or rough bony edges and prominences can be removed with a side-cutting rongeur. The ridge is then smoothed with a bone file. Care must be taken to avoid removing too much bone, since there is a deficiency of bone to begin with. The incision is closed without tension by interrupted sutures, with caution exercised not to reduce the depth of the vestibular sulcus.

Maxillary Tuberosity Reduction

An increase in the vertical dimension of the maxillary tuberosity is frequently encountered. When of sufficient degree, this increase will impinge upon the intermaxillary space required for successful denture construction. It may also be pendulous, inhibiting denture stability and palatal bony undercuts may be present. Pneumatization of the maxillary sinus may proceed into the elongated tuberosity.[46]

Causes

- Gingival fibromatosis.
- Loss of the lower molar teeth permitting over eruption of the upper molar teeth with an accompanying bony alveolar hyperplasia when the teeth are extracted the enlarged bony tuberosity may remain.
- The resection of a maxillary 3rd molar.
- An enlarged maxillary antrum.

Hyperplastic tuberosity is recontoured by wedge resection.[47] Two elliptical incisions are made over the crest of the tuberosity and carried down to bone. The resulting wedge of tissue is grasped with a hemostat and dissected free and sutured in position.

Reduction of the Mylohyoid Ridge

Extreme alveolar atrophy sometimes accentuates the mylohyoid ridge, which can be palpated along the lingual surface of the mandible in the second and third molar area. Occasionally the mylohyoid ridge and external oblique ridge are the highest points of the atrophic mandible, since the alveolar process has been reduced to a groove by resorption.

Gillies[48] states that the mylohyoid ridge should be reduced whenever the ridge is found to be at the same level as or at a higher level than the alveolar process. Frequently, the lingual mucoperiosteum overlying the mylohyoid ridge becomes traumatized, ulcerates, and fails to heal. In such a case the bony shelf must be removed in order to permit closure of the ulcerated tissue with sutures.

Howe[49] states that reduction of the mylohyoid ridge is the most useful single operation available for the grossly resorbed mandible, for not only is the painfully sharp bony edge reduced, but the lingual sulcus is also lowered at the same time.

The incision is made in the residual gingiva on the crest of the alveolar process from the bicuspid to the third molar region. In cases in which a mucosal ulcer overlies the bony prominence the incision is adapted to include the ulcer. In this way the lingual flap does not have a 'button hole' perforation. The lingual mucoperiosteum is reflected carefully, exposing the mylohyoid ridge and muscle. The mylohyoid muscle is attached to the edge and inferior surface of the mylohyoid ridge and must be carefully incised with a scalpel, keeping the blade directed laterally toward the mandible. Once the muscle has been reflected, the bony ridge can be reduced with rongeurs and bone file. Interrupted sutures close the wound and complete the operation. The detached mylohyoid muscle will reattach to the mandible at a lower level. If the patient already has a denture, the lingual flange can be border trimmed with impression compound and relined temporarily with a soft denture-lining material. The recontoured denture flange serves to hold down the mylohyoid muscle, resulting in a deeper lingual sulcus.

Elimination of Labial Mandibular Undercut

Many patients experience resorption of the mandibular alveolar process, resulting in a marked labial and buccal undercut due to more resorption in the apical areas than at the alveolar crest. With such a ridge it is extremely difficult for a patient to wear a denture successfully.

Two methods of treatment are available:

1. Excision of the overhanging bone at the alveolar crest can be performed.
2. The undercut area can be filled and recontoured with a bone graft or some biologically inert foreign material.

If the alveolar process is broad, the patient usually can afford to sacrifice a little buccal overhanging bone. Even if the posterior ridge is narrow, the support offered by the oblique line will compensate for the narrow ridge. Anteriorly the problem is more acute, if the anterior ridge is reduced in size, it must bear a larger share of the masticatory load per unit area and eventually undergo additional resorption.

In such cases it is useful to fill out the undercut rather than reduce the surface area. Tantalum mesh and cartilage have been used to fill an undercut extending from the right molar area around to the left molar area with favorable results.[50]

Transplantation of autogenous alveolar bone can produce very satisfying results and should be considered whenever bone is being removed for alveoloplasty.

Genial Tubercle Reduction

Genial tubercles give attachment to genioglossus superiorly and geniohyoid inferiorly. One may note that the separation between the genioglossi and geniohyoids can often be identified by a layer of fat between these muscles. Approximately one-half or less of the genioglossi are sectioned at the genial tubercle on the superior and lateral portions. Obwegeser reported that difficulty in swallowing will occur for several months, if the genioglossi are sectioned completely. The dimensions of the genial tubercle are highly variable. Like the mylohyoid ridge, sharp edges may be trimmed, but do not require trimming as they will usually resorb.

Torus Palatinus

Torus palatinus, or palatal torus, is a benign, slowly growing, bony projection of the palatine processes of the maxillae and occasionally of the horizontal plates of the palatine bones. It occurs bilaterally along the median suture on the oral surface of the hard palate. The etiology is unknown. Heredity, superficial trauma, malocclusion, and functional response to mastication have been suggested as possible factors.[51]

Palatal tori serve no useful purpose. Generally no treatment is indicated unless:

- They become as large as to interfere with speech.
- The mucosa becomes traumatized due to trauma from occlusion, ulcerates, and fails to heal because of its poor vascularity.
- The patient cannot otherwise be convinced that he or she does not have a malignant tumor.
- The torus interferes with the design and construction of a removable dental prosthesis.

A median palatal incision is made in the mucosa the full length of the torus with two short, obliquely diverging incisions at the anterior and posterior ends, avoiding the vascular foramina. If the torus extends to the posterior border of the hard palate, care must be exercised to avoid penetration through the soft palate into the nasal cavity (Figs 13.16A to D). Each flap is reflected with a periosteal elevator and is sutured to the mucosa of the alveolar process to keep it out of the operative field.

If the torus is small and pedunculated and if the palatal bone is thick, it is possible to cleave the torus from the palate with a sharp blow of a mallet on a sharp, single-beveled chisel. In a broad based torus, a no. 703 carbide fissure bur or another bone bur of comparable size, can be used to cut crisscross grooves, dividing the torus in multiple small segments, giving it the appearance of a waffle. Once the torus has been divided, the pieces can be removed with rongeur forceps or with a mallet and chisel, without the hazard of fracturing the palate.

The stump of the torus then is smoothed with bone files, chisels or large bone burs. The torus need not be reduced to the extent that a concave palatal contour

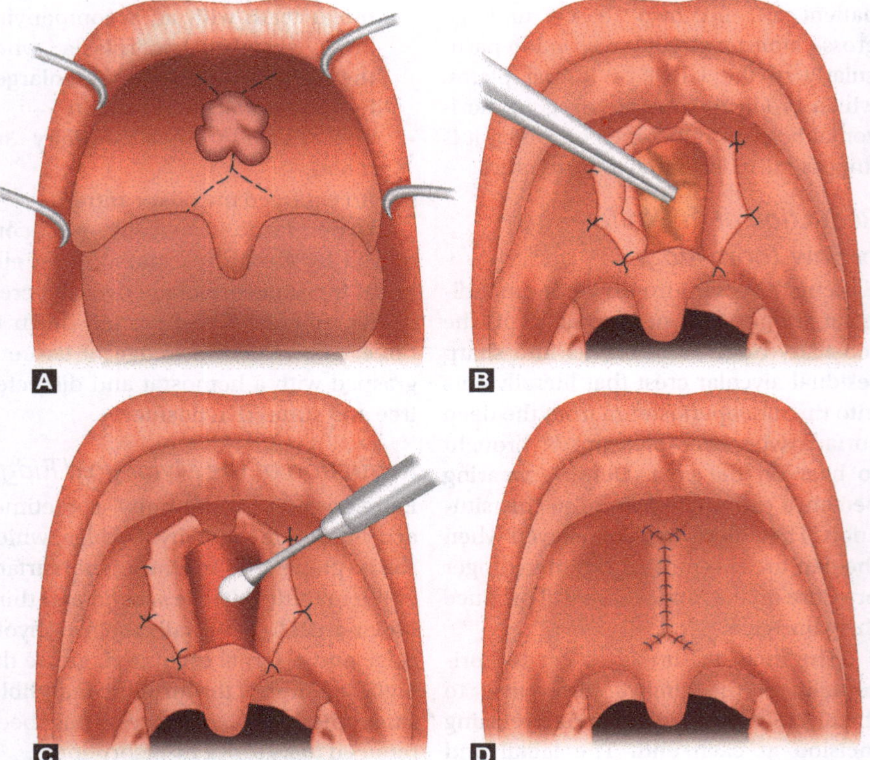

Figs 13.16A to D: Removal of palatal tor: (A) Transverse incision; (B) Division of large tori into multiple fragments; (C) Smoothening the palatal bed; (D) Closure

results. A flat palate, or even one with a slight residual median ridge, is adequate in most cases.

There is often a surplus of palatal mucosa that can be trimmed with scissors, if desired and then the mucosa is closed over the bony wound with non-absorbable suture. Great care must be exercised in suturing, as the thin mucosa tears quite easily. Some surgeons prefer to save all or most of the surplus mucosa. In such cases, the mucosa is replaced with the edges everted and held with mattress sutures so that the raw surfaces of the two flaps are in contact. This results in a thicker mucosal covering in the midline of palate.

The most important postoperative care is prevention of hematoma formation by the use of a rubber drain or by a splint or stent. A stent is used to adapt and support the mucosal flaps in contact with the bone, thus eliminating dead space into which blood and serum can accumulate.

Several complications of torus removal are possible and all can be avoid or controlled.[52]

- Hemorrhage.
- Hematoma.
- Sloughing of the palatal mucosa.
- Perforation of the floor of the nose.
- Fracture of the palate.

Buccal Exostoses

For the prosthetic patient there are two problems. Reduction of the buccal exostosis is necessary for the accuracy of the denture impression and the stability and retention of the denture; and yet this bone reduction could result in excessive loss of cortical bone, thus leaving the cancellous bone covered only by mucosa. As a result, excessive resorption of the alveolar process could occur, substantially reducing not only the size of the alveolar process, but also the transverse width of the entire maxilla.

The incision is placed on the crest of the ridge. An anterior, oblique or relaxing, incision is made, if necessary, to gain sufficient access to the area. The mucosal flap is reflected to a level immediately above the exostosis, which is removed with rongeurs, burs, or a sharp chisel. After removal of the exostosis the alveolar process is smoothened, and the mucosa replaced and sutured. Only routine postoperative care is necessary.

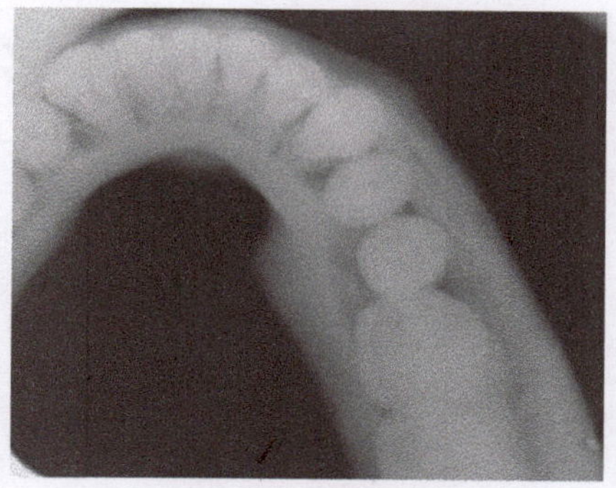

Fig. 13.17 : Torus mandibularis as seen on occlusal radiograph

Torus Mandibularis

Torus mandibularis, or mandibular torus, is an exostosis, usually occurring bilaterally on the medial surface of the body and alveolar process in canine-premolar region (Fig. 13.17). Mandibular tori are composed of dense, cortical bone with minimal amounts of a medullary core. The overlying mucoperiosteum is very thin, as it is on the entire medial surface of the mandible. Laceration or traumatic ulceration of the mucosa is not uncommon. Mandibular tori are removed.

- When they become so large that they cause speech impairment or difficulty in eating.
- When the covering mucosa ulcerates as a result of trauma and fails to heal.
- To facilitate the construction of removable partial and complete dentures.

Removal of mandibular tori is not difficult. It is easily accomplished in the office with local anesthesia, frequently at the same time as the removal of the posterior teeth.

The incision is made on the crest of the alveolar process from the molar to the incisor region (Figs 13.18A and B). Most mandibular tori can be removed by a sharp blow of a mallet on a sharp chisel. In the case of a large, fusiform torus, it is helpful to use a dental bur to establish a plane of cleavage before using the mallet. Water tight closure is done to prevent any hematoma formation. A stent can also be used to protect the thin lingual mucosa.

Ridge Augmentation Procedures

Patients suitable for ridge augmentation should:

- Have gross mandibular atrophy, that is the vertical symphyseal height of 2 cm or less.
- Be middle aged or younger and medically fit.
- Be aware that a subsequent vestibuloplasty may be required.
- Be grossly dissatisfied with their existing dentures.

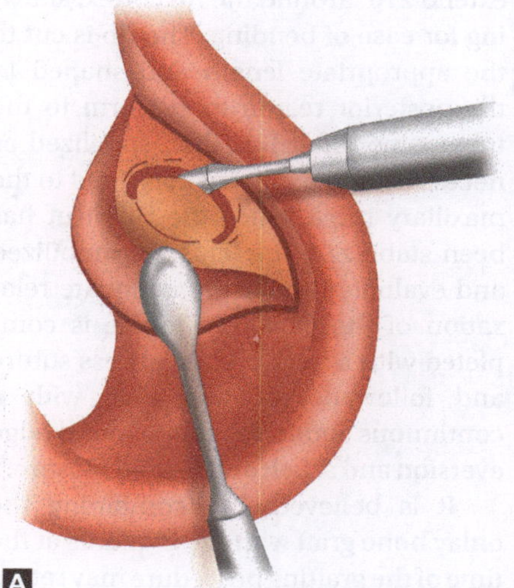

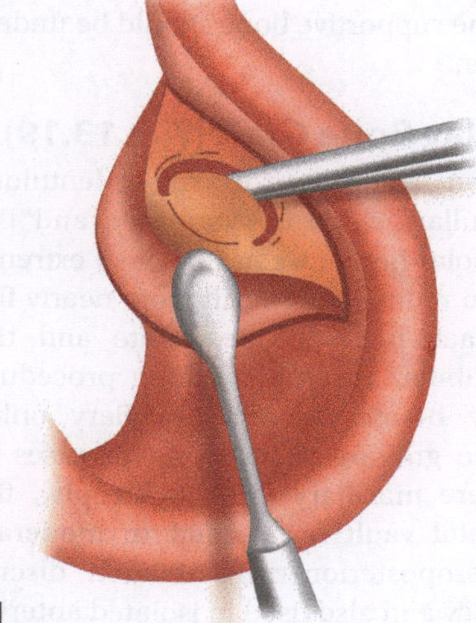

Figs 13.18A and B: Lingual tori excision: (A) Incision and flap elevation; (B) Removal of tori using chisel/bur

Maxillary Ridge Augmentation

Surgical preprosthetic reconstruction of the maxilla is complicated by several unique anatomic features. The proximity of the maxillary sinus to the nasal cavity, the contour of the zygomatic buttress, the position of the hamulus, and the nature of the alveolar bone of the maxilla make surgical augmentation more difficult than it is in the mandible. Contributing aspects (such as periodontal disease, malnutrition, and menopause) and systemic disease states (such as osteoporosis) should be evaluated and corrected preoperatively whenever possible.

Clinical examination should be conducted systematically. Radiographic examination will require panoramic radiographs to evaluate the jaws for pathology, sinusitis, retained teeth and roots, residual bone height of the mandible, proximity of the maxillary antrum to the alveolus, and position of the inferior alveolar neurovascular bundle. Lateral cephalograms with the head in a natural position and the lips in an unrestrained position will allow for evaluation of the anteroposterior relationship of the maxilla and the mandible as well as general shape of the anterior maxilla and mandible. Vertical height, position of the genial tubercles, and proximity of the sinuses and nasal floor can also be evaluated. An occlusal radiograph of the mandible can permit evaluation of mandibular width.[53] When a nearly flat surface exists between the palate and the vestibule, replacement of the supportive bone should be undertaken.

Onlay Bone Graft (Fig. 13.19)

When resorption of the edentulous maxillary ridge is symmetric and the alveolar bone loss has been so extreme as to reduce the maxilla to a nearly flat surface between the palate and the vestibule, an onlay grafting procedure may be considered. Maxillary onlay bone grafting is indicated in cases of severe maxillary alveolar atrophy, flat palatal vault form, mild to moderate anteroposterior ridge relation discrepancy and also used in isolated anterior ridge loss.

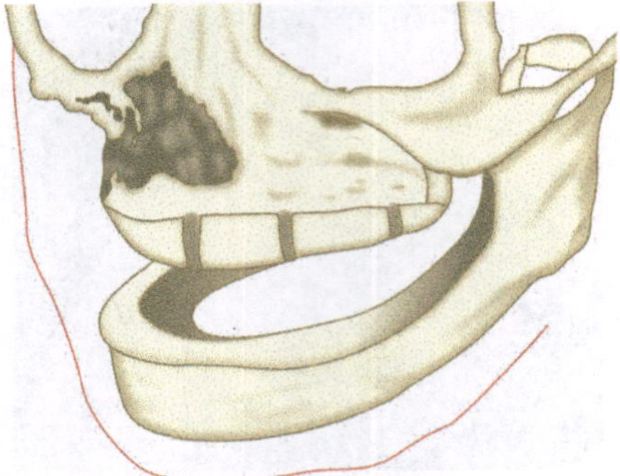

Figs 13.19: Total maxillary onlay bone grafting

Once the ribs have been harvested, the orofacial region is approached. An incision is made through the crestal tissue from tuberosity to tuberosity. A facial mucoperiosteal flap is reflected, exposing the zygomatic crest of the maxilla, the piriform apertures and, if necessary, the infraorbital foramen. Depending on the amount of facial tissue available for closure, a limited palatal flap may be developed. The rib graft may be fixed by a variety of techniques, including stainless steel wires and miniplates. Preparation of the rib for grafting is performed on a separate table, while the maxilla is prepared. Using a cast of the maxilla, poured in acrylic and gas sterilized for use in the surgical field, one rib is despined and kerfed (notched) on the inner aspect (lesser curvature), allowing it to bend to the contour of the residual maxilla. The notching should extend 270° around the rib cortex, allowing for ease of bending. The rib is cut to the appropriate length and shaped in the posterior region to conform to the tuberosity. The rib is then stabilized as necessary and the rib strut is fitted to the maxillary ridge. Once the rib strut has been stabilized, the flaps are mobilized and evaluated to ensure adequate relaxation of the closure. Closure is completed with a horizontal mattress suture and followed by oversewing with a continuous suture for good wound edge eversion and a 'belt and braces' closure.[54]

It is believed that combining the onlay bone graft with the implants at the time of the grafting procedure may retard the bone resorption often associated with onlay bone grafts by allowing for earlier and better functional loading of the bone graft.[55]

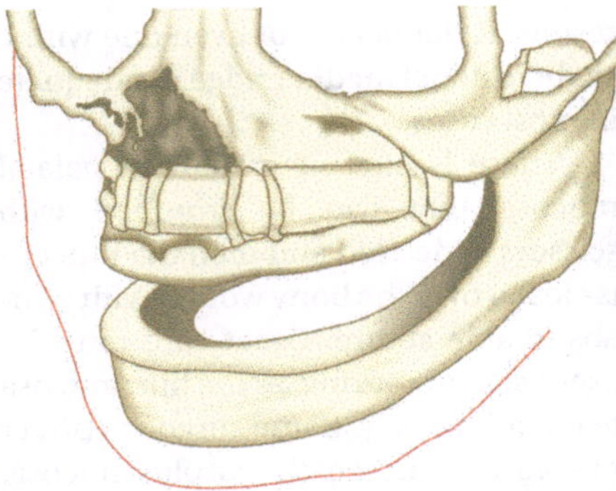

Fig. 13.20: Total maxillary interpositional bone graft

Total Interpositional Bone Graft (Fig. 13.20)

Owing to the rapid resorption of the onlay graft system, Farrell et al.[56] preferred the interpositional bone graft for the atrophic maxilla with good palatal vault form.

Patients with Class III relationships, usually secondary to the edentulous alveolar bone loss of both the maxilla and the mandible, can also benefit from anterior repositioning of the mobilized segment.

After the maxilla is down fractured, an interpositional bone graft is performed with an allogeneic strut of bone between the lateral antral walls. The bone graft, which has been shaped to the proper height and dumbbell-mortised for insertion along the lateral antral wall, is positioned and retained in place with transosseous wires through the previously placed bur holes.

Total Maxillary Osteotomy with Advancement (Fig. 13.21)

Maxilla has a natural tendency to resorb to a smaller more posterior position, while the mandible seems to become more prominent with edentulous alveolar bone loss. This combined with vertical over closure, gives the appearance of mandibular prognathism. If patient is deemed to have a deficiency in the anterioposterior relationship or in the transverse dimension, it can be corrected

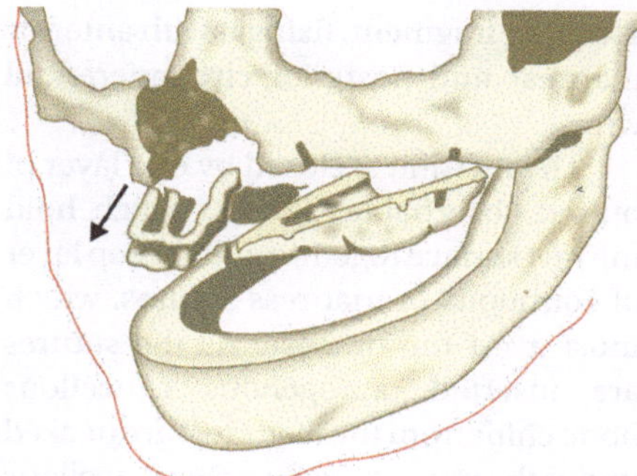

Fig. 13.21: Advancement of total osteotomized maxilla

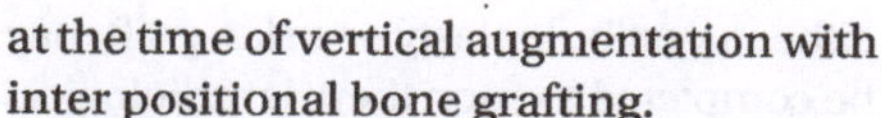

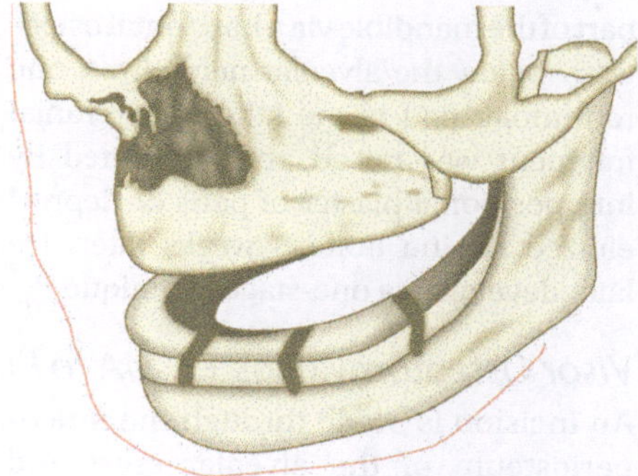

Fig. 13.22: Total mandibular onlay bone grafting

at the time of vertical augmentation with inter positional bone grafting.

The maxilla can be positioned forward for a predetermined distance and stabilized with the transosseous wires and interpositional bone grafts. Graft should be used if the advancement is greater than 5 mm or if there is an anomaly that would increase the chances of relapse. Stabilization is easily accomplished by placing a block of allogeneic bone, hydroxyapatite,[57] or autologous bone in the posterior section and wedging the posterior aspects of the maxilla apart. However, this amount of movement is generally not necessary in these patients.

Mandibular Procedures

A common pattern of mandibular EBL involves the generalized loss of alveolar bone, uniformly throughout the arch. This tends to produce a mandible in which the genial tubercles and mylohyoid ridges remain elevated and the rest of the ridge is flat. The basal bone is all that remains, leaving a mandible that may appear pencil-thin on panoramic radiographs. Clinically, a 'negative ridge' exists where the muscle attachments have actually elevated above the region available for denture bearing.

The height of remaining mandibular bone may be measured at the mental foramen region. The area should be evaluated for height and width.

The goal of surgical treatment to augment the mandibular ridge include:

- Providing optimum ridge from for the support of a prosthesis.
- Improvement of the maxillomandibular relationship.
- Increasing the bony bulk of the mandible.
- Providing adequate bone for implant placement in selected patient.

Several procedures are available for augmentation of edentulous mandible.[58] There is less chance of infection from an autogenously bone graft because of rapid healing.

Total Onlay Graft (Fig. 13.22)

For the mandible with generalized atrophy that measures less than 3 to 6 mm at the mental foramen region, there are few viable treatment alternatives. The patient usually is unable to wear a lower prosthesis, has Class III ridge relationships, and is at risk for injury from minor trauma. The total onlay graft is one of the few surgical options feasible for these patients.

The graft material of choice for the total onlay graft should be autologous bone. Rib or ileum is satisfactory. Pulmonary disease is a relative contradiction for removal of an endogenous rib use as a graft. The sharp spine on the superior edge of rib is removed by nears of rongeur. If ileum is to be used, the medial cortex and cancellous marrow can be harvested and contoured to appropriate shape. The placement of the rib should be slightly toward the lingual surface of the mandible, this is an attempt to reproduce the position of the resorbed alveolar ridge. Anteriorly the rib should rest on the mandible toward the lingual

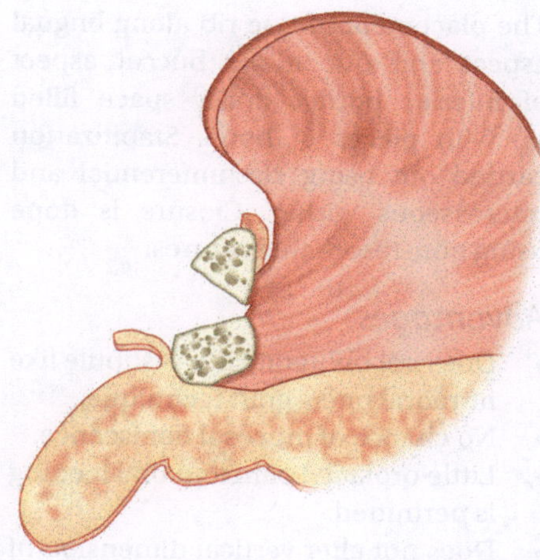

Fig. 13.23: Horizontal osteotomy for interpositional bone graft augmentation

surface. If ileum is used, the graft should fit over the basal bone of the mandible.

Alternative Method

By splitting both ribs and removing the cancellous bone, four sections of ribs are placed so that each inner cortex is next to an outer cortex. The cancellous bone and any chips from the excess length of rib may be packed around the rib. The total on lay graft to augment the mandible can achieve an immediate increase in the mandible height equal to the height of the graft place.

Augmentation to Inferior Border of Mandible (Fig. 13.23)

The procedure was suggested by Saunders and Cox[59] (1976). While as Beumer[60] (1979), in their study showed that inferior border grafting is superior to superior border grafting. Quinn[61] (1992) gave a new technique for inferior border augmentation and gave following indications:

- Augmentation of severely atrophic edentulous mandible.
- Prevention of pathologic fracture.
- Management of non-union/malunion of severely atrophic mandible.

Ribs are harvested and kerfing of ribs is done. A deep submandibular incision on both sides is taken. Subplatysmal dissection is done to expose lower border done protecting the mental bundle.

The placement of one rib along lingual aspect and one along buccal aspect of inferior border done, space filled up with pieces of bone. Stabilization carried out using circumferential and interosseous wiring. Closure is done using non-resorbable sutures.

Advantages

- Does not obliterate the vestibule like intraoral onlay graft technique.
- No chance of mucosal dehiscence.
- Little orofacial pain and oral feeding is permitted.
- Does not alter vertical dimension of occlusion.
- Secondary lingual sulcoplasty is not needed as mylohyoid muscle is lowered in initial surgery.
- Excellent for fracture stabilization and splints are not needed.
- Lesser bone resorption as direct masticatory forces are not applied.
- Patients with a history of sulcoplasty with skin graft placement—no violation of the SSG.
- Patients with a functioning subperiosteal implant with atrophic ridge—strengthening of mandible with salvage of implant.
- Augmentation of pencil thin mandibles where interpositional grafting/ visor osteotomy is not possible.
- Skin graft vestibuloplasty is easier in inferior border grafting than superior border grafting.

Disadvantages

- Large extraoral incision with extraoral scarring.
- Redundant, loose tissue required to avoid distortion of facial appearance.
- Does not correct superior border irregularities.

Interpositional Bone Graft Augmentation

In an attempt to overcome the disadvantage of subperiosteal onlay grafting (i.e. rapid resorption), interpositional bone graft techniques were developed. Barros-Saint-Pasteur,[62] a pioneer in the field, initially described a two-stage procedure. This involved mobilization of the alveolar part of the mandible via a horizontal osteotomy below the alveolar nerve from one retromolar pad to the other. The cranial fragment was raised and supported by interpositional plaster of paris or deproteinized bovine bone 3 weeks later. He later developed a one-stage technique.[63]

Visor Osteotomy (Figs 13.24A to F)

An incision is made through the mucoperiosteum of the alveolar crest and flaps raised.

Harle[64] made the osteotomy cut midway between the labial and buccal cortices between the mental foramina and on the lingual third posteriorly to them so as to avoid the inferior dental canal. This produces a weak and often small lingual portion of bone, which is easily fractured. The inferior dental bundle should be mobilized adequately. A groove is cut in the posterior molar area in the external oblique ridge and the bundle is reflected laterally and fixed onto the soft tissues of the cheek adjacent to the mandible by a loose catgut suture.

There are disadvantages to bundle mobilization:

- The blood supply of the mandible is further reduced (Oikarinen[65]). However, there is evidence that the supply may not have been of significance (Bradley[3]).
- The bundle is attached to the lateral surface of the mandible by scar tissue after wound closure. This may increase the difficulty of subsequent vestibuloplasty.

After reflection of the bundle, a continuous vertical cut through the mandible is made by a surgical burr or oscillating saw midway between the lingual and labial cortices from one side to the other as far as the reflected nerve bundle. The assistant's finger placed beneath the jaw give warning that the lower border has been reached. After completion of the vertical section, two cuts are made with the oblique saw blade at right angles through the lingual cortices in the vertical plane to complete the osteotomy.

Harle[64] advised placing the lower 20% of the lingual bone in contact with the main fragment, fixing it with anterior mattress and posterior circumferential wires.

The incision is closed by one layer of buried absorbable sutures, which hold the raw surface together and the top layer of continous or mattress sutures, which must avert the mucosa. As the sutures are inserted, autogenous cancellous bone chips from the iliac crest are packed under the mucosa against the cancellous surface of the lingual bone as far back as the ramus.

Dentures may be inserted three months postoperatively and, if necessary, either a vestibuloplasty or a skin graft may be completed as soon there is radiological evidence of the consolidation of the bone graft. The procedure has the two important drawbacks—width of mandible is reduced to half, no more than twice its height can be gained and a potential damage to inferior alveolar nerve (IAN).

Visor Osteotomy with Bone Grafting

The visor osteotomy doubles the mandibular height and is therefore suitable, where the mandible is approximately 2 cm or more in height. However, if the vertical height of the jaw is less or there is subsequent resorption the long term gain will not be sufficient. In this event the required gain can be achieved by the interposition of blocks of corticocancellous bone.

Sandwich Osteotomy (Fig. 13.25)

A corticocancellous bone graft is harvested from iliac crest (5 cm^2 cortical and 15 mL cancellous). The recipient site preparation is as usual. Full thickness mucoperiosteal flap elevated by giving incision between two retromolar pad areas. Mental nerve is identified and freed. A lingual subperiosteal tunnel in retromolar region is made. A horizontal osteotomy inferior to inferior alveolar canal (IAC) with inferior angulation of saw is done lingually. Superior segment is fractured upwards. Bone flap is pedicled to genioglossus and suprahyoid muscles. Superior segment is repositioned superiorly. Cortical bone from

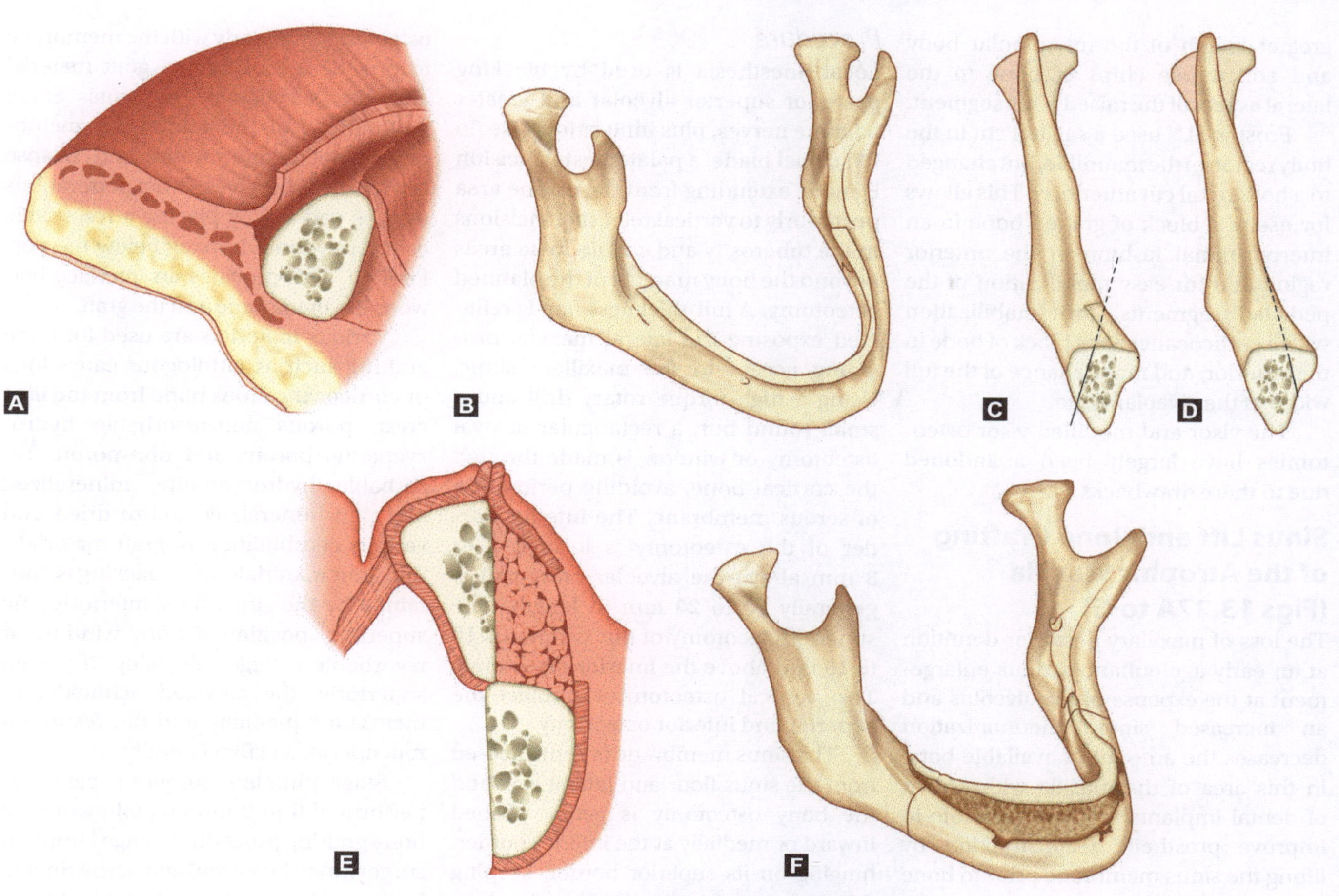

Figs 13.24A to F: Technique for visor osteotomy

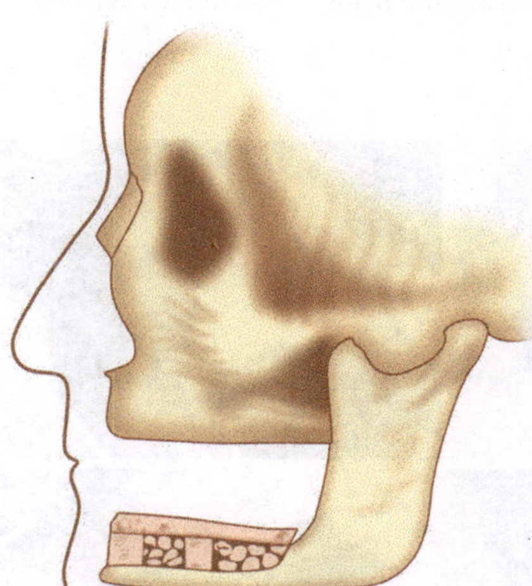

Fig. 13.25: Sandwich technique for mandibular ridge augmentation

ilium is harvested and placed in canine and molar areas on both sides. Superior segment is secured to inferior with thick resorbable sutures. Cancellous marrow is packed around cortical struts and a water tight closure of soft tissue is achieved.

The procedure suffers in that not enough space is present between the crest and foramina for horizontal cut, if only anterior area is addressed the posterior remains deficient and if done below mental nerve, the risk of fracture and damage to mental nerve from overlying denture is present.

Modified 'Visor' Osteotomy (Fig. 13.26)

The combination of the 'visor' and the 'sandwich' techniques was designed to overcome the aforementioned disadvantages of both methods. A modification of the visor osteotomy has been recommended for patients with at least 8 mm of bone height as measured at the mental nerve region. This procedure involves a parasagittal split of the mandible from the midbody on one side to the same position on the opposite side. The lingually pedicled segment is raised in visor fashion and wired into position. This procedure has been modified in various reports. Peterson and Slade,[66] raised the lingual segment along a

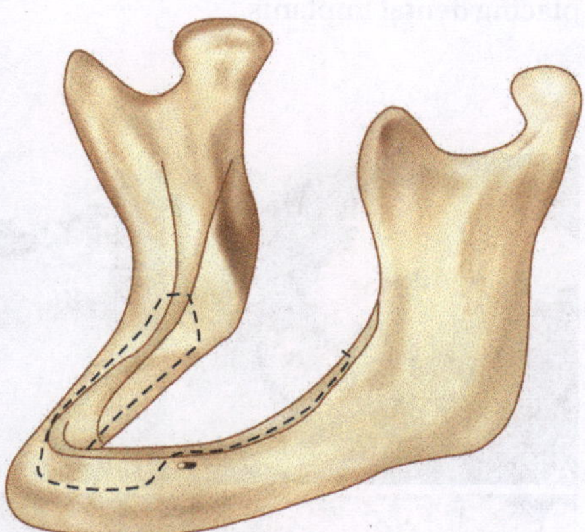

Fig. 13.26: Ostetomy cut for modified visor osteotomy

greater length of the mandibular body and added free chips of bone to the lateral aspect of the raised bony segment.

Frost et al.[67] used a sagittal cut in the body region of the mandible, but changed to a horizontal cut anteriorly. This allows for use of a block of grafted bone in an interpositional fashion in the anterior region and for easy mobilization of the pedicled segments, firm stabilization with a corticocancellous block of bone in the anterior, and maintenance of the full width of the alveolar ridge.

The visor and modified visor osteotomies have largely been abandoned due to there drawbacks.

Sinus Lift and Bone Grafting of the Atrophic Maxilla (Figs 13.27A to G)

The loss of maxillary posterior dentition at an early age enhances sinus enlargement at the expense of the alveolus and an increased sinus pneumatization decreases the amount of available bone in this area of the maxilla with ardent of dental implants it is now possible to improve prosthetic reconstruction by lifting the sinus membrane prior to bone grafting of this region and subsequently placing dental implants.

Procedure

Local anesthesia is used by blocking posterior superior alveolar and greater palatine nerves, plus infiltration. Use no 15 scalpel blade, a palatocrestal incision is made extending from the canine area posteriorly to vertical releasing incisions in the tuberosity and canine fossa areas beyond the bony margins of the planned osteotomy. A full-thickness flap is reflected exposing the lateral maxilla, providing access to the maxillary sinus. Using a high-torque rotary drill and a small round bur, a rectangular or oval osteotomy or window is made through the cortical bone, avoiding perforation of serous membrane. The inferior border of the osteotomy is located 2 to 3 mm above the alveolar crest and is generally 10 to 20 mm in length. The superior osteotomy of this window is 10 to 15 mm above the inferior osteotomy. Two vertical osteotomies connect the superior and inferior osteotomy.

The sinus membrane is gently teased from the sinus floor and lateral wall and the bony osteotomy is gently pushed inward or medially at the inferior border, hinging on its superior border, keeping the sinus membrane away from the sinus floor at the same time, elevating the osteotomy superiorly with the membrane to provide a roof for the graft material and the subsequent implants. Small perforations of the underlying membrane do not require suturing and collapse inward on themselves. Other perforations may be covered by placing a resorbable collagen wound dressing below the perforation. This provides an interface between the membrane and the graft.

Various materials are used for bone grafting such as autologous cancellous or corticocancellous bone from the iliac crest, porous non-resorbable hydroxyapatite, porous and non-porous resorbable hydroxyapatite, mineralized and non-mineralized freeze dried and various combination of graft materials. The graft materials, after packing is contained by the sinus floor inferiorly, the superiorly positioned bony window or resorbable collagen dressing, if placed superiorly, the elevated Schneiderian membrane medially and the resutured mucoperiosteal flap laterally.

Stage I implant surgery is generally performed 6 to 9 months following the bone grafting procedure. Stage I implant surgery may be performed at the time of bone grafting, if adequate residual bone is available prior to grafting (3–6 mm).

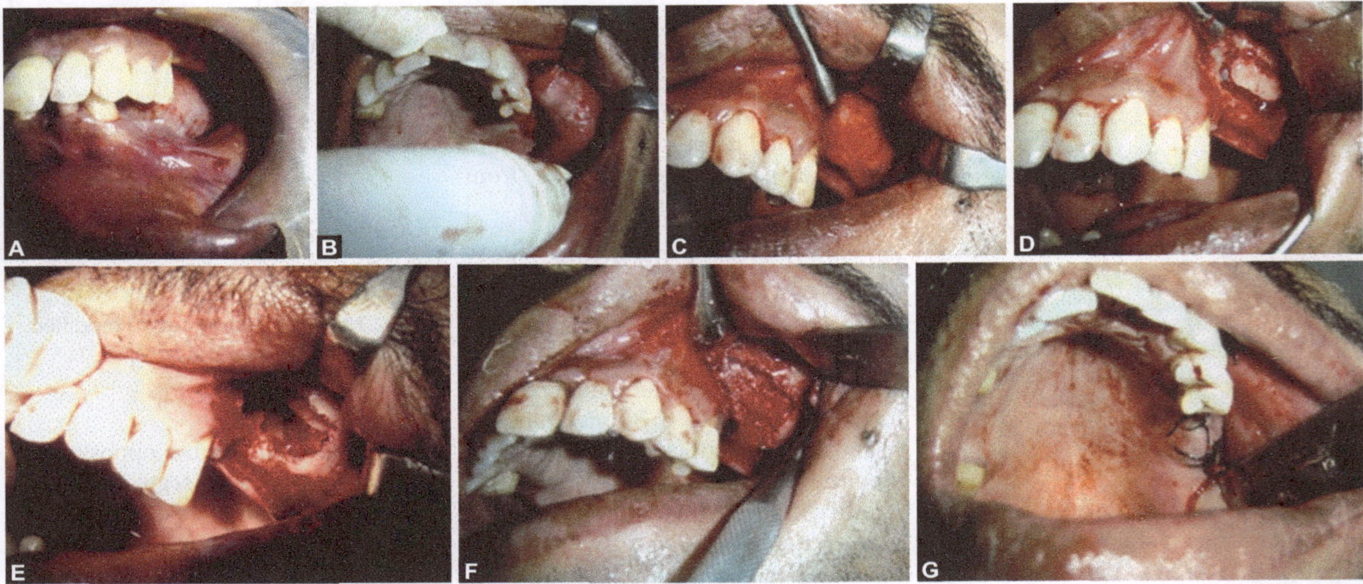

Figs 13.27A to G: Sinus lift procedure

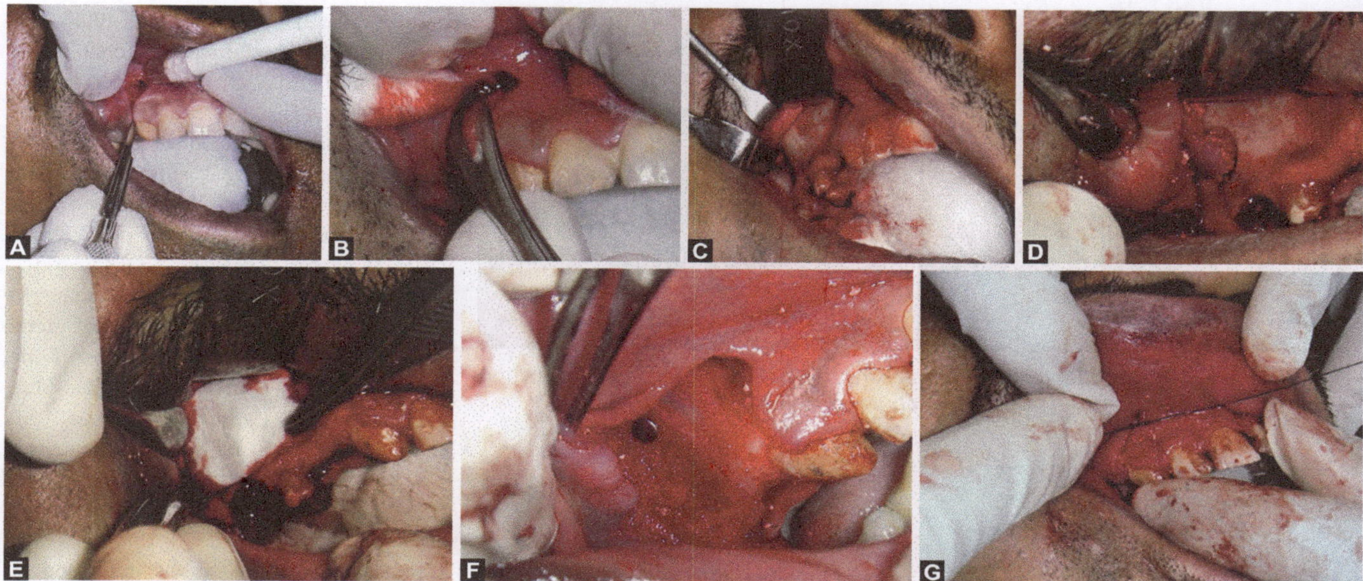

Figs 13.28A to G: Sinus lifting procedure with autogenous bone graft and coverage with allographic membrane: (A) Incision; (B) Flap reflection; (C) Exposure of the wall of sinus; (D) Bone grafting; (E) Membrane to cover the area; (F) Membrane fixed with titanium track; (G) Closure

Sinus lifting procedure with autogenous bone graft and coverage with allographic membrane (Figs 13.28A to G).

Alveolar Ridge Distraction

The Russian orthopedic surgeon, Gavriel Ilizarov, pioneered the reconstruction technique of distraction osteogenesis for managing a variety of limb deformities.[68] In distraction osteogenesis bone transport is done with help of distractor. Retention of complete denture in patient with severe atrophy of alveolar processes is extremely difficult (Figs 13.29A and B). It overcomes the disadvantages of autogenous grafting such as additional surgical site morbidity and graft failure due to infection or improper healing.

Technique

In this procedure a horizontal incision on the vestibular surface is made followed by exposure of alveolar process by reflecting mucoperiosteal flap. Lingually mucosa remains attached to the bone, providing blood supply to transport bone segment during distraction. After identification of mental nerves bilaterally and preparation of adequate space in soft tissues, vertical distraction system is fitted submucosally and temporarily attached with single screw. Then osteotomy site is marked and distractor is removed. Osteotomy is performed with divergent vertical cuts to prevent undercuts at the inferior osteotomy margins. After completion of cuts the transport segment should be mobilized carefully using an osteotome. The distractor is then placed and secured with screws and acute activation of distractor is done to check for functioning of distractor. Then mucosa is closed with nut of distractor exposed so that it can be used later to transport the segment.

After 5 to 7 days of latency, distraction begins at the rate of 0.5 mm two times per day, thereby displacing the upper segment to desired height. The amount of augmentation can be assessed radiographically at regular intervals intervals (Figs 13.30 and 13.31).

After desired amount of distraction is achieved, the consolidation period is initiated and continued for 8 to 12 weeks. After completion distractor is removed, preferably under local anesthesia.

The complications of this procedure are as follows:

- There are chances of mandibular fracture in severely resorbed mandible, while distraction.
- If during surgery the osteotomy cuts result in improper vector for distraction, then it will lead to formation of undesirable shape of alveolar process.
- If blood supply of the transport segment is hampered during surgery by accidental stripping of lingual mucosa attached then necrosis of bone segment can occur.

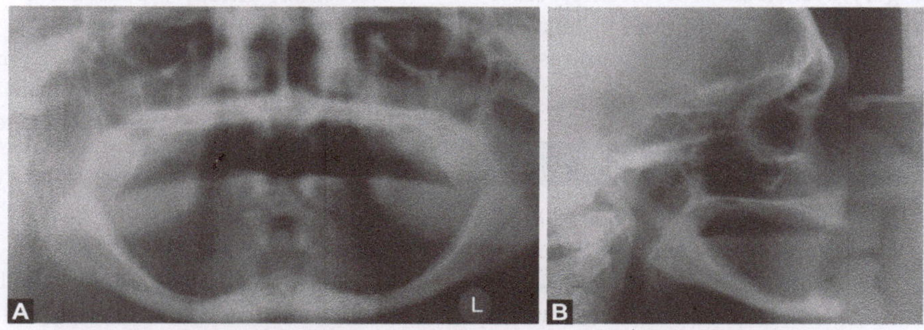

Figs 13.29A and B: Resorbed mandible (*Source:* Craniofacial distraction osteogenesis 2001 Mosby)

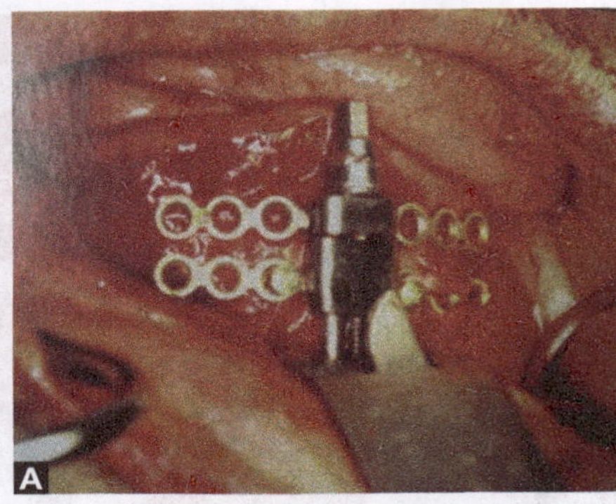

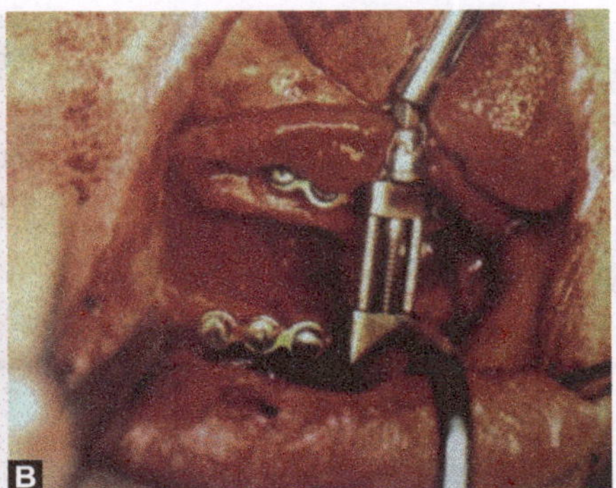

Figs 13.30A and B: Surgical procedure with distraction *in situ* and activated distraction. (*Source:* Craniofacial distraction osteogenesis 2001 Mosby)

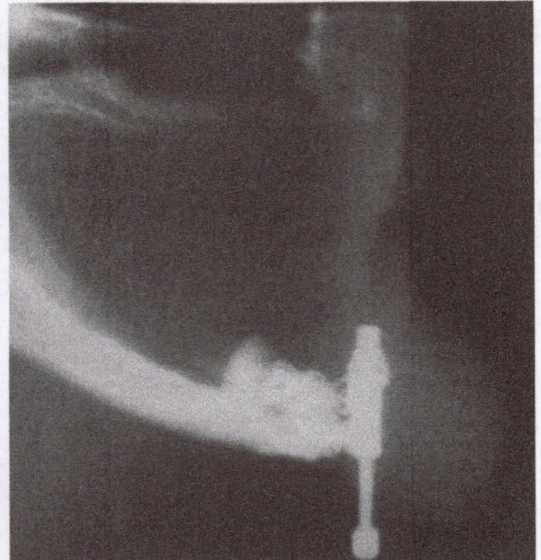

Fig. 13.31: Postoperative radiograph with distractor placed anteriorly on mandible. (*Source:* Craniofacial distraction osteogenesis 2001 Mosby)

- In severely resorbed ridge there are chances of damage to the inferior alveolar nerve.

Distraction osteogenesis is a valuable method of augmentation of the alveolar process when performing preprosthetic surgery, even in cases of extremely resorbed mandible. In addition, it decreases additional morbidity and requires only single operation.

REFERENCES

1. Willard AT. Ridge preparation for edentulous cases. Am J Dental Science. 1853;4:134.
2. Atwood DA. Bone loss of edentulous alveolar ridges. J Periodontol. 1979;50: 11 (4 Special Issue).
3. Bradley JC. Age changes in the vascular supply of the mandible. British Dental Journal. 1972;132:142.
4. Branzi A, Quintarelli G. Ulteriore contribute allo studio anastomoistologico delle modificazioni dellarteria muscellare interna nelle varie eta dell'uomo. Riv Ital Stomat. 1956;11:1.
5. Robling AG, Castillo AB, Turner CH. Biomechanical and molecular regulation of bone remodeling. Annu Rev Biomed Eng. 2006;8:455-98.
6. Enlow DH. The remodeling of the edentulous mandible. The Journal of Prosthetic Dentistry. 1976;36(6):685-93.
7. Jaime Pietrokovski, et al. Morphologic characteristics of bony edentulous jaws. Journal of Prosthodontics. 2007;16(2): 141-7.
8. Lammie GA. The reduction of the edentulous ridges. The Journal of Prosthetic Dentistry. 1960;10(4):605-11.
9. Schweitzer JM. The telescoped complete denture: A research report at the clinical level. The Journal of Prosthetic Dentistry. 1971;26(4):357-72.
10. Dhir RC. Clinical assessment of the overdenture therapy. J Indian Prosthodont Soc. 2005;5:187-92.
11. Helsham RW. Some observations on the subject of roots of teeth retained in the jaws as a result of incomplete exodontia Aust Dent J. 1960; 5:70-7.
12. Casey DM, Lauciello FR. A review of the submerged root concept. J Prosthet Dent. 1980;43:128-32.
13. Garver DG, Fenster RK, Baker RD, et al. Vital root retention in humans: a preliminary report. J Prosthet Dent. 1978; 40(1).
14. Garver DG, Fenster RK. Vital root retention in humans: A final report. The Journal of Prosthetic Dentistry. 1980;43(4):368-73.
15. Garver DG, Theodore E. Muir: The retention of vital submucosal roots under immediate dentures: A surgical procedure. The Journal of Prosthetic Dentistry. 1983;50(6):753-6.
16. Boyne PJ, Rothstein SS, Gumaer Kl, et al. Long-term study of hydroxylapatite implants in canine alveolar bone. Journal of Oral and maxillofac Surg. September 1984;42(9):589-94.
17. Ashley, et al. Preprosthetic Surgeries. In: Carl Kruger (Ed). Textbook of Oral and Maxillofacial Surgery. WB Saunders.
18. Obwegeser H. On the indication for the various methods of vestibuloplasty and plastic surgery of the floor of the mouth. Fortschr Kiefer Gesichtschir. 1965;10:1-8.
19. Obwegeser H. Die submukoese Vestibulumplastik Dtsch Zahnaerztl Z 1959;14: 629-39.
20. Fouad Al-Mahdy Al-Belasy. Mandibular Anterior Ridge Extension: A modification of the kazanjian vestibuloplasty technique. Oral Maxillofacial Surgery. 1997;55.
21. Wallenius K. Ridge extension: A modified operative technique. J Oral Surg Anesth Hosp Dent Serv. 1963;21:54.
22. Kazanjian VH. Surgery as an aid to more efficient service with prosthetic dentures. J Am Dent Assoc.1935;22: 566.
23. Godwin JG. Submucous surgery for better denture service. J Am Dent Assoc. 1947;34:678.
24. Cooley DO. A method for deepening the mandibular and maxillary sulci to correct deficient edentulous ridges. J Oral Surg. 1952;10:279-89.
25. Collett HA. Immediate maxillary ridge extension. Dent Digest. 1954;60:104-6.
26. Clark HB Jr. Deepening of labial sulcus by mucosal flap and vancement: Report of a case. J Oral Surg. 1953;11:165.
27. Edlan A. Prosthetic repair of the vestibule of the maxilla. Cesk Stomatol. 1953;53(5):271-6.
28. Caldwell JB. Lingual Ridge Extension. J Oral Surg. 1955;13:287.

29. MacIntosh RB, Obwegeser HL. Preprosthetic surgery: A scheme for its effective employment. J Oral Surg. 1967; 25;397-413.
30. In: Fonseca R, Davis W, (Eds): Reconstructive preprosthetic oral and maxillofacial surgery, Philadelphia, WB Saunders. 1985;64-9.
31. Obwegeser HL. Die Totale Mundbodenplastik. Schweiz Mschwr Zahnheilk. 1963;73(7):565-72.
32. Steinhauser E, Obwegeser H. Rebuilding the alveolar ridge with bone and cartilage autografts. Trans Congr Int Assoc Oral Surg. 1967. pp. 203-8.
33. Trauner R, Eskici A, Kurhajec P. Alveoplasty with ridge extension. British Journal of Oral Surgery. 1970;8(1):70-6.
34. Black EE, Moore JR. Modified technics in mandibular pre prosthetic surgery. J Oral Surg. 1970;28:184.
35. Miller EL. Sometimes overlooked: preprosthetic surgery. JPD. 1976;36.
36. Cutright DE. Morphogenesis of inflammatory papillary hyperplasia. The Journal of Prosthetic Dentistry. 1975; 33(4):380-5.
37. Ettinger RL. The etiology of inflammatory papillary hyperplasia. The Journal of Prosthetic Dentistry. 1975; 34(3):254-61.
38. Steven A, Rathofe. A comparison of healing and pain following excision of inflammatory papillary hyperplasia with electrosurgery and blade-loop knives in human patients. Oral Surgery, Oral Medicine, Oral Pathology. 1985; (2):130-5.
39. Getter L, Perez B. Controlled cryotherapy in the treatment of inflammatory papillary hyperplasia. Oral Surgery, Oral Medicine, Oral Pathology. 1972; 34:178-86.
40. Desjardins RP. Etiology and management of hypermobile mucosa overlying the residual alveolar ridge. JPD. 1974; 32.
41. Gongloff RK, Woodard KL. A surgical technique for the correction of the hypermobile anterior maxillary ridge. J Oral Surg. 1981;39:340-2.
42. Hickey JC, Zarb GA. Boucher's prosthodontic treatment for edentulous patients (8 edn). The CV Mosby Co., St Louis (1980).
43. Dean OT. Surgery for the denture patient. J Am Dent Assoc. 1936;23:2124.
44. Thoma KH, Holland DJ: Atrophy of the mandible. Oral Surg. 1951; 4:1477.
45. Hopkins R. Alveolectomy and alveolotomy, in Moore JR: Surgery of the Mouth and Jaws. Oxford, Blackwell Scientific, 1985. pp. 449-50.
46. Leonard M. The maxillary tuberosity: indications and simple technique for reduction. Dent Today. 2001;20(2):52-5.
47. Hernandez A. Maxillary tuberosity ridge reduction. Dent Surv. 1978;54(3): 43-4.
48. Gillies RJ. A surgical aid to a prosthetic problem. Aust dent J. 1956;1:329.
49. Thomas J. Starshak, Bruce Sanders editors: Preprosthetic Oral and Maxillofacial Surgery. pp. 99-101.
50. Guernsey LH. Preprosthetic surgery in Textbook of Oral and Maxillofacial Surgery Gustav O Kruger. 5th edn. St Louis, Toronto, London, The CV Mosby Company, 1979.
51. Rezai RF, Jackson JT, Salamat K. Torus palatinus, an exostosis of unknown etiology: review of the literature. Compend Contin Educ Dent. 1985; 6(2):149-52,147.
52. Ghalichebaf M, Bycroft B, Graves R. An unpredictable result from a torus palatinus removal and its treatment: a clinical report. J Prosthet Dent. 1992; 68(3):397-8.
53. MacIntosh RB, Obwegeser HL. Preprosthetic surgery: a scheme for its effective employment, J Oral Surg. 1967;25:397-413.
54. Terry BC, Albright JE, Baker RD. Alveolar ridge augmentation in the edentulous maxilla with use of autogenous ribs, J Oral Surg. 1974;32: 429-34.
55. Kahnberg KE, Nystrom E, Bartholdsson L. Combined use of bone grafts and Branemark fixtures in the treatment of severely resorbed maxillae. Int J Oral Maxillofac Surg. 1989;4:297-304.
56. Farrell CD, Kent JN, Guerra LR. One-stage interpositional bone grafting and vestibuloplasty of the atrophic maxilla. J Oral Surg. 1976;34(10):901-6.
57. Albert RM. Wittkampf: Augmentation of the Maxillary Alveolar Ridge With Hydroxylapatite and Fibrin Glue; JOMS. 1988;46.
58. Mercier P. A comparative study of the efficacy and morbidity of five techniques for ridge augmentation of the mandible; JOMS. 1952;50.
59. Sanders, Cox R. Inferior border rib grafting for augmentation of the atrophic edentulous mandible. J Oral Surg. 1976;34:897.
60. Beumer J. Complete dentures for patients with mandibular inferior border rib grafts. J Oral Surg. 1979;37:301.
61. Quinn PD, Kent K, MacAfee KA. Reconstructing the atrophic mandible with inferior border grafting and implants: A preliminary report. Int J Oral Maxillofac Implants. 1992;7(1):87-93.
62. Barros-Saint-Pasteur J. Plastic restoration of the alveolar crest of the mandible. Acta Odontol Venez. 1966;4(1):3-21.
63. Barros-Saint-Pasteur J. Plastic reconstruction of the alveolar crest. Clinicosurgical investigation. Acta Odontol Venez. 1970;8(2):168-82.
64. Harle F. Visor osteotomy to increase the absolute height of the atrophied mandible. J Maxillofac Surg. 1975;3:257.
65. Ylikontiola L, Kinnunen J, Oikarinen K. Factors effecting neurosensory disturbance after mandibular bilateral sagittal split osteotomy. J Oral Maxillofac Surg. 2000;58:1234.
66. Peterson LJ, Slade EW. Mandibular ridge augmentation by a modified visor osteotomy: A preliminary report. J Oral Surg. 1977;35:999.
67. Frost DE, Gregg JM, Terry BC, et al. Mandibular interpositional and onlay bone grafting for treatment of mandibular bony deficiency in the edentulous patient. J Oral Maxillofac Surg. 1982;40(6):353-60.
68. Samchukov ML, Cope JB, Cherkashin AM. Craniofacial diteraction osteogensis, 2001, Mosby.

Section 4

Maxillary Sinus

14 Diseases of Maxillary Sinus

Borle Rajiv M, Arora Aakash, Nimonkar Pranali V

The maxillary sinus is of great applied importance to an oral surgeon due to its anatomical proximity to the teeth. It is commonly involved in inflammatory disorders of dental origin, especially from the upper premolars and molars. Injudicious instrumentation in this area during the exodontia procedures can lead to oroantral communications. The malignant lesions originating from maxillary sinus involve the teeth. Similarly, pain originating from the sinus may be referred to the teeth (*referred odontalgia*) and can be mistaken as dental pain. The dental surgeon may be the first person to see the patient in both the latter conditions and is expected to diagnose these conditions correctly.

APPLIED SURGICAL ANATOMY[1,2]

The maxillary sinus is the largest of all the paranasal sinuses. The size of the maxillary sinus is variable even in two sides of a same skull. It has an average height of about 3.5 cm in molar area, an average transverse width of about 2.5 cm and an average anteroposterior depth of about 3.2 cm.[3] The maxillary sinus is pyramidal in shape with its base towards the lateral nasal wall and apex directed towards the zygomatic process of maxilla. It is the largest and the most important of all the paranasal sinuses.

It has got a roof, which is the floor of the orbit and is ridged by the presence of infraorbital canal, floor (alveolar process) which is about 1.25 cm below the nasal floor, anterolateral wall, posterolateral wall and the posterior wall. The posterolateral wall forms the medial boundry of the infratemporal fossa. The roof of the sinus is very thin and the infraorbital nerve may lay hanging in the sinus (Figs 14.1A and B). The floor has several bony projections, which correspond to the roots of the maxillary teeth and the sinus may have incomplete bony septae. It opens in the middle meatus of the nose in the *hiatus semilunaris*, through an opening called *ostium maxillare*, which is present in anteriosuperior part of the base of hiatus semilunaris (Fig. 14.2). The clinical ostium is smaller than the bony ostium. Thus, its opening is situated at a higher level than the base of the sinus. The sinus is lined by pseudostratified, columnar, ciliated epithelium and goblet cells, which secrete the mucous. The rhythmic beating of the cilia is responsible for the drainage of the sinus against the gravity. The posterosuperior part of lateral wall of inferior meatus is the thinnest area and is the preferred site for the nasal antrostomy.

AGE CHANGES IN THE MAXILLARY SINUS

At birth the maxillary sinus is an oblong cavity longer anteroposteriorly than

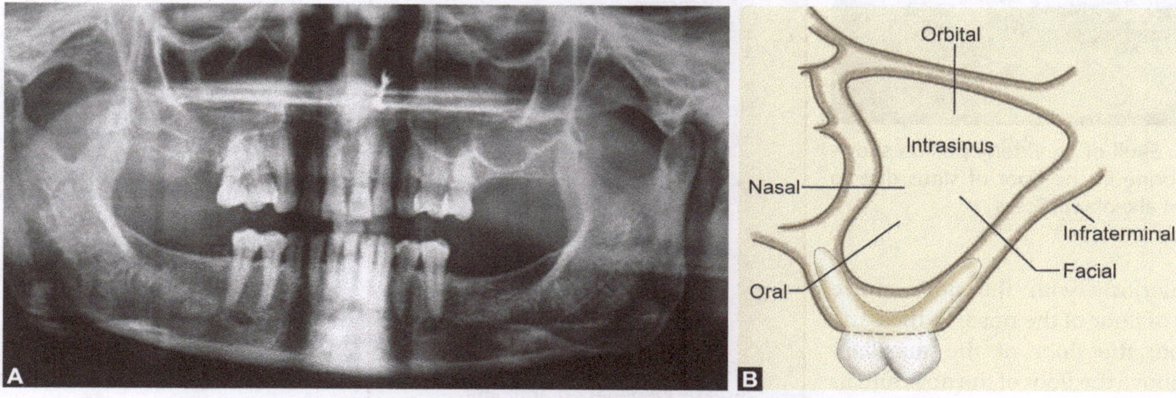

Figs 14.1A and B: Various walls of the maxillary sinus

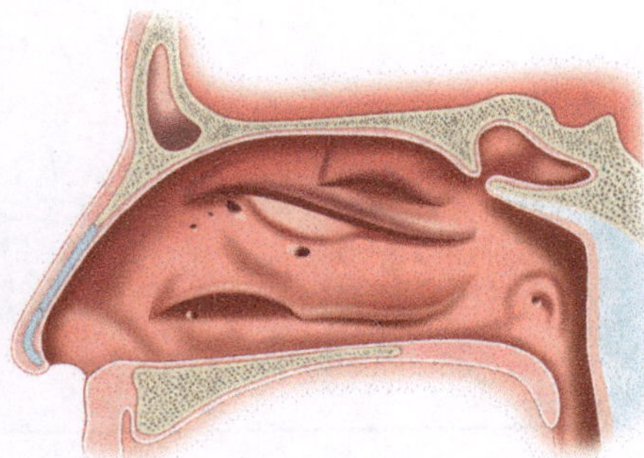

Fig. 14.2: Conchi and meati on the lateral nasal wall with ostium maxillary in the middle meatus

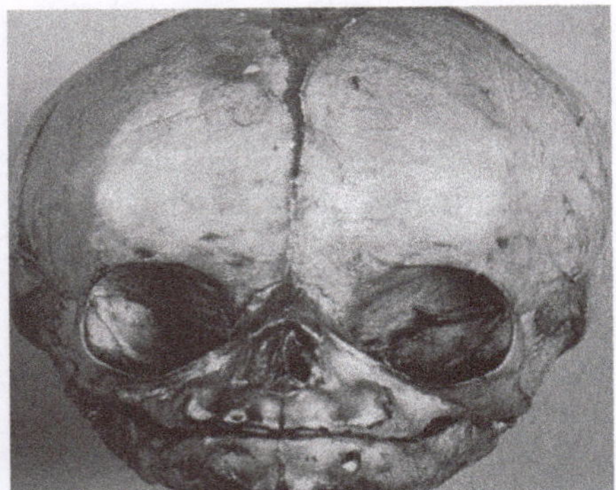

Fig. 14.3: Fetal skull showing floor of maxillary sinus above the floor of nose due to underdeveloped alveolar process

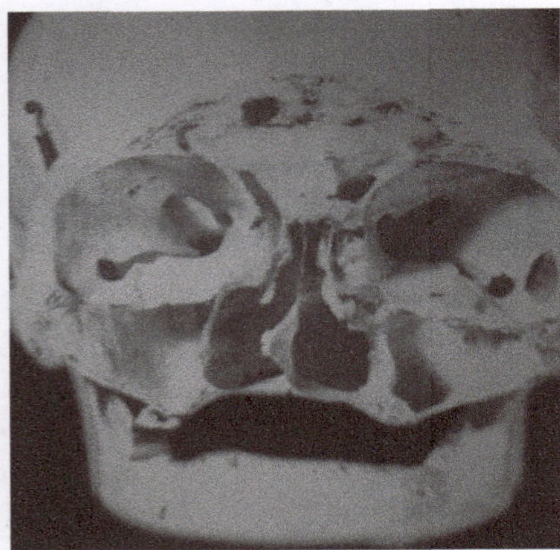

Fig. 14.4: Skull of an elderly person showing thin bone in the floor of sinus due to atrophy of alveolar process

superoinferiorly with the floor above the level of floor of the nose. In the early childhood, the floor of the maxillary sinus is above the floor of the nose and as the teeth develop, the growth of alveolar process takes place and the floor also starts descending down, (Fig. 14.3). At around 12 years, the floor of the sinus is at level with the floor of the nose.

In the elderly persons, as there is a loss of the teeth and atrophy of the alveolar process occurs, the bone separating the oral cavity and the floor of maxillary sinus becomes thin and the chances of oroantral fistula are increased (Fig. 14.4).

The sinus depends on the action of the cilia for its drainage. The lack of ciliary action leads to stasis of secretions, which leads to infections. The blood supply of the sinus is from facial, infraorbital and greater palatine vessels[4] and its lymphatic drainage is to submandibular lymph nodes. The nerve supply to the sinus is from infraorbital, anterior, middle and posterior superior alveolar nerves. The sinus attains its full growth with the eruption of permanent teeth. At the old age, the teeth are exfoliated and the alveolar process becomes resorbed and atrophic and thus the floor is close to the oral cavity. The diseases of the maxillary sinus can be classified as shown in (Box 14.1).

MAXILLARY SINUSITIS

The maxillary sinusitis is usually secondary to allergy or infection.[5] The inhaled pollens get deposited on the lining of the upper airway, including the maxillary sinus.[6] The sinus lining becomes edematous, inflamed and congested. This leads to excessive secretion of mucous, loss of ciliary action, stasis of secretions and secondary infection. The primary infection of the sinus occurs when the sinus gets exposed to the exogenous microorganisms, e.g. when there is an oroantral fistula or a foreign body in the sinus.[7]

Box 14.1: The classification of the diseases of the maxillary sinus

- Developmental disorders
- Inflammatory diseases
  - Allergic
  - Infective
  - Odontogenic
  - Degenerative
  - Traumatic
- Neoplastic diseases
  - Primary tumors – carcinoma, papillomas
  - Tumors, originating from oral cavity and secondarily involving the sinus, like oral squamous cell carcinoma, odontogenic tumors and cysts, minor salivary gland tumors, etc.
- Cysts—mucoceles
- Granulomatous diseases—Hansen's disease, Wegener's granuloma

The exposure of the sinus during trauma may also lead to the sinusitis. The sinus can also get infected secondary to the odontogenic pathology. The apices of maxillary molars and the premolars are very close to the floor of the sinus. A chronic periapical infection leads to destruction of intervening bone and the infection enters the sinus (*odontogenic sinusitis*). The destruction of the floor of the sinus by tumors can also lead to the infection of the sinus.

Etiology of Maxillary Sinusitis

- Overwhelming infection.
- Interference with antral drainage:
  - Congenital anatomical abnormalities leading to decreased drainage.
  - Deviated nasal septum (DNS), causing obstruction to the drainage.
  - Paradoxical turbinates.
  - Malformed uncinate process.
- Alteration in quality of mucosa—cystic fibrosis.
- Ciliary dysfunction:
  - Kartagener syndrome[8]—combination of *situs inversus*, chronic sinusitis and bronchiectasis.
  - Smooth cilia syndrome
  - Young syndrome[9]—bronchiectasis, rhinosinusitis and reduced fertility.
  - Samter's triad[10]—combination of asthma, aspirin sensitivity and nasal/ethmoidal polyposis.
  - Rhinitis medicamentosa.
- Nasal obstruction:
  - Choanal atresia.
- Odontogenic sinusitis:
  - Dentoalveolar abscess.
  - Periapical granuloma or infected periapical cyst communicating with the sinus.

Box 14.2: Classification of the sinusitis as per duration

- Acute (< 4 weeks)
- Subacute (4–12 weeks)
- Chronic (> 12 weeks)

- Involvement of the sinus during surgeries (OAF):
  - Facial trauma.
  - Tumors of maxillary sinus or nasal cavity.
- Fungal sinusitis:[11]
  - Common fungal infections are *Aspergillus*, mucormycosis, candidiasis.
  - *Aspergillus* infection occurs in healthy patients without relationship to pulmonary aspergillosis.
  - Mucormycosis occurs in uncontrolled diabetes mellitus.
  - Candidal infection occurs in patients with long-term antibiotics.

The maxillary sinusitis can be further classified according to duration as (Box 14.2).

In the chronic sinusitis although the clinical signs and symptoms are mild, there are degenerative changes in the lining which leads to loss of ciliary action, stasis of secretions and acute exacerbation of the infection.

Clinical Features

- Pain and tenderness over the maxillary sinus, which is usually associated with headache. The headache is often due to involvement of other sinuses, especially the frontal and sphenoid sinuses. In pansinusitis, the headache is a consistent feature. The headache often gets aggravated on bending forward and radiates to the eye. The pain also radiates to the teeth and is often mistaken as dental pain (*referred odotalgia*) and the dental surgeon may be the first person to be consulted by the patient for the same.

  This pain can be differentiated from dental pain by absence of acute septic focus in the area, tenderness over the sinus, increased and foul smelling secretions from the nose and presence of congestion in the nasal mucous membrane, which are absent in dental pains. Classical tenderness can be elicited over the involved sinus and all the maxillary posterior teeth may be tender to percussion in absence of any obvious pathology. The sinus tenderness is associated with erythema and flushing of the cheek and the patient often complains of heaviness over the sinus. Thus, the clinician must be careful while examining such cases (Box 14.3).

Box 14.3: Clinical signs of sinusitis

- Pain
- Fever
- Headache aggrevated on bending
- Nasal stuffiness
- Nasal discharge–mucoid, purulent, foul smelling
- Anosmia
- Negative transillumination test
- Haziness of sinus on X–ray
- Epistaxis
- Referred odontalgia
- Cough

- **Nasal discharge:** The mucous discharge from the nose on the involved side increases. The discharge is increasingly foul smelling in chronic cases and purulent in nature in cases where there is suppuration (empyema antri).[12] The edema of the nasal lining and the thick secretions lead to nasal stuffiness and blockade.
- **Epistaxis:** The inflamed sinus lining bleeds on blowing of nose or spontaneously. In chronic sinusitis, polyp formation occurs which also bleeds readily.
- **Fever:** In acute sinusitis the patient has fever, malaise, bodyache and other systemic signs of infection.
- **Anosmia:** The temporary loss of smell sensation results due to edema of the nasal lining and nasal blockade due to secretions.
- Nasal stuffiness due to edema, secretions or polyps.
- Purulent/foul smelling discharge due to infection.
- **Cough:** The trickling of secretions to the lower respiratory passage (nocturnal postnasal drip) leads to infection of lower respiratory tract and productive cough.
- Spread of infection to other paranasal sinuses leads to signs of pansinusitis. The maxillary sinus is usually the first to be involved as its opening is at a higher level than the floor. As the drainage is nondependent, the drainage basically depends on the functioning of cilia. The inflammation of the sinus lining leads to loss of ciliary function, stasis of secretions and secondary infection.
- Radiological examination reveals haziness of the maxillary sinus (Fig. 14.5A) on X-ray paranasal sinuses (PNS also called PA Water's sinus view). In the cases of chronic sinusitis the entire sinus appears hazy and the sinus lining may show thickening (Figs 14.5B and C). When polypoidal growth is present, a soft tissue shadow of the polyps may be seen. In case of empyema antri, when the X-ray PNS is taken in sitting position, a clear cut fluid level is seen, which is not seen if the X-ray is taken in the lying position as the fluid spreads in the sinus in this position[13] (Figs 14.6A and B). The fluid level also shifts on tilting of the head.
- Antroscopy done using an endoscope passed through a nasal antrostomy could be useful in studying the polypoid growths, mucoceles or foreign bodies in the sinus and for taking biopsies of the intra-antral growths.[14]
- Transillumination test is negative when the sinus is grossly inflamed, occupied with pus, hematoma or tumor.

Management

The management of sinusitis can be divided into (Flow chart 14.1):

- Medicinal treatment.
- Surgical treatment.

Medicinal Treatment[15]

- In cases with allergic sinusitis, antihistaminics and decongestants are prescribed. Antibiotics are often prescribed to prevent secondary

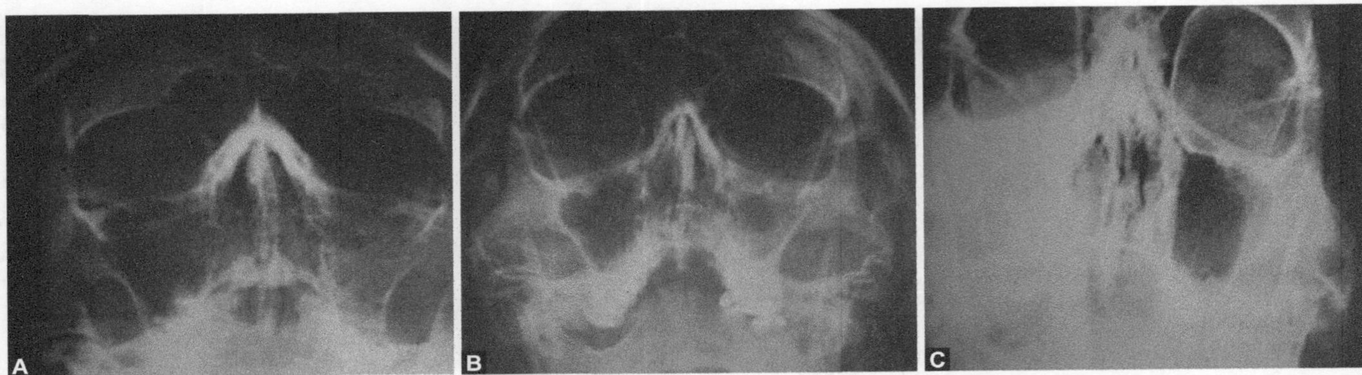

Figs 14.5A to C: (A) Early sinusitis showing mild haziness of the left sinus; (B) Chronic sinusitis showing thickening of the left sinus lining; (C) Chronic sinusitis showing complete haziness of right sinus

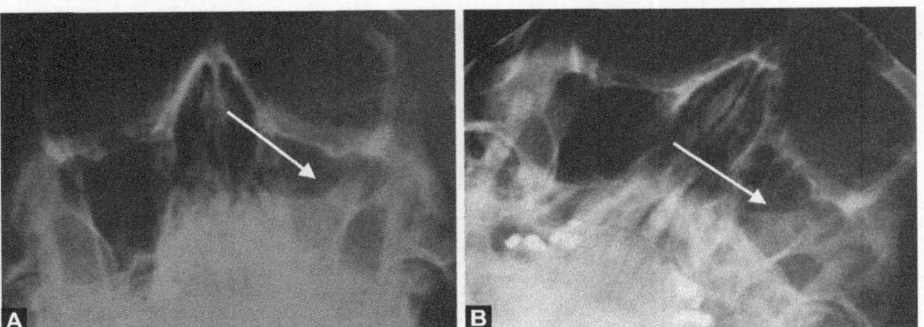

Figs 14.6A and B: Fluid level note the shifting of the fluid level on tilting of the head

Flow chart 14.1: Treatment of maxillary sinusitis

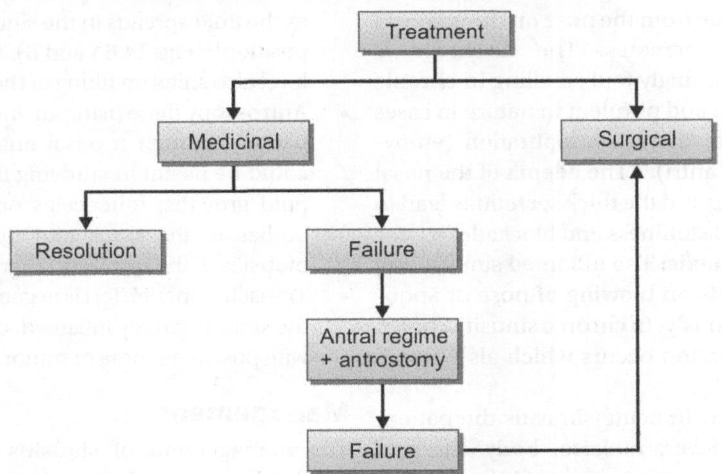

infection. Macrolide of antibiotics are preferred as they cover gram positive organisms, which are commonly seen in upper respiratory tract infections. Erythromycin, Roxithromycine or Azithromycin are the commonly used macrolaids. Cephalosporins, penicillin group of antibiotics are also commonly used drugs. The analgesics and antipyretic drugs are prescribed to relieve the pain and fever.

- The use of antihistaminic tends to dry up the secretions and can lead to further stasis. Hence, mucolytic drugs like bromhexine in a dose of 8 mg, three times a day can be prescribed. The steam inhalation is particularly useful as it has decongestant and mucolytic action. Mucolytics and decongestants like tincture benzoin, camphor, chlorbutol and menthol are commonly used. However, some clinicians believe that these agents may cause rebound congestion.
- The topical decongestants (Ephedrine sulfate 0.5% or 1% in normal saline, Xylometazoline HCl 0.1%) should be used judiciously as their excessive use can lead to rhinitis medicamentosa and lead to further loss of ciliary action. Instead the plain normal saline drops are safe. The systemic decongestants like phenylpropanolamine and pseudoephidrine are often useful.

The above mentioned treatment comprising of antibiotics, antihistaminics and decongestants and steam inhalation are collectively called '*sinus regime*'.

Surgical Treatment

Nasal Antrostomy

The nasal antrostomy done in the inferior turbinate is very useful in establishing a dependent drainage for the sinus, especially when the ciliary function is comprised and the normal opening is blocked by edema, congestion or by a polyp or a tumor. It helps in clearing the stasis, drainage and in relieving the pain. It is a simple procedure done under local anesthesia using a trochar and cannula on outdoor basis. Antral lavage can also be done through this site with the help of normal saline solution.

The resolution should occur normally with medicinal treatment and the antrostomy. The resistant cases, which do not respond to this treatment and change to a chronic sinusitis require further surgical treatment in the form of Caldwell-Luc operation.

Caldwell-Luc Operation[16]

It is the surgical procedure for accessing the maxillary sinus. It can be done for diagnostic (biopsies of intra-antral growths) or for therapeutic purposes (Fig. 14.7A).

Indications

- Chronic sinusitis with severe degeneration of lining, polypoid growths, mucoceles in the lining.
- Foreign bodies in the sinus.
- For diagnostic purpose
- For elevating the fractures of zygoma and the floor of the orbit.

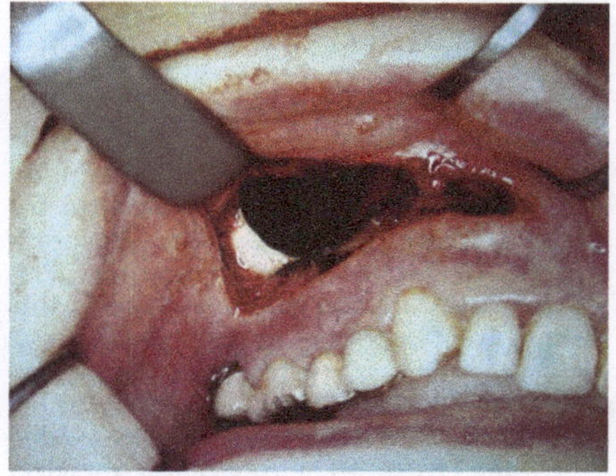

Fig. 14.7A: A Caldwell–Luc operation

Procedure

The Caldwell-Luc operation is performed under general anesthesia. An intraoral degloving incision is taken in the labial vestibule over the canine fossa (Fig. 14.7B1). The bone is exposed. The round bony cut is marked over the canine fossa using a round bur (post stamp incision) and the incision is completed with a fissure bur or an ossisector. When a preexisting oroantral fistula is present, the same bony defect is widened to create an access to the sinus. The opening should be wide enough to permit adequate access to the sinus (approximately of the size of the index finger). Under good illumination the sinus lining is inspected. Any foreign body present should be picked up. The diseased lining is gently curetted. As the lining is inflamed, it tends to bleed on provocation, which is cleared by suction or intermittent packing using roller gauze. Care should be taken while curetting the posterior and the superior walls, as they are thin and fragile and may further be eroded by the pathology. If these walls are perforated accidentally, hemorrhage and damage to the orbital contents can occur, respectively. After all the diseased lining is curetted out, hemostasis is achieved by packing with roller gauze. As the lining is removed, the ciliary action is absent due to removal of the lining. So to facilitate free gravity dependent drainage nasal antrostomy is done. The pack left *in situ* for achieving hemostasis, the end of the pack is taken out through the nasal antrostomy site and intraoral incision is closed primarily. The sinus regimen is started and continued for 8 to 10 days. The excised lining is submitted for histopathological examination.

The alternative procedure for the Caldwell-Luc operation is Denker's procedure in which in addition to Caldwell-Luc surgery a slit of bone is removed from the anterior bony angle of the antrum right up to the lateral nasal aperture so as to render continuous, free, unimpeded drainage of the sinus from the canine fossa and the nasal cavity (Fig. 14.7B2).

CARCINOMA OF MAXILLARY SINUS[17,18]

The carcinoma of maxillary sinus is the tumor classically originating from its lining. The oral squamous cell carcinoma originating from the maxillary gingiva or the malignant minor salivary gland tumors originating from the palatal minor salivary glands may secondarily involve the sinus, but are not true carcinomas originating from the antral lining. In advanced cases, it is difficult to say where the tumor has originally started from.

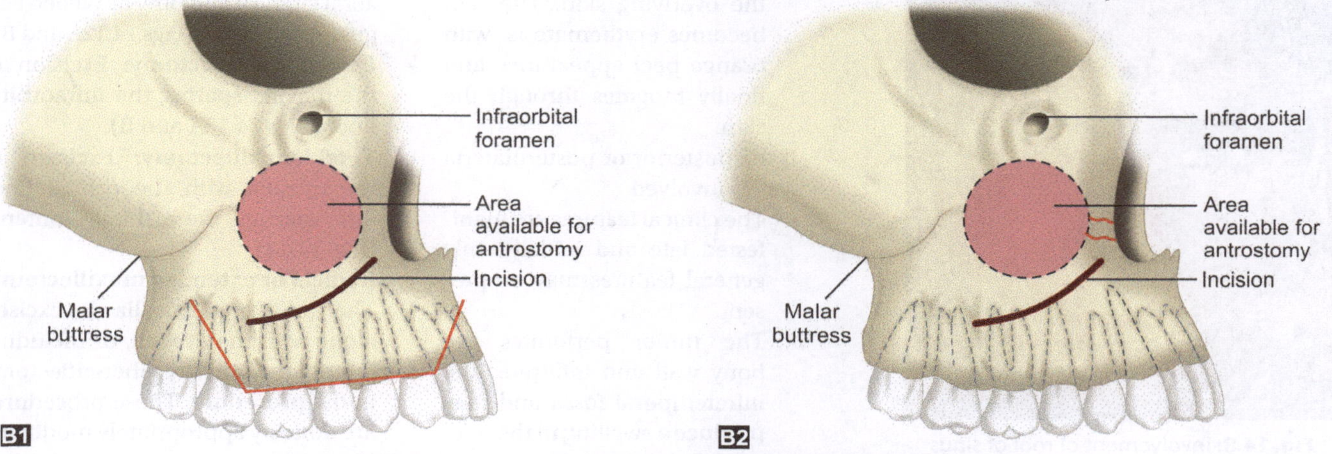

Fig. 14.7B: (B1) Incisions for Caldwell-Luc operation; (B2) Denker's procedure

Etiology

- Smoking.
- Snuff inhalation.
- People working in hardwood furniture industry, nickel refining, leather work and manufacture of mustard gas.
- Chronic maxillary sinusitis.
- In some cases no etiological factor is detected.

Clinical Features

- General
  - Signs of chronic sinusitis.
  - Foul smelling nasal discharge.
  - Nasal stuffiness.
  - Epistaxis.
  - Loss of transillumination.
- The clinical features depending upon the wall involved:
  - If the floor is involved.
    - i. Loosening of the teeth.
    - ii. Spontaneous exfoliation of teeth and fungation of tumor, intraorally.
    - iii. Pain on mastication as the teeth are loose.
    - iv. Heaviness in the teeth due to the involvement of the superior dental plexus.
  - If the roof is involved (Fig. 14.8)
    - i. Neurological deficit in the distribution of infraorbital nerve, anterior and middle superior alveolar nerves as they are present in the floor of the orbit.

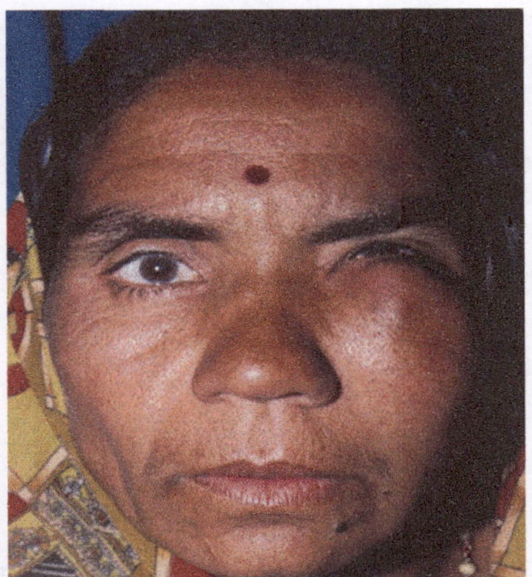

Fig. 14.8: Involvement of roof of sinus

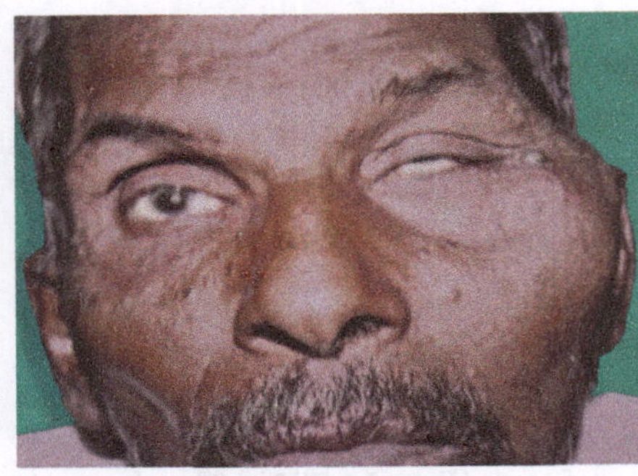

Fig. 14.9: Involvement of anterolateral wall

    - ii. The involvement of the inferior rectus and inferior obliques muscles will produce diplopia.
    - iii. As the tumor encroaches upon the orbital cavity initially there is proptosis and destruction of the eyeball.
  - If the medial wall is involved
    - i. Bulging of the lateral nasal wall towards the septum.
    - ii. Nasal blockage.
    - iii. Obstruction to the drainage of the sinus as the opening gets blocked, leading to recurrent sinusitis.
  - If the anterolateral wall is involved (Fig. 14.9)
    - i. Involvement of the infraorbital nerve leads to neurological deficit in the distribution of its branches, i.e. inferior palpebral, superior labial and lateral nasal nerves.
    - ii. Swelling in the infraorbital area, which gets adherent to the overlying skin. The skin becomes erythematous, with orange peel appearance and finally fungates through the skin.
  - If the posterior or posterolateral wall is involved
    - i. The clinical features are manifested late and initially only general features may be present.
    - ii. The tumor perforates the bony wall and infiltrates the infratemporal fossa and may produce a swelling in the buccal area posteriorly below the zygomatic bone.
    - iii. Trismus due to muscle infiltration.

The X-ray picture on the X-ray PNS shows haziness and irregular destruction of the walls. The CT scans are very useful in giving complete information about the extent of the tumor (Figs 14.10A to C).

Management[19,20]

The diagnosis must be established by taking a biopsy and histopathological examination. The carcinoma of maxillary sinus is usually less radio responsive. Surgery is the most preferred treatment modality when the tumor is operable and the patient is fit to undergo surgery. The contraindications for the surgery are, tumor extending to infratemporal fossa by perforating the posterior wall, full thickness involvement of anterior wall including the overlying skin, nasoethmoidal extensions and medically compromised patients. The carcinomas of the sinus are not known to metastasize to the cervical lymphatics in the earlier stage of the disease, but in advanced cases neck node metastasis must be carefully evaluated and treated.

Surgical Treatment[21]

- **Segmental maxillectomy:** In this lower level of the maxilla or only the involved segment is excised. The procedure can be accomplished intraorally, through a degloving incision in the buccal vestibule (Figs 14.11A to C). Some surgeons prefer the extraoral lateral rhinotomy or Weber-Fergusson approach (Figs 14.12A and B).
- **Partial maxillectomy:** Excision of the maxilla sparing the infraorbital floor (Figs 14.12A and B).
- **Total maxillectomy:** Excision of the maxilla with the orbital floor but sparing the orbital contents (Fig. 14.13).
- **Radical or extended maxillectomy:** The unilateral maxilla is excised along with the eyeball, or including ethmoidectomy, sphenoidectomy in the procedure. These procedures are done by appropriately modifying

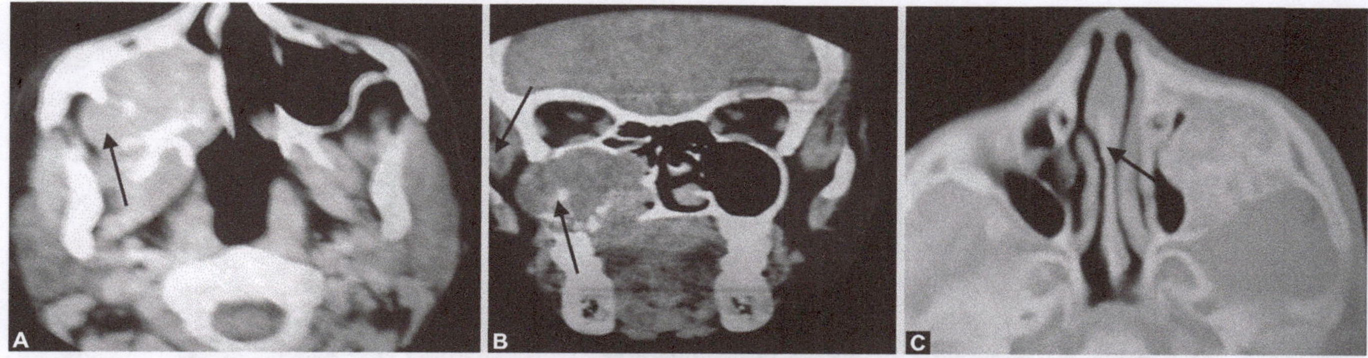

Figs 14.10A to C: CT scans showing growth in the maxillary sinus: (A and B) Malignant tumors causing destruction of the walls; (C) Benign tumor causing expansion of the walls

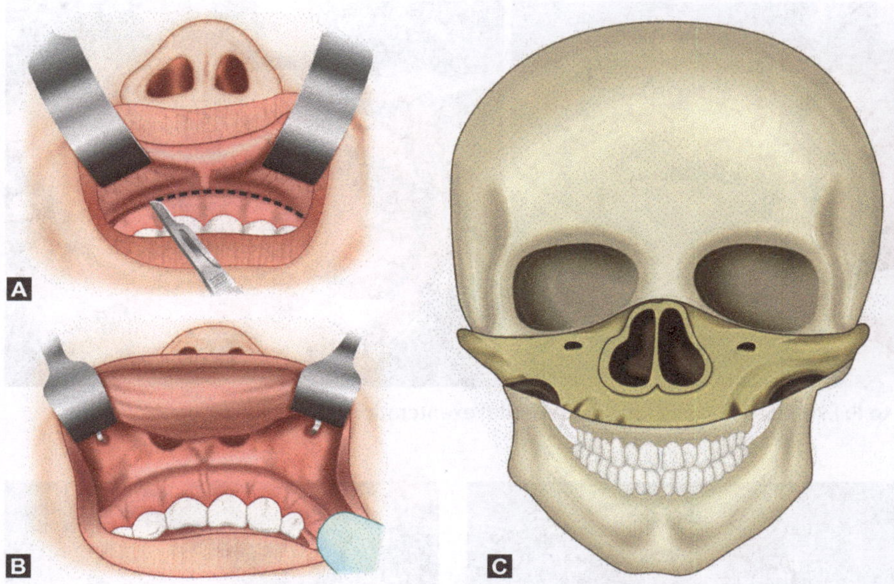

Figs 14.11A to C: Intraoral degloving incision

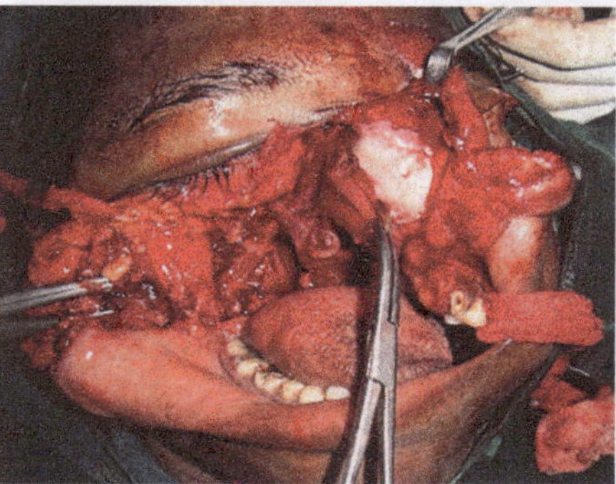

Fig. 14.13: Total maxillectomy, orbital floor removed

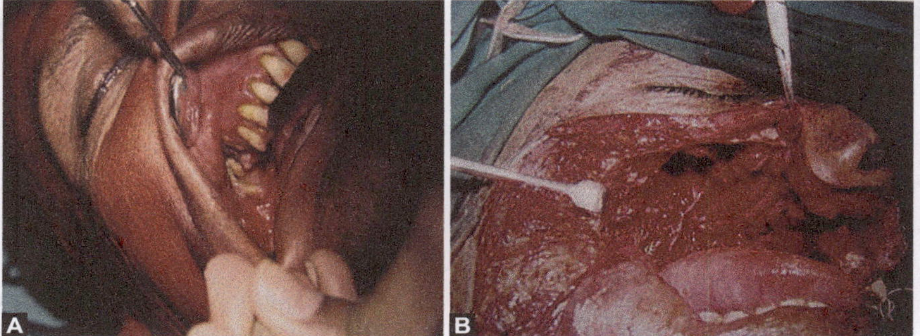

Figs 14.12A and B: Weber-Fergusson incision for partial maxillectomy

the Weber-Fergusson incision (Figs 14.14A to F).

When the tumor shows metastasis in the cervical lymph nodes, neck dissection along with the maxillectomy is required.

The reconstruction of the defect is done with temporalis muscle-fascia flap, laterally rotated nasal septal flap, free fibular flap or by placing obturators which cover the defect.

OROANTRAL FISTULA

The oroantral fistula (OAF) is a pathological communication between the oral cavity and the maxillary sinus, which is lined by epithelium. It is the chronic version of the acute communication of the maxillary sinus into the oral cavity. It facilitates the regurgitation of fluids from the oral cavity into the maxillary sinus and contamination of the sinus with the oral microbial flora, which leads to chronic sinusitis.

Etiology

- Traumatic extraction of maxillary molars or premolars teeth, which are in close anatomical proximity with the sinus.

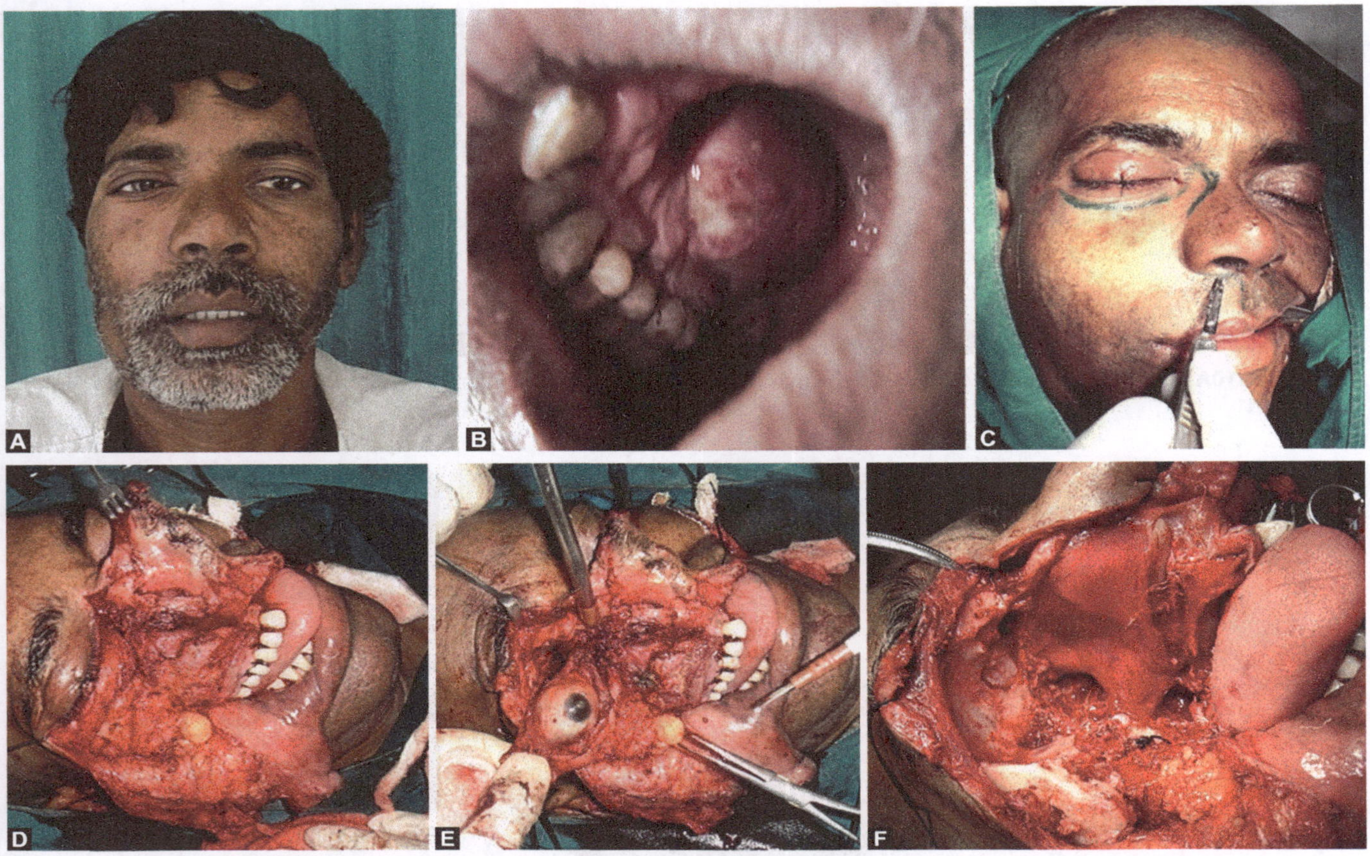

Figs 14.14A to F: Extended maxillectomy with orbital exenteration

- Accidental dislodgement of a root in the maxillary sinus.
- Fracture of maxilla passing through the wall of the sinus (dentoalveolar Le-Fort I, II).
- Malignant tumors of sinus or oral cavity.
- Gummatous lesions of the maxilla like tuberculosis and leprosy.
- Osteomyelitis of maxilla.
- Wegener's or Stuart's granulomatosis.
- Following the resection of the cysts and tumors of the maxilla.

Clinical Features

- Regurgitation of fluid in the sinus when the patient tries to drink the water (Fig. 14.15).
- Loss of resonance and nasal twang to the voice.
- When the patient's nostrils are compressed and he is asked to blow through the nose it produces frothing or bubbling in the blood present in the socket of the extracted tooth, when the bleeding stops or the patient reports late, the same procedure will produce abnormal leakage of the air in the oral cavity, which is demonstrated by deflection of the cotton wool filaments held below the socket and cause the fogging of the mouth mirror held below the socket (Fig. 14.16). This will occur due to escape of air into the oral cavity through the communication/fistula.
- Unilateral epistaxis following the trauma.
- Transillumination test is positive.

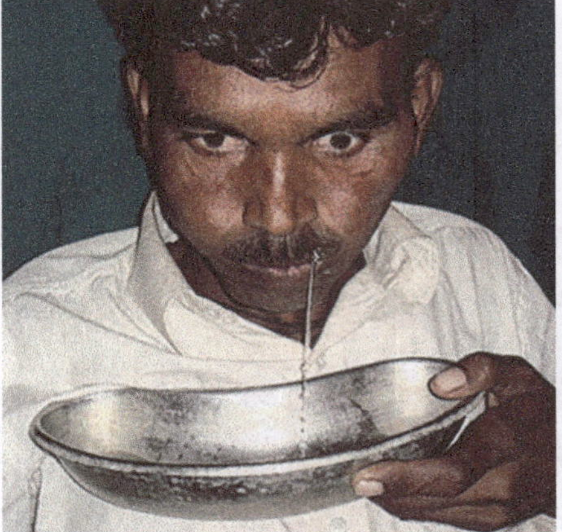

Fig. 14.15: Nasal regurgitation of fluid

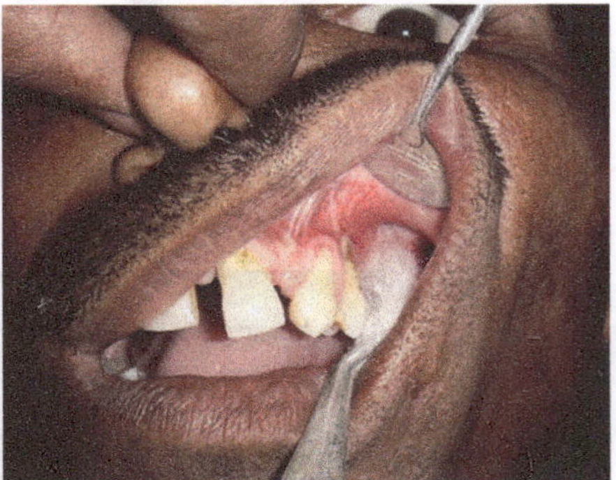

Fig. 14.16: Deflection of the cotton wool filaments

- In chronic cases unilateral, foul smelling pus discharge may be present and signs of maxillary sinusitis are present due to secondary infection from the oral flora.
- Inability to whistle.

Diagnosis

The diagnosis is based on the clinical history, demonstration of above mentioned signs and symptoms and on the X-ray findings. The X-ray PNS shows haziness of the sinus when the sinusitis sets in or when there is bleeding in the sinus. Dislodged foreign body, if it is large may also be seen on the X-ray. The intraoral periapical radiographs show the defect in the bone above the apices of the roots with loss of cortication of the floor of the sinus. If the fistula is large, clear cut communication between the socket and the sinus is seen.

General Management

Once the diagnosis is established, the treatment should be started as early as possible to prevent infection in the sinus. An average dental surgeon lacks adequate skill and training to deal with such problems and hence, it is desirable that he gives the first aid treatment and refers the patient to the maxillofacial surgeon for definitive treatment. The first aid treatment comprises of –

- Gentle packing of the socket with wet gauze to control the bleeding. This is effective in controlling the bleeding from the socket only. The antral bleeding needs the packing of the sinus with roller gauze and sometimes anterior nasal packing.
- To follow Do's and Don'ts like:
  - Do not ask the patient to blow the nose forcefully and repeatedly.
  - Do not probe the sinus with sharp instruments.
  - Do not curette the socket.
  - Place loose wet gauze pack in the socket and place a suture across the socket engaging the buccopalatal gingival.
  - Prescribe antibiotics and other symptomatic treatment.
  - Refer the patient to the competent person for the further management.

Definitive Management[22]

The small communications do not require any specific treatment as the blood clot seals off the communication. The surgeon must ensure that the clot is not dislodged. It can be achieved by approximating the buccal and palatal gingiva, across the socket with sutures after reducing the height of the alveolar bone (Fig. 14.17). Instructions should be given to the patient against blowing the nose forcefully, vigorous gargling and smoking. The moderate and large-sized fistulas require definitive treatment.

The definitive treatment comprises of plastic closure of the OAF by taking various flaps. The flaps can be classified as follows:

- Buccal flap (Burger's flap, Moczair's flap,[23] Rherman's flap[24]).
- Palatal flap (Ashley's palatal pedicle flap[25]).
- Combition of buccal and palatal flap (advancement flaps).
- Distant flaps like lingual pedicle flap. Buccal mucosal pedicle flaps, Buccal fat pad graft,[26] etc.
- Bone grafts.
- Alloplastic implants like titanium, silastic, silicon or membranes.
- Simple procedures like providing an obturator fabricated in acrylic resin to cover the defect (Box 14.4).

Box 14.4: Different methods of closure of OAF

Management of OAF
If the OAF is small (< 5 mm)
Advancement of buccal and palatal gingiva and closure
If the OAF is large
Buccal flaps
Burger's flap
Rehrmann's flap
Moczair's flap
Palatal flaps
Ashley's pedicle flap
Others
Schuchardt's Transversal flap
Regional flaps
Tongue flaps
Buccal fat pad
Randomized cheek flaps
Distant flaps
Temporal muscle fascia flaps
Bone grafts
Alloplastic material–silastic, titanium
Obturators

When the oroantral fistula is associated with the displacement of the root fragment into the sinus simple maneuvers can be performed in an attempt to remove it. These are compressing the nostrils and asking the patient to blow forcefully through the nose. The pressure of the air may sometimes drive the root piece out through the same fistula. The antrum is packed with a roller gauze and then the gauze is pulled out abruptly, the root piece may get entangled with it and come out along with the gauze. The root piece can sometimes enter in the plane between the bone and the antral lining, rather than entering into the sinus and remain asymptomatic for time. However, the root fragments which are in the antrum serve as source of infection and should be removed by performing Cardwell-Luc operation, if the simpler methods described earlier

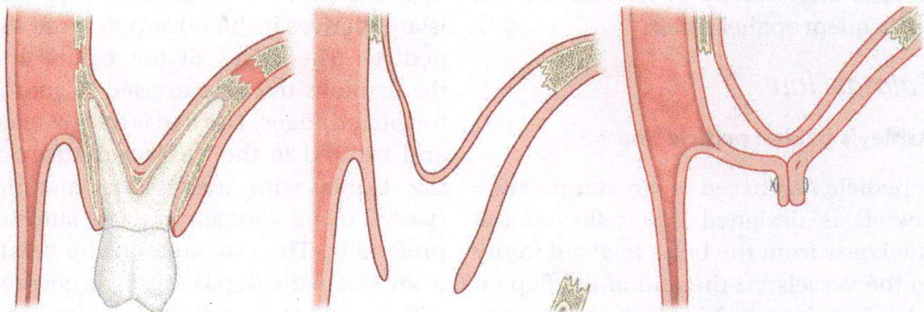

Fig. 14.17: Simple closure of small OAC by approximating buccal and palatal flaps

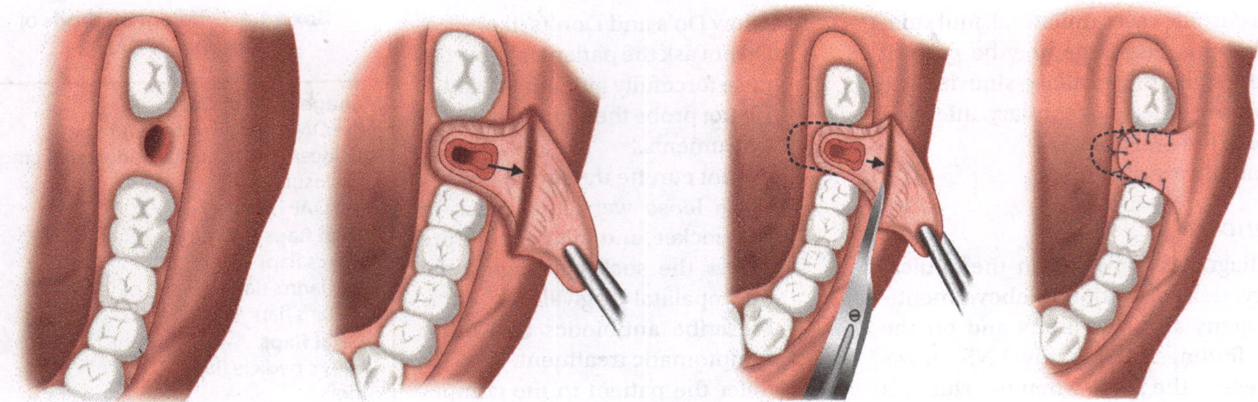

Fig. 14.18: Burger's flap

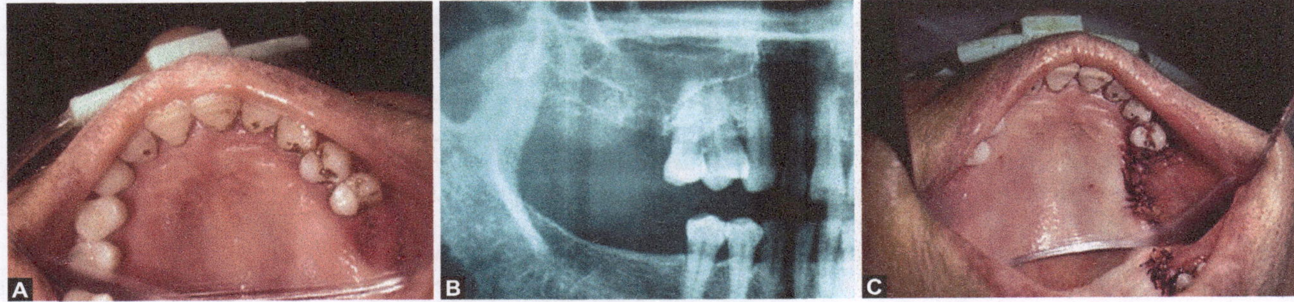

Figs 14.19A to C: Rehrmann's technique used to close OAF

fail. The indications for Caldwell-Luc operation in OAF are root piece in the sinus and chronic OAF causing chronic sinusitis and producing polypoid degenerative changes in the lining.

Buccal Flaps

Burger's flap

The edges of the socket are trimmed and rounded off. A full thickness mucoperiosteal trapezoid flap is designed and reflected on the buccal side. The periosteum is tough and nonelastic and thus, limits the advancement of the flap. The periosteum is selectively incised from inside of the flap carefully. This enhances the elasticity of the flap as the mucosa is elastic. The flap is then advanced to the palatal side and sutured with the palatal gingival margin. This flap is an example of advancement flap (Fig. 14.18). The similar procedure was described by Rehrmann (Figs 14.19A to C).

However, the Rehermann's flap is a broad based flap and rather than the periosteal scoring, liberal undermining is done to advance the flap. This results into obliteration of the buccal vestibular depth.

Moczair's flap[23]: It is also described as a buccal sliding trapezoidal flap procedure for closure of alveolar fistulas. The change in the vestibular sulcus is negligible by shifting the flap one tooth distally. The main disadvantage of this flap being that it necessitates greater amount of dentogingival detachment in order to facilitate the shift (Fig. 14.20). The distal shifting of the flap covers the OAF but leaves gap/defect, medially on the buccal alveolus. As the raw area lies on the healthy bone it heals uneventfully by granulation and subsequent epithelization.

Palatal Flap

Ashley's palatal pedicle flap[25]

A pedicle flap based on greater palatine vessels is designed and reflected full thickness from the bone to avoid injury to the vessels. At the end of the flap an island is designed in such way that is covers the defect created by excision

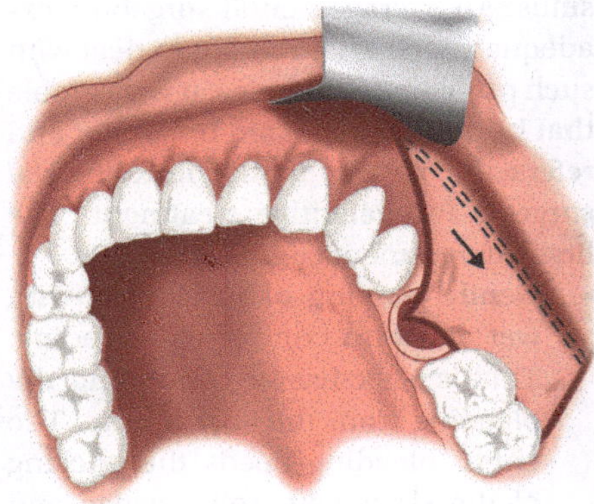

Fig. 14.20: Moczair's flap

of the fistula adequately. Thus, this flap is called island pedicle flap. The island derives its blood supply from the pedicle. The edges of the fistula and the fistulous tract are excised to get the freshened edges. The flap is then rotated and sutured to the freshened edges of the fistula with absorbable material (vicryl) using vertical mattress sutures, preferably. The raw area on the palate from where the flap is raised, is covered with a gauze soaked in antiseptic solution like acriflavin or povidone

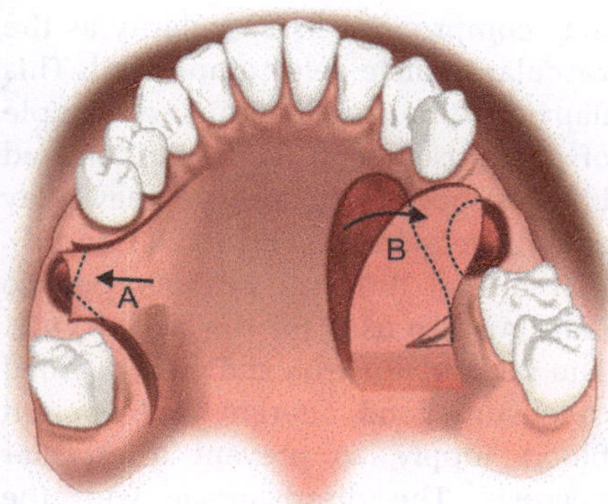

Fig. 14.21: Straight advancement flap (A). Palatal rotational-advancement flap (B); (Ashley's palatal flap)

iodine, which is secured in place using stay sutures. This pack is removed after 24 hours as contamination with food makes it foul smelling and unhygienic. It is preferable to use a nonadhesive material like Vaseline gauze but, it is not well-accepted by the patient when used intra-orally owing to its unpleasant taste. The island heals and unites with the edges of the fistula. The palatal raw bone gradually gets epithelized. Once the flap heals and the fistula gets closed, the pedicle can be detached from the palatal end and can be returned back to the palate and sutured back in its original position after freshening the edges of the palatal raw area and curetting the underlying granulation tissue. This second stage procedure is usually done after two weeks, as early attempt may lead to avascular necrosis of the flap as the collateral circulation is not well established. The Ashley's flap is an example of rotation flap (Fig. 14.21).

Palatal rotational-advancement flap: This technique in contrast, provides adequate mobility and tissue bulk to the flap (Figs 14.22A to C). It requires the mobilization of large amount of palatal tissue. The flap often kinks following the rotation of the flap and can cause venous congestion. Kruger suggested a V-shaped excision of the lesser curvature of the flap to minimize folding (Fig. 14.23).

Pedicle island flap: Its use for closure of oroantral defect was mentioned by Hendersen in 1974.

Advantages: It can be used in closure of large fistula. It is a one-stage local procedure that provides a flap with an excellent bulk, blood supply and mobility. Necrosis of the palatal bone of the donor site is not a problem with this procedure, as there is ample blood supply from the nasal mucosa. This procedure is suitable for closure of posterior fistula, which is pedicled on the greater palatine vessels (Fig. 14.24). Its application is limited in closure of anterior defect. Gullan and Arena described a modification of island flap to obtain approximately 1 cm extra length of the flap by freeing the vessels at the greater palatine foramen. This provides an additional mobility for anterior advancement of the flap.

Palatal hinged flap: This flap is utilized for closure of small to moderate size fistulas (Fig. 14.25).

The procedure is simple to perform with minimum morbidity.

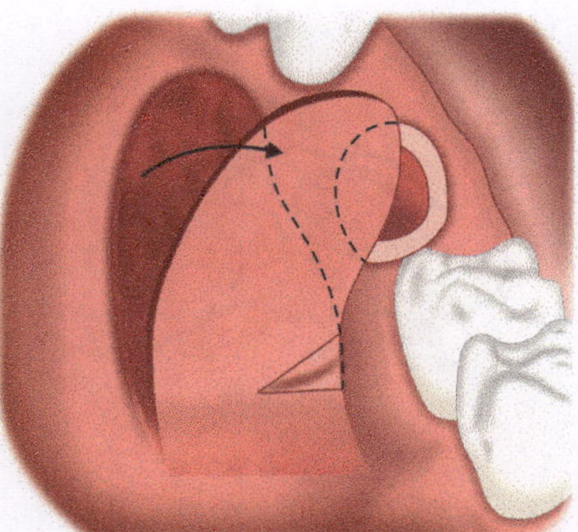

Fig. 14.23: Kruger's modification

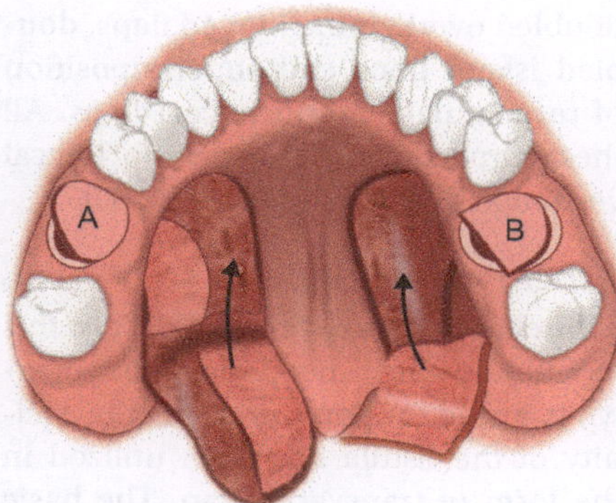

Fig. 14.24: Island flap based on greater palatine vessel

Both island and hinged flaps leave a small raw area for granulation.

Combined Local Flaps

These include the combination of inversion and rotational-advancement flaps,

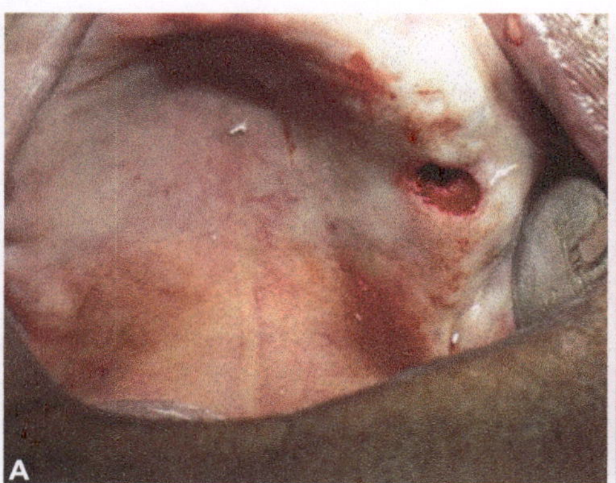

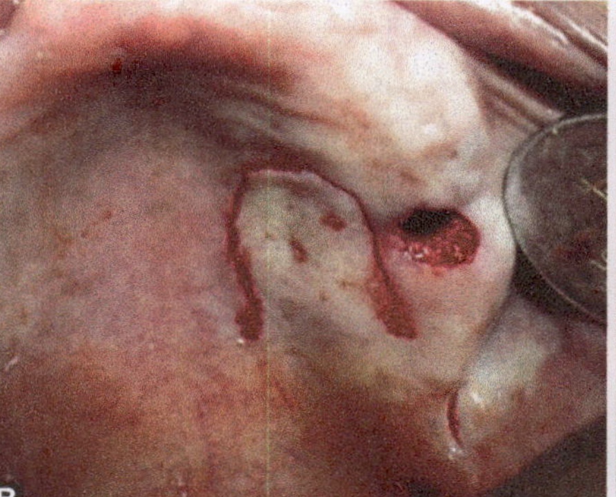

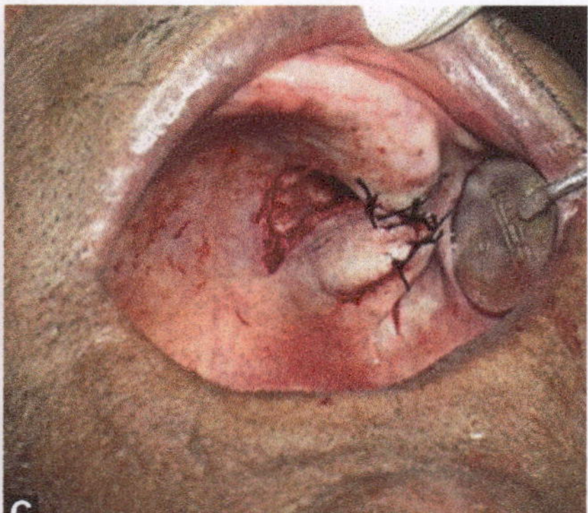

Figs 14.22A to C: Closure of fistula by palatal rotational-advancement flap

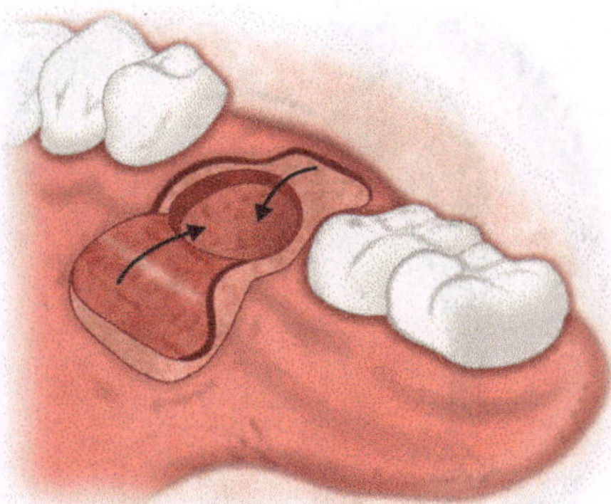

Fig. 14.25: Palatal hinged flap

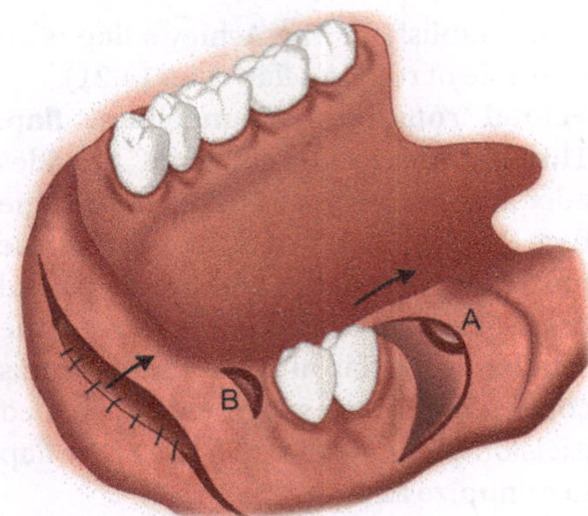

Fig. 14.27: Schuchardt's transversal flap (A), Modification by Egyedi (B)

doubled overlapping hinged flaps, doubled island flaps and superimposition of reverse palatal and buccal flaps. All these procedures preserve the buccal vestibular height (Figs 14.26A to C).

Other Procedures

Schuchardt's transversal flap[27]: In this technique, the mucoperiosteum overlying an edentulous ridge in the vicinity of the fistula has been utilized in the form of transversal flap. The basic advantage of this technique is the buccal vestibular height is not affected following the closure. However, it does not offer greater mobility and results in a raw area over the donor site (Fig. 14.27). Modification of Schuchardt method was described by Egyedi. He utilized a labial vestibular bipedicle flap to close a fistula in the anterior region.

Advantages

- Bilateral blood supply.
- Donor site closed by primary closure.
- Favorable for closure of minor anterior fistula in association with missing anterior teeth.

Disadvantages

- Reduces the labial sulcular height.
- Presence of two pedicles on top of the alveolus.

Distant flaps

The most commonly used distant flap is lingual myomucosal pedicle flap. This flap could be either on anteriorly or posteriorly based pedicle. The anteriorly based pedicle flap is preferable due to its ease in handling. The posteriorly based pedicle flaps are required to be rotated for proper placement which may compromise its vascularity as the vascular pedicle gets compressed. This flap is myomucosal and thus an example of composite flap with randomized blood supply as it does not have any feeding vessel in it (Figs 14.28A and B). The buccal mucosal random pedicle flaps are also used for closing the OAF. The pedicle must be sufficiently broad to ensure good afferent and efferent blood supply, to prevent a vascular necrosis. The disadvantage with the lingual pedicle flap is its instability as the movements of the tongue tend to cause dehiscence of its margins.

Use of buccal pad of fat: The buccal fat pad can be effectively used to close moderate sized oroantral communications, especially in the posterior areas. The buccal fat pad is easy to harvest and provides adequate tissue to cover moderate defects. The buccal fat pad can reach anteriorly up to the premolar area. It is reliable and heals by secondary epithelization. The morbidity to the donor site is negligible (Figs 14.29A and B).

Use of temporalis muscle fascia: The temporalis muscle fascia flaps can be used for the repair of large oroantral fistulas, which generally result following ablative tumor surgeries or tissue loss secondary to trauma. The temporalis muscle fascia flap is pedicled on the deep temporal vessels. The flap is tunneled below the zygomatic arch and drawn into the oral cavity. The reach of the flap is not adequate anteriorly and can be used to close the defects in the molar area.

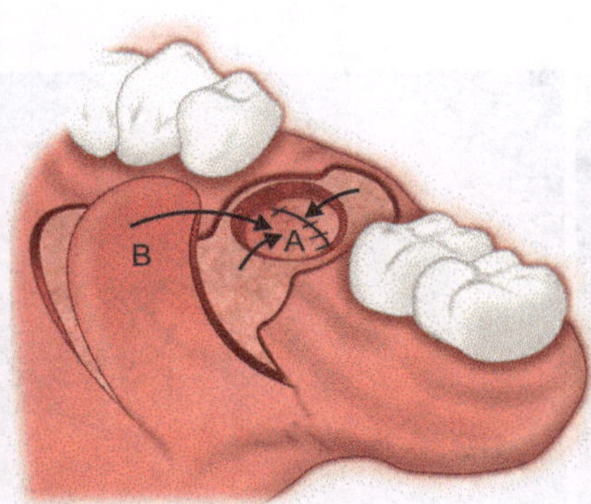

A Hinged and palatal rotational advancement flap

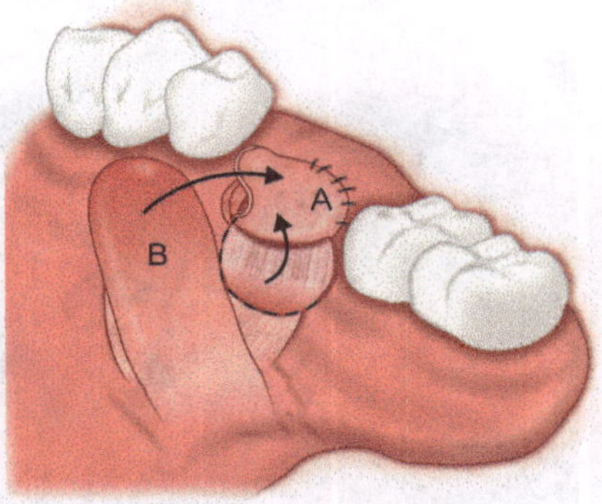

B Inversion flap (A) and palatal rotational advancement flap (B)

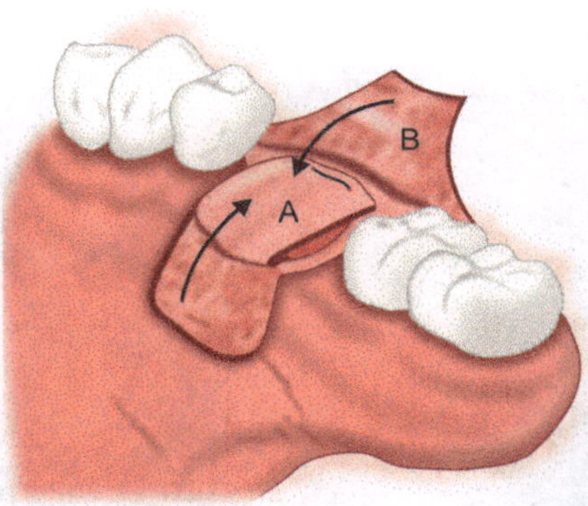

C Reverse palatal and buccal advancement flap

Figs 14.26A to C: Combined local flaps

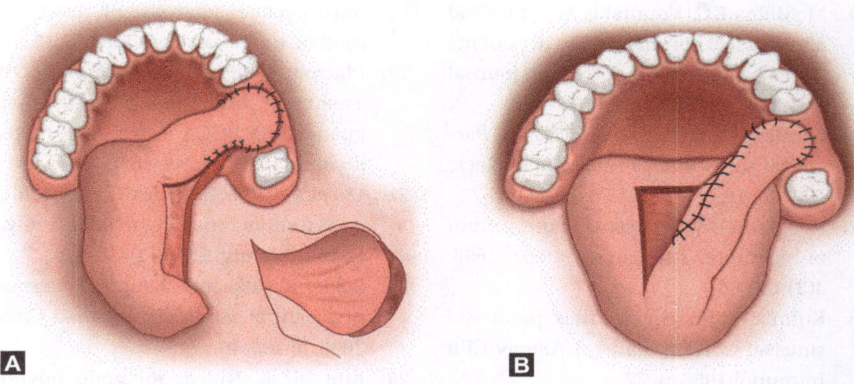

Figs 14.28A and B: Posteriorly and anteriorly based tongue flaps

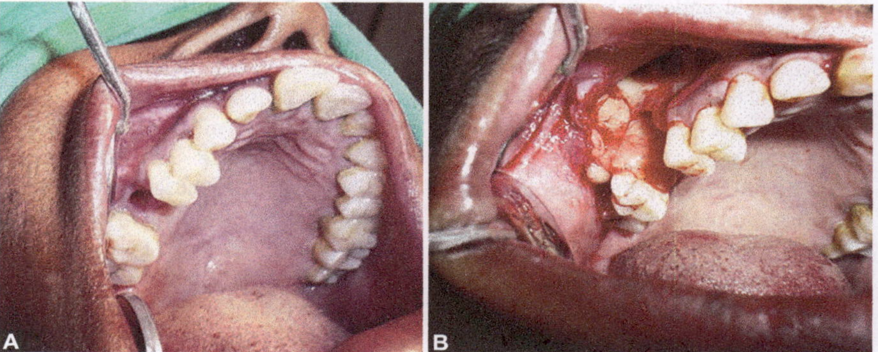

Figs 14.29A and B: Use of buccal fat pad for the closure of OAF

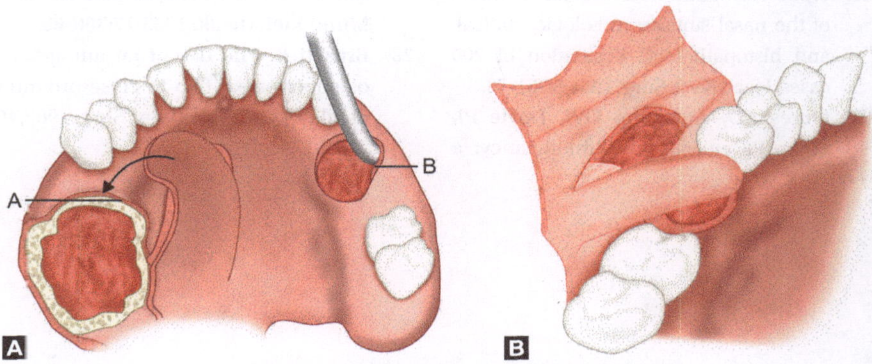

Figs 14.30A and B: Bone grafting to close OAF; (A) Bone graft; (B) Buccal osteoperiosteal flap

Use of bone grafts[28]: The OAF has two ways compounding, i.e. in oral cavity and the maxillary sinus. Hence, primary bone grafting is not advisable as good soft tissue cover cannot be provided on both the ends in spite of using any technique for closure of OAF. If the defect is large then in the primary state attempt should be made to close the OAF using a soft tissue flap and once the antral lining is healed and established, second surgery should be performed for bone grafting. The bone graft is placed between the antral lining and oral mucosa. The use of an autogenous cancellous bone in the closure of palatal defect is a well known procedure (Figs 14.30A and B). Cockerham et al. in 1976 suggested that, when a conservative method fails or when the size of the defect is too large, bone graft should be indicated in the closure. Whitney et al. advocated bone grafts in cases where there is need to recontour the alveolar ridge. The disadvantage with this technique is that an additional surgical procedure is needed to obtain the bone graft, this increases the length of the procedure and morbidity.

A single stage and simpler surgical procedure was given by Brusati in 1982. In this, he took the bone from the lateral wall of the antrum and pedicled on the periosteum to close the alveolar defect (Figs 14.30A and B). The disadvantage with this procedure was that the buccal vestibular height was reduced as a result of the use of the buccal flap as a soft tissue coverage and in case of dehiscence chances of additional oroantral communication are there.

Acrylic Obturators

When the fistula is very large, e.g. due to tumor is fabricated to rehabilitate the patient.

Alloplastic Material

Alloplastic material can be used in conjunction with the soft tissue flaps. They are placed below the flap to cover the bony defect.

Various alloplastic materials used are:

- Gold foil
- Gold plate
- Tantalum plate
- Soft polymethylmethacrylate
- Lyophilized collagen.

By using alloplastic materials, it does not require raising of a large amount of local tissue. The procedure does not affect the buccal vestibular height and there is no raw area left behind for granulation following the closure.

REFERENCES

1. McGowan DA, Baxter PW, James. The maxillary sinus and its Dental implications. Oxford: Wright, Butterworth-Heinemann Ltd. Chapter 1. 1993.
2. Ritter FN, Lee D. The paranasal sinuses, Anatomy and surgical techniques. St Louis, The Mosby company. 1978.
3. Harneja NK, Hukmani P: A study of the maxillary sinus in Indian subjects; Indian Journal of Otolaryngology. 1980; 32(4):101–2.
4. Traxler H, Windisch A, Geyerhofer U, et al. Arterial blood supply of the maxillary sinus. Clin Anat. 1999;14(6):417-21.
5. Aust R, Drettner B. Oxygentension in human maxillary sinus under normal and pathological conditions. Acta Otolaryngol; 1973. p. 78.
6. Furukawa CT. The role of allergy in sinusitis in children. J Allergy Clin Immunol;1992. p. 90.
7. Brook I. Microbiology and management of sinusitis. J Otolaryngol;1996. p. 25.
8. Kartagener M. Zur pathogenese der bronchiectasien. I Mitteilung: bronchiectasien bei situs viscerum inversus. Betr Klin Tuberk. 1933;83:498-501.
9. Handelsman DJ, Conway AJ, Boylan LM, Turtle JR. "Young's syndrome. Obstructive azoospermia and chronic sinopulmonary infections". N Engl J Med. 1984;310(1):3-9.
10. McMains KC, Kountakis SE. "Medical and surgical considerations in patients with Samter's triad". American journal of rhinology. 2006;20(6):573-6.
11. Ferreiro JA, Carlson BA, Cody T. Paranasal sinus Fungal Balls. Head Neck; 1997. p. 19.
12. Roughton EW. Empyema of the antrum of highmore. The Laryngoscope. 1898; 4(3):159-63.
13. Kuhn JP. Imaging of the paranasal sinuses: Current status. J Allergy Clin Immunol;1986. p. 77.
14. Menlhelm ER, Oliverio TJ, Benson ML, et al. Optimal CT evaluation for functional endoscopic sinus surgery. Am J Neuro Radiol;1991. p. 12.
15. Benninger MS, Anon J, Mabry RS. The medical management of rhino sinusitis. Otolaryngol Head Neck Surg. 1997;117 (3 Pt 2):S41-9.
16. Mabry RL, Marple BF. Open maxillary sinus procedures. In: Kennedy DW, Bolker WE, Zinreich SJ, (Eds). Diseases of sinuses: Diagnosis in management. Hamilton: BC Decker. Inc 2001.
17. Lewis JS, Castro EB: Cancer of the nasal cavity and paranasal sinuses. J Laryngol Otol. 1972;86:255-62.
18. Weber AL, Stanton AC. Malignant tumors of the nasal sinuses: radiologic, clinical, and histopathologic evaluation of 200 cases, Head Neck Surg. 1984;6:761-76.
19. Flores AD, Anderson DW, Doyle PJ, et al. Paranasal sinus malignancy: a retrospective analysis of treatment methods, J Otolaryngol.1984;13:141-6.
20. Macnab T, Flores AD, Anderson DW. Treatment of paranasal sinus malignancy: the BCCA experience, J Otolaryngol. 1992; 21:244-48.
21. Yucel A, Cinar C, Aydin Y, et al. Malignant tumors requiring maxillectomy. J Craniofac Surg. 2000;11:418-29.
22. Sokler K, Vuksan V, Lauc T. Treatment of oroantral fistula. Acta Stomat Croat. 2002;36:135-40.
23. Moczair L. Nuovo methodo operatiopela chisura delle fistole del seno mascellase di origina dentale. Stomatol (Roma). 1930;28:1087-88.
24. Rehrmann A. Eine methode zur Schliessung von Kieferhohlenperforationen. Dtsch. Zahnarztl. Z. 1936:39:1136-9.
25. Ashley REA. A method of closing antroalveolar fistulae. Ann. Otol Rhinol. Laryngol. 1939;48:632-5.
26. Poeschl PW, Baumann A, Russmmeller G, Poeschl E, Klug C, Ewers R. Closure of Oroantral Communications with Bichat's Buccal Fat Pad. J Oral and Maxillofac Surg. 2009;67(7):1460-6.
27. Schuchardt K. Methodik des Verschlusses von Defekten im alveolarforsate zalm lose oberkiefer. Dtsch. Zahn Mund Kieferheilk. 1953;17:366-69.
28. Brusati R. The use of an autogenous osteoperiosteal flap to close oroantral fistulas. J Oral Maxillofac Surg. 1982;40: 250-51.

Section 5

Salivary Glands Pathologies

15 Diseases of Salivary Glands

Borle Rajiv M, Agni Nishit, Arora Aakash

Salivary glands may be classified as major and minor glands. Major glands are paired glands. They include parotid, submandibular and sublingual salivary glands. There are numerous minor salivary glands that are widely distributed in the oral cavity in the submucosal layer. They include labial, buccal, palatine, lingual and incisive glands. Based on the type of secretions, salivary glands are classified as:

- Mucous salivary glands
- Serous salivary glands
- Mixed salivary glands.

Salivary glands are often involved in a wide variety of disorders that frequently require surgical treatment. These glands can be involved with acute and chronic inflammatory processes, give rise to benign and malignant tumors, manifest congenital abnormalities or represent involvement of a systemic disorder. Amongst all the disorders, the most common are problems with neoplasms and infections.

The rate of secretion of individual glands ranges from barely perceptible during sleep to as high as 4 mL/min on maximal stimulation. In a 24 hours period, the submandibular gland produces 70 percent of the saliva, parotid gland 25 percent and minor glands another 5 percent.

EMBRYOLOGICAL DEVELOPMENT

The salivary glands arise from the epithelial lining of the oral cavity.[1] They arise as a proliferation of oral epithelial cells forming a focal thickening that grows into the underlying ectomesenchyme. Continued growth results in the formation of a small bud connected to the surface by a trailing cord of epithelial cells, with mesenchymal cells condensing around the bud. Clefts develop in the bud, forming two or more new buds and this process is continued and is known as branching morphogenesis. This produces successive generations of buds and a hierarchical ramification of the gland.

Several factors control the branch points and the overall structure of the glands. Members of the fibroblast growth factor protein family along with transforming growth factor-β play a major role in the branching. The differential contraction of actin filaments at the basal and apical ends of the epithelial cells probably provides the physical mechanism underlying cleft formation. The deposition of extracellular matrix components within the clefts apparently serves to stabilize them. The specific mesenchyme associated with the salivary glands seems to provide the optimum environment for gland development.

The development of lumen within the branched epithelium occurs first in the distal end of the main cord and in branch cords, then in proximal end of the main cord and finally in the central portion of the main cord. Lumina form within the ducts before they develop within the terminal buds. A few studies have hypothesized that apoptosis of centrally located cells in the cell cords may be responsible for lumen formation.

Following the development of the lumen in the terminal buds, the epithelium consists of two layers of cells. The cells of the inner layer differentiate into secretory cells of the mature gland. They may be mucous or serous depending on the gland type. Few cells of the outer layer form contractile myoepithelial cells that are present around the secretory end pieces and intercalated ducts. As the epithelial parenchymal component increases in size and number, there is a decrease in the associated mesenchyme. However, a thin layer of connective tissue remains around each secretory end piece and duct of the adult gland. Thicker partitions of connective tissue (septa), which are continuous with the capsule invest the excretory ducts and divide the gland into lobes and lobules. They contain the nerves and blood vessels, which supply the gland.

The parotid gland is the first to appear and begins development at 4th to 6th week of intrauterine life. They develop from the buds that arise from the oral ectodermal lining near the angle of the stomodeum and later grow towards the ear. The ducts are formed by 10 weeks of intra uterine life. Secretions commence by 18 weeks. The capsule and connective tissue develop from the surrounding mesenchyme.

The submandibular glands appear late in the 6th week. They develop from the endodermal buds in the floor of the stomodeum. Acini begin forming at 12 weeks and secretory activity begins at 16 weeks. The growth continues after birth also.

The sublingual glands appear in the 8th week. They develop from endodermal buds in the paralingual sulcus. The minor salivary glands too develop at 8 to 12 weeks of gestation.

The cells of the secretory end pieces and ducts attain maturity during last 2 weeks of intrauterine life. The glands continue to grow postnatally with the volume proportion of acinar tissue increasing and that of ducts, connective tissue and vascular tissue decreasing up to 2 years of life.

SURGICAL ANATOMY OF PAROTID GLAND

The parotid gland is the largest of the salivary glands weighing approximately about 15 to 30 g (avg. 25 g).[2] It is an irregular, lobulated, yellowish mass lying largely below the external acoustic meatus in a deep hollow between the mandible and sternocleidomastoid muscle. It lies in the retromandibular fossa and reaches medially to the styloid process and muscles arising from it. Upwards it extends up to external acoustic meatus, which is situated in a groove of the gland. Surrounding the acoustic meatus on its inferior surface, the gland reaches posteriorly to the mastoid process and sternocleidomastoid muscle. Anteriorly, it is in contact with the posterior border of medial pterygoid muscle and mandibular ramus. A part of the gland extends anteriorly on the outer surface of the mandibular ramus and masseter muscle as thin, triangular layer.[3] Outer surface of the gland is situated superficially covered by capsule, superficial fascia and skin. Upper lobules of the superficial part of gland cover the craniomandibular articulation in front of the ear, but never transgress the lower border of the zygomatic arch (Fig. 15.1).

A dense fibrous capsule derived from the investing layer of the deep cervical fascia and incompletely invests the gland. The capsule is tight and firmly connected with strong septa dividing the lobes and lobules of the gland from one another. It is closely adherent to the gland. The toughness of the fascia/capsule on the external surface of the gland restricts a massive swelling in parotid space infections, which are very painful due to the unyielding nature of the capsule. As the parotid abscess is non-fluctuant due to the presence of the tough fascial covering, once the abscess is diagnosed one should not wait for the fluctuations to develop and then drain the abscess, but drain it at the earliest. The delay tends to mount more pressure and induces ischemic necrosis of the gland parenchyma, which can be avoided by early drainage/decompression. If the drainage is delayed the chances of bursting the abscess in the external auditory canal are high. Similarly, the benign tumors are slow to project outwards to any great extent and hence take years to present as conspicuous bulges. The parotid fascia continues anteriorly as the masseteric fascia and thus it is collectively referred to as parotidomasseteric fascia.

Parotid gland is like an inverted, flat, three-sided pyramid, presenting a small superior and superficial, anteromedial and posteromedial surfaces. It tapers inferiorly into a blunt apex. The facial nerve and its branches pass within the parotid gland and divide it into superficial and deep parts or lobes. About 80 percent of the Parotid gland lies superficial to the nerve, thus comprising the bulk of the gland and 20 percent of the gland lies deep to the nerve entering the parapharyngeal space. A narrow isthmus connects the superficial and deep lobes. The other structures that lie within the gland are lymph nodes, external carotid artery and retromandibular vein. The tumors of the parotid involving both the superficial lobe and the deep lobe are often described as '*dumbbell tumor*' due to its peculiar appearance.

Duct of the parotid gland, i.e. the Stensen's duct is about 5 cm (*2 inches*) long and passes forward across the masseter about a finger breadth below the zygomatic arch.[4] It crosses the masseter at junction of upper and middle one-third. At its anterior border it turns medially almost at right angle, traversing the buccal fat pad and the buccinator muscle. It then runs obliquely forwards for a short distance between the buccinator and oral mucosa to open upon a small papilla (*salivary caruncle*) opposite the crown of 2nd maxillary molar. The duct

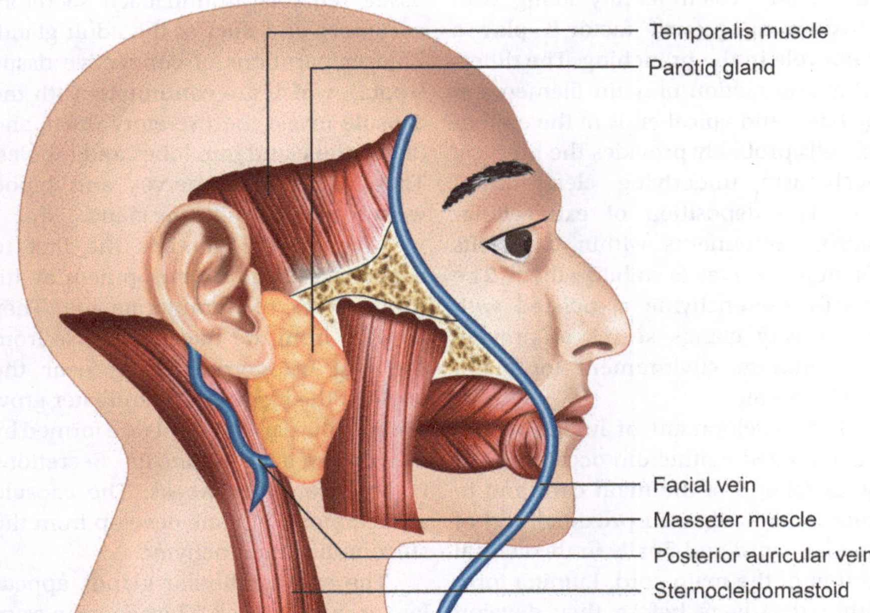

Fig. 15.1: Relation of parotid gland with surrounding structures

is relatively straighter and the secretions are serous in nature thus, the chances of the salivary calculus are very low in the Stensen's duct. If the calculus is formed in the duct it is usually found near the point where the duct bends acutely at the anterior border of the masseter muscle. The duct can be palpated over the clenched masseter muscle. During the inflammatory pathologies the duct is well felt and is chord-like in consistency and tender.

The structures passing through the gland are the terminal part of the external carotid artery, retromandibular vein and the lymph nodes. Hence the pathologies of the gland could be parenchymal or non-parenchymal in origin.

IDENTIFICATION OF THE FACIAL NERVE

Isthmus of the gland (part behind the ramus of the mandible joining the superficial and deep lobes) is most often found in the bifurcation of the facial nerve into upper temporofacial and lower cervicofacial divisions. There can be anatomical variations in the branching of the nerve (Fig. 15.2).

The facial nerve can be identified either proximally or distally. Proximally the main trunk of the nerve is identified before it enters the gland. Distally it is identified as branches after the nerve leaves the gland. It is ressected only when function is impaired preoperatively. Identification for the preservation of the facial nerve is carried out in three ways:

- Early direct identification of the main trunk where it exits through the stylomastoid foramen.
- Retrograde approach to the trunk from either the mandibular branch, where it passes over the retromandibular vein or the peripheral branches alongside the parotid duct.
- Supravital staining of the parotid gland, contrasting the blue normal gland from the unstained tumor and the gleaming white facial nerve branches.

There are four facial nerve pointers at the stylomastoid foramen.

1. The cartilaginous pointer described by Conley[5] (1978) is an artificially created landmark at its anterior-inferior border formed by posterior traction on the external auditory canal. The backward pull on the cartilage causes the meatus to assume the shape of a horn, the curved extremity of which allegedly points to the position of the facial nerve (Fig. 15.3). The nerve is located medial and inferior to the pointer. This is probably the least reliable as it depends on the configuration of the cartilaginous meatus.
2. The segment of the nerve, which lies in the interval between the stylomastoid foramen and parotid gland is extremely short, but is an ideal location to find the facial nerve before the parotidectomy commences. It is best found by searching in the tympanomastoid sulcus, which is formed by the edge of the bony external meatus on one hand and the anterior face of the mastoid process on the other. The tympanomastoid sulcus lies at the apex of the vaginomastoid angle, which is formed by meeting of the vaginal process of tympanic portion of the temporal bone and mastoid process. The nerve emerges from the stylomastoid foramen some 3 to 4 mm deep to the outer edge of the bony external canal. However; the groove is filled with fibrofatty lobules that mimic the trunk of the facial nerve, which may lie as deep as 1 cm to this landmark.
3. The most reliable landmark for finding the nerve is the posterior belly of the digastric muscle, which lies just inferior to the nerve. The anterior superior aspect of the posterior belly of the digastric muscle is inserted just behind the stylomastoid foramen.
4. The styloid process is a useful confirmatory landmark. The facial nerve courses lateral to the styloid process near the base of the styloid. However, to depend on it for finding the nerve is to court trouble, since it lies medial and anterior to the point of emergence of the nerve from the mastoid. The posterior auricular artery bleeds frequently, while looking for the facial nerve, since it lies below and just lateral to the nerve.

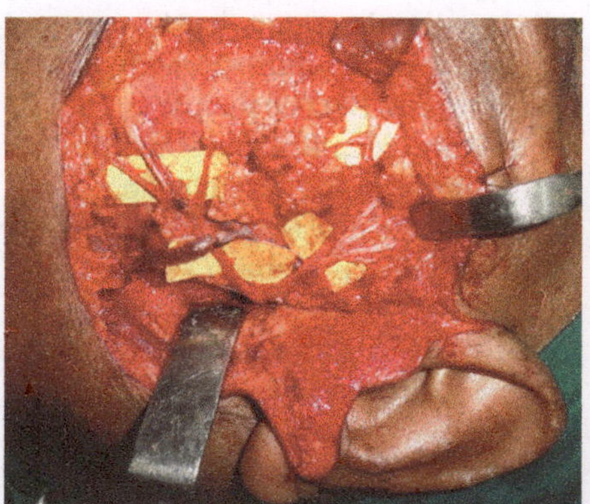

Fig. 15.2: Branches of facial nerve

Fig. 15.3: Cartilaginous pointer of Conley

SURGICAL ANATOMY OF SUBMANDIBULAR GLAND

Submandibular gland is irregular in shape and of the size of a walnut. It has a mixture of serous and mucous acini, but is chiefly serous. The upper pole lies on the medial surface of the mandible in the submandibular fossa and lower pole extends beyond boundaries of the digastric triangle covering intermediate tendon of the digastric muscle. The gland is palpable between the index finger placed on the floor of the mouth and thumb placed anteromedial to the angle of mandible below the floor.

Inferiorly the gland approaches the greater cornu of the hyoid, which serves as a useful landmark when marking

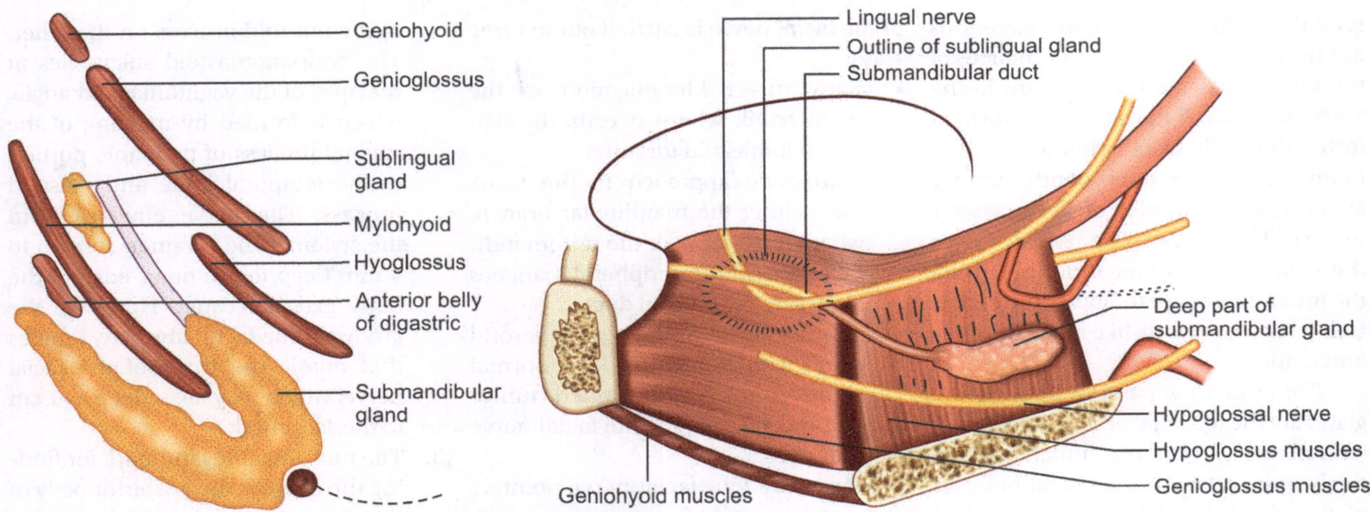

Fig. 15.4: Submandibular gland and its relation to deeper structure

the incision for the operation to remove the gland. The marginal mandibular branch of the facial nerve and its subsidiary branches lie plastered to the outer aspect of the deep cervical fascia and never make contact with the gland or its capsule. So the dissection should be done in a plane deep to the fascia overlying the submandibular gland. Any dissection limited to a plane within the capsule does not harm these structures. However, most inferior of the branches of the marginal mandibular nerve lies close to the lower border of the submandibular gland and could be damaged when gaining entry to the plane of dissection at the beginning of the surgery. The hypoglossal nerve with its venae comitantes lies on the hyoglossus, but is separated from the deep aspect of the gland by a potential space (Fig. 15.4). Escape of disease from the deep aspect of the gland would be the only likely circumstance to put the nerve at risk when removing benign tumors. The lingual nerve arches gently downwards just above the deep part of the gland to which it is attached by a ganglionic connection, alongside which is a small blood vessel. The nerve subsequently passes below the duct then round its outer aspect in the form of a broad loop before heading for the mucosa of the tongue. It is at risk when the deep part of the gland is being mobilized. The duct of the submandibular gland is longer and has a tortuous course. In addition, it has an uphill course. Thus the secretions have to be emptied against gravity and there are increased chances of retention. Also, the mineral content of the secretion is high, especially calcium content,[6] which along with increased retention of secretions result into higher incidence of calculus formation and inflammatory pathologies.

SURGICAL ANATOMY OF SUBLINGUAL GLAND

Sublingual glands are the smallest of the major salivary glands. They lie beneath the mucosa of the floor of the mouth causing an elevation, salivary eminence, on the floor of the oral cavity. The gland is narrow, flat, shaped like an almond and weighs 3 to 4 g.[4] There are 8 to 20 ducts of the sublingual gland. The smaller ducts mostly open separately on the summit of the sublingual fold and a few into submandibular duct. From anterior part of the gland, small rami arise from the major salivary duct and known as Bartholin's duct. Smaller or minor sublingual glands may be subdivided into two groups. One group lies at the superior surface of the gland. They release short ducts 5 to 15 in number, which open at the crest of sublingual eminence on the floor of the oral cavity. These minor ducts are known as ducts of Rivinus. The excretory ducts of the sublingual glands are very superficially located and hence easily get damaged. They result into mucous retention cysts the '*ranula*'.

Incidence

In most parts of the world the incidence of salivary gland tumors, both benign and malignant, varies from 1 to 2 per 100,000 populations per year.[7] Because of the rarity of tumors of the salivary glands, they are often included as "miscellaneous" or "other" head and neck tumors in epidemiologic surveys of neoplasia. The annual incidence of salivary gland tumors varies around the world from approximately 0.4 to 13.5 cases per 100,000 people.[8]

Salivary gland neoplasms do not exhibit any strong predilection for a particular sex nor is there any distinct racial incidence pattern. Patients of all ages can be affected.[9] However, the majority of salivary gland tumors are diagnosed between fourth and seventh decade.

Historically, an exception to the low incidence of salivary gland neoplasms is its incidence in Inuit population living in the western and central Canadian Artic. From 1950 to 1966 salivary gland neoplasms, predominantly lymphoepithelial carcinoma accounted for approximately 25 percent of all cancers affecting this population. These tumors were so prevalent that the term 'Eskimomas' was coined to denote them. The mortality rate arising from these tumors was 100 and 400 times greater among Inuit men and women respectively as compared to Canadian men and women.

In the United States, data on salivary gland tumors is limited to incidence of salivary gland carcinomas. In 1959, Dorn and Cutler reported a higher incidence of salivary gland carcinoma in nonwhites than whites. Recent data (May 1989) from surveillance, epidemiology and end results (SEER) registries of the National Cancer Institute show the age-adjusted incidence of salivary gland cancer from 1982 to 1986 in all races and both sexes to be 0.9 cases per 100,000 people. Since malignant tumors comprise between 35 to 40 percent of all salivary gland tumors, it is estimated that annual incidence of salivary gland tumors in the United States is between 2.2 and 2.5 cases per 100,000 people. It accounts for 650 deaths per year in the USA. In USA 3 to 4 percent of all neoplasms of the Head and Neck are salivary gland neoplasms. In UK it comprises of 40 cases per year.

AT CRI, Varanasi; 1 to 4 new cases per year are diagnosed as salivary gland tumors. They account for less than 1 percent of all registered malignancies. Table 15.1 gives the site-wise incidence of salivary gland tumors.

Incidence of Salivary Gland Tumors According to Site[10]

Age and sex predilection for major salivary gland tumors is as follows: Benign: 40 years and Malignant: 55 years. Male predominance is seen in Warthin's tumor and female predominance in Acinic cell tumors.

Site Wise Distribution[11]

The site-wise distribution of the salivary gland tumors is tabulated in Table 15.2.[12]

General Classification of Salivary Gland Pathologies

The salivary gland pathologies can be broadly classified as shown in the Box 15.1.

WHO Histological Classification of Tumors of the Salivary Glands 2005

Because of the low incidence of the salivary gland tumors their classification has emerged slowly. The WHO classified the salivary gland tumors first in 2002, which was subsequently modified in the year 2005 as shown in Box 15.2.

TNM Classification and Staging of the Salivary Gland Neoplasms

The first clinical staging system was developed by Spiro and co-workers at the Memorial Hospital. The TN (Tumor, Nodes) system and TNM modification (Tumor, Nodes, Metastases) was developed for the parotid gland and gland neoplasms.

The American Joint Commission on Cancer in 2002, staged the salivary gland neoplasms. The staging system follows the tumor, node, metastasis (TNM) system of staging like other parts of the body. Primary tumor stage depends primarily on: (a) the size of the primary tumor, (b) extraparenchymal extension and (c) involvement of the seventh cranial nerve or skull base. Minor salivary gland tumors staged according to the system used to classify primary tumors of the particular sites of origin, e.g. oral cavity, oropharynx, etc.

Box 15.1: Classification of the salivary gland pathologies

- Developmental
  - Aplasia—absence of gland
  - Atresia—absence of duct
  - Aberrancy—ectopic gland
- Enlargement of gland
  - Inflammatory
    - i. Viral: Mumps, Coxsackie-A, CMV, influenza, parainfluenza virus
    - ii. Bacterial
    - iii. Allergic
    - iv. Sarcoidosis
    - v. Obstructive
  - Non-inflammatory
    - i. Autoimmune: Sjögren's syndrome, Mikulicz's disease
    - ii. Alcoholic cirrhosis
    - iii. Diabetes mellitus
    - iv. Nutritional deficiency
    - v. HIV associated
- Cysts
  - Extravasation cysts
  - Retention cysts
  - Ranula
- Tumors of salivary glands
  - Benign
  - Malignant
- Necrotizing sialometaplasia
- Salivary gland dysfunction
  - Sialorrhea
  - Xerostomia

Table 15.1: Site wise incidence of salivary gland tumors

Type	Parotid	Submandibular	Sublingual	Minor glands[11] (Palate)
Benign	80%	60%	30%	53%
Malignant	20%	40%	70%	47%

Table 15.2: Site wise distribution of the salivary gland tumors

Site	Distribution %	Malignant %
Parotid	75–80	17–20
Submandibular	5–10	50
Sublingual	1–2	80
Minor glands	10–20	50

Box 15.2: WHO classification of salivary gland tumors 2005

Tumor categories	Code
• **Malignant epithelial tumors**	
– Acinic cell carcinoma	8550/3
– Mucoepidermoid carcinoma	8430/3
– Adenoid cystic carcinoma	8200/3
– Polymorphous low-grade adenocarcinoma	8525/3
– Epithelial–myoepithelial carcinoma	8562/3
– Clear cell carcinoma, not otherwise specified	8310/3
– Basal cell adenocarcinoma	8147/3
– Sebaceous carcinoma	8410/3
– Sebaceous lymphadenocarcinoma	8410/3
– Cystadenocarcinoma	8440/3
– Low-grade cribriform adenocarcinoma	
– Mucinous adenocarcinoma	8480/3
– Oncocytic carcinoma	8290/3
– Salivary duct carcinoma	8500/3
– Adenocarcinoma, not otherwise specified	8140/3
– Myoepithelial carcinoma	8982/3
– Carcinoma ex-pleomorphic adenoma	8941/3
– Carcinosarcoma	8980/3
– Metastasizing pleomorphic adenoma	8940/1
– Squamous cell carcinoma	8070/3
– Small cell carcinoma	8041/3
– Large cell carcinoma	8012/3
– Lymphoepithelial carcinoma	8082/3
– Sialoblastoma	8974/1
• **Benign epithelial tumors**	
– Pleomorphic adenoma	8940/0
– Myoepithelioma	8982/0
– Basal cell adenoma	8147/0
– Warthin's tumor	8561/0
– Oncocytoma	8290/0
– Canalicular adenoma	8149/0
– Sebaceous adenoma	8410/0
– Lymphadenoma	
i. Sebaceous	8410/0
ii. Non-sebaceous	8410/0
– Ductal papillomas	
i. Inverted ductal papilloma	8503/0
ii. Intraductal papilloma	8503/0
iii. Sialadenoma papilliferum	8406/0
– Cystadenoma	8440/0
i. Soft tissue tumors	
– Hemangioma	9120/0
i. Hematolymphoid tumors	
ii. Hodgkin lymphoma	
– Diffuse large B-cell lymphoma	9680/3
– Extranodal marginal zone B-cell lymphoma	9699/3
i. Secondary tumors	

Behavior is coded as follows:
0- benign tumors
1-borderline or uncertain behavior
3-malignant tumors

Primary Tumor (T) (Box 15.3)

Box 15.3: Primary tumor (T)

- TX—Primary tumor cannot be assessed
- T0—No evidence of primary tumor
- T1—Tumor 2 cm or less in greatest dimension without extraparenchymal extension
- T2—Tumor > 2 cm but not > 4 cm in greatest dimension without extraparenchymal extension
- T3—Tumor > 4 cm and/or tumor having extraparenchymal extension
- T4a—Tumor invades skin, mandible, ear canal, and/or facial nerve
- T4b—Tumor invades skull base and/or pterygoid plates and/or encases carotid artery.

(Extraparenchymal extension—clinical or macroscopic evidence of invasion of soft tissues or nerve, except those listed under T4a and T4b. Microscopic evidence alone does not constitute extraparenchymal extension for classification purposes)

Regional Lymph Nodes (N) (Box 15.4)

Box 15.4: Nodal metastasis N

- NX—Regional lymph nodes cannot be assessed
- N0—No regional lymph node metastasis
- N1—Metastasis in single ipsilateral lymph node, 3 cm or less in greatest dimension
- N2—Metastasis in single ipsilateral lymph node, > 3 cm but not > 6 cm in greatest dimension; or in multiple ipsilateral lymph nodes, none > 6 cm in greatest dimension; or in bilateral or contralateral lymph nodes, none > 6 cm in greatest dimension
- N2a—Metastasis in single ipsilateral lymph node, > 3 cm but not > 6 cm in greatest dimension
- N2b—Metastasis in multiple ipsilateral lymph nodes, none more than 6 cm in greatest dimension
- N2c—Metastasis in bilateral or contralateral lymph nodes, none more than 6 cm in greatest dimension
- N3—Metastasis in a lymph node more than 6 cm in greatest dimension

(Regional nodes are the cervical nodes. Midline nodes are considered ipsilateral nodes.)

Distant Metastasis (M)(Box 15.5)

Box 15.5: Distant metastasis (M)

- MX—Presence of distant metastasis cannot be assessed
- M0—No distant metastasis
- M1—Distant metastasis

The malignant salivary gland neoplasms can be staged as shown in Table 15.3.

DIAGNOSTIC AIDS

In salivary gland disease a careful history and examination will usually provide a correct diagnosis, but the major salivary glands may pose a diagnostic challenge because they are not only affected by specific local pathology, but also by systemic disease. A meticulous history leads to the determination of the nature of the lesion in the salivary glands. It must include the onset, duration, progress and rapidity of growth, extent of growth, presence of associated symptoms like paresthesia, pain, cystic enlargement, infection. A history of sudden growth or ulceration usually suggests malignancy.

Inspection and palpation are most important diagnostically. Any palpable enlargement is abnormal. The major salivary glands are palpated and the orifices of the ducts are observed for saliva output. Bimanual palpation is done to differentiate the major salivary glands from lymph node enlargement (Fig. 15.5).

Table 15.3: Staging of the malignant salivary gland neoplasms

Stage 1	T1	N0	M0
Stage 2	T2	N0	M0
Stage 3	T3	N0	M0
	T1	N1	M0
	T2	N1	M0
	T3	N1	M0
Stage 4A	T4a	N0	M0
	T4a	N1	M0
	T1	N2	M0
	T2	N2	M0
	T3	N2	M0
	T4a	N2	M0
Stage 4B	T4b	Any N	M0
	Any T	N3	M0
Stage 4C	Any T	Any N	M1

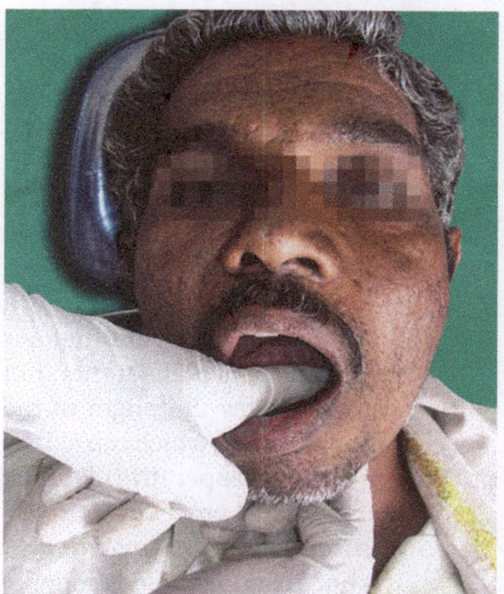

Fig. 15.5: Bimanual palpation of the submandibular gland and its duct

Mobility denotes that the lesion has not infiltrated the surrounding tissues. A malignant tumor and its lymphatic spread except early lymph node metastasis are not readily movable. If the tumor is fluctuant, the tumor probably is cystic. However regardless of the sites both benign and malignant tumors resemble each other clinically. Histopathology is the gold standard to final diagnosis. It is important to document function of the facial nerve when evaluating parotid tumors, because the nerve runs through the gland and evidence of decreased motor function of the nerve thus has diagnostic significance. Facial nerve paralysis (Bell's palsy) is usually indicative of malignancy.

Investigations

The investigations that can be performed to aid in diagnosing the salivary gland neoplasms are as follows:

- **Diagnostic imaging:**
  - *Routine radiographs:* It is not of much value except for diagnosing radiopaque sialoliths and parenchymal calcification. Salivary gland enlargements are not seen on plain radiographs.
  - *Ultrasonography:* It is a non-invasive technique, utilizes non-ionizing radiation, gives good soft-tissue discrimination, has excellent sensitivity for mass lesions and can be repeated as frequently as required. It helps to distinguish a cystic lesion from a solid mass in space occupying lesion. Normal salivary gland is homogeneously relatively hyperechogenic on USG than adjacent muscle. Tumors and cysts are more hypoechoic than normal parenchyma.[13] It is a more sensitive scan than CT for identification of small lesions less than 1 cm in diameter. Neoplasms appear as solid masses. A relatively well-defined capsule with a homogeneous central area is indicative of a benign or low-grade malignant tumor. An irregular or ill-defined capsule with complicated heterogeneous center indicates malignant or inflammatory changes.[14] Overall sensitivity of USG in detecting parotid tumors is very high. The drawbacks of USG include its inability to demonstrate the facial nerve in relation to the parotid gland and to define the extent of tumors extending outside the deep surface or of extraglandular lesions such as nasopharyngeal tumors invading the deep aspect of the gland. In addition, it is difficult to image the deep lobes of the major salivary glands.
  - *Doppler ultrasound and color-flow imaging:* It enables immediate recognition of vascular structures and allows confident discrimination between small vessels and ducts and rapid assessment of the vascularity of the mass lesions.
  - *Sialography:* It involves intubation of the principal duct of the salivary gland and instillation of radiopaque contrast medium to

delineate the ductal system and any other spaces in continuity. Its chief value is in assessment of obstructive pathology.

- *Radionucleotide scanning:* It is a valuable diagnostic tool in the evaluation of salivary gland physiology and pathology. These scans are useful in differentiating between acute obstructive and non-obstructive sialadenitis, showing presence of parenchymal masses greater than 1 cm in diameter and in few cases in identification of specific types of tumors. It includes static and dynamic scanning.
- *CT scan:* It provides excellent soft tissue details that show not only the lesion, but also involvement of the surrounding structures. It can be used to evaluate masses involving the parotid gland and adjacent structures and their relation to the facial nerve. The criteria of nerve involvement in parotid neoplasms on CT rely on bony changes along the course of the facial nerve, which include bone erosion, sclerotic margins and widening of the normal diameter of the fallopian canal or stylomastoid foramen.
- *MRI scan:* MRI differs from CT in its apparent sensitivity to calcification. The soft tissue contrast obtained with MRI allows very good assessment of majority of the salivary masses. Benign or low-grade neoplasms have well defined margins with relatively homogeneous low signal intensity on T1-weighted images and high signal on T2-weighted images, which is thought to reflect high proportion of serous and mucinous products present. By contrast, high-grade malignancies have poorly defined margins and tend to have heterogeneous low signal on both T1 and T2-weighted images, reflecting the high nuclear-cytoplasm ratio and lack of serous and mucinous material. Perineural spread can be diagnosed early on MRI due to better soft tissue delineation. The criteria of nerve involvement include replacement of normal perineural fat with tumor, enhancement with gadolinium (regardless of size) and increased size of the nerve in question (regardless of enhancement).
- *Arteriography:* It not only defines the vasculature of the tumor, but also delineates the origin of the vascular supply, which can aid the surgeon in preoperative planning of the surgical procedure.
- *Positron emission tomography*[15]*:* It is not a routinely used modality for diagnosis of salivary gland disorders because salivary glands have a variable and inconsistent uptake of Fluorodeoxyglucose (FDG), which is a radiotracer most commonly used with positron emission tomography (PET) scans. Hence, FDG-PET is unreliable both in tumor detection and in distinguishing benign from malignant tumors. The FDG-PET is too expensive and is not cost-effective. However FDG-PET measures the metabolic activity in various tissues and hence is superior to CT and MRI in diagnosing recurrence and differentiating it from post-operative fibrosis.[16] Since it can measure tumor metabolism, it can be used to evaluate tumor proliferation rates or tumor hypoxia, which can be used to optimize treatment strategy such as fractionation scheme for radiotherapy or sequence for combined therapy.

• **Histopathology:**

- *Fine needle aspiration cytopathology (FNAC):* It has a fairly high accuracy in the diagnosis of salivary gland lesions. The diagnostic accuracy of FNAC is 98 percent for benign tumors, 93 percent for malignant tumors and 88 percent for metastatic tumors. It has a minimal chance of tumor implantation along the needle tract. However, the aspirate may show limited histological architectural features and the tumor-stroma interface, which is of importance in diagnosis of many salivary tumors. Also, the status of invasion by the tumor, which is the most important criteria in predicting biologic behavior, is not disclosed by FNA.
- *Incisional biopsy:* It plays a minor role in diagnosis of salivary gland lesions. The tumors of the parotid are seldom biopsied as there are chances of seeding of the tumor cells and fungation through the skin at the site of biopsy.
- *Frozen sections* during surgery are helpful to determine the benign or malignant nature of the tumor, surgical clearance, however the accurate histopathological diagnosis of the tumor may not be possible on frozen sections.

Histopathological diagnosis of salivary gland tumors is often challenging, especially when it is done with FNAC. Clinicians make fanatic efforts to diagnose these lesions preoperatively. It is often difficult to make the subtyping of the salivary tumors on the basis of cytology or histopathology alone but may require special immunohistopathological techniques. Open biopsies are not always indicated. The salivary gland contains parenchyma and non-salivary inclusions such as lymphatic tissue, blood vessels and nerves. The tumors of parenchymal origin comprise of 95 to 96 percent of salivary tumors and the tumors of the interstitial tissue origin comprise of 4 to 5 percent salivary tumors. The salivary gland swellings could be inflammatory or neoplastic in origin. Hence, the clinician needs to know preoperatively the nature of the swelling rather than the subtyping. A simple approach to salivary gland swellings can simplify the approach to their diagnosis and management. The clinician should try to know if the swelling is salivary or nonsalivary in origin. If it is salivary in origin,

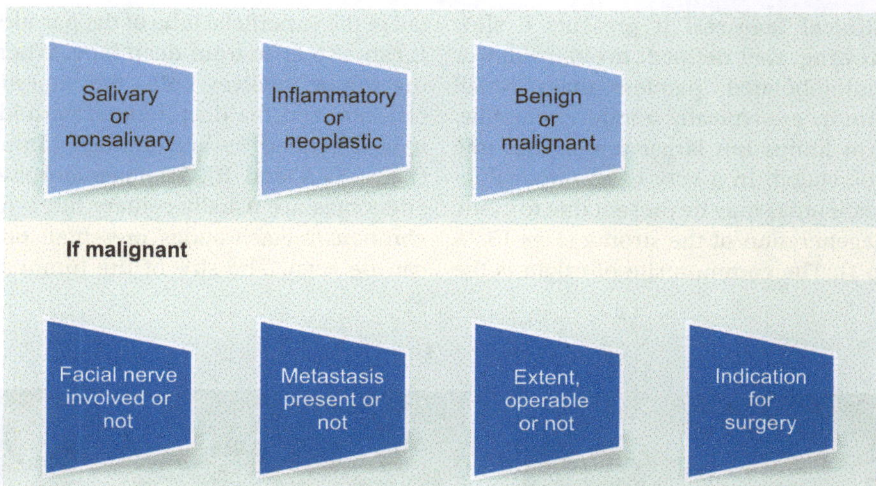

Fig. 15.6: The diagnosis and evaluation of salivary gland swellings

then whether it is inflammatory or neoplastic. If it is neoplastic, then it should be known whether it is benign or malignant. A subtyping beyond this need not be known because it will usually not affect the treatment plan. All malignant tumors are locally infiltrative and tend to metastasize to the regional lymph nodes. It may be argued that the Adenoid cystic carcinoma spreads perinurally, but the fact remains that several other malignant tumors are also known to spread perinurally and perivascularly (Fig. 15.6).

Salivary gland swelling chronology for diagnosis should be as shown in Fig. 15.6.

If the tumor is malignant, then the clinician should know the extent of the tumor, whether facial nerve is involved or not and if the regional lymph node metastasis or distant metastasis is present or not. These factors will guide the surgeon about the operability of the tumor, reconstruction modalities, preservation or sacrifice of the facial nerve, regional lymph node dissection required or not. It will also prompt the choice of the treatment as to whether it should be surgery alone or surgery plus chemoradiations or just chemoradiation.

ETIOLOGY OF TUMORS

The etiology of salivary gland tumors is unknown. However, investigations have been carried out to link salivary gland neoplasms to etiologic factors like viruses, radiation, occupation, lifestyle, hormones, etc.

Viruses

Epstein-Barr viruses have been implicated in the etiology of malignant lymphoepithelial lesion,[17] a form of malignant salivary gland carcinoma. The interrelationships of immunity, environmental factors and genetic constitution of the host may all play a role in malignant transformation of salivary gland epithelial cells. The other viruses suspected as possible etiologic agents are *Polyomavirus*, *Cytomegalovirus*, type C particles similar to those associated with murine leukemia, type B particles similar to those associated with murine breast tumors and human papilloma virus types 16 and 18.

Radiation

Evidence exists for the relationship between exposure to ionizing radiation and the later development of salivary gland tumors.[18] The substantial lymphoid component of the parotid gland may be more susceptible to low-dose radiation damage than the parenchyma. It seems that doses as low as 140 Rad may increase the risk of developing salivary gland neoplasms. Ultraviolet radiation may also be associated with an increased risk of salivary gland cancer.

Occupation

People in occupations such as asbestos mining,[15] manufacturing of rubber products leading to increased exposure to nitrosamines, industries that use these rubber products such as shoe manufacturing, plumbing (exposure to metals) and woodworking in the automobile industry are more prone to develop salivary gland carcinoma. Similarly people associated with an increased exposure to silica dust are more prone to salivary gland tumors.[19]

Lifestyle

Researchers could demonstrate no association of salivary gland tumors with heavy smoking or heavy alcohol consumption. However, cigarette smoking may play a causative role in the development of epidermoid carcinomas. Warthin's tumor is strongly associated with cigarette smoking.[20] Although severe malnutrition such as kwashiorkor causes enlargement of salivary glands, increased incidence of salivary gland tumors have not been observed.

Endogenous Hormones

They have a role in carcinogenesis of salivary gland tumors. Studies have indicated the presence of estrogen receptors in 80 percent of normal salivary glands and prolactin-binding activity in both normal and neoplastic salivary gland tissue. There has been an increased incidence of salivary gland tumors in patients with breast cancer.[21]

COMMON SALIVARY GLAND NEOPLASM

Pleomorphic Adenoma or Benign Mixed Tumor

Definition: It is a tumor of variable/incomplete, encapsulation, characterized microscopically by architectural rather than cellular pleomorphism. Epithelial and myoepithelial elements intermingle most commonly with tissue of mucoid, myxoid or chondroid appearance.

It is also called mixed salivary gland tumor due to presence of variety of components such as mucoid, myxoid, chondroid and sometimes osseous tissue.

Epidemiology: Most common salivary gland tumor (60% of all salivary gland tumors).[22] Mean age of presentation is 46 years (ranges from 1st–10th). Slight female preponderance.

Localization: 84 percent in parotid, 8 percent in submandibular gland and 0.5 percent in sublingual gland.[23] Lower pole of parotid is most common location.

Clinical features: It presents a slow growing, well defined, ovoid, round or multilobulated, painless mass. Small tumors are typically smooth, immobile, firm lumps but larger tumors become bosselated. In a very large tumor fluctuant areas may be present due to cystic degeneration of the stroma (Figs 15.7A to J). The common site of origin is the tail of the superficial lobe of the parotid. It can also arise from deep lobe. When the tumor involves both, the superficial lobe and the deep lobe of parotid, it is described as a Dumbbell tumor (Figs 15.8A and B). The pleomorphic adenomas are usually solitary but synchronous/metachronous presentati ons can be seen. The size of the tumor is

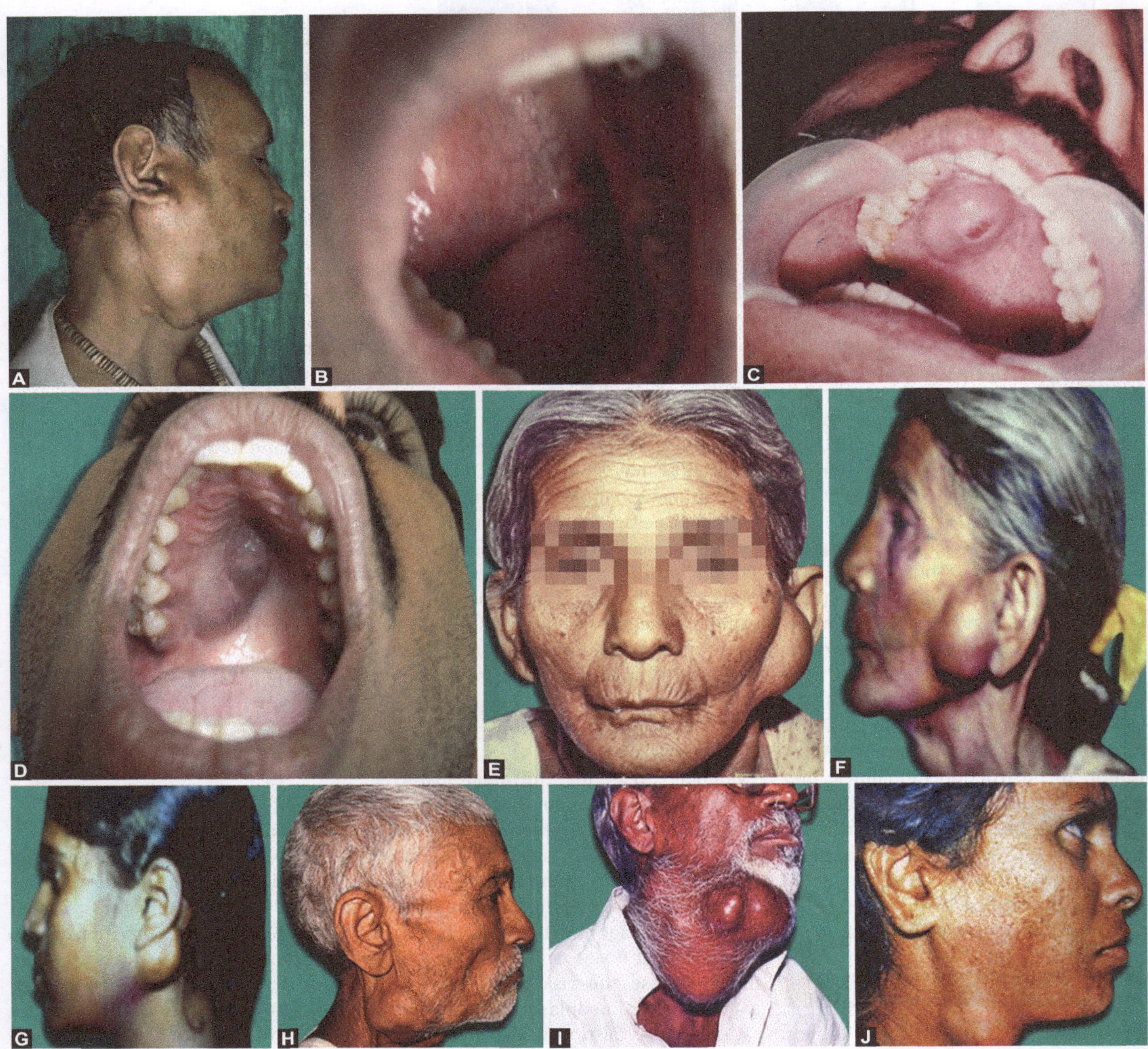

Figs 15.7A to J: Various presentations of pleomorphic adenomas in major and minor salivary glands

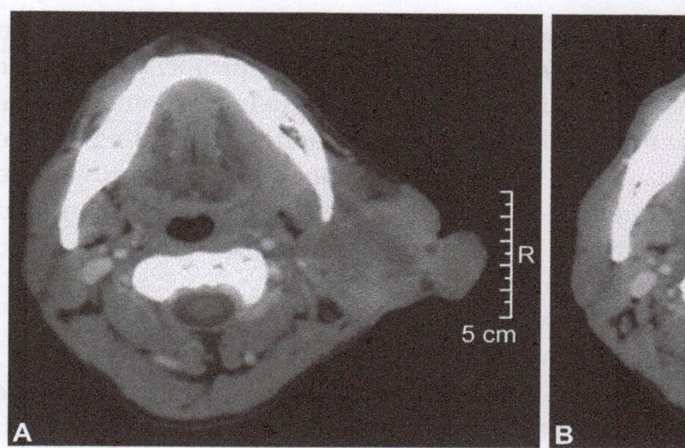

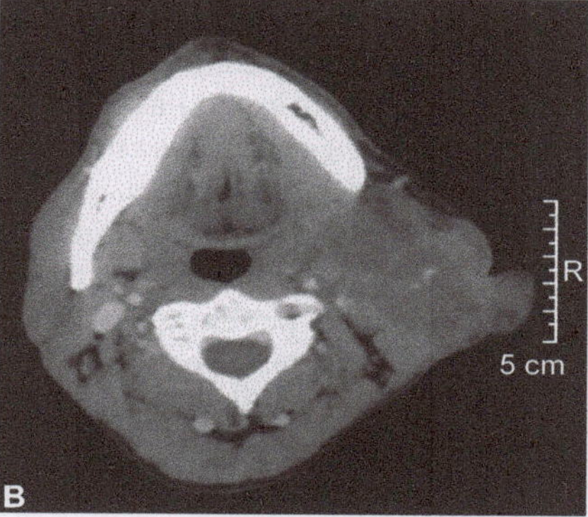

Figs 15.8A and B: CT scan of extensive pleomorphic adenoma of parotid involving the superficial and deep lobes (Dumbbell tumor)

variable at the time of first diagnosis. The tumor is usually asymptomatic and thus, the patients tend to ignore it and the tumor grows slowly, but steadily to a large size. Inspite of large size the involvement of the facial nerve does not occur. The larger tumors have a typical multilobulated appearance and it does not sag down, but stands out inspite of its large size and weight due to the presence of the chondroid tissue. The facial nerve is not involved in benign variants even if the tumor is large (Fig. 15.9). The encapsulation is incomplete and thus the tumor tends to recur even after surgery, if the resection is not adequate.

Histopathology: The pleomorphic adenoma has remarkable degree of morphological diversity. The essential components are capsule (usually incomplete), epithelial and myoepithelial cells and mesenchymal or stromal elements. The epithelial component shows a wide variety of cells including cuboidal, basaloid, squamous, spindle, plasmacytoid and clear cells. The cells are cytologically bland and have vacuolated nuclei without prominent nucleoli and low mitotic frequency. The epithelium usually forms sheets or duct like structures, duct show cuboidal luminal cells and there may be abluminal layer of myoepithelial cells. Mesenchymal component is usually mucoid/myxoid, cartilaginous or hyalinized. Due to the presence of diversified tissue it is often called a mixed tumor. Deposition of homogeneous eosinophilic hyaline material between tumor cells and within stroma can be striking feature of some tumor.

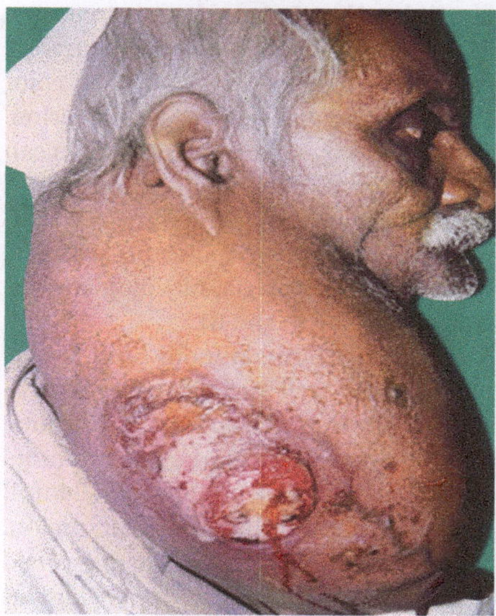

Fig. 15.9: Large lipoma in the parotid area note the tumor surface is not lobulated and is sagging down. The tumor is not standing out like the pleomorphic adenoma

Warthin's Tumor (Papillary Cystadenoma Lymphomatosum)

Warthin's tumor represents the second most common benign salivary gland neoplasm, comprising approximately 6 to 10 percent of all parotid tumors. Warthin's tumors rarely occur in the submandibular or minor salivary glands. Warthin's tumors affect men more commonly than women, with a male-to-female ratio of 5:1[24] and they typically appear between the 4th and 7th decades of life. The prevalence is increased among tobacco smokers.[25] Warthin's tumors are bilateral in 12 percent of cases. Warthin's tumors have a smooth capsule. When incised, multiple cystic spaces that contain mucinous material are appreciated. On microscopic evaluation, multiple papillae are present, projecting into the cystic spaces. The papillae consist of double-layered epithelium. The outer layer consists of granular eosinophilic cells. The stroma beneath the epithelium is lymphoid, often containing germinal centers.[26]

Warthin's tumors are best treated by means of superficial parotidectomy, which spares the facial nerve.[27,28]

Oncocytoma

Oncocytomas are unusual benign neoplasm that arises from the granular oncocytes within the salivary glands. These tumors account for less than 1 percent of all salivary gland tumors. They occur more commonly in older patients and affect men and women equally. Malignant oncocytomas do occur, but they are extremely rare.[29]

Benign oncocytomas are smooth and firm with a rubbery consistency. The tumors are cellular, containing round eosinophilic cells with a granular cytoplasm. The nuclei are small and have indentations. The granular appearance of this electron microscopy is used to identify this ultrastructural feature, which can be diagnostically helpful.

These tumors most commonly arise in the superficial portion of the parotid gland, they are best treated with superficial parotidectomy with preservation of the facial nerve. Tumors that occur outside the parotid gland should be excised with a cuff of normal tissue.

Monomorphic Adenoma

Monomorphic adenomas are often grouped with pleomorphic adenomas. These are distance tumors histologically, however and lack pleomorphic features. Basal cell adenomas and clear cell adenomas are included in this group to tumors. Monomorphic adenomas are benign, slow growing and the least aggressive of the salivary gland tumors.

They probably represent fewer than 2 percent of salivary gland neoplasms.[30]

The most common variety of monomorphic adenomas is the basal cell adenoma. Basal cell adenomas occur most commonly in the minor salivary glands, usually the upper lip.[31] Of the major salivary glands, the parotid gland is the usual location of occurrence.

Macroscopy: The tumors are encapsulated and are smooth.

Microscopic appearance: The tumors contain epithelial parenchyma, which is sharply demarcated from the scant stroma by a thick, prominent basement membrane. The epithelial cells have a palisading appearance at the periphery of the tumor parenchyma. The appearance can be confused with adenoid cystic carcinoma, but the distinction is clearly important, as the biologic behavior of the two tumors is vastly different.

Treatment: It consists of surgical excision with a margin of normal tissue for these benign and non-aggressive tumors.

Mucoepidermoid Carcinoma

Definition: It is a malignant glandular epithelial tumor, characterized by mucus, intermediate and epidermoid cells with columnar, clear cells and oncocytoid features.

Epidemiology: Most common primary salivary gland malignancy in both adults and children. Mean patient age is approx 45 years. The M: F ratio is 3:2.

Localization: Half of the tumors occur in major glands, 89.6 percent involved the parotid, 8.4 percent submandibular and 0.4 percent sublingual gland.[32] The central mucoepidermoid carcinomas in the mandible, especially at the angle due to entrapment of glandular tissue during embryonic fusion have been reported. The mucoepidermoid carcinoma is also seen in the tongue.[33]

Pathogenesis: Four possible origins have been described:[34]

1. Entrapment of retromolar mucous glands within the mandible, which subsequently undergo neoplastic transformation.
2. Developmentally included embryonic remnants of the submaxillary gland within the mandible.
3. Neoplastic transformation of the mucus secreting cells commonly found in the pluripotential epithelial lining of dentigerous cysts associated with impacted third molars.
4. Neoplastic transformation and invasion from the lining of the maxillary sinus. Our patient gave a prior history of cyst enucleation in the same region as the tumor, which may indicate the possibility of neoplastic transformation of the cyst wall into a malignant non-odontogenic tumor.

Clinical features: Most tumors present as firm, fixed and painless swellings. Sublingual gland lesions may demonstrate pain in spite of small size. Superficial intraoral neoplasms may exhibit a blue-red color and mimic a mucocele or vascular lesion. The mucosa overlying palatal tumors can be papillary. Cortical bone is sometimes superficially eroded. Symptoms can include pain, otorrhea, paresthesia, facial nerve palsy, dysphagia, bleeding and trismus (Figs 15.10A and B).

Macroscopy: Firm, smooth often cystic, tan or pink, well defined or infiltrative edges.[35] The tumor often has slimy stroma.

Tumor spread: Parotid gland tumors spread to adjacent preauricular lymph nodes, then to submandibular region. Submandibular gland neoplasms spread to submandibular and upper jugular lymphatic chain.

Histopathology: Mucoepidermoid carcinoma is characterized by squamoid (epidermoid) mucus producing cells and cells of intermediate type. Proportion of different cell types and their architectural configuration varies in and between tumors. They are usually multicystic with solid component and sometime the latter predominates. According to the clinical behavior and the severity of the dysplasia the tumor can be subgraded as low grade, moderate grade or severe grade tumors.

Adenoid Cystic Carcinoma

Adenoid cystic carcinoma (ACC) is the second most common malignant salivary gland tumor, representing approximately 10 percent of all salivary gland neoplasms.[36] It is the most common malignancy in the submandibular gland and usually appears as slow-growing painless mass. It has a tendency for early ulceration (Figs 15.11 to 15.14).

The most common symptom is a slow growing mass followed by pain due to the propensity of these tumors for perineural invasion. Facial nerve paralysis may also occur in parotid tumors.

Metastasis to regional lymph nodes is uncommon, but distant metastasis, (usually to the lung) is more common. Adenoid cystic carcinoma is unique in the survival at 5 years is approximately 65 percent, but 15-year survival is only 12 percent. Because of the slow growth of this tumor, patients may remain free of disease after initial treatment for 10 years or longer, only to develop metastases.[37-39] Local recurrence is also common. The tendency for this tumor to grow along perineural[40] and perivascular planes, often with skip lesions, helps explain the generally poor success of treatment.

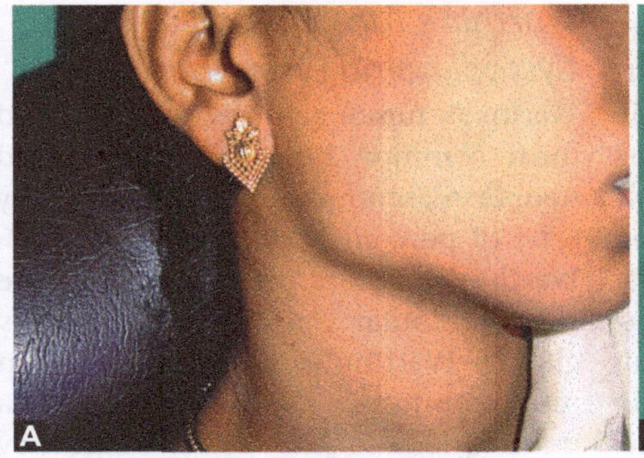

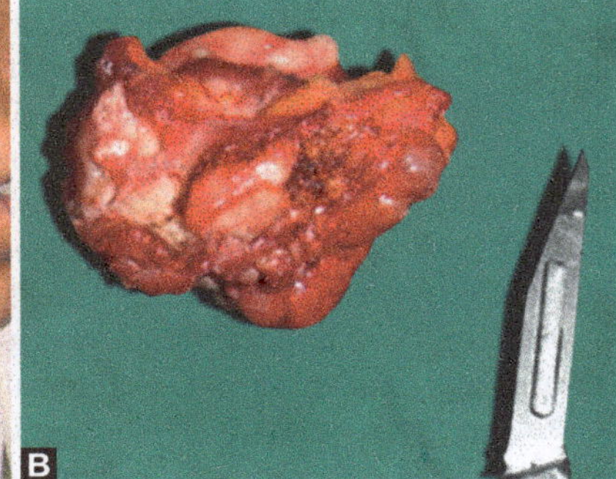

Figs 15.10A and B: Mucoepidermoid carcinoma of the submandibular salivary gland treated with excision of the affected gland

Gross findings: Adenoid cystic carcinomas are usually monolobular and non-encapsulated. They have a gray-pink color and infiltrate the surrounding normal tissue.

Microscopically: The tumors consist of basaloid epithelial elements that from cylindrical structures. Tumors are classified by the general architecture into the following three type: Cribriform, Tubular and Solid.[41] The cribriform pattern has the classic '*swiss cheese*' appearance with basophilic mucinous substance filling the cystic spaces. In the tubular pattern, the cells are arranged in smaller ducts and tubules with less prominent cystic spaces. The solid type is characterized by sheets of neoplastic cells with few cystic spaces. Any given, tumor may contain all three patterns, but common to all types is the propensity for perineural invasion.[42] Perineural extension accounts for the difficulty in eradicating adenoid cystic carcinoma despite extent of excision.

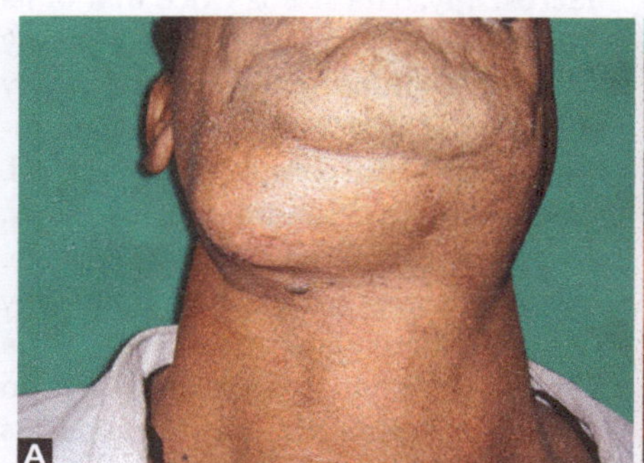

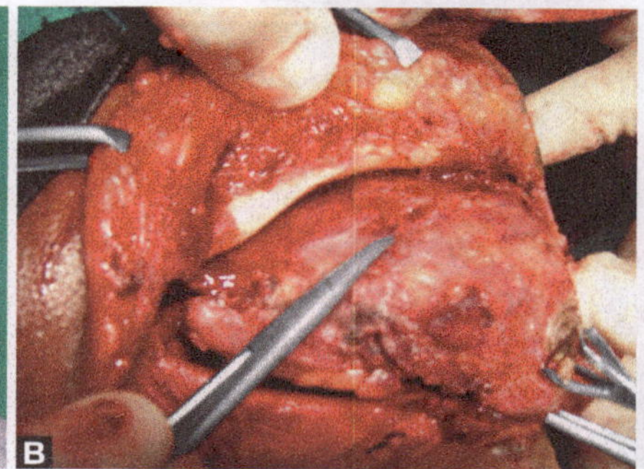

Figs 15.11A and B: ACC involving the sublingual salivary gland

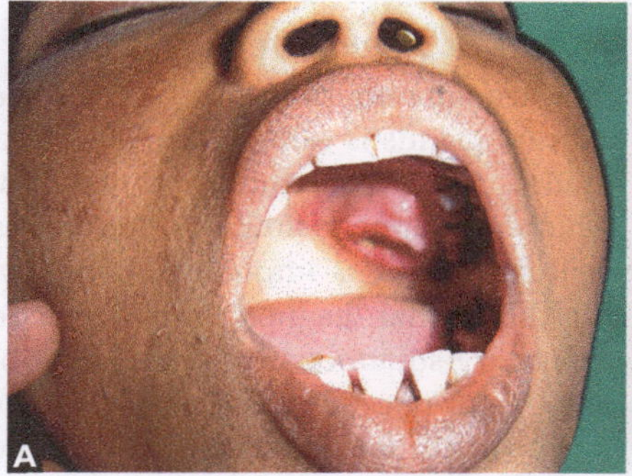

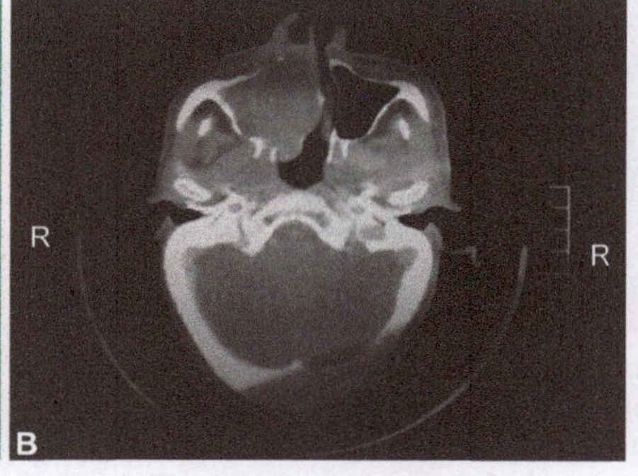

Figs 15.12A and B: ACC involving minor salivary gland of palate

Acinic Cell Carcinoma

Definition: Malignant epithelial neoplasm of salivary glands characterized by cytoplasmic zymogen granules.

Epidemiology: Slightly more women are affected than men.[43] Affected patients are ranging from young children to elderly adults, but is seen especially in 2nd decade.

Localization: Overwhelming majority 80 percent parotid gland 17 percent intraoral salivary gland, 4 percent submandibular gland, 1 percent submental gland.[44]

Clinical features: Slowly enlarging/ solitary unfixed mass, some patients experience pain which is often described as vague and intermittent.

Macroscopy: 1 to 3 largest dimension, circumscribed solitary nodules, lobular and tan red. Firm to soft, solid to cystic.

Tumor spread: Acinic cell carcinoma initially metastasizes to cervical lymph nodes.

Histopathology: Several cell types and growth patterns are recognized. Acinar, intercalated ductal, vacuolated, clear, glandular, solid/lobular, microcystic, papillary, follicular, (solid, solid-lobular, acinar-microcystic, papillary cystic, tubuloductal, follicular/macrocystic and dedifferentiated[45]).

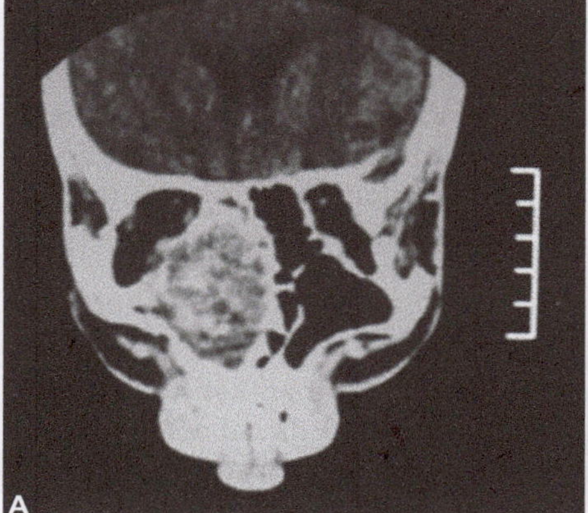

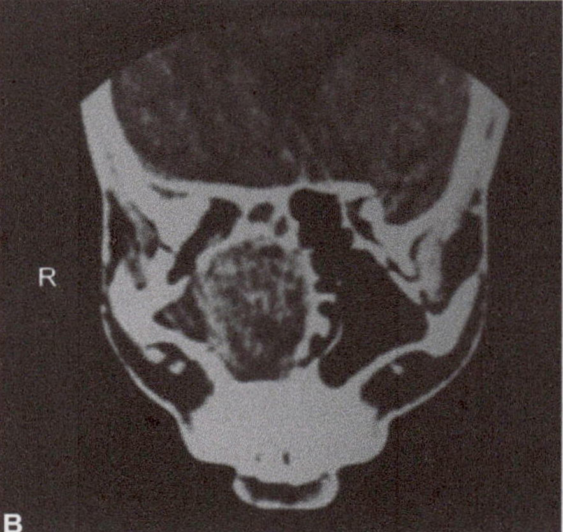

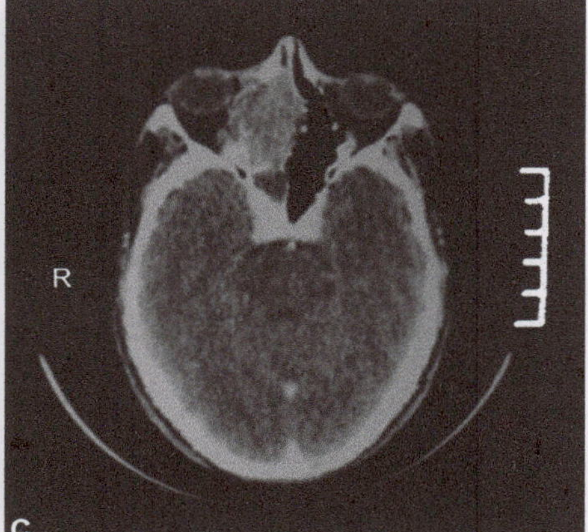

Figs 15.13A to C: ACC CT scan showing extension of the tumor to the skull base

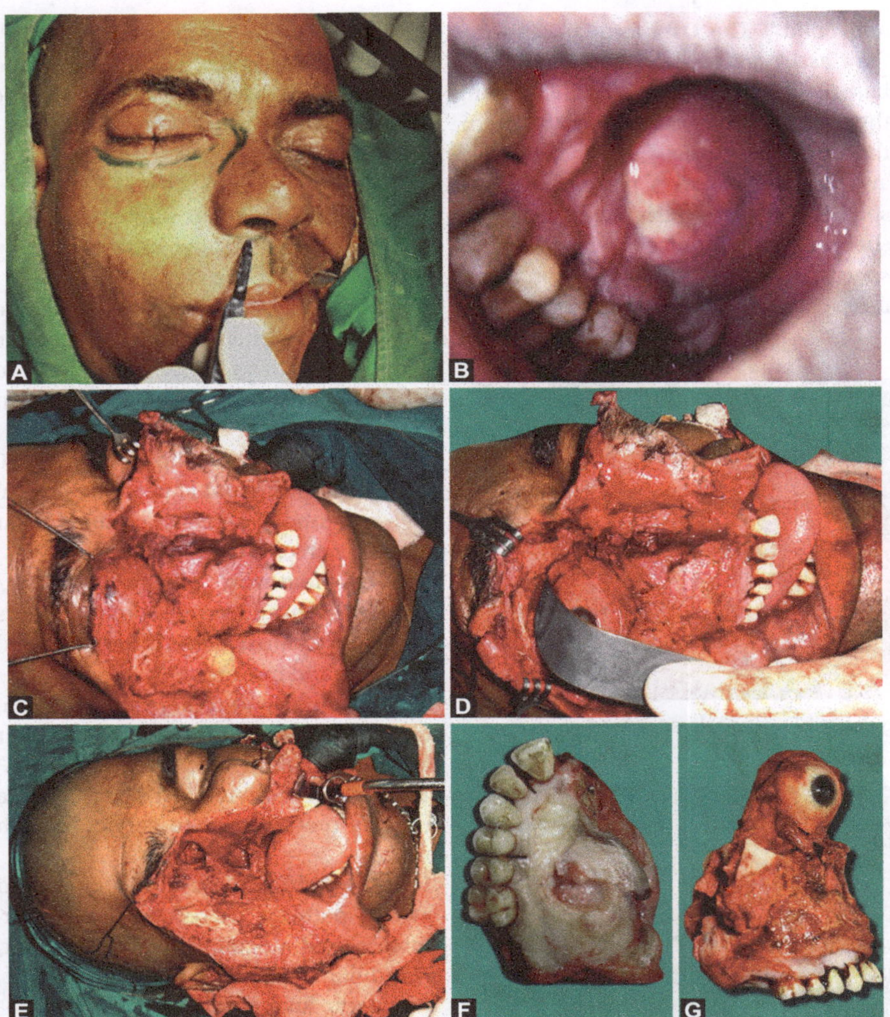

Figs 15.14A to G: Case of ACC involving minor salivary gland, extending to orbit, sphenoidal and ethmoidal air sinuses: (A) Approach to tumor with Weber Fergusson incision; (B) Intraoral presentation of the tumor; (C) Intraoperative photograph showing hemi-maxillectomy with ethmoid and sphenoidal sinus clearance; (D) Removal of the orbital contents; (E) Surgical defect created after wide local excision of tumor; (F and G) Excised specimen

Acinar cells are large polygonal with light basophilic, granular cytoplasm, round eccentric nuclei, cells are enlarged in sheets nodules/lobules, cystic microcystic, papillary projections, lymphoid infiltrate positive.[46]

Carcinoma Ex-pleomorphic Adenoma

Definition: Pleomorphic adenoma (PA) from which an epithelial malignancy has derived.

Epidemiology: They comprise 3.6 percent of all salivary gland tumors, 12 percent of all salivary malignancy and 6.2 percent of all pleomorphic adenomas.[47]

Etiology: Accumulation of genetic instabilities in long-standing pleomorphic adenomas.[48] Carcinoma ex-PA usually presents in 6th to 7th decades,[49] approximately 1 decade later than patients of pleomorphic adenoma.

Localization: Carcinoma ex-pleomorphic adenoma most frequently arises in the parotid gland, may originate in submandibular gland and minor salivary glands.[50,51]

Clinical features: Long-standing mass (> 3 years) with recent history of rapid growth over previous few months.[52] The earliest sign could be paresthesia of the overlying skin and subsequently the signs of involvement of the nerves in the area[53] (facial nerve in case of the parotid gland) may follow (Figs 15.15A to H and 15.16A and B). Like other carcinomas it has tendency to metastasize to the cervical lymph nodes.

Macroscopy: The size is twice that of its benign counterpart (1.5–2.5 cm), poorly circumscribed and many are extensively infiltrative. Occasionally are well circumscribed scar-like or completely capsulated.

Histopathology: Proportion of benign vs. malignant components are quite variable. Malignant component is most frequently a poorly differentiated adenocarcinoma or an undifferentiated carcinoma.[54] An infiltrative, destructive growth pattern is most reliable diagnostic criteria. Nuclear hyperchromatism and pleomorphism are important diagnostic criteria.

Squamous Cell Carcinoma

Primary squamous cell carcinoma of the salivary glands is rare. Ruling out high-grade mucoepidermoid carcinoma, which may appear similar to squamous cell carcinoma, is important. Similarly, the differential diagnosis must exclude a primary squamous cell carcinoma of the skin or upper respiratory squamous mucosa with regional metastasis to the salivary glands. Excluding these two possibilities, true primary squamous cell carcinomas likely represent 0.3 to 1.5 percent of salivary gland tumors.

As in other head and neck squamous cell carcinomas, local and regional recurrence occurs frequently. Treatment comprised of wide local excision, cervical neck dissection where ever merited and chemoradiations, if needed.

Adenocarcinoma (Not Otherwise Specified)

Definition: Malignant salivary gland tumor that exhibits ductal differentiation, but lacks any of the histomorphological features that characterize the other defined types of salivary carcinoma.

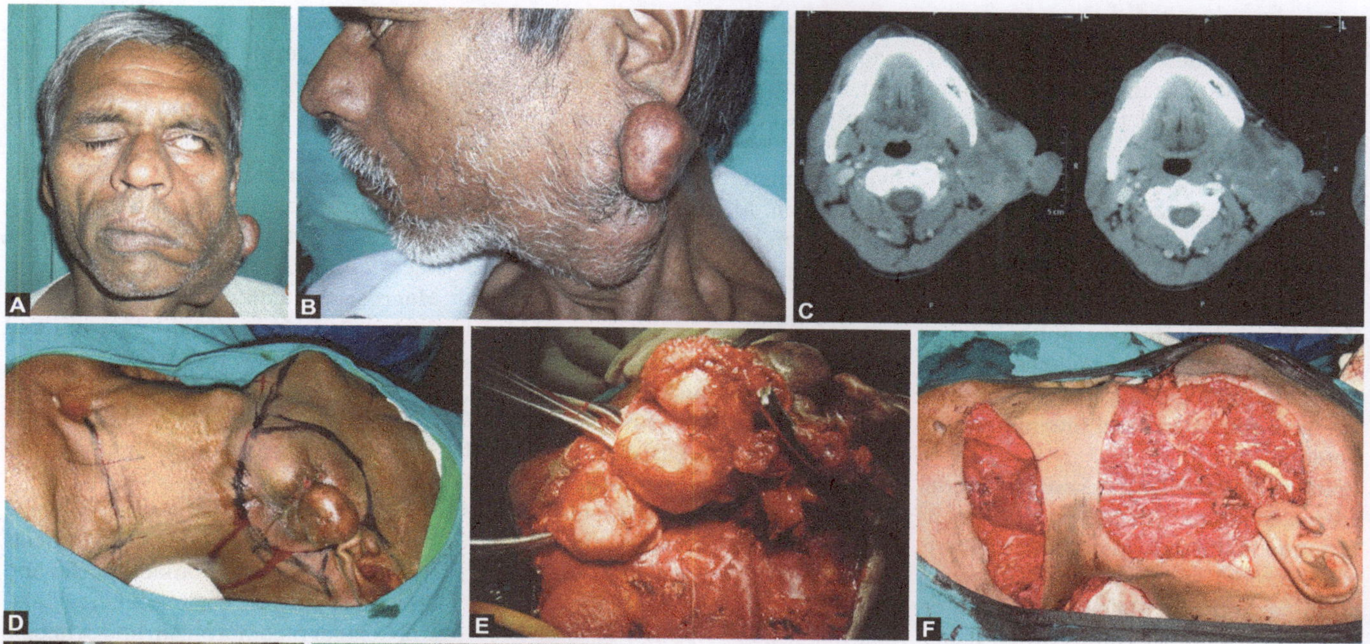

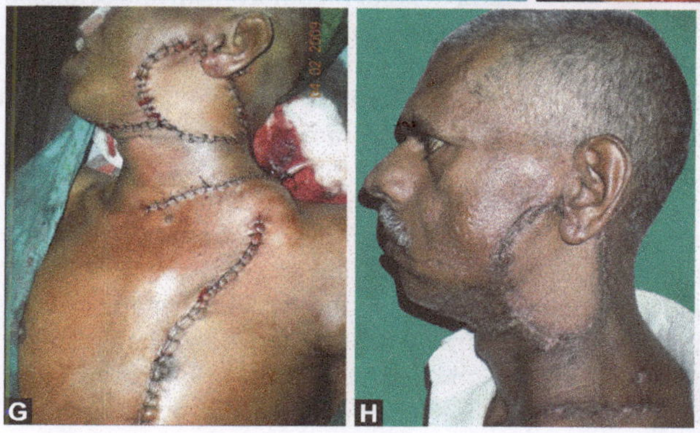

Figs 15.15A to H: Malignant pleomorphic adenoma of left parotid gland: (A) Bell's palsy due to facial nerve involvement; (B) Fixity to skin; (C) CT scan; (D) Marking of incision; (E) Exposed tumor; (F) Tumor excision with radical neck dissection; (G and H) Reconstruction with PMMC flap

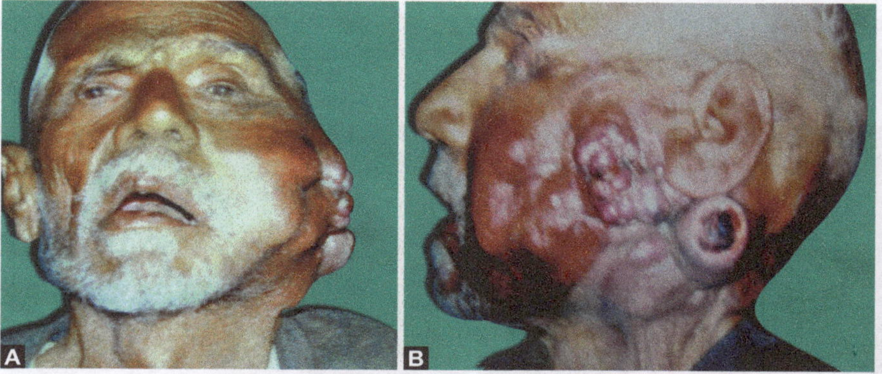

Figs 15.16A and B: Carcinoma ex-pleomorphic adenoma

Epidemiology: It is second only to mucoepidermoid carcinoma in occurrence, accounts for 17 percent of salivary carcinomas. Women outnumber men slightly. Average patient age is 58 years.

Localization: About 60 and 40 percent respectively occur in major and minor glands. Major gland involved is parotid, minor glands are from the hard palate, buccal mucosa.

Clinical features: Most patients with tumors of major glands present with solitary, asymptomatic masses, but 20 percent have pain or facial weakness. Pain is often associated with submandibular glands. Minor salivary glands are often ulcerated and about 20 percent of palatal tumors involve the underlying bone.

Macroscopy: Adenocarcinoma partially circumscribed, but in many areas the periphery is irregular and ill defined. Areas of hemorrhage and necrosis may contract with white or yellowish cut surface.

Histopathology: All tumors have presence of glandular or duct like structures, infiltrative growth into parenchyma or surrounding tissues. Tumor cells are in nests and cords or large discrete islands with intervening trabeculae of fibrous connective tissue.

Prognosis: Minor salivary gland tumors have better survival than major gland tumors. Fifteen years survival rate for low intermediate and high-grade tumor was 54, 31, and 3 percent respectively.[55]

Polymorphous Low-grade Adenocarcinoma

Definition: A malignant epithelial tumor characterized by cytologic uniformity, morphologic diversity, an infiltrative growth pattern and low metastatic potential.

Epidemiology: Polymorphous low-grade adenocarcinoma (PLGA) is the most common intraoral malignant salivary gland tumor[56] accounting for 26 percent of all carcinomas. Male:Female ratio is 2:1. Patient age ranges from 16 to 94 years. Mean age is 59 years.

Localization: Approximately 60 percent of the cases involve palate. Other intraoral localization are buccal mucosa, retromolar region, upper lip and base of tongue.[57]

Clinical features: It presents as a painless mass in the palate. Duration of lesion varies from weeks to as much as 40 years. Bleeding telangiectasia or ulceration of the overlying mucosa occasionally occurs.

Macroscopy: PLGA usually appear as a firm circumscribed, but nonencapsulated, yellow-tan lobulated nodule up to several centimeter.

Histopathology: It is characterized by cytologic uniformity, histologic diversity and an infiltrative growth pattern. The tumor cells are small to medium size and uniform in shape with bland, minimally hyperchromatic oval nuclei and occasionally nucleoli. Main microscopic features are lobular, papillary, papillary-cystic, cribriform, trabecular or small duct-like structures. Cells form concentric whorls or targetoid arrangements around blood vessels or nerves. Stroma may show areas of hyalination or mucinosis.

Prognosis: Overall survival rate of patients with PLGA is excellent. Local recurrence rate varies between 9 and 17 percent and a regional metastasis rate is 9 to 15 percent. The distant metastasis have been seldom reported.

Sebaceous Carcinoma (Figs 15.17A to C)

Definition: Sebaceous carcinoma is a malignant tumor composed of sebaceous cells of varying maturity. They are arranged in sheets and/or nests with different degrees of pleomorphism, nuclear atypia and invasiveness.

Epidemiology: There is a bimodal age distribution with a peak incidence in the third decade and the 7th and 8th decades of life (range 17–93 years). The male and female incidence is almost equal. Unlike sebaceous neoplasms of the skin there is no increased risk of developing a visceral carcinoma in patients with a salivary gland sebaceous tumor.

Localization: Approximately 90 percent arise in the parotid area, with occasional tumors in the oral cavity, vallecula, sublingual gland, submandibular gland and epiglottis.

Clinical features: Patients typically present with a painful mass with varying degrees of facial nerve paralysis and occasional fixation to the skin.

Macroscopy: Tumors have ranged from 0.6 to 8.5 cm in greatest dimension and vary from yellow, tan-white, grayish-white, white, to pale pink. They are well circumscribed or partially encapsulated, with pushing or locally infiltrating margins.

Histopathology: Tumors are composed of multiple large foci and nests or sheets of cells with hyperchromatic nuclei and abundant clear to eosinophilic cytoplasm. Cellular pleomorphism and cytologic atypia are present to varying degrees and are much more prevalent than in sebaceous adenomas. Squamous differentiation is common. There may be areas of basaloid differentiation, particularly at the periphery of cellular nests. Areas of necrosis and fibrosis are common. Perineural invasion is seen in greater than 20 percent of tumors; vascular invasion is infrequent. Rare oncocytes and foreign body giant cells with histiocytes may be observed, but lymphoid tissue with follicles or subcapsular sinuses is not seen.

Prognosis and predictive factors: The treatment of choice is wide surgical excision for low stage carcinomas.

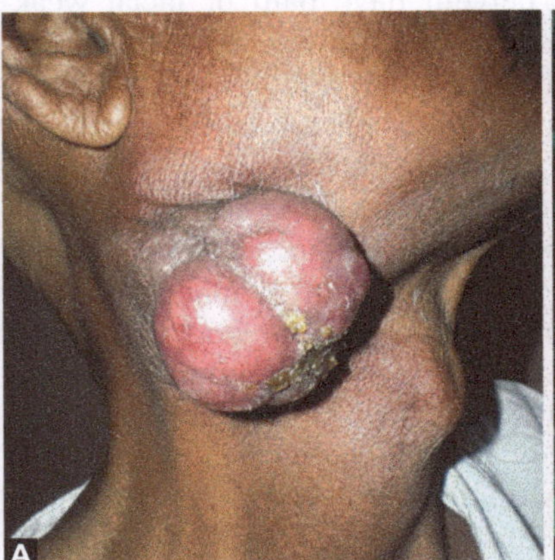

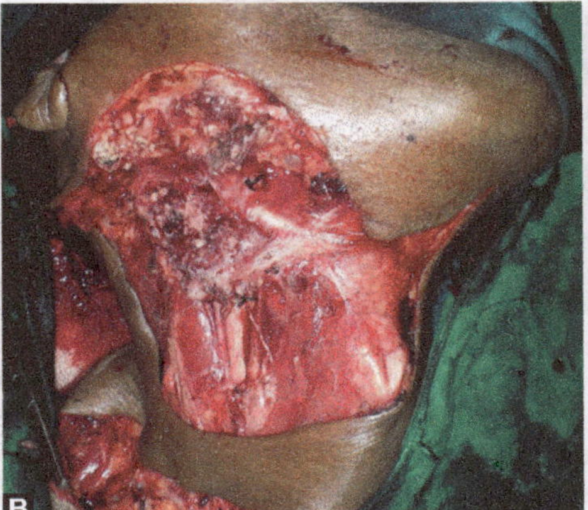

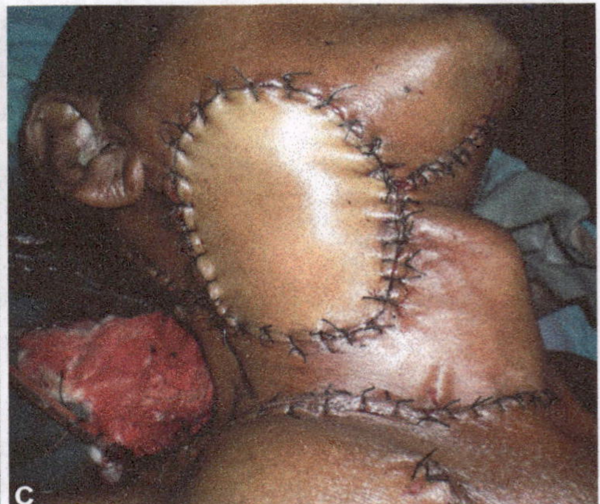

Figs 15.17A to C: Sebacious carcinoma of parotid gland: (A) Preoperative photograph; (B) Intraoperative photograph showing excision of tumor with neck dissection; (C) Closure and reconstruction with PMMC flap

Adjunctive radiation therapy is recommended for higher-stage and grade tumors. The overall 5-year survival rate is 62 percent, slightly less than the survival for similar tumors arising in the skin and orbit.

APPROACH TO THE MANAGEMENT OF SALIVARY GLAND TUMORS

- Try to know whether it is benign or malignant—Usually clinical examination and FNAC is adequate to determine the same. The subtyping of the tumor does not affect the treatment planning and thus it is not necessary.
- If it is malignant the grade, i.e. whether it is low, intermediate or high-grade malignancy.
- If it is malignant remove the total gland. Address the neck nodes if indicated.
- The facial nerve should be preserved unless it is distinctly indicated to be sacrificed in cases where:
  - There is clinical evidence of nerve involvement.
  - It is difficult to dissect the nerve free due to the tumor infiltration.
  - Tumors known to spread perinurally, e.g. adenoid cystic carcinoma.

Management of Parotid Tumors

The various procedures that are commonly practiced are:

- Local excision of the parotid gland
- Superficial parotidectomy with preservation of the facial nerve
- Functional superficial parotidectomy
- Total parotidectomy with preservation of the facial nerve
- Radical parotidectomy with or without neck dissection in continuity
- Parotidomandibulectomy
- Temporoparotidectomy.

Surgical technique most commonly used is partial or total parotidectomy with facial nerve preservation. Routine patient preparation is done such as shaving of the hair, i.e. one fingerbreadth all around the pinna followed by shampoo bath and scrubbing of the surgical site. It is preferred that the side of the face to be operated is not covered by drapes to visualize the twitching of the facial muscles. Adrenaline diluted with saline is infiltrated locally along the incision site to reduce bleeding. Blair's incision is commonly used for access. The incision in the neck crease is deepened first exposing and dividing the platysma and identifying the thick deep fascia, at the angle of the mandible. The greater auricular nerve is identified and preserved. Facial nerve injury is avoided at this stage due to its position deep to the deep fascia but some subcutaneous fat should be left on the fascia near the zygomatic bone due to superficial location of the facial nerve. The branches of the facial nerve are visible through the translucent fascia as they emerge from the anterior border of the gland. Facial nerve identification is carried out using the various facial nerve pointers[58] or using facial nerve monitoring. As each branch is identified, it is labeled by under running it with a length of black silk, the ends of which are clamped in mosquito artery forceps. The facial nerve and its branches are invested by loose connective tissue and lie in tunnels within the parotid into which the tips of the blades of curved mosquito artery forceps may be insinuated. The blades are then opened a little to stretch the tissues and raised, so as to lift the gland substance off the surface of the nerve, a short length of which may then be exposed by cutting through the gland with scissors. At all times when a cut is made the adjacent nerve must be seen clearly. The facial nerve splits into an upper temporofacial and a lower cervicofacial division at the level of the condylar neck. Each branch is dissected free of the parotid gland so as to mobilize the entire gland. Tissue adjacent to tumor is compressed into a thin capsule. Where the tumor, reaches the surface of the gland some overlying subcutaneous fat should be left to cover it as the flap is raised. Penetration on the deep surface will bring it into contact with the muscle such as masseter or loose connective tissue. The former can be excised in continuity with the mass; the latter should be divided under direct vision some little distance from the tumor and allowed to collapse on to its surface. Filamentous structures passing horizontally or radiating from the region of the main trunk are likely to be nerves and should be conserved. The branches decrease in diameter as they are traced peripherally in contrast to the main duct that increases in size to reach 2 to 3 mm in cross-section as it emerges from the gland anteriorly. Further it passes diagonally upwards and forwards. Blood vessels, except for the transverse facial generally run up from below and unlike nerves, have elasticity, so that with care they can be distinguished. Branches from the great auricular nerve differ from those of the facial by remaining on the surface of the gland as they are traced posteriorly. The branches of the facial nerve should be preserved as far as possible until visible infiltration by malignancy is seen or facial nerve weakness is present preoperatively. In general, the nerves pass superficial to the retromandibular vein, but some may pass deep to it.[59] Careful mobilization of both nerve and vein with division and ligation of the latter is necessary. Tiny vessels should be sealed with diathermy by accurately grasping them with fine artery forceps and touching briefly with the electrode, avoiding damage to adjacent nerves. The mobilization and excision of the superficial lobe containing the tumor mass is carried out.

Complications

- Facial paresis or paralysis often result from poor technique and failure to preserve small nerve branches
- Bleeding and hematoma formation, which can significantly compromise the airway
- Rarely, persistent salivary leakage or sialocele formation occurs

- Frey's syndrome
- Skin flap necrosis.

Functional Superficial Parotidectomy

Functional superficial parotidectomy involves preservation of the stensen's duct and its connection to the deep lobe. This is possible if the duct is deep to the facial nerve and does not obstruct dissection of the nerve. Here, the function of the gland is preserved.

Advantages of functional superficial parotidectomy:

- It is a simpler surgery than conservative superficial parotidectomy.
- It preserves partial function of the parotid gland.
- It avoids the influence of subsequent gland atrophy on facial contour.
- It decreases postoperative complications.

Partial Superficial Parotidectomy

It is excision of only that portion of the superficial lobe containing the tumor with preservation of the facial nerve. It results into lesser incidence of Frey's syndrome. So also, gland function is preserved due to more parenchyma being preserved (Figs 15.18A to C).

Total Parotidectomy with Facial Nerve Preservation

Total parotidectomy with facial nerve preservation or sacrifice involves complete excision of the entire gland parenchyma with preservation of the facial nerve wherever possible (Figs 15.19A to E, 15.20A and B). The nerve is sacrificed only if there is malignant infiltration or preoperative facial nerve paresis. However, in such a situation it is immediately reconstructed with microneurosurgical transfer from greater auricular nerve or sural nerve.

Other extended surgeries such as parotidomandibulectomy or temporoparotidectomy or parotidectomy with neck dissection can be performed depending on the extent of local or regional invasion by the tumor.

Management of Submandibular and Sublingual Gland Tumors

Extracapsular excision of the submandibular gland is done, if tumor is confined to the gland proper. If the tumor has spread beyond the confines of the gland, an extended surgical procedure for resection of the involved areas of the floor of the mouth should be carried out with marginal or segmental mandibulectomy, depending on the extent of the tumor.

An approximately 7 cm long incision is made in the submandibular skin crease around two finger breadths below the lower border of the mandible and a subplatysmal dissection is done to raise a flap. The capsule of the gland and surrounding soft tissue must be left intact over the gland when the surgical procedure is being carried out for a neoplastic growth. The gland is removed together with its investing fascia, which is separated from the anterior and posterior bellies of the digastric and the stylohyoid muscle. The facial artery and vein are identified early in their course as close to the inferior posterior pole of the gland and deep to it and are ligated (Figs 15.21A and B). After transection of these vessels they are elevated superiorly to identify and reflect the marginal mandibular nerve from the field. After safeguarding the mandibular nerve, the fascia is divided at the inferior mandibular border. The superficial part of the gland is dissected from the muscle up to the posterolateral border where three vital structures are identified here viz. lingual nerve, hypoglossal nerve and Wharton's duct. When the free edge of the mylohyoid is retracted medially the attachment of the lingual nerve to the gland that represents its parasympathetic supply is evident. The Wharton's duct is inferior to lingual nerve and is often surrounded by sublingual glands. As fascia and gland are mobilized upwards from the surface of the hyoglossus, the hypoglossal nerve is identified more inferiorly. It is accompanied by ranine vein, which may aid in its identification. The vena comitans that accompany the nerve are inevitably damaged. Posteriorly the angular tract of fascia has to be cut with scissors to allow the gland in its fascial envelope to be drawn down.

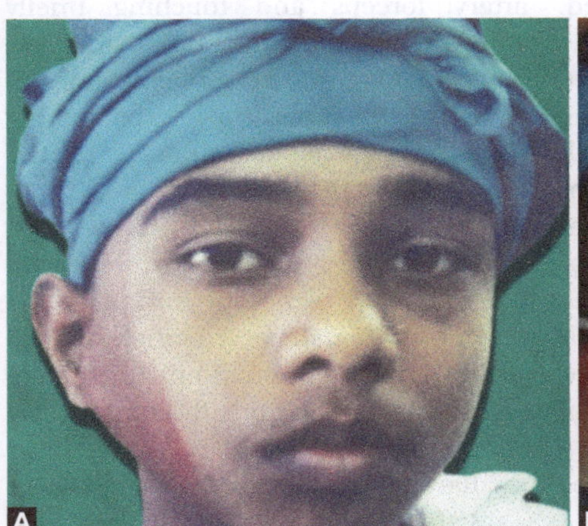
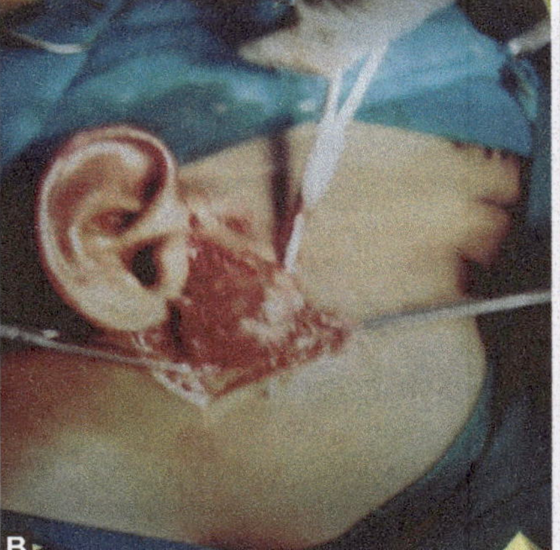
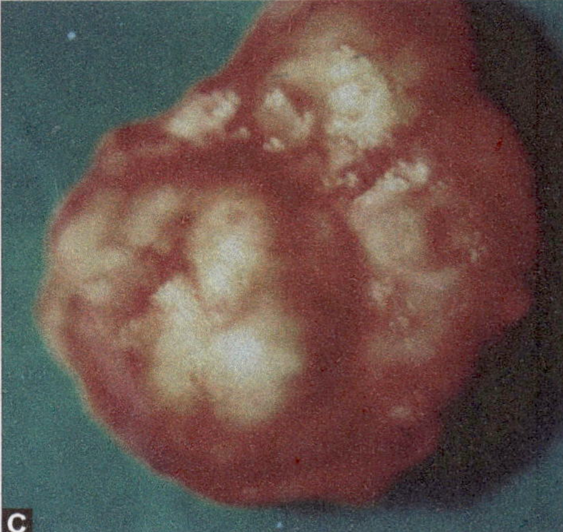

Figs 15.18A to C: Partial superficial parotidectomy

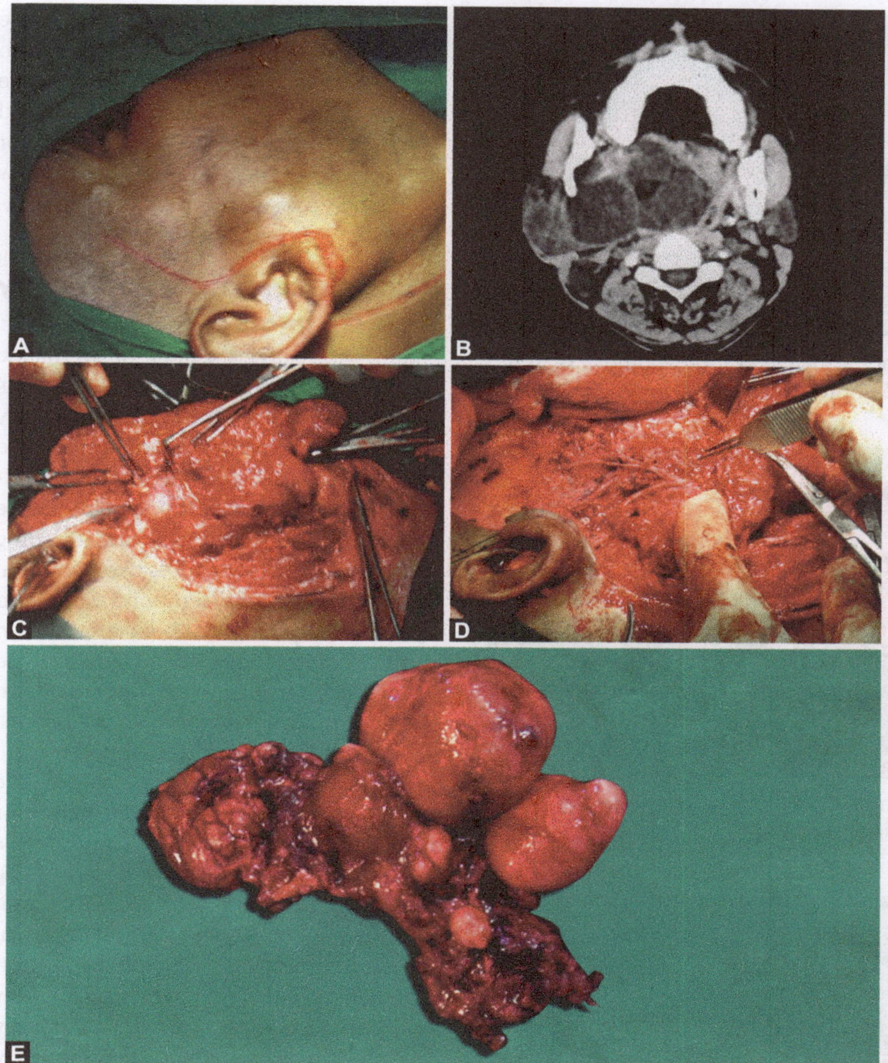

Figs 15.19A to E: Pleomorphic adenoma involving both deep and superficial lobes of parotid (Dumbbell tumor). Note the tumor has also involved the submandibular gland. Treated by parotidectomy and excision of the submandibular glands. Preserving the facial nerve

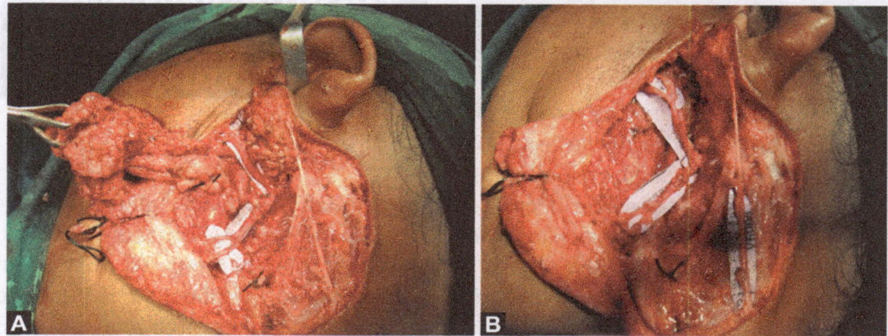

Figs 15.20A and B: Pleomorphic adenoma of the parotid. Tumor removed by performing total paratidectomy, preserving the facial nerve

This step is the most difficult because it is important not to grasp the gland with instruments, particularly tissue forceps lest the tumor be ruptured. Where necessary the upper pole may be mobilized via the mouth. An assistant can then depress the gland towards the submandibular wound to enable the operation to be concluded. The duct and the branch of the lingual nerve supplying the submandibular gland are ligated and transected. The duct is divided close behind the papilla. During excision for inflammatory disease the nerve is always separated from the gland with knife or scissors. However, if the nerve appears to be involved in a tumor it is sectioned in front of and behind the gland and the cut ends sutured. Should a greater margin of tissue than the immediate capsule be required laterally, the periosteum of the mandible is divided along the lower border and stripped up from the submandibular fossa. It must be divided at the level of the mylohyoid line, so that the lingual nerve can be found and freed as described above. The wound is closed in layers with drainage in the usual way (Figs 15.22A and B).

For the sublingual gland excision intraoral incision is placed parallel to the floor of the mouth lateral to the submandibular duct, with care taken not to extend the incision more posteriorly than the first molar tooth, so as to avoid damage to the lingual nerve. When sublingual gland excision is necessary for a tumor, it should be removed with a wide margin including a rim resection of the mandible. The larger tumors may require the extraoral submandibular incision for their excision.

Complications

- Hematoma in the dead space is avoided by proper hemostasis and compression dressing or placement of drain in the postoperative period.
- Trismus is a result of masseter muscle spasm or inflammation of the TMJ capsule secondary to trauma. It is self-limiting, but long-standing cases may require intra-articular steroid injections.

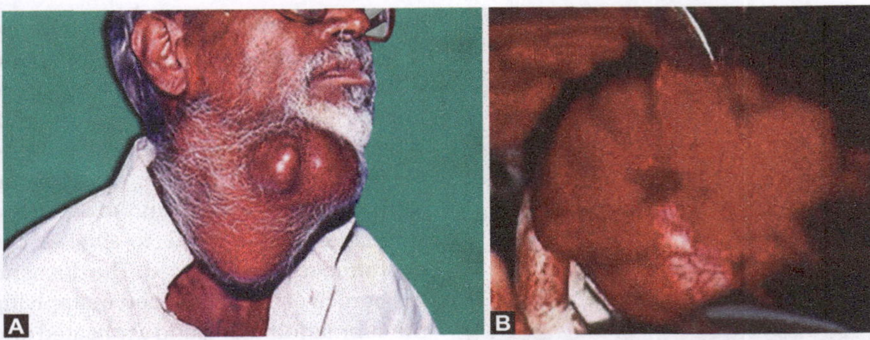

Figs 15.21A and B: (A) Pleomorphic adenoma involving submandibular gland; (B) Intraoperative photograph

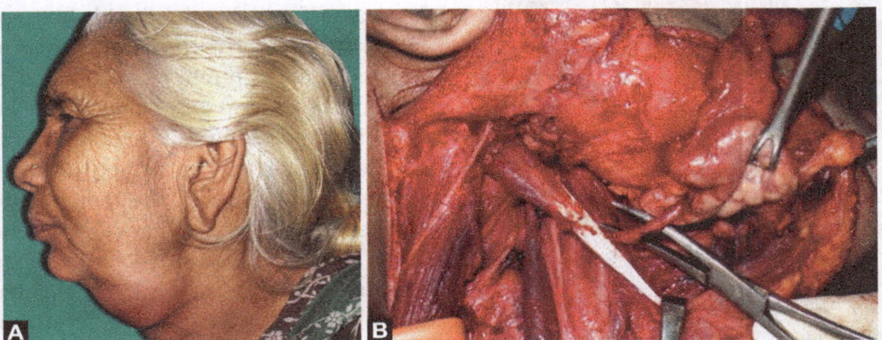

Figs 15.22A and B: (A) Pleomorphic adenoma involving submandibular gland; (B) Mobilization of the gland superficially to identify the facial artery

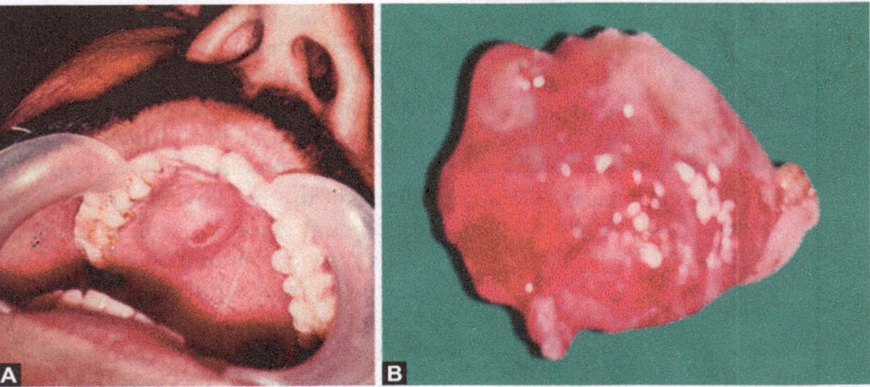

Figs 15.23A and B: Pleomorphic adenoma of the palate treated with wide local excision

- Salivary fistula or a sialocele occurs due to discontinuity between the remaining gland parenchyma and the duct. It is self-limiting and is managed by repeated aspiration, pressure dressing, wound care and patience. The patient can even be prescribed antisialagogue medication.
- Facial nerve paresis can be temporary or permanent. Temporaray facial nerve paresis results from neuropraxia due to stretching and handling of the nerve during surgery. Permanent damage occurs usually if the nerve is transected or sacrificed.
- Frey's syndrome[60] is associated with gustatory sweating. During surgery if the auriculotemporal nerve is damaged, secretomotor parasympathetic nerves from the otic ganglion supplying the parotid gland and sympathetic nerves supplying the sweat glands traveling in the same nerve are transected. During regeneration there is cross-innervation of the nerve endings. Hence, while eating food due to activity of the secretomotor parasympathetic nerves, which now supply the sweat glands, there is sweating.

Management of Minor Salivary Gland Tumors

The minor salivary glands of the palate are the most commonly involved glands due to salivary gland tumors. Majority of the minor salivary gland tumors are malignant. Thus, they involve the investing bone and due to the spongy nature of maxilla spread fast into the adjoining vital anatomical structures like paranasal sinuses, orbit, infra-temporal fossa and subsequently the skull base and can produce intracranial involvement. The tumor seen outside may be small but rapidly infiltrates the deeper structures. They often require radical excision.

The benign tumors like pleomorphic adenomas are also present in the minor salivary glands and may require less radical excision without compromising the surgical margins (Figs 15.23A and B and 15.24A to D). Various surgical procedures like shelling of the tumor, segmental resection of the maxilla, low level maxillectomy, hemimaxillectomy and radical/extended maxillectomy may be required to treat the neoplasm depending on their size, site of involvement, type of underlying pathology.

RADIOTHERAPY AND CHEMOTHERAPY IN THE MANAGEMENT OF SALIVARY GLAND TUMORS

Radiotherapy

Traditionally salivary gland tumors were considered to be radioresistant, however management of malignant salivary gland neoplasms has changed in recent years. Research over a period of years suggests that postoperative photon irradiation improves local control rates in patients with high

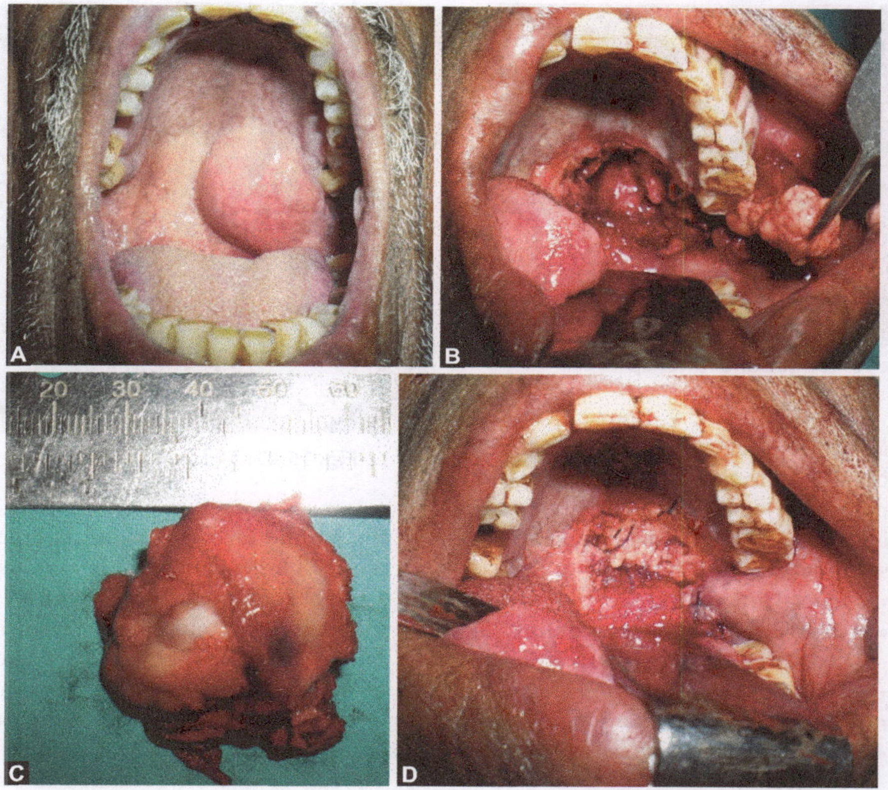

Figs 15.24A to D: (A) Pleomorphic adenoma of palate; (B) Intraoperative photograph showing excision of the tumor and harvestion buccal pad of fat (BFP); (C) Excised specimen; (D) Reconstruction of the surgical defect with BFP

risk of residual microscopic disease. Postoperative radiotherapy has shown to improve locoregional control for patients with advanced-stage gland cancer. Reports suggest that use of adjuvant radiotherapy in conjunction with surgery is superior to surgery alone in treatment of high-grade and/or advanced cancers of the parotid gland.[61] Adenoid cystic carcinoma has been reported to be the most consistent radioresponsive tumor type. In cases of adenoid cystic carcinoma wherein there is perineural spread radiotherapy should also be directed along the path of the cranial nerve at risk for involvement. A postoperative radiation dose of 60 Gy (50 – 75 Gy) in 30 fractions to the operative bed is thought to be beneficial. In cases of named nerve invasion, the path of the nerve should be treated electively up to its ganglion.

Wide-field radiation therapy to the parotid glands may result in significant complications, including severe xerostomia, sensorineural hearing loss, osteoradionecrosis of the temporal bone and radiation injury to the temporal lobe. Recent advances in the delivery of radiation therapy including three-dimensional conformal radiotherapy (3DCRT) and intensity-modulated radiotherapy (IMRT) have led to better tumor dosimetry and relative sparing of surrounding normal structures such as the oral cavity, cochlea and brain.

Neutron beam therapy has also shown to improve locoregional control rates (67%) for advanced stage tumors.[62,63] Fractionated neutron irradiation has high relative biologic effectiveness in many salivary gland histologic types as compared to conventional radiation.

In cases of inoperable tumors, fast-neutron radiation therapy provides higher rates of locoregional control of the unresectable salivary gland cancer as compared to photon or electron radiation therapy.[64]

Chemotherapy

The role of chemotherapy in the management of salivary gland cancers is under study and in the budding stages.[65,66] Various chemotherapeutic regimens are used currently for palliation of advanced tumors and there is no benefit for use in the induction or adjuvant setting. The overall response rate to chemotherapy is found to be 42 percent. Generally combination therapy is more effective against salivary gland tumors as compared to single-drug therapy. The most effective drug regimens include cisplatin, paclitaxel, doxorubicin, 5-fluorouracil and epirubicin in different combinations. Although salivary gland cancers show some response to various chemotherapeutic agents, these responses are rarely complete, are usually short-lived, and have not resulted in significant improvement in long-term survival. A recent study indicated that the frequent expression of multidrug resistant genes by carcinoma of the salivary glands might be responsible for the low response rates to conventional chemotherapy.

CYSTIC CONDITIONS

The mucocele (mucus retention cyst) is the most common cystic lesion of the minor salivary glands (Figs 15.25A and B). The vast majority presents the extravasation phenomenon and has no epithelial lining. The common site is lower lips of young people and the etiology is usually minor trauma.[67] Up to 20 percent lesions may represent true retention cyst secondary to obstruction or microliths. The cyst may burst and drain spontaneously and occasionally lead to complete resolution following scarring. The simple removal of cyst leads to recurrence of mucocele. The vertical incision over the cyst and complete removal of the underlying mucus gland is almost always curative.

In the sublingual salivary gland, the mucous retention cyst occurs due to retention of the saliva beneath the thin mucous membrane of the floor of the mouth, which is called ranula. The bluish color gives it is resemblance to the belly of the frog and thus the name, ranula (Fig. 15.26). The cyst is

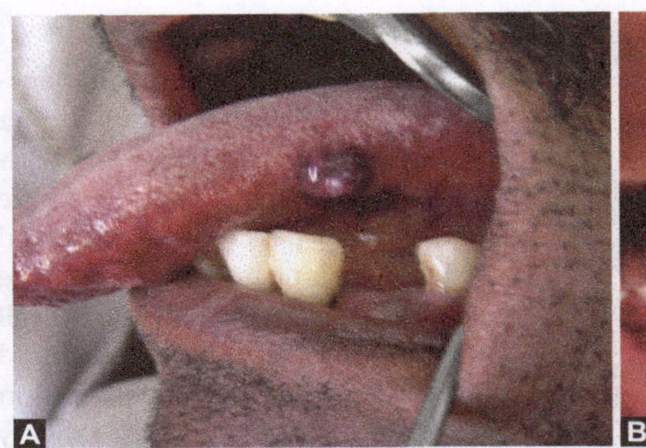

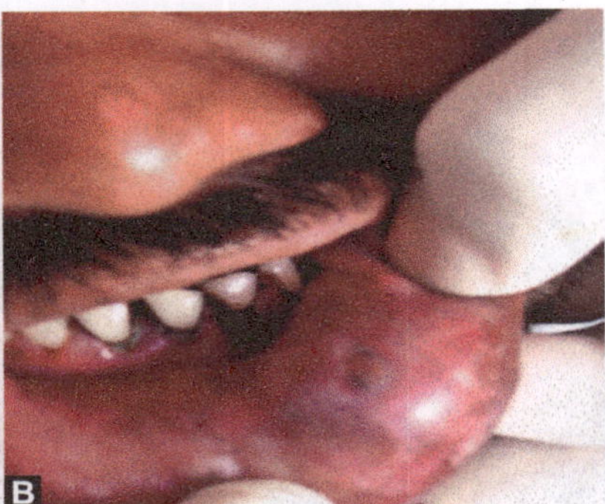

Figs 15.25A and B: Mucoceles of tongue and lower lip

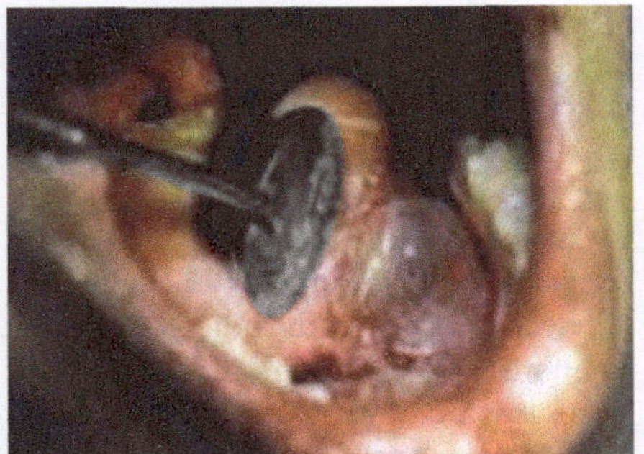

Fig. 15.26: Sublingual 'ranula'

usually present above the mylohyoid curtain, but then mylohyoid does not always from a complete diaphram and allows the leakage of the saliva below the mylohyoid allowing the lesion to present in the upper part of neck, which is called a 'plunging ranula'. The treatment modalities are deroofing the cyst and marsupialization to the over lying oral mucosa or total excision of the sublingual salivary gland.

The cystic lesions are uncommon in the submandibular salivary gland. The cystic lesions involving the parotid gland, the hereditary polycystic disease, parotid duct cyst, retention cyst, lymphoepithelial cyst. The later is most common and warrants differentiation from solitary tumors like cystic pleomorphic adenoma, mucoepidermoid tumor. Multiple, bilateral lymphoepithelial cysts of the parotid gland are seen in AIDS.

INFLAMMATORY DISEASES

The inflammatory disorders (sialadenitis) can be classified into bacterial, viral and fungal. The bacterial diseases are further classified into specific (Tuberculosis Actinomycosis) or no-specific like suppurative infections. The bacterial diseases can be secondary to the following:

- Ductal anamolies
- Obstructive ductal conditions like sialolithiasis (calculus) or strictures.
- Hematogenous infections.
- Secondary to dehydration (uremia, liver failure, diabetes, exanthematous fevers)
- Immunosuppressed states
- Secondary to viral infections like mumps.

The infections result secondary to stasis of salivary flow, which in turn facilitates the retrograde spread of the bacteria from oral cavity in the gland through the duct. Poor oral hygiene is one of the predisposing factors for the suppurative sialadenitis.

Suppurative Parotitis

Suppurative parotitis is the acute bacterial infection of the parotid gland (Fig. 15.27). The predisposing factors are mentioned above. The causative organisms are staphylococci or streptococci. The predisposing factors are states of dehydration, strictures of the duct, calculus, exanthematous fevers and immunosuppression.

The clinical features are as follows:

- General constitutional signs and symptoms like, high-grade fever, malaise, body ache, leukocytosis. The signs of dehydration may be present.
- The local signs are diffuse inflammatory swelling and tenderness over the parotid area. The skin becomes tense, glossy and erythematous. The ear lobule gets lifted, which is the pathognomonic sign of parotid swelling as there is no other anatomical structure in this region except the parotid, which can cause this sign (Fig. 15.27).
- The salivary caruncle situated on the buccal mucosa opposite the maxillary second molar is inflamed and milking of the gland leads to purulent discharge from the orifice. The salivary flow is diminished.
- Due to the presence of the dense fascia the swelling are not fluctuant and are extremely painful due to the mounting pressure as the fascia is non-yielding. The mounting pressure leads to ischemic necrosis of the gland parenchyma and the abscess may spontaneously burst in the external auditory canal.
- The duct when palpated over the clenched masseter muscle feels cord like.

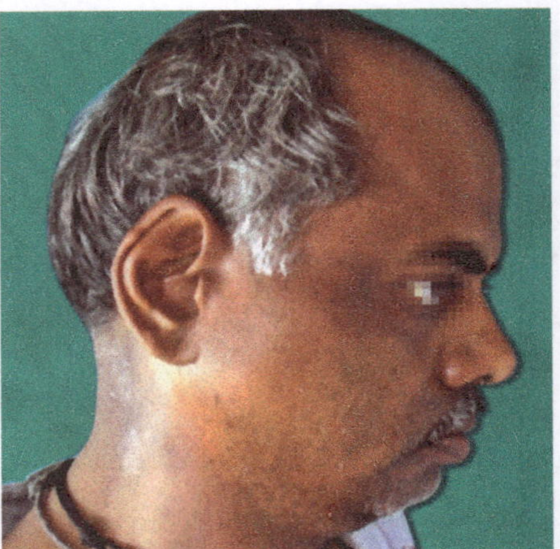

Fig. 15.27: A case of parotitis

The investigations comprise of plain X-ray to rule out calculus. Sialography is strictly contraindicated in acute parotitis as it may aggravate the infection and lead to the necrosis of the gland. The culture of the pus from the duct by taking a swab after milking the gland may help in planning the antibiotic therapy.

Management

The management comprises of the medicinal treatment, supportive treatment and the surgical treatment. The medicinal treatment comprises of prescription of parenteral antibiotics like ampicillin 1 to 2 g/day or crystalline penicillin 10 to 20 Lac IU, 6 hourly.[68] Anti-inflammatory and analgesics may be prescribed for symptomatic relief. The supportive treatment in the form of maintaining the hydration of patient by oral or parenteral rehydration therapy is given. Maintenance of good oral hygiene by antiseptic gargles is advocated. The infection may resolve with this treatment. One should not wait for the localizing signs of the infection such as fluctuations to occur and the prompt drainage/decompression should be undertaken to prevent ischemic necrosis of the gland. The best way of draining the parotid abscess is by placing an incision parallel to the branches of the facial nerve to avoid injury to them. The preauricular incision and blunt dissection to drain the abscess gives good cosmetic results.

The infection if not managed may get suppressed and pass into subacute or chronic form. The gland becomes fibrotic and degenerated.

Once the acute stage has resolved then dilatation of duct by using blunt probe may help in removing any mucus plug and facilitates the free flow of the saliva. Sialogogue may also be helpful.

Submandibular Gland

The cause of sialadenitis of the submandibular salivary gland is more commonly due to obstructive pathology, as the sialolithiasis is more common in it. The gland becomes inflamed, painful and tender. A swelling appears below the lower border of the mandible. The skin becomes tense, glossy and erythematous, the constitutional signs and symptoms are present. The gland becomes palpable on bimanual examination be placing one finger on the external surface and the other in the lingual sulcus intraorally. This examination helps in differentiating the salivary gland swelling from the lymph node swelling. The lymph nodes are not commonly palpable bimanually, unless they are sizably enlarged, during bimanual palpation effort should be made to feel any hard calculus in the gland or its duct. The milking of the gland results in purulent discharge from the opening of the duct.

The investigations are plain occlusal X-ray of the mandibular arch to rule out any calculus in the duct or the gland. The treatment is similar to that of acute parotitis, however if the calculus is present it should be removed once the acute symptoms subside.

Obstructive Pathologies

Sialolithiasis

Sialolithiasis is the condition characterized by formation of the calculus in the gland or the duct. It is commonly seen in the submandibular gland than the parotid. It is also reported rarely in the sublingual gland, but almost non-existing in the minor salivary glands. The calculus or a sialolith causes obstruction to the flow of the saliva, stasis and paves the way for retrograde spread of the infection in the gland from the oral cavity and thus infection secondary to the obstruction is hall mark of the sialolithiasis. In the submandibular gland 85 percent stones are radiopaque and more commonly present in the duct. Sometimes the submandibular gland calculus is present in the promotion of the duct that lies posterior to the mylohyoid muscle, i.e. in the hilum of the gland. On the other hand 85 percent of the parotid stones are radiolucent (mucus plugs) in nature and are commonly present in the duct distal to its bend where it turns acutely at the anterior border of the masseter and pierces the buccinator muscle. The cause for larger incidence of the calculus in the submandibular gland is the mixed and viscid nature of the secretions, more inorganic contents, uphill and tortuous course of the duct. The clinical manifestations of sialolithiasis are:

- **Pain and swelling:** The pain has classical relation with the meals. The pain is aggrevated during the meals as the salivary flow increases during the meals and the salivary clearance is slow. It leads to distension of the gland and feeling of discomfort, tightness in the gland. The gland gets swollen due to salivary retention. The phenomenon is labeled as sialoangiectasis (*dilation of the salivary duct*) (Figs 15.28 to 15.30).
- The obstruction invariably leads to retrograde infection in the gland and the clinical signs of chronic sialadenitis like, purulent discharge, diminished flow of saliva are present.
- On palpation calcified, hard calculus may be palpable. In the submandibular gland bimanual palpation of the gland and duct may show presence of calculus. In cases of the parotid, on palpation of the gland and the duct over the clenched masseter the calculus may be felt.
- Plain radiographs show the calcified body in the gland or the duct. The calculus in the submandibular duct is best seen on the mandibular occlusal radiographs and the calculus in the phylum is seen on lateral oblique view of mandible. The calculus in the parotid superficial lobe is seen on the PA view of the skull and mandible and that in the deep lobe are seen on the lateral oblique view of the mandible. The calculi in the parotid duct can be visualized by placing the dental film in the upper buccal vestibule (Figs 15.31A to C).

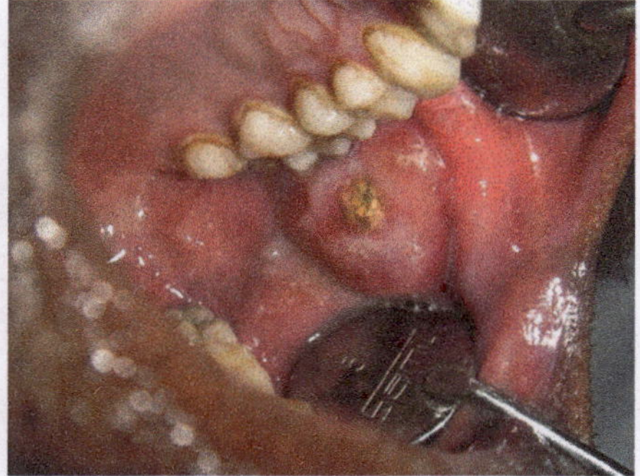

Fig. 15.28: Sialolith in the orifice of the Stensen's duct

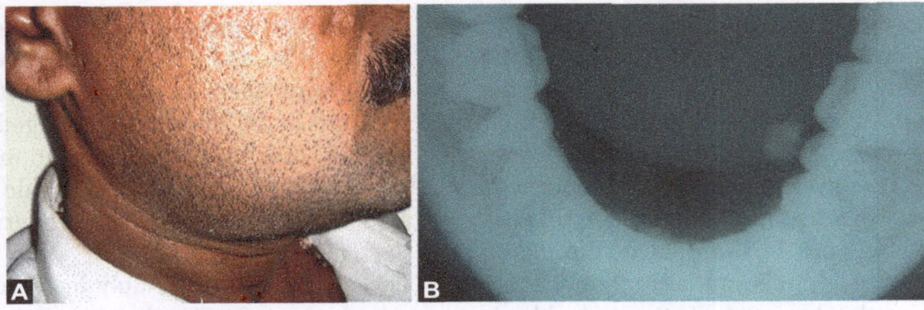
Figs 15.29A and B: Submandibular swelling in a case of sialolithiasis, occlusal view shows sialolith

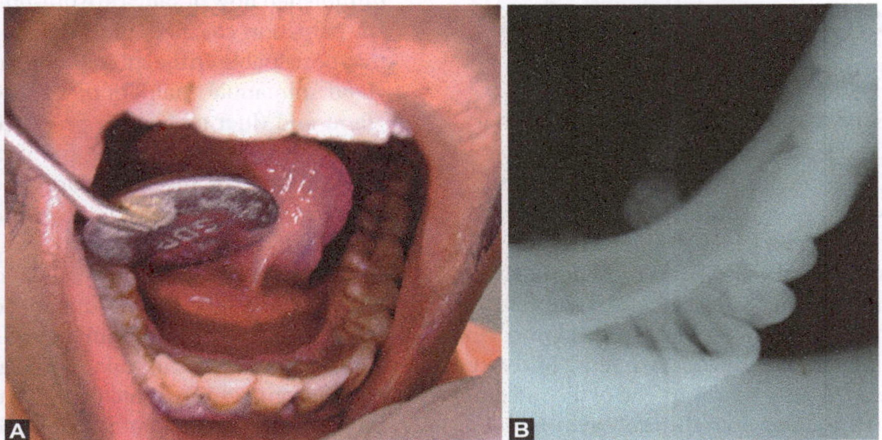
Figs 15.30A and B: Inflamed duct due to calculus

- The hypocalcified calculi or the mucus plugs may not be seen on plain radiographs and sialography in such cases may show a classical filling defect.
- The chronic infection in the gland secondary to obstruction may lead to degenerative changes and fibrosis in the gland.

Management

The calculus needs to be removed surgically in order to relieve the obstruction and prevent infection. The small stones may get ejected spontaneously. The small stones situated near the orifice of the duct can be removed by massaging and milking of the gland. The calculus in the submandibular duct is removed transorally under local anesthesia (Figs 15.32A and B). A suture is placed around the duct distal to the calculus to prevent posterior slipping of the calculus. An incision is placed directly on the calculus in the floor of mouth, parallel to the lingual vestibule. The duct is also incised over the stone and the stone is removed. The duct is irrigated to remove microliths. The incised ends of the duct are sutured to the mucosa of the floor of mouth to create new opening. The stones, which are situated posteriorly to the mylohyoid, i.e. in the phylum of the gland are difficult to be removed transorally and such stones are managed by existing the gland itself through the submandibular incision. The duct of the excised gland is traced above the masseter as anteriorly as possible and then ligated. The ligation of the duct prevents communication between the oral cavity and neck. If the duct is ligated too far posteriorly, the backflow of saliva from the sublingual gland, on rare occasions may lead to formation of calculus in it.

The calculus in the parotid duct in the portion that lies below the buccinator can be removed transorally. But, the calculus that lies in the part of the duct over the masseter is removed through an extraoral incision placed on the skin. The incision is placed parallel to the branches of the facial nerve to avoid damage to them. After the calculus is removed, the duct is repaired over the canula.

The stones can also be removed by other modalities like, endoscopic removal, lithotripsy.

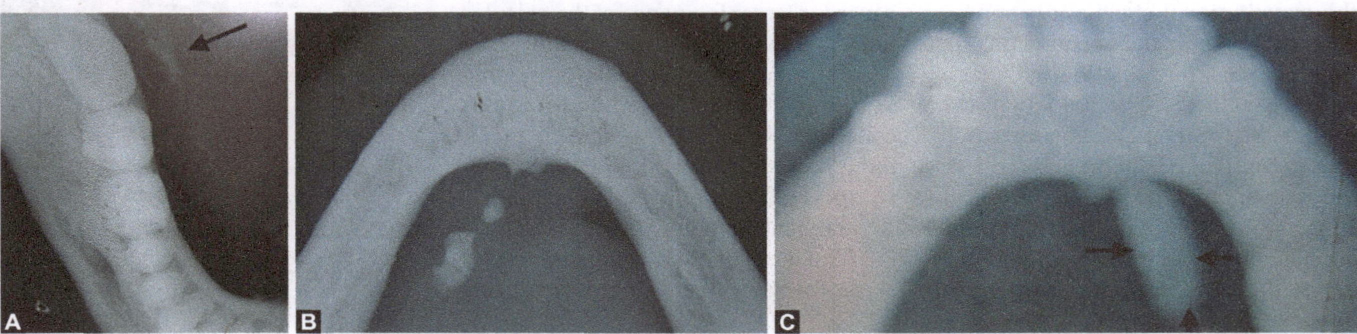
Figs 15.31A to C: Radiographs showing sialolith in the Warton's duct

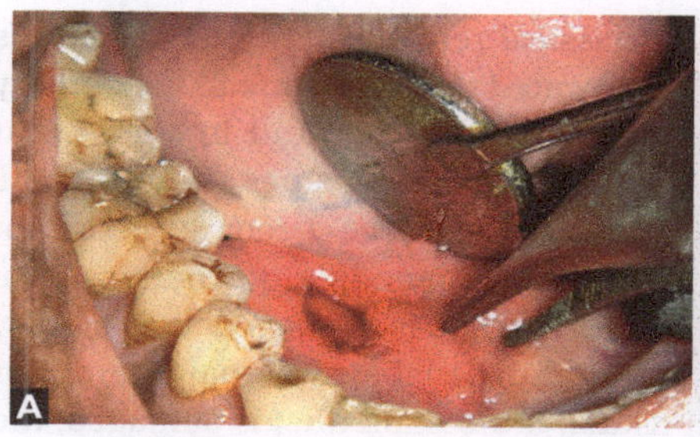

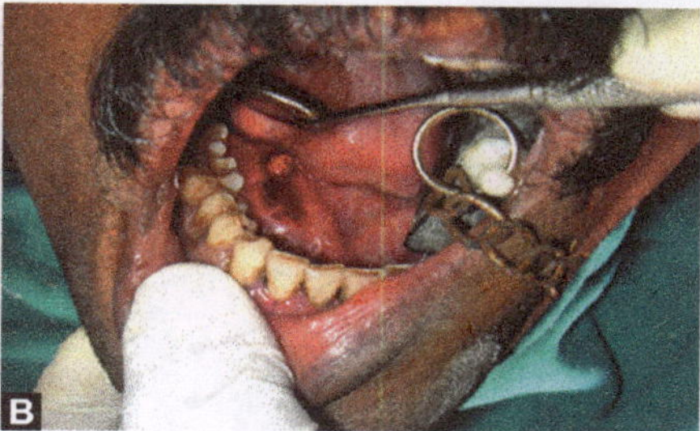

Figs 15.32A and B: Transoral removal of calculus in the duct of the submandibular salivary gland

Sialography

Sialography is a specialized radiological technique for visualizing the salivary gland with a contrast medium. This technique is no more popular due to advent of newer technology like ultrasonography and MRI scans.

Contrast Medium

Contrast medium are iodine based solutions. They are classified as follows:

- **Ionic aqueous solution:** This is an aqueous (water soluble) solution and is available in two types viz. lothalamate (Conray 480) and metrizoate (Triosil).
- **Oil-based solution:** This is water insoluble and is available in two types: Iodized poppy seed oil-lipiodol and water insoluble organic iodine compounds such as pantopaque (Table 15.4).

Indications

The indications for sialography are as follows:

- Obstructive pathologies like stricture, mucus plugs, hypocalcified calculi, external compressions.
- Degenerative conditions.
- Chronic inflammatory conditions (chronic sialodentis, Sjögren's syndrome).
- Intra and extraglandular tumors.
- Ductal anamolies (perforations, sialoceles, fistulas).

Contraindications

The contraindications for sialography are:

- Allergy to the dye.
- Acute inflammatory conditions. The injection of dye in acute inflammation will cause severe pain and can lead to necrosis of the gland.

Procedure

- The orifice of the duct is identified and isolated.
- Local anesthesia is infiltrated around the opening.
- The duct opening is dilated by probing with a blunt probe like a lacrimal probe.
- The duct is cannulated using a 22 no. cannula and the cannula is secured in place with a circumferential suture around the duct.
- The dye is loaded in a Luer lock syringe and the syringe is attached to the cannula. The dye is slowly pushed, with simultaneously massaging the gland. The injection is continued until the patient feels discomfort due to pressure.
- If the piston, the syringe is released the dye tends to flow back due to increased pressure in the gland, to prevent back flow of the dye the piston is held in place with the help of adhesive tape.
- The X-rays are taken at regular interval as the die is filled and flows out of the duct.
- The salivation is stimulated to empty the gland of the dye after the procedure.

Interpretation

- The normal salivary gland shows a 'winter tree' or 'leaf less tree' appearance, because in the functional gland the saliva present in the acini prevents the entry of the dye in them and thus only the ductules and the duct are seen (Figs 15.33A to E).
- In case of the chronically inflamed gland and in Sjögrens syndrome, the gland has the 'leafy tree' or the 'blossom tree appearance' as the non-functional acini are empty and the eye enters in them and thus at the end of the ductules a round ball is seen.
- When there is a stricture of mucus plug in the duct a filling defect is seen. In case of multiple strictures, a sausage-string appearance is seen.
- In case of intraglandular tumors the normal glandular structure surrounds the tumor and thus a 'cannon ball' appearance is produced.
- The extraglandular tumor displaces the glandular structure is displaced to one side and produces a 'ball in hand appearance'.
- In case of perforation of the duct or sialocele the spillage of the dye in the soft tissue is seen.

Table 15.4: Various dye agents, their advantages and disadvantages

Dye type	Advantages	Disadvantages
Oil based	Densely radiopaque	Extravasated dye may remain in tissues for months
	Good contrast	Foreign body reaction
	High viscosity – slow excretion from gland – adequate time for the procedure	Requires increased pressure for introduction into duct—may force calculi deeper into the duct
Water based	Less viscosity – easily introduced	Less radiopaque—less contrast medium is needed
	Rapidly excreted	Rapid excretion
	Easily absorbed and excreted if extravasated	

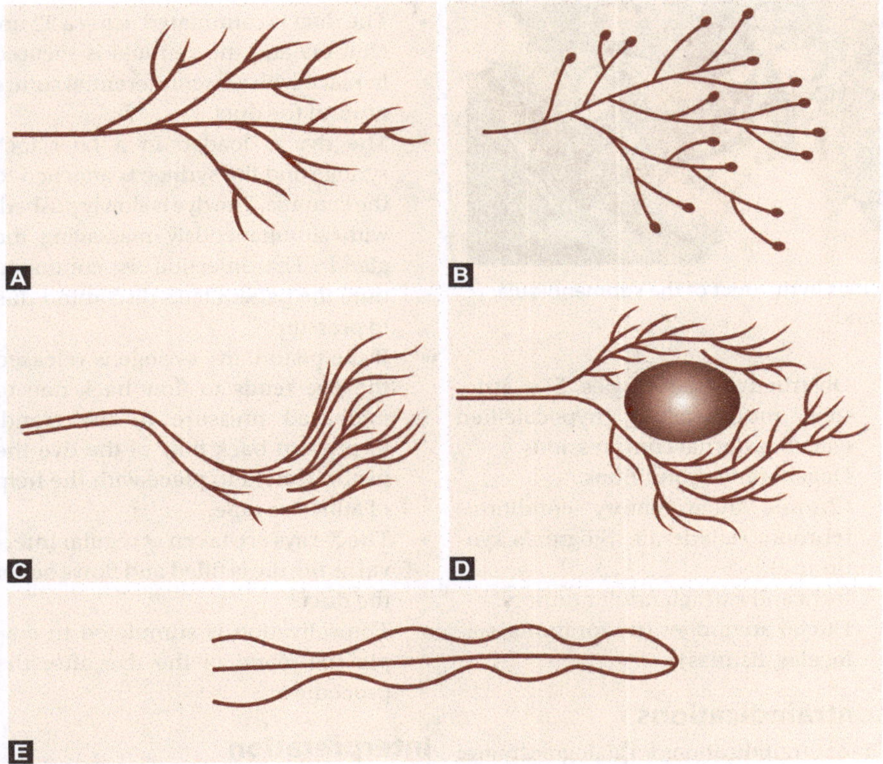

Figs 15.33A to E: Diagrammatic representation of the different sialographic pictures: (A) Winter tree appearance; (B) Blossom tree appearance; (C) Ball in hand appearance; (D) Cannon ball appearance; (E) Sausage string appearance

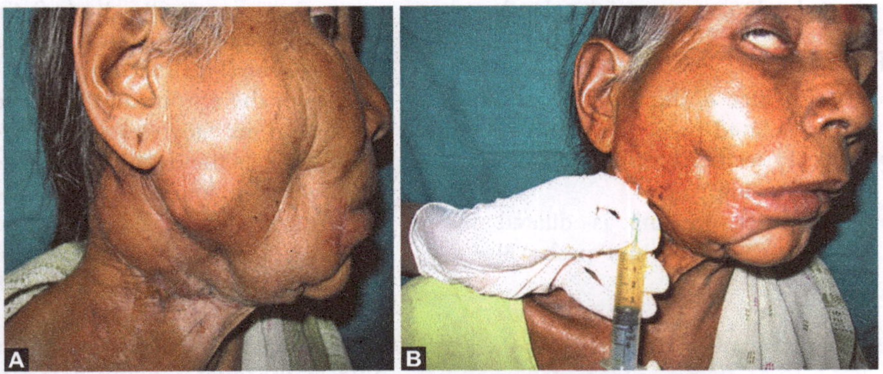

Figs 15.34A and B: Sialocele following ablative tumor surgery

SALIVARY FISTULA

The injuries to the duct of the salivary gland lead to extravasation of the saliva in the soft tissue. The saliva fails to drain in the oral cavity. The injuries could be due to penetrating injuries on the check or as a result of the accidental damage during the surgical procedure. The saliva collects in the adjoining soft tissue and produces asymptomatic swelling unless there is secondary infection. The collection of the saliva is the soft tissue plane is termed as sialocele (Figs 15.34A and B). The swelling gradually erodes the overlying skin and forms a fistula, which drains saliva. The discharge is watery in nature and has a classical relation to the meals as it is aggravated during the meals. Secondary infection can set in and in such event the condition becomes symptomatic and the discharge becomes purulent in nature. Depending on the nature of the duct that is damaged the salivary fistula can be labeled as major or minor fistula. If the main duct is damaged, the major fistula is formed and if the small collecting duct is severed then the minor salivary fistula results.

The management of this condition comprises the following:

- **Conservative management:** It is generally done for the minor fistulas. A compression dressing is given, which prevents the cutaneous drainage of the saliva and the mounting pressure of saliva within the tissue finds a way out in the oral cavity through the transected distal end of the duct. The pressure is maintained till the tract is formed between the two severed ends of the duct. The minor salivary fistulas close with the conservative treatment and the cutaneous drainage of the saliva stops spontaneously.
- **Anastomosis of the severed duct:** If the fistula is of recent onset then the area is explored surgically and the two severed ends are identified and anastomosed over the peripheral venous catheter (PVC) cannula (Fig. 15.35).
- **Total excision** of the involved gland in case of the persistent major fistula which fails to respond to conservative treatment and where the anastomosis of the duct is not possible due to loss of tissue, the involved gland may be excised.

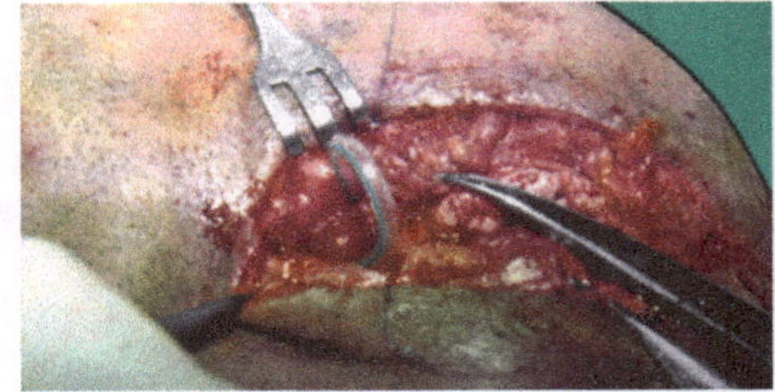

Fig. 15.35: Anastomosis of the duct over the canula

- **Irradiation of the gland:** Irradiation renders the gland fibrotic and non-functional and the fistula gets obliterated.

REFERENCES

1. Antonio Nanci. Ten Cate's Oral Histology: Development, Structure, and Function. Mosby. Missouri; chap 11. 2005. pp. 299-328..
2. Berkovitz S, Hackney BKB, Ruskell CM. IGL Gra's Anatomy. The anatomical basis of clinical practice. 39th Churchill and Livingtone, Edinburg. 2005,pp.1290..
3. DuBrul EL. The oral viscera. In: DuBrul EL (Ed). Sicher and DuBrul's Oral Anatomy, 8th edn. Ishiyaku EouroAmerica, St Louis. Chapt 6. 1988. pp. 161-78..
4. Snell RS. Clinical anatomy. 7th edn. Philadelphia (PA): Lippincott Williams and Wilkins. 2004; Chapter 11:719-922..
5. Conley J. Search for and identification of the facial nerve. Laryngoscope. 1978;88: 172-6..
6. Harrison JD. Histochemical and biochemical determination of calcium in salivary glands with particular reference to chronic submandibular sialadenitis. Virchows Archiv. 1993;423(1).
7. I Van Der Waal. Salivary gland neoplasms. I Van Der Waal, Prabhu SR, Wilson DF, Daftary DK, Johnson NW, (Eds). Oral diseases in the Tropics. Oxford University Press, Delhi; Chap 41. 1993. pp. 478-486.
8. Spitz MR, Batsakis JG. Major salivary gland carcinoma. Arch Otolaryngol. 1984;110:45.
9. Sharma D. Salivary gland tumors. Text of Smt. Radha Devi Memorial Oration delivered on 29th December, 99 at Madurai during ASICON. Indian association of surgical oncology. (www.indiandoctors.com/iaso/htm. Accessed on 18th July,05)
10. Eneroth CM. Salivary gland tumors in the parotid gland, submandibular gland and the palate region. Cancer. 1971;27:1415-8.
11. Walker NI, Gobe GC. Cell death and cell proliferation during atrophy of the rat parotid gland induced by duct obstruction. J Pathol. 1987;152:333-44.
12. Cornog JL, Gray SR. Surgical and clinical pathology of salivary gland tumors. Rankow RM, Polayes IM, (Eds). Diseases of Salivary glands. WB Saunders, Philadelphia. Chap 5. 1976.pp. 99-142.
13. Bialek EJ, et al. US of the Major Salivary Glands: Anatomy and Spatial Relationships, Pathologic Conditions, and Pitfalls. RadioGraphics. 2006;26: 745-63.
14. Lee YYP, Wong KT, King AD, Ahuja AT. Imaging of salivary gland tumors. European journal of radiology. 2008; 66(3):419-36.
15. Graham S, Blanchet M, Rohrer T. Cancer in asbestos-mining and other areas of Quebec. J Natl Cancer Inst. 1977;59(4): 1139-45.
16. Jong-Lyel Roh. Clinical Utility of 18F-FDG PET for Patients with Salivary Gland Malignancies. Journal of Nuclear Medicine. 2007;48(2):240-6.
17. Tsai CC, Chen CL, Hsu HC. Expression of Epstein-Barr virus in carcinomas of major salivary glands: a strong association with lymphoepithelioma-like carcinoma. Hum Pathol. 1996;2 7(3):258-62.
18. Schneider AB, Favus MJ, Stachura ME, et al. Salivary gland neoplasms as a late consequence of head and neck irradiation. Ann Intern Med. 1977;87(2):160–4.
19. Zheng W, Shu XO, Ji BT, et al. Diet and other risk factors for cancer of the salivary glands:a population-based case-control study. Int J Cancer. 1996 17;67(2):194-8.
20. Sadetzki S, Oberman B, Mandelzweig L, et al. Smoking and risk of parotid gland tumors: a nationwide case-control study. Cancer. 2008;112(9):1974-82.
21. In der Maur CD, Klokman WJ, van Leeuwen FE, et al. Increased risk of breast cancer development after diagnosis of salivary gland tumor. Eur J Cancer. 2005;41(9):1311-5.
22. Johns M, Nachlas N. Salivary gland tumors Paperella. Shumrick, Gluckman, Meyerhoff editors. Otolaryngology; WB Saunders Company. Philadephia. 3rd edn. 1991;3:2099-127.
23. Rankow RM, Polayes IM. Diseases of the Salivary Glands Pennsylvania: WB Saunders. Chapter 5: 1976. pp. 99-142.
24. Chung YFA. Epidemiology of Warthin's tumor of the parotid gland in an Asian population. British Journal of Surgery. 1999;86(5):661-4.
25. Jens Peter Klussmann. High risk for bilateral Warthin's tumor in heavy smokers – review of 185 cases. Acta Otolaryngologica. 2006;126(11): 1213-7.
26. Kumar V, Abbas AK, Fausto N. Robbins and Cotran pathologic basis of disease, 7 edn. St. Louis, MO: Elsevier Saunders 2005.
27. Nussbaum M. Superficial parotidectomy with facial nerve preservation. In: Nussbaum M, (Ed), Modern Technics in Surgery, Futura, Mount Kisco, NY (1981).
28. Moshe Harell. Superficial parotidectomy for benign parotid lesions. Operative techniques in otolaryngology. 1996; 7(4): 315-22.
29. Mahnke, Christoph, Janig, et al. Malignant oncocytoma of the parotid gland: Case report and review of the literature. Australian Journal of Oto-Laryngology, 1998.
30. Batsakis JG, Brannon RB, Sciubba JJ. Monomorphic adenomas of major salivary glands: a histologic study of 96 tumors. Clin Otolaryngol Allied Sci. 1981;6(2):129-43.
31. Minicucci EM, de Campos EB, Weber SA, et al. Basal cell adenoma of the upper lip from minor salivary gland origin. Eur J Dent. 2008;2(3):213-6.
32. Eversole LR. Mucoepidermoid Carcinoma: Review of 815 reported cases. Oral Surg Oral Med Oral Pathol. 1970;28:490–5.
33. Heidelberger KP, Batsakis JG. Mucoepidermoid carcinoma of the tongue. J Laryngol Otol. 1973;87(12):1239-42.
34. Shafer WG, Hine MK, Levy BM. Text book of Oral Pathology. Philadelphia WB Saunders, 3 edn. 1974. pp. 225-31.
35. Luna, Mario A. Salivary Mucoepidermoid Carcinoma: Revisited. Advances in Anatomic Pathology. 2006;13(6):293-307.
36. Spiro RH, Huvos AG, Strong EW. Adenoid cystic carcinoma of salivary origin. A clinicopathologic study of 242 cases. Am J Surg. 1974;128(4):512-20.
37. Spiro RH. The controversial adenoid cystic carcinoma. Clinical considerations. In: McGurk M, Renehan AG

(Eds). Controversies in the Management of Salivary Gland Disease. Oxford, UK: Oxford University Press. 2001. pp. 207-11.

38. Speight PM, Barrett AW. Salivary gland tumors. Oral Dis. 2002;8(5):229-40.
39. Friedrich RE, Bleckmann V. Adenoid cystic carcinoma of salivary and lacrimal gland origin: localization, classification, clinical pathological correlation, treatment results and long-term follow-up control in 84 patients. Anticancer Res. 2003;23(2A):931-40.
40. Hoffman H, Funk G, Endres D. Evaluation and surgical treatment of tumors of the salivary gland. In: Comprehensive management of head and neck tumors Thawley SE, Panje WR, Batsakis JG, Lindberg RD (Eds). Philadelphia: WB Saunders Company; 1999. pp. 1147-81.
41. Batsakis JG, Luna MA, el-Naggar A. Histopathologic grading of salivary gland neoplasms: III. Adenoid cystic carcinomas. Ann Otol Rhinol Laryngol. 1990;99(12):1007-9.
42. Dale H Rice. Malignant Salivary Gland Neoplasms. Otolaryngologic Clinics of North America. 1999;32(5).
43. Abrams AM, Corayn J, Scofield HH and Hansen LS. Acinic cell adenocarcinoma of the major salivary glands—a clinicopathologic study of 77 cases, Cancer. 1965;18:1145-62.
44. Hoffman HI, Kannell LH, Robinson RA, Pinkston JA, Menck HR. National Cancer Data Base Report on cancer of the head and neck—ACC (Multi-institution report). Head and Neck, 1999.
45. Amisha Shah. Acinic cell carcinoma, papillary-cystic variant of the parotid gland: A case report with review of literature. Oral Oncology Extra. 2005; 41(7):137-41.
46. Lewis JE, Olsen KD, Weiland LH. Acinic cell carcinoma Clinicopathologic review. Cancer. 1991;67(1):172-9.
47. Olsen KD, Lewis JE. Carcinoma ex pleomorphic adenoma: a clinicopathologic review. Head Neck. 2001;23: 705-12.
48. Eneroth CM, Zetterberg A. Malignancy in pleomorphic adenoma. A clinical and microspectrophotometric study. Acta Otolaryngol. 1974;77(6):426-32.
49. Beahrs OH, Woolner LB, Kirklin JW, et al. Carcinomatous transformation of mixed tumors of the parotid gland. ALH. AMA Arch Surg. 1957;75(4):605-13; discussion 613-4.
50. Gnepp DR. Malignant mixed tumors of the salivary glands: a review. Pathol Annu. 1993;28 Pt 1:279-328.
51. Gnepp DR, Wenig BM. Malignant mixed tumors. In: Ellis GL, Auclair PL, Gnepp DR. Surgical pathology of salivary the glands. Philadelphia: Saunders; 1991. pp. 350-68.
52. LiVolsi VA, Perzin KH. Malignant mixed tumors arising in salivary glands. I. Carcinomas arising in benign mixed tumors: a clinicopathologic study. Cancer. 1977;39(5):2209-30.
53. Seifert G, Mehlkle A, Haubrich J, et al. Diseases of the Salivary Glands: Diagnosis, Treatment, Facial Nerve Surgery. Stuttgart: Georg Theime Verlag; 1986. pp. 222-81.
54. Gnepp DR. Malignant mixed tumors of the salivary glands: a review. Pathol Annu. 1993;28 Pt 1:279-328.
55. Spiro RH. Factors affecting survival in salivary gland cancers. In: McGurk M, Renehan AG (Eds). Controversies in the Management of Salivary Gland Disease. Oxford, UK: Oxford University Press; 2001.pp. 143-50.
56. Yih WY, Kratochvil FJ, Stewart JC. Intraoral minor salivary gland neoplasms: review of 213 cases. J Oral Maxillofac Surg. 2005;63(6):805-10.
57. Luna MA, Wenig BM. Polymorphous low-grade adenocarcinoma. In: Barnes L, Eveson JW, Reichart P, Sidransky D(Eds). Pathology and Genetics Head and Neck Tumors. World Health Organization Classification of Tumors. Lyon: IARC Press; 2005.pp. 223-4.
58. Pather N. Landmarks of the facial nerve: implications for parotidectomy. Surgical and Radiologic Anatomy. 2006; 28(2).
59. Neil Bhattacharyya. Anomalous relationship of the facial nerve and the retromandibular vein: A case report. JOMS. 1999;57(1):75-6.
60. Frey L. Le syndrome du nerf auriculo-temporal. Rev Neurol. 1923;2:92-104.
61. Guillamondegui OM, Byers RM, Luna MA, et al. Aggressive surgery in treatment for parotid cancer: the role of adjunctive postoperative radiotherapy. Am J Roentgenol Radium Ther Nucl Med. 1975;123(1):49-54.
62. Krüll A, Schwarz R, Engenhart R, et al. European results in neutron therapy of malignant salivary gland tumors. Bull Cancer Radiother 1996; 83 (Suppl): 125-9s, 1996.
63. Douglas JG, Lee S, Laramore GE, et al. Neutron radiotherapy for the treatment of locally advanced major salivary gland tumors. Head Neck. 1999;21(3): 255-63.
64. Wang CC, Goodman M. Photon irradiation of unresectable carcinomas of salivary glands. Int J Radiat Oncol Biol Phys. 1991;21(3):569-76.
65. Suen JY, Johns ME. Chemotherapy for salivary gland cancer. Laryngoscope 1982;92(3):235-9.
66. Posner MR, Ervin TJ, Weichselbaum RR, et al. Chemotherapy of advanced salivary gland neoplasms. Cancer. 1982; 50(11):2261-4.
67. Re-Cecconi D, Achilli A, Tarozzi M, et al. Mucoceles of the oral cavity: a large case series (1994-2008) and a literature review. Med Oral Patol Oral Cir Bucal. 2009.
68. Schmitt W, Ortel S, Blume H. Clinical and experimental contribution to the penicillin therapy of acute suppurative parotitis. Zentralbl Chir. 1954;79(38): 1589-1601.

Section 6

Infections of Maxillofacial Region

16 Management of Periapical Infections

Borle Rajiv M, Garg Ketan

The periapical infections are commonly seen in the clinical practice. The periapical infections result secondary to pulpal pathologies and the involved tooth is invariably non-vital and discolored. The exposure of the pulp to the external (oral) environments secondary to caries, attrition/abrasion leads to contamination and subsequently infection of the pulp (Box 16.1). Similarly, the thermal or chemical insult of the pulp also leads to inflammatory changes in the pulp. The pulp is enclosed in an inexpansile chamber (tooth) and inflammation and edema of the pulp leads to increased pressure within the chamber leading to its compression and ischemia. The pain of pulpitis is very severe and the involved tooth becomes to hot and cold. In fact, the hot and cold could be the aggravating and/or relieving factors for the pain in this condition. The mounting pressure within the pulp chamber compresses the periapical blood vessels and the lymphatics and the ischemic necrosis of the pulp takes place. The tooth which had pulpitis and was very painful and sensitive to hot and cold becomes less painful and insensitive owing to the necrosis of the pulp. The necrotic pulp serves as a good nidus for the microbial proliferation. The infection leads to liquefactive necrosis of the pulp and the necrotic, infected material escapes into the periapical area of the tooth leading to periapical infection. The mounting periapical pressure due to infection and inflammation causes extrusion of the tooth. The tooth has premature contact due to extrusion and patient feels pain during mastication. The tooth also becomes tender on vertical percussion and the mobility sets in due to lysis of periodontal fibers. The infection initially produces widening of lamina dura and mild periapical rarefaction on radiographs and endodontic therapy is good enough to drain and manage the periapical infection. However, the long standing periapical infection leads to changes like chronic periapical granuloma, periapical cyst and it may not be amenable to the endodontic treatment alone and to prevent recurrent episodes of infection and to remove the periapical pathological tissue completely, the endodontic treatment needs to be followed by the periapical surgery.

Box 16.1: The common causes of the pulpal pathologies

- Carious lesions leading to pulp exposure and infection.
- Regressive conditions like abrasion, attrition, erosion leading to pulp exposure.
- Fractures of the tooth involving the pulp.
- Dentoalveolar injuries which lead to luxation of the tooth and render it non vital which serves as a nidus for the infection.
- Extension of the periodontal infections to the periapical area.

CAUSES

The common causes of the pulpal pathologies are:

- Carious lesions leading to pulp exposure and infection.
- Regressive conditions like abrasion, attrition, erosion leading to pulp exposure.
- Fractures of the tooth involving the pulp.
- Dentoalveolar injuries which lead to luxation of the tooth and render it non-vital, which serves as a nidus for the infection.
- Extension of the periodontal infections to the periapical area.

FATE OF THE PERIAPICAL INFECTION

- Complete resolution, if the cause is treated.
- Transition to the chronic form leading to PA granuloma or cyst formation.
- Spread to adjoining bone.
- Extension in the adjacent soft-tissue spaces.

The periapical infection (abscess) can be drained through the root canal or through the socket of the tooth by extracting the offending tooth. This is very important in the management of the pain due to acute periapical infection/abscess. The common mistake done by the clinician is the attempt to treat the periapical infection by prescribing heavy doses of analgesics and antibiotics. The pain never gets relieved satisfactorily with medication as the cause of the pain is pressure and the decompression of the area will give lasting relief to the patients rather than the antibiotics and analgesics alone.

The history of the periapical surgeries also reveals the procedure called 'trephination' (creating the hole in the buccal cortical plate) to decompress the infection.[1] The infection should be promptly drained by opening the root canal and then the drugs should be prescribed. Endodontic therapy will lead to satisfactory remission of the infection. However, the chronic infections may not be treated by endodontic therapy alone. The periapical cyst, granuloma or the extension of the infection in soft tissue leading to a chronic cutaneous or gingival sinus may require further surgical intervention in the form of periapical curettage, apicoectomy and excision of cutaneous sinus along with the tract (Figs 16.1 to 16.3).

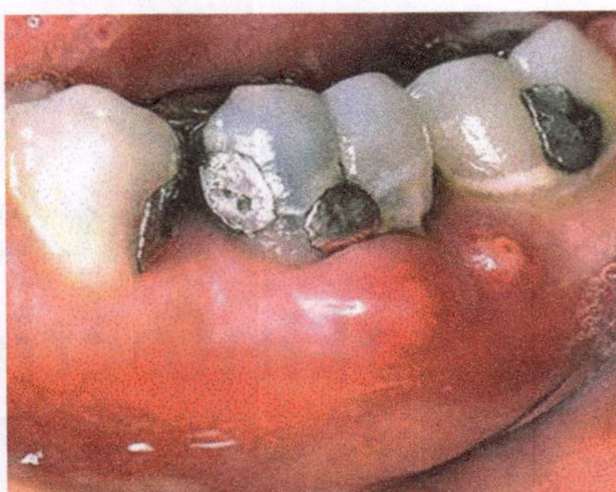

Fig. 16.1: Case of periapical abscess

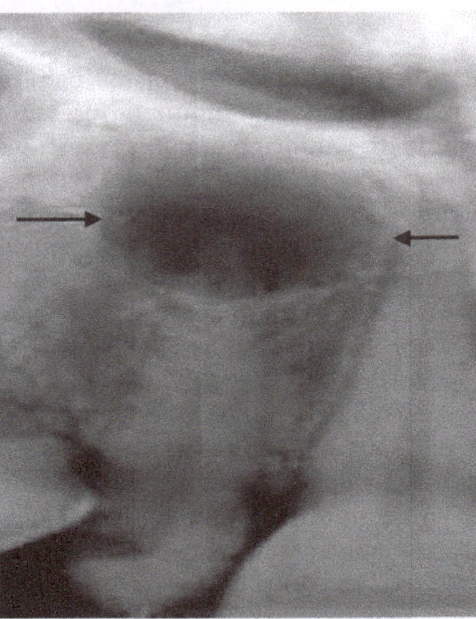

Fig. 16.2: Radiological picture

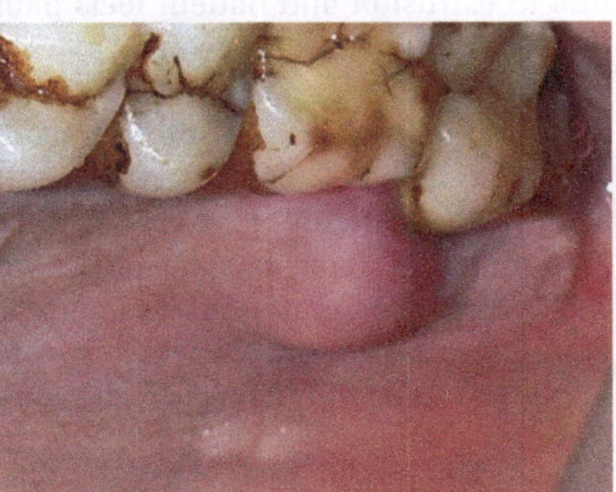

Fig. 16.3: Peridontal abscess

PATHOGENESIS OF PERIAPICAL LESIONS

Fish[2] described the reaction of periradicular tissues to noxious products of tissue necrosis, bacterial products and antigenic agents from root canal by establishing experimental foci of infection in the jaws of guinea pigs by drilling openings in the bone and packing in wool fibers saturated with broth culture of microorganisms. Four well-defined zones of reaction were found:

Zone of Infection

This zone was found in the center of the lesion and characterized by polymorphonuclear leukocytes. The microorganisms not disposed off by polymorphonuclear leukocytes are found in Haversian canals.

Zone of Contamination

This zone is characterized by round cell infiltration around the central zone. Fish observed an area of cellular destruction by the toxins released from the central zone. The nature of the toxins however could not be established (tissue-breakdown products or exotoxins). Prevalence of lymphocytes was noted. Autolytic death of bone cells with empty lacunae is seen.

Zone of Irritation

This zone is characterized by macrophages and osteoclasts. Fish found irritation evidences further from the central lesion as the toxins became more diluted. In this zone, normal bone cells and osteoclasts just managed to survive in the presence of small, round cells. These osteoclasts activated the bone tissue, while the collagen framework was destroyed by macrophages. This opens up a gap in the bone around the center of the lesion; as trees are felled to isolate a forest fire, and this space is then subsequently filled with polymorphonuclear lymphocytes and until this has taken places a danger of widespread of necrosis remains. The histologic picture is of starting of reparative activity.

Zone of Stimulation

This zone is characterized by fibroblasts and osteoblasts. At the periphery, the toxin is mild enough to be stimulant according to Fish's observations. Fibroblasts lay down collagen fibers, which act like a wall of defense around the zone of irritation and act like a scaffold on which osteoblasts build new bone. This newly built bone is deposited in irregular fashion.

APICOECTOMY/ APISECTOMY

Apicoectomy is the surgical procedure done to resect the diseased apex of an infected root of a tooth. This term is often interchanged with the term apicoectomy. The history of this surgery dates back to late 18th century when a hole was drilled in the buccal cortex of the alveolar bone to drain the periapical abscess. The surgery is often done to eliminate the periapical pathology, which can not be treated by endodontic

Box 16.2: The indications for the periapical surgery or the apicoectomy

- Periapical cysts
- Periapical granulomas
- Over extended root canal fillings
- Dilacerated, calcified or curved root canals, which can not be adequately obturated by anterograde method and remain under filled.

Box 16.3: Indications for periradicular surgery (According to Europian Society of Endodontics 1994)[3]

- Obstructed canal with radiologic findings and/or clinical symptoms.
- Extruded material with radiologic findings and/or clinical symptoms.
- Failed root canal treatment when retreatment is inappropriate (isthmus tissue, persistent acute symptoms or flare-ups, risk of root fracture).
- Perforations with radiologic findings and/or clinical symptoms, and where it is impossible to treat from within the pulp cavity

Box 16.4: Contraindications for periradicular surgery (According to Europian Society of Endodontics 1994)[2]

- Local anatomical factors (e.g. inaccessible root end).
- Tooth with inadequate periodontal support.
- Nonrestorable tooth, without function (no antagonist, no pillar for removable or fixed prothesis).
- Uncooperative patient.
- Compromised medical history.

means alone. The indications and contraindications for the periapical surgery are summarized in Box 16.2 to 16.4.

Indications for the Periapical Surgery or the Apicoectomy

- Periapical cysts
- Periapical granulomas
- Over extended root canal fillings
- Dilacerated, calcified or curved root canals, which can not be adequately obturated by anterograde method and remain under filled.

Indications and Contraindications for Periradicular Surgery

Indications for Periradicular Surgery (According to Europian Society of Endodontics 1994)[3]

- Obstructed canal with radiologic findings and/or clinical symptoms.
- Extruded material with radiologic findings and/or clinical symptoms.
- Failed root canal treatment when retreatment is inappropriate (isthmus tissue, persistent acute symptoms or flare-ups, risk of root fracture).
- Perforations with radiologic findings and/or clinical symptoms and where it is impossible to treat from within the pulp cavity.

Contraindications for Periradicular Surgery (According to Europian Society of Endodontics 1994)[2]

- Local anatomical factors (e.g. inaccessible root end).
- Tooth with inadequate periodontal support.
- Nonrestorable tooth, tooth without function (no antagonist, no pillar for removable or fixed prosthesis).
- Uncooperative patient.
- Compromised medical history.

ANATOMICAL CONSIDERATIONS

The anatomical structures, which are to be considered while performing periapical procedures include:

- Maxillary sinus[4] (Fig. 16.4)
- Inferior alveolar neurovascular bundle and mental nerve as it emerges from the mental foramen[5]
- Facial artery
- Floor of the nose with anterior nasal spine

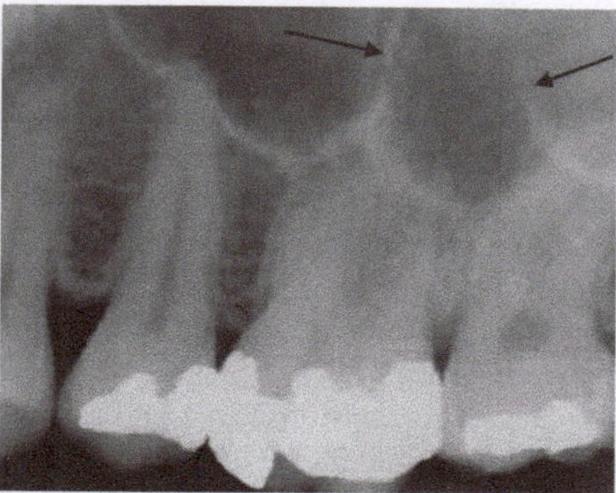

Fig. 16.4: Maxillary sinus

- Nasopalatine nerve and vessels
- Greater palatine neurovascular bundle
- Floor of the mouth.

Each of these should be kept in mind and taken into consideration, while performing surgery in the involved region so as to avoid damage to them.

The standard armamentarium required for the periapical surgery is shown in Box 16.5 and Figure 16.5.

Box 16.5: Instruments required

- Local anesthetic solution containing vasoconstrictor
- No. 3 BP handle with No. 15 Surgical blade
- Molt periosteal elevator
- Cawood-Minnesota retractor
- Standard dental high speed handpiece No. 6 round bur and No. 557 long fissure bur
- Mayo-Hegar needle holder
- Dean's surgical dissecting scissors
- Black silk or Vicryl suture (3 '0' or 4 '0') on cutting needle. The instruments required for periapical surgery are shown in the Figure 16.5.

Steps

- Soft tissue access via a mucoperiosteal flap
- Cortical ostectomy to approach the root apex
- Apical curettage
- Apicoectomy
- Retrofilling.

Flap Designing

Basic principles to be followed, while reflecting the mucoperisteal flap. The flap should be wider at the base than the apex to ensure proper blood supply and drainage of the flap (Figs 16.6A and B, Fig. 16.7).

The incisions recommended for this procedure are[6,7]

- Degloving incision (Figs 16.8A and B)
- Submarginal flap (Figs 16.9A to C)
- Semilunar incision (Figs 16.10A and B)
- Trapezoid incision (Figs 16.11 and 16.12)
- Triangular incision (Figs 16.13A and B)
- Envelope incision (Figs 16.14A and B)
- Palatal flap for maxillary posteriors (rare) (Fig. 16.15).

Surgical Procedure

The routine patient preparation is done prior to the surgery. Good quality post root canal treatment (RCT) radiographs are obtained to assess the size of the lesion to facilitate proper planning and reflection of the mucoperiosteal flap. Under all aspectic precautions like part preparation, draping, etc. the procedure is usually carried out under the local anesthesia. The general anesthesia is indicated in extensive lesions and where the patient compliance is poor. After taking one of the above mentioned incisions suitable in the given case a full thickness mucoperiosteal flap is designed and reflected. Selection of the appropriate flap design should be based on the following principles:

- Incision should lie on healthy bone so that after closure the suture line lies on solid healthy bone, as incisions closed over a dead space tend to breakdown.
- Healing is initiated by epithelial migration across the suture line and this is four times faster in attached gingiva as compared to alveolar mucosa and this advantage should be taken by placing horizontal incision over the attached gingival.
- The horizontal incision should extend atleast one tooth on the either

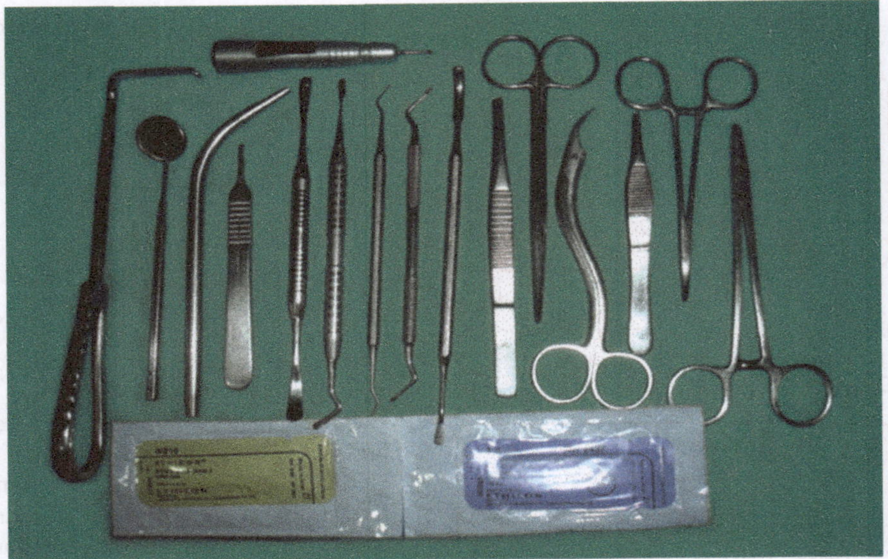

Fig. 16.5: Instruments required for periapical surgery

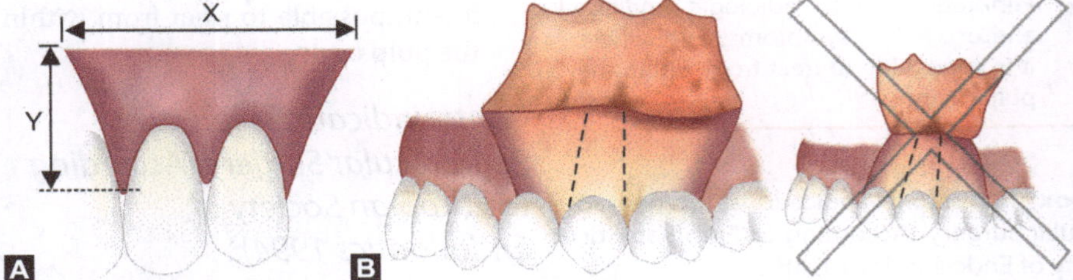

Figs 16.6A and B: Flap designing: (A) Dimensions of flap (x>y); (B) Correct and incorrect way of designing of flap

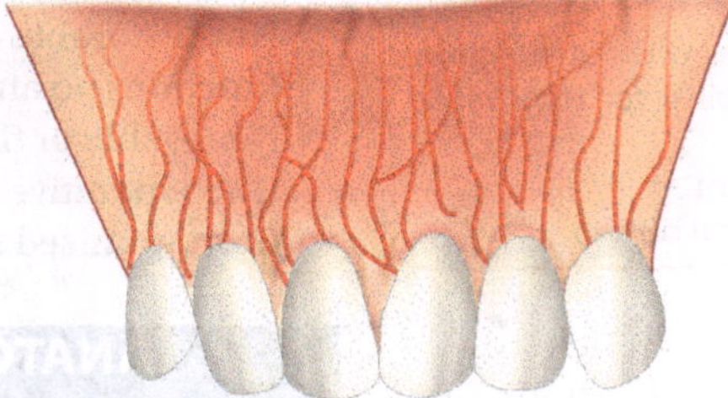

Fig. 16.7: Direction of blood supply in the anterior maxillary region

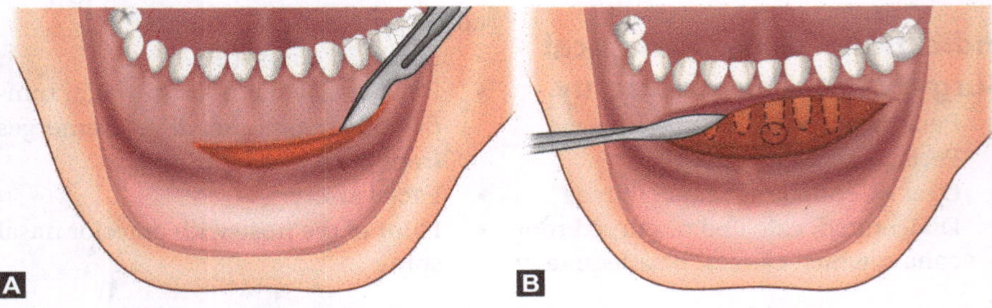

Figs 16.8A and B: Flap design for lower anteriors degloving incision

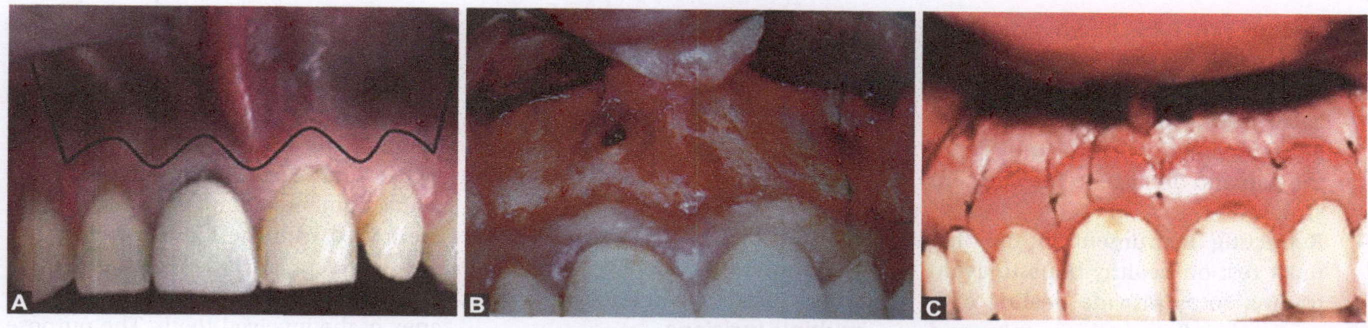

Figs 16.9A to C: Luebke-ochsenbein (scalloped) submarginal flap

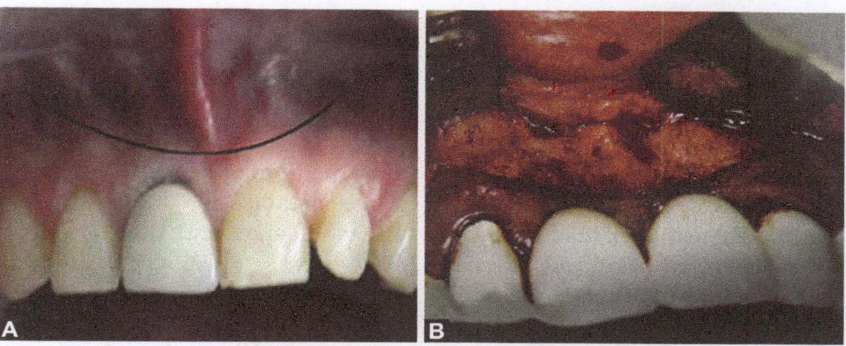

Figs 16.10A and B: Semilunar incision

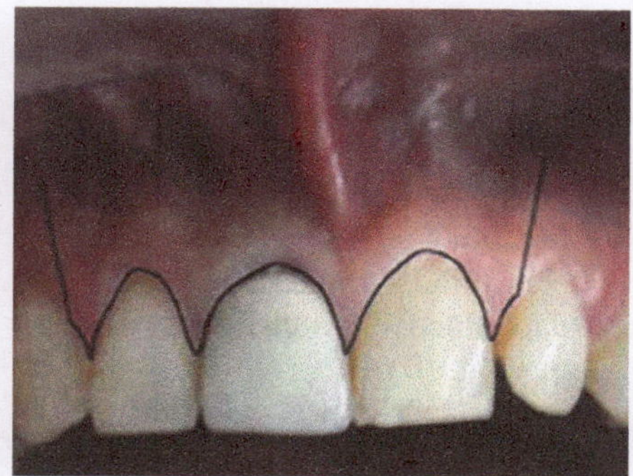

Fig. 16.11: Trapezoid flap

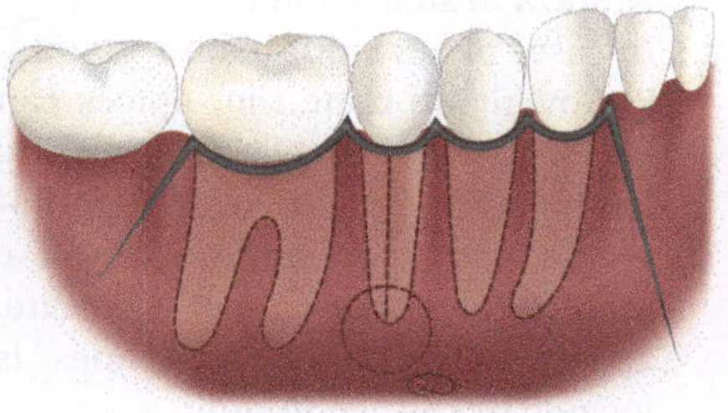

Fig. 16.12: Triangular/trapezoidal flap for posterior mandible with release in the lateral incisor-canine area to avoid damage to the mental nerve and vessels

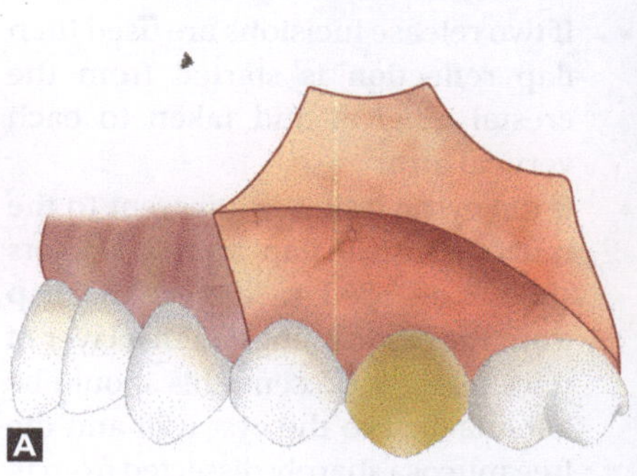

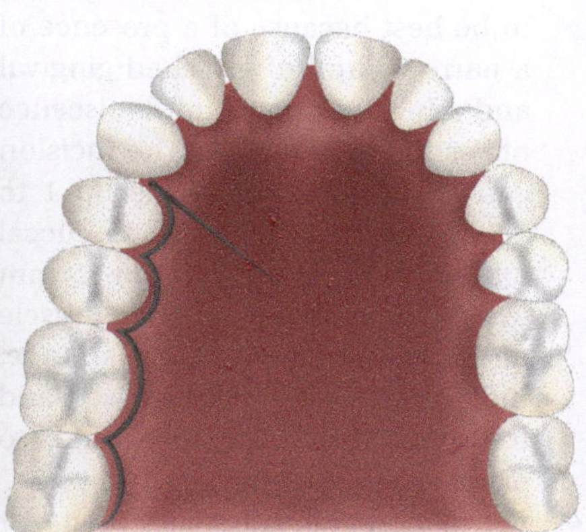

Figs 16.13A and B: Triangular incision

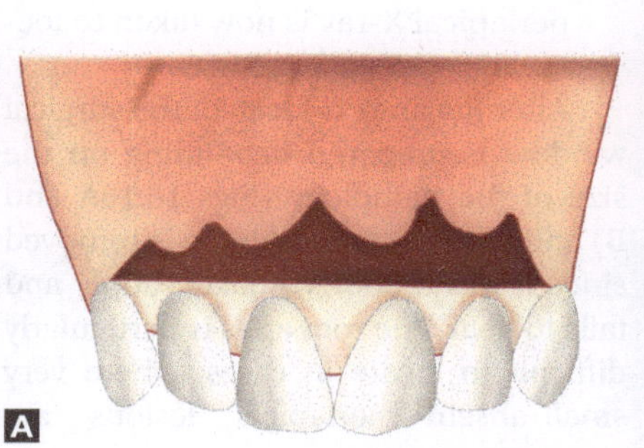

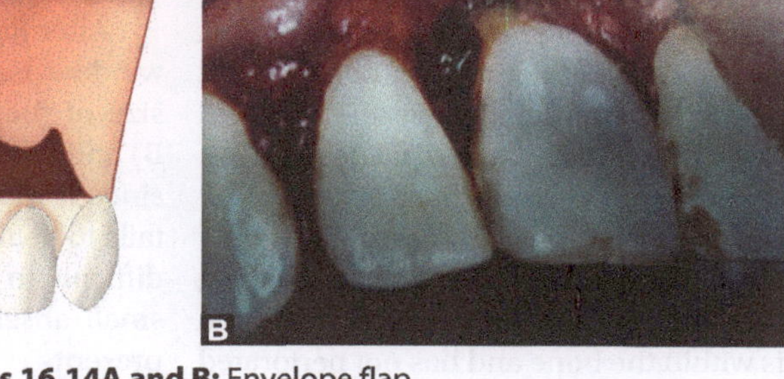

Figs 16.14A and B: Envelope flap

Fig. 16.15: Palatal flap design

side of the tooth/teeth on which apicoectomy is to be performed.

- The flap must provide adequate access and visualization of the surgical site without tearing/bruising of the flap and damage to the adjacent structures.
- Retracting instrument of the flap must rest on healthy bone to avoid trauma so as provide healing with minimal inflammation, pain and subsequent scarring of tissues and subsequent carrying of the tissue.
- The primary blood supply for the free alveolar mucosa is derived from the supraperiosteal vasculature that runs parallel to the long axis of the tooth and any horizontal incision in this unattached mucosa will greatly compromise the blood supply of the flap, which will result in compromised healing. Therefore, only vertical release incisions should be made in the alveolar mucosa (*see* Fig. 16.7).
- The vertical release incision should be made at an obtuse angle to the horizontal one so as to have a flap with a broad base with respect to the apex.
- Horizontal incision is to be placed in the gingival sulcus in cases of severe periodontal disease.
- Fixed and removable prosthetic restorations if present should be considered with the incision being placed on the attached gingival in visible smile zones and under the denture base, in cases of presence of removable prostheses.
- In cases of mandibular anterior teeth, the sulcular incision is considered to be best because of a presence of a narrow band of attached gingival and a high incidence of dehiscence of vestibular incisions. The incision can also be placed in the lip 1 to 1.5 cm anterior to the mucobuccal fold, this incision goes for 2 mm into the orbicularis oris muscle and a myocutaneous flap is made, the periosteum is then incised and the superior flap is then elevated to expose the root apex.
- For mandibular molar and premolar regions sulcular incisions with anterior release in the lateral incisor-canine area are indicated. Never place the incision in the buccal mandibular vestibule. If additional access is required then a posterior release incision can be given.

Technique

- Horizontal incision is made first with a sharp, clean stroke avoiding multiple incisions.
- The vertical arm or arms are then added to it.
- Intactness of papilla should be maintained as it will serve as an anchoring point for sutures.
- The entire length of the incision should then be scored with a periosteal elevator to assure its completeness to the bone and avoid accidental tearing of the flap.
- The flap is then raised with the sharp end of the periosteal elevator starting with the horizontal incision and the blunt end is then used to reflect the flap.
- With the sulcular incision, the elevation is started at the incisal papilla farthest from the release incision.
- If two release incisions are used then flap reflection is started from the crestal gingival and taken to each vertical arm.
- If the cystic lesion is adherent to the mucoperiosteal flap then a scissors should be used to dissect the flap from the cystic lining. Often a layer of thick tissue is present, this should be left attached to the cyst wall and the free mucosa sharply dissected from it.

To access the palatal root of the maxillary molars a sulcular incision with a vertical release in the region of the canine is indicated. These areas require a large soft-tissue flap to provide adequate access through the dense palatal bone. The vertical releasing incision should extend just short of midline and be tapered posteriorly. It may involve the terminal branches of the greater palatine artery. The buccal cortical plate is exposed. If a sinus is present previously, then perforation in the cortex is noticed along with the gingival sinus tract. If the lesion is within the bone and has not perforated through the bone then the intact cortical plate is seen. If the cortical perforation is present, the same is widened with the help of the flat fissure bur to expose the periapical pathology. If the cortex is intact a post stamp incision is taken in the bone with a number 8 round bur and the holes are joined with the flat fissure bur and the intervening bone is removed to expose the periapical pathology and the apex of the involved tooth. The purpose of creating a window in the bone is to gain working access to the tooth being treated. The size of the bone window should be large enough to provide complete removal of the periapical pathology.

The root apex of the offending tooth should be located precisely to prevent injury to the apices of the adjacent teeth. Three methods may be used to locate the tooth apex and thus the area of ostectomy:

1. In most cases the cortical plate may be thin because of underlying pathology and may show fenestrations or fistulae. A periosteal elevator or curette is used to start the access window in such situations.
2. In cases of posterior teeth with thicker overlying bone root apices can be located by establishing working length of the tooth over a radiograph and then transposing the measurement with a file or curette, approximate site of root apex is located by this technique.
3. If still not located as in cases of mandible molars then it can be done by using a round bur to drill a hole into the buccal cortical plate as close to the estimated apex as possible; a medium sized gutta-percha point is then placed into the hole and a periapical X-ray is now taken to locate the apex accurately.

After the apex is located, the surgical window is prepared depending on the size of the pathology (Figs 16.16A and B) and all unsupported bone is removed since it has a poor vascular supply and fails to heal. The root apex is particularly difficult to locate in cases, where very small/absent periapical lesions are present.

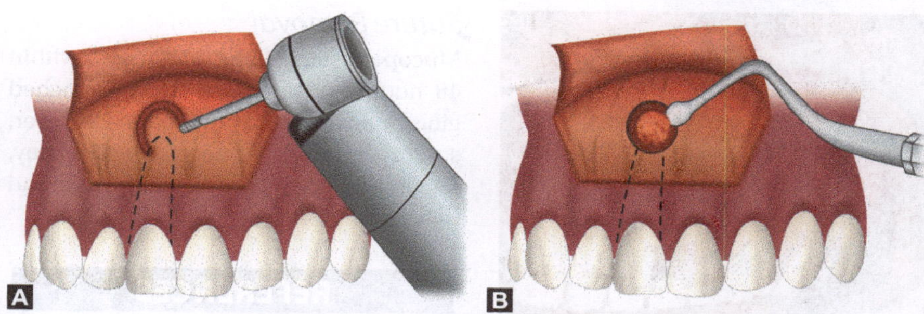

Figs 16.16A and B: Preparation of the bony window

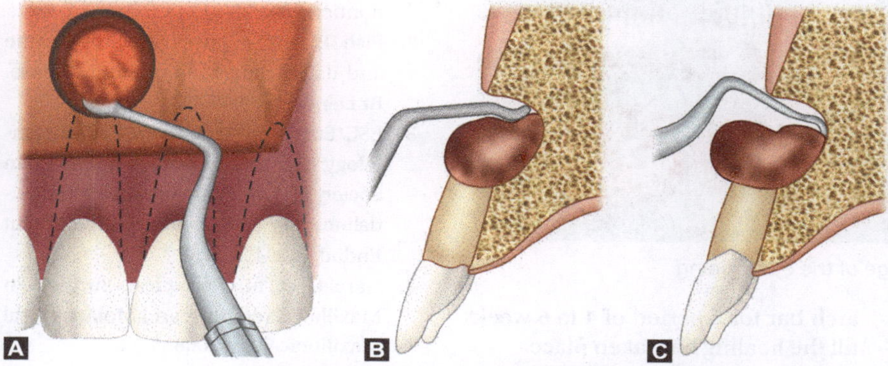

Figs 16.17A to C: Apical curettage (periapical cyst)

Apical Curettage

Two types of pathosis are associated with endodontically treated teeth (Figs 16.17A to C):

- Granulation tissue
- Radicular cyst

Granulation tissue is removed with curette (*see* Figs 16.16A and B). Complete removal is advised in cases of smaller radiographically confined lesions. In cases of large lesions, any communications with the nasal cavity, maxillary sinus, lingual plate defects, adjacent roots, inferior alveolar neurovascular bundle should be ruled out.

If no communications are present then complete removal of the lesion should be done.

A periapical cyst differs from granulation tissue in terms of tissue characteristics, organization and structure. The cysts are well-encapsulated structures and should be removed *in toto* as a single unit. After delineation of the bony soft-tissue border, a curette is used to gently disengage the sac from the bone by placing the sharp edge against the bone and convex surface against the cystic membrane to avoid perforation of the cystic lining (Figs 16.17A to C, 16.18A to D). On the other hand the granuloma is composed of fragile, friable tissue, which bleeds and fragments readily on instrumentation. It is often removed in piece meal. The stoppage of the bleeding from the bone should be taken as a sign of complete removal of the granuloma. The lining of the cyst also tends to fragment and bleed if it is grossly infected.

In cases of large lesions, which are close to the vital structures and are likely to result in large defects and damage to the adjacent vital structures, an alternative treatment plan comprising of elimination of the source of infection and creation of an effective periapical seal by endodontic therapy, preoperatively, then the residual cystic lining or granulation tissue will resolve and the magnitude of the periapical surgery will be reduced and morbid complications can also be avoided. All the tissue that are removed should be submitted to the pathologist for histopathological examination.

Apicoectomy

Purpose

To create an apical bevel permitting the operator to access the apex

The angle of bevel should be kept minimum to minimize leakage through dentinal tubules. The ideal angle of resection is flat (0°) cut since it minimizes apical leakage (Fig. 16.19).[8] The technical requirement for good surgical access to place a retrograde filling means that some bevel is necessary, which should be kept to the smallest angle possible.

Factors

The factors affecting inclination of bevel are[9]:

- Anatomy of the root.
- Surgical visibility and access to the site.
- Size of instrument used to prepare the root end for retrofilling.

The cut through the apex should bevel the root so that it gives a lateral/forward inclination toward the operator. This permits an adequate view of the apical foramen. The projecting Gutta-percha point should be identified while performing apicoectomy.

Retrograde Filling[10]

If the apical seal of the root canal filling is inadequate then the chances of micro-leakage and the recurrent infections are very high. To avoid these complications, apical seal can be achieved by doing the retrograde filling.

Wound Closure and Postoperative Care

- Wound should be thoroughly irrigated with sterile normal saline solution before closure.
- Closure should not be too tight.
- First suture after repositioning the flap in proper alignment is to be

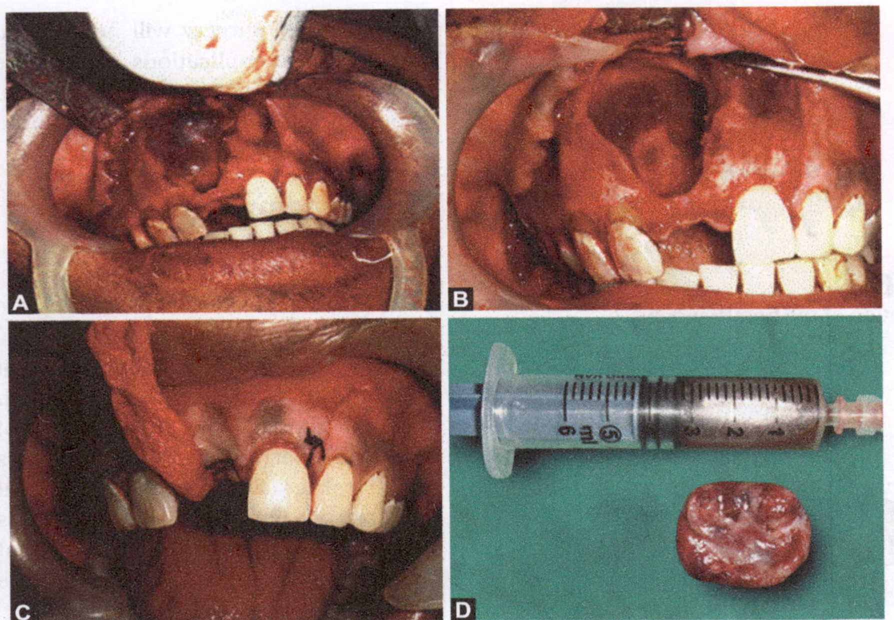

Figs 16.18A to D: Curettage of the cystic lining

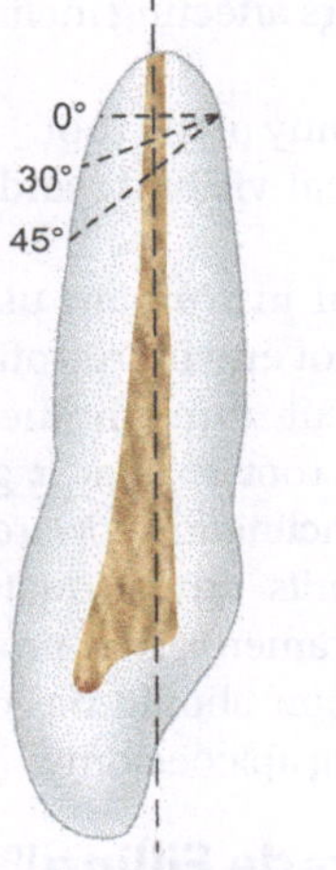

Fig. 16.19: Direction of the bevel

placed at the point of convergence of the vertical and horizontal incisions. This is the positional suture, once this is done, then the vertical and lastly the horizontal incisions are closed.

- Periodontal sling or simple interrupted sutures can be placed.
- Some portion of the vertical incision can be left open to facilitate drainage of the collected hematoma/exudate.
- If the teeth are found to be mobile then they can be splinted using an arch bar for a period of 4 to 6 weeks till the healing has taken place.

Pain

The postoperative pain is managed by non-steroidal anti-inflammatory drugs (NSAID's) or any other suitable analgesic.

Antibiotics[11]

Generally not required, but depends on:

- Medical history.
- Length of time the wound was open.
- Surgical contamination.
- Clinical findings.

Usually the beta lactum group of antibiotics are adequate to provide good cover (e.g. penicillin, amoxicillin, ampicillin and cephalosporins).

Swelling

A mild to moderate postoperative swelling is expected and can be managed by use of icepacks and anti-inflammatory drugs. Routine use of steroids is not advocated for periapical procedures. Application of the cold packs in first 24 hours of surgery help in reducing the inflammatory edema by inducing vasoconstriction.

Suture Removal

Mucoperiosteal flap reattaches within 48 hours and incisions in the attached gingiva heal within 4 to 5 days. However, suture removal is done on 7th day, depending upon clinical judgement and patient comfort.

REFERENCES

1. Brian M. Henry. Trephination for acute pain management. Journal of endodontics. 2003;29(2):144-6.
2. Fish EW. The physiology of dentine and its reaction to injury and disease. Br Dent J. 1928;49:593.
3. ESE/European Society of Endodontology: Consensus report of the European Society of Endodontology on quality guidelines for endodontic treatment. Int Endod J. 1994;27:115.
4. Garcia, et al. Periapical Surgery in Maxillary Premolars and Molars. J Oral Maxillofac Surg. 2008.
5. Martí, et al. Distance Between Periapical Lesion and Mandibular Canal as a Factor in Periapical Surgery in Mandibular Molars. J Oral Maxillofac Surg. 2008.
6. Gutmann JL, Harrison JW. Surgical Endodontics. 1994;123-299.
7. Vreeland DL, Tidwell E. Flap design for surgical endodontics. Oral Surg. 1982; 54:461-5.
8. Gagliani M, Taschieri S, Molinari R. Ultrasonic root-end preparation: influence of cutting angle on the apical seal. J. Endod., Baltimore, 1998. v.24, n.11, pp.726-30.
9. Hirsch JM, Ahlstrom U, Hendrikson PA, Periapical surgery. Int J Oral Surg. 1979;8:173-85.
10. Obón-Arroyave, SI, et al. *Ex vivo* microscopic assessment of factors affecting the quality of apical seal created by root-end fillings. Int. Endod. J. 2007; 40(8):590-602.
11. Baumgartner JG, Bakland LK, Sugita EI. Microbiology of endodontics and asepsis in endodontic practice. In John Ingle, Leif Bakland (Eds) Endodontics, 5th edn, BC Becker, London, Chapter 3, pp. 63-94.

17 Odontogenic Infections

Borle Rajiv M, Angik Richa

The infections of the maxillofacial area are of great importance to the oral and maxillofacial surgeon. They are not only common in clinical practice, but are also challenging and can lead to fatal complications if not treated timely. The common causes of odontogenic infections are dental caries and periodontal infections. The oral cavity is a highly contaminated cavity. The oral flora exists in such a way that some microorganisms suppress the growth of the others. The fungal growth is usually suppressed. However, with long-term antibiotic therapy the bacterial flora gets disturbed and the fungi get an opportunity to proliferate and produce fungal infections, e.g. candidiasis (*opportunistic infection*). The saliva and its composition also keep in control the growth and pathogenicity of microorganisms by virtue of its pH and secreted antibodies. There is a delicate balance between the virulence of the microbes and the host resistance. Whenever there is imbalance between these two factors, the infection is caused by the normal oral inhabitants. The infection may remain confined to the dentoalveolar area in a healthy host, but when the microorganisms are highly virulent and the host resistance is severely depleted, the infection spreads to the adjoining tissue planes. The lymphatic and hematogenous spread of the infection can lead to the systemic complications which could be fatal. Usually it is being said that to cause the infection 10^6 million microorganisms are required in health, but this number gets reduced in patients with immunosuppression.

The tissues around the teeth, bone, periosteum, muscles and fascia serve as the anatomical barriers for the spread of the infection to the adjoining tissue planes. The maxillofacial infections are restricted to the particular area by these anatomical barriers; however more virulent organisms are capable of breaking these anatomical barriers by producing toxins and the infection spreads to the other adjacent areas. The odontogenic infection arises from the tooth and is initially confined to the alveolar bone, which serves as the first barrier. The spongy bone offers least resistance and the infection spreads along this path of least resistance to the cortical plates which are the second barrier, which get eroded and perforated more readily where they are thin. If the cortical plate gets perforated above the muscle attachment, the infection forms intraoral abscess on the gingiva called gingival abscess or the parulis, e.g. mandibular anterior teeth. If the cortical plates are eroded below the muscle attachment then an extraoral swelling is produced, e.g. the mandibular posterior teeth. The third barrier is the periosteum covering the bone which is tough, nonelastic and firmly adherent to the bone. The infection after perforating the cortex forms the subperiosteal infection which leads to the accumulation of the inflammatory edema or pus below the periosteum, raising the pressure and the periosteum is forcefully stripped out producing severe pain. As the periosteum is eroded and perforated, the infection comes in the soft tissue around the bone which is elastic and resilient and the pressure drops and the severity of the pain also drops. The next barrier is the muscle attachment to the bone and the fascia, investing layer of the cervical fascia and they try to limit the further spread of the infection. However, if they are also broken the infection spreads further to the adjoining tissue planes. The infection has two fates; first it will localize, suppurate and form an abscess and the second it may spread locally and systemically. It is usually seen that the staphylococcal infections have tendency for early localization and the streptococcal infections tend to spread without getting localized as the microorganisms produce hyaluronidase which breaks down the intercellular cementing substance and facilitate the further spread without suppuration (cellulitis). The anaerobic infections are not primary in occurrence and will be precipitated if the environments are favorable to the growth of anerobic organisms such as hypoxic tissue, large hypoperfused cavities, slough or necrotic material. They occur as opportunistic infections. The orofacial infections are usually gram positive and the causative organisms are usually staphylococci or streptococci. The staphylococci are the inhabitants of the skin, while as streptococci are the primary organisms of the oral cavity. The bacteroids and the *Escherichia coli* are the next in frequency. The gram-negative infections are commonly seen in the peritonial cavity, genitourinary passage, but they can occasionally occur in oral cavity as a result of *nosocomial* or *hospital acquired infections*. The odontogenic infections spread to the adjoining fascial spaces formed by the deep cervical fascia.

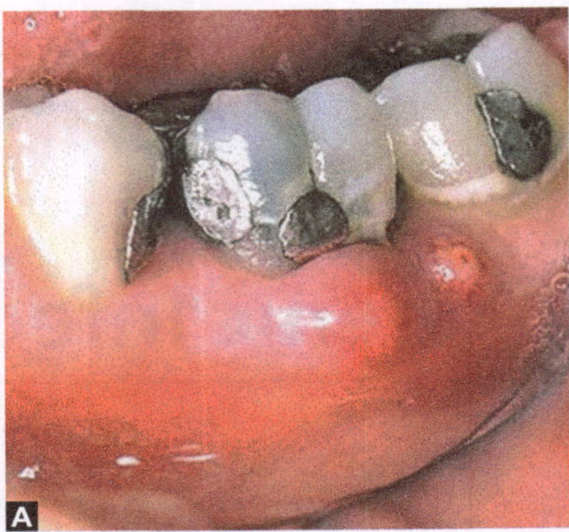

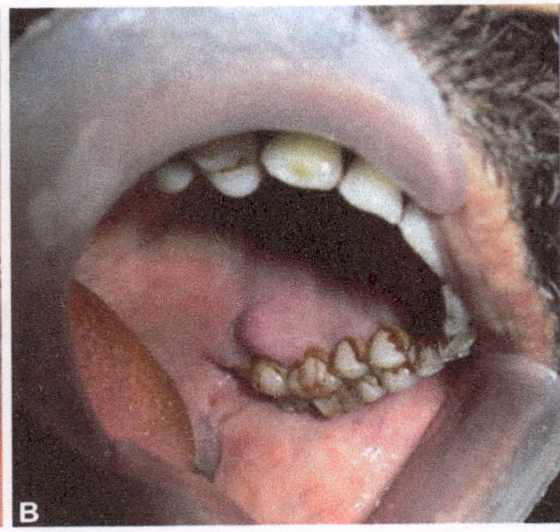

Figs 17.1A and B: Gingival abscess or a 'Parulis'

APPLIED SURGICAL ANATOMY

The bacterial quantity and virulence determine the clinical course of the infection. The microorganisms produce lytic enzymes, potent endotoxins and exotoxins and interference with or resistance to host humoral and cellular defences.

The infection once set has three fates:

1. The body's defence systems overpower the microorganisms and either completely eliminate them or the infection gets localized to form an abscess which drains spontaneously on the surface.
2. The infection changes from acute to chronic form and persists. It undergoes acute exacerbations intermittently whenever the environments are conductive.
3. It spreads in an aggressive manner and produces local and systemic complications which could be life threatening.

The anatomical barriers present in the body tend to restrict the spread of the infection and try to localize it.

LOCAL BARRIERS

Alveolar Bone

Most of the odontogenic infections originate in the alveolar bone, which forms the first barrier for the spread of the infection. The alveolar bone has components like spongy bone, cortical bone, periosteum and the muscles and fascia attached to it. As the infection progresses within the bone, it spreads in the radial manner through the spongy bone and extends to the cortical plates. Once the cortical plates are perforated the infection comes to lie below the periosteum to form the subperiosteal abscess. If the cortex is perforated above the muscle attachment (e.g. mandibular anterior teeth) then the infection localizes intraorally to form a gingival abscess (*parulis*) (Figs 17.1A and B). If the infection perforates the cortex below the muscle attachment (e.g. mandibular posterior teeth), then the infection extends in the anatomical spaces around the bone and presents extraorally.

Periosteum

Periosteum is the next local barrier. This structure is better developed in mandible and hence can delay further spread of infection leading to development of a subperiosteal abscess. The periosteum is tough, non-elastic and is tenaciously adherent to the bone and thus when the pressure mounts due to subperiosteal infection; it gets stripped from the bone. As the periosteum is non-yielding, the pressure does not get relieved and the subperiosteal abscess is very painful. It does not provide much resistance and the infection spreads into adjacent surrounding soft tissues.

The adjacent Muscles and Fascia are the next barriers for the localization of infection.

Anatomy of the Cervical Fascia

The fibrous connective tissue that constitutes the cervical fascia varies from loose areolar tissue to dense fibrous bands. This fascia serves to envelope the muscles, nerves, vessels and viscera of the neck, thereby forming planes and potential spaces that serve to divide the neck into functional units. The cervical fascia functions to both direct and limit the spread of disease processes in the neck.

The cervical fascia was first described by Burns in 1811. It is now generally agreed upon that the cervical fascia can be divided into a simpler superficial layer and a more complex deep layer that is further subdivided into superficial, middle and deep layers.

Superficial Fascia

The superficial layer of cervical fascia ensheaths the platysma in the neck and extends superiorly to the face to cover the muscles of facial expression. Below the mouth, the muscles of facial expression are deep to it whereas above the mouth they are superficial to this layer. It is the equivalent of subcutaneous tissue elsewhere in the body and forms a continuous sheet from the head and neck to the chest, shoulders and axilla.

Deep Cervical Fascia

The deep cervical fascia can be divided into anterior, middle and posterior layer (Fig. 17.2).

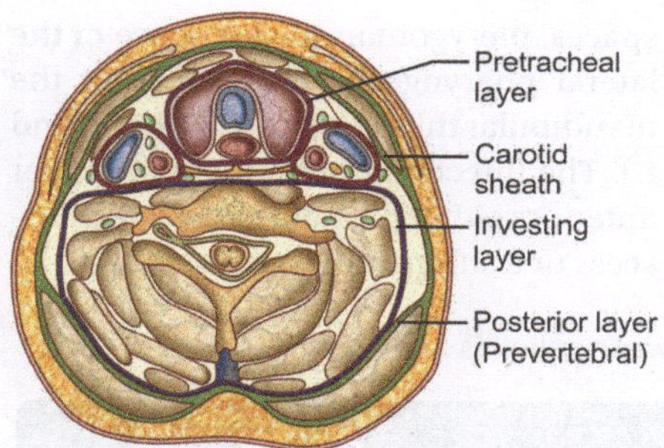

Fig. 17.2: Different layers of the cervical fascia in cross section of the neck

A. Anterior layer:
- Parotidomassetric fascia
- Temporal fascia

B. Middle layer:
- Muscular division:
  - Sternohyoid—omohyoid
  - Sterothyroid—thyrohyoid
- Visceral:
  - Buccopharyngeal fascia.

C. Posterior layer:
Anterior—Alar fascia
Posterior—Prevertebral layer.

Anterior Layer

The anterior layer of the deep cervical fascia is also known as the investing layer or the enveloping layer or the external layer or the superficial layer of the deep fascia. It has been described using the *'rule of twos'*—it envelops two muscles, two glands and forms two spaces. This layer originates from the spinous processes of the vertebral column and spreads circumferentially around the neck and splits to cover the sternocleiodomastoid and trapezius muscles. In the midline, inferiorly it splits 2 centimeters above the manubrium forming the suprasternal space of Burns. The space of burns contains anterior jugular vein, lymph nodes and the loose connective tissue. Superiorly, it attaches to the hyoid bone and continues superiorly to enclose the submandibular and parotid glands. The portion of the fascia covering the masseter muscle and enclosing the parotid gland is known as the 'Parotideomassetric fascia'. It also covers the anterior bellies of the digastrics and the mylohyoid, thereby forming the floor of the submandibular space. At the mandible, the fascia splits into an internal layer, which covers the medial surface of the medial pterygoid and attaches to the skull base and an outer layer that covers the masseter and inserts on the zygomatic arch.

Middle Layer

The middle layer of the deep cervical fascia is also known as the visceral fascia, the prethyroid fascia and the pretracheal fascia. It can be thought of in two subdivisions, the muscular division, which surrounds the infrahyoid strap muscles and the visceral division, which envelops the pharynx, larynx, esophagus, trachea and thyroid gland. The superior extent of the muscular division is the hyoid and thyroid cartilage, inferiorly it inserts on the sternum and clavicle. Its surgical significance is that this layer of deep cervical fascia should be divided in the midline to approach the thyroid gland and trachea. It does not have any significance regarding spread of infection from orofacial region. However, it is responsible for the movement of the thyroid swelling on deglutition.

The visceral division attaches to the hyoid bone above and surrounds the trachea, esophagus and thyroid gland. Above the hyoid, the fascia surrounds the pharynx on the lateral and posterior sides lying on the superficial side of the constrictor muscles of the pharynx where it is known as the buccopharyngeal fascia. It extends inferiorly into the upper mediastinum where it is continuous with the fibrous pericardium and covers the thoracic trachea and esophagus. The retropharyngeal, pretracheal and lateral pharyngeal spaces lie superficial to this layer. A specialized condensation of the fascia forms around the carotid arteries on either side which is called carotid sheath which encloses common carotid artery, internal jugular vein and the vagus nerve.

Posterior Layer

The deep layer of the deep cervical fascia originates from the spinous processes

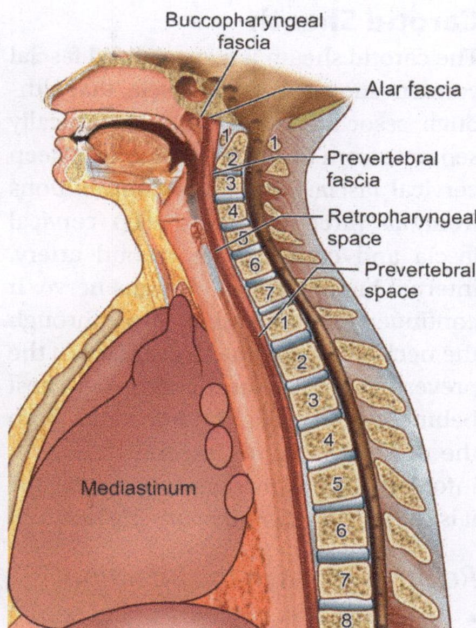

Fig. 17.3: Posterior Lincoln's highway

of the cervical vertebra and the ligamentum nuchae. At the transverse processes of the cervical vertebra, it divides into an anterior alar layer and a posterior prevertebral layer.

The alar fascia extends from the base of the skull to the second thoracic vertebra (T2). It lies between the visceral layer of the middle fascia and the prevertebral layer. It fuses with the retropharyngeal fascia between C6 and T4. This fusion forms the bottom of the retropharyngeal space and infections of the retropharyngeal space may rupture the alar fascia and enter the danger space which is continuous with the posterior mediastinum (*Posterior Lincoln's highway*) (Fig. 17.3).

The prevertebral fascia lies just anterior to the vertebral bodies and extends the entire length of the vertebral column. It travels circumferentially around the neck and covers the paravertebral muscles, the deep muscles of the posterior triangle of the neck and the scalene muscles. This layer of fascia surrounds the brachial plexus and subclavian vessels and continues laterally as the axillary sheath. It may be involved by infections of the vertebral bodies and is not involved in maxillofacial infections.

Carotid Sheath

The carotid sheath is a specialized fascial condensation of cervical fascia, that although associated with, but anatomically separate from the other layers of the deep cervical fascia. It receives contributions from all three layers of deep cervical fascia and contains the carotid artery, internal jugular vein and vagus nerve. It continues from the skull base through the neck along the anterior surface of the prevertebral fascia and enters the chest behind the clavicle. The infections from the neck region can descend through it into the anterior mediastenum and thus it is called *'Anterior Lincoln's highway'*.

Relative Terms in the Infection

- **Abscess:** It is defined as 'a localized collection of the pus' or an abscess is 'a pathological cavity lined by granulation tissue and contains pus'. The suppuration is a hallmark of an abscess and the common organisms that are responsible to form an abscess are staphylococci, predominantly present in the skin. Differences between cellulitis and abscess is given in Table 17.1.
- **Cellulitis:** It is in literal sense the inflammation of the cells. A cellulitis is a nonsuppurative, spreading inflammation (Figs 17.4A and B). The causative microorganisms are streptococci, predominantly present in the oral flora.
- **Bacteremia:** Transient presence of viable bacteria in the circulating blood.
- **Septicemia:** Systemic toxicity due to invasion by virulent microorganisms or their toxins in the bloodstream coming from a local seat of infection.

The clinical presentation of the infection changes with the duration as depicted in the Table 17.2.

FASCIAL SPACES

The fascial spaces are divided into:
- Those around the mandible.
- Those around the maxilla.

The facial spaces are also named by other names and the synonyms are summarized in Table 17.3. The infection from the tooth spreads to various fascial spaces adjacent to the jaw (Table 17.4). Commonly the infections from the mandibular molars spread to the sublingual or submandibular space. While as the infection to the buccal, submasseteric spaces, pterygomandibular space or the lateral pharyngeal space are from the mandibular third molars (Figs 17.5A and B). The infections from the mandibular anteriors either produce the gingival abscess or a submental space abscess.

Table 17.1: Differences between cellulitis and abscess

Characteristics	Cellulitis	Abscess
Duration	Acute phase	Chronic phase
Pain	Severe and generalized	Localized
Size	Large	Small
Localization	Diffuse borders	Well-circumscribed
Palpation	Doughy to indurated, pitting edema	Fluctuant
Presence of pus	Absent	Present
Degree of seriousness	Greater	Less
Bacteria	Aerobic	Mixed

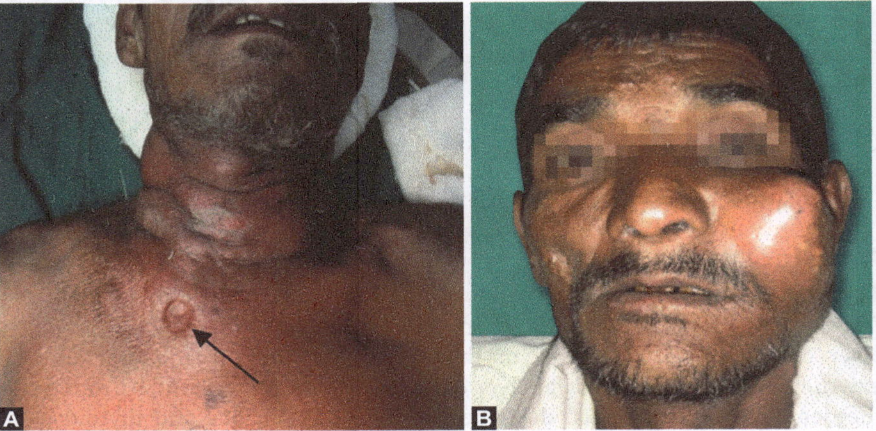

Figs 17.4A and B: Cellulitis. (A) Note the pitting edema; (B) Localized abscess.

Table 17.2: Various stages of infection

Characteristic	Inoculation	Cellulitis	Abscess
Time	0–3 days	3–7 days	> 5 days
Pain	Mild-moderate	Severe and generalized	Moderate-severe and localized
Size	Small	Large	Small
Localization	Diffuse	Diffuse	Circumscribed
Palpation	Soft, doughy, mildly tender	Hard, exquisitely tender	Fluctuant, tender
Presentation	Normal color	Reddened	Peripherally reddened
Skin quality	Normal	Thickened	Centrally undermined and shiny
Temperature	Slightly heated	Hot	Moderately heated
Loss of function	Minimal or none	Severe	Moderately severe
Tissue fluid	Edema	Serosanguineous, flecks of pus	Pus
Levels of malaise	Mild	Severe	Moderate-severe
Severity	Mild	Severe	Moderate-severe
Percutaneous bacteria	Aerobic	Mixed	Anaerobic

Table 17.3: Different spaces around the jaw bones

Spaces around the mandible	Spaces around the maxilla
Submasseteric space	Buccal space
Submandibular space	Canine fossa/infraorbital space
Submental space	Infratemporal space
Sublingual space	Lateral pharyngeal space
Masticator space	Retropharyngeal space
	Superficial and deep temporal pouches

The infections originating from the maxillary anterior teeth spread to the infraorbital space while as that from the molars spread to the buccal space, the infratemporal space and the maxillary sinus. The infections originating from the palatal root of the maxillary molars may form a localized palatal abscess. (Fig. 17.6).

Table 17.4: Probable etiology, contents and the related spaces

Space	Likely causes	Contents	Neighbouring spaces
Buccal	Upper premolars Upper molars Lower premolars	Parotid duct Anterior facial artery and vein Transverse facial artery and vein Buccal fat pad	Infraorbital Pterygomandibular Infratemporal
Infraorbital	Upper canine	Angular artery and vein Infraorbital nerve	Buccal
Submandibular	Lower molars	Submandibular gland Facial artery and vein Lymph nodes	Sublingual Submental Lateral pharyngeal Buccal
Submental	Lower anteriors Symphysis fracture	Anterior jugular vein Lymph nodes	Submandibular (on either side)
Sublingual	Lower premolars Lower molars Direct trauma	Sublingual glands Whartson's duct Lingual nerve Sublingual artery and vein	Submandibular Lateral pharyngeal Visceral (trachea and esophagus)
Pterygomandibular	Lower third molars Fracture of mandible angle	Mandibular division of trigeminal nerve Inferior alveolar artery and vein	Buccal Lateral pharyngeal Submasseteric Deep temporal Parotid
Submasseteric	Lower third molars Fracture of mandible angle	Masseteric artery and vein	Buccal Pterygomandibular Superficial temporal Parotid
Infratemporal and deep temporal	Upper molars	Pterygoid plexus Interior maxillary artery and vein Mandibular division of trigeminal nerve Skull base foramina	Buccal Superficial temporal Inferior petrosal sinus
Superficial temporal	Upper molars Lower molars	Temporal fat pad Temporal branch of facial nerve	Buccal Deep temporal
Lateral pharyngeal	Lower third molars Tonsils Infections in neighboring spaces	Carotid artery Internal jugular vein Vagus nerve Cervical sympathetic vein	Pterygomandibular Submandibular Sublingual Peritonsillar Retropharyngeal

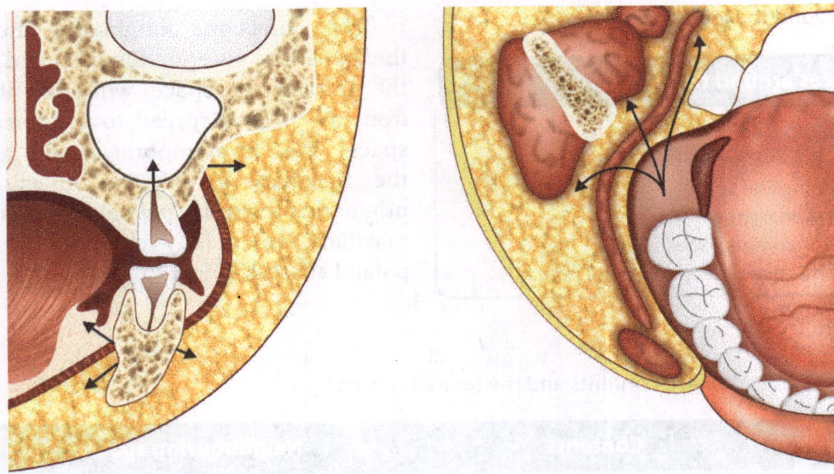

Fig. 17.5A: Spread of infection from the teeth to various spaces

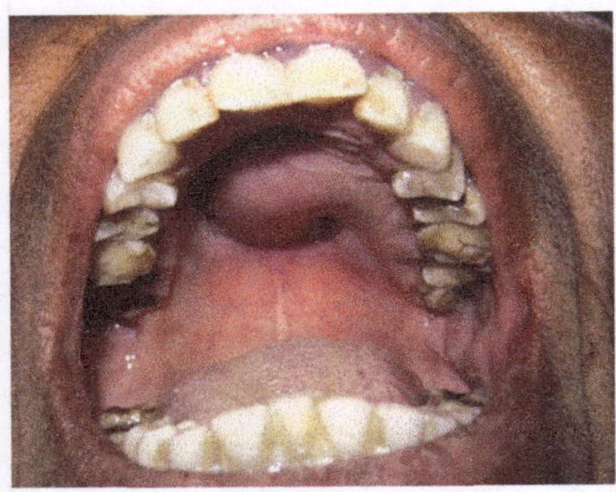

Fig. 17.5B: Palatal abscess due to periapical infection originating from the palatal root of maxillary molar

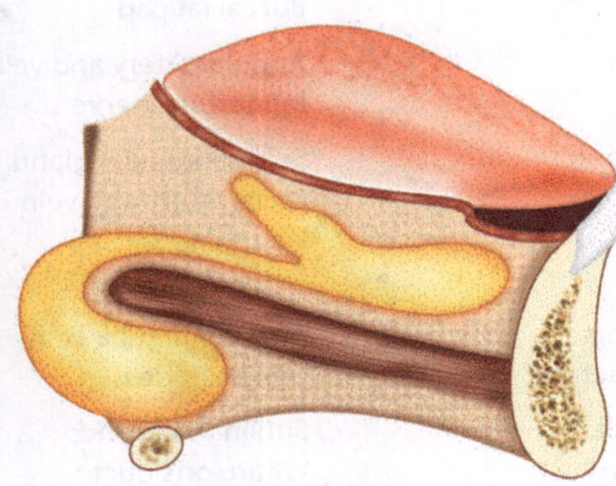

Fig. 17.6: Spread of infection from sublingual to submandibular space behind the mylohyoid muscle

Although the involvement of the particular space commonly occurs due to a specific tooth, it is not a rule of thumb (Table 17.5). Moreover, the infection when aggressive rapidly spreads to the adjacent spaces. If we carefully look at the spaces it will be noticed that the superficial temporal pouch freely communicates with the submasseteric space, inferiorly, while as the deep temporal pouch communicates inferiorly with infratemporal fossa, the lateral pharyngeal space and with the pterygomandibular space. Similarly due to the presence of loose spaces between the instrinsic muscles of the tongue, a unilateral sublingual space infection rapidly becomes bilateral. As the sublingual space is separated from the submandibular space by an incomplete partition of the mylohyoid, the infection from one space extends to the other from the posterior border of this muscle. In short although these anatomical compartments try to limit the spread of the infection, they are liable to breakdown and the infection can still spread to the adjacent area by breaking down of these barriers. Apart from the virulence of the microorganisms and the effects of their toxins on the intercellular cementing substance, the other major determinant is pressure generated within the tissue by inflammatory edema, which causes breakdown of these barriers and facilitates the lateral spread of the infection.

SPACES AROUND THE MANDIBLE

Submandibular Space Infection

Surgical Anatomy

The submandibular space is present below the mandible. It is also called as the digastric triangle as it is bound anteroposteoriorly by the anterior and the posterior bellies of the digastric muscle, respectively. The medial wall is formed by the mylohyoid muscle and the hyoglossus muscle while the lateral

Table 17.5: Various space infection and their synonyms

Name	Synonym
Space of the body of the mandible	Mandibular space
Submandibular space	Submaxillary space Submylohyoid space
Masticator space	Masticatory space Masseteric space
Temporal space	Temporal pouches
Infratemporal spaces	Postzygomatic space
Buccal space	Buccinator space
Infraorbital space	Canine space
Lateral pharyngeal space	Parapharyngeal space Pharygomaxillary space
Retropharyngeal space	Retroesophageal space
Pretracheal space	Perivisceral spaces Paravisceral spaces Paratracheal spaces
Carotid space	Visceral vascular space Anterior Lincoln's highway

Box 17.1: Boundaries of the space

Anterior	Anterior belly of digastric muscle
Posterior	Posterior belly of digastric muscle, stylohyoid muscle stylopharyngeous muscle
Superior	Medial aspect of mandible and attachment of mylohyoid muscle
Inferior	Anterior and posterior bellies of digastric muscle
Medial	Mylohyoid, hyoglossus, styloglossus
Lateral	Skin, superficial fascia, platysma, superficial, layer of deep cervical fascia Anterior bellies of digastric muscles

wall is formed by the skin, superficial fascia and the platysma. The base of the submandibular space is situated at the lower border of the mandible and the apex is at the common tendon of the digastric muscle at the greater cornu of the hyoid bone (Box 17.1). The contents are the submandibular lymph nodes, the submandibular salivary gland, facial artery and anterior facial vein.

Applied Anatomy

The space lies between the anterior and posterior bellies of digastric muscles. The mylohyoid muscle which forms the floor of the oral cavity separates this space from the sublingual space below, is the key to diagnosis and surgical management of this space infections. This muscle attaches to the lingual surface of mandible along the mylohyoid ridge which runs obliquely and downward from posterior to anterior. Odontogenic infections of this space are commonly caused by 2nd and 3rd molar teeth and rarely by 1st molar as their root apices lie inferior to mylohyoid line of muscle attachment. Only loose connective tissues separate one side of floor of mouth from other permitting bilateral spread of infection with ease (Figs 17.6 and 17.7).

Diagnosis is established by brawny or soft swelling in the submandibular region along with an associated diseased mandibular molar. Infectious process commonly spreads across the midline into contralateral submandibular space.

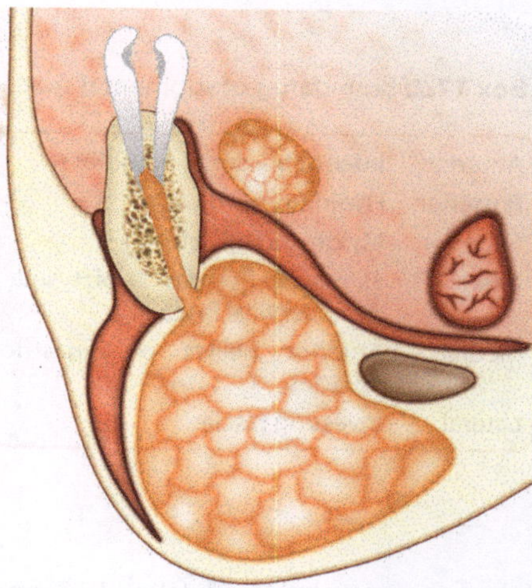

Fig. 17.7: Spread of periapical infection from the molar to submandibular space below the mylohyoid line

Source of Infection

- The common sources of infection are the odontogenic infections from the mandibular posterior teeth,[1] either by direct spread or spread through the lymphatics. The involved lymph nodes breakdown due to suppuration and the septic material is discharged in the adjoining tissue space.
- Septic fractures of the mandible,[2] osteomyelitis of mandible.
- The infections originating from the submandibular salivary gland due to sialoithiasis and the other suppurative glandular pathologies.[3]
- Rarely hematogenous infections, extension from adjacent tissue spaces like submasseteric space, sublingual space can also lead to the submandibular space infection.

Clinical Features

- There is a swelling involving the submandibular area, which is diffuse in the beginning and tends to get localized and extends from the lower border of the mandible to the hyoid bone, superioinferiorly. More virulent infections break the tissue barriers and spread to the adjoining space.
- The muscles become spastic and there may be trismus.
- The swelling shows all the classical signs of inflammatory swelling like redness, raised local temperature, tenderness and pain. Initially, the diffuse swelling is firm in consistency and pits on pressure due to cellulites, but as the abscess gets localized bimanual palpation elicits fluctuations.
- Constitutional sign and symptoms are present in the acute phase.
- The submandibular lymph nodes are enlarged, tender and firm in consistency, but they are difficult to assess in presence of swelling.

Management

The primary management is surgical drainage. The incision and drainage is done through a standard submandibular incision taken 1 cm below and behind the inferior border of the mandible to avoid the damage to the marginal mandibular branch of facial nerve (Figs 17.8A and B). Superficial abscesses are drained through a stab incision, but the deep seated abscess is drained by dissecting the tissue layer wise to open the skin, superficial fascia, platysma and deep fascia. In deep seated abscess, sometimes the fluctuations are difficult to be elicited and thus to confirm the presence of the pus in deeper planes it is a good idea to insert a wide bore needle and aspirate. The incision is always placed on the dependent part to facilitate gravity assisted drainage, however when the abscess is pointing

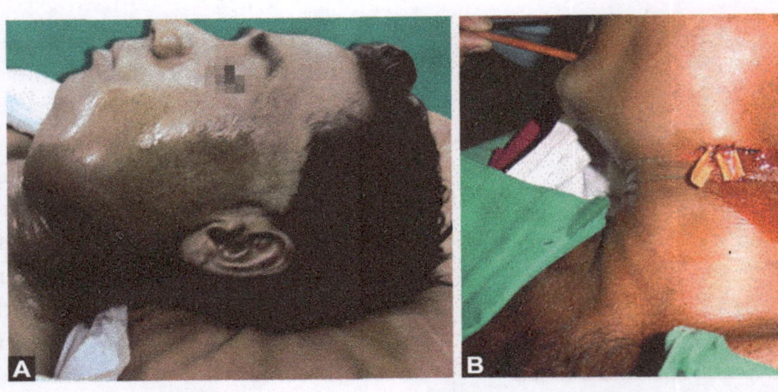

Figs 17.8A and B: A case of submandibular abscess drained by incision and drainage, corrugated rubber dam drain in place

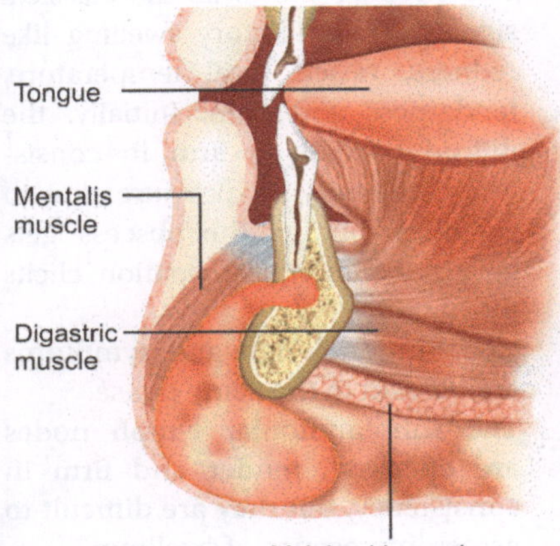

Fig. 17.9: Anatomical boundaries of the submental space

on skin, the incision may be placed on the most prominent part to drain the abscess and to achieve the gravity assisted drainage, especially in the large abscess cavities, another counter incision is placed at the dependent site. The drainage of the septic material helps in reducing the edema, prevent further spread of infection due to reduced tension in the tissue planes and prevent further absorption of the septic material. The septic focus like offending tooth should also be removed simultaneously to prevent the infection from slipping into chronic phase from the acute phase (Fig. 17.9).

Submental Space

A potential space exists in the chin. If the infection from the incisors exits labially through the mandibular bone, inferior to the muscle attachments, the submental space gets involved (Box 17.2 and Fig. 17.9). The chin appears grossly swollen and is quite firm and erythematous. Submental infection may spread easily to either or both submandibular spaces (*see* Fig. 17.6).

Box 17.2: Boundaries of submental space

Anterior	Inferior border of mandible
Posterior	Hyoid bone
Superior	Mylohyoid muscle
Inferior	Skin, superficial fascia, platysma, deep cervical fascia
Medial	Anterior bellies of digastric muscles
Lateral	Investing fascia

Source of Infection

- Infections from the lower anterior teeth
- Infected symphyseal or parasymphyseal fractures
- Extension of submandibular space infection
- Suppuration in the submental lymph nodes.

Clinical Features

- The submental space infection produces a swelling below the chin producing a classical double chin appearance (Figs 17.10A and B).
- The skin is erythematous, tense, glossy and tender to touch.
- The local temperature is raised.
- Once the infection gets localized, the fluctuations may be elicited.

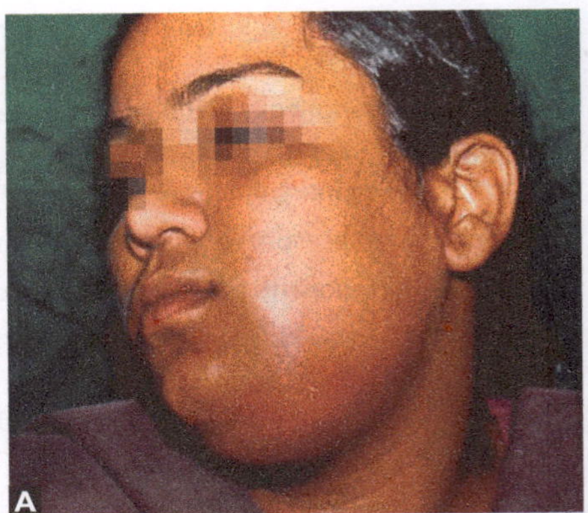

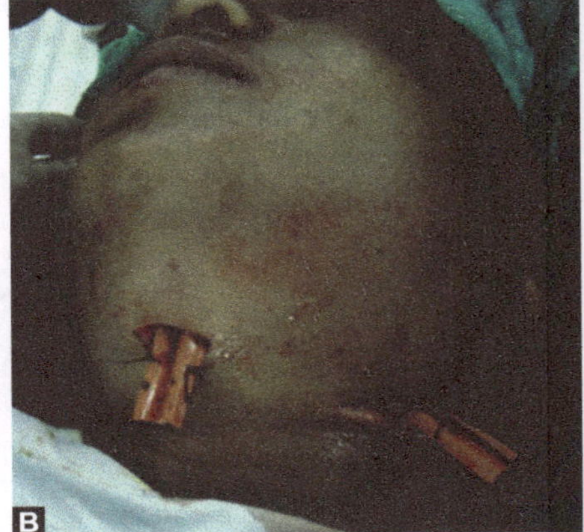

Figs 17.10A and B: Submental space infection drained by incision and drainage

Management

Percutaneous surgical drainage is the most effective approach. Transverse incision is given in the skin below the symphysis of the mandible provides dependent drainage and the most cosmetically acceptable scar. Blunt dissection is carried out by inserting a sinus forceps in upward and backward direction. Drain is inserted. Space may be drained orally through the mentalis muscle through the labial vestibule, but dependent drainage cannot be established (Figs 17.11A and B).

Sublingual Space Infection

The sublingual space is located within the mandibular body, extending from the genial tubercles anteriorly up to the base of the tongue, at the body of the hyoid bone. It is a 'V'-shaped space lying lateral to muscles of tongue, including hyoglossus, genioglossus and geniohyoid. The roof is formed by the mucosa of the floor of the mouth. The

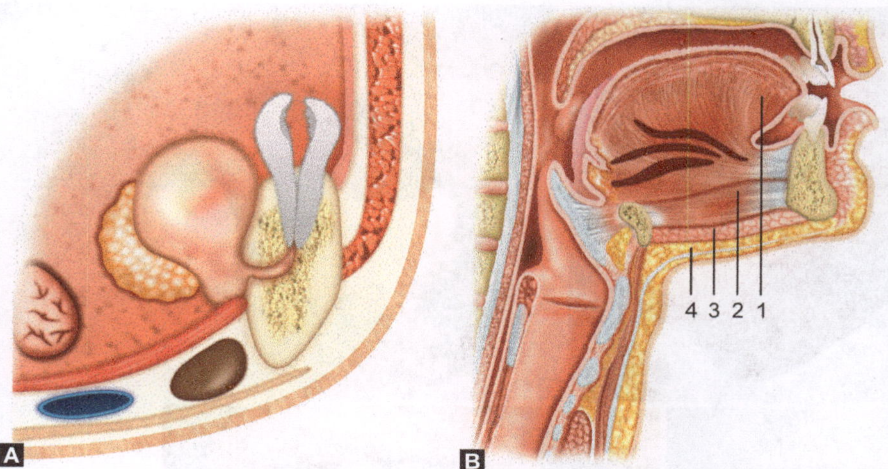

Figs 17.11A and B: Sublingual space infection: (A) Showing sublingual spread of the infection through the perforation of the lingual cortex, as the root tip is above the attachment of mylohyoid resulting in sublingual space infection; (B) Loose spaces in the floor of mouth (2) and around the intrinsic muscles (1) of the tongue facilitate the bilateral spread of the infection. (3) Geniohyoid muscle and (4) Deep cervical facial

floor is formed by the mylohyoid anteriorly and the hyoglossus posteriorly (Box 17.3). The space contains the duct of the submandibular gland and the part of the gland which lies superior to the mylohyoid. The sublingual gland is also enclosed in this place. The lingual nerve and the submandibular ganglion are also present within this space.

Applied Anatomy

Anteriorly the sublingual space communicates with submental space. In this area, the sublingual space may be invaded by infection from incisor teeth especially from periodontal infections. Posteriorly, it is continuous with the submandibular space at posterior edge of mylohyoid muscle and the infection can traverse into submandibular space.

Box 17.3: Boundaries of the sublingual space

Anterior	Lingual aspect of mandible
Posterior	Body of hyoid
Superior	Mucosa of floor of mouth
Inferior	Mylohyoid muscle
Medial	Anterior bellies of digastric muscles
Lateral	Investing fascia

Elevation of tongue is clinical hallmark of sublingual space infection. Patient is usually unable to protrude his tongue to or beyond vermillion border of upper lip.

Source of Infection

- Odontogenic infections from mandibular teeth which drain above the mylohyoid muscle (Fig. 17.11).
- Infection of the sublingual or submandibular salivary glands.
- Extension of the submandibular, submental or pterygomandibular spaces.

Clinical Features

The initial clinical feature of the sublingual space infection is the congestion and edema of the floor of the mouth (Figs 17.12C and D). The edema increases rapidly to cause elevation and protrusion of the tongue (Figs 17.12A to C). This sign is the warning sign of the impending laryngeal edema as the sublingual space extends right up to the hyoid bone and can induce the laryngeal edema. This emergency drainage must be undertaken to prevent respiratory embarrassment due to the laryngeal edema. The earliest warning sign of the laryngeal edema is complaint of breathlessness in supine position and the patient prefers to stay in the sitting position.

Management

An incision is made close to the lingual cortical plate, lateral to the sublingual plica, as lingual nerve, which is deeply placed, is less likely to be damaged by this approach. The other important structures lie medial to the plica is Wharton's duct, sublingual artery and veins (Figs 17.12E). The sinus forceps is then inserted and opened to evacuate the pus. If the space is drained extraorally, a submandibular incision is taken and a sinus forcep is introduced to pierce the mylohyoid muscle, which forms the floor of the sublingual space. This approach provides gravity dependent drainage.

Masticatory Space

Masticatory space is formed by splitting of investing fascia into superficial and deep layers. The superficial layer lies along lateral surfaces of masseter and lower half of temporalis muscles.

Applied Anatomy

Superiorly the superficial layer fuses with periosteum of zygoma and temporalis fascia. The deep layer passes along the medial surface of pterygoid muscles before attaching to base of skull superiorly. Like the perimandibular spaces, masticatory space is one anatomical compartment enclosed by splitting of the anterior layer of deep cervical fascia around the muscles of mastication (Fig. 17.13). Infections of this space occur more frequently from third molars, the pericoronitis associated with it and caries induced dental abscesses, contaminated inferior alveolar nerve blocks, direct trauma or through surgery in the area.

The clinical features comprise of swelling around the ramus of mandible, pain, tenderness, fever and difficulty in deglution. The hallmark of masticatory space infection is trismus.

The masticatory space comprises of following four spaces:

1. Pterygomandibular space.
2. Submasseteric space.
3. Temporal space.
4. Infratemporal space.

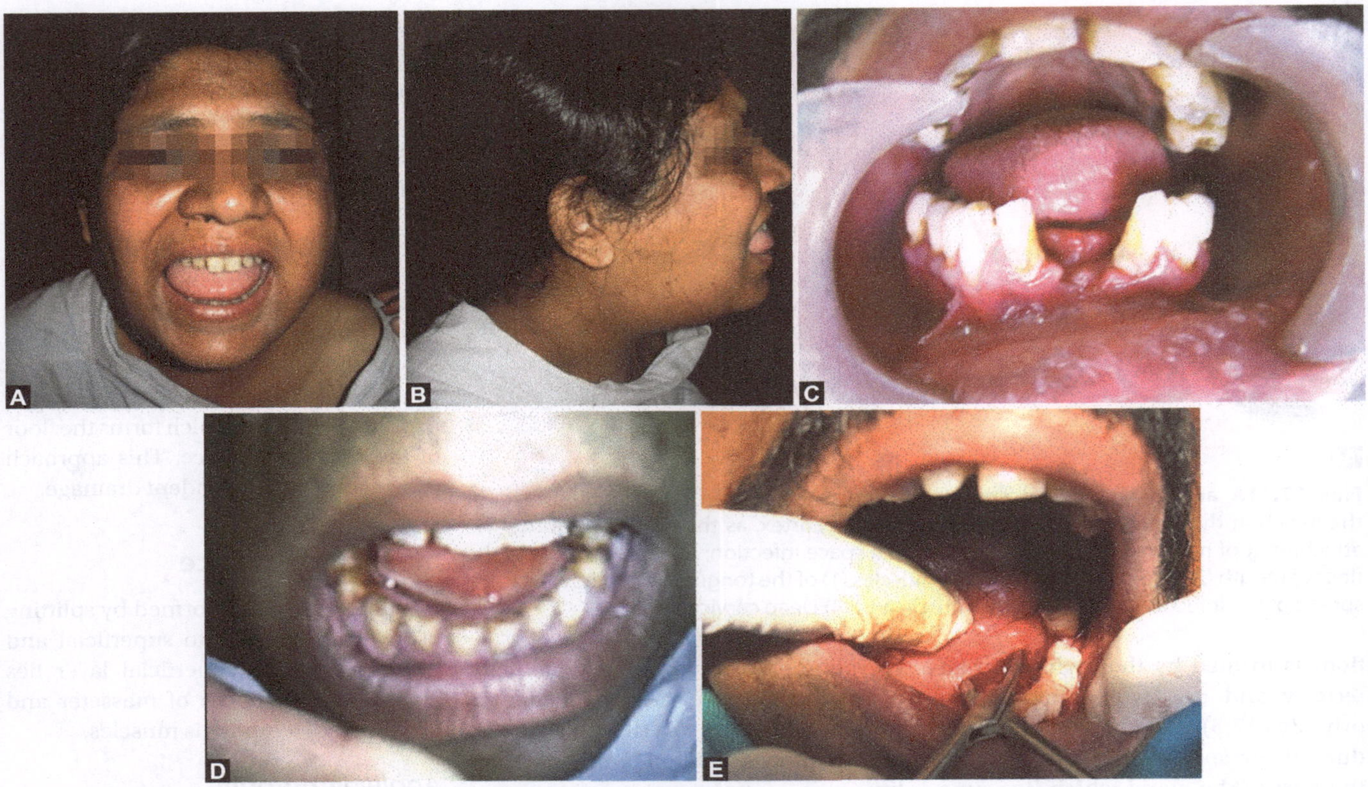

Figs 17.12A to E: Sublingual space infection: (A and B) Protrusion and lifting of the tongue; (C and D) Elevation of the floor of mouth; (E) The space drained by a transoral incision

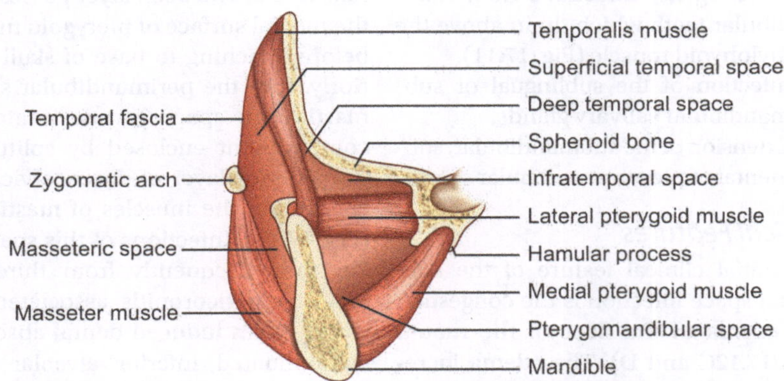

Fig. 17.13: Masticator space and its communicating spaces

Management

Masseteric and pterygoid compartments may be entered by superficial, sharp and deep blunt dissection at the external angle of the mandible avoiding the mandibular branch of facial nerve. This approach allows dependent drainage of both the spaces at the insertion of muscle sling on inferior border at mandibular angle. Extraoral incision and drainage is a more technical and prudent than intraoral approach.

Pterygomandibular Space

Of all the severe odontogenic infections, it is the most frequently affected anatomical compartment. Infections of this space are correlated highly with pericoronitis of mandibular 3rd molar. Trismus caused by edema and inflammation of the medial pterygoid muscle hinders the view of swollen anterior tonsilar pillar and the deviation of uvula to opposite side that are characteristic of infection in this space. Infection may spread into infratemporal portion of the deep temporal space by passing superiorly around lateral pterygoid muscle. More commonly infection spreads to the lateral pharyngeal space.

The pterygomandibular space lies medial to the ramus of the mandible and its boundaries are shown in Box 17.4 and Fig. 17.14.

Contents

Mandibular nerve, lingual nerve, inferior alveolar artery and vein mylohyoid nerve and vessels.

- **Teeth involved:** Buccal roots of maxillary second and third molars.
- **Spread:** Superficial temporal, parotid spaces.

Box 17.4: Boundaries of pterygomandibular space

Laterally	Anterior border of ramus of mandible
Medially	Medial pterygoid muscle
Superiorly	Infratemporal surface of greater wing of sphenoid and zygomatic arch, lateral pterygoid muscle
Inferiorly	Pterygomasseteric sling
Anteriorly	Buccinator and superior pharyngeal constrictor muscles as they meet at the pterygomandibular raphe
Posteriorly	Deep portion of parotid gland

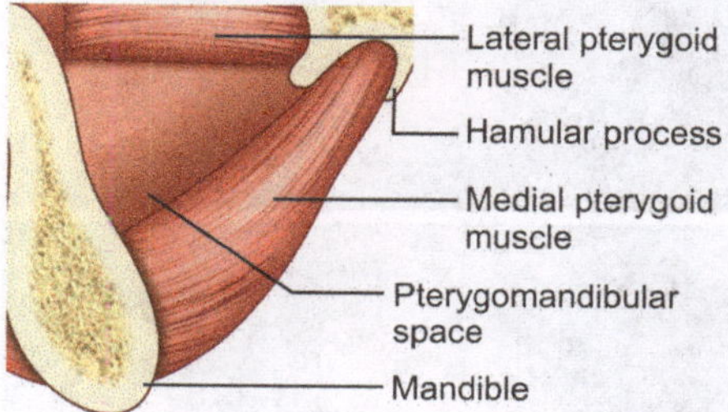

Fig. 17.14: Boundaries of the pterigomandibular space

Fig. 17.15: Drainage of pterygomandibular space through Risdon's approach

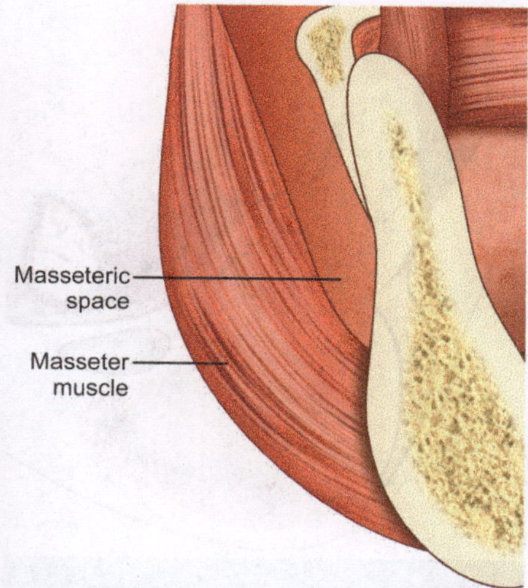

Fig. 17.16: Anatomic boundaries of the submasseteric space

Applied Anatomy

Needle track infections occur most often in the pterygomandibular space because of attempts to anesthetize inferior alveolar nerve before dental procedures. Incision is given in the buccal vestibule opposite second and third molars. The exploration is carried out medial to coronoid process and temporalis muscle upwards and backwards with a sinus forceps. The space is entered and drained and drain is secured.

Sources of Infection

- Due to contaminated needles/solution used while giving pterygomandibular block.
- Septic fractures of mandibular ramus.
- Infections from mandibular third molars.

Management

An incision is placed along the anterior border of the coronoid process and the sinus forcep is passed medial to the ramus of the mandible to enter and drain the pterygomandibular space, transorally. However, in presence of severe trismus when transoral drainage is not possible an extraoral submandibular 'Risdon's incision' is placed and the dissection is carried out medially to detach the insertion of the medial pterygoid muscle from the angle of the mandible to drain the pterygomandibular space (Fig. 17.15). The drain is placed *in situ*. Jaw exercises (active moth opening) are necessary to prevent the trismus post operatively.

Submasseteric Space Infection

Surgical Anatomy

The submasseteric space is present lateral to the ascending ramus of the mandible (Figs 17.16 and 17.17A). It is bounded laterally by the masseter muscle and the fascia covering it, medially by the lateral surface of the ascending ramus. Inferiorly, it extends up to the insertion of the masseter at the angle of the mandible and superiorly it extends up to the origin of the masseter at the inferior border of the zygomatic arch and thus the submasseteric space infection can also extend to the infratemporal fossa.[4]

Source of Infection[5,6]

- Mandibular third molar infections are the most common source of infection as the infection can extend subperiosteally in the submasseteric space. The infections from the mandibular posterior teeth can also lead to the submasseteric space infections.
- Septic fractures at the angle of the mandible are also the cause of the submasseteric space infection.
- The minor causes are the extension of the infection from the adjoining tissue planes in the infratemporal space, temporal pouch abscess, sublingual space infection, etc. Suppurative parotitis can also secondarily involve the submasseteric space as the parotid fascia after covering the parotid gland goes on to cover the masseter muscle (parotidomasseteric fascia) and the infection can extend into the sub masseteric space.
- Hematogenous spread of the infection can also lead to submasseteric space infection in cases of septicemia.

Clinical Presentation

- The first sign of the submasseteric space infection is trismus due to the spasm of the masseter.[7] The swelling is inconspicuous as the infection lies below the muscle. The mild swelling

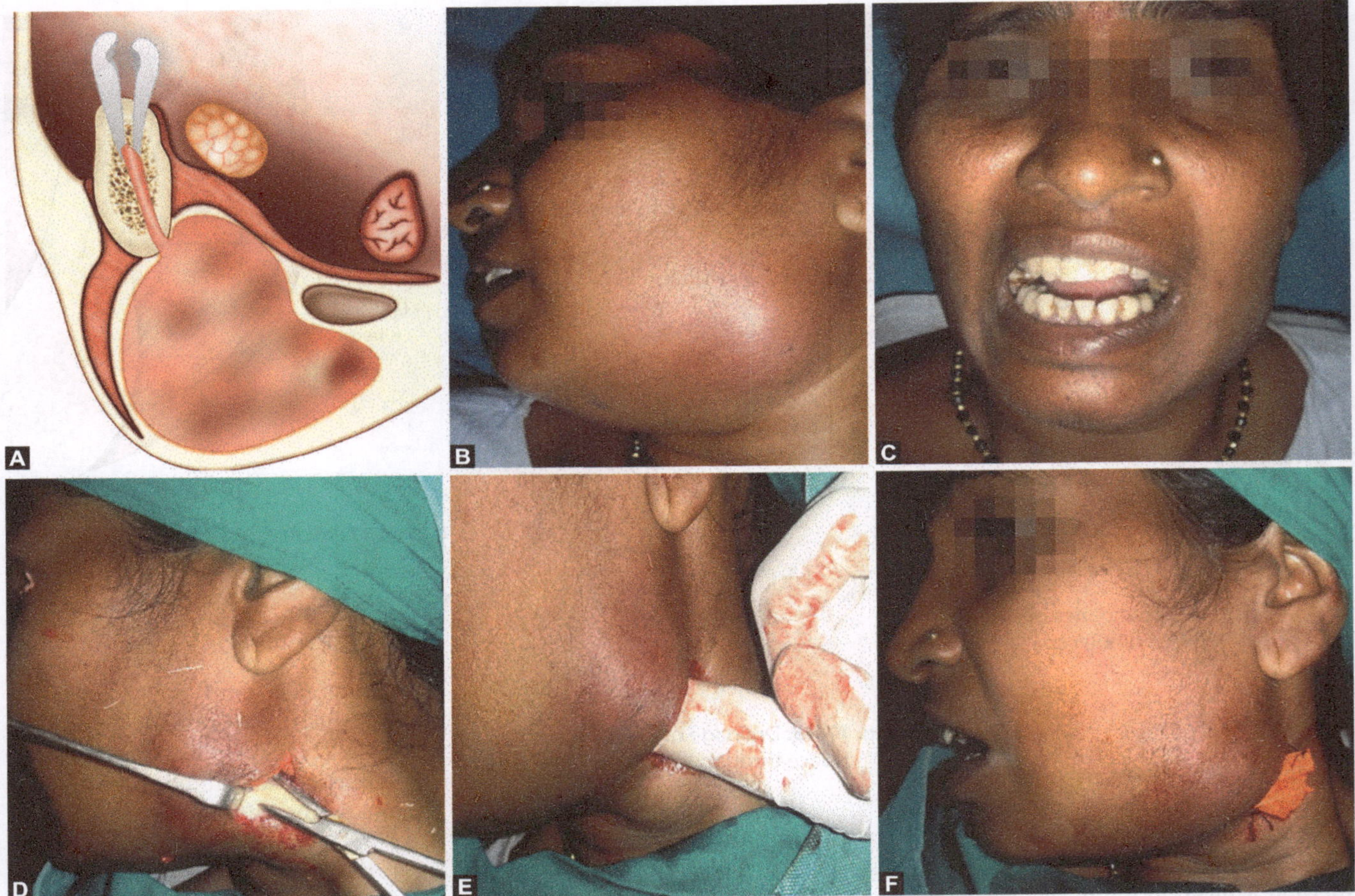

Figs 17.17A to F: Submasseteric space abscess, note the trismus, the abscess is superficial plane leading to dusky appearance to skin, treated with incision and drainage

over the angle of the mandible which is relatively a late occurrence and is diffuse in nature. The infection gets localized due to the anatomical barrier formed by the muscle (Figs 17.17B and C). The swelling sometimes mimics the parotitis and may be misdiagnosed as parotitis. The differentiating feature is that classical parotid swelling is posteriorly present over the parotid area and is associated with lifting of the ear lobule. The more virulent infections rapidly breakdown the tissue barriers and extend to the adjacent tissue planes.

- The infection leads to irritation and spasm of the muscle and leads to trismus.
- The infection when diffuse is firm in consistency and tender to touch the local temperature is also raised.
- When the infection gets localized and still present below the masseter, deep seated fluctuations can be elicited by bimaunal palpation. When the infection becomes superficial by perforating through the fibers of the masseter and comes to lie below the superficial fascia and the skin, the swelling becomes fluctuant due to laudable pus.
- The intraoral septic focus in the form of carious tooth, pericoronitis is usually present.
- General constitutional signs and symptoms like fever, malaise, body ache, etc. are present.

The submasseteric space infection can extend to the submandibular space due to the direct extension.

Management

The medicinal treatment comprises of prescription of antibiotics and anti-inflammatory drugs which help in localizing the infection. The application of glycerine and magsulf dressing during the diffuse state of the infection is also helpful in localizing the infection. Once the infection is localized, surgical treatment like drainage is indicated.

Surgical Management

The surgical treatment comprises of incision and drainage of the abscess. The submassertic space infection/abscess can be drained intraorally as well as extraorally. In the intraoral procedure, an incision is placed in the retromolar area along the anterior border of the ramus and the dissection is done along the lateral border of the ramus. An artery forcep is introduced between the ramus and the masseter muscle to drain the abscess. A guaze drain is placed to facilitate the drainage of the pus along it. The disadvantage of this procedure is that the incision site is not dependent and the gravity assisted drainage is not present.

The extraoral procedure consists of placing a standard Risdon's submandibular incision 1 cm below and behind the inferior border of the mandible and curling around the angle. The incision avoids damage to the marginal mandibular branch of the facial nerve and the scar is hidden. The superficial abscess gets drained with only a stab incision. But, the deep seated abscess is drained by dissecting the tissue layer by layer and after incising and reflecting the fibers of the masseter muscle at its insertion at the angle of the mandible, taking precaution not to damage the facial artery (Figs 17.17D to F).

A sinus forceps or a gloved finger is passed through the incision and moved in different directions to break all the loculi and achieve full drainage. A corrugated rubber dam drain is inserted and kept in place to facilitate drainage. If there is bleeding from the absess cavity then an iodoform, acriflavine or the glycerine-magsulf tape gauze is gently packed in abscess cavity to achieve the hemostasis and keep the drainage site patent.

SPACES AROUND MAXILLA

Buccal Space

Buccal space is the potential space between buccinator muscle and masseter muscle[8] (Box 17.5 and Fig. 17.18).

Infection of this space is identified easily because of marked cheek swelling associated with a diseased molar or premolar tooth. Because the buccal space is a portion of the subcutaneous space, buccal infections can spread through the subcutaneous space into the periorbital space and pass the inferior border of mandible to the subcutaneous tissue lying superficial to the submandibular space, this spread may confuse the diagnosis of submandibular space abscess.

Box 17.5: Boundaries of buccal space

Superior	Zygomatic arch, infraorbital space
Inferior	Lower border of mandible
Anterior	Zygomaticus major muscle above and depressor anguli oris muscle
Posterior	Anterior edge of masseter muscle, pterygomandibular space
Medial	Buccinator muscle, buccopharyngeal fascia
Lateral	Skin, subcutaneous tissue

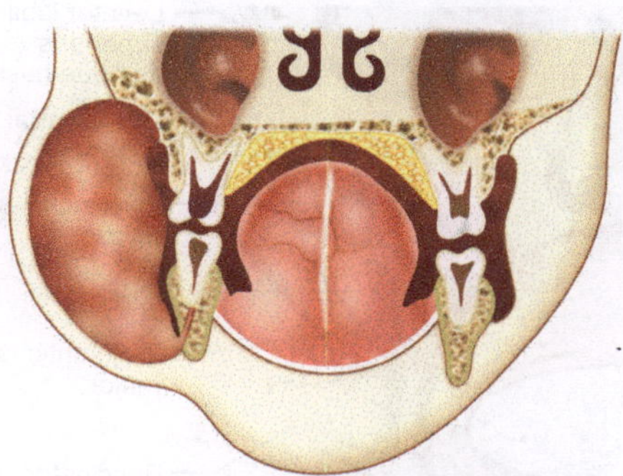

Fig. 17.18: Buccal spread of infection via periapical infection of maxillary and mandibular teeth

Source of Infection[9]

- Maxillary premolars and molars if root apices are above the attachment of the buccinator muscle.
- Mandibular premolars and molars if root apices are below the attachment of the buccinator muscle.

Clinical Features

- Extraoral swelling of the cheek from lower border of mandible to infraorbital rim (Figs 17.19A and 17.20) and from anterior border of masseter to corner of mouth when the lower compartment is involved. When the upper compartment is involved (due to maxillary teeth) the swelling extends from the zygomatic bone to the corner of the mouth. As the face has plenty of loose areolar spaces the adjoining area is edematous and presents like a diffuse cellulitis.
- The obliteration of the buccal vestibule occurs due to bulging swelling in the buccal vestibule of the maxilla or the mandible, depending on whether the upper or lower compartment is involved.

Management

The management comprises of drainage of the abscess transorally, by placing

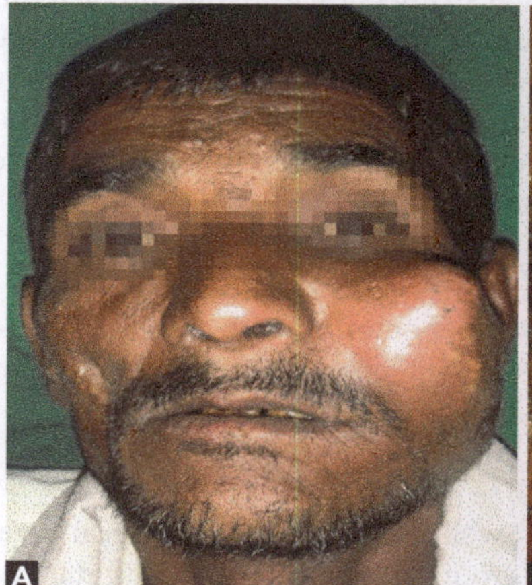

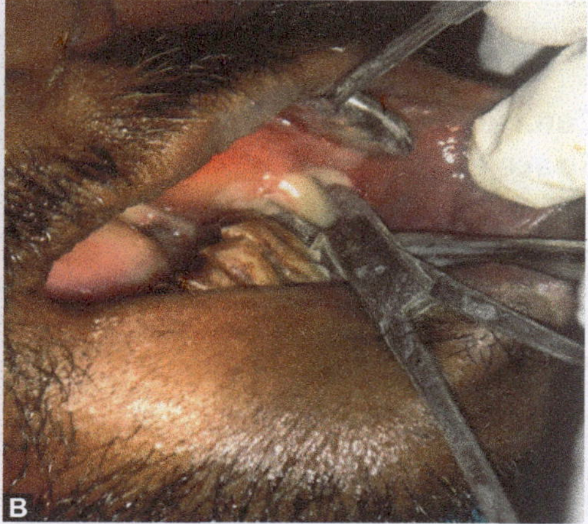

Figs 17.19A and B: (A) Localized buccal space abscess; (B) Drained intraorally at dependent site although the prominent part was extraorally

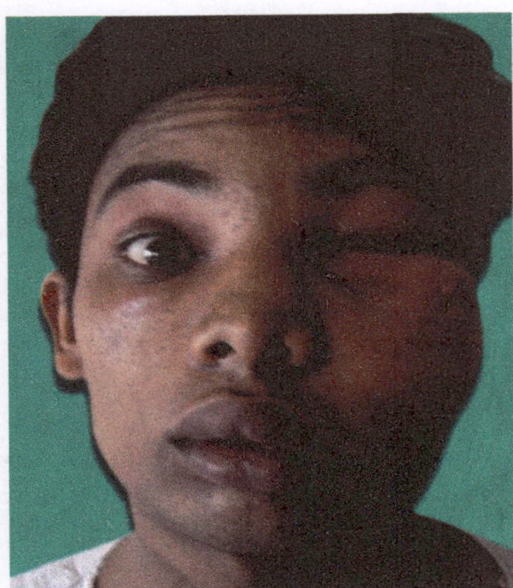

Fig. 17.20: Diffuse cellulitis due to buccal space infection

the incision in the respective buccal vestibule (Fig. 17.19B). Even if the abscess is localized and the prominent part is on the skin incision should be avoided to prevent unsightly scar on the face. The drain is left *in situ*. The maxillary buccal space drains passively with a vestibular incision as it is facilitated by gravity. But for the mandibular buccal space as the gravity assisted drainage is not possible, libral incision should be taken and the collection should be periodically evacuated by compressing the tissue extraorally. Even if the infection is not localized and is in the stage of cellulitis decompression by way of placing incision produces rewarding results by causing early resolution.

Canine Space or Infraorbial Space Infection

The canine space or infraorbital space is situated over the anterior surface of the maxilla in the infra orbital area and its boundaries are as shown in (Box 17.6 and Fig. 17.21).

Box 17.6: Boundaries of canine space

Superior	Levator labii superioris alaeque nasi, levator labii superioris, zygomaticus minor
Inferior	Caninus (Levator anguli oris), oral mucosa
Anterior	Orbicularis oris, nasal cartilages
Posterior	Buccinator and buccal space
Medial	Anterolateral surface of maxilla

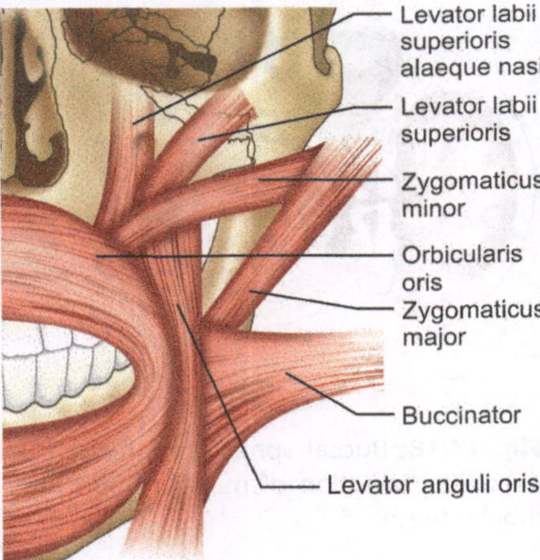

Fig. 17.21: Anatomical boundaries of the canine space

Clinical Features

Odontogenic infection enter the canine space from the periapical abscess of the maxillary canine that erode through the buccal cortex superior to the attachment of the levator anguli oris muscle. The levator of the upper lip (quadratus labii superioris) originates from the face of the maxilla by several heads to insert into the angle of the mouth. Medially, a potential space exists between the infraorbital and zygomatic heads, as well as between it and the caninus muscle arising from the bone above the canine fossa. This represents a plane along which an infection from the canine tooth can track superiorly. Alternatively, there may be direct extension from maxillary vestibular infections and from buccal space infection that pass freely into the canine space.

Source of Infection

- Upper anterior teeth and bicuspid
- Skin infection from nose and upper lip.

Signs and Symptoms

- Swelling is present from lateral nasal groove to the anterior boundary of the buccal space and from upper lip to the preseptal area of the lower eyelid (Fig. 17.22).

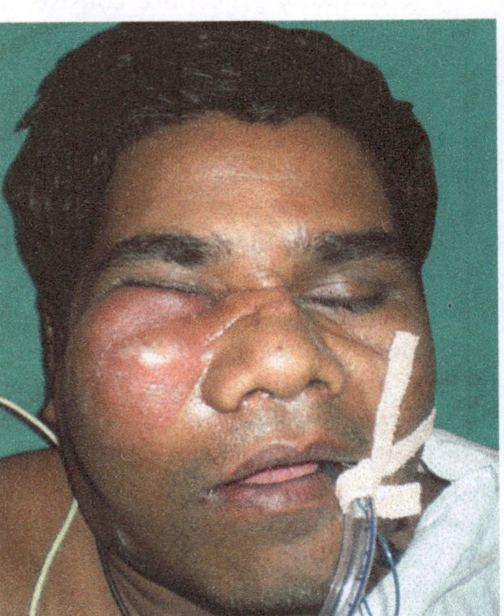

Fig. 17.22: Infraorbital space infection, note edema of eyelids

- Cheek swelling and redness.
- Obliteration of nasolabial folds.
- Obliteration of the labial vestibule due to the swelling.
- Edema of upper and lower eyelid.
- Tenderness and severe pain secondary to infraorbital nerve edema and inflammations.

The swelling of the eyelids is a common occurrence due to the presence of the loose areolar tissue. The edema is more conspicuous in the morning when the patient gets up from sleep (dependent edema) and it gradually gets reduced over a period of time, as the patient is upright. The edema sometimes extends to upper eyelid closing the eye completely. The abscess tends to point intraorally in the labial vestibule.

Surgical Treatment

Treatment is by dependent drainage intraorally or percutaneously if the abscess is pointing there. The transoral

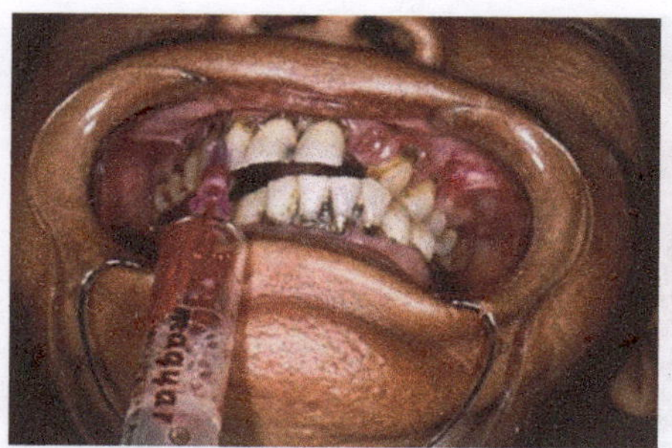

Fig. 17.23: Aspiration of the blood stained, purulent material in a case of canine space infection

dissection is preferred as the percutaneous drainage leaves an unsightly scar on the face. As with all infections from pulpally involved teeth, extraction or root-canal therapy of the offending tooth is also necessary.

Drainage of the canine space abscess is made by making incision parallel to and in depth of the maxillary vestibule adjacent to the abscessed tooth (Fig. 17.23). Blunt dissection is carried superiorly through the levator anguli oris muscle into the canine space. Careful dissection is necessary to preserve the infraorbital nerve and its branches. A drain is positioned into the infected space and secured in position by suture.

Aggressive antibiotic therapy is important to aid in resolution of the local infection and to prevent the extension into the orbit and the brain as it lies in the '*Danger zone*' of the face.

Angular vein, an ascending branch of the facial vein, courses through the canine space. Canine space infection may give rise to septic thrombi in the angular vein, which can travel to the cavernous sinus by way of superior and inferior ophthalmic vein of the orbit.[10]

Temporal Space

Temporal pouches are fascial spaces in relation to temporalis muscle. They are two in number—superficial and deep temporal space.

Superficial Temporal Space

Superficial temporal space lies between the deep temporal fascia which is continuation of parotideomasseteric fascia and the temporalis muscle.

Box 17.7: Boundaries of the superficial temporal space

Laterally	Skin, temporal fascia
Medially	Squamous temporal bone and skull base
Inferiorly	Superior surface of lateral pterygoid muscle
Superiorly and posteriorly	Attachment of temporalis to cranium, anterior border
Anteriorly	Posterior wall of maxillary sinus, pterygomandibular fissure

Box 17.8: Boundaries of the deep temporal space

Laterally	Temporalis muscle
Medially	Lateral surface of the temporalis muscle
Inferiorly	Superior surface of lateral pterygoid muscle
Superiorly and posteriorly	Attachment of temporal fascia to cranium, anterior border
Anteriorly	Attachment of the fascia to the orbital process of the zygoma

Boundaries (Boxes 17.7 and 17.8)

Anteriorly: Posterior surface of lateral orbital rim.

Posteriorly: Fusion of temporal fascia with pericranium.

Inferiorly: Zygomatic arch (Fig. 17.24).

Applied anatomy

Temporal fascia splits into two layers that pass lateral and medial to zygomatic arch. This compartment contains leaflet of buccal fat pad and three small veins that drain temporal region. Buccal space infection may follow buccal fat pad into this space.

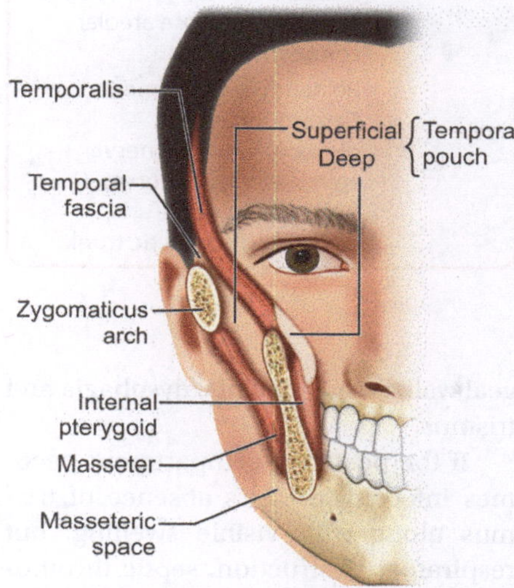

Fig. 17.24: Anatomical boundaries of the temporal pouches

Deep Temporal Space

Deep temporal space lies deep to temporalis muscle and skull. Below the level of zygomatic arch, superficial and deep space communicate directly with the infratemporal and pterygopalatine fossa.

Contents

Terminal division of internal maxillary artery and mandibular division of trigeminal nerve

Clinical Features

The temporal space infections produce a mild swelling in the temporal area (Fig. 17.25A). The swelling is not very conspicuous due to the presence of the tenacious temporal fascia in case of superficial pouch involvement and in case of the deep pouch, due to the presence of the temporalis muscle and overlying fascia. The hallmark of the temporal pouch infection is trismus due to the spasm of the temporalis muscle.[11] The superficial pouch infection extents below the zygomatic arch in the massetric area producing a classical 'dumbbell'-shaped swelling (Fig. 17.25C). The deep pouch infections can extend to the infratemporal, lateral pharyngeal and pterigomandibular spaces.

Management

Extraoral incision is placed in the temporal region, well above the hairline,

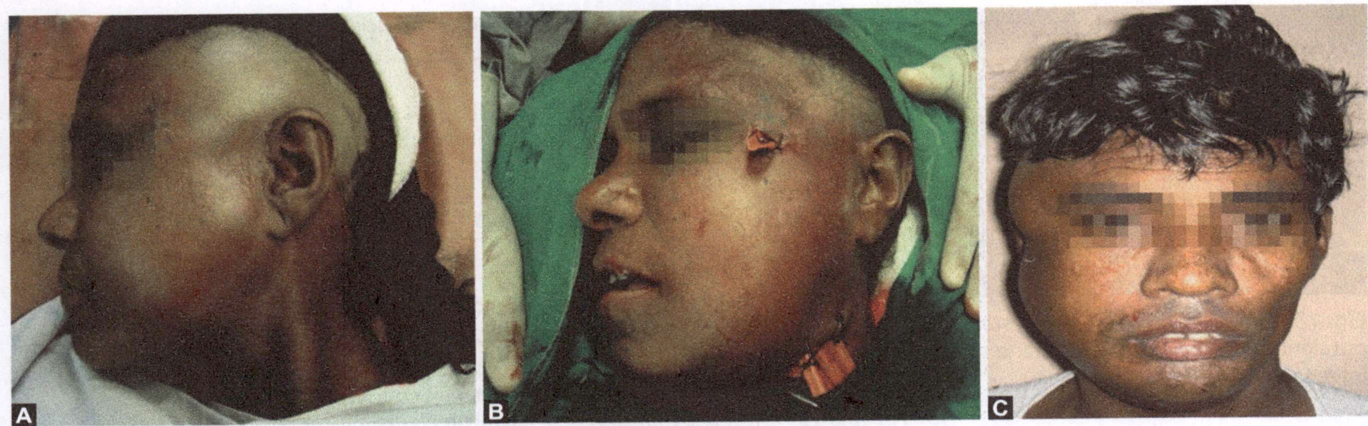

Figs 17.25A to C: Typical dumbbell-shaped swelling in temporal pouch infection

45 degrees to zygomatic arch. The hemostat is inserted above and below the temporalis muscle. The care should be taken not to damage the branches of facial nerve. The incision can be placed above and parallel to the zygomatic arch (Fig. 17.25B). The temporal fascia is divided to evacuate the contents of the superficial pouch and the temporalis muscle is pierced open to drain the contents of the deep pouch. As the abscess cavity heals by fibrosis there can be persistant trismus and hence postoperative physiotherapy should be given to prevent the muscle fibrosis and trismus.

Parapharyngeal Spaces

Parapharyngeal spaces include lateral pharyngeal and retropharyngeal spaces. They form a ring around pharynx and together form a pathway for spread of orofacial infections in neck and mediastinum.

Lateral Pharyngeal Space (Pharyngomaxillary Space)

Lateral pharyngeal space is a potential, inverted cone, shaped space with its base at the skull and its apex at the greater cornu of hyoid bone (Box 17.9). It is divided into anterior and posterior compartments by styloid process and a short layer of condensed fascia called aponeurosis of *Zuckercandl and Testut.* If the anterior compartment becomes infected, the patient exhibits pain, fever, chills, medial bulging of lateral pharyngeal wall, deviated uvula, dysphagia and trismus.

Box 17.9: Boundaries and contents of the lateral pharyngeal space

Superiorly	Base of skull, petrous part of temporal bone with foramen lacerum and jugular foramen
Inferiorly	Hyoid bone
Anteriorly	Pterygomandibular raphe
Laterally	Ascending ramus of mandible, medial pterygoid muscle, medial surface of deep lobe of parotid gland.
Medially	Pharyngeal wall, superior and middle constrictors and stylopharyngeus
Posteriorly	Stylohyoid muscle, upper part of carotid sheath, prevertebral fascia with foramen lacerum and jugular foramen
Contents	Anterior compartment: Lymph nodes, ascending pharyngeal, facial artery, loose areolar connective tissue. Posterior compartment: Carotid sheath, glossopharyngeal nerve, spinal accessory nerve, hypoglossal nerve and cervical sympathetic trunk.

If the posterior compartment becomes infected, there is absence of trismus along with visible swelling, but respiratory obstruction, septic thromophlebitis of IJV may ensue in late stages.

Applied anatomy

Relations of lateral pharyngeal space explain its most common involvement in maxillofacial infections. Infections may encircle the airway by spreading from one lateral pharyngeal space to other through retropharyngeal space. Contrast enhanced CT is valuable aid in confirmation of diagnosis, determination of extent and stage of deep cervical space infections.

Infections in the parapharyngeal spaces have sometimes been associated with morbid vascular or neurologic problems and occasionally with mortality. Knowledge of the anatomy of the discrete anterior and posterior compartments of the lateral pharyngeal space provides information for accurate diagnosis, ensures correct treatment and thus, affects eventual outcome of the infection.

The styloid process divides the space into an anterior muscular compartment closely related to the tonsillar fossa and a posterior vascular compartment.[12]

The *anterior compartment* contains fat, muscle, lymph nodes and connective tissue.

The *posterior compartment,* also called the post-styloid or retro-styloid compartment, contains cranial nerves IX to XII[13,14] and the carotid sheath and its contents (the internal carotid artery, internal jugular vein, vagus nerve and lymph nodes). The carotid sheath extends from the base of the skull down through the lateral pharyngeal space, runs along the prevertebral fascia below the hyoid bone, and then enters the chest below the clavicle. The sympathetic trunk lies behind the sheath in a fascial reflection from the deep surface of the posterior wall.[15]

The possibility that the strongest fascial plane in the head and neck is the stylopharyngeal aponeurosis of Zuckerkandel and Testut, formed by the confluence of the alar, buccopharyngeal and stylomuscular fascia. This aponeurosis is a barrier against direct spread of anterior compartment infections to the vital structures of the posterior compartment.[16]

Pathophysiology and etiology of infection

Common sites of origin of parapharyngeal infection include the teeth, tonsils and adenoids; parotid gland and lymph glands draining the nose and the pharynx.[17] Thrombosis of the internal jugular vein or of peritonsillar veins, metastatic tumors with secondary infection of the internal jugular lymph node chain, iatrogenic introduction of organisms during infiltration for a mandibular nerve block[18] or administration of an anesthetic during tonsillectomy are documented causes of spread of infection. The most common origin of a lateral pharyngeal space infection, however, is odontogenic, secondary to a grossly carious molar, pericoronitis or tooth extraction. Usually involvement is by direct extension over the mylohyoid muscle and into the anterior lateral pharyngeal space, although sometimes infection may first occur in the pterygomandibular space and subsequently spread to the lateral pharyngeal space (Fig. 17.26).

Every peritonsillar space abscess (quincy) can become a lateral pharyngeal space abscess by local spread. Infection in such a patient is much more severe than the classic peritonsillar abscess in that it not only presents with tonsillar inflammation and swelling of the lateral pharyngeal wall, but also extreme trismus and occasional parotid swelling.

The deep fascia of the parotid gland is not complete at the base of the skull and it fails to cover the upper inner surface of the gland.[19] On the other hand, the lateral aspect of the gland forms a rather dense capsule. Therefore, parotid infections readily pass medially into the lateral pharyngeal space.[20]

Parapharyngeal infections may occur from lymphatic drainage of surrounding tissues such as the periodontal region. Idiopathic cervical abscesses may spread across fairly large areas of uninvolved tissues through lymph vessels from the portal of entrance directly to the lymph nodes of the neck. In such cases, the glands may breakdown and form an abscess. Involvement of the posterior compartment of the lateral pharyngeal space may be secondary to rupture of lymph nodes draining an odontogenic infection. Theoretically, in such cases, the anterior compartment may not become involved in the infection. With inflammatory swelling of the lymph glands for more than several weeks, an abscess frequently results. Suppuration without high fever may develop.

Middle ear infections with associated mastoiditis can develop into an internal Bezold' s abscess,[21] the result of the infection breaking through the bone and creating a subperiosteal abscess on the inner aspect of the mastoid tip in the region of the digastric groove. Further progression of this abscess will directly involve the lateral pharyngeal space.

Clinical features

The symptoms of lateral pharyngeal infections will vary according to whether the anterior, posterior or both compartments are involved.

There are four cardinal signs of involvement of the *anterior lateral pharyngeal compartment*:[22]

1. Trismus.
2. Induration and swelling at the angle of the jaw.
3. Fever.
4. Pharyngeal bulging (Fig. 17.27).

Trismus is the most important sign and results from the close relationship of the infection to the medial pterygoid muscle.[23]

Because the anterior compartment ends at the level of the angle of the

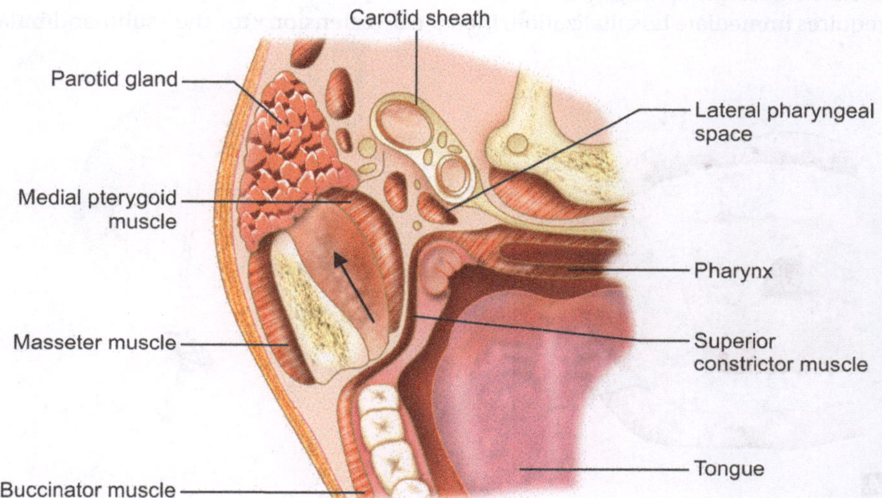

Fig. 17.26: Spread of odontogenic infection from pterygomandibular space to the lateral pharyngeal space

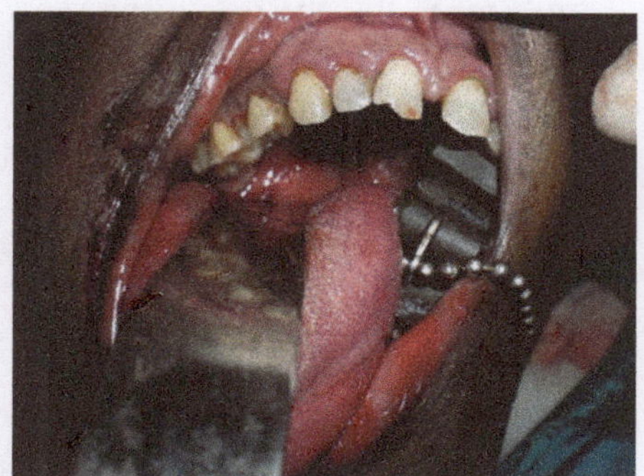

Fig. 17.27: Medial displacement of lateral pharyngeal wall

jaw, induration and swelling is evident medial to the angle of the mandible.

At this point, the most superficial part in the neck, the anterior compartment is separated from the skin surface by two thick complete fascial layers—the superficial layer of the deep cervical fascia, and the blind end of the anterior lateral pharyngeal space or fascial fold.[22] Fluctuation, therefore, can be felt late or may not be detected at all.

Fever usually occurs concomitantly with infection that is localized in the fascial space. Pharyngeal bulging is due to the thin fasciomuscular wall between the pharynx and the compartment.

Because of the relation to the tonsillar area, there is usually bulging of the posterolateral pharyngeal wall and tonsillar region as well. It is relatively easy to differentiate isolated peritonsillar infections from lateral pharyngeal space infections. A hoarse voice and a usual lack of trismus are associated with peritonsillar abscess.[24] It is often difficult to differentiate a pterygomandibular space abscess from lateral pharyngeal space abscess. Sometimes they are confluent.

Infections in the *posterior compartment* will show:

- Posterior tonsillar pillar deviation and retropharyngeal swelling due to the proximity of the two areas.
- May show neurologic involvement of cranial nerves IX through XII and of the cervical sympathetic chain, with ipsilateral Horner's syndrome.[25]
- Thrombosis of the internal jugular vein with sepsis may cause abrupt rises and falls in temperature and chills.
- Blood cultures are often positive.
- Venous blowouts are more common than arterial. Even though the tightness of the vascular sheath resists intrusion, erosion of the common, external, or internal carotid artery may occur within the carotid sheath.
- In infections limited to the posterior compartment, the muscles of mastication are not involved and minimal trismus or tonsillar prolapse occurs.
- Because of the close relationship with the parotid space, however, swelling of the lateral posterior pharyngeal wall and the parotid space do occur.

Complications

Shapiro[26] lists a number of complications that may ensue with any parapharyngeal space infection, including mediastinitis, jugular thrombosis, edema of the larynx, Ludwig's angina, hemorrhage from erosion and blowout the large vessels, osteomyelitis of the mandible, pneumonia, vagus involvement (sudden death), meningitis and parotid abscess.

Lifschutz[27] states that the blood vessels are usually the last to yield in the case of an abscess or sloughing infection in the deep cervical space. Sudden spontaneous rupture of the abscess into the throat may rarely produce fatal consequences due to aspiration.

The erosion and rupture of major vessels like internal jugular vein and the internal carotid artery in the posterior compartment leads to fulminating hemorrhage which is invariably fatal.

The infection can spread upwards through foramen lacerum, ovale, jugular foramen producing brain abscess, meningitis or sinus thrombosis. It spreads downward into carotid sheath towards mediastinum, a pathway called 'anterior Lincoln's highway' of the neck.

Management

Treatment of parapharyngeal infection requires immediate hospitalization, incision and drainage, maintenance of airway, removal of the causative agent and antibiotic therapy initiated empirically and adjusted when results of culture and antibiotic sensitivity tests have been obtained.

Incision and drainage is most important to decompress the lateral pharyngeal space and avoid the dreaded complications of major vessel erosion, airway embarrassment, and sepsis.

There are multiple approaches to the lateral pharyngeal space: intraoral,[28] extraoral and a combination of both (Figs 17.28A and B). The intraoral incisions can be either transpharyngeal[13] or lateral.[29]

The transpharyngeal approach is made through the tonsillar fossa. This approach is not recommended because adequate drainage is very difficult to obtain and because there is absolutely no exposure of the vessels.

The lateral approach is most easily performed by making an incision lateral to the pterygomandibular raphe and dissecting bluntly with a Kelly clamp medial to the medial pterygoid muscle into the parapharyngeal space.

All peroral incisions are contraindicated when there has been prior hemorrhage.

The extraoral submandibular incision is the safest approach and should be used if there is any involvement of the posterior compartment. A vertical extension to the submandibular

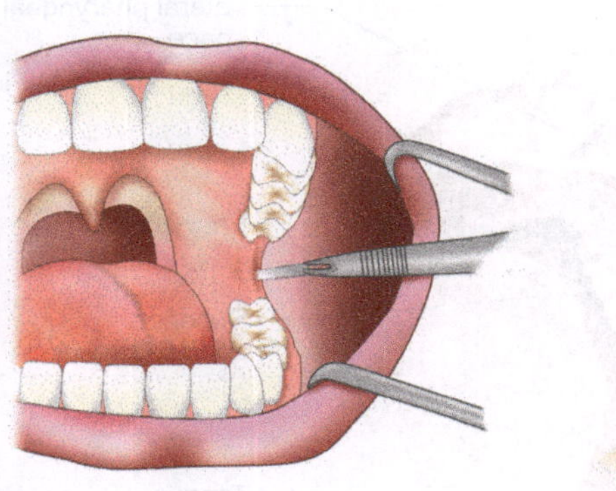

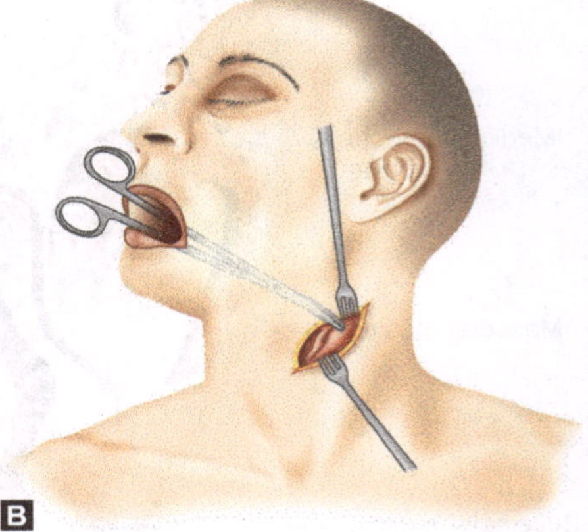

Figs 17.28A and B: Incision and drainage of lateral pharyngeal space: (A) Intraoral mucosal incision; (B) Kelly clamp anterior to the sternocleidomastoid muscle

incision may be given to form a T shaped incision, which may rarely be necessary to have adequate exposure for control of major vessels.[30]

In the combined intraoral and extraoral approach, the mucosal incision is made lateral to the pterygomandibular raphe.[29] A large curved Kelly clamp is then passed lateral to the superior constrictor muscle and medial to the medial pterygoid muscle. The blunt dissection is carried posteroinferiorly below the angle of the mandible. When the tip of the instrument is palpated extraorally anterior to the sternocleidomastoid, a cutaneous incision is made over the tip (Fig. 17.29). This technique affords direct access into the lateral pharyngeal space and aids correct placement of the external incision in a patient with gross edema. Blunt dissection behind the posteriorly retracted sternocleidomastoid allows direct entrance into the inferior aspect of the posterior compartment. Finger dissection is carried out to identify such landmarks as the hyoid bone and the posterior belly of the digastric muscle. Loculations of pus are broken up. The presence of old blood clots should alert one to the possibility of major vessel erosion and subsequent severe hemorrhage. Examination by vascular surgeon and an arteriogram should be obtained. If one encounters only purulent material, the wound should be irrigated and a large drain is inserted.

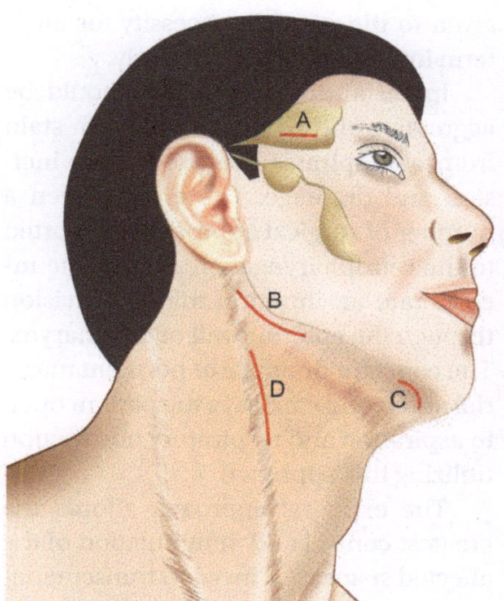

Fig. 17.29: Various incisions for draining the fascial space infections; (A) For temporal pouches; (B) Submandibular, submasseteric and pterigomandibular space; (C) Submental space; (D) Lateral pharyngeal space

Intubation, elective tracheostomy or cricothyrotomy should be contemplated in cases involving airway compromise or vascular complications. Significant tongue elevation, severe dysphagia and rapid speed of infection, all suggest need for airway protection. Should these signs present prior to elective tracheostomy, muscle relaxants should not be given, because intubation via the oral route may not be impossible.[29] Fiberoptic laryngoscopy, with the patient awake and comfortable, may be a useful adjunct. Should doubt occur during control of the airway, emergency cricothyroid puncture may be difficult, because landmarks are masked by the swelling. If the anesthesiologist wishes to attempt intubation, the neck should be marked for a tracheotomy incision and injected with local anesthesia prior to such attempts. If an immediate tracheotomy is needed, a vertical midline incision will provide the quickest and most bloodless access.

Retropharyngeal Space

Retropharyngeal space is a potential midline space between the pharyngobasilar fascia, which attaches the pharyngeal constrictors to the base of the skull and prevertebral fascia. This space is continuous with retroesophageal space into the posterior mediastinum to the level of sixth thoracic vertebra. The anatomical boundries of the retropharyngeal space are as shown in Box 17.10.

Dyspnea, dysphagia, nuchal rigidity, esophageal regurgitation and fever characterize retropharyngeal space infections.

Applied anatomy

Retropharyngeal and lateral pharyngeal spaces contain a rich supply of lymph nodes that drain Waldeyer's ring. When these nodes necrose, fascial space infection may develop.

Box 17.10: Boundaries of retropharyngeal space

Laterally	Carotid sheath, lateral pharyngeal space
Superiorly	Base of the skull
Inferiorly	Fusion of retropharyngeal fascia
Anteriorly and posteriorly	Deep cervical fascia and alar fascia
Medially	Midline septum

Infections of these spaces may prove fatal owing to their ability to impinge on the airway directly and potential involvement of danger space.[31]

The deep layer of the deep investing fascia encloses the vertebra and paravertebral musculature. This deep layer is further subdivided into the prevertebral and alar layers.

- The prevertebral layer lies anterior to the vertebral column from the base of the skull to the coccyx.
- The alar layer of the deep layer of the deep cervical fascia lies posterior to the middle layer and pharynx and fuses with the transverse processes. This fascia extends from the base of the skull to the posterior mediastinum (Fig. 17.30).

The retropharyngeal abscess is an abscess in the potential space of loose connective tissue posterior to the pharyngeal wall and anterior to the middle layer of the deep investing fascia; or between the middle layer of the deep investing fascia and the alar layer of the investing fascia, or between the alar and prevertebral layers of the deep layer of the deep investing fascia. This extends from the base of the skull to the mediastinum. Because of the interconnecting nature of the layers of the deep fascia, retropharyngeal abscesses may communicate with the lateral pharyngeal space, the pretracheal space and the mediastinum.

Pathophysiology and etiology

The incidence of retropharyngeal abscess is greatest in the 3 to 4 year-old age group. Even though only a low incidence has been reported since the introduction of antibiotics, the retropharyngeal abscess does occur in adults.

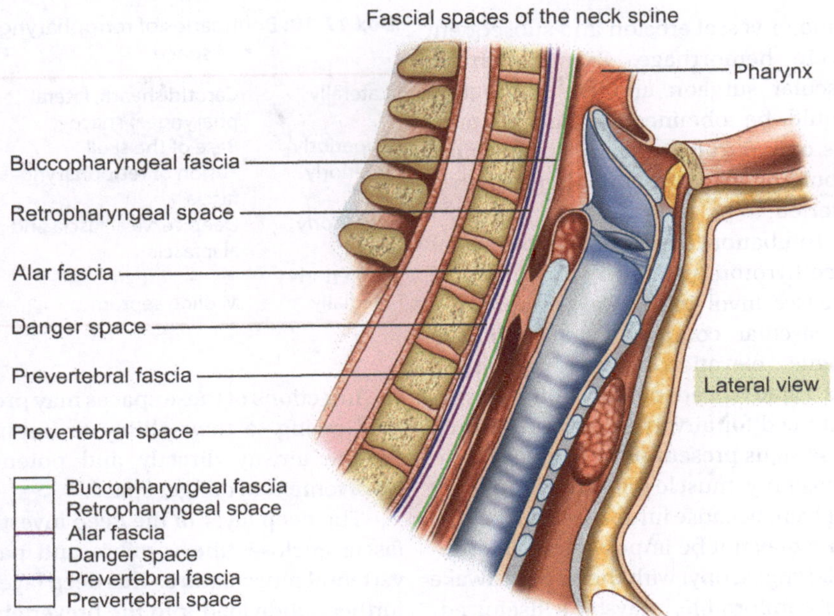

Fig. 17.30: Retropharyngeal space and fascial boundaries

These are usually due to[32-35]

- Otologic
- Pharyngeal or nasopharyngeal infections can directly spread to the retropharyngeal space
- Upper respiratory infections
- Odontogenic infections
- Cervical osteomyelitis
- Foreign body introduction
- Regional trauma
- Spread by the lymphatics.

It is well known that the parotid, submandibular and masticator spaces communicate with the lateral pharyngeal space. Infections originating in any of these spaces may then ultimately progress to affect the retropharyngeal region via the lateral pharyngeal space.[36]

The organisms identified with infections of the retropharyngeal space are consistent with the specific etiology. Odontogenic or oropharyngeal infections frequently yield combinations or anaerobic and aerobic gram-positive and gram-negative bacteria, predominantly *Bacteroides fragilis* or *Streptococcus* species. Sinusitis, otitis media and mastoiditis most frequently reveal anaerobes of a mixed variety. *Staphylococcus aureus, Coccidioides immitis* and *Mycobacterium tuberculosis* are most implicated in retropharyngeal abscesses secondary to vertebral osteomyelitis.[35,36]

Clinical Features

The signs and symptoms of retropharyngeal abscess include:[32,33,35,37]

- Fever
- Sialorrhea
- Stiff neck
- Sore throat
- Dysphagia
- Possible stridor
- Leukocytosis
- Occasional lateral neck erythema and swelling.

Each of these, however, are not diagnostic and must be correlated with radiographic findings. Soft tissue radiographs are invaluable in identifying abnormalities of the retropharyngeal region. Hay[38] in 1930 was the first to correlate soft tissue radiographs and posterior pharyngeal pathosis. In his review of 50 'soft tissue lateral neck' radiographs of adults, he measured the distance between cervical vertebrae and the posterior pharyngeal wall from C_1 to C_5 as being representative of the thickness of soft tissue in the retropharyngeal region. The retropharyngeal soft tissue regional average was 2.0 mm in males and 1.9 mm in females, with a range in both from 1.5 to 4.0 mm. Wholey et al.[39] in 1958 reviewed 480 soft tissue radiographs of the neck in adults. Retropharyngeal region was identified from the base of the skull to C_5. The representative distance between C_2 and the posterior pharyngeal wall was used as a standard. This distance averaged 3.4 mm in adults and ranged from 1.0 to 7.0 mm. The representative distance for the retrotracheal region was from C_6 to the posterior tracheal wall and this average was 14.0 mm with a range of 9.0 to 22.0 mm. Using these studies as standards, soft tissue radiographs of the neck in adults that lie beyond the accepted range and are correlated clinically will be diagnostic.

The use of the CT scan[40] has proved to be more effective in diagnosing the retropharyngeal region abscess.

Treatment

The most important initial consideration is maintenance of a patent airway. Possible airway compromise must be addressed early in the treatment plan. Elective tracheostomy, fiberoptic intubation or blind, awake nasotracheal intubation are all viable alternatives for initial airway maintenance. Consideration must be given to the possible necessity for long-term intubation postoperatively.

Initial antibiotic therapy should be aggressive and based on the gram stain from an aspirate or a productive incision and drainage. There have been a number of surgical approaches reported to the retropharyngeal region. Some incorporate an intraoral midline incision through the anterior wall of the pharynx. The constant drainage of purulent material and blood can leave the patient open to aspiration and respiratory obstruction utilizing this approach.

The extraoral approach affords the greatest control and manipulation of the affected spaces. An incision transcutaneously anterior to the sternocleidomastoid muscle from the level of the angle of the mandible to the level of the hyoid bone will allow retraction of the sternocleidomastoid muscle. The carotid sheath with its contents can then be inspected for possible erosion. Retraction of both the muscle and the sheath allows for a blunt dissection into the lateral pharyngeal and retropharyngeal space, the latter verified by palpation of the anterior processes of the cervical spine posteriorly and the endotracheal tube anteriorly. Appropriate drains may then be placed. These drains are then irrigated and advanced in accordance with the individual postoperative course.

Complications

The most frequent complication of the retropharyngeal abscess is dissection to the posterior mediastinum with resultant mediastinitis, pleuritis and pericarditis.[34,41] Spontaneous rupture of the abscess into the pharynx may result in aspiration pneumonia or empyema.[32,33] Erosion of the great vessels of the neck have been reported and are potentially fatal.[42] Upper airway obstruction is a potential threat and close observation is required.

GENERAL PRINCIPLES OF INFECTION MANAGEMENT (BOX 17.11)

Although the antibiotics are useful in the management of the infections, the role of surgical intervention is very important, in the early resolution and preventing further complications. The specific infections like tuberculosis, syphilis, typhoid, etc. are primarily treated with drugs and surgery has a minor role in specific situations only.

Box 17.11: Principles of abscess drainage

- Place the incision on the most dependent part
- If the incision is placed on the prominent part, place the counter incision on the dependent part
- Liberal, dependent, passive drainage should be achieved
- Use sinus forcep or index finger to break the locules
- Break all locules to change multiloculated cavity into a uniloculated one
- Use drain
- Send the sample for C and ST.

But the primary line of treatment for the pyogenic infection is surgical, comprising of decompression or drainage. One should not always wait for the signs of the localization of the infection and formation of the localized abscess, but should proceed with surgical decompression at the earliest. The decompression helps in reducing the mounting pressure within the tissue planes and thus helps in:

- Preventing lateral spread of the infection due to pressure.
- Prevents pressure/ischemic necrosis of the tissue.
- Improves the local circulation by decompressing the pressure.
- Improves the drainage of the part by opening up the lymphatic and venous cannels which were blocked by edema and pressure and thus reduces tissue edema, congestion and stasis of local circulation due to reabsorption of interstitial edema.
- Improves delivery of the antibiotics to the local site and thus helps in controlling the infection rapidly.
- Prevents further complications like laryngeal edema, mediastenitis, etc.

If the signs of localization such as fluctuations are present, the drainage must be undertaken promptly. In the maxillofacial area due to presence of loose areolar tissue a deep seated abscess will invariably be accompanied by the edema or cellulitis of the overlying skin. Thus, classical fluctuations may sometimes get masked. It is particularly true in cases of submasseteric, deep temporal pouch and the parotid abscess where the overlying muscle or thick fascia will mask the fluctuations. In such cases, diagnostic aspirations with the help of wide-bore needle may be done to demonstrate a deep seated pus pocket. The USG or CT scan may also be helpful in locating pus pockets so that the drainage can be adequately planned and undertaken. Once the diagnosis of an abscess is arrived at, the drainage can be done by any of the documented methods, i.e. Hiltons method or modified Hiltons method. The surgical procedure is often referred to as an Incision and Drainage (I and D). While incising the abscess, the incision must be placed on the most dependent site to facilitate gravity assisted drainage. However, if the most prominent part of the abscess is chosen and it is not the most dependent part then a counter incision should be placed on the dependent site to facilitate gravity assisted drainage. The incisions taken for the drainage of an abscess or the decompression of the cellulitis should always be liberal to achieve free and passive drainage. While draining large abscess or multiple fascial space involvement, the incision should be liberal enough to allow passage of the index finger. When the index finger is introduced in an abscess the finger being blunt does not damage the vital structures and palpates the anatomical landmarks, simultaneously. It also breaks the locules in the abscess and converts a multiloculated abscess into a uniloculated cavity thus helps in complete drainage of the septic material and reduces further absorption of the bacterial toxins. The chances of missing any pocket or locules are minimum as the infected tissue is often fragile and easily gives way with pressure applied by the inserted finger. The healthy tissue offers resistance to the finger and thus the operator is in position to know the completeness of the procedure.

While draining any abscess one must remember three golden rules:

1. The incision should be at dependant site.
2. It should be liberal.
3. It should facilitate, free passive drainage.

If the presence of necrotic granulation tissue is noticed lining the abscess, such tissue should be gently curetted out. If the infected, necrotic granulation tissue is left *in situ*, it will bleed for a long time being friable in nature. Secondly, such tissue will breakdown and liquify to produce pus subsequently and thirdly leaving such tissue will increase the load on the scavenging mechanisms of the body. The abscess cavity should be gently irrigated with normal saline or diluted povidone iodine solution to flush out the septic material and necrotic tissue tags. Use of hydrogen peroxide is debated as some clinicians feel that the effervescence produced by it will drive out the debris of necrotic tissue and deliver the nascent oxygen which helps in inhibiting the growth of anaerobic microorganisms and facilitate formation of the granulation tissue, while others feel that the effervescence will drive the microorganisms in deeper tissue planes to cause flaring of the infection.

The drained pus should be carefully collected in a sterile bulb and should be submitted to microbiology lab for culture and sensitivity to determine specific antibiotic therapy. Usually the midstream of the drained pus is collected.

After the drainage the most suitable material used as a drain is a corrugated rubber dam drain. The tube drains or vacuum drains are not ideal unless the irrigation of the abscess cavity is planned subsequently. The drain facilitates the free drainage of pus and exudates and keeps the opening (incision) patent. Gauze drains should not be used ideally as the gauze has capillarity. It absorbs fluid, swells and impedes the drainage. It should be used as a pack cum drain to achieve hemostasis, only when the abscess cavity bleeds and should be removed after 24 hours and replaced by rubber dam drain. The appropriate time for removal of the drain is variable and depends on the given case and condition. If the pus discharge gets reduced and is minimal in last 24 hours then it could be either because of the infection getting controlled or it could be due to blockade of the corrugations due to fibrin. In such cases, the drain should be displaced to break adhesions and the soakage should again be observed for next 24 hours and if the soakage is still minimal then the drain should be discontinued. It is also recommended to withdraw the drain gradually daily so that

- The drain does not get blocked due to fibrinous adhesions.
- The abscess cavity and gets filled gradually from the base and shrinks.
- While doing the gradual withdrawal the fixing stitch is removed which may lead to falling of the drain in the cavity to prevent this, a sterile safety pin is used to fix the drain.

Similarly the drain should not be kept for long after the purpose of drainage is achieved as:

- It can introduce retrograde infection.
- It may be in contact with major vessel and may erode it.
- It may get biodegraded and may become difficult to remove.

The local care of the incision wound and the abscess cavity is required following the drainage. Although abscess is an infected cavity, the daily dressings must be done under aseptic care. The abscess cavity may be gently irrigated with sterile normal saline to flush out the necrotic tissue tags, thick pus, etc. Povidon iodine 5 percent solution can be used for irrigation.

When the cellulitis is present the use of glycerin magnesium sulfate (glycerin magsulf) dressing is helpful (Figs 17.31A to C). It is the gauze soaked in the saturated solution of the magnesium sulfate in glycerine. It has following effects:

- The magsulf is hygroscopic and thus helps in drawing the interstitial fluid thus reduces edema, reduces tissue pressure, improves local circulation and drainage and facilitates healing.
- The glycerin magsulf produces exothermic reaction and produces heat which causes vasodilatation and reduces congestion due to improvement of local circulation.
- Glycerin has soothing action on tissue.

MEDICINAL TREATMENT IN OROFACIAL INFECTIONS

The supportive management comprises of antibiotics and anti-inflammatory drugs. The antibiotics usually prescribed in the management of the odontogenic infection are penicillin or cephalosporin group of antibiotics (*beta-lactam group*) as the infection of odontogenic origin is caused by the oral microorganisms, which predominantly are gram-positive and respond well to the penicillin group of antibiotics. In severe infections or where the patient has compromised immunity, higher doses should be prescribed. Cloxacillin can be added

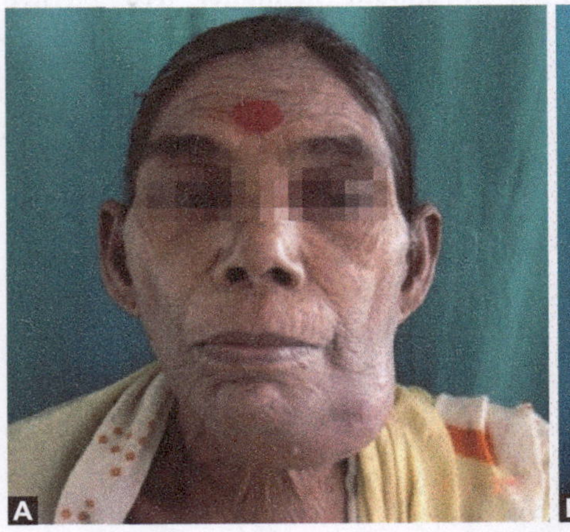

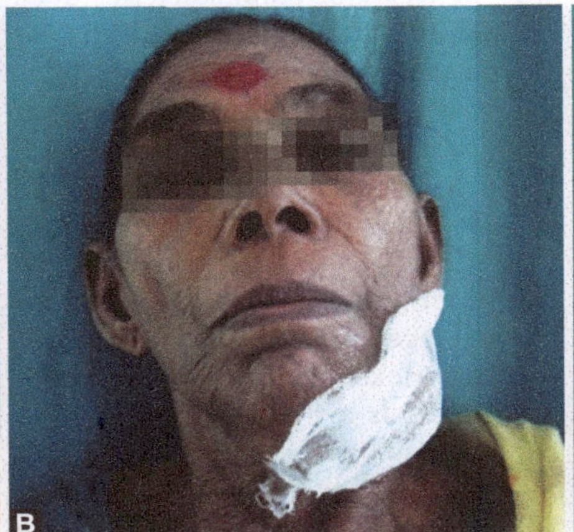

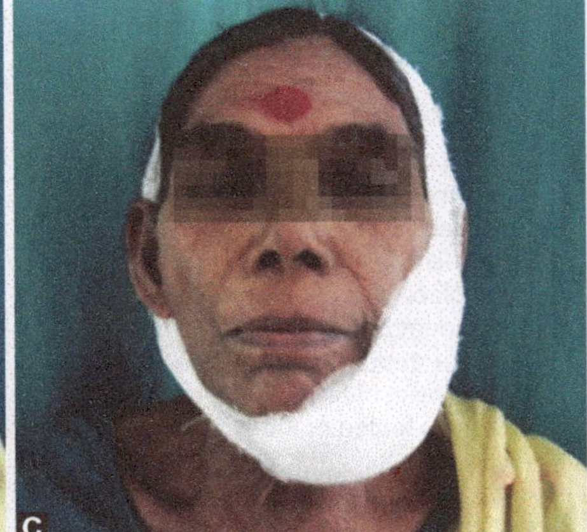

Figs 17.31A to C: Glycerine and magsulf dressing is used in the diffuse and acute stage

to ampicillin or amoxicillin as the later two may not be effective in the presence of (*penicillinase*) beta-lactamase producing organisms. Cloxacillin has a property of resisting the beta-lactamase (*penicillinase*) and thus is more effective in such situation and is known to potentiate the action of the ampicillin and amoxicillin. The addition of the clavulanic acid also potentiate the action of amoxicillin (Augmentin) in presence of beta-lactamase-producing microorganisms (Table 17.6).

In the mixed infections, to give wider spectrum of coverage against the gram-negative organisms aminoglycosides (gentamycin, amicacin) may be given. However, gram-negative infections are seldom present in the orofacial area and are more common in the genitourinary and lower gastrointestinal tract infections and hence the aminoglycosides are of limited value in the management of odontogenic infections. The aminoglycosides may be added to beta-lactam antibiotics, if the gram-negative microorganisms are detected on the culture of the pus sample. The gram-negative organisms may sometimes be present in the postoperative nosocomial infections in the maxillofacial area.

When evidence of anaerobic infection like slough, crepitus, gas, foul-smelling, thick greenish black pus is present, then metronidazole in appropriate dose should be added. The anaerobes are facultative organisms and will cause the infection only when the conductive environments for their growth and proliferation are present such as, hypoperfused cavities, dead or devitalized tissue.

Definitive antibiotic therapy can be started after the culture and sensitivity test. Glycerine and magsulf dressing is used in the diffuse and acute stage.

SELECTION OF ANESTHESIA

The superficial, minor abscess can be drained comfortably under the local anesthesia. However, deep seated abscess cannot be drained completely under local anesthesia alone. The skin can be infiltered with local anesthetic and the incision may be painless, but while draining large, deep seated,

Table 17.6: Various antibiotics used in the management of odontogenic infection

Name	Group	Dose	Adverse effects
Amoxicillin Ampicillin Ampiclox/Amoxyclox Clavulanate	Penicillin Penicillin Penicillinase resistant Penicillin Beta lactamase inhibitor	40–45 upto 80–95 mg/kg/wt Used orally and injection With clavulanate it is 1.2 g in which 1 g is ampicillin and 0.2 g is clavulanic acid	• Bone marrow depression • Granulocytopenia • Rarely hepatitis • Pain at site of IM injection • Phlebitis/thromobophlebitis at site of IV injection • Hypersensitivity
Cefazolin Cephalexin Cefadroxil	Cephalosporin first generation	1–1.5 g every 6 hourly 1 g every 6 hourly 1 g every 12 hourly	• Nephrotoxic, but not as aminoglycosides • Diarrhea • Hypersensitivity
Cefoxitin Cefaclor	Cephalosporin second generation	2 g every 4 hourly or 3 g every 6 hourly 1 g every 8 hourly	
Cefotaxime	Cephalosporin third generation	2 g every 4–8 hours	
Ceftriaxone		2 g every 12–48 hours	
Cefepime	Cephalosporin fourth generation	2 g every 8 hourly	
Gentamicin	Aminoglycoside	2 mg/kg loading and then 3–5 mg/kg/day in adults For children upto 2 years 2–2.5 mg/kg every 8 hours	• Ototoxicity • Nephrotoxicity
Amikacin		15 mg/kg/day	
Clindamycin	Lincosamide	150–600 mg in divided doses for adults 10–30 mg/kg in 4–6 divided doses	• Abdominal pain • Diarrhea • Blood in stools
Metronidazole	Nitroimidazole	750 mg to 2 g/day in divided doses	• Headache • Nausea • Metallic taste • Dry mouth • Rarely vomiting, diarrhea

multilucolated abscess drainage will be very painful while draining. Moreover just the placement of the incision is not synonymous with drainage, the loculi within are required to be broken to achieve complete drainage. Attempting to drain such abscess under local anesthesia may be incomplete job. Sedating the patient, giving intravenous anesthetic agents like thiopental sodium and ketamine carry a high risk of aspiration of pus as the airway is often unguarded. Although the abscess is drained by extraoral incision during the manipulation, the eroded or thinned out loculi may rupture intraorally leading to aspiration. The cases of trismus, large abscesses, lateral or retropharyngeal abscesses pose a great threat of aspiration. It is therefore advisable to guard the airway by intubation and packing of the pharynx. Most of the perianal abscesses produce pronounced trismus and endotracheal intubation may be difficult. In such cases blind intubation is risky. Thus, intubating fiberoptic bronchoscope or laryngoscopically guided intubation should be attempted. If there is pronounced laryngeal edema as in cases of Ludwig's angina, cricothyroidotomy or tracheostomy should be done to secure the airway and intubate the patient for administration of anesthesia.

COMPLICATIONS OF MAXILLOFACIAL INFECTIONS

Ludwig's Angina

Ludwig's angina is defined as *acute, 'non-suppurating, necrotising cellulitis' involving the submandibular, sublingual and submental spaces, bilaterally.* It is a life-threatening complication caused due to infection.

Etiology

- Odontogenic infections are by far the most common cause of this condition, the infection spreads to the adjoining tissue planes either by direct spread or through the lymphatics, which in turn suppurate and breakdown and the septic material is discharged in that tissue plane which spreads to the adjacent tissue planes.
- Septic fractures
- Salivary gland infections
- Hematogenous infections.

Predisposing Factors

- Immunosuppression
- Steroid therapy
- Diabetes
- Debilitating conditions
- Due to advent of the antibiotics the occurrences of this condition is uncommon, but in the above mentioned patients the Ludwig's angina can be precipitated.

Causative Organisms

It is primarily caused by the beta-hemolytic streptococci.[43] The hallmark of the streptococcal infection is that the infection tends to spread rather than localizing, due to liberation of exotoxins by the streptococci which breakdown the intercellular cementing substance which facilitates the spread of the infection along the tissue planes. Apart from streptocci, *E. coli* has also been isolated from the cultures taken in the cases of Ludwig's angina.[44] Anaerobic organisms are also isolated when there are gangrenous changes in the tissue due to combined effect of increased interstitial pressure, hypoxia and the effects of the bacterial exotoxins. The devitalized tissue serves as the nidus for proliferation of the anerobic organisms. However, the predominant organisms are the streptococci.

Clinical Features

- It is characterized by acute course producing, bilateral swelling due to cellulites of the submandibular, sublingual and submental spaces. The skin is tense, glossy and hyperemic. The consistency is often described as '*wood like*' or called brawny induration.[43]
- The swelling of the submental space produces a classical double chinned appearance.
- Skin is tense due to accumulation of the inflammatory exudates in the interstitial compartment which makes the tissue to pit and blanch on pressure (Fig. 17.32A and B).
- Tenderness on palpation is present.
- Due to mounting interstitial fluid pressure, the edema rapidly spreads along the fascial plane, breaking the tissue barriers and go on to involve the adjoining spaces.
- The involvement of the sublingual space leads to edema and congestion of the floor of mouth and the tongue gets lifted and protrudes out (Figs 17.33A to D, 17.34A to C).
- The infection of the sublingual space rapidly spreads along it to its base which is present at the hyoid bone. Posterior inferior to the base of the

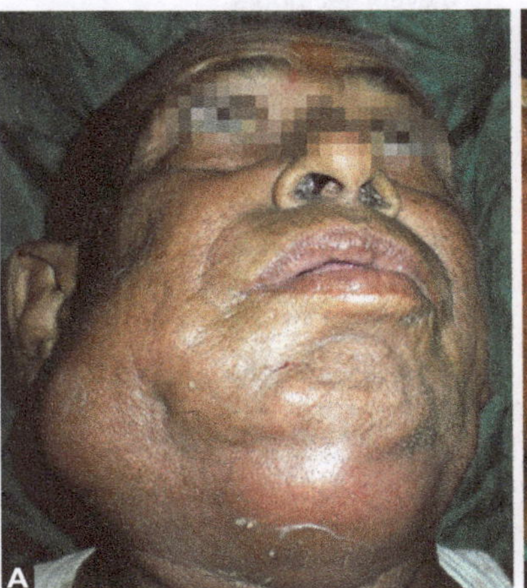

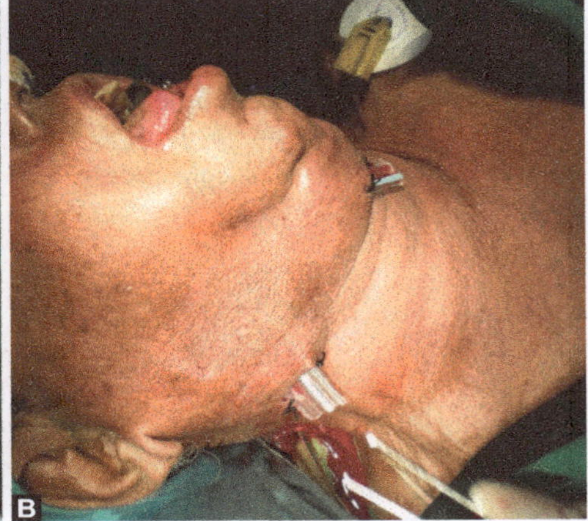

Figs 17.32A and B: (A) Unilateral submandibular, submental and sublingual space infection not falling in definition of Ludwig's angina, but it is potentially dangerous; (B) Surgical decompression accomplished and drains in place

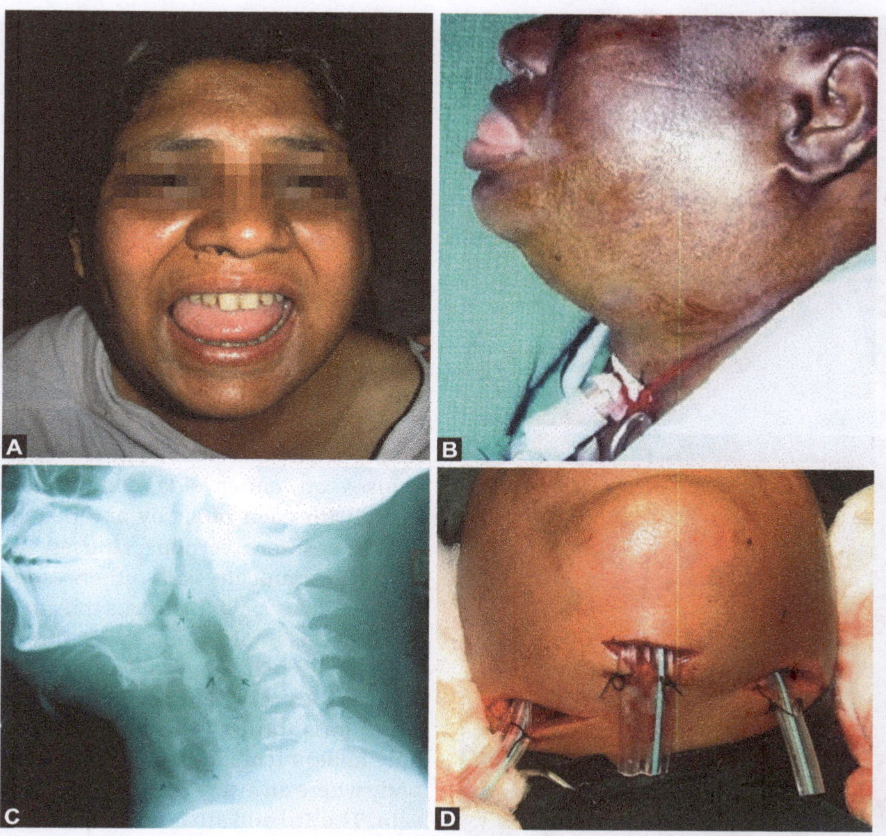

Figs 17.33A to D: (A and B) Ludwig's angina clinical picture, patient looks toxic, tongue is elevated, tracheostomy in place; (C) X-ray shows distended neck shadow due to cellulitis; (D) Separate incisions for decompression of the submandibular, sublingual and submental spaces

sublingual space lays the larynx and the edema extends to the larynx causing the edema of the epiglottis and the cords, which leads to acute respiratory obstruction, due to which death can occur due to asphyxia. Thus, an acute respiratory emergency situation is created which warrants immediate attention. The early signs of the laryngeal edema are dyspnea which gets aggravated when the patient lies down. The dyspnea in supine position should be regarded as the warning sign of impending laryngeal edema. As the edema increases the dyspnea worsens and progresses into asphyxia. The lateral X-ray of the neck shows edematous soft tissue shadow and if the laryngeal edema is present then the epiglottis may look like a raised thumb (thumb sign of epiglotitis).

- The patient has often dysphagia and saliva may dribble from the corner of the mouth.
- The patient is extremely toxic with high-grade fever (> 104°F), malaise, body aches, leukocytosis and all the classical constitutional features of septicemia are present. The peripheral blood smear may show intracellular eosinophilic toxic granules and presence of band cells.

Management

The treatment of Ludwig's angina is primarily surgical. The first priority in the management is always the lifesaving measures. If the patient has signs of the laryngeal edema like dyspnea, to save the life of the patient emergency tracheostomy should be performed promptly. Endotracheal intubation is nearly impossible in these patients due to severe laryngeal edema, elevation of the tongue and trismus (Fig. 17.34D).

Even if the signs of laryngeal edema and the respiratory embarrassment are not conspicuously present, the surgical decompression of the tissue planes must be undertaken immediately, to relieve the pressure within the tissue so that the edema does not increase further and does not spread laterally. This is achieved by giving a liberal incision on the skin and opening the tissue planes—layer-by-layer dissection. In the older literature, a horse shoe-shaped incision is described in the submandibular area along inferior border of the mandible.[45] Two separate incisions are given bilaterally in the submandibular area and one in the submental area is commonly practiced (Fig. 17.34E). The decompression of the sublingual space is most important which is achieved by piercing open the *mylohyoid muscle*, which in fact is a must in case of Ludwig's angina. The sublingual space can also be decompressed by placing an incision on the floor of the mouth; parallel to the lingual vestibule. The term decompression is often used as the purpose of the incision is to open the tissue plane to reduce the mounting pressure within the tissue planes and to prevent the further spread of the edema. As the condition is usually non-suppurating, the pus is absent. In some cases, there may be deep seated small pocket of pus, which is surrounded by area of cellulites. After placing the incision, a corrugated rubber drain may be left *in situ* to keep the incisions patent and to drain the exudate (*see* Fig. 17.32B). The decompression serves three purposes:

1. It reduces the tension within the tissue plane and prevents the further spread of the edema and infection.
2. As the pressure in the tissue drops the circulation of the tissue improves which facilitates reabsorption of the edema.
3. It drains the septic material, if any and prevents further bacteremia. The edema reduces gradually.

The medicinal supportive treatment comprises of prescription of parenteral

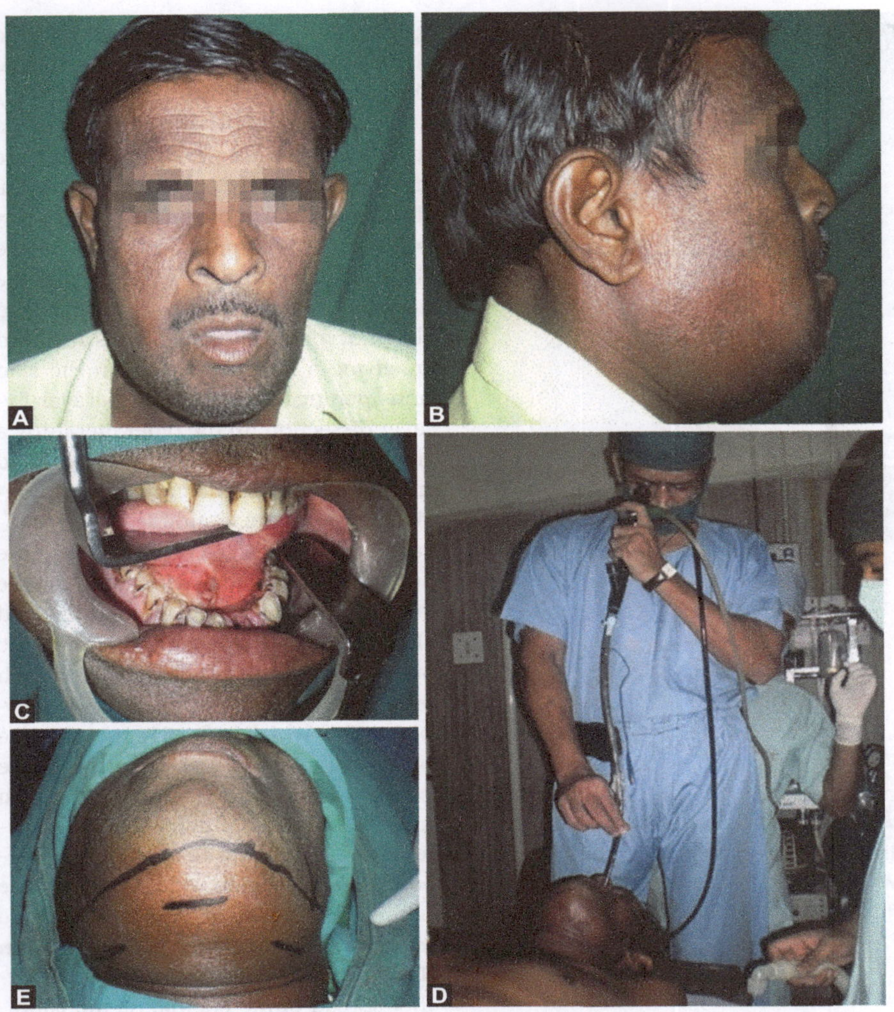

Figs 17.34A to E: Ludwig's angina: (A) Cellulitis of submental and submandibular spaces with elevation of the tongue; (B) Lateral view; (C) Congestion and swelling of the floor of mouth; (D) Intubated with fiberoptic broncoscope; (E) Marking of incisions for decompression

antibiotics. As the patient has dysphagia, oral antibiotics are not prescribed. The choice of the antibiotic is usually the penicillin group of antibiotics is high therapeutic doses, as the infection is caused by streptococci. Crystalline penicillin in a dose of 10 to 20 lacs IU IV, every 6 hourly is given. Alternatively, ampicillin 2 to 4 g/day is divided doses or third generation cephalosporins can be prescribed to make the spectrum of the antibiotics wider aminoglyconsides like gentamycin 1 to 4 mg/kg of body weight or amikacin 500 mg every 8 hourly may be prescribed.[46,47] Metronidazole is not the primarily prescribed antibiotic unless gangrenous tissue is present. As the circulatory impairment occurs and the environments are ischemic and hypoxic, due to mounting pressure within the tissue plains, as prophylactic major against the anaerobic infection metronidazole may be prescribed. Intravenous fluids are administered to maintain proper fluid and electrolyte balance and to fulfill the nutritional requirement of the patient as the patient has difficulty in deglutition. Other symptomatic treatments like analgesics, anti inflammatory drugs may be prescribed. The local care of the wound is taken by dressings. The drain should be maintained until the edema regress substantially. The septic focus precipitating this complication should be eliminated either simultaneously or subsequently.

Cavernous Sinus Thrombosis

The cavernous sinuses are the venous sinuses situated in the middle cranial fossa, which are situated on either side of sella turcica. They are formed by splitting of dura and are traversed with numerous fibrous septae, thus giving it a cave-like appearance and thus the name, '*cavernous sinus*'. The cavernous sinuses on either side communicate freely with each other by anterior and posterior intercavernous sinuses they also communicate with other venous sinuses like sagital sinus, transverse sinus and sigmoid sinus either directly or indirectly. The internal carotid artery and the VIth carnial nerve, i.e. abducent nerve pass through this sinus. It is the only anatomical location in the human body where an artery passes through the vein. The 3rd and 4th cranial nerves and the mandibular and maxillary branches of the 5th cranial nerve pass through the lateral wall of the cavernous sinus.[48] The cavernous sinus communicates extra cranially with the neck veins.

- The ophthalmic and angular veins into the anterior facial vein (*anterior connection*).
- Through emissary veins with the pteygoid plexus of veins (*posterior connection*).

The facial veins, unlike the veins of the extremities lack valves as the blood flow through these veins is along the gravity and the valves are not required to prevent the back flow of the blood. Due to this, any septic thrombophlebitis in these veins is capable to travel in a retrograde manner and can extend intercranially through them in the cavernous sinus. The area of the face between the inner canthi of the eye and the corners of the mouth is called 'danger triangle' of the face as severe sepsis in this area can lead to septic thrombophlebitis and the infection can spread in the retrograde manner and can extend in the cavernous sinus through the angular and the ophthalmic veins into the carvernous sinus[49] (Fig. 17.35A). This is the anterior root of spread of infection. The other route is through the emissary veins at the base of the skull which communicate with cavernous sinus. Any infection in the infratemporal fossa at the base of the skull can lead to spread of infection to the cavernous sinus.[50] The third route is direct spread of extra cranial infection into the cavernous sinus as a result of osteomyelitis of the base of the skull (Fig. 17.35B).

The carvernous sinus thrombosis is a rare complication of maxillofacial infections.[51,52] The predisposing factors are:

- Immunocompromised patients
- Malnourishment
- Diabetes
- Leukemia
- Angranulocytosis
- HIV infection.

Clinical Features

- The patient is fibrile with body temperature elevated to 104°F to 105°F and the patient is extremely toxic.
- The level of consciousness is altered as a result of increased intracranial pressure.
- There is severe infection in the above mentioned sites in the form of canine space infection, boil, cellulites or carbuncle in the nasal area, etc.
- The veins are blocked due to septic thrombophlebitis and the ensuing venous stasis leads to the edema of the face especially around the eyes (Figs 17.36A and B).
- The fundus appears congested on fundoscopy and it could be the initial sign of the cavernous sinus thrombosis. Sometimes, the edema of the eyelids is so severe that fundoscopy may not be possible.
- The eyeball is pushed out due to increased intraorbital pressure owing to the edema and proptosis results.
- The 6th cranial nerve passes through the cavernous sinus and thus it is the first nerve to be involved producing paralysis of the lateral rectus muscle and diplopia results.
- The 3rd and the 4th cranial nerves lie in the lateral wall of the sinus and are involved later, producing complete external opthalmoplagia, diplopia on all gazes. The pupil becomes fixed and dilated and does not respond to light. Thus, a superior orbital fissure syndrome is precipitated.
- Next due to thrombosis of the cavernous sinus spreads intracranially in the other venous sinuses producing severe venous stasis and cerebral edema is precipitated. The signs of the raised intracranial pressure develop. The papilledema developes.

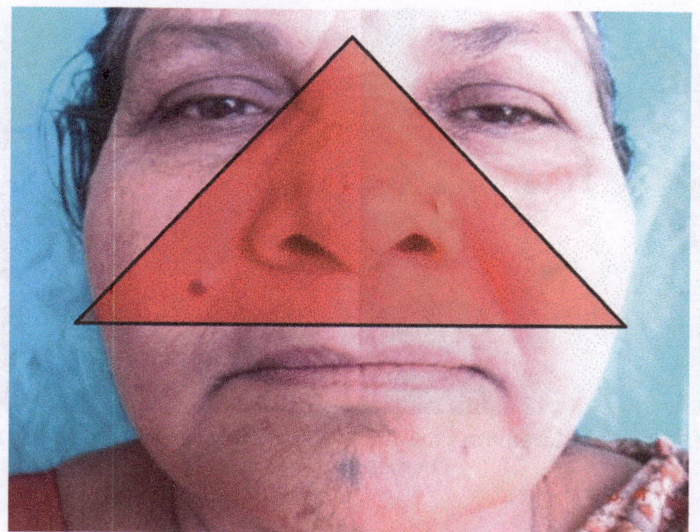

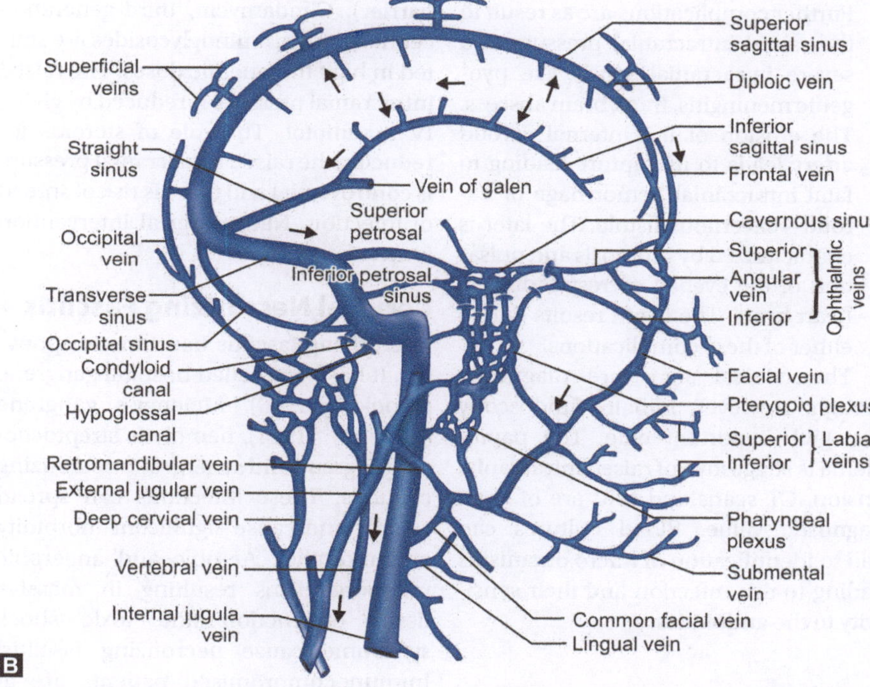

Figs 17.35A and B: (A) Danger triangle' of the face; (B) Venous network connecting with the cavernous sinus;

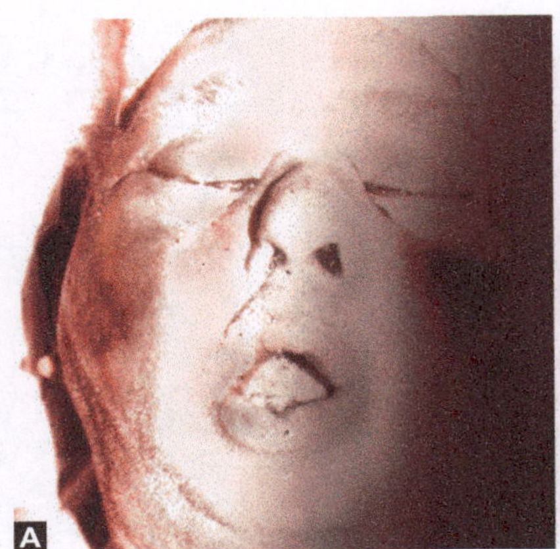

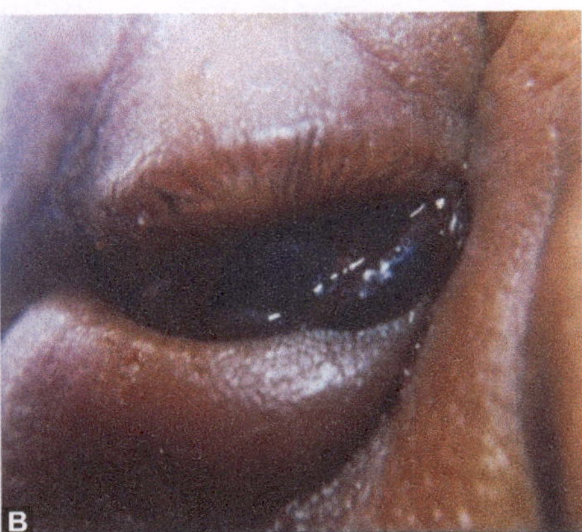

Figs 17.36A and B: Cavernous sinus thrombosis, note massive facial edema and severe chemosis of conjuctiva

- Further complications are as result to the raised intracranial pressure and severe intracranial sepsis like pyogenic meningitis, frank brain abscess. The erosion of the internal carotid artery leads to its rupture leading to fatal intracranial hemorrhage or carotid—cavernous fistula. The later is characterized by proptosis and pulsation of the eyeball corresponding to heart beats. The death results due to either of these complications.

The clinical signs are diagnostic enough. However, initially fundoscopy may give important clue. The papilledema is suggestive of raised intracranial tension. CT scans and MRI are of great diagnostic value. Blood cultures can lead to identification of micro organisms leading to this infection and their sensitivity to the antibiotics.

Management

The best management is prevention. In the patients who have the predisposition to this condition or spread of infection, the infections in the anterior facial area and at the base of the skull should be managed with broad spectrum antibiotics and active surgical intervention in time. Once the cavernous sinus thrombosis sets in, the mortality is high. The patient is given broad spectrum parenteral antibiotics preferable those which cross the BBB (blood brain barrier). Clindamycin, third-generation cephlosporins, aminoglycosides are started in high therapeutic doses. The raised intracranial pressure is reduced by giving IV manniotol. The role of steroids for reducing the raised intra cranial pressure is controversial and there is risk of spread of infection. Neurosurgical intervention is mandatory.

Cervical Necrotizing Fasciitis

Necrotizing fasciitis has various eponyms. It has been called hospital gangrene (Brooks,[53] 1966), Meleney's gangrene (Meleney[54] 1924), hemolytic streptococcal gangrene and synergestic necrotizing cellulitis. These infections can spread rapidly and cause significant morbidity and mortality. Aerobic and anaerobic microorganisms resulting in massive tissue destruction and toxic shock syndrome cause necrotizing fasciitis. Immunocompromised patients are at an increased risk of developing necrotizing fasciitis. Necrotizing fasciitis may affect any part of the body; however it most commonly affects the extremities, abdominal wall and the perineum.

Definition

Necrotizing fasciitis is an uncommon rapidly spreading soft tissue infection of polymicrobial origin characterized by extensive necrosis and gas formation in the subcutaneous tissue and superficial fascia.

Pathophysiology

Necrotizing fasciitis is a severe and potentially fatal infection of the dermal, fascial and subcutaneous layers of the skin. These infections are marked by the absence of clear local boundaries or palpable limits. This explains the frequent delay in recognizing the surgical nature of the infection. These infections could be clostridial or nonclostridial.

It is classically associated with clostridial infections, but organisms such as *Escherichia coli, Klebsiella, Peptostreptococcus* and *Bacteroides* may also produce subcutaneous emphysema. The more common anaerobic organisms seen in necrotizing fasciitis of the head and neck include *Peptostreptococcus, Bacteroides melaninogenicus* and *Fusobacterium.*[55]

The most common cause of cervical necrotizing fasciitis (CNF) is dental infections. Immunocompromised patients and those suffering from systemic illnesses such as diabetes mellitus are at an increased risk of developing this infection. It may also affect previously healthy individuals (13–31%). It is in these patients who are infected with Group A beta hemolytic streptococci that the infection spreads with a speed to produce massive tissue infection. The causative organism may be a single agent, commonly Group A beta hemolytic streptococci or Staphylococcal Aureus or may be a polymicrobial infections. Polymicrobial infections are caused by mixed aerobic and anaerobic pathogens. Synergy between them contributes to the pathogenesis of polymicrobial fasciitis, i.e. synergistic gangrene.

In most cases, the pathogen gains entry through a disruption of the skin caused by trauma or surgery. Initially, there is cellulitis which leads to invasion of the deeper tissues. Clinically, at this stage skin changes of erythema and edema are seen. Progressive tissue necrosis causes an invasion by the normal flora. Continuous bacterial overgrowth and synergy, causes a decrease in oxygen tension and development of local ischemia and proliferation of anaerobic organisms. In 4 to 5 days gangrene is evident and after 8 to 10 days necrotic tissue separates from the underlying ischemic, but viable tissue. Staphylococci and streptococci produce extracellular enzymes that damage connective tissue. Bacterial metabolism may produce insoluble hydrogen, nitrogen, nitrous oxide and hydrogen sulfide gases that result in subcutaneous emphysema. Obliterative endarteritis and thrombosis of the subcutaneous vessels along with necrotic superficial fascia and microbial colonization of the skin and fascia is seen. The necrosis of the fascia and obliteration of the blood vessels renders the overlying skin ischemic and undergoes gangrenous changes and sloughing. Myonecrosis is rarely seen except in clostridia infections.

Clinical Features

Systemic

- High fever
- Tachycardia
- Weakness
- Nausea
- Sepsis
- Hemolysis
- Intravascular volume depletion.

Local

- Affected area becomes swollen and erythematous
- Sudden pain, edema and generalized toxicity (Fig. 17.37A)
- The skin overlying becomes dusky with purple mottling
- Gas formation under the skin
- Frank gangrene of skin with sloughing, exposing the underlying necrotizing fascia and subcutaneous fat (Fig. 17.37B).

Diagnosis: Is made on the basis of:

- Clinical history/features
- Radiographs
- CT scan
- Frozen section.

Investigations

The routine investigations show leukocytosis, band cells and toxic granules in the leukocytes. The USG of the neck shows the collection in the superficial planes and the superficial necrotic foci and the CT scans are useful in detecting the deep seated collections and the necrosis.

Management

The critical step in management is the recognition of the condition and early, aggressive surgical intervention.[56] These infections require a rapid diagnosis as mortality rates up to 76 percent have been reported without early intervention. Mortality is higher in patients over 50 years of age, those with associated systemic illnesses like diabetes mellitus or peripheral vascular diseases and when there is a delay in diagnosis. Pain out of proportion to other clinical findings is an important clue to the diagnosis of this condition. Treatment involves wide local and serial surgical debridement supported by intravenous antibiotics and other supportive treatment[57] (Figs 17.38 to 17.40). It is essential that all areas of necrotic tissue be debrided. Excision to the point of bleeding tissue is a useful guide for debridement. There are certain centers which advocate the use of hyperbaric oxygen for treating this condition.[58]

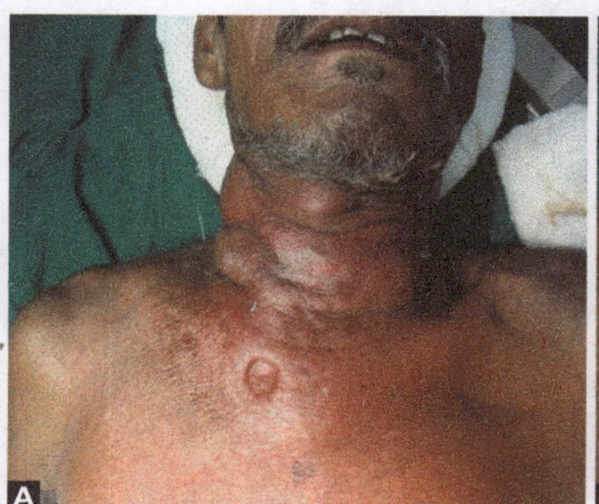

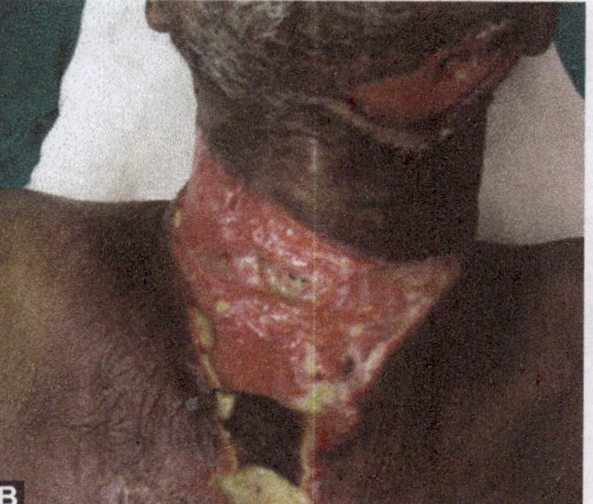

Figs 17.37A and B: CNF: (A) Pitting edema due to extensive cellulitis; (B) Subsequently resulting into gangrene of the skin

FUNGAL INFECTIONS OF THE MAXILLOFACIAL AREA

Mucormycosis

Mucormycosis represents most fatal, acute, opportunistic fungal infection. It is caused by fungi belonging to Mucoraceae family and includes *Rhizopus*, *Mucor*, and *Absidia*; the *Mucor* is the most common. The terms phycomycosis and mucormycosis are used interchangeably to denote infection by class phycomycetes. *Mucor* is found in soil like *Aspergillus*, but the source of infection in mucormycosis is mucor found in oral cavity, which is a part of normal oral microbial flora.

It presents in six clinical forms:[59]

1. *Rhinoparanasal and rhinocereberal*: The entry portals of this variant are mucosa of mouth, nose, paranasal sinuses.
2. *Pulmonary:* It is seen in patients with malignancy.
3. *GIT:* It is seen in malnourished patients.
4. *Cutaneous:* It is most often seen in burns patients.
5. CNS.
6. *Disemminated:* It is rare, but very severe.

Pathogenesis

Mucormycosis is a rare opportunistic infection that usually affects patients who have a depleted immunological status or uncontrolled diabetes. Depending on the immunological status of the host it may present in any of the above six forms. Rhinicerebral and pulmonary variants are most commonly seen in diabetic patients whereas the GIT variant is seen in malnourished patient. Inhalation of spores of this fungus is the primary portal of entry. However, in cases of cutaneous variant, the entry portal is breach in the skin. After its entry, the fungus grows and invades the tissues, especially blood vessels and elastic lamina of arterioles which further leads to thrombosis and tissue necrosis. The fungus has affinity for adipose tissue and spreads along the buccal fat pad and the periorbital fat leads to widespread maxillary and orbital involvement. Once the infection enters the orbit, it can enter the cranial cavity either through the blood vessels or by direct extension through the superior orbital fissure.

Disseminated disease is due to extension of the primary disease in severely immunocompromised patients.

Figs 17.38A to E: CNF managed with decompression, serial debridement and skin grafting

Rhinocerebral Mucormycosis

Symptoms

- Facial pain/headache.
- Impaired mental state.
- Fever.
- **Orbital involvement:** Orbital cellulitis, loss of extraoccular muscle function followed by proptosis, conjunctival swelling, loss of vision due to retinal artery stenosis (Figs 17.41A to F).
- Cranial nerve involvement manifested as pupillary dilation, ptosis. This is a marker of poor prognosis.
- **CNS involvement:** Meningoencephalitis, brain abscess, cavernous sinus thrombosis.
- **Involvement of nasal cavity:** Rhinorrhea, bloody discharge, necrosis of nasal turbinates and septum, necrotic lesions of hard and soft palate which appear as sharply demarcated black eschars on mucosa. The mucosa might also appear ischemic and cyanotic before ulceration is produced. Anesthesia of the mucosa might also be present.

Pulmonary Mucormycosis

Pulmonary mucormycosis is predominantly seen in patients with malignancies. It shows a significant neutropenia due to the chemotherapy taken for the hematologic malignancies. Many patients are on broad-spectrum antibiotics.

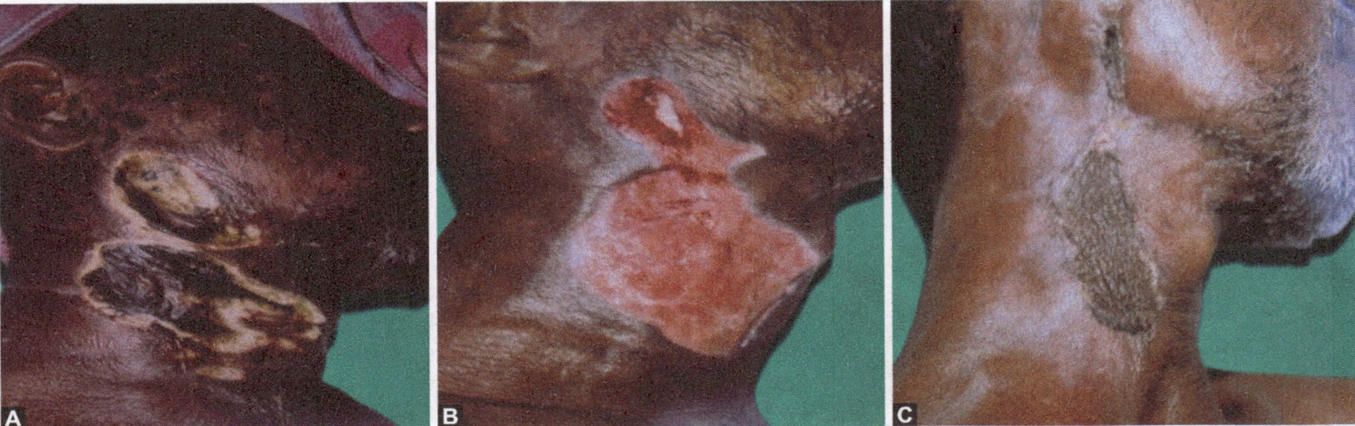

Fig. 17.39A to C: CNF treated with serial debridement and skin grafting

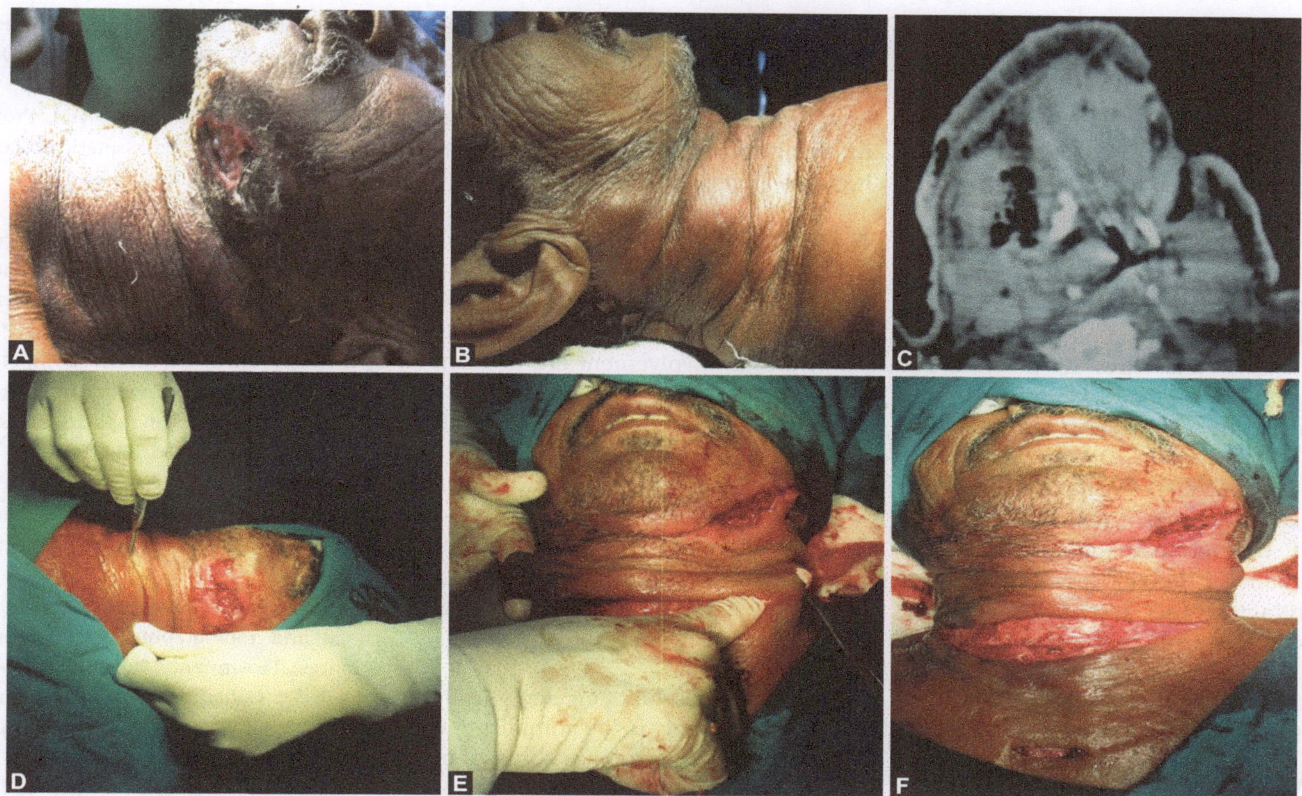

Figs 17.40A to F: CNF treated with liberal fasciotomy incision (surgical decompression) and debridement of necrotic fascia

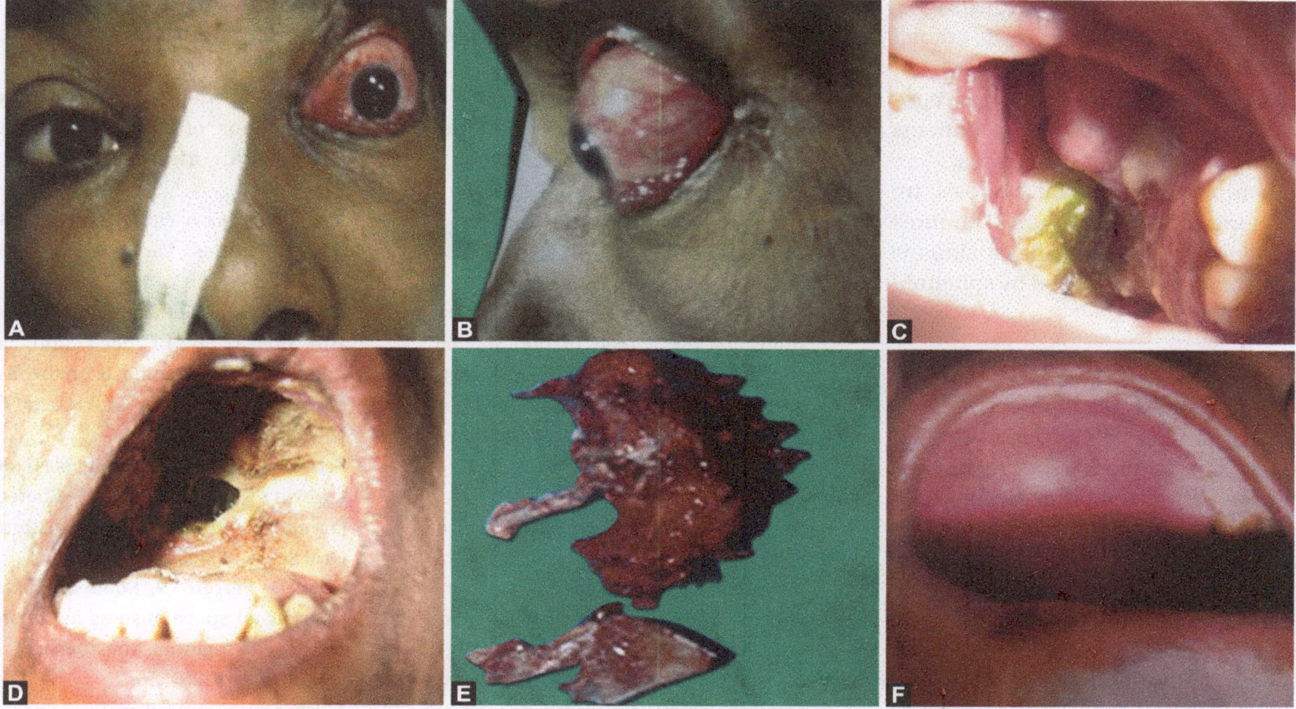

Figs 17.41A to F: Rhinocerebral mucormycosis in a 55-year-old, diabetic woman, treated with surgical debridement and amphotericin B

They present with fever, dyspnea, cough followed by hemoptysis and pulmonary infarcts. Fatal pulmonary hemorrhage due to erosion of major blood vessels can also occur. Pulmonary infiltration, consolidation and cavitation occur in high percentage of patients.

Cutaneous Mucormycosis

Primary lesion appears as superficial, painful, erythematous patches with central necrosis showing pustules and papules. Secondary lesions are a result of disseminated disease.

GIT Mucormycosis

This arises from organisms that enter GIT through contaminated food. All portions of the GIT are susceptible to contracting this lesion. Usually, this disease presents in the acute form and is rapidly fatal. Initial manifestations include abdominal pain and distension, nausea, vomiting and fever.

CNS Mucormycosis

Usually it occurs due to primary disease of nasal cavity and paranasal sinuses. It is characterized by decreasing level of consciousness, focal neurological signs, hemiplegia, hemiparesis and cranial nerve involvement.

Isolated brain involvement is reported in IV drug abusers in patients suffering from AIDS and leukemia.

Hemiplegia and facial necrosis are indicators of poor prognosis. The most commonly involved paranasal sinus is the ethmoid sinus followed by sphenoid and maxillary sinus.

Diagnostic Procedures

"*Early diagnosis is key to saving patient*" Hallmark of diagnosis is demonstration of organisms on biopsy specimens. The specimen is stained immediately with Hematoxylin and Eosin stain. However, more specific staining is done by Gomori Methanamine Silver (GMS) stain. Culture of the fungus is done using Saboraud's glucose agar. The *mucor* shows irregularly shaped, non-septate hyphae with branching at 90 degree angle.

Diagnostic tools include CT scan of paranasal sinuses, which might also include the study of intracranial contents in case of changes in mental status. Angiography of ICA can be done if its involvement is suspected. However, its involvement is associated with an increased mortality rate.

Management

- Debridement of all necrotic tissue (*see* Figs 17.41A to F).
- Orbital excenteration if the signs of orbital involvement are present, i.e. ophthalmoplegia, retinal artery stenosis, invasion of periorbital soft tissue, orbital apex syndrome.
- Correct acidosis and neutropenia
- After the identification of fungus, start IV amphotericin B. After giving a test dose of 0.3 mg/kg, a daily dose of 0.5 to 0.7 mg/kg and a total dose of 2500 to 4000 mg can be given.
- Monitor renal function periodically as renal toxicity is the complication of prolonged therapy with amphotericine. Lipid formulation of amphotericin B causes increased blood levels of the drug with decreased renal toxicity.
- Concomitant use of 5 fluorocytosine acts as synergistic and has a kidney sparing effect.
- Hyperbaric oxygen can be used.
- Overall survival is poor, i.e. less than 50 percent.

REFERENCES

1. Aya Ohshima. Anatomical considerations for the spread of odontogenic infection originating from the pericoronitis of impacted mandibular third molar: Computed tomographic analyses. OOOOE. 2004;98(5):589-97.
2. Parhiscar A, Har-El G. Deep neck abscess: A retrospective review of 210 cases. Ann Otol Rhinol Laryngol. 2001;110(11):1051-4.
3. Joacim Stalfors. Deep neck space infections remain a surgical challenge. A study of 72 patients. Acta Oto-laryngologica. 2004;124(10):1191-6.
4. Bransby-Zachary GM. The submasseteric space. Br Dent J. 1948;84:10-3.
5. Mandel L, Baurmash H. Submasseteric abscess. Oral Surg Oral Med Oral Pathol. 1958;11:1210-9.
6. Balatsouras DG, Kloutsos GM, Protopapas D, et al. Submasseteric abscess. J Laryngol Otol. 2001;115:68-70.
7. Nishimura T, Okabe Y, Furukawa M. A chronic organized masseter abscess causing trismus resolved by hemimasseter myotomy. Auris Nasus Larynx. 1996;23:140-2.
8. Tart RP, Kotzur IM, Mancuso AA, et al. CT and MR imaging of the buccal space and buccal space masses. RadioGraphics. 1995;15:531-50.
9. Smoker WRK. Oral cavity. In: Som PM, Curtin HD, (Eds). Head and neck imaging. 3rd edn. St. Louis: Mosby. 1996; pp. 488–544.
10. Felice O'ryan. Orbital infections: Clinical and radiographic diagnosis and surgical treatment. 1988;46(11):991-7.
11. Ash C, Cohen MA. Temporal-space infections: report of three cases. J Otolaryngol. 1996;25(6):416-20.
12. Mattucci K, Samet C. Pterygomaxillary space abscess. New York State Journal of Medicine. NY State J Med. 1974;74: 1409.
13. Zangenbrunner DJ, Dajani S. Pharyngomaxillary space abscess with carotid artery erosion. Arch Otolaryngol. 1971;94:447.
14. Granite EL. Anatomic considerations in infections of the face and neck: review of the literature. J Oral Surg. 1976;34:34.
15. Levitt GW. Cervical fascia and deep neck infections. Laryngoscope. 1970; 80:409.
16. Paonessa DF, Goldstein JC. Anatomy and physiology of head and neck infections (with emphasis on the fascia of the face and neck). Otolaryngol Clin North Am. 1976;9561.
17. Schwarti HC, Bauer RA, Davis NJ, et al. Ludwig's angina: use of fiberoptic laryngoscopy to avoid tracheostomy. J Oral Surg. 1974;32:608.
18. Kitay D, Ferraro N, Sonis ST. Lateral pharyngeal space abscess as a consequence of regional anesthesia. J Am Dent Assoc. 122(6):56-9.
19. Mosher HP. Submaxillary fossa approach to deep pus in the neck. Trans Am Acad Opthalmol Otolaryngol. 1929;34: 19.

20. Collier FA, Yglesias L. The relation of the spread of infection to fascial planes in the neck and thorax. Surgery. 1937;1:323.
21. Bezold F. Ein neuer Weg fFCr die Ausbreitung eitriger EntzFCndung aus den RE4umen des Mittelohrs aus die Nachbarschaft. Deutsche medizinische. Wochenschrift. 1881;28:381-4.
22. Hall C. The parapharyngeal space: an anatomical and clinical study. Ann Otol Rhinoi Laryngol. 1939;43:793.
23. Alaani A. Parapharyngeal abscess: diagnosis, complications and management in adults. European Archives of Oto-Rhino-Laryngology. 2005;262(4).
24. William R. Dzyak. Diagnosis and treatment of lateral pharyngeal space infections. 1984;42(4):243-9.
25. Petri Koivunen. Internal carotid artery thrombosis and Horner's syndrome as complications of parapharyngeal abscess. 1999;121(1): 160-2.
26. Shapiro SL. Deep cervical infection following tonsillectomy. Arch Otolarvnuol. 1930;11:701.
27. Lifschutz J. Fatal hemorrhage resulting from retropharyngeal abscess. Arch Otolaryngol. 1931;14:149.
28. Yannick G Amar. Intraoral drainage: recommended as the initial approach for the treatment of parapharyngeal abscesses. 2004;130(6):676-80.
29. Archer WH. Oral Surgery. Philadelphia: WB Saunders, 1966; pp. 362.
30. Mosher HP. Submaxillary fossa approach to deep pus in the neck. Trans Am Acad Opthalmol Otolaryngol. 1929; 34:19.
31. Ridder GJ, Technau-Ihling K, Sander A, et al. Spectrum and management of deep neck space infections: an 8-year experience of 234 cases. Otolaryngol Head Neck Surg. 2005;133(5):709-14.
32. Frank I. Retropharyngeal abscess. J Am Med Assoc. 1921;77:517.
33. Richards L. Retropharyngeal abscess. New England J Med. 1936; 215:1120.
34. Janecka IP, Rankow RM. Fatal mediastinitis following retropharyngeal abscess. Arch Otolaryngol. 1971; 93(6): 630-3.
35. Bryan CS, King BG, Bryant RE. Retropharyngeal infection in adults. Arch Int Med. 1974;134:127.
36. Dzyak WR, Zide MR. Diagnosis and treatment of lateral pharyngeal space infections. J Oral Maxillofac Surg. 1984; 42:243.
37. Greene JS, Asher IM. Retropharyngeal abscess: a previously unreported symptom. Annal Emerg Med. 1984;13:615.
38. Hay PD. The neck. Annal Roentgeonolo. 1930;9:5.
39. Wholey MH, Bruwer AJ, Baker HL. The lateralm roentgenogram of the neck. Radiology. 1958;71:350.
40. Endicott JN, Nelson RJ, Saraceno CA. Diagnosis and management decisions in infections of the deep fascial spaces of the head and neck utilizing computerized tomography. Laryngoscope. 1982;92:630.
41. Levine TM, Wurster CF, Krespi YP. |Mediastinitis occurring as a complication of odontogenic infections. Laryngoscope. 1986;96:747.
42. Alexander DW, Leonard JR, Trail ML. Vascular complications of deep neck abscesses. Laryngoscope. 1968;78:361.
43. Srirompotong Somchai. Ludwig's angina: A clinical review. European Archives of Oto-Rhino-Laryngology. 2003; 260(7):401-3.
44. Burt R. Meyers Ludwig's angina: Case report, with review of bacteriology and current therapy. AMJ Med. 1972;53(2): 257-60.
45. Lieutenant Colonel Thomas R. Gaines. Penicillin in the treatment of patients with deep infections of the neck. Arch Otolaryngol. 1945;42(1):1-5.
46. Esquivel Bonilla D, Huerta Ayala S, Molina Moguel JL. Report of 16 cases of Ludwig's angina: 5-year review. Pract Odontol. 1991;12(4):23-4, 28.
47. Daniel Bross-Soriano. Management of Ludwig's angina with small neck incisions: 18 years experience. Otojournal. 2004;130(6):712-7.
48. Ramanand Y. An atypical presentation of cavernous sinus thrombosis. Indian J Otolaryngol Head and Neck Surg. 2007;59:2.
49. David Goldenberg. Facial vein thrombophlebitis: A rare but potentially lethal entity. Otolaryngol Head Neck Surg. 2000;122(5):769-71.
50. Herbert G Childs Jr. Thrombosis of the cavernous sinus secondary to dental infection. Am J Orthodont Oral Surg. 1942;28(7):B402-B413.
51. Deji A. Ogundiya. Cavernous sinus thrombosis and blindness as complications of an odontogenic infection: report of a case and review of literature. JOMS. 1989;47(12):1317-21.
52. M Wen-Der Yun. Cavernous sinus thrombosis following odontogenic and cervicofacial infection. European Archives of Oto-Rhino-Laryngology. 1991; 248:7.
53. Brooks S. Civil War Medicine. Springfield, 111, Charles C Thomas Co. 1966.
54. Meleney FL. Hemolytic streptococcus gangrene. Arch Surg. 1924;9:317-64.
55. Dunbar NM. Necrotizing fasciitis: manifestations, microbiology and connection with black tar heroin. J Forensic Sci. 2007;52(4):920-3.
56. John D Urschel. Necrotizing soft tissue infections. Postgrad Med J. 1999;75:645-9.
57. De Backe. Management of necrotizing fasciitis in the neck. J Cranio Maxillofac Surg. 1996; 24(6): 366-71.
58. Jallali N, Withey S, Butler P. Hyperbaric oxygen as adjuvant therapy in the management of necrotizing fasciitis. Am J Surg. 189(4):462-6.
59. Baker RD, Seabury JH, Schneidau JD Jr. Subcutaneous and cutaneous mucormycosis and subcutaneous phycomycosis. Lab Invest. 1962;11:1091-1102.

18 Osteomyelitis of the Facial Bones

Borle Rajiv M, Yadav Abhilasha, Arora Aakash

Osteomyelitis is defined[1] as *'an inflammatory condition of bone that begins as an infection of medullary cavity and Haversian systems of the cortex and extends to involve the periosteum of the affected area'*. The meaning of the word osteomyelitis is '*osteon*' meaning bony, '*myelos*' is marrow and the word '*itis*' means inflammation.

APPLIED SURGICAL ANATOMY

The bone has essentially three structures, a cortical bone, a cancellous bone and the periosteum. The cortical bone is present outside and is covered by the periosteum, while the cancellous bone lies within the cortical bone. The facial bones are the flat bones and unlike the long bones the blood supply to these bones is predominantly through the nutrient vessels that enter the bone through the foramina and then they branch out to form a network in the cancellous bone. The other source of the blood supply is through the periosteum. The periosteum has two layers, the outer is fibrosed and provide the attachment to the muscles and derives blood supply through these attachments. The vessels giving the periosteal supply run parallel to cortical surface of bone giving off nutrient vessels, which penetrate cortical bone and anastomose with the dominant nutrient vessel (*e.g. the inferior alveolar artery in mandible*). The inner layer of the periosteum is cellular and is called cambium. The cambium helps in reparative and remodeling functions. As the age progresses the periosteum becomes less cellular and fibrosed thus, the periosteal source of blood supply diminishes and so is the reparative potential. The bone, marrow is enclosed in the cancellous bone. The bone, marrow is made up of cancellous bone which is rich in osteoblastic precursor cells, reticuloendothelial cells, erythrocytes, granulocytes and platelets and is highly vascular. The cortical bone is made up of dense bone, which contains a well-organized trabecular system connecting the bone marrow with the cortical bone. It consists of longitudinally oriented canals, the Haversian system, which is the central canal having nutrient blood vessel. It gives blood supply to osteocytes, which are lodged in lacunae (Figs 18.1A and B).

There are communicating canals called the Volkmann's canals. The Volkmann's canals connect the Haversian systems with each other. The Volkmann's canals also connect the bone marrow to the periosteum, which envelops the cortical bone (Figs 18.1C and D). These well organized complex interconnected systems provide nourishment for repair and regeneration of bone. As the age progresses the bone marrow becomes less cellular and fibrosed and its vascularity is also diminished. This brings down the reparative potential of the bone.

The facial bones by and large have an excellent vascularity and thus, the incidence of osteomyelitis is fairly less as compared to the long bones. Out of all the facial bones, the mandible is the most common bone to be involved by osteomyelitis due to the presence of more of compact bone and relatively less cancellous bone. The lesser amount of cancellous bone leads to lesser blood supply unlike the other facial bones. The other facial bones (e.g. the maxilla) have thin cortical bone and more cancellous bone leading to more blood supply and less chances of the osteomyelitis. The osteomyelitis of maxilla or other facial bones is very rare and whenever it occurs, the other predisposing conditions like immunosuppression,[2] uncontrolled diabetes,[3] sickle cell disorders,[4] etc. are usually present and they should always be ruled out. The osteomyelitis of the jaw bones is more common as compared to rest of the facial bones as the odontogenic infections are the most common source of infections in the maxillofacial area. The jaw bones provide anchorage to the teeth and are also commonly affected by odontogenic infections and the osteomyelitis.

PATHOPHYSIOLOGY OF OSTEOMYELITIS

The process leading to osteomyelitis (OML) is initiated by acute inflammation, hyperemia, increased capillary permeability and infiltration of granulocytes. Tissue necrosis occurs as proteolytic enzymes are released and vascular thrombosis ensues. As the pus accumulates, the intramedullary pressure increases resulting in vascular collapse, venous

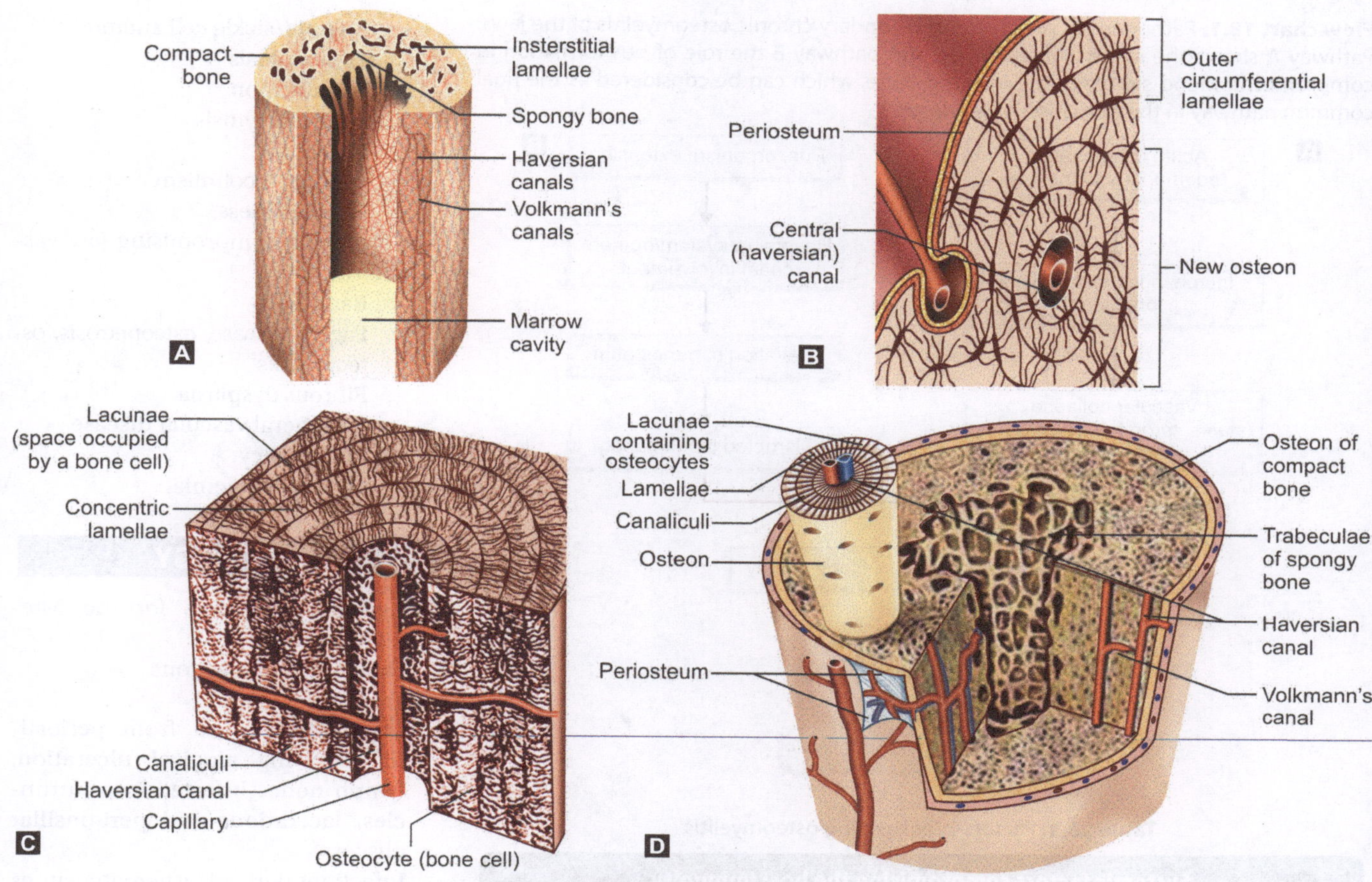

Figs 18.1A to D: Haversian system of the bone

stasis and ischemia. Pus travels through the Haversian and nutrient canals and accumulates beneath the periosteum, elevating it from the bone and thereby further reducing the vascular supply.

Compression of the neurovascular bundle accelerates thrombosis and ischemia and results in osteomyelitis induced (*inferior alveolar in case of mandible*) nerve dysfunction. Extensive periosteal elevation occurs more frequently in children, presumably because the periosteum is bound less firmly to bone than in adults. If pus continues to accumulate, the periosteum is penetrated and mucosal and cutaneous abscesses and fistulas may develop. If this condition is treated with antibiotics alone, without appropriate surgical intervention, the condition may progress to chronic form.

Inflammation regresses, granulation tissue forms, and new blood vessels lyse the bone, thus separating fragments of necrotic bone (*sequestra*) from viable bone (Flow chart 18.1). Small sections of bone may be lysed completely, whereas larger ones may be isolated by a bed of granulation tissue encased in a sheath of new bone (*involucrum*). Sequestra may be revasularized, remain quiescent, reabsorb or be infected chronically and require surgical removal before the infection subsides completely. Occasionally the involucrum is penetrated by channels (*cloacae*), through which pus escapes to an epithelial surface. Bone surrounding a sequestrum sometimes appears radiographically as less densely mineralized than the sequestrum itself, because increased vascularity of adjacent vital bone creates a relative demineralization. Ischemia causes increase in CO_2 level, which attracts calcium due to change in pH. The calcium deposition leads to increase in mineralization of the sequestrum (*dystrophic calcification*). Secondly, the calcium mobilization from the devitalized bone does not take place and hence, the sequestrated bone appears more opaque on the X-ray. As reparative mechanism the periosteal bone apposition also takes place and the periosteal reaction is evident on the X-ray. The lifting of the periosteum at the edges of the bony defect produces a triangular elevation called the *Codman's triangle*.[5] The initial radiological picture of an acute osteomyelitis is alteration and thinning of the trabecular pattern. While as the more opaque sequestrum is separated from normal bone by radiolucent area (*involucrum*) and associated periosteal reaction is the picture in chronic osteomyelitis. The sequestra formation leads to undermining of the bone and renders it weak. Such a weak bone is liable to fracture even during functional movements or on application of mild stress (*pathological fracture*).

Flow chart 18.1: Pathogenesis of acute and secondary chronic osteomyelitis of the jaws. Pathway A shows the role of inflammation and pathway B the role of pus formation in compromising blood supply of the infected bone, which can be considered as the final common pathway in the formation of sequestra

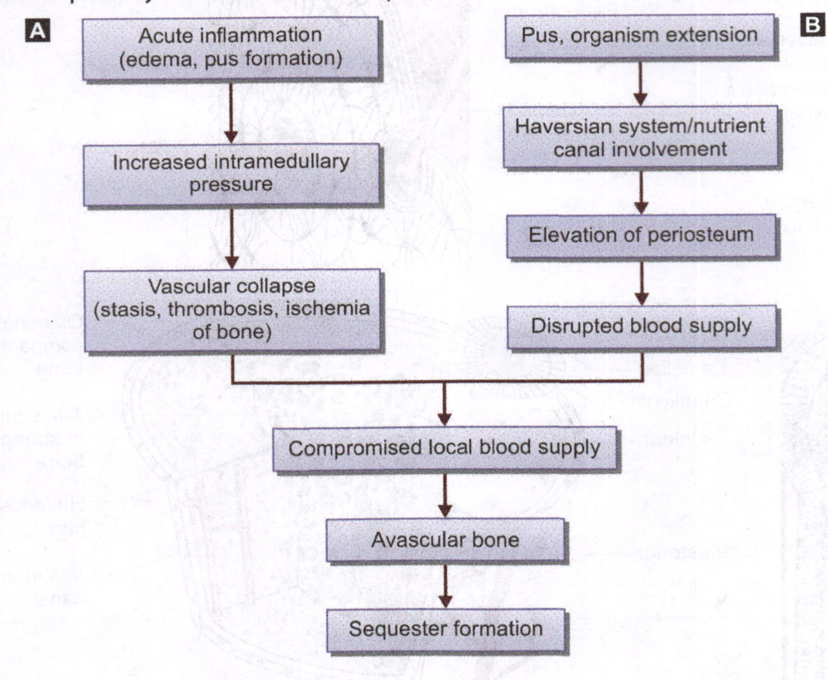

Table 18.1: Factors-predisposing osteomyelitis

Systemic factors compromising the host immunity	
Diabetes mellitus	Malnutrition
Autoimmune disorders	Chemotherapy
AIDS	Corticosteroid and other immunosuppressive therapy
Agranulocytosis	Alcohol and tobacco
Anemia (especially sickle cell)	Drug abuse
Leukemia	Prior major surgery
Syphilis	Herpes simplex virus (zoster) and cytomegalovirus infection
Local and systemic factors altering bone vascularity	
Smoking	Osteoporosis
Diabetes mellitus	Bisphosphonate-induced osteochemonecrosis
Florid osseous dysplasia	Other forms of osteonecrosis (mercury, bismuth, arsenic)
Fibrous dysplasia	Tobacco
Paget's disease	Radiation therapy and osteoradionecrosis
Osteopetrosis (Albers-Schonberg disease)	Bone malignancy (primary or metastatic)

PREDISPOSING FACTORS

The odontogenic infections are common in occurrence, however majority of them do not lead to osteomyelitis. The chances of precipitation of osteomyelitis are enhanced if there is an underlying local or systemic pathological of condition (Table 18.1).

- Conditions compromising the Host defense are (Fig. 18.2):
  - Diabetes
  - Anemia/sickle cell anemia
  - Tuberculosis
  - Malnutrition
  - Agranulocytosis
  - Leukemia
  - Chronic alcoholism
  - Febrile illness.
- Conditions compromising jaw vascularity are:
  - Radiation
  - Paget's disease, osteopetrosis, osteoporosis
  - Fibrous dysplasia
  - Peripheral vascular disease
  - Malignancy
  - Sickle cell anemia.

ETIOLOGY

The etiological factors for the osteomyelitis are[6]:

- Odontogenic infections
- Trauma
- Infections derived from periostitis following gingival ulceration, lymph nodes infected from furuncles, lacerations and peritonsillar abscess.
- Infections derived by hematogenous route—furuncle on face, wound on the skin, upper respiratory tract infection, middle ear infection, mastoiditis, systemic tuberculosis.

The mechanisms of systemic diseases/conditions predisposing to osteomyelitis (Adapted from Marx 1991) are as under (Box 18.1).

Many authors have tried to classify the osteomyelitis in different ways. The basic classification as per the duration is acute, sub acute or chronic osteomyelitis. The osteomyelitis can also be classified as per the specific or non specific infective organisms precipitating infection and subsequently the osteomyelitis, as specific or non specific infective osteomyelitis (Box 18.2).

Huddson's classification is as given in (Box 18.3).

CLINICAL FEATURES

The clinical features of osteomyelitis can be enumerated as per the type of osteomyelitis as follows:

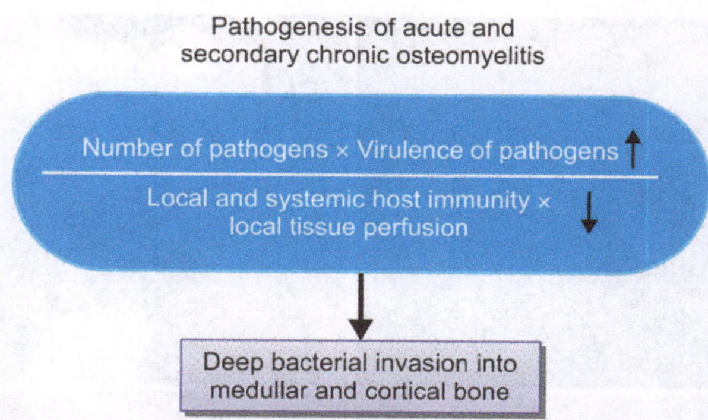

Fig. 18.2: Interaction of host and pathogens. If the balance is shifted to the advantage of the aggressor, deep bone infection will be established

Box 18.1: Mechanism of precipitation of osteomyelitis due to various factors

Disease	Mechanism facilitating bone infection
Diabetes	Diminished leukocyte chemotaxis, phagocytosis and lifespan; diminished vascularity of tissue due to vasculopathy thus reducing perfusion and the ability for an effective inflammatory response; slower healing rate due to reduced tissue perfusion and defective glucose utilization
Leukemia	Deficient leukocyte function and associated anemia
Malnutrition	Reduced wound healing and reduction of immunological response
Cancer	Reduced wound healing and reduction of immunological response
Osteopetrosis (Albers-Schonberg disease)	Reduction of bone vascularization due to enhanced mineralization, replacement of hematopoietic marrow causing anemia and leukopenia
Severe anemia (particularly sickle-cell anemia)	Systemic debilitation, reduced tissue oxygenation, bone infarction (sickle cell anemia), especially in patients with a homozygous anemia trait
IV drug abuse	Repeated septic injections, spreading of septic emboli (especially with harboring septic vegetation on heart valves, in skin or within veins)
AIDS	Impaired immune response
Immunosuppression (steroids, cytostatic drugs)	Impaired immune response

Box 18.2: Classification

Historically accepted classification based on clinical course
- Acute
- Subacute
- Chronic

Infective
- Specific
  - i. Tuberculosis
  - ii. Syphillis
  - iii. Actinomycosis
- Non-specific
  - i. Pyogenic
  - ii. Necrosis

Acute Suppurative Osteomyelitis

- Deep intense pain.
- High grade, intermittent fever.
- Constitutional signs of the acute infection such as bodyache, malaise, leukocytosis, raised ESR, etc.
- Paresthesia or anesthesia of lower lip due to involvement of the inferior alveolar nerve.
- The cause is usually, clearly identifiable in the form of acute infection associated with the tooth.

Box 18.3: Hudson's classification[7]

- Acute forms of OML (suppurative and non-suppurative include:
  - Contiguous focus:
    - i. Trauma
    - ii. Surgery
    - iii. Odontogenic infections
  - Progressive:
    - i. Burns
    - ii. Sinusitis
    - iii. Vascular insufficiency
  - Hematogenous (metastatic): Developing skeleton (children)
- Chronic forms of OML
  - Recurrent multifocal:
    - i. Developing skeleton (children)
    - ii. Escalated osteogenic activity (age < 25 years)
  - Garre's:
    - i. Unique proliferative subperiosteal reaction
    - ii. Developing skeleton (children to young adults)
  - Suppurative or non-suppurative:
    - i. Inadequately treated forms
    - ii. Systematically compromised patients
    - iii. Chronic refractory OML
  - Diffuse sclerosing:
    - i. Fastidious organism
    - ii. Compromised host/pathogen interface

- Pus discharge from the gingival crevice.
- Mobility of the teeth in the involved area.
- Acute osteomyelitis may not show pronounced radiological features, because to develop the same more than 30 percent calcium has to be mobilized from the bone. The radiological picture may range from simple rarefaction of the bony trabeculae (Fig. 18.3) to '*moth eaten*' radiolucency (Fig. 18.4). The offending tooth is present, which may show periapical rarefaction.
- A strongly positive radionucleotide scan along with the above.

Subacute Suppurative Osteomyelitis

The clinical signs and symptoms are less severe as compared to the acute condition and some of the signs are well established. The duration of the disease

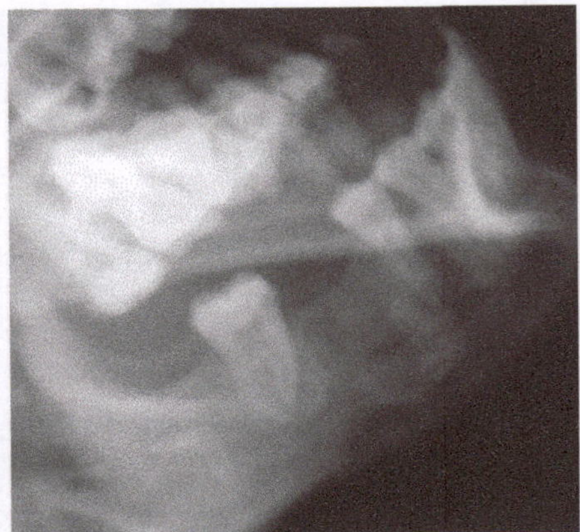

Fig. 18.3: Patchy rarefied radiolucent lesion

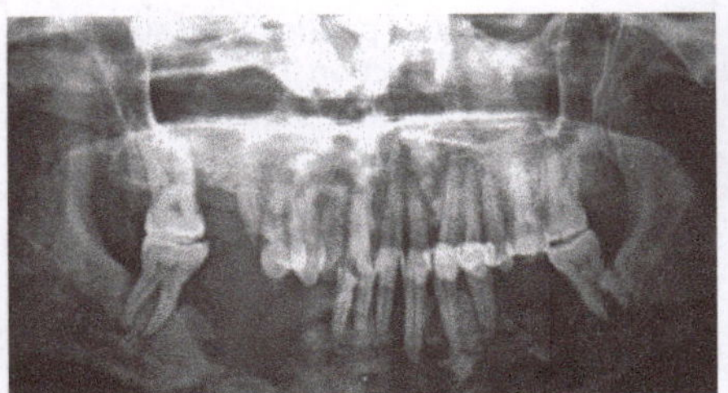

Fig. 18.4: Osteomyelitis moth-eaten appearance on X-ray

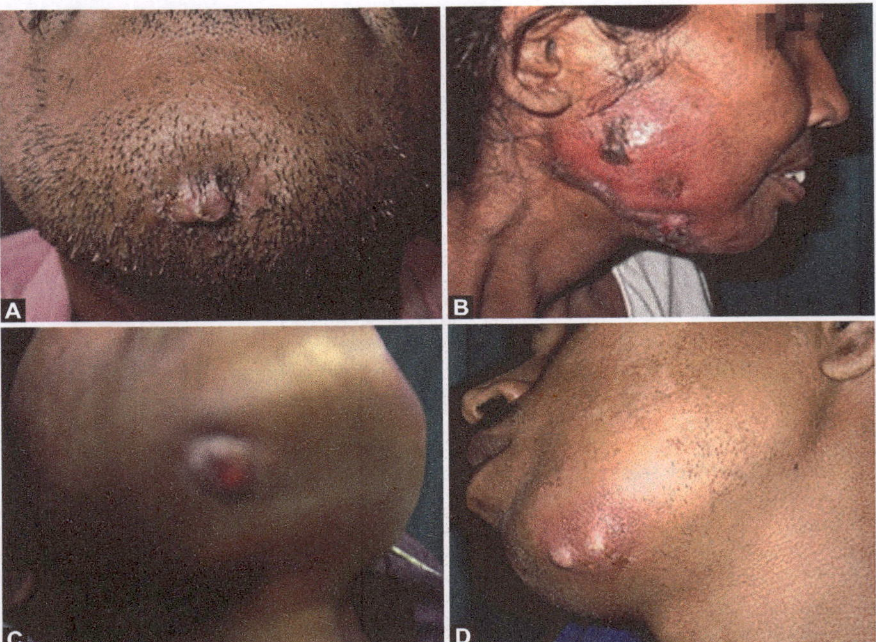

Figs 18.5A to D: Cutaneous sinus secondary to chronic osteomyelitis

is longer as compared to the acute variety.

- There is a deep seated, dull, pain, anorexia and fever (101°F to 102°F).
- The teeth in the involved area become loose and are tender on percussion.
- The pus exudates through gingival and cutaneous fistulas.
- Fetid oral odor may be present due to pus.
- The cellulitis of the cheek may be present over the involved area.
- The expansion of the bone due to periosteal reaction.
- The infection gets localized to form an abscess in the adjoining soft tissue.
- The regional lymph nodes get enlarged and are discrete, soft and tender.
- Leukocytosis is not a consistent finding.

Chronic Osteomyelitis

As the acute symptoms subside, due to antibiotic therapy without surgical treatment or due to the immunity controlling the infection, the condition slips into a chronic form wherein the symptoms are less severe, intermittent and persistent unless comprehensive treatment is undertaken. The abscess drains spontaneously on the skin or gingival surface leading to a chronic pus discharging sinus, which is adherent to the bone through an epithelized sinus tract and drains pus intermittently (Figs 18.5A to D). The infected bone undergoes necrosis and gets separated from the normal bone, the necrotic bone is called as the sequestrum. It serves as the nidus of infection and the pus collects inside the bone and the tissue plane intermittently. When sufficient pressure is generated, it drains through the sinus. As the pus is drained out, the sinus becomes non-draining. The sinus opening shows exuberant granulation tissue and as the sinus tract is epithelized, it fails to heal even after the septic focus is eliminated. The cutaneous sinus may sometimes be formed at a distance from the bony lesion. Sometimes more than one sinus tracts are present. As the surrounding soft tissue is indurated, sometimes it becomes difficult to differentiate between fungating malignancy, which is secondarily infected and an osteomyelitis if the patient is seen in this stage for the first time and where the past history is not reliable.

The surrounding soft tissue is indurated, thickened or woody in consistency. Pain and tenderness are usually mild and non-significant.

RADIOLOGICAL FEATURES

Worth's Criteria (1969)[8]

- *'Moth-eaten'* appearance (enlargement of medullary spaces and widening of Volkmann's canals) (Fig. 18.4)
- Islands that is *'seqeustrum'* (avascular necrotic bone, which harbors microorganisms) with evidence of trabecular pattern and marrow spaces (Figs 18.6A and B).

The computerized tomography scans are very informative and useful in detecting and assessing the osteomyelitis. It gives accurate indication of:

i. Bone destruction
ii. Periosteal reaction (Fig. 18.7)
iii. Medullary destruction
iv. Cortical involvement.

The MRI scan is more accurate compared to CT scans, which gives information about the bone marrow changes and the soft tissue changes.

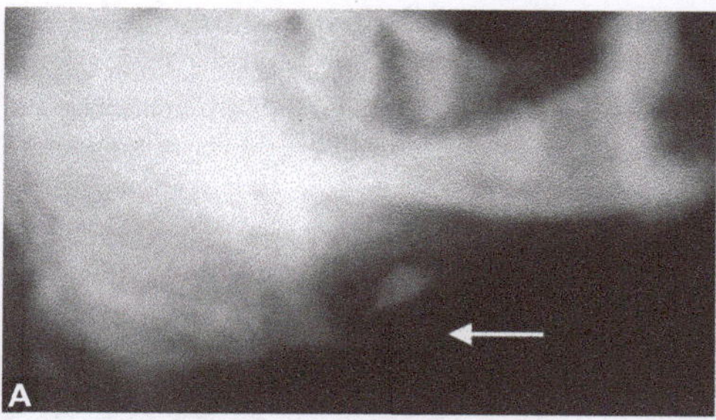

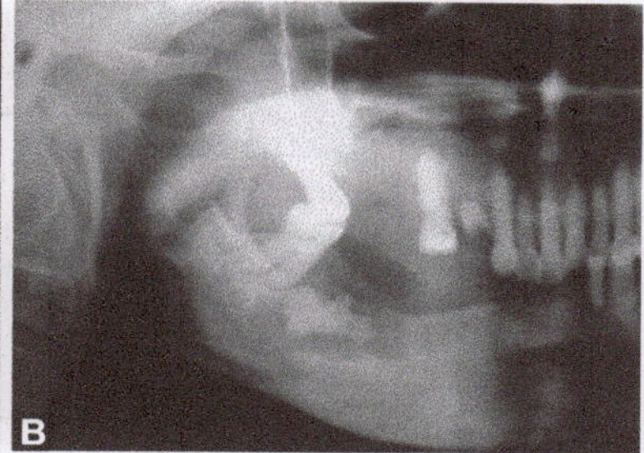

Figs 18.6A and B: Radiopaque sequestrum

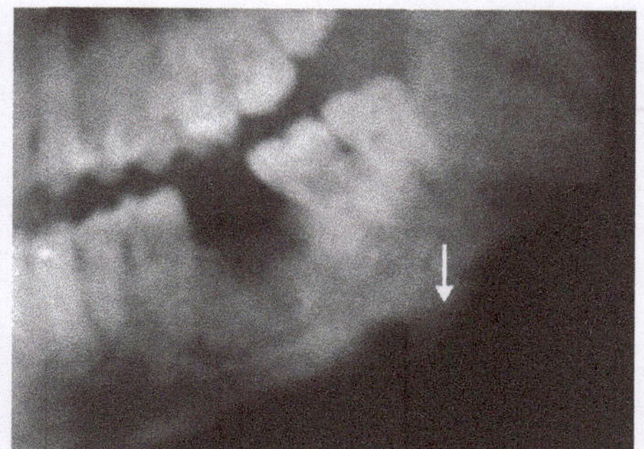

Fig. 18.7: Periosteal reaction

Specialized Investigations

In the borderline cases, the specialized investigations are carried out to detect the bony changes at an early stage, which helps in detection of the osteomyelitis, vascularity and reparative activity in the bone.

Bone Scintigraphy

Bone scanning (*scintigraphy*), radionuclide imaging, or skeletal scintigraphy is useful in determining the presence of reactive bone thus, it is particularly helpful in the diagnosis of bone disease. It helps in the diagnosis and management of osteomyelitis of the jaws, which is based on reactive bone formation rather than demineralization. The changes are seen as early as 3 days after the onset of symptoms of OML.

In this bone is scanned using Tc-labeled ethylene diphosphonate,[9] which is administered intravenously. The radioisotope is distributed to the entire skeleton and concentrated in areas of increased blood flow and osteoblastic activity. A rectilinear scanner or scintillation camera, both of which contain sodium iodide, a crystal nuclide that emits light, is then used to obtain images of the isotope containing areas. The resulting image shows the distribution of radionuclide in areas of increased bone activity. The complete bone scan has three phases:

- Flow study consists of serial images at the intervals of 3 to 4 seconds during 1 to 2 minutes after injection of the drug.
- Blood pool study consists of a single image obtained 5 to 10 minutes after injection.
- Delayed study includes multiple views obtained 2 to 4 hours after injection.

Positive Tc scan results can be useful in confirming the diagnosis of acute OML, although bone scan findings may be negative very early in the disease.

Addition of gallium 67 to technetium (Tc) 99 aids in distinguishing OML from malignancy and trauma.[10]

If neoplastic disease is not suspected as the cause of symptoms due to the age, clinical findings or laboratory studies, a positive Tc scan result alone is sufficient to diagnose OML. When the patient's age and clinical findings make the diagnosis equivocal, as when a neoplasm is suspected, the Tc scan may be followed by a gallium scan (Ga). Positive findings on both tests usually confirm the infectious nature of the disease. When the Tc scan result is positive and the Ga scan results are negative, OML probably is not the primary disease. Ga uptake that exceeds Tc uptake indicates active inflammatory disease. In chronic OML reduced Ga accumulation in the follow-up scan is useful indicator for termination of therapy in OML.

Recently positron emission tomography (Figs 18.8A and B) using radioisotopes of physiologically active compounds such as glucose,[11] ammonia and flouride have shown greater promise in mapping out varying margins of metabolic activity.

PRINCIPLES OF TREATMENT OF OSTEOMYELITIS

- Thorough clinical evaluation and correction of host defense deficiencies.
- Administration of empirical antibiotics.
- Imaging to rule out bone tumors.
- Removal of the septic foci such as loose teeth and sequestra.
- Administration of culture guided antibiotics; repeated cultures
- Possible placement of irrigating drains/polymethylmethacrilate–antibiotic beads

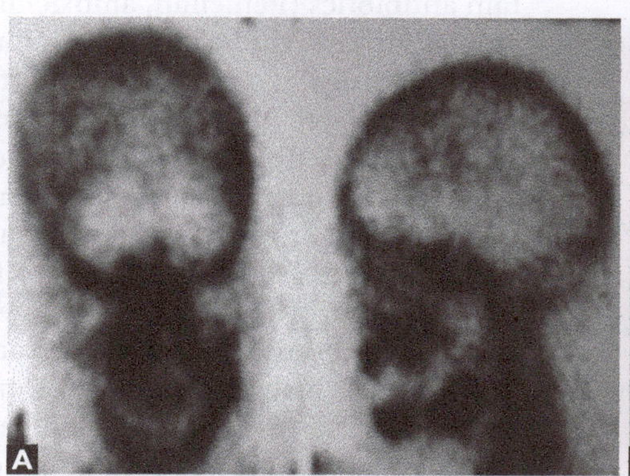

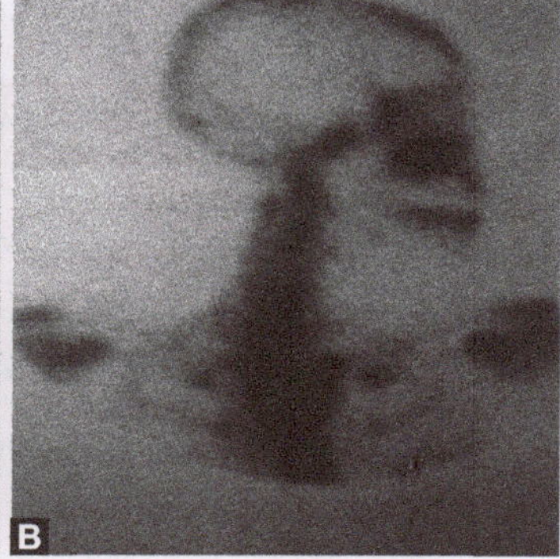

Figs 18.8A and B: Positron emission tomographic scan in case of osteomyelitis

- Surgical management by sequestrectomy, debridement, decortication, resection, reconstruction
- Hyperbaric oxygen therapy

Marx (1992) has proposed certain guidelines for three management of osteomyelitis as given in Box 18.4.

By and large the diagnosis of osteomyelitis on clinical and radiological findings is easy. But, in the early, borderline and cases with atypical presentation the evaluation of the cases should be undertaken as depicted in the Box 18.5.

Decision Tree[12]

Decision tree for diagnosis of osteomyelities is illustrated in Flow chart 18.2.

Flow chart 18.2: Decision tree for diagnosis of osteomyelitis

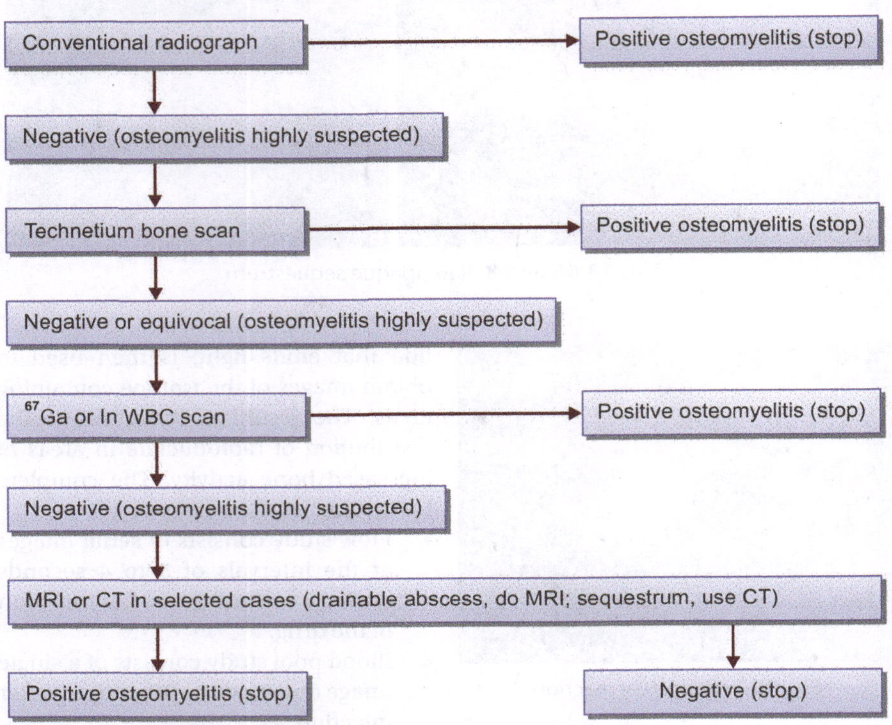

Medicinal Treatment

The medicinal treatment of osteomyelitis comprises of administration of antibiotics, supportive treatment, dietry suppliments and other symptomatic interventions such as administration of analgesics, antipyretics and anti inflammatory drugs. The osteomyelitis of the jaw bones is commonly secondary to odontogenic infections and thus, the microbial flora is similar to oral flora comprising of gram positive microorganisms such as streptococci, staphylococci. These organisms are sensitive to beta lactam antibiotics. Owing to the hypoperfused environments and the necrotic tissue, the facultative anerobes also invade making it a mixed infection. Thus, routinely the beta lactam antibiotics (Penicillin, amoxicillin, ampicillin and cephalosporins) along with the drugs like metronidazole (for anerobic infections) are suited for empirical antibiotic therapy. However, upon the culture and sensitivity if other organisms such as gram negative are detected then aminoglycosides can be administered. The chances of infections from the other organisms apart from those which are the part of oral flora, increase in case of osteomyelitis secondary to grossly contaminated fractures of the jaw, hospital acquired infections or hematogenous infections in a compromised host. The selection of the specific antibiotics depends upon the culture and sensitivity report of the pus samples taken from the lesion. The antibiotic regimen for osteomyelitis of the jaws recommended by Topazian[13] is as shown in Box 18.6.

Box 18.4: Treatment guidelines for acute and chronic osteomyelitis (Marx 1992)

- Disrupt the infectious foci
- Debride any foreign bodies, necrotic tissues, or sequestra
- Culture and identify specific pathogens for eventual definitive antibiotic treatment
- Drain and irrigate the region
- Begin empiric antibiotics based on Gram's stain
- Stabilize calcified tissue regionally
- Consider adjunctive treatments to enhance microvascular reperfusion: Trephination, decortication, vascular flaps HBO therapy
- Reconstruction: as necessary following resolution of infection.

Box 18.5: Decision tree

- Conventional radiograph-Positive-OML stop
  Negative OML highly suspected
- Technetium bone scan Positive-OML-stop
  Negative OML highly suspected
- Ga67 or IN111 WBC scan-Positive-OML stop
  Negative OML highly suspected then
- MRI or CT-Positive-OML stop
  Negative-OML stop

Local Antibiotic Therapy

Closed wound irrigation suction: After intraoral debridement, sequestrectomy and saucerization or decortications, two small pediatric nasogastric feeding tubes, catheters or polyethylene drain tubes, 3 to 4 mm in diameter and 6 to 10 inches long in length are placed against the bony bed through separate skin incisions at some distance and secured with sutures.

One tube is connected to low pressure suction to allow drainage of pus and serum and another is kept patent to provide a route through which local antibiotics are instilled in very high concentrations.[14]

Box 18.6: Topazian protocol for antibiotic regimen for osteomyelitis

Regimen I	For hospitalized/medically compromised patients or when intravenous therapy is indicated	Aqueous penicillin, 2 million units IV q4h, plus metronidazole, 500 mg IV q6h. When improved for 48–72 hours, switch to: Penicillin V, 500 mg PO q4h, plus metronidazole 500 mg PO q6h, for an additional 4–6 weeks. OR Ampicillin/salbactum 1.5–3 g IV q6h, When improved for 48–72 hours switch to: Amoxicillin/clavulanic acid (Augmentin) 875/125 mg PO bid, for an additional 4–6 weeks.
Regimen II	For out patient treatment	Penicillin V 2 g, plus metronidazole 0.5 g q8h PO, for 2–4 weeks after last sequestrum removed and patient without symptoms. OR Clindamycin, 600–900 mg q6h IV; then clindamycin 300–450 mg q6h PO OR Cefoxitin 1 g q8h IV or 2 g q4h IM or IV, until no symptoms, then switch to: Cephalexin 500 mg q6h PO, for 2–4 weeks ***For penicillin allergic patients:*** Clindamycin (as above) Cefoxitin as above, for allergy not of anaphylactoid type.

Negative Pressure Healing[15]

Negative pressure healing occurs by three mechanisms:

1. **Altered blood flow:** Vacuum increases the vascularity of wound edges by increasing blood flow diameter, velocity, blood volume, endothelial proliferation and angiogenesis and thus promotes healing.
2. **Mechanical deformation:** Because of the negative pressure there is stretching of the cells which causes disturbances in the extracellular and intracellular skeleton. To overcome this there is increased mitotic activity, which in turn promotes healing.
3. **Pressure gradient:** Pressure itself pulls cytotoxic substances, bacteria, normal cells towards infected site, reduces interstitial edema and thus promotes healing.

Antibiotic Impregnated Beads

Used in the treatment of OML to deliver high concentrations of antibiotics into the wound bed and in immediate proximity to the infected bone.

Gentamycin-PMMA beads[16]: The unique advantage of using antibiotic impregnated PMMA beads is in the fact that a very high local concentration of antibiotics can be delivered with minimal concomitant systemic levels. Antibiotic should be bacteriostatic, or preferably bactericidal and be sufficiently stable in the face of high temperatures to prevent degradation during the curing the process of the cement.

Indications for using beads:

- Infection that is refractory to traditional treatment.
- Decreased blood flow to the infected area.
- Immunocompromised host.
- Medically compromised patient.

Surgical Management

Surgical management of acute and chronic osteomyelitis is depicted in Fig. 18.9.

Sequestrectomy and Saucerization

Sequestrum formation is a classical sign of secondary chronic and advanced acute osteomyelitis cases. Usually a time frame of at least 2 weeks after onset of infection is necessary until presentation. In general, sequestra are confined to the cortical bone, but may also be cancellous or cortico-cancellous. Once a sequestrum is fully formed, it may persist for several months in untreated cases before being resorbed or spontaneously expelled through the oral mucosa or the facial skin. Resorption of sequestrum is achieved by lytic activity of the osteoclast cells in the surrounding granulation tissue. Gradually the granulation tissue may ingrow the

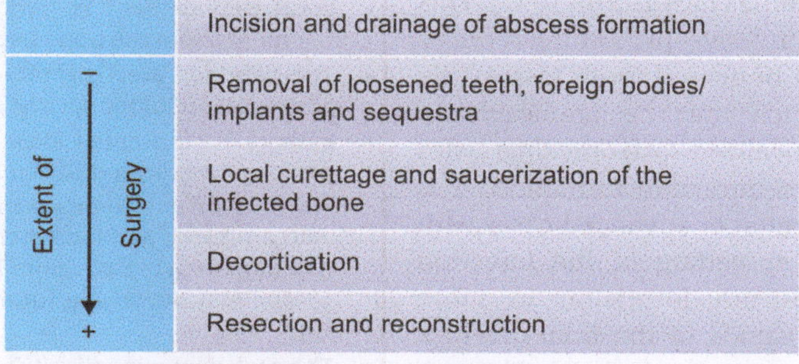

Fig. 18.9: Surgical management of acute and secondary chronic osteomyelitis. Depending on the extent of the infected bone, surgery has to be adapted, resulting in a smaller or larger procedure

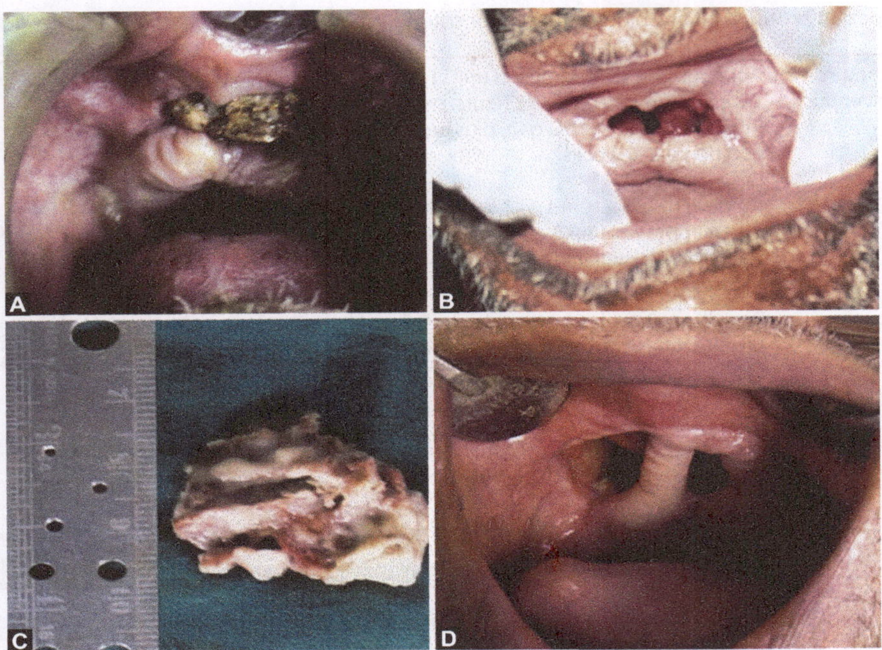

Figs 18.10A to D: Maxillary osteomyelitis in an uncontrolled diabetic patient treated with sequestrectomy

sequestrum and promote its degradation. If sequestra are not fully removed in treatment, partial, superficial healing may occur. Because sequestrum are avascular, they are poorly penetrated by antibiotics or HBO and hence, are ideal breading grounds for bacteria. They serve as sources of exacerbations of the osteomyelitis when pus and granulation tissue accumulates around them. In rare cases of osteomyelitis of the jaws, a sterile abscess formation around the sequestrum (Brodie's abscess), common to long bone osteomyelitis, occurs.[13]

Once the sequestrum is formed completely, it may be removed with minimal surgical trauma (Figs 18.10A to D). This minimally invasive procedure reduces subsequent bone and tooth loss. While this approach may be applicable in cases of localized osteomyelitis with superficial sequestrum formation, it is contraindicated in advanced cases with protracted spreading of the infection and sequestrum formation in more profound regions of the bone. Here a more aggressive surgical debridement is necessary, which clearly must exceed the sole removal of sequestrum.

Saucerization describes the 'unroofing' of the oral-faced jawbone to expose the medullary cavity for subsequent thorough debridement. The margins of necrotic bone overlying the focus of osteomyelitis are excised creating direct visualization of the infected medullary cavity. This allows direct access to be formed and forming sequestra, granulation tissue, and affected bone (Box 18.7).

Saucerization can be useful in early acute osteomyelitis cases and cases of limited extent. In early stages of the infection, it helps in decompression of the medullary cavity and allow ready extrusion of pus, debris, granulation tissue and avascular fragments. Since the removal of bone by this procedure is limited, the strength of the mandible is not critically jeopardized and healing by secondary intention is suffcient. While the saucerization procedure is frequently used in mandibular osteomyelitis, it is rarely needed in the maxilla. Because of its thin cortex, sequestra usually form more rapidly and are exposed to the oral cavity, creating wider defects and possibly causing oroantral fistulas (Figs 18.11, 18.12 and 18.13).

- Surgical removal of dead necrotic bone is sequestrectomy.
- Helps in establishment of local microvascular proliferation.
- Saucerization is the unroofing of the bone to expose the medullary cavity for thorough debridement (Box 18.5).
- Permits removal of formed and forming sequestra.

Box 18.7: Surgical technique for saucerization

- Access to the bone by creating a mucoperiosteal flap, usually using a gingival crest incision
- Refection of fap should be as limited as possible to preserve local blood supply
- Affected teeth (loosened and other dental foci within the affected area) are extracted
- The lateral cortex of the mandible is reduced using burs or rongeurs, until the sufficient bleeding bone is encountered at all margins, approximately to the level of the unattached mucosa, thus producing a saucer-like defect
- Local debridement is performed by removing granulation tissue and loose bone fragments from the bone bed using curettes
- The debrided area is thoroughly irrigated with sterile saline solution with or without additional antibiotic such as neomycin
- If there is substantial local bleeding due to hyperemia caused by the inflammatory process, a medicated pack may be placed and serve as local compression device
- The buccal flap is trimmed and a medicated pack (such as iodoform gauze lightly covered with antibiotic and local steroid ointment is placed for hemostasis and to maintain the flap in a retracted position. The pack is placed firmly without pressure and retained by several non-resorbable sutures, extending over the pack from the lingual to the buccal flap
- The pack is remained *in situ* for several days up to 2 weeks or even more in some instances and may be replaced several times, until the surface of the bed of granulation tissue is epithelialized and the margins have healed

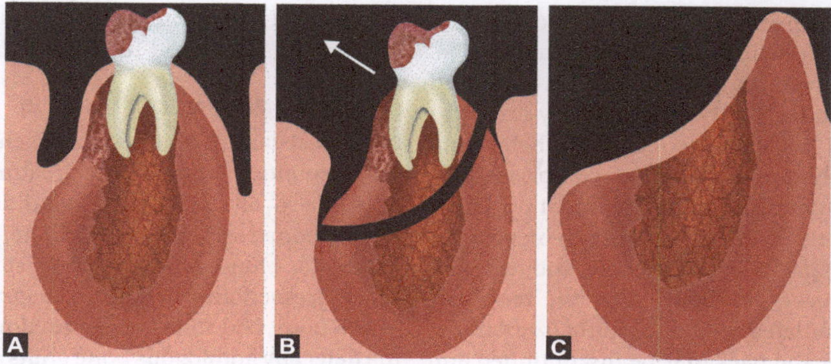

Figs 18.11A to C: Sequestrectomy and saucerization

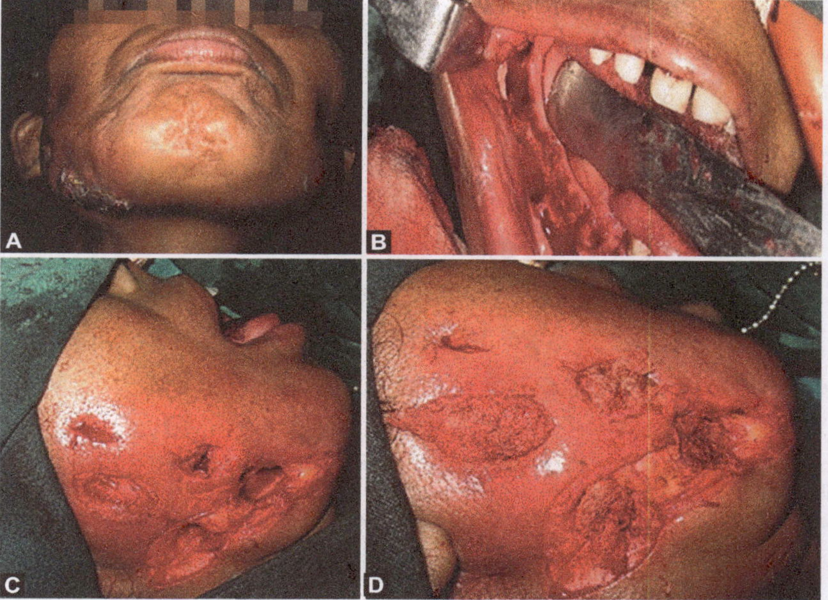

Figs 18.12A to D: Chronic osteomyelitis treated with sequestrectomy and curettage (Case 1)

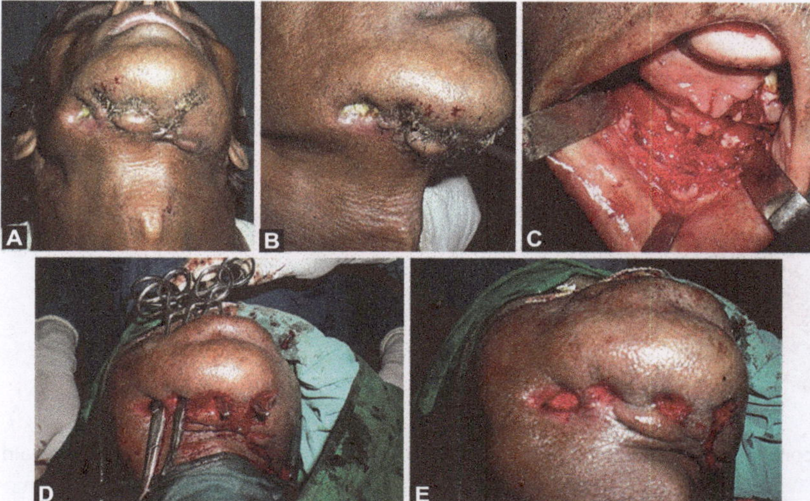

Figs 18.13A to E: Chronic osteomyelitis treated with sequestrectomy and curettage (Case 2)

Decortication

Decortication was first advocated for treatment of osteomyelitis of the mandible in 1917 and further described by Mowlem.[17] In advanced acute and secondary chronic osteomyelitis of the jaws, especially the mandible, use of decortication promotes resolution based on the premise that the affected cortical bone is avascular and harbors microorganisms. The medullary cavity shows destruction and is largely replaced by granulation tissue and pus. Parenteral or per oral administered antibiotics cannot reach the affected region. Waiting for sequestrum formation and reducing surgery to sequestrectomy is not an option because of the advanced stage of the infection with risk for further spread, abscess formation and cellulitis. Furthermore, the disadvantages associated with prolonged antibiotic therapy may become more prominent with time.

The major purpose of the decortication procedure is to remove the chronically infected cortex of the jawbone and gain access to affected medullary cavity to allow a sufficient decompression of intramedullary pressure and meticulous surgical debridement under direct visualization (Figs 18.14 to 18.16). Furthermore, this procedure allows bringing well-perfused tissue (e.g. masseter muscle) into contact with bone, promoting further healing.

- Lateral and inferior cortex removed.
- Irrigation and debridement.
- Trimming up to bleeding point in vital bone.
- Refers to removal of chronically infected cortex of bone.
- The lateral and inferior border cortex is removed 1 to 2 cm beyond the affected area, thus providing access to the medullary cavity.
- Used as initial treatment of primary and secondary chronic OML or when initial conservative regimens have failed.

After the surgical procedures such as sequestrectomy, saucerization or corticotomy are undertaken, the ensuing surgical defect is not closed primarily and is packed open leaving *in situ* the

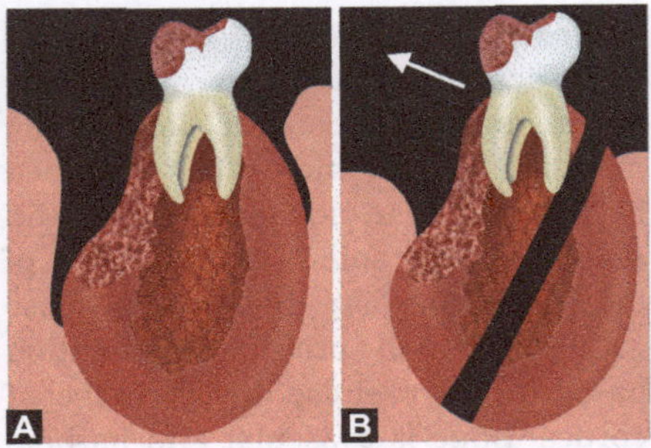

Figs 18.14A and B: Lateral and inferior cortex removal

gauze pack impregnated in the 5 percent povidone iodine solution or acriflavine. The wound is an infected wound and is unlikely to heal by primary intention and heals by secondary epithelization. Daily care of the wound comprises of irrigation with saline, 5 percent povidone iodine solution and hydrogen peroxide. The pack is changed daily and its size is reduced gradually. After the base gets granulated and the epithelization begins, the pack may be discontinued and only wound hygiene maintenance is indicated (Figs 18.15 and 18.16).

Resection and Reconstruction

In the resistant cases of OML, which do not respond to the routine treatment or if there are associated conditions like osteopetrosis, irradiated bone, for complete, elimination of the infective process resection of the involved segment of the bone and then reconstruction of the defect by autologous bone grafts and

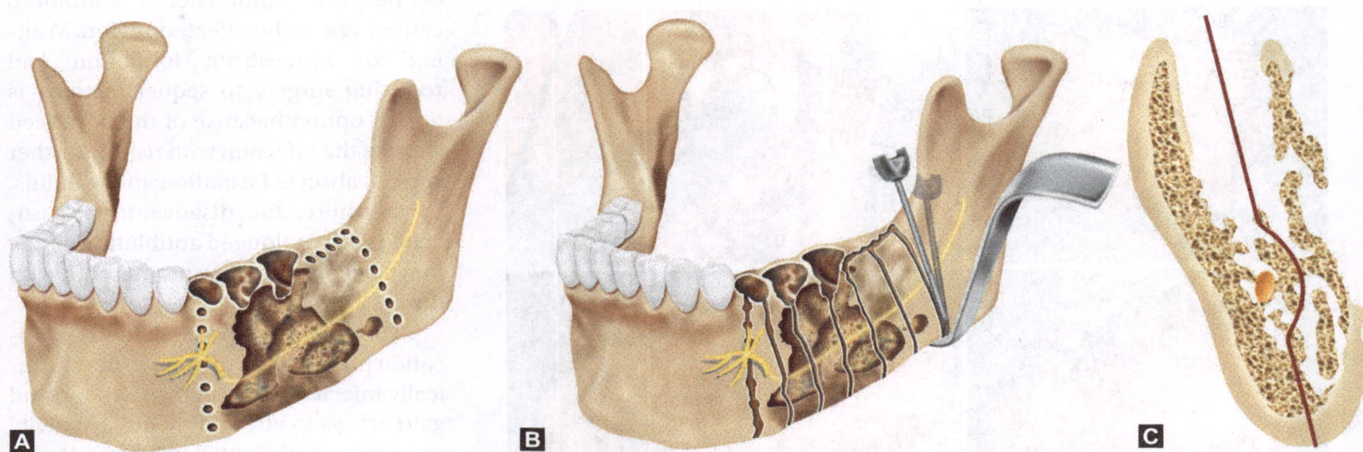

Figs 18.15A to C: Decortication: The margins of the intended area of decortication are marked with a burr. Note that the distal and mesial borders are selected in an area, where well-vascularized and healthy bone are assumed, usually 1–2 cm beyond the affected area. When performing the osteotomies, it should be stressed that they are strictly limited to the buccal cortex of the mandible to avoid damage to the inferior alveolar nerve

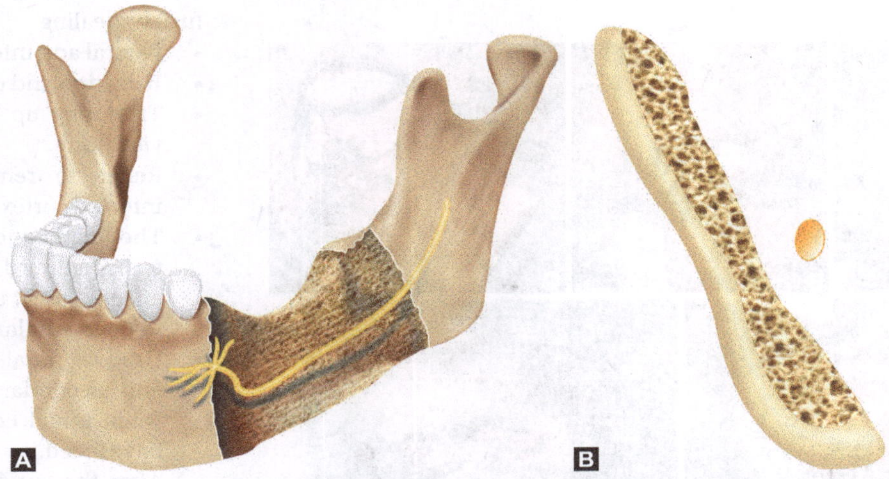

Figs 18.16A and B: Mandible after completed decortication and surgical debridement. The remaining bone represents the remaining vital bone tissue

the reconstruction plates is advocated. However, unless the infection has totally resolved the reconstruction should be differed as the chances of rejection of the graft or the implant due to infection are optimum.[18]

Trephination

Trephination is the creation of holes or windows in the overlying cortical bone adjacent to the infectious process for the decompression of the medullary compartment. It provides multiple surgical transcortical ports that allow transudative weeping and vascular communication between the periosteum and the medullary cavity.[19]

Hyperbaric Oxygen Therapy

The hyperbaric oxygen (HBO) therapy is indicated in the cases of osteomyelitis, which do not respond to routine treatment due to presence of certain associated conditions like irradiated jaw, osteosclerosis, osteopetrosis, and geriatric patients. It facilitates the healing of the bone and also helps in combating the infection. The HBO therapy involves the intermittent, twice daily, inhalation of 100 percent humidified oxygen under 2 atmospheric pressure (ATA) for 90 minutes. HBO reduces the hypoxia within the affected tissues and stimulates angiogenesis in the hypovascular tissues.[20] It enhances phagocytic activity of leukocytes to stimulate fibroblast growth, increase in collagen formation and promote growth of new capillaries.

Five aspects of HBO beneficial in the treatment of OML of jaws.[21]

- Enhances the lysosomal degradation potential by enhancing the development of intracellular halides in PMN's and oxygen radicals that are major components of the catabolic enzymes of the macrophage lysosome. Formation of these enzymes is depressed in hypoxic environment such as found in osteomyelitic foci.
- Free radicals of oxygen are formed during HBO therapy that is toxic to many pathogenic anaerobes that do not have protective intracellular superoxide scavenging enzymes.
- Many exotoxins liberated by the pathophysiologic activity of microorganisms are rendered inert by exposure to elevated partial pressures of oxygen.
- Tissue hypoxia is intermittently reversed by the HBO therapy, mimicking the tissue level during wound healing by saturating the interstitial plasma above the normal levels produced by the hemoglobin oxygen transport mechanism.
- Positive enhancement of neoangiogenesis in the aerobic portion of the proliferative phase of wound healing.

Hyperbaric Oxygen Chamber

The patient is placed in a chamber. Oxygen is given by mask or by hood. It is given for 5 days per week for 30, 60, or more dives at 2.4 ATA for 90 minutes, while breathing 100 percent oxygen twice daily.

Hart and Mainous[22] (1976) and Marx[23] (1983) protocol (Box 18.8) recommends 60 sessions with 2 ATA of oxygen.

The complications of hyperbaric oxygen therapy are summarized in Box 18.9.

The hyperbaric oxygen therapy is contraindicted in the conditions mentioned in the Box 18.10.

DIFFERENT TYPES OF OSTEOMYELITIS AND THEIR CLINICAL PRESENTATIONS

Different types of osteomyelitis and their clinical presentations is given in Box 18.11.

Box 18.8: Marx protocol (1983)

- 30 initial dives, if improved then 60 dives completed
- Otherwise, sequestrectomy + 30 dives
- If wound dehiscence, resection + 60 dives and 20 dives after 10 weeks
- Patient with pathological fracture, orocutaneous fistula are given 30 dives more prior going to resection.

Box 18.9: Complications of HBO therapy

- Most of the complications associated with HBO delivery result from barometric pressure changes or oxygen toxicity
- Eustachian tube dysfunction
- Tympanic membrane rupture
- Oxygen toxicity
- Ear sinus, or tooth pain
- Decompression sickness
- Pneumothorax

Box 18.10: Contraindication for hyperbaric oxygen (HBO) therapy

- Pneumothorax
- COPD
- Optic neuritis
- Acute viral infection
- Acute seizures
- URI
- Pregnancy
- Thoracic surgery
- Ear surgery
- Malignant disease

Box 18.11: Types of osteomyelitis

- Infantile osteomyelitis
- Acute pyogenic osteomyelitis
- Chronic suppurative
- Chronic non-suppurative
- Garre's osteomyelitis
- Actinomycosis
- Tubercular osteomyelitis
- Syphilitic osteomyelitis

Infantile Osteomyelitis

(*Synonym: Osteomyelitis maxillaries neonatorum*)

Infantile osteomyelitis was first described by Rees[24] in 1847. It can occur within first 9 months of life and as early as 1 week after birth.

Etiology

- Hematogenous infection.
- Perinatal trauma to the oral mucosa from obstetrician's finger, mucus suction bulb and unhygienic condition during the child birth.
- Infection involving maxillary sinus.
- Unhygienic human or artificial nipples.

Clinical Features

- Sudden onset, very acute course.
- General constitutional symptoms, high grade fever.
- Facial cellulitis centered around orbit, intercanthal swelling, palpebral edema, closure of eye, conjunctivitis, proptosis.
- Inability to suckle and signs of dehydration.
- Subperiosteal abscess in alveolar region.
- Fistulae or pus draining tracts on alveolar mucosa.
- Sloughing out of bone and teeth buds.

Microorganisms

- *Staphylococcus aureus*
- *Haemophilus influenzae*
- Streptococci
- Pneumococci
- *Neisseria gonorrhoeae*
- Coliform bacilli

Radiographic findings are noticed in late stages, sequestra and necrotic tooth germs.

Differential Diagnosis

The condition needs be differentiated from the infantile cortical hyperostosis.

Treatment

- Broad spectrum antibiotics.
- Culture and sensitivity test for specific antibiotic therapy.
- Incision and drainage of fluctuant abscess.
- Irrigations of sinus tracts with normal saline, 5 percent povidone iodine and hydrogen peroxide.
- Supportive therapy such as parenteral feeding.
- Sequestrectomy as indicated by clinical and radiographic findings.
- Two weeks postoperative intravenous antibiotics, followed by an additional 6 weeks administration of oral antibiotics.
- Children, who have undergone sequestrectomy, should be followed up by an orthodontist to aid in the development of arch and maintenance of occlusion.

Chronic Sclerosing Osteomyelitis

Chronic sclerosing osteomyelitis is an inflammatory, non-suppurative, painful disease with a protracted course. It commonly affects basal bone and alveolar process of mandible. It is usually unilateral and produces recurrent swelling and pain.[25] It is usually caused by a low-grade infection.

Radiographic Findings

Diffuse intramedullary sclerosis with poorly defined margins is noted with occasional focal areas of radiolucency and radiopacity.

Treatment

- Antibiotics
- Removal of source of infection
- Wound irrigation
- Debridement.

Garre's Osteomyelitis

Garre's osteomyelitis is irritation induced focal thickening of periosteum and cortical bone. It is usually caused in the children as a result of low-grade infection.[26] The infection leads to periosteal irritation and it stimulates the proliferation and bone apposition.[27] The characteristics of this type of osteomyelitis are:

- It is a non-suppurative inflammatory process.
- It is characterized by peripheral subperiosteal bone deposition.
- It occurs primarily in children and young adults.
- The common etiological factors are carious tooth, soft tissue infections.
- It produces a localized, hard, nontender swelling of lateral and inferior cortices of the mandible.
- As it is a low-grade infection, the lymphadenopathy, hyperpyrexia and leukocytosis are seldom present.

Radiological Features

A focal area of well-calcified bone proliferation may be seen that is smooth and has *'onion skin'* appearance.[28]

Differential Diagnosis

- Infantile cortical hyperostosis:[29] It occurs in young infants and involves a number of bones. The clavicles and ulnae are usually involved, but the mandible is invariably involved. The condition is uninfluenced with antibiotics. The disease usually is self- limiting and eventually regresses.
- Ewing sarcoma.
- Osteosarcoma.
- Fibrous dysplasia: Clinically it is indistinguishable from Garre's osteomyelitis. The only differentiating feature is radiological appearance of 'onion skin appearance' in Garre's osteomyelitis.

Treatment

The treatment comprises of removal of infected tooth and curettage of the socket. Surgical recontouring of the expanded bone is undertaken at a later stage. If the teeth are to be conserved then the endodontic therapy should be started to treat the offending teeth.[30] As it is the low-grade infection, the antibiotic therapy is not aggressive unlike the pyogenic osteomyelitis.

Actinomyces Osteomyelitis

Introduction

Actinomycosis is an infectious disease caused by a slender gram positive, rod-shaped bacterium, *Actinomyces israelii*, that exhibits a number of simple fungus like characteristics, such as tendency to grow as a mass of rounded bodies (clubs) and filaments in tissues (hence the term *ray fungus*), low virulence and a property of eliciting suppuration, necrosis and a chronic granulomatous response.

Clinical Presentation

- It may involve soft tissue or bone (actinomyces osteomyelitis) or both.
- It presents as a chronic, persistent, infection with induration and nodularity of the tissues due to fibrosis and intermittent, spontaneous occurring draining sinuses.

- A variation of this description is another presentation in which the most prominent finding is limited mouth opening, often months or years after removal of posterior tooth or after some trauma. This is mainly attributed to fibrosis of one of the muscles of mastication or from chronic deep seated focus of infection. This presentation is often termed as '*Lumpy jaw*'. (Lumpy jaw is more common in cattle's than humans).
- The disease forms external sinuses that discharge distinctive '*sulfur granules*' (the colonies of the organism) and spread unimpeded by anatomic barriers when endogenous oral commensals invade the tissues of the oral-cervicofacial, thoracic, pelvic and abdominal regions.[31] Tissues may be invaded by direct extension or by hematogenous spread.
- Cervicofacial disease may affect the mandible and overlying soft tissues, parotid gland, tongue and maxillary sinus. Nearly every structure and space of head and neck may be an initial site of involvement. Secondary spread to other areas of the head and neck readily occur.
- Firm soft tissue masses are present on the skin; they have purplish, dark red, oily areas with occasional small zones of fluctuations. Spontaneous drainage of serous fluids containing granular material may occur.
- Regional lymph nodes may be occasionally involved.
- The patient usually has no fever and constitutional symptoms.
- Delayed healing of extraction sockets can be noted.

Microbiology

Actionomyces is not a fungus, but rather a gram positive, microaerophilic, non-spore forming, non-acid-fast bacteria. The morphologic characteristics vary with filamentous cocci or bacillary forms. They are not sensitive to antifungal drugs and unlike fungi, are sensitive to antibiotics. The cell wall electron microscopy and other studies confirm their bacterial nature.

A. israelii is mostly responsible for the human actinomycosis. *A. naeslundii, A. odontolyticus* and *A. meyeri* are less common causes of the disease. Most infections are accompanied by other organisms, such as *Actinobacillus actinomycetemcomitans, Bacteroides* species, *Eikenella corrodens*, Enterobacteriaceae, *Fusobacterium* species, *Porphyromonas* species, *Prevotella* species, staphylocci and streptococci, and may be potential copathogens that aid in the inhibition of host defenses or reduce oxygen tension.[32]

Investigations

Radiolucency of varying size can be seen on radiographs (OPG). The focus of infection may be difficult to locate. Orthopantomogram may be supplemented by a CT scan or MRI. Sometimes a scan with ^{67}Ga, which is taken up by inflammatory cells, or a scan using 99-technetium methylene diphosphonate, which is taken up by osteoblasts, will locate the focus of infection, which CT scan and plain radiographs cannot detect. Laboratory investigations show increased ESR and leukocytosis.

Treatment

The management comprises of surgical management with incision and drainage and debridement. The administration of the antibiotics and supportive treatment are recommended. The penicillin group of antibiotics are the drug of choice like crystalline penicillin 5 to 10 lac U 6 hourly or penicillin V 1 g 6 hourly or ampicillin 500 mg to 1 g 6 hourly or amoxicillin 500 mg 8 hourly can be given.[33] Antibiotics must be administered for a prolonged period as the condition may recur. For patients who are allergic to penicillin, Doxycillin 100 mg twice a day for 6 months can be used. Imaging should be done intermittently, throughout the treatment to monitor healing of bone and possible need of additional surgical procedures like sequestrectomy and saucerization.

Nocardial Osteomyelitis

Nocardial osteomyelitis resembles the actinomycosis to a large extent in its clinical presentation.[34] The causative organism is *Nocardia asteroides.* It can occur without a dental injury. It presents as suppurative lesion with necrosis and abscess formation. The treatment is incision and drainage and sulphonamides for 6 to 8 weeks.

Tuberculous Osteomyelitis

Tuberculosis of bone is an uncommon form of chronic osteomyelitis, occurring more often in young individuals and usually in late stages of the disease. The sites of predilection are dorsal and lumbar vertebrae and epiphysis and diaphysis of long bones and the flat bones, including those of the skull and mandible, which are rarely affected. Tubercular osteomyelitis of the mandible is found to be more among children than adults. Tuberculosis in the oral and maxillofacial region is five times more prevalent in males than in females. However, isolated tuberculosis of mandible in the absence of active pulmonary tuberculosis is an uncommon clinical entity. Due to the rarity of tuberculosis of mandible, it seldom arises clinical suspicion, especially when a positive history of a systemic infection or therapy is denied. The diagnosis, therefore, is variable and established after biopsy.[35] The involvement of the mandible by tuberculous infection is extremely rare as it contains less cancellous bone though the mandibular involvement is more frequent than maxilla and the alveolar and angle regions have greater affinity. The infection may extend to the mandible by:[36]

- Direct transfer from infected sputum or infected raw milk of cow through
  - An open pulp in carious tooth.
  - An extraction wound.
  - Gingival margin or perforation of an erupting tooth.
- Regional extension of soft tissue lesion to involve the underlying bone.
- Hematogenous route: Bacilli are possibly transferred from a primary focus in another part of the body and localized in the jaw, after trauma. Tuberculosis of the jaw causes slow necrosis of the bone and may involve the entire mandible. The destruction of the bone in

radiographs appears as blurring of trabecular details with irregular areas of radiolucency. Two types of clinical presentation of the disease are seen, closed lesions, which is devoid of any draining sinuses and is not open to oral environment and open lesions, presence of multiple draining sinuses. There is erosion of the cortex with little tendency to repair. Gradually the bone is replaced by soft tuberculous granulation tissue without sequestra formation as is typically seen in other bacterial and viral osteomyelitis. Caseation appears at places followed by softening and liquefaction. A subperiosteal abscess then forms presenting as a painless, soft and cold (devoid of signs of inflammation) swelling. This cold abscess may burst either intraorally or extraorally forming single or multiple sinuses. Pathological fracture of mandible and sequestration may also occur. Usually tuberculosis of the mandible presents as multifocal lesion elsewhere in body, involving other bones and lungs. The diagnosis of a case of tuberculosis of mandible is extremely difficult as there are no specific signs pathognomic of infection. The only manifestation may be a localized swelling of the jaw and it may be misdiagnosed as a pyogenic abscess or if sinuses are present, or it may be confused with actinomycosis. The diagnosis must be established by histological examination of tissue and demonstration of the organisms in the lesion. Although it is rare, the differential diagnosis of tubercular osteomyelitis must always be kept in mind by clinicians, when routine therapy fails to bring about an improvement in the lesions of mandible. Since the involvement of bone occurs in late stages of the disease, the prognosis is poor and death from involvement of internal organs or from tubercular meningitis is common. However, if the lesion is primary and detected early, the disease is completely curable and can lead to reversal of all destructive bony changes.

Diagnosis and Management

The hematological picture is of lymphocytosis, monocytosis, raised ESR and the Montoux test may be positive. In case of open jaw lesions, AFB may be positive in saliva.

Diagnosis of the lesion is generally confirmed on aspiration for smears, biopsy and culture studies. Radiography, scintigraphy, CT scan aid in diagnosis. However, histopathology is the most common modality of reaching the confirmatory diagnosis.

Management consists of surgical treatment based on pathological studies.

Unlike the pyogenic osteomyelitis, the management of tubercular osteomyelitis is primarily with chemotherapy with antitubercular (anti-Koch's) drugs such as streptomycin, isoniazide, rifampicin, ethambutol and pyrazinamide. The surgical management is marginal and restricted to debridements and drainage after the chemotherapy is started.

- **Closed lesions:** *Positive aspirate for AFB:* In these cases, patient is started on a suitable anti-tubercular regimen, that is, isoniazid, rifampicin, ethambutol and pyrazinamide.
  Negative aspirate for AFB: A complete excisional biopsy and debridement is advocated.
- **Open lesions:** For open lesions, incisional biopsy is done for histopathological studies. If found positive for tuberculosis, anti-tubercular regimen is started and no surgery is performed immediately to prevent dissemination of the disease, that is, miliary spread of tuberculosis by hematogenous route. After 6 to 9 weeks of anti-tubercular treatment, patient is reassessed clinically, as well as radiographically to decide upon the need for surgery.

Syphilitic Osteomyelitis

The syphilitic osteomyelitis or the gumma is commonly seen in the tertiary syphilis. With the advent of better modalities of diagnosis, awareness and better treatment modalities, the disease is not so common now-a-days. The maxilla is more affected than mandible in this condition. The gummatous perforation of the palate can lead to oroantral or oronasal communication. The sequestra are called filiary sequestra, because they are fine.

Age Incidence

Syphilitic osteomyelitis can be congenital, but it usually occurs between the ages of 30 to 40 years.

Site

Syphilitic osteomyelitis usually occurs in shaft of long bones and it affects the skull. In majority of cases, there is hyperostosis.

Radiographic Features

The affected bone shows marked periosteal changes, the outline of medulla becomes obliterated.[37] In old cases, gumma may be formed or in the form of filiary sequestra may be present.

Clinical Features

Gummatous osteomyelitis forms *bone dependent bone destruction* and new bone formation in which there are areas of mottling.

The diagnosis is the basis of history of exposure, presence of primary chancre previously, positive KTVDRL test. The treatment comprises of crystalline penicillin 10 to 20 lacs IU 6 hourly for 2 weeks and later with long acting penicillin (Penidure) 6 to 12 lac IU, once in a week or biweekly for 3 to 4 months. Surgery has marginal role in the management condition.

Osteomyelitis of Mandible in Sickle Cell Disease

Pathogenesis

Sickle cell disease is an inherited hemoglobinopathy. It occurs when hemoglobin SS is deoxygenated and the molecules polymerize to form pseudocrystalline structures known as 'tactoids'. This leads to the characteristic sickle-shaped red cell. The polymerization is reversible when reoxygenation occurs. However, distortion of the red cell membrane may be permanent (irreversible sickling). The greater the concentrations of sickled hemoglobin, the more easily the tactoids are formed. This process may be enhanced or retarded by the presence of other hemoglobins. Because of the sickled cells, there is increased viscosity and loss of plasticity. Sludging occurs in the microvasculature, which causes obstruction to blood flow and leads to tissue ischemia (Flow chart 18.3). The ischemic tissue subsequently becomes edematous and painful.[4] Involvement of the bones in sickle cell disease has been reported in the literature.[38] In the long bones, the head of femur is commonly involved and facial bone involvement may occur on rare occasions. The pathophysiology for such involvement involves trauma or infection in bone, which leads to inflammatory changes, stasis of circulation and hypoxia. The hypoxia serves as a stimulus for inducing sickling, which clogs the lumena of the capillaries and the tissues are rendered ischemic, with subsequent infarction. Such ischemic bones become necrotic and can become secondarily infected. In the long bones, this secondary infection is usually caused by various strains of salmonella. However, in the jaw bones, the organisms that are cultured from such lesions belong to the flora of the oral cavity such as streptococci, staphylococci and *Escherichia coli.*

Flow chart 18.3: Pathophysiology of sickle cell osteomyelitis

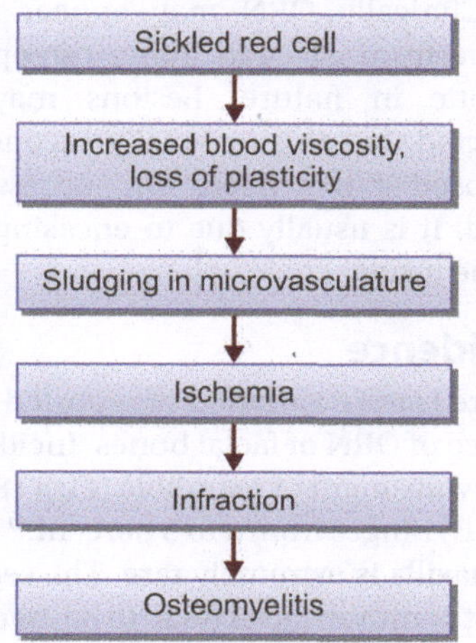

The factors that precipitate the sickle cell osteomyelitis of the bone are periapical infection and periodontal infections.[39] In the event of sickling, if the avascular necrosis of the bone occurs, it can get secondarily infected and the osteomyelitis is the end result.

The sickle cell osteomyelitis follows the pattern of osteomyelitis of the jaws in patient with normal hemoglobin concentration and rest of the course of the disease is similar to that of pyogenic osteomyelitis. The mandible is the common bone to be involved in this condition, however, the involvement of maxilla can also occur. As the maxilla is not commonly involved in osteomyelitis, whenever it is seen other predisposing conditions should be suspected and ruled out. In the central India, sickle cell disorders are common amongst the tribal population and so is the incidence of sickle cell related complications, including osteomyelitis. Hence, all maxillary osteomyelitis cases must be thoroughly evaluated and predisposing medical conditions such as diabetes (due to microangiopathies) and sickle cell disease must be ruled out (Figs 18.17A and B).

Diagnosis

The diagnosis of sickle cell disease can be made on the basis of:

- Demonstration of early and late sickling on the peripheral blood smear.
- Hemoglobin electrophoresis to detect SS pattern.

Whenever a patient with sickle cell disorder needs the surgery following precautions must be taken during the surgery and anesthesia.

- Maintain proper hydration and prevent dehydration.
- Prevent hypoxia and acidosis.
- Prevention of hypothermia.
- Follow aseptic principle and avoid infection.
- Tissue to be handled gently and excessive trauma should be avoided as these factors can precipitate the sickling.

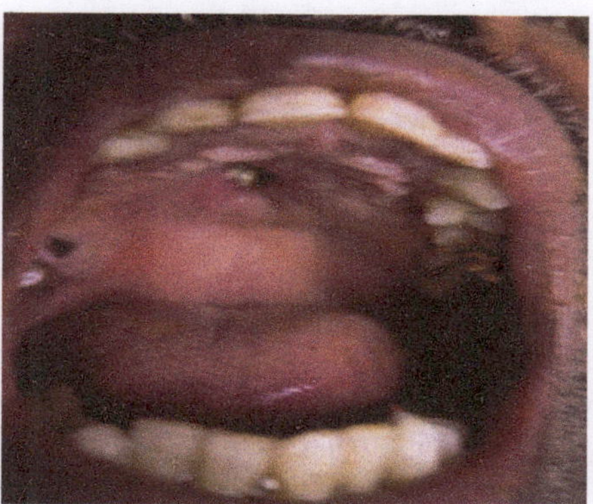

Fig. 18.17A: Case of sickle cell OM of maxilla

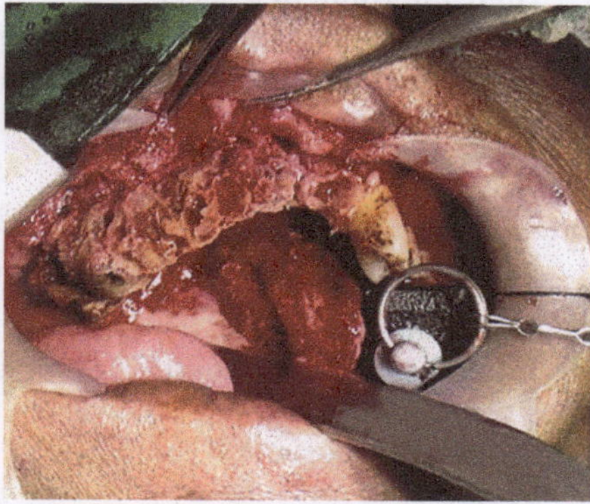

Fig. 18.17B: Total maxillary sequestration in a patient with sickle cell anemia

Treatment

Treatment of sickle cell osteomyelitist comprises of[40]:

- Antibiotic therapy.
- Surgery comprising of sequestrectomy, saucerization or decortications.
- Precautions during the anesthesia as mentioned above.
- Prevention of infection.
- Gentle tissue handling.

Post-traumatic Osteomyelitis

Post-traumatic osteomyelitis is the osteomyelitis of the mandible following an infected fracture.

Risk Factors[41]

- Ineffective fixation, reduction and immobilization.
  - Delay in treatment (old fracture).
  - Delay in administration of antibiotic therapy or inadequate antibiotic therapy.

- More than 50 percent of a tooth root exposed in a fracture.
- Devitalized segments of bone in the fracture site because of excessive stripping of periosteum, overzealous use of transosseous wiring, or overheating of bone by burs.
- Decreased host resistance or increased susceptibility to infection.

Signs and Symptoms

Early signs:

- Deep, intense pain.
- High, intermittent fever.
- Paresthesia or anesthesia of the mental nerve (arising after trauma and reduction of fracture).
- A clearly defined cause.

Late signs:

- Cellulitis over the involved portion of mandible.
- Intraoral or extraoral draining sinuses.
- Mild leukocytosis.
- Fever.

Radiologically, a moth-eaten appearance and sequestrum formation may be present.

Treatment[42]

- Removal of non-vital tissue, foreign bodies and associated teeth.
- Debridement of infected areas.
- Establishing drainage.
- Continuous irrigation and drainage systems.
- Local and systemic antibiotics.
- Immobilization of the mandible.
- HBO therapy.

The rigid fixation of the fracture and bone grafts is not advisable, until the infection is controlled for the fear of loss of graft due to infection and rejection of the implant.

OSTEORADIONECROSIS

Malignancies of maxillofacial region are treated by (i) radiation therapy, (ii) surgery, (iii) chemotherapy, (iv) combination therapy. Radiation often has serious effects on hard and soft tissues. Because of its inorganic composition, bone absorbs more energy than soft tissue and is more susceptible to secondary radiation. The effects of radiation on bone depend on the following four factors, viz:

1. Quality of radiation
2. Quantity of radiation
3. The location and extent of lesion
4. Condition of teeth and periodontium.

Mucositis, atrophic mucosa, xerostomia, and radiation caries are common. An additional late and major complication of therapeutic radiotherapy for head and neck cancer is osteoradionecrosis. For many years osteoradionecrosis was considered an infection initiated by injury to irradiated bone leading to marked pain, bone loss, functional and cosmetic disability. In recent times studies by Marx[43,44] (1983) has shown that it is a chronic, non-healing wound caused by ***hypoxia, hypocellularity and hypovascularity*** of irradiated tissue.

Before 1960s, orthovoltage was routinely used for therapeutic radiation, but was found to be highly deleterious to bone and resulting in incidence of jaw bone necrosis ranging from 17 to 37 percent.[45] In recent years orthovoltage has been replaced by megavoltage and other techniques such as dose fractionization, collimation, shielding of normal tissues and maintenance of pre-irradiation and postirradiation health, which are found to be bone sparing reduced the incidence of osteoradionecrosis to 2 to 5 percent.[46]

Complication of osteoradionecrosis (ORN) is dependent on the radiation dose to bone. Radiation dose in excess of 50 Gy have been seen to elevate the risk of ORN.[47] Radioactive implants within a tissue tumor also show a higher incidence of ORN.

The mandible is affected more commonly than maxilla, because most oral tumors are perimandibular, moreover the absence of dense cortical plates and the presence of a dense vascular network in maxilla lessens the likelihood of radiation necrosis effects compared with the mandible.

Ionizing radiation destroys neoplastic cells by damaging chromosomes and thus, causing impaired cell division. Irradiation induces inflammatory response in soft tissue erythema, desquamation and pigmentation of overlying skin. Radiation results in progressive obliterative arteritis (endarteritis, periarteritis, hyalinization and fibrosis and thrombosis of vessels), devitalization of tissues. The periosteal vessels and larger vessels such as inferior alveolar artery are markedly affected. As long as overlying soft tissues do not breakdown, irradiated bone may function normally.[48] Previously ORN was thought to be a triad of radiation, trauma and infection. Marx et al.[48] have shown that microorganisms are merely contaminants and trauma is only one of several factors involved in the disease.

Definition

Osteoradionecrosis is the exposure of nonviable, nonhealing, nonseptic lesion of irradiated bone, which fails to heal without intervention.[49]

The ORN is a radiation induced, non-healing, hypoxic wound rather than true osteomyelitis of irradiated bone. The viable, radiation damaged cells are not replaced by cells of similar type resulting in less cellular and more of collagen. This fibrotic and poorly vascularized tissue has reduced or absent healing ability. Tissue breakdown occurs due to inability of tissues to maintain normal cell turnover and collagen synthesis and such tissues are susceptible to spontaneous breakdown from minor injury.[50]

Clinically ORN may appear as a sequestrum of dead bone, osteopenic fibrotic in nature. Lesions may be infected, but this is usually secondary. Exposed bone need not necessarily dead. It is usually due to encasing soft tissue insult.

Incidence

There is wide variation of reported incidence of ORN of facial bones. Incidence of involvement of mandible (Figs 18.18A and B) ranges from 2 to 3 percent.[51] ORN of maxilla is extremely rare. The second most common facial bone to be involved is temporal bone. Tooth extraction is reported to be a triggering factor for

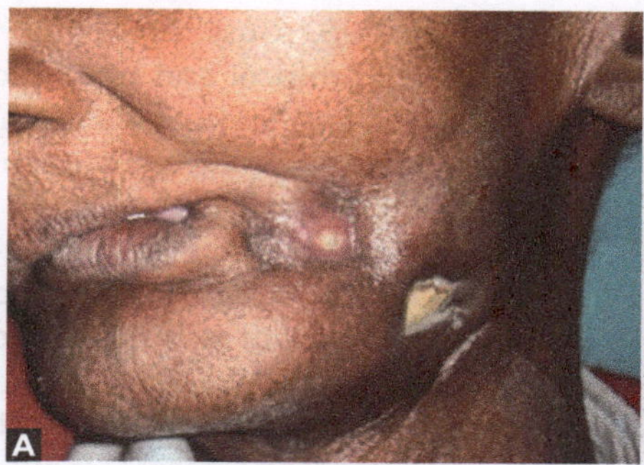
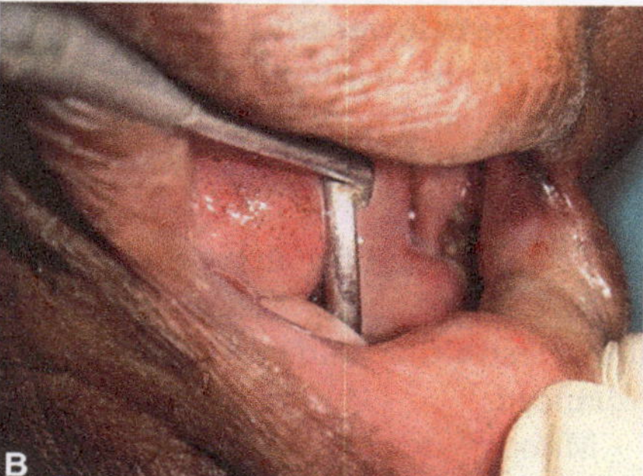

Figs 18.18A and B: Osteoradionecrosis of the mandible

ORN in 60 to 89 percent of cases.[52-54] The mean time period between RT and development of ORN has been reported to be between 7.5 to up to 20 years.

Effects of Radiation

Effects of radiations on various tissues is illustrated in Table 18.2.

Clinical Features

The ORN has varied clinical presentations. It is usually painful, debilitating and frequently refractory to treatment.

The signs and symptoms vary depending upon the condition:

- Pain (severe, deep and boring) and evidence of exposed bone are the chief presenting features.
- Initially patient may develop trismus, fetid breath, pyrexia, soft tissue abscesses and persistently draining sinuses.
- Exposed bone with intraoral/extraoral fistulae (Figs 18.18A and B). The exposed bone often has rough surface that abrades adjacent soft tissue and causes further discomfort.
- There is slow sequestration, because not only osteoblastic, but also, osteoclastic activity is destroyed.
- Pathologic fractures may also occur.
- The tissues surrounding exposed bone may be indurated or ulcerated.
- If induration persists after infection has been controlled by irrigation and antibiotics, or if ulceration is present, a biopsy should be performed.

Radiographic Features

Little radiographic change occurs in early stages of disease. The characteristic changes seen in osteomyelitis of non-irradiated bone (sequestra and involucra) occur late or not at all in irradiated bone because of severely compromised blood supply.

Treatment

There is no universally accepted protocol for management of ORN. Two treatment modalities are:

Conservative Method

- Administration of systemic antibiotics.
- Selective rinsing with topical antiseptics.
- Removal of small sequestra.
- Local debridement.
- Use of narcotic analgesics and nerve blocks (bupivacaine or alcohol), nerve avulsion or rhizotomy for effective pain control.
- Other supportive care such as adequate hydration and nutrition.
- Maintenance of good oral hygiene by oral rinses of 1 percent sodium fluoride gel, 1 percent chlorhexidine gluconate and plain water help reduce xerostomia, mucositis and radiation caries.

Ultrasound therapy: Use of ultrasound combined with local debridement. Ultrasound treatment is non-invasive and reportedly promotes neovascularity and neocellularity of ischemic tissues and has been used successfully in treating ORN of jaws.[55] An ultrasound program of 1 watt/cm^2, 3 mega Hz, pulsed 1:4, 15 min a day for 60 days is proposed to be optimum.

Radical Method

Treatment methodology is aimed at supporting and salvaging viable, but compromised tissue and not attempting to resurrect dead tissue. The treatment is directed at reversing the hypoxia and increasing the vascularity and cellularity of tissues.

Definitive treatment should be directed towards either revascularization of bone or excision of affected bone, with or without reconstruction. Adjunctive treatment with HBO or other modalities

Table 18.2: Effects of radiations on various tissues

Tissue	Radiation induced changes	Complications
Oral mucosa	Atrophy	Mucositis, recurrent ulcerations, intolerance to hot and spicy food, loss of taste sensation
Skin	Atrophy, inflammation	Diminished healing potential, painful ulceration
Bone marrow	Hypovascularity, diminished cellularity, myelofibrosis	Diminished healing potential
Periosteum	Hypovascularity, fibrosis, diminished cellularity	Diminished healing potential
Dental pulp	Hypovascularity, fibrosis, diminished cellularity	Brittleness of tooth structure, diminished reparative potential
Salivary gland	Atrophy, diminished salivary flow	Burning sensation in oral cavity, radiation caries, increased chances of odontogenic infections

may be necessary and feasible in select patients.

The overall treatment comprises of:

- Local debridement
- **Adequate pain control:** Use of narcotic analgesics and nerve blocks (bupivacaine or alcohol), nerve avulsion or rhizotomy
- Control of infection by administration of systemic antibiotics (as decided on culture and sensitivity) and local irrigation of wounds by topical antibiotics
- Supportive treatment such as adequate hydration, nutritional supplements
- Hospitalization, if required
- Maintenance of good oral hygiene by oral rinses of 1 percent sodium fluoride gel, 1 percent chlorhexidine gluconate and plain water help reduce xerostomia, mucositis and radiation caries
- Sequestrectomy
- **Pathologic fractures:** These do not heal readily. The best form of treatment is excision of necrotic ends of both fragments with or without reconstruction
- **Bone resection:** It is performed when there is persistent pain, infection or pathological fractures. Preferentially done intraorally to avoid orocutaneous fistula in radiation compromised skin
- Adjunctive therapy with hyperbaric oxygen (HBO) (Flow chart 18.4).

Hyperbaric Oxygen Therapy in Osteoradionecrosis

The HBO therapy consists of breathing 100 percent oxygen through a face mask or hood of monoplace or large chamber at 2.4 absolute atmospheric pressure for 90 minutes session or dives for as many as 5 days a week totaling 30 or more sessions, often followed by another 10 or more sessions.

The HBO treatment causes increase in arterial and venous oxygen tension. Oxygen under increased tension enhances healing by direct bacteriostatic effect on microorganisms that renders them susceptible to lower antibiotic concentration and by enhancing phagocytic killing. In addition, neoangiogenesis, fibroblastic proliferation and collagen synthesis occur. As resorption and replacement of devitalized bone with healthy tissue progresses, formation of sequestra that undergo resorption is enhanced.

Marx[44,56] described a protocol for its effective use in several situations, especially for prevention, treatment, reconstruction of mandible, where reconstruction is indicated. It accounts for marked decrease in pain, trismus, and closure of fistulas.

Marx-University of Miami Protocol[57]

All patients entering this protocol receive 30 sessions of HBO (stage I). Those with a pathological fracture, orocutaneous fistula or osteolysis of inferior border of mandible (as viewed by panoramic radiographs or a CT scan) are placed in group III category and have a continuity resection of mandible.

Stage I: If individuals with ORN have none of the criteria to place them in stage III, they undergo initial 30 HBO sessions. If softening of the exposed bone results (an attempt at spontaneous sequestration and formation of healthy granulation), the wound is debrided and 10 more HBO sessions provided. If no changes occur in exposed bone, patients are reclassified as stage II.

Stage II: Non-continuity resection of exposed bone to bleeding margins by alveolar bone resection or decortication followed by 10 HBO sessions. If the tissue heals spontaneously with no exposed bone, the patient is considered a stage II respondent. If wound dehiscence results in exposure of non-viable bone, the individual is considered a stage II non-respondent and together with stage I non-responders enters stage III treatment.

Stage III: Patients whose condition does not respond to either stage I or II, treatment undergo a continuity resection and 10 postoperative sessions of HBO and reconstruction after 3 months.

Vudiniabola S, Goss AN et al.[58] modified Marx protocol and proposed staging depending upon its clinical presentation plus response to treatment with HBO as follows:

Stage I: Exposed bone with non-healing wound 30 HBO sessions and review. Those patient who respond well, further 10 HBO sessions. Non-respondents considered as stage II ORN.

Stage II: Local debridement to induce fresh bleeding, followed by 10 HBO sessions.

Stage III: Non-respondent stage II ORN or those with orocutaneous fistula, pathologic fracture or inferior border resorption, total 30 HBO sessions, followed by resection and stabilization of remaining jaw by external fixation or IMF.

Stage III R: If reconstruction is required, then they are reclassified as stage III R with 10 sessions of HBO further.

Prevention of Osteoradionecrosis

Preirradiation Dental Care

- **Extraction of teeth:** The teeth in direct beam of radiation, non-restorable, periodontally compromised should be extracted. Radiation therapy is delayed by 10 to 14 days to allow initial healing.
- Alveoloplasty.
- Restoration of teeth, topical fluoride application and periodontal therapy should be completed.
- **During therapy:** Mouth rinses with 0.2 percent aqueous chlorhexidine, supervised cleaning of all teeth, oral hygiene instructions, dietary counseling.

Postirradiation Dental Care

- Avoidance of denture use.
- Use of saliva substitutes.
- Restoration of teeth with postirradiation pulpitis.
- Limit any extractions (if needed) to 1 or 2 per appointment under proper antibiotic cover followed by meticulous wound care.

Flow chart 18.4: Treatment of ORN

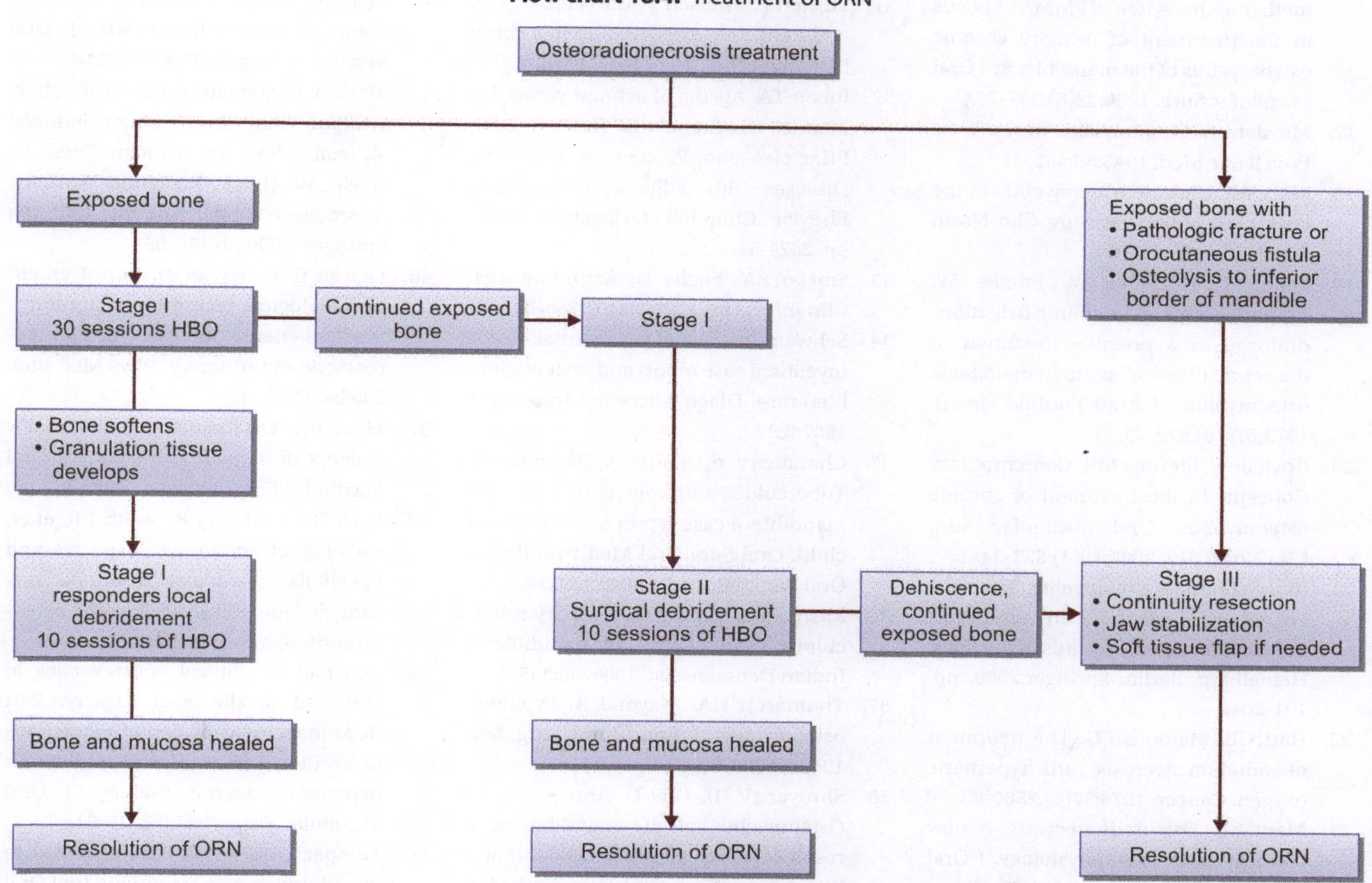

REFERENCES

1. Richard G Topazian, Morton H Goldberg, James R Hupp. Oral and Maxillofacial Infections, 4th subedition. WB. Saunders Company; 2002; p. 214.
2. Hovi L, Saarinen UM, Donner U, et al. Opportunistic Osteomyelitis in the jaws of children on immunosuppressive chemotherapy. Pediat Hematol/Oncol. 1996; 18(1):90-94.
3. Bachalli PS. Incidence of chronic non-suppurative osteomyelitis of the maxilla in diabetic adult patients and its management. Int J Oral Maxillofac Surg. 2007;36(11):1039.
4. Borle RM, Prasant MC, Badjate SJ, et al. Sickle cell osteomyelitis of the maxilla: a case report. J Oral Maxillofac Surg. 2001;59(11):1371-73.
5. Desai RV, Jain V, Katariya S. Codman's triangle in tubercular osteomyelitis. J Postgrad Med. 2002;48(2):157-8.
6. Koorbusch GF, Fotos P, Gall KT. Retrospective assessment of osteomyelitis: Etiology, demographics, risk factors, and management in 35 cases. Oral Surg, Oral Medi, Oral Pathol. 1992;74(2):149-54.
7. Hudson JW. Osteomyelitis of the jaws: a 50-year perspective. J Oral Maxillofac Surg. 1993;51(12):1294-1301.
8. Worth HM. Principles and Practice of Oral Radiologic Interpretation. Chicago: Year book Medical Publisher Inc. 1969.
9. Gold R. Diagnosis of osteomyelitis. Pediatr Rev. 1991;12:292.
10. Tsuchimochi M, Higashino N, Okano A, et al. Study of combined technetium 99m methylene diphosphonate and gallium 67 citrate scintigraphy in diffuse sclerozing osteomyelitis of the mandible: case reports. J Oral Maxillofac Surg. 1991;49:887-97.
11. Termaat MF, Raijmakers PG, Scholten HJ, et al. The accuracy of diagnostic imaging for the assessment of chronic osteomyelitis: a systematic review and meta-analysis. J Bone Joint Surg Am. 2005;87(11):2464-71.
12. Aliabadi P, Nikpoor N. Imaging osteomyelitis. Arthritis Rheum. 1994; 37(5):617-22.
13. Richard G Topazian, Morton H Goldberg, James R Hupp. Osteomyelitis of jaws in Oral and Maxillofacial Infections, 4th subedition. WB Saunders Company; 2002.
14. Turlington EG. Transactions of the IV International Conference on Oral Surgery. Copen hagen, Denmark: Munksgaard; 1973.
15. Wee Leon Lam, Anselmo Garrido, Paul RW Stanley. Use of topical negative pressure in the treatment of chronic osteomyelitis. J Bone Joint Surg Am. 2005;87:622-24.
16. Grime PD, Bowerman JE, Weller PJ. Gentamicin impregnated poly-

methylmethacrylate (PMMA) beads in the treatment of primary chronic osteomyelitis of the mandible. Br J Oral Maxillofac Surg. 1990;28(6):367-74.
17. Mowlem R. Osteomyelitis of the jaws. Proc R Soc Med. 1945;38:452.
18. Marx RE. Chronic osteomyelitis of the jaws. Oral Maxillofac Surg Clin North Am. 1991;3(2):367-81.
19. Laube J, Honscha W, Franke W. Trephination and antibiotic irrigation-drainage as a possible treatment of the septic phase of acute hematogenic osteomyelitis. Z Arztl Fortbild (Jena). 1973;67(19):972-73.
20. Coviello V, Stevens MR, Contemporary Concepts in the treatment of chronic osteomyelitis. Oral Maxillofac Surg Clin North Am. 2007;19(4):523-34.
21. Jörg Schmutz. Osteomyelitis Therapy-Hyperbaric Oxygen as an Adjunct in Treatment of Osteomyelitis of the Jaws. Heidelberg, Berlin: Springer;2008. pp. 191-204.
22. Hart GB, Mainous EG. The treatment of radiation necrosis with hyperbaric oxygen. Cancer. 1976;37(6):2580-85.
23. Marx RE. Osteoradionecrosis: a new concept of its pathophysiology. J Oral Maxillofac Surg. 1983;41:282-88.
24. Rees GA. On uncommon forms of abscess in childhood. London Med Gaz. 1847;4:859.
25. Shafer WG. Chronic sclerosing osteomyelitis. Oral Surg. 1957;15:138-42.
26. Oulis C, Berdousis E, Vadiakas G, et al. Garre's osteomyelitis of an unusual origin in a 8-year-old child. A case report. Int J Pediatr Dent. 2000;10:240-44.
27. Eversole LR, Leider AS, Corwin JO, et al. Proliferative periostitis of Garre's: its differentiation from other neoperiostoses. J Oral Surg. 1979;37: 725-31.
28. Eswar N. Garré's osteomyelitis: a case report. J Indian Soc Pedod Prev Dent. 2001;19(4)157-59.
29. Caffey J. Infantile cortical hyperostoses. J Pediatr. 1946;29:541-59.
30. Batcheldor GD Jr, Giansanti JS, Hibbard ED, et al. Garré's osteomyelitis of the jaws: a review and report of two cases. J Am Dent Assoc. 1973;87(4):892-7.
31. Thisted E, Poulsen P, Christensen PO. Actinomycotic osteomyelitis in a child. J Laryngol Otol. 1987;101(7): 746-8.
32. Russo TA. Agents of actinomycosis. In: Mandell GL, Bennett JE, Dolin R (Eds). Principles and Practice of Infectious Diseases, 6th edition. Philadelphia Elsevier Churchill Livingstone 2005. pp. 2924-34.
33. Smego RA, Foglia G. Actinomycosis. Clin Infect Dis. 1998;26(6):1255-61.
34. Schwartz JG, Tio FO. Nocardial osteomyelitis: a case report and review of the literature. Diagn Microbiol Infect Dis. 1987;8:37.
35. Chaudhary S, Kalra N, Gomber S. Tuberculous osteomyelitis of the mandible: a case report in a 4-year-old child. Oral Surg Oral Med Oral Pathol Oral Radiol Endod. 2004;97:603-6.
36. Mishra YC, Bhoyar SC. Primary tuberculous osteomyelitis of mandible. J Indian Dental Assoc. 1986; 58:335-9.
37. Thomason HA, Mayoral A. Syphilitic osteomyelitis. J Bone Joint Surg Am. 1940;22:203-6.
38. Shroyer JV III, Lew D, Abreo F, et al. Osteomyelitis of the mandible as a result of sickle cell disease. Report and literature review. Oral Surg Oral Med Oral Pathol. 1991;72(1):25-8.
39. Girasole RV, Lyon ED. Sickle cell osteomyelitis of the mandible: report of three cases. J Oral Surg. 1977;35(3):231-34.
40. Dietrich R Lawrenz. Sickle cell disease: a review and update of current therapy. J Oral Maxillofac Surg. 1999;57(2):171-78.
41. Merritt K. Factors increasing the risk of infection in patients with open fractures. J Trauma. 1988;28:823.
42. Robert M Kellman, Darin L Wright. Management of post-traumatic osteomyelitis of the mandible. In: Alex M Greenberg, Joachim Prein (Eds). Craniomaxillofacial Reconstructive and Corrective Bone Surgery; Principles of Internal Fixation Using the AO/ASIF Technique. Springers; 2002. pp. 433-8.
43. Marx RE. Chronic osteomyelitis of jaws, Oral Maxillofac Surg Clin North Am. 1991;3:367.
44. Marx RE. A new concept in the treatment of osteoradionecrosis. J Oral Maxillofac Surg. 1983;41(6):351-7.
45. Mark A Engleman, Gayle Woloschak, William Small Jr. Radiation-induced skeletal injury. In: William Small Jr, Gayle W (Eds). Radiation Toxicity: A practical Guide, Volume 128. US: Springer. 2006.pp.155-69.
46. Lauren O'Malley, et al. Improvement of radiological penumbra using intermediate energy photons (IEP) for stereotactic radiosurgery. Phys Med Biol. 2006;51:2537-48.
47. Marx RE. Osteoradionecrosis: a new concept of its pathophysiology. J Oral Maxillofac Surg. 1983;41(5):283-8.
48. Marx RE, Carlson ER, Smith BR, et al. isolation of actinomyces species and Eiikenella corrodens from patients with chronic diffuse scelerosing osteomyelitis. JOMS. 1994;52:26.
49. Clayman L. Clinical controversies in oral and maxillofacial surgery: Part II. Management of dental extractions in irradiated jaws: a protocol without hyperbaric oxygen therapy. J Oral Maxillofac Surg. 1997;55:275-81.
50. Tompach PC, et al. Cell response to hyperbaric oxygen treatment. Int J Oral Maxillofac Surg. 1997;26:82-86.
51. Bras J, de Jonge HK, van Merkesteyn JP. Osteoradionecrosis of the mandible: pathogenesis. Am J Otolaryngol. 1990;11(4):244-50.
52. Marx RE, Johnson SP. Studies in the radiobiology of ORN and their clinical significance. Oral Surg Oral Med Oral Pathol. 1987;64:379-90.
53. Beumer J III, Silverman S Jr, Berak SB Jr. Hard and soft tissue necrosis following radiation therapy for oral cancer. J Prosthet Dent. 1972;27:640-7.
54. Murray CG, Daly TE, Zimmerman SO. The relationship between dental disease and radiation necrosis of the mandible. Oral Surg Oral Med Oral Pathol. 1980;49:99-104.
55. Harris M. The conservative management of osteoradionecrosis of the mandible with ultrasound therapy.

Br J Oral Maxillofac Surg. 1992; 30:313.

56. Marx RE. Hyperbaric oxygen: its role after radiotherapy. In: Booth PW, Schendel SA, Hausamen JE (Eds). Maxillofacial Surgery. New York: Churchill Livingstone; 1999.
57. Marx RE. Osteoradionecrosis of the jaws: Review and update. HB02 Rev. 1984;5:78-128.
58. Vudiniabola S, Pirone C, Williams J, et al. Hyperbaric oxygen in the prevention of osteoradionecrosis of the jaws. Aust Dent J. 1999;44(4):243-7.

BIBLIOGRAPHY

1. Hudson JW. Osteomyelitis of the jaws. JOMS. 1993;51:1294-1301.
2. Laskin DM. Oral and Maxillofacial Surgery, Illinois, Chicago. Mosby CV. 1999;256-76.
3. Olaitan AA, Amuda JT. Osteomyelitis of mandible in sickle cell disease. BJOMS. 1997;35:190-2.
4. Sano K, Yoshida Shin-ichi. Preauricular mass presenting as a sign of osteomyelitis of the temporal bone. JOMS. 1998;56:1364-52.
5. Sato M, Yamaguchi S. Osteomyelitis of the mandible in a patient with acquired systemic analgia. JOMS. 1997;55:97-9.
6. Topazian RG, Goldbery MH. Oral and Maxillofacial Infections, USA, Saunders WB. 2002;214-42.

Section 7

Maxillofacial Trauma

- Management of Soft Tissue Injuries
- Fractures of Mandible
- Fractures of Middle Third of Facial Skeleton
- Facial Burns
- Medicolegal Aspects of Injury

19 Management of Soft Tissue Injuries

Jajoo Suhas N, Yadav Abhilasha, Garg Rajat

INTRODUCTION

Injuries to the face commonly result in a significant psychological response. The face is the most prime possession of an individual and everybody wants to look good and presentable. The disfigurement of the face due to injuries or ablative surgeries causes a big psychological dent and undermines the self-esteem of the person. The management of the facial hard and soft tissue injuries is often very challenging as the patients are very demanding and want the function and the esthetics to be restored to its preinjury status, which may not be always possible. Injuries to the head occur in over 70 percent of all automobile accidents and nearly 70 percent cases of assaults. The management of facial lacerations is not the priority, especially if it is associated with grievous injuries like head injury or acute respiratory obstruction.

DEFINITION OF WOUND

The acute wound is a breakdown of the integrity of the soft tissue envelope surrounding any portion of the body. It is defined by size, depth and involved anatomic structures. The time course between an acute versus chronic wound is a continuum between 4 and 6 weeks. It is during this time that if an acute wound has not healed spontaneously, it is likely to become a chronic, 'problem wound' that requires further intervention.

EXAMINATION AND HISTORY

The time spent in the examination of the injury and treatment planning is never wasted and is ultimately beneficial for the patient. In the soft tissue injuries, which are without bony injuries, the minimal and esthetically acceptable scar can be achieved if the wound is first thoroughly cleaned, debrided and meticulously sutured, using an appropriate technique and material. But, when there is a bony injury treatment plan changes, hence, a careful examination and evaluation is warranted. Apart from general aspects of the history that are common to all trauma patients, a complete history of the incidence leading to the injury should be taken. A careful history reveals presence of any foreign bodies in wounds by understanding the mechanism of the injury (such as splinters, glass pieces). Particular attention should be paid to the wounds, which have been in contact with caustic substances such as the wounds during the industrial accidents. In a typical road traffic accident (RTA) injury the dirt, foreign bodies are embedded in the wound, but are obscure initially because of blood. Foreign bodies in automobile accidents may be glass, plastic or metal. A careful examination should be done for the presence of any foreign body such as glass, which not detected on radiographs.

The specialized nature of the different anatomical structures of the face demands special attention to be paid to the facial injuries like the injuries to brow, eyelid, nose; lip and ear require careful assessment and treatment to avoid deformity and potential interference with function. Injuries to eyelid and orbit require ophthalmic evaluation to establish visual status and presence of any corneal damage. Facial injuries can be superficial, but may extend to involve adjacent structures including bones, nerves, ducts, muscles, vessels, glands and/or dentoalveolar structures. A thorough head and neck examination determines the extent of associated facial wounds.

The involvement of cranial nerves (Vth and VIIth) may be associated with lacerations that involve the face. The facial nerve exits the stylomastoid foramen and divides into five branches within the parotid gland dividing the gland into superficial and deep lobes. Any injury to the gland, preauricular area or cheek should arouse suspicion for associated facial nerve injury. Facial nerve is deep when it exits stylomastoid foramen then gradually become superficial, that is why involvement of facial nerve injury depends on location of wound and extent of wound (Fig. 19.1). Injury to the parotid gland or its main duct can lead to salivary fistula. The parotid duct is approximately 5 cm in length and 5 mm in diameter. It exits the gland and runs along the superficial surface of the masseter muscle and then penetrates the buccinator muscle to enter the oral cavity opposite the upper second molar. The treatment of parotid duct injuries

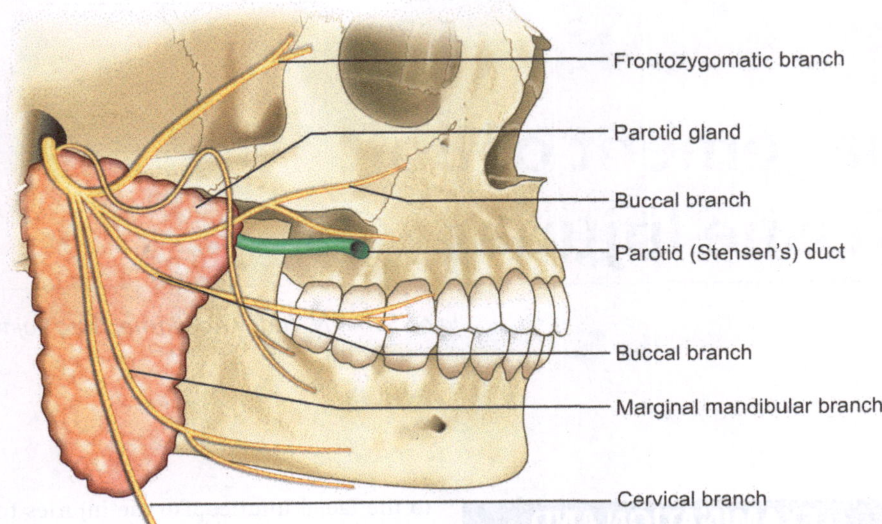

Fig. 19.1: Facial nerve and its branches

depends upon the location of the injury. If the injury involves the proximal duct, while it is still in the gland, the parotid capsule should be closed and a pressure dressing is placed. If the injury is present in the mid-region of the duct, the duct should be repaired. Injuries involving the terminal portion of the duct should be drained directly into the mouth. Lacerations are closed primarily and a pressure dressing is placed to prevent fluid accumulation. If the deep soft tissue injuries are present in the infraorbital area the branches of the infraorbital nerve may get involved producing sensory deficit in the area of distribution of the nerve.

If the penetrating injuries are present on the neck, face and temporal bone, critical evaluation of the wound should be done to rule out injuries to the underlying vital structures.

The lines of minimal tension, also called relaxed skin tension lines, are result of the adaptation of the skin to the function and are also related to the elastic nature of the underlying dermis. The intermittent and chronic contractions of the muscles of facial expression create depressed creases in the skin of the face. These creases become more visible and deepen with the growing age (Fig. 19.2). For instance, the supraorbital wrinkle lines and the transverse lines of the forehead are caused by the contraction of the frontalis muscles, which is inserted into the skin of the lower forehead. In the upper eyelids, many fine perpendicular strands of fibers of the elevator aponeurosis terminate in the dermis of the skin and along the tarsus to form the supratarsal fold. Similar insertions in the lower lid create fine horizontal lines, which are accentuated by the circumferential contraction of the orbicularis oculi muscle.

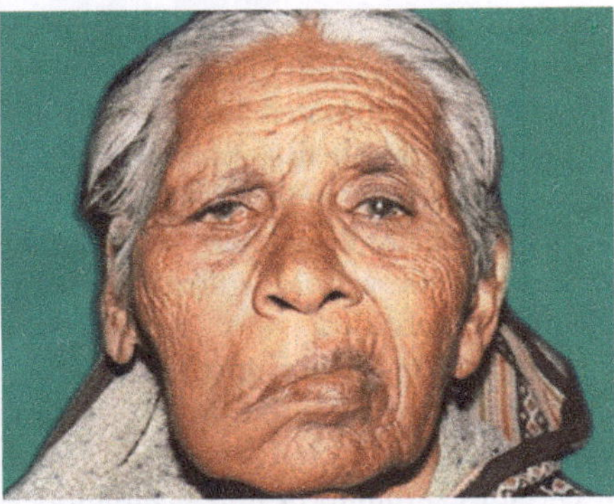

Fig. 19.2: Lines of minimal tension seen on face in old age

Incision should be preferably made along or within the lines of minimal tension as the ensuing scar is inconspicuous and gives excellent esthetic results. Any incision or portion of an incision that crosses such a crease often produces unsightly and conspicuous scars.

TYPES OF INJURY

Wounds can be classified into tidy and untidy wounds (Box 19.1). The surgeons aim is to convert untidy wounds to tidy wounds by removing all contaminated and devitalized tissue.

Primary repair is possible with tidy wounds, but contaminated wounds require debridement on one or several occasions before definitive repair can be carried out.

It also can be classified according to level of tissue insult:

Abrasions

- Contusions

Incised wounds

- Lacerations
- Avulsions
- Bites (animals and humans)
- Crush injury
- Penetrating injuries

These all types may be associated with or without tissue loss.

Abrasions

Shear forces that remove a superficial layer of skin cause abrasions such as sliding along pavement, dirt or glass that removes the epithelial layer and papillary layer of dermis leaving the raw bleeding reticular layer of dermis exposed. This type of wound may be painful because of exposed free nerve endings. Abrasions can be superficial and deep. The age of the abrasion can be ascertained by clinical appearance of the wound as depicted in Figs 19.3A to C. The wound should be gently cleansed with a mild soap solution and irrigated with normal saline. These superficial injuries usually heal with local wound care and can be left exposed for healing, but deep abrasions are never left open as it can lead to contamination of the wound. It is important to determine whether foreign bodies have been

Box 19.1: Types of wound

Tidy wounds	Untidy wounds
Incised	Crushed or avulsed
Clean	Contaminated
Healthy tissue	Devitalized tissue
Seldom tissue loss	Often tissue loss

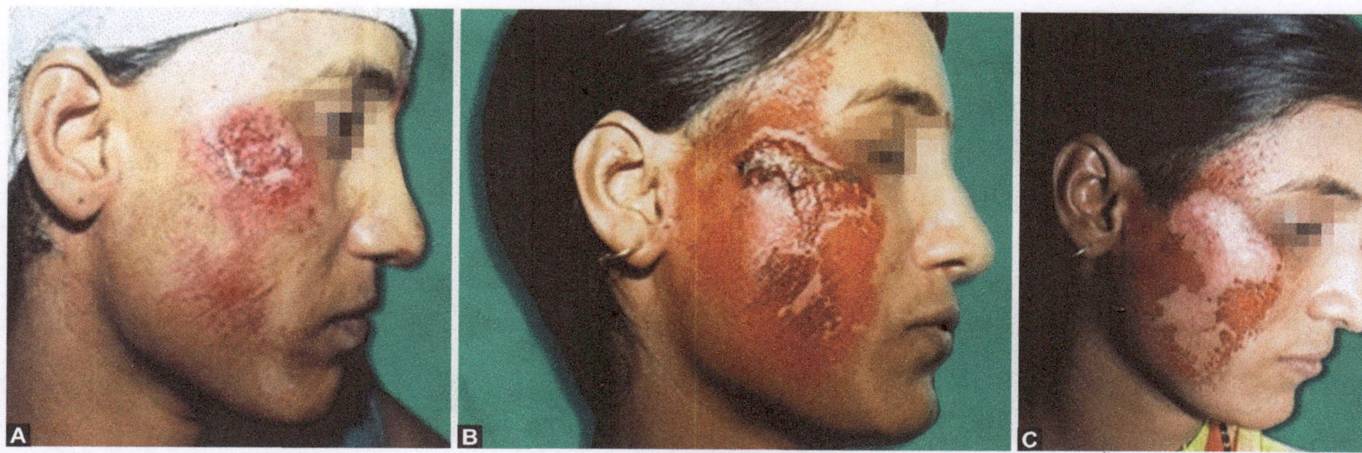

Figs 19.3A to C: Healing of abrasion: (A) On 1st day with dark red scab; (B) After 3–5 days brownish red scab; (C) After 5–7 days falling off of scab

embedded in the wound. Failure to remove all foreign material can lead to permanent 'tattooing' of the soft tissue. After the wound is cleansed the abrasion is covered with a thin layer of topical antibiotic ointment like bacitracin to minimize desiccation and secondary crusting of the wound and dressed with cotton gauze or covered with antibiotic coated cellulose acetate gauze.

The epithelialization without significant scarring is complete in 7 to 10 days, if the epidermal pegs have not been completely removed. At 14 days, fibroblast and capillary formation in the dermis increases and new elastic fibers develop by 3 months. If the abrasions significantly extend into the reticular dermal layer, significant scarring from granulation tissue formation will result (Fig. 19.4). For this compression can be given over injury to avoid hypertrophy of the granulation tissue.

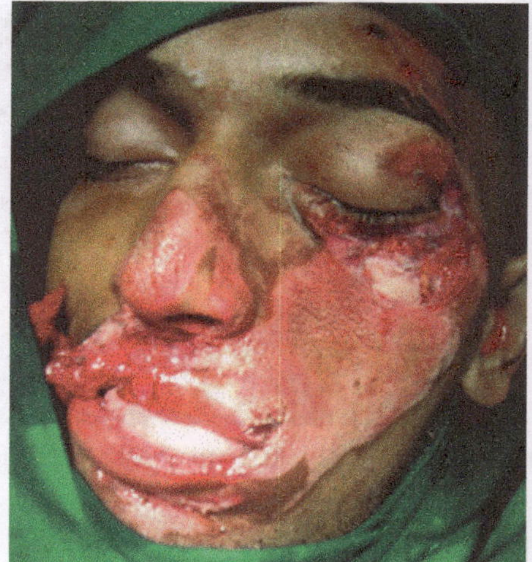

Fig. 19.4: Abrasion on cheek region with laceration on lip and infraorbital region

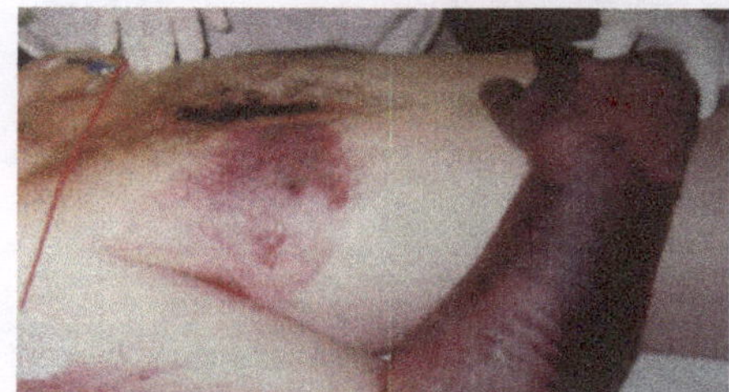

Fig. 19.5: Contusion on chest due to blunt injury

Contusions

Contusions are caused by blunt trauma that causes edema and hematoma formation in the subcutaneous tissues (Fig. 19.5). It occurs variably depending upon the area involved (eyelids or lip) will develop a relatively greater amount of swelling than forehead or cheek, as it has more loose aerolar tissue. Small hematomas usually resolve without treatment; hypopigmentation or hyperpigmentation of the involved tissue can occur, but is rarely permanent. Large hematomas should be drained (evacuated) to prevent permanent pigmentary changes and secondary subcutaneous atrophy. Usually the overlying skin and mucosa are intact, but if the contusion is associated with a laceration, the contused margins should be excised before closure. If contused margins involve vital structures like eye than delayed closure should be done until the contusion resolves. In general there is no specific treatment for most facial contusions with the exception of ear or septal hematomas, which requires immediate evacuation.

Incised Wound

These wounds have sharp and clear cut margins and are caused by a sharp object drawn across the skin/mucosa. Sharp instruments may be like knife, razor, scissors or sword, axe, hatchet. Incised wound is always broader than the edge of the weapon causing it owing to the retraction of the divided tissues. It is somewhat spindle shaped; it's length greater than depth and width. As the edges of the wound are sharp and healthy, without any devitalization they can be closed primarily after irrigation with sterile normal saline solution and diluted antiseptics line 5 percent povidone iodine solution. They heal fast and the ensuing scars are acceptable (Figs 19.6A to D).

Lacerations

Lacerations are caused by blunt to semi sharp and hard objects to the soft tissue. Lacerations can have sharp,

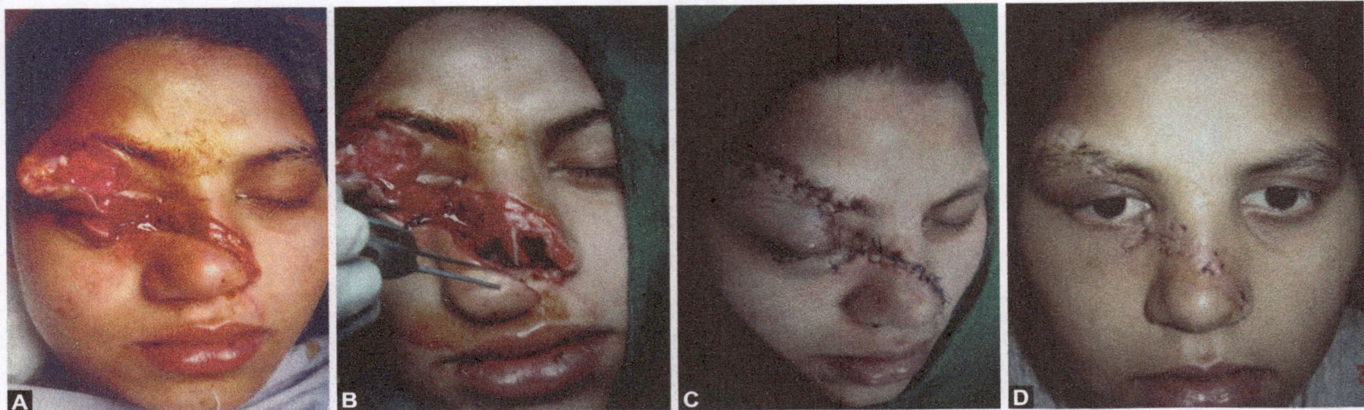

Figs 19.6A to D: (A) Incised wound over the nose and eyelid caused by a razor; (B) Clear division of the alar and septal cartilages; (C) Primary closure of the wound; (D) Clinical photograph on 8th postoperative day showing good healing and minimum scarring

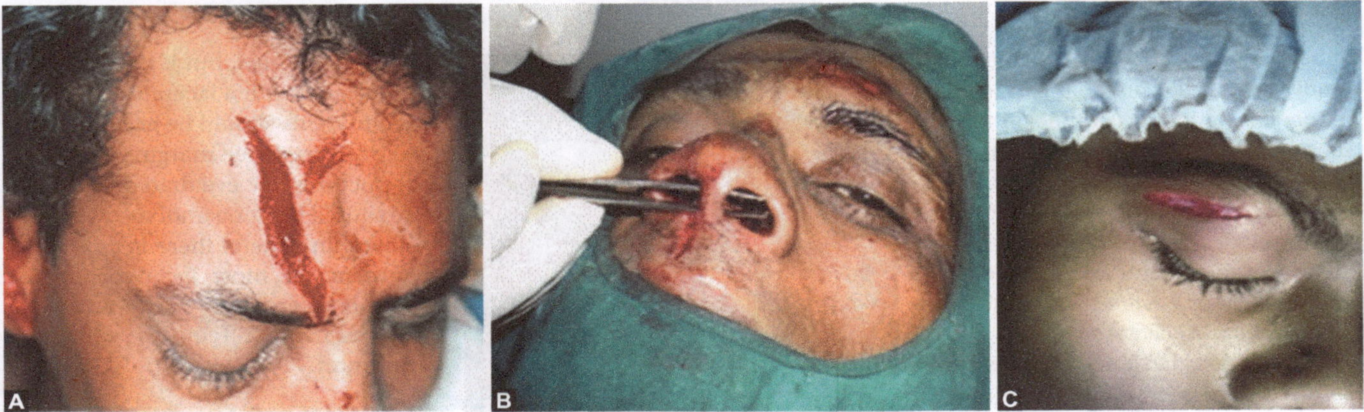

Figs 19.7A to C: Different types of simple laceration seen: (A) On forehead; (B) On lip with nasal injury; (C) On upper eyelid

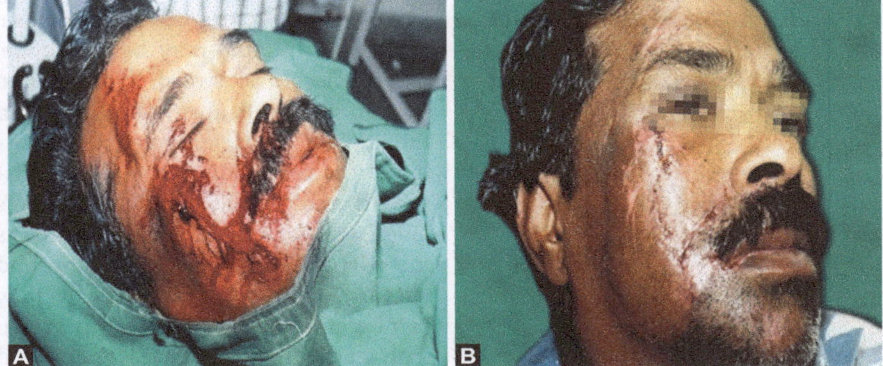

Figs 19.8A and B: (A) Laceration with ragged borders; (B) Scar of stellate laceration

contused, ragged or stellate margins as seen in crushing type of injury or they may involve partial avulsion of tissues that remain pedicled to surrounding structures. Closure is performed using a layered technique. Laceration can be simple, stellate or flap-like.

Simple Laceration

Simple laceration may be clean, contaminated or contused. Clean lacerations may be repaired with little debridement. Contaminated wounds should be cleansed and closed primarily; it can be delayed if necessary for 5 to 7 days. Similarly, contused wounds should be evaluated if enough tissue is available after excising the margins it should be closed primarily with loose, approximating sutures, otherwise treatment should be delayed until contusion resolves (Figs 19.7A to C).

Stellate Laceration

If the margins are bevelled or ragged they should be conservatively excised to provide perpendicular skin edges to prevent excessive scar formation[1] (Figs 19.8A and B). Undermining of the soft tissue wound margins is helpful in suturing of tissue without excessive tension at the wound margin. But, extensive undermining leads to contraction of wound and scarring. Interrupted sutures should be used to close the wound as far as the stellate portion of the wound margin. Rarely there

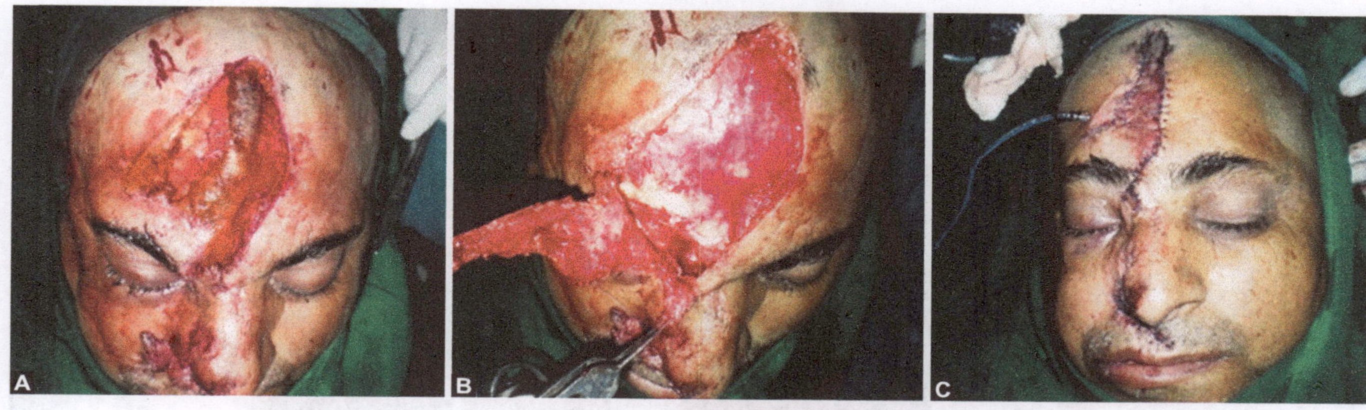

Figs 19.9A to C: Flap-like laceration: (A) Preoperative; (B) After debridement; (C) Closure

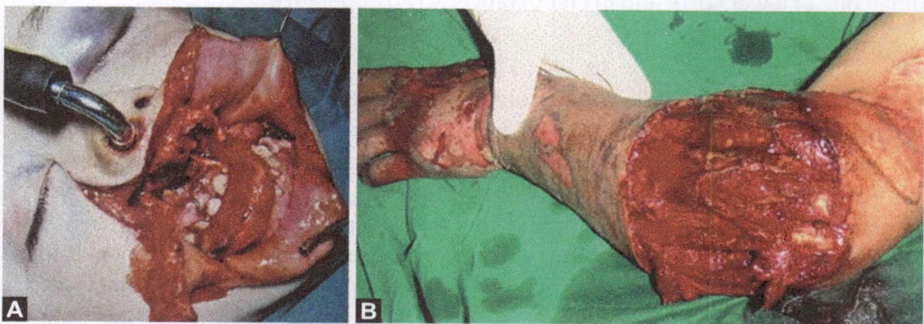

Figs 19.10A and B: Avulsions: (A) Cheek; (B) Forearm

is an indication for changing the direction of the wound margins by Z-plasty at the time of primary wound repair. These procedures should be done as secondary revision procedures if indicated. Use of adhesive strips can assist in relieving tension on the wound margin.

Flap-like Lacerations

It is a laceration with significant undermining of the soft tissues without loss of tissue (Figs 19.9A to C). Debris is very commonly found in deep tissues under the flap. Pressure dressings play an important role in minimizing dead space and limiting hematoma formation or fluid collection within the deep tissue.[2] The use of drains may be helpful in achieving the desirable cosmetic results and ensuring proper healing.

Avulsions

Avulsive injures are characterized by the loss of segments of soft tissue. These injuries are relatively uncommon, occurring mostly due to gunshot wounds or weapon injuries[3] (Figs 19.10A and B). Sometimes initial examination may show apparent loss of tissue, but thorough examination reveals that the tissue margins have been retracted or rolled under the wound margin. Undermining the adjacent tissue, followed by primary closure, can close small defects. When primary closure is not possible, other options are considered. These include local flaps, skin grafts or apposition of the skin margin to the mucous membrane. Facial wounds should not be allowed to heal by secondary intention (granulation tissue formation) because of excessive scar formation.

Animal and Human Bites

Animal and human bite wounds have a significant risk of infection as they are highly contaminated. These can be animal and human bites. Animal bites particularly from dogs, are polymicrobial and are more avulsive due to the 'pull back' response of the victim where as human bites are mostly on lip, nose and ear. Most wounds are thoroughly irrigated with minimal debridement and primary closure, but when wounds are more than 24 hours old than closure is controversial. Some prefer primary closure so that minimal risks of infection, but other prefer delayed primary closure. An adjunctive broadspectrum antibiotic with tetanus and rabies prophylaxis is necessary (Figs 19.11 and 19.12).

Crush Injury Syndrome

Crush injury syndrome can be described as prolonged severe compression of one or several compartments of the body (Fig. 19.13). As a consequence of multiple compartment involvement and extensive myonecrosis, there is excessive formation of myoglobin and potassium, which enters into the systemic circulation and cause hyperkalemia, cardiac arrhythmia, shock, renal failure and death.

Clinical Features

In patients those are subjected to massive crush injury that has been prolonged for several hours, following features can be seen:

- Sudden massive swelling, marked edema with variable degree of local hemorrhage.
- Paralysis of involved limb is seen. The peripheral pulses may be

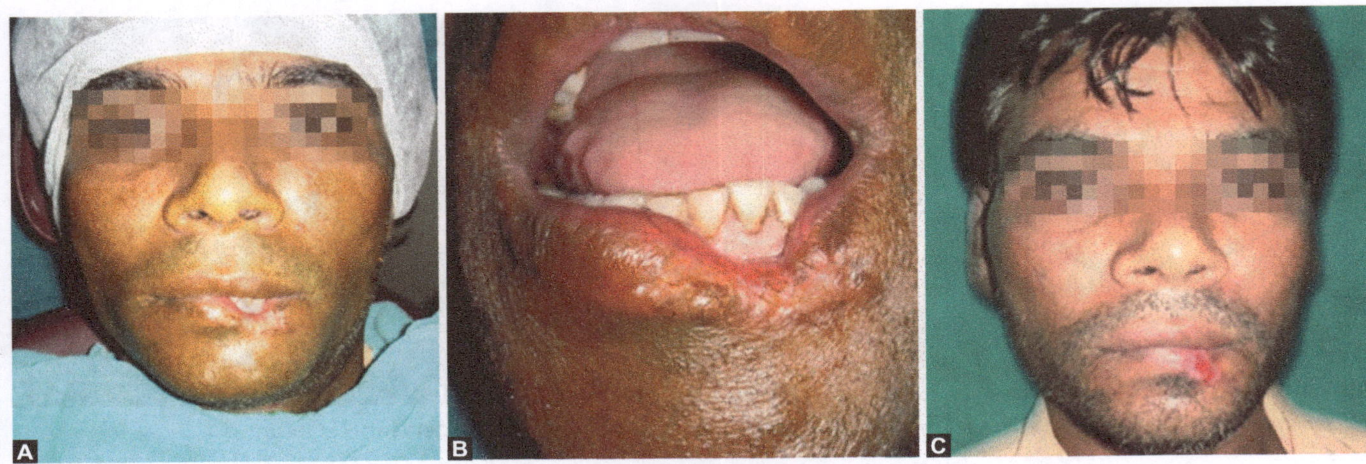

Figs 19.11A to C: Human bite of lower lip: (A and B) Preoperative; (C) Postoperative

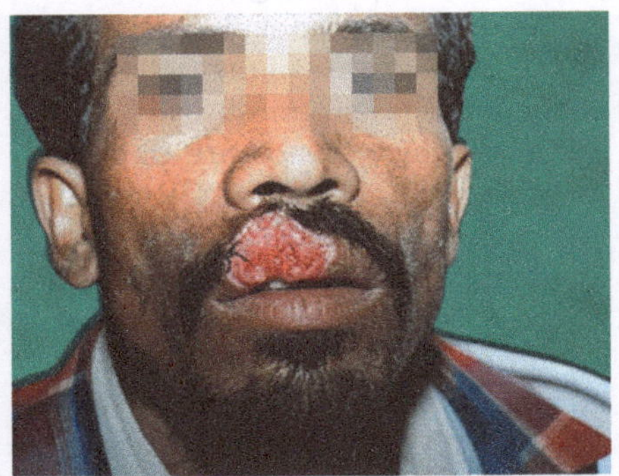

Fig. 19.12: Pig bite present on upper lip

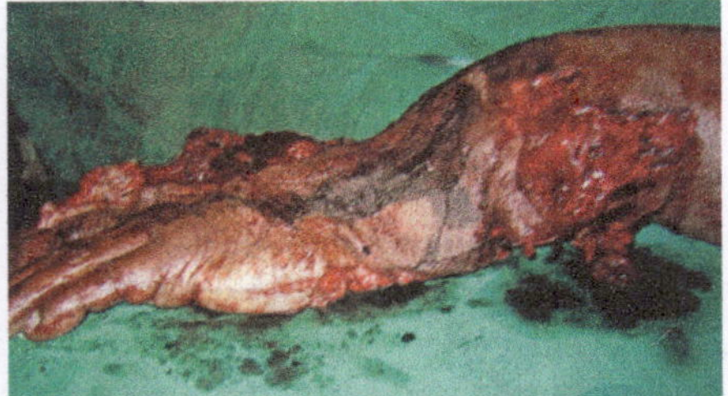

Fig. 19.13: Crush injury of a hand

misleading as the main arterial supply is damaged due to extensive involvement of muscle.

- Patient will have pale, cold and moist skin, while maintaining normal blood pressure.

Due to prolonged compression there will be anoxia, which will lead to increased capillary permeability and massive transudation, leading to extravasation of plasma and electrolyte bearing fluid. This is the first phase of shock, which is compensated by peripheral vasoconstriction; this compensatory mechanism is capable to keep up with the fluid loss. But, once blood pressure falls then the second stage of shock will develop, which is a life-threatening situation. To prevent hypovolemic shock in patients with crush injuries intravenous (IV) isotonic saline and crystalloids solution is most important to prevent shock.

Penetrating Injuries

Penetrating injury occurs when an object pierces the skin and enters the deeper tissues of the body, creating an open wound. The penetrating object may remain embedded in the tissues, come out the way it entered in, or may pass through the tissues and exit from another area (surface) like knife, bullet or splinters of the blast injuries. The bullet injuries may look simple or the entry wound at the penetrating site may look small, but it may have an exit wound site on the other side, which will be massive due to rotation of the bullet in the tissues in concentric manner.

Penetrating trauma can be serious because it can damage internal organs, vital organs and presents a risk of shock and infection. The severity of the injury varies widely depending on its site, the characteristics of the penetrating object and the amount of energy transmitted to the tissues. Assessment of the penetrating injury may involve X-rays or computed tomography (CT) scans and treatment comprises of repair of the damaged structures and removal of foreign objects.

As a missile passes through tissue, it decelerates, dissipating and transferring kinetic energy to the tissues; which causes the injury. The velocity of the projectile is a more important factor than its mass in determining how much damage is done; kinetic energy increases with the square of the velocity. The amount of energy transferred to tissue by a missile depends on the square of its velocity, the density of the tissue and the presenting area of the missile, for example the denser the tissue, the greater the amount of energy transmitted to it.[4] The path of a projectile can be estimated by imagining a line from the entrance wound to the exit wound, but the actual trajectory may vary due to differences in tissue density.

While penetrating facial trauma can pose a risk of airway obstruction due to edema or bleeding. Penetrating injury to the eye can cause the rupture of the globe or leakage of the vitreous humor posing a serious threat to eyesight. Penetrating head injury accounts for only a small percentage of all traumatic brain injuries and it is associated with a high mortality rate. Penetrating head trauma can cause cerebral contusions and lacerations, intracranial hematomas, pseudoaneurysms and arteriovenous fistulas.

Assessment can be difficult because much of the damage is often internal and not visible. The patient is thoroughly examined. X-ray and CT scanning may be used to identify the type and location of potentially lethal injuries. Sometimes before an X-ray is performed on a person with penetrating trauma from a projectile, a paper clip is taped over entry and exit wounds to show their location on the film.

MANAGEMENT OF SOFT TISSUE INJURIES

Before the 17th century, it was a common practice to pour hot oil on the wounds in order to cauterize damaged blood vessels to achieve the hemostasis, but the French surgeon Ambroise Pare[5] challenged the use of this method in 1545 and he was the first to propose using ligature to control the bleeding.

During the American Civil War, chloroform was used during surgery to reduce pain and allow more time for operations. As the sterile technique was not practiced in the hospitals, infection was the leading cause of death for wounded soldiers. During the World War I, doctors began replacing patients lost fluid with salt with parenteral fluid therapy. The practice of blood transfusion became more popular during the World War II to replace lost fluids. The use of antibiotics also came into practice during World War II.

The management of the soft tissue injury can be divided as:

- Primary general management
- Specific/definitive management.

Primary General Management

The initial examination involves evaluating and stabilizing the trauma patient. Any life-threatening conditions should be identified and managed immediately. The assessment of airway, breathing and circulation is made, which is followed by a general neurologic assessment with particular attention to cervical spine and head injuries before evaluation of facial soft tissue wounds. The fractures of supporting facial bones must be excluded by careful clinical and radiographic examination. Facial lacerations do not require immediate treatment because of the excellent blood supply to the facial region. During the assessment of other injuries, the wounds should be kept moist with sterile dressings of gauze soaked in an antibiotic solution until final management.

It is important to simultaneously achieve hemostasis, while stabilizing and evaluating the patient who has sustained trauma. The bleeding from most of the sites will respond to application of a pressure dressing. The bleeding from the lacerations involving the scalp can occasionally be difficult to control with pressure and may require clamping, ligation or electrocautery. The face is well supplied with blood vessels, which are generally small in diameter and supplied with elastic fibers. When blood vessels of face are completely transected, they tend to contract and collapse and bleeding stops spontaneously because the vessels become occluded with thrombi and compressed by the enveloping hematoma. However, partially transected vessels have a propensity for continued hemorrhage. Tough tissues of scalp do not allow vessels to retract due to the presence of aponeurosis and the scalp lacerations can bleed excessively for a long time.

In the soft tissue injuries other than those involving the face, the time-lapse from initial injury to treatment is important. Secondary risk of infection increases with the lapse of time. Because of the rich vascularity of the face there is no 'golden period' for the suturing or repair of facial wounds and the healing of facial wounds is unaffected by the interval between injury and repair. That is why primary closure of facial wounds, can be delayed, if there is underlying bone fracture. Treatment of the fracture should be completed before final soft tissue closure, because the wound itself may provide an access to the fracture site and if is undertaken prior to fracture reduction the suture line may get disrupted. Prophylactic antibiotics should be given in all contaminated wounds as well as for clean wounds, if there is any delay in repair. Betalactlam antibiotics are mostly used as a prophylactic antibiotic, but when the wounds are deep, soiled and have plenty of crushed or devitalized tissue, Metronidazole should be added to cover the anaerobic microorganism. The aminoglycosides can also be used along with beta-lactam antibiotics, if the wounds are badly soiled and likely to be invaded by gram negative organisms to provide broader spectrum of coverage.

A history of tetanus immunization status is essential as part of medical history. Facial wounds often appear clean, but they are at risk and require tetanus prophylaxis. Although the face has excellent vascularity and the anaerobic environments are rare, the badly soiled wounds with devitalized tissue require prophylaxis against tetanus with administration of tetanus toxoid (active immunity).

The American College of Surgeons Committee on Trauma Recommendations on Tetanus Care[6] (1987) are as follows Box 19.2.

However, in Indian circumstances as the immunization status of the patient is not known or reliable due to

Box 19.2: Tetanus prophylaxis

Fully immunized individuals
If the last dose of tetanus toxoid was given within 10 years, administer 0.5 mL absorbed tetanus toxoid for tetanus prone wounds. If < 5 years have elapsed since last dose, then this booster may be omitted.

Partially immunized individuals
When the patient has received two or more injections of tetanus toxoid and last dose was received more than 10 years ago, 0.5 mL absorbed toxoid is administered for both tetanus prone and nontetanus prone wounds.

Individuals not adequately immunized
For nontetanus prone wounds administer 0.5 mL of absorbed toxoid.
For tetanus prone wounds

- Administer 0.5 mL absorbed toxoid
- Administer 250 units TIG
- Administer antibiotics.

ignorance and illiteracy, especially in rural population it is always safe to administer tetanus toxoid, prophylactically following an injury.

Specific Management for Wounds

The decision is made first whether to repair the wound in the casualty department under local anesthesia or to perform the repair in the operating room under a general anesthesia. Large complicated, extensive lacerations involving deep structures demand ideal lighting and patient cooperation. General anesthesia offers the best opportunity for exploration and repair. The patient may require repair of other traumatic injuries in the operating room and on many occasions, definitive repair of associated facial soft tissue injuries can be performed at the same time. Facial injuries in pediatric patients must be repaired under general anesthesia as the patients do not cooperate.

A thorough evaluation of the 7th cranial nerve should be undertaken prior to injection of local anesthetic or administration of a general anesthetic. Injecting local anesthetic prior to cleaning the wound will allow more effective wound cleaning and preparation. One should avoid injecting the local anesthetic directly into the wound as important landmarks could get distorted. Regional nerve blocks are beneficial in minimizing the amount of local anesthesia required and also prevent distortion of the tissues. However, the local infilteration of local anesthetic solution containing adrenaline provides good hemostasis and dry field during the surgery.

WOUND DEBRIDEMENT

Debridement is the most fundamental principle in surgical wound preparation before the closure. Inadequate debridement is the surgical corollary to a postoperative infectious complication after acute wound bed closure.[7] It is a plastic surgery dictum.

Under adequate anesthesia the wound is thoroughly debrided (Figs 19.14A to C). All the nonvital tissue is excised with an attempt to salvage the tissue as much as possible, as radical debridement on the face is not recommended due to the excellent vascularity. Devitalized tissue impedes phagocytosis and often works as a nidus of infection. Persistent infection at a wound site leads to the release of inflammatory cytokines from monocytes and macrophages, which delays wound healing. An anaerobic environment results and limits leukocyte function. Soft tissue wounds are often contaminated with bacteria and foreign material. Treatment of these injuries involves copious irrigation and is aimed at minimizing the bacterial wound flora and removing any foreign bodies. With respect to infection rates, studies have shown no statistical difference in wounds irrigated with normal saline when compared to other antimicrobial solutions.

Soaps do not harm the intact skin surfaces when used in proper concentration, as the thick layer of epidermis protects the underlying tissue, but soaps may enter the wound and cause cellular damage and necrosis. Hydrogen peroxide produces effervescence and is known to flush out small dirt particles from the wound bed. It also releases nascent oxygen however; it impedes wound healing and has poor bactericidal activity. A good rule is to avoid irrigating the wound with any solution that would not be suitable for irrigating the eye. Toxic materials like alcohol, hydrogen peroxide, benzalkonium chloride, strong soaps like hexachlorophene and povidone-iodine should not have direct contact with open wound as these agents induce cellular necrosis on contact. If these agents are used around the wound, they should be used in dilute form (povidone-iodine 1 mL/L can be used) and the wound should be thoroughly irrigated with balanced salt solutions. Normally, 0.5 percent cetrimide or savlon is considered to be best solutions for wounds.

Lacerations that are extending into the scalp or any hair bearing area that should be shaved to provide good

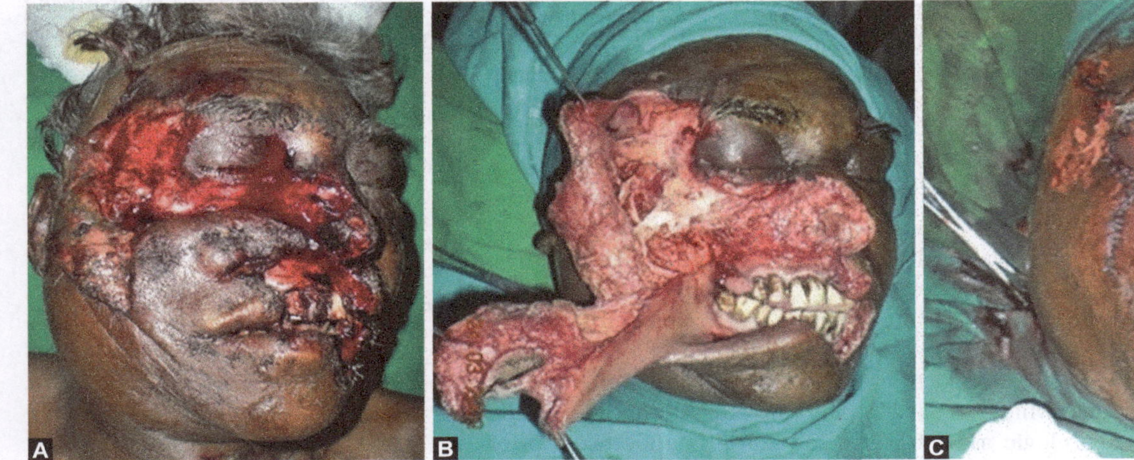

Figs 19.14A to C: Wound debridement: (A) Preoperative laceration; (B) Thoroughly debrided laceration; (C) Closure

access for debridement and repair. However, areas such as eyebrows and eyelashes should never be shaved rather clipped closely to provide landmark for positioning of soft tissues during closure.

Careful and meticulous cleaning of the wounds primarily will avoid unfavorable results such as 'tattooing,' infection, hypertrophic scarring and granulomas. A pulsatile type of irrigating device is useful for removing debris, necrotic tissue and loose material. An abrasive wound having debris and dirt should be scrubbed with a soft scrub brush and detergent soap to remove deeply imbedded foreign material. However, soaps may cause cellular damage and necrosis. A surgical blade may be helpful to scrape foreign material that is deeply embedded. Polymyxin B sulfate can be used to remove residual grease or tar in wounds. Proper cleaning and good surgical technique are imperative in minimizing infection. Infections are rare when the wound is closed so that no dead space, devitalized tissue, or foreign bodies remain beneath the sutured skin.

Conservation should be the rule in debridement of facial wounds and debridement should be limited to devitalized tissue that either is stained by road tar or contains dirt or other particles that cannot be removed with meticulous scrubbing.

Primary Closure

After meticulous cleaning and debridement the closure/repair of the wound is undertaken. If there is no tissue loss or if with mobilization of the tissue by undermining of the skin or mucosa, if the wounds can be closed primarily it should be undertaken. Care must be taken not to approximate the tissue under tension as the incision line can break producing dehiscence of the wound. One has to anticipate the subsequent inflammatory edema that can ensue in these wounds due to trauma and heavy contamination. Thus, the closure should be passive and tension free and should be able to accommodate the edema. The too tight sutures may stop bleeding from the skin flap margins, but invariably strangulate the wound edges producing ischemic necrosis of the wound margins and dehiscence (gaping) of the suture line. The sutures should be tied loose, so that the suture line itself should serve as drainage channel for the collected exudates under the skin flaps. In case gross collection is detected below the skin flaps it is advisable to open one or two sutures to drain the collection.

In the grossly contaminated wounds ideal material for closure of the deeper tissue is not catgut, but material like vicryl should be used. Similarly, multifilament material is having capillarity like linen or silk are not ideal for the closure of the skin and in such situation monofilament, inert material having minimum capillarity like prolene should be used for better cosmetic results.

If the wound cannot be closed primarily due to tissue loss then closure with the help of local flaps should be planned.

Local Flaps

A flap is a unit of tissue that may be transferred from a donor to a recipient site, while maintaining its blood supply.[8]

A flap is different from a graft; it has an intrinsic blood supply that is responsible for its viability. A graft must rely on diffusion until its vascularity becomes re-established. The anatomy of macrocirculation is used to define and design a flap. The major arterial inflow and venous outflow of a flap constitute the foundation from which the microcirculatory beds then provide nutrition and oxygen and carry away CO_2 and waste products, thus forming the basis of cellular metabolism throughout the flap. Vascularity of a flap can be determined either by excising small margin of flap or by needle prick method at various sites of flap to check bleeding. If bleeding is present it means flap is having good vascularity. The major disadvantages of flap are additional incision and later more scar formation on face, but at the same time local flaps are the best to close the avulsive defect. Facial flaps do best when the pedicle is based laterally and inferiorly. Basic flaps used on face are advancement, rotational, transposition and free vascularized flaps.

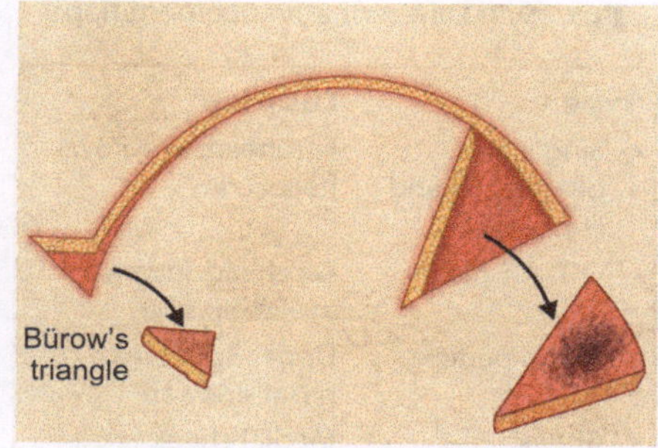

Fig. 19.15: Rotational flap technique

Rotational Flap

Basic rotation flap is a simple pivotal flap, which is curvilinear in shape and which rotates around a pivotal point near the defect (Fig. 19.15). It is best suited for triangular defects, designed immediately adjacent to defect—so one side of the defect is the advancing edge of the flap.

Advantages

- The flap has two sides, both edges can be placed in borders of esthetic units of face
- It has broad base and reliable vascularity
- It has great flexibility in design and positioning
- Arterial and venous disruptions may be minimized and sensory innervations can be maximized by good positioning of flap base.

Disadvantages

- Defect has to be triangular.
- It creates a right angle at the distal tip thus, care should be taken, while positioning the tip to avoid compromised vascularity.
- Effective length becomes progressively less as flap moves through its arc of rotation; hence, care should be taken, while designing.

Advancement Flaps

Advancement flaps it involves making of two parallel incisions from the defect and undermining the tissue until the flap can be advanced into the defect under minimal tension. The various types of

Box 19.3: Different advancement flaps

Type	Location
• Single and bilateral (U-and H-plasty)	Forehead, eyebrow, helical rim
• O-T, A-T plasty	Forehead, lower eyelid, lip, chin
• Island pedicle	Upper lip, cheek, nasal sidewall
• Cheek advancement	Medial cheek
• Mucosal advancement	Lower lip
• Wedge resection with advancement	Lip, ear

advancement flaps and their utility in different anatomical regions is shown in Box 19.3.

- **Single-pedicle advancement flap:** It is the most basic flap, also called U-plasty. Ratio of defect the length to the flap length is 3:1 (Figs 19.16A and B).
- **Bilateral advancement (H-plasty):** It is typically made when a single-pedicle advancement flap does not allow sufficient tissue for closure of the defect. The major disadvantage of this flap is the potentially long suture line (Figs 19.17A and B).
- **O-T plasty or A-T plasty:** This flap represents a type of bilateral advancement flap where a triangular defect is closed by advancing tissue from either side of the defect (Figs 19.18A and B). The advantage of this flap is that the defect can be divided in half by the use of the two flaps allowing placement of the incisions in natural creases, junctions of esthetic units or in the hairline. It works very well in the forehead and temple with the horizontal component placed in the hairline and along the lip with the horizontal limb at the vermilion.
- **V-Y plasty:** This is a unique flap where a V-shaped flap is moved into a defect with primary closure of the donor area leaving a final Y-shaped suture line (Figs 19.19 and 19.20).
- **Cheek advancement flap:** These flaps are optimally used in the cheek where the increased elasticity and mobility of the skin allows wide undermining and closure of medium to large defects along the lateral nasal wall and infraorbital area (Figs 19.21 and 19.22).

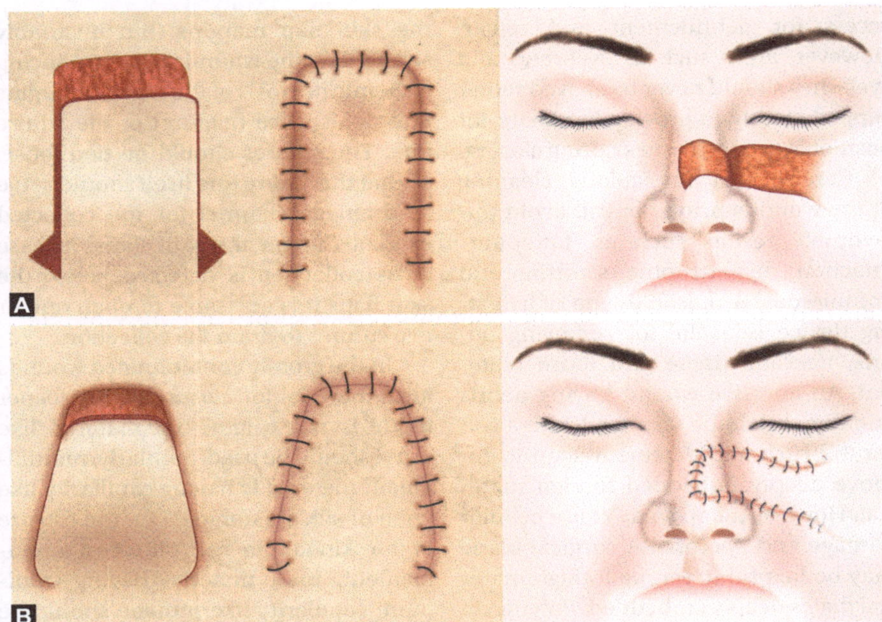

Figs 19.16A and B: U-plasty

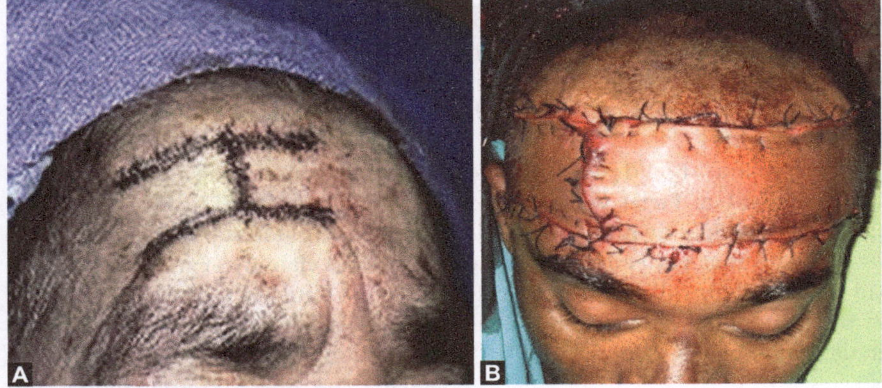

Figs 19.17A and B: Bilateral advancement flap on forehead

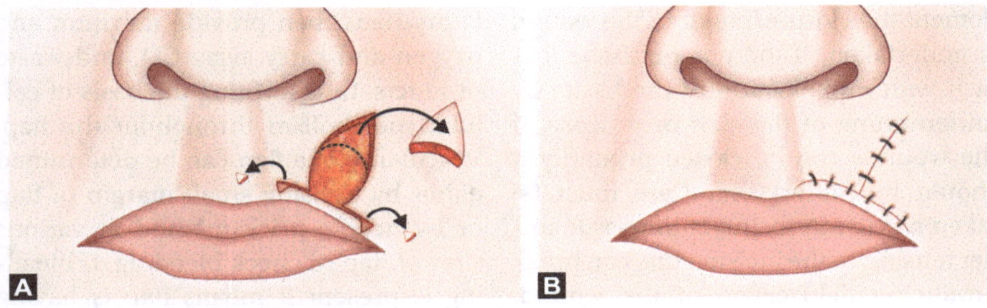

Figs 19.18A and B: O-T plasty to close defect on upper lip

Transposition Flaps

Transposition flaps involves swinging the flaps into areas of defect over healthy tissue, with a secondary defect at the donor site that is closed primarily

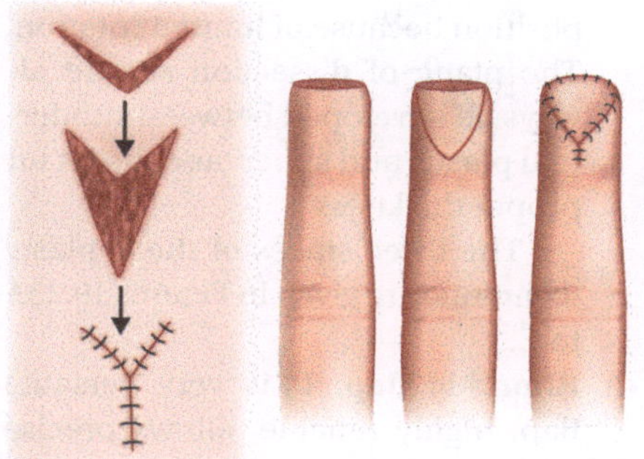

Fig. 19.19: V-Y plasty in which V- shaped defect is created and sutured to form a Y-shape

by undermining adjacent tissue or by coverage with a free skin graft.

Various transposition flaps are:

- **Z-plasty:** Z-plasty is a method of surgical revision of a scar or closure of a wound using a Z-shaped incision to reduce contractures of the adjacent skin. A straight line closure may result into more scar contracture and hence a Z-closure is useful to minimize contractures when used primarily (Figs 19.23A to C). It can elongate a contracted scar or rotate scar tension line. The middle segment of the Z-shaped incision is made along the line of greatest tension or contraction and the flaps are raised on opposite sides of the two ends and then transposed, the length and angle of each flap must be precisely the same to avoid mismatched flaps that may produce bad scar. It requires a proper skin thickness, a thin flap contracts readily and give unesthetic scar and a flap with too much subcutaneous tissue is difficult to

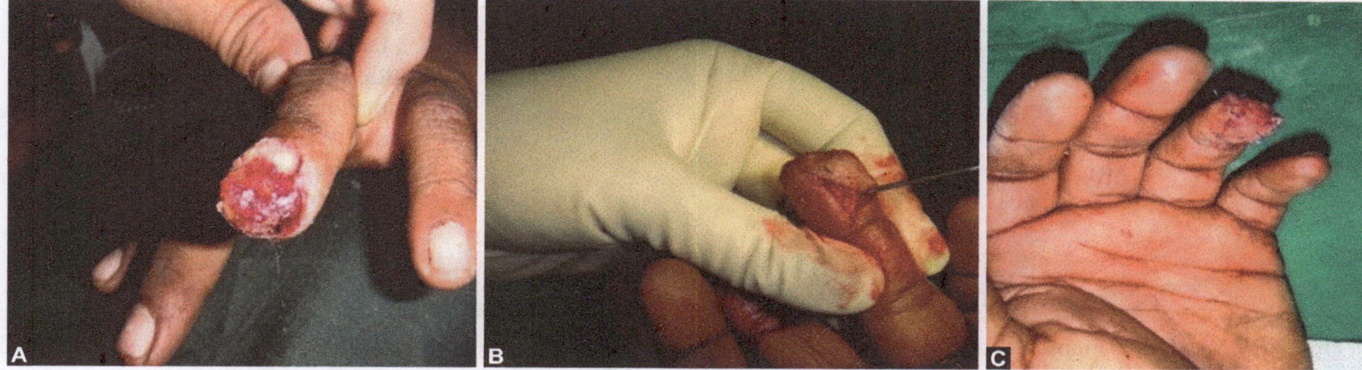

Figs 19.20A to C: A defect on finger in which V-shaped defect is created and sutured to form a Y-shape

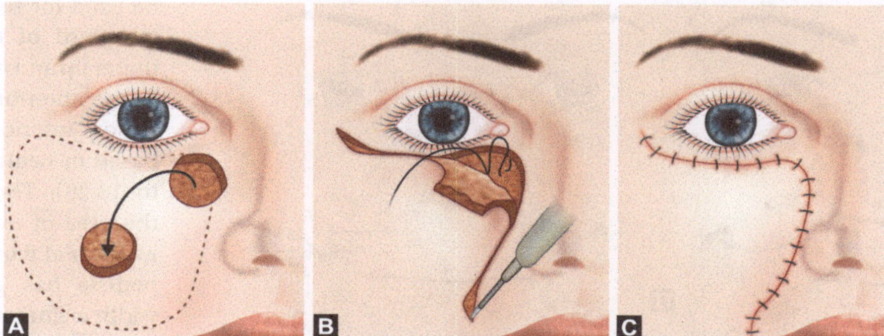

Figs 19.21A to C: Cheek advancement flap

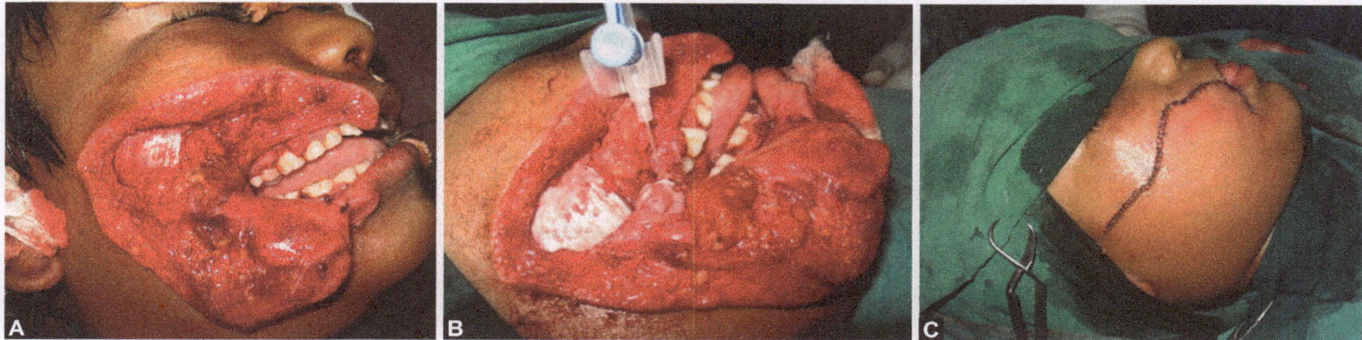

Figs 19.22A to C: Cracker burst injury: (A) After debridement; (B) Canulation of parotid duct; (C) Final closure

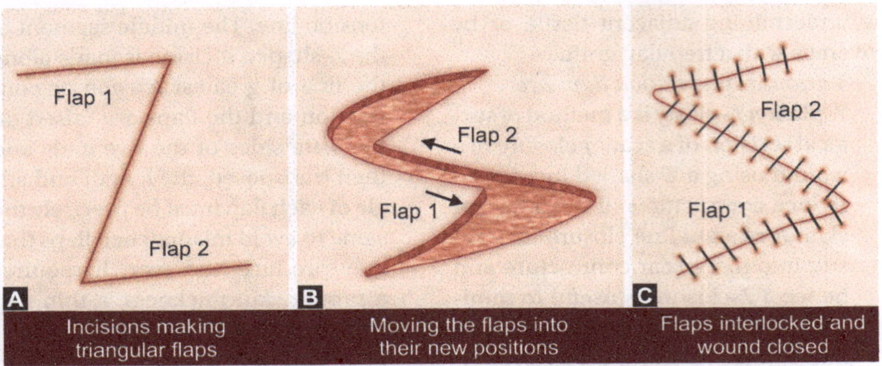

Figs 19.23A to C: Stages of Z-plasty technique

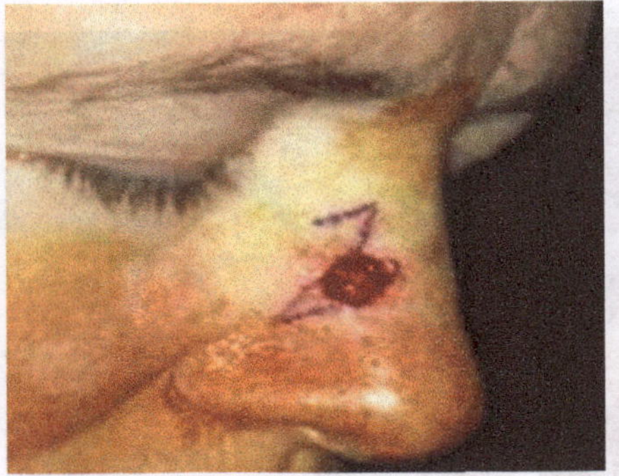

Fig. 19.24: Marking for rhombic flap to close defect

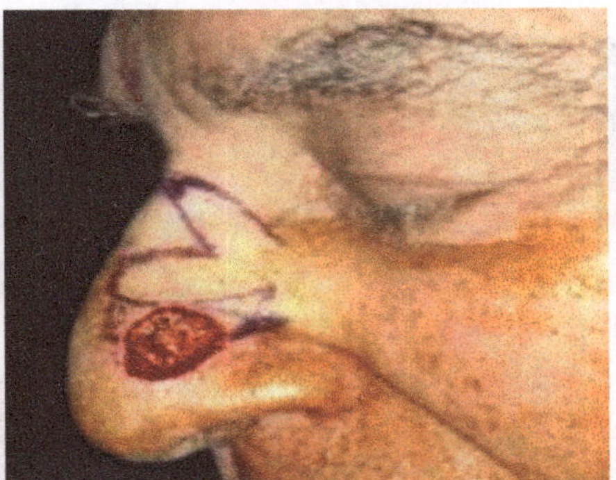

Fig. 19.25: Marking for bilobed flap to close the defect

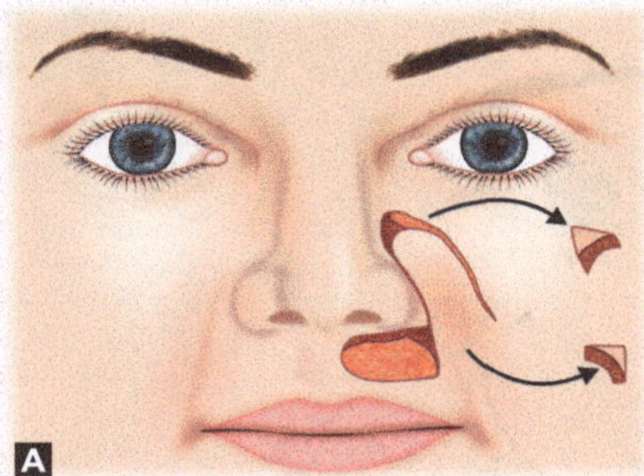

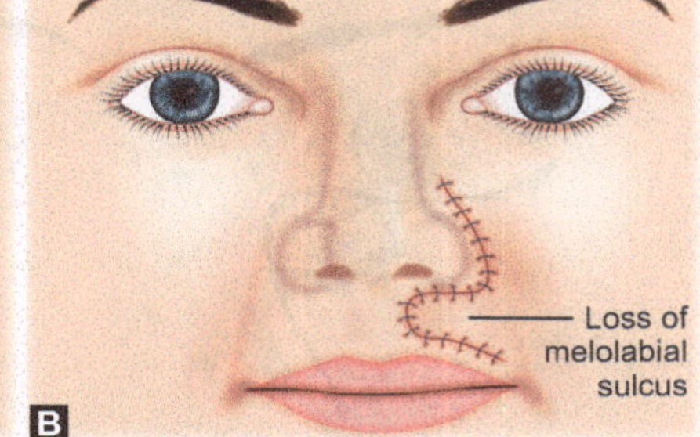

Figs 19.26A and B: Inferiorly based nasolabial flap

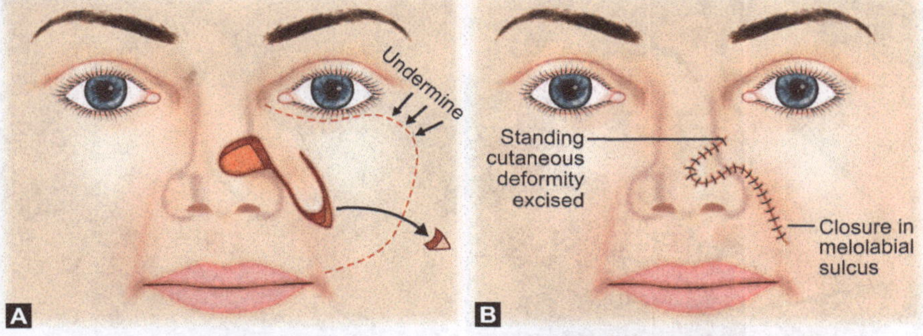

Figs 19.27A and B: Superiorly based nasolabial flap

position because of limited rotation. The plane of dissection should always be developed between subdermal plexus and subcutaneous fat for proper thickness.

The three stages of the Z-plasty technique are given in Figures 19.23A to C.

- **Rhombic flap:** It is very versatile flap, highly reliable, allows precise incisions and wound closures resulting in predictable straight line scars. Major disadvantage is risk of necrosis is more with this flap. It consists of two equilateral triangles placed base to base to form a rhombus (Fig. 19.24).
- **Bilobed flap:** It is a double transpositioned flap that shares a single base. It is used extensively for nasal reconstructions. The primary flap is to repair the surgical defect and the secondary flap is used to repair the flap donor site. The secondary flap defect is then closed primarily. It is used extensively for nasal reconstruction (Fig. 19.25).
- **Nasolabial flap:** It is an axial pattern flap based on angular artery. It can be used for reconstruction of lower two-third of nose, perinasal area, upper lip and minor intraoral defects in the anterior area. The flap could be on inferiorly based, superiorly based or central pedical (Figs 19.26 to 19.28). The flap is reliable but the area of average is limited. The nasolabial flap based on the central pedicle has good length but the width is limited.

Whenever tissue loss is extensive, which cannot be repaired using local flaps, distant flaps can be taken in such cases- such as pectoralis major myocutaneous flap, deltopectoral flap, trapezius flap. Free tissue transfer using microvascular anastomosis have increased the flexibility in the soft tissue and osseous reconstruction, e.g. radial forearm flap, fibular flaps, lateral scapular flap.

Free Grafts

Graft is something that is potentially dead and its survival depends on recipient site

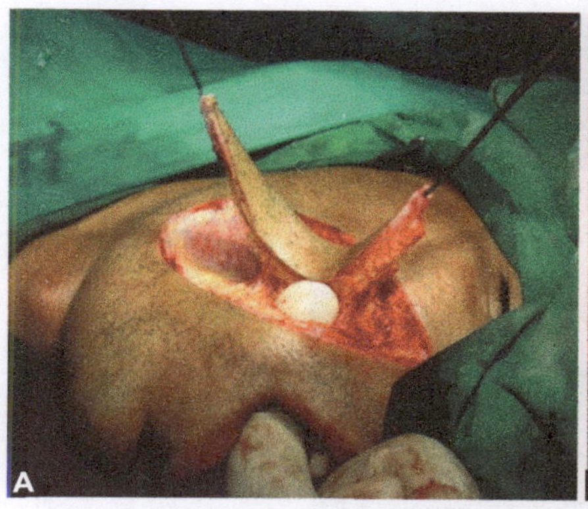
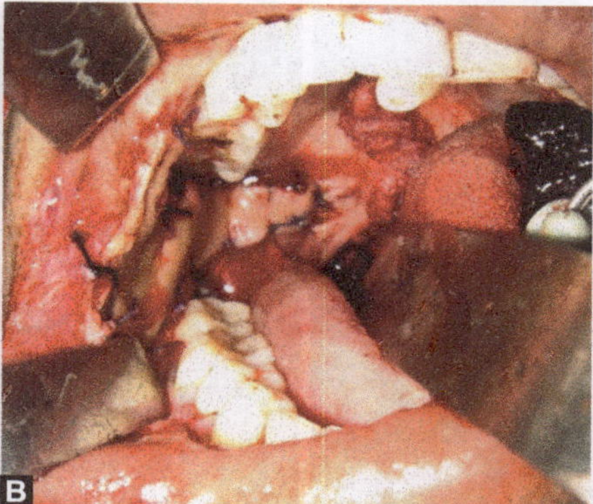

Figs 19.28A and B: Bi-peddled nasolabial flap for intraoral closure

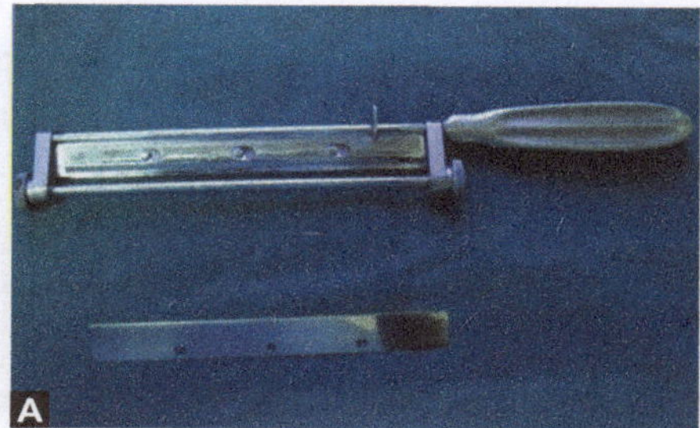
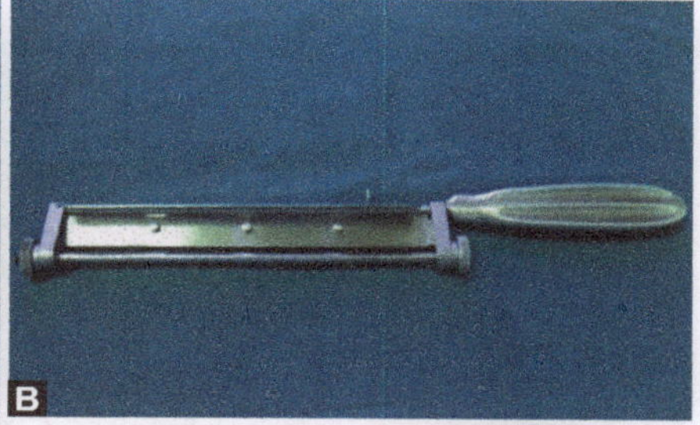

Figs 19.29A and B: Humby knife used for harvesting the skin grafts

whereas flap is attached to a pedicle, which provides an arterial blood supply with venous and lymphatic drainage.

Following are some of the free grafts:

- Split-thickness skin grafts
- Full-thickness skin grafts (Wolf graft)
- Composite full-thickness skin and cartilage grafts
- Pinch grafts (Free skin grafts)
- Dermal and fat grafts
- Fascial grafts
- Chondromucosal grafts.

The first four receive their blood supply from recipient site and last three are avascular.

A free skin graft consists of entire thickness of the epidermis and a variable amount of the dermis. A split skin graft consists of entire epidermis with variable amount of dermis, where as full thickness skin grafts consists of entire epidermis and dermis. When there is full thickness defect of the cheek or lip, mucosa can be closed to the skin. Split skin graft will preserve the original size and shape of the defect, which can be repaired later, till then it will provide sterile cover and minimize fibrosis.

A skin graft adheres to its new bed by fibrin. This diffuses from the plasma bed and supplies the immediate nutritional requirements in the form of plasmatic circulation. This is enhanced by the outgrowth of capillary buds such that a circulation of blood in the graft can be demonstrated at 48 hours. At the same time, fibers grow into the fibrin, which convert the adhesive clot into a more definite fibrous tissue attachment that increases over the ensuing days, so that by 5 days reasonable anchorage has occurred and that is why we keep pressure dressing over skin grafts for at least 5 days after which anchorage has occurred and chances of any hematoma formation beneath the graft would be minimal.

Instrument required for split skin grafts is Humby knife (Figs 19.29A and B).

Salient Features for Harvesting Skin Graft

- Skin graft should have a good vascular bed at the recipient site for better uptake and support.
- Donor site and recipient site should be free of pathogens deleterious for graft.
- Graft should be in closest possible contact with the bed to prevent hematoma, air bubble, which does not allow proper healing.
- Graft should be totally immobile over the bed for which it should be covered with pressure dressing for first 5 days till anchorage of graft has occurred at the recipient site.
- The raw surface of donor site after graft harvesting should be covered with vaseline gauze pieces, then with burn pads and then tightly tied roller bandage. Dressing is kept for 15 days till it gets loose its own.

INJURIES REQUIRE SPECIAL CONSIDERATION

Lip

Injuries of lip require special care because of the peculiar anatomy of the region of the vermilion border. Even a mismatch of 1 mm of vermilion border can be noticeable. After the trauma as the edema sets in and approximation of margins may result in irregular vermilion margin, which may become conspicuous after the edema subsides. The nerve blocks for establishing local anesthesia are preferred rather local infiltration to avoid distortion of the tissue. The wound on the lip should be closed in layers; the re-approximation of orbicularis oris muscle is very important as any disruption will leads to scar formation and compromised function.

Ear

The ear has a very good blood supply and can maintain large portion of tissue on very small pedicles. Injuries on ear

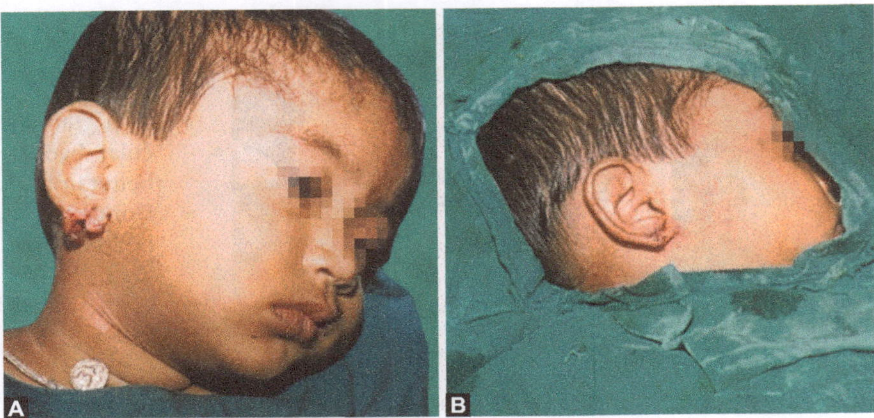

Figs 19.30A and B: Ear lobule repair

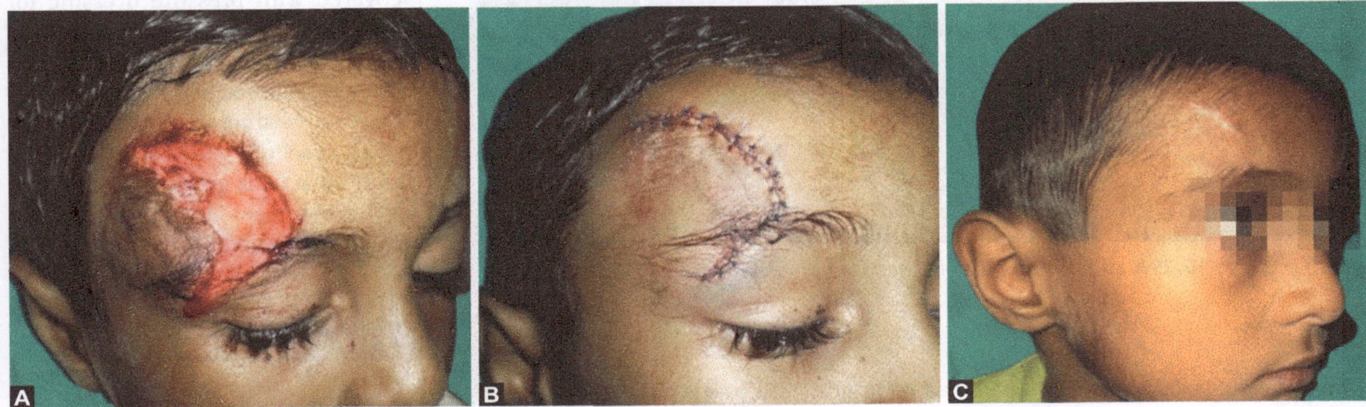

Figs 19.31A to C: Injury of eyebrow closed primarily

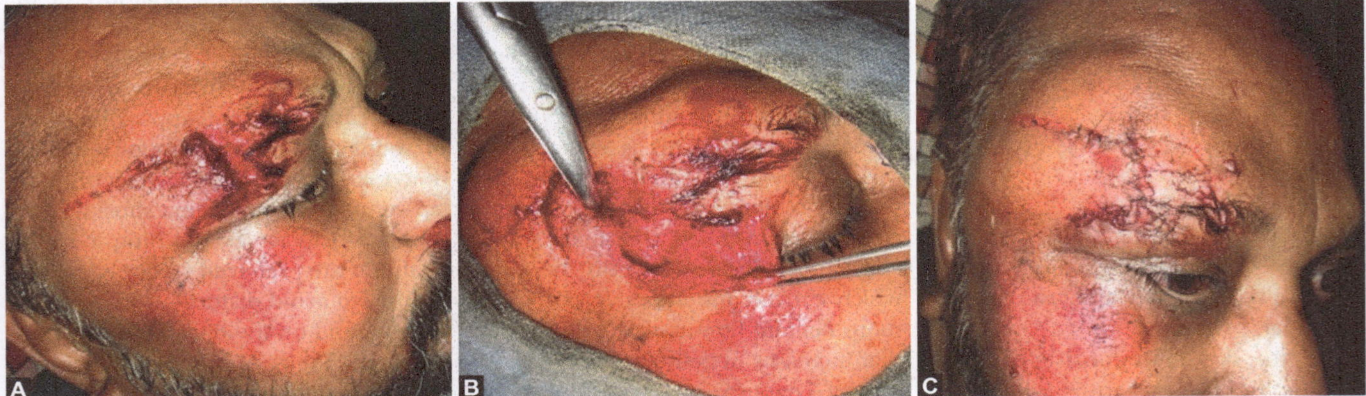

Figs 19.32A to C: Injury of eyebrow and upper eyelid

require conservative debridement and manipulation to maintain as much tissue as possible. The cartilage of the ear does not require suturing as the manipulation and undermining of skin over it can devitalize the cartilage. Minimal sutures should be used to close ear defects and the sutures should be placed through the skin establishing good skin closure (Figs 19.30A and B).

Eyebrow

Reconstruction of eyebrows is extremely difficult as it can lead to esthetic and functional deformity. Eyebrows are never shaved for part preparation and incision given on eyebrows should be oblique and parallel to the hair follicles to avoid injury to hair follicle, which leads to loss of hair and unsighty scar (Figs 19.31 and 19.32). Sutures should not be secured

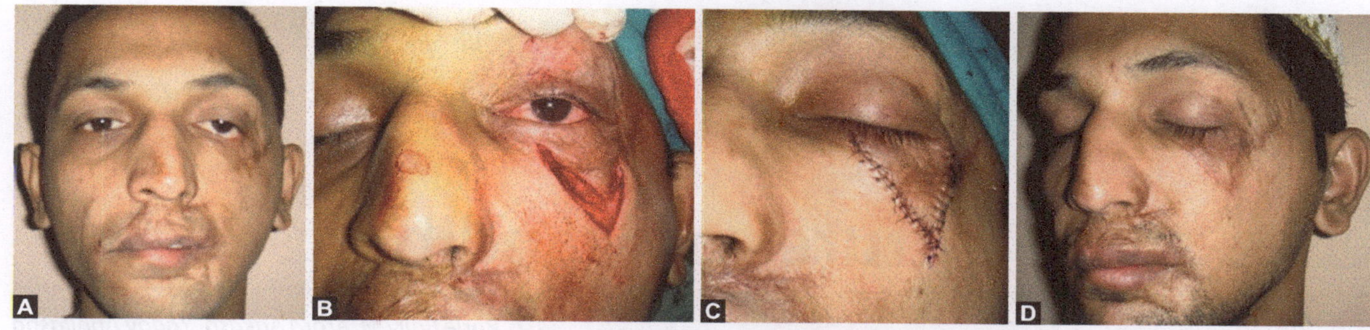

Figs 19.33A to D: Correction of post-trauma ectropion: (A) Preoperative view; (B) V-shaped incision given; (C) V to Y closure done; (D) Postoperative view showing corrected ectropion

tightly as it causes decrease blood supply to hair follicles. Single layer closure is never justified for eyebrows.

Eyelid

Eyelids are composed of very thin skin, alveolar tissue, orbicularis oculi muscle, tarsus, tarsal glands and conjunctiva. Eyelid is thin and contains containing so many structures and during reconstruction these all should be sutured individually. Levator muscle inserts in skin of upper lid and is responsible for elevation of the eyelid. If closure is not done in layers it can lead to formation of scar and ectropion (Figs 19.33A to D). Injuries to the nasolacrimal apparatus must be addressed properly facing to which epiphora may result. Hence, a careful examination and these special considerations should be taken during any management of soft tissue injury on face.

SUGGESTED READING

1. Craniomaxillofacial Trauma by David DJ and Simpson DA.
2. Maxillofacial Surgery Vol. 2, 2nd edition-Peter Ward Booth.
3. Maxillofacial Trauma and Esthetics Facial Reconstruction by Peter Ward Booth.
4. Oral and Maxillofacial Trauma 3rd edition Vol. 2 edited by Raymond J. Fonseca.
5. Peterson's Principles of Oral and Maxillofacial Surgery 2nd edition Vol. 1 edited by Michael Miloro.
6. Rowe and William's Maxillofacial Injuries edited by William's JLI Vol. 1.
7. Stell and Maran's Head and Neck Surgery 4th edition by John C Watkinson.
8. Surgical Clinics of North America.
9. Textbook of Plastic surgery 6th edition Grabb and Smith.
10. Textbook of Plastic Surgery Vol 2-McCarthy.

REFERENCES

1. Ochs M, Tucker M. Current concepts in management of facial trauma. Journal of Oral and Maxillofacial Surgery. 1993; 51(1):42-55.
2. Singer AJ, Hollander JE, Quinn JV. Evaluation and Management of Traumatic Lacerations. N Engl J Med. 1997;337:1142–8.
3. Haug RH. Etiology, Distribution, and Classification of Craniomaxillofacial Deformities: Traumatic Defects. Craniomaxillofacial reconstructive and corrective bone surgery. Springer New York. 2002.
4. Bartlett, et al. Ballistics and Gunshot Wounds: Effects on Musculoskeletal Tissues. J Am Acad Orthop Surg. 2000;8:21-36.
5. Ambroise Pare La Méthod de traicter les playes faites par les arquebuses et aultres bastons à feu 1545.
6. Advisory Committee: Centers for Disease Control: Tetanus—United States, 1987 and 1988. MMWR. 1990; 39:7-41.
7. Lee C, Hansen S. Management of Acute Wounds. Clinics in Plastic Surgery. 2007; 34(4):685-96.
8. Charles H Thorne. Grabb and Smith's Plastic Surgery. Lippincott Williams and Wilkins. 2002.

20 Fractures of Mandible

Borle Rajiv M, Arora Aakash, Yadav Abhilasha

The mandible forms the lower third of the face. It is the most prominent part of the lower third of the face at the symphyseal area and thus, most vulnerable site to be traumatized during the road traffic accidents (RTA). Similarly it is the most tempting site to be hit during the assault and thus, the fractures of the mandible are most common in the symphyseal or the para symphyseal area.

APPLIED SURGICAL ANATOMY OF MANDIBLE

The mandible is the strongest of all the facial bones and it is the only mobile bone of the facial skeleton. It is roughly horseshoe shaped with the symphysis being its most prominent part. It has thick cortical plates. The condyles articulate with the glenoid fossa of the temporal bone, superior to which the middle cranial fossa is located. The condylar neck is thin, slender and weak. This is a natural protection provided by the nature. When there is trauma to the symphyseal area, the forces are transmitted to the condyle and the base of glenoid fossa along the bone, if the condylar necks were strong structures, the forces would have been transmitted to the base of the glenoid fossa, resulting in the fracture and the condyles would have entered in the middle cranial fossa creating a grievous head injury. To prevent such grievous injuries, the nature has made the condylar process thin, slender and weak. Whenever there is trauma to the symphysis, the condyles tend to get pushed upwards and posteriorly and they strike against the glenoid fossa. The condylar neck fractures readily, owing to its weakness and absorbs all the shock and prevents it from being transmitted to the base of the skull.

The ramus of the mandible is thin as compared to the body. Whenever a thick portion of the bone unites with the thin portion, it constitutes a line of weakness. Further, the third molars are located in the angle region and when they are impacted they occupy lot of space in the bone and undermine it. The bone grains, which are oriented vertically in the ramus change their course at the angle of mandible as they enter the body of mandible. This abrupt change in the course of the bone grains also makes the bone weak. All these factors make the mandible vulnerable for fracture at this site.

In the canine area also the mandible is weaker as the canine has a longest and the stoutest root and it occupies lot of space in the bone and undermines and weakens it. Thus, the mandible has a tendency to fracture at this site.

The symphyseal area as stated earlier is most prominent and most vulnerable to trauma. There is compression of the outer cortex and expansion of the inner cortex and the fracture will result when the forces are beyond the capacity of the bone to withstand them.

There is a pair of genial tubercles on the lingual cortical plate in the midline, situated superoinferiorly, which give origin to the genioglossus and geniohyoid muscles, respectively. Whenever there is a bilateral fracture at the parasymphysis area, the tongue tends to loose its anchorage on the bone and the patient looses control and the tongue tends to fall back. It is especially true for the unconscious patient, where the tongue fall blocks the airway and it could be fatal if not prevented. The inferior alveolar neurovascular bundle passes through the bone and in case of fracture it may get traumatized and can lead to hematoma and neurological deficit.

CLASSIFICATION OF FRACTURE MANDIBLE

The fracture is defined as a breach in the continuity of the bone. The general classification of fractures of the bone is as follows:

- **Simple fracture:** Simple fracture is the fracture of the bone, where the fracture line is not exposed to external environments as the overlying soft tissue cover is intact (Figs 20.1A and B).
- **Compound fracture:** Compound fracture is that, where the fracture line is exposed to the external environments (Internal—oral cavity, external—atmosphere) (Figs 20.2A and B).
- **Comminuted fracture:** Comminuted fracture is that fracture, where there are multiple fracture lines and more than two fragments of the bone are present (Fig. 20.3).
- **Simple comminuted fracture:** When the comminuted fracture is not exposed to the external environments.

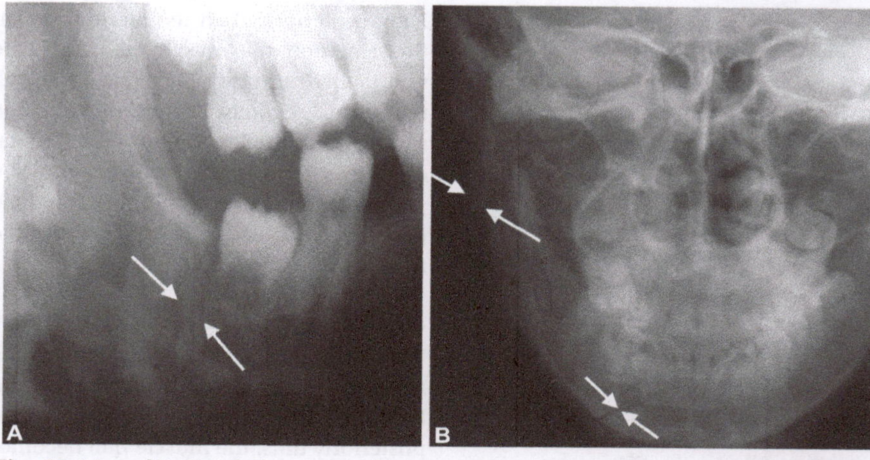

Figs 20.1A and B: Simple fracture, in figure A although the tooth is involved the fracture is simple because the tooth is unerrupted

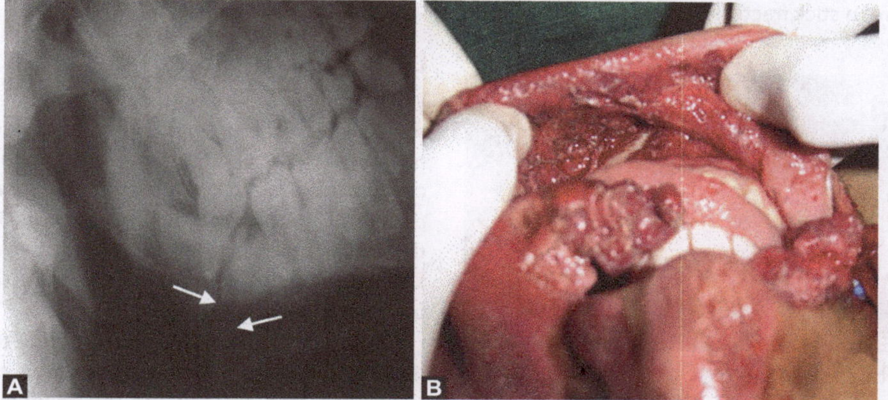

Figs 20.2A and B: (A) Compound fracture due to involvement of the erupted tooth and fracture of the tooth; (B) Degloving laceration is present, compounding the fracture intraorally

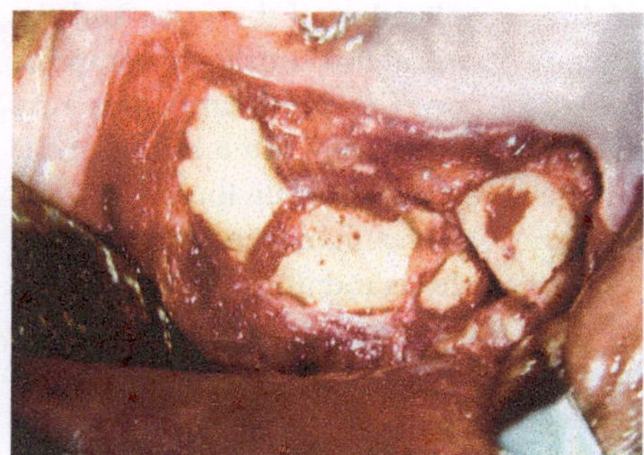

Fig. 20.3: Comminuted fracture

- **Compound comminuted fracture:** When the comminuted fracture is exposed to the external environment.
- ***Green stick fracture:*** Green stick fracture is the incomplete fracture and often presents like a cortical bending rather than breaking. It is commonly seen in the children, where the bones are elastic and resilient. The children are susceptible to fall and thus this is a natural protection against the fracture. This type of fracture is commonly seen in the long bones. In the facial skeleton the condylar neck is the most common site to show this fracture (Figs 20.4A and B).
- **Pathological fracture:** When the bone is undermined by any pathology and has become significantly weak, can fracture readily with physiological function, trifle trauma or normal functional pressure or movement (Figs 20.5A and B).

According to the Site

The fractures can be classified according to the site of fracture and its incidence as follows[1] (Figs 20.6A and B):

- Symphyseal fractures and parasymphyseal fractures (including the canine area fracture) (14%)
- Body fractures (21%)
- Gonial area or angle fractures (20%)
- Condylar fractures (intracapsular) and subcondylar fractures (high and low) (36%)
- Coronoid process fractures (2%)
- Dentoalveolar fractures (3%).

According to Displacement and Ability to Prevent Displacement due to Muscle Pull

The fracture fragments are liable to displacement according to unfavorable muscle pull leading to difficulty in the management of these displaced fractures. The elevators of the mandible are attached to the ramus (masseter, temporalis, lateral pterygoid), while as the depressors of the mandible, i.e. the suprahyoid muscles (digastricus, geniohyoid) are attached to the body and the genial tubercles, respectively. The lateral pterygoid is attached on the pterygoid fovea at the neck of the condyle, which commonly displaces the subcondylar fractures medially and sometimes the fractured condyle gets dislocated in the infratemporal fossa (Fig. 20.7).

Vertically Favorable

When the fracture line is viewed from the superior aspect of the mandible (alveolar border) and is passing from buccal cortical plate to the lingual cortical plate with the buccal end lying mesially and the lingual end of the line lying distally. In such a situation, the distal fragment will be drawn closer to the proximal fragment due to the pull of the medial pterygoid muscle and the fracture segments will come closer rather than getting separated in bucco-lingual plane and thus the fracture is called vertically favorable (BALP).

Vertically Unfavorable

In vertically unfavorable case, the fracture line passes buccolingual with the buccal end lying mesially, when viewed from superior border. The distal fragment

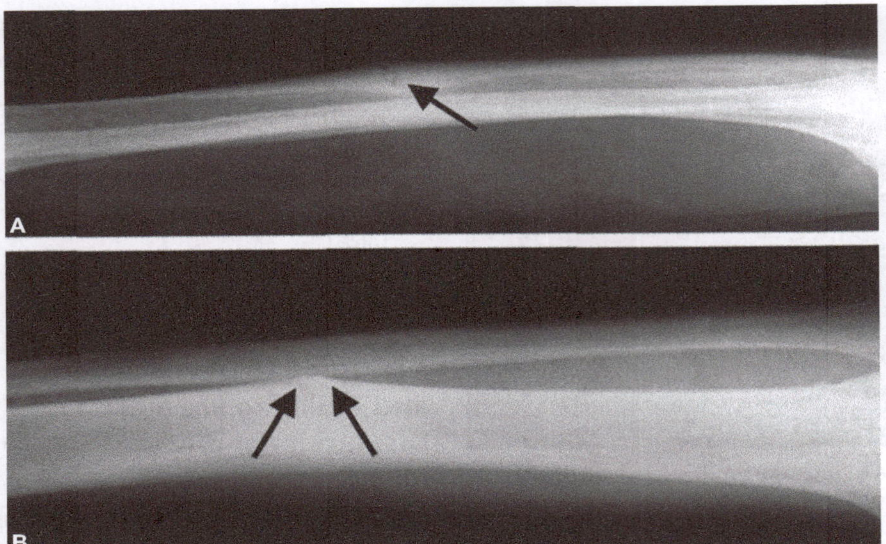

Figs 20.4A and B: Green stick fracture

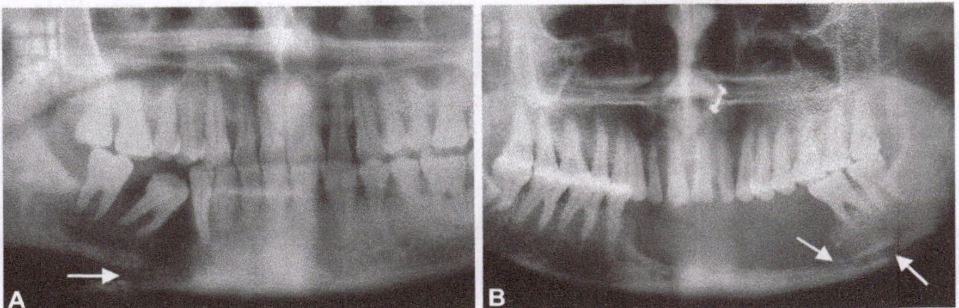

Figs 20.5A and B: Pathological fracture

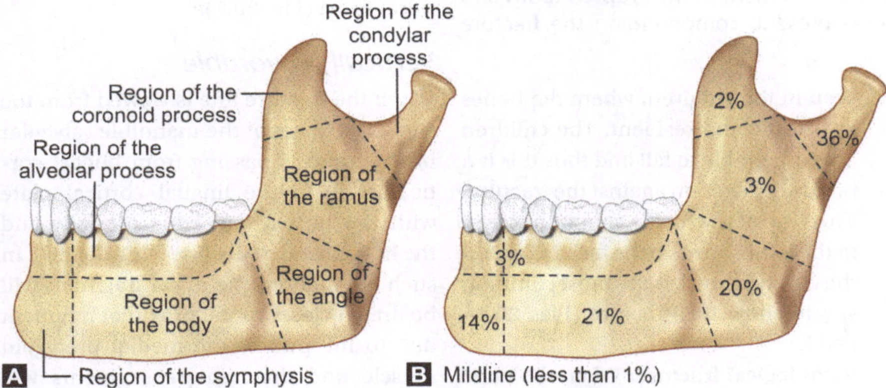

Figs 20.6A and B: Fracture sites and incidence

in this case will be easily viewed from superior border. The distal fragment in this case will easily get drifted lingually due to the pull of the medial pterygoid muscle, thus there will be separation of the fragments in the buccolingual plane due to the unfavorable muscle pull, and the fracture is said to be vertically unfavorable (Figs 20.8A and B).

Horizontally Favorable

When viewed from the buccal side (horizontally), the fracture line runs superoinferiorly with its superior end lying posteriorly than its inferior end. In this situation the muscle pull from the temporalis and masseter muscle will pull the distal segment superiorly and the suprahyoid muscles will put the proximal segment inferiorly, thus drawing both the segments closer to each other. This type of fracture is called horizontally favorable fracture.

Horizontally Unfavorable

When viewed horizontally, the fracture line runs superoinferiorly with its superior and lying anteriorly and the inferior end lying posteriorly thus, the muscle pull becomes unfavorable and drifts the proximal and distal fracture segments apart. This is described as a horizontally unfavorable fracture (Figs 20.9 and 20.10).

Direct and Indirect Fracture

When the force is applied to the bone, the cortex (*buccal cortex*) at the site of application of the force undergoes compression and the other cortex (*lingual cortex*) of the bone undergoes tension. If the force is greater than the compressive and the tensile strength of the bone a fracture ensues.

Similarly, when the force is applied to the mandible, the point of application of the force is compressed and the resultant vector travels along the bone and applies tensile force on the point intersected by this vector. The fracture occurs at the site of direct application of the force and the fracture occurs at this site due to compression of the bone (*direct fracture*). A fracture also occurs at the site intersection of the resultant vector by tensile forces (*indirect fracture*). For example, the force applied to the symphysis menti results in a direct fracture at the symphysis. The vector travels to the condylar necks bilaterally and induce indirect fractures of subcondylar areas bilaterally, as the condylar necks are weak. This is called *'Tripod fracture'* (*as the fracture is at three points*) or *'parade ground fracture'* or *'guardsman's fracture'*. The later terms are used because when the soldier at the parade ground stand upright for a long time and faints, falls on the chin and the fracture occurs at symphysis and condylar necks, bilaterally (Figs 20.11A and B).

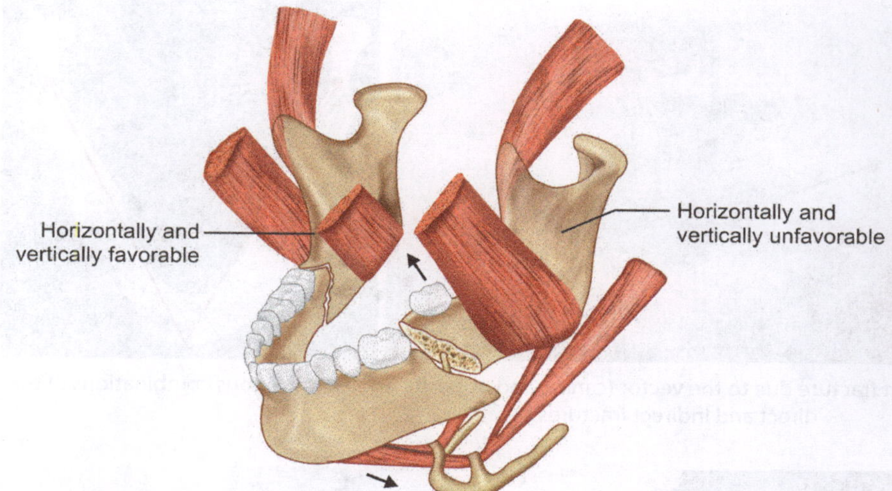

Fig. 20.7: Muscle attachments of the mandible, causing displacement of the fractured segments due to unfavorable pull

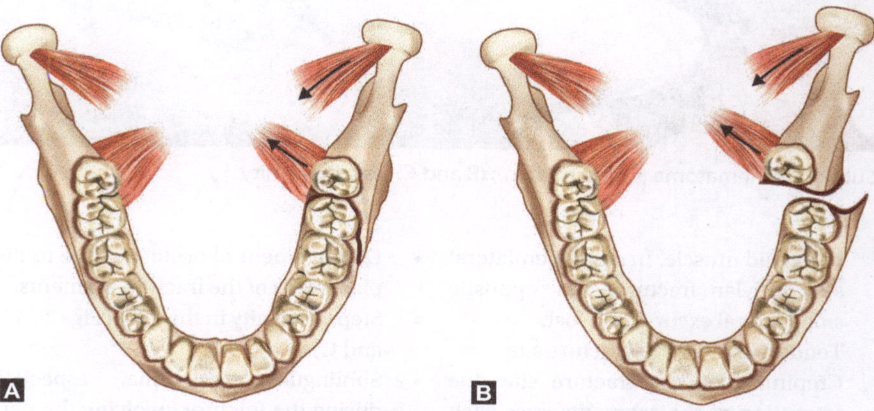

Figs 20.8A and B: Vertically favorable and unfavorable fractures

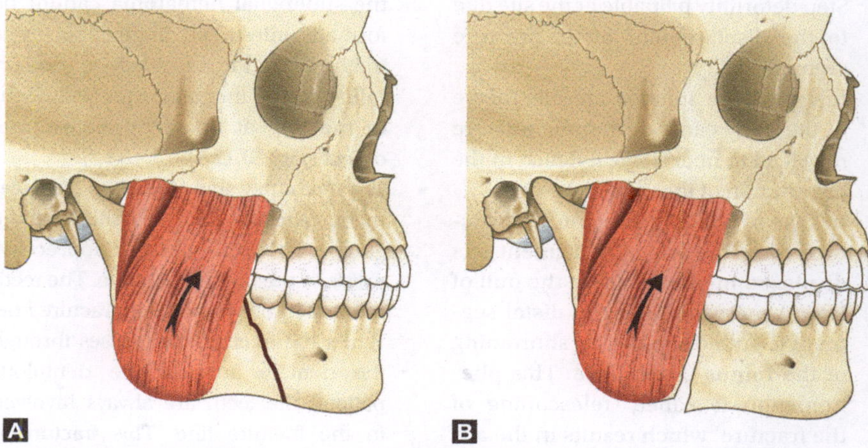

Figs 20.9A and B: Horizontally favorable fracture (A); Unfavorable fracture (B)

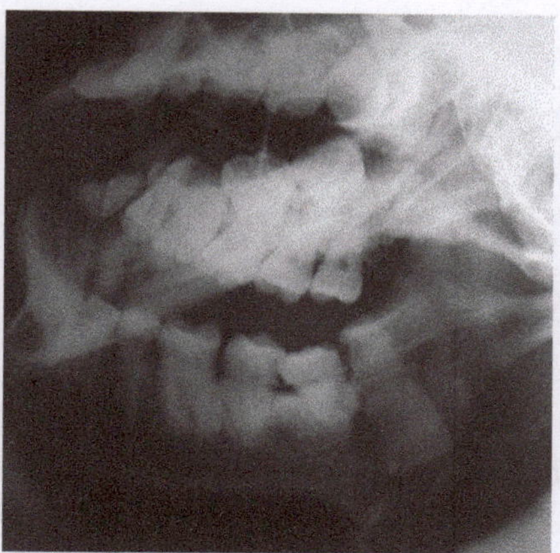

Fig. 20.10: Horizontally unfavorable fracture of the proximal segment has been displaced superiorly

Box 20.1: Combination of direct and indirect fractures

Direct	Indirect
Symphysis	Bilateral subcondylar
Parasymphysis	Contralateral subcondylar fracture
Canine region	Contralateral angle
Body	Contralateral angle or subcondylar

The other common examples of direct and indirect fractures are shown in Box 20.1 and Fig. 20.11C.

It is necessary to know this combination because as a rule of thumb, when ever a direct fracture is seen at the site of primary impact, one must examine the corresponding indirect fracture site and rule out the indirect fracture. If this principle is followed during the examination of the patient, the chances of missing the indirect fracture are minimized. Although, no two traumas are identical, no two fractures are identical. These are the standard combinations, which are commonly encountered in the clinical practice, but occasionally different patterns of injuries can be seen due to varied nature of the trauma (Figs 20.11B).

CLINICAL FEATURES OF THE FRACTURE

The clinical features of the fractures are as follows:

- Pain, inability to masticate and swallow leading to dribbling of saliva.
- Swelling and hematoma.

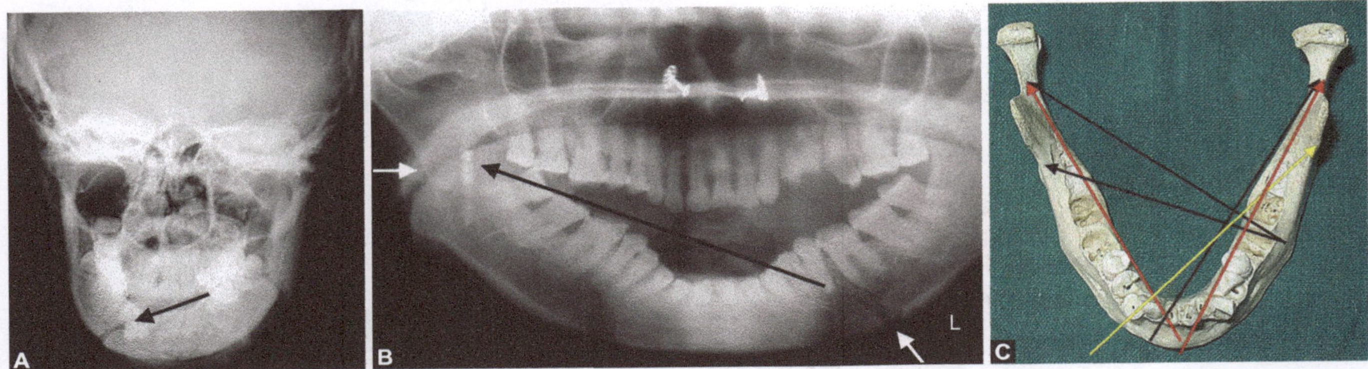

Figs 20.11A to C: (A and B) Direct and indirect fracture due to the vector (canine and opposite angle); (C) Various combinations of the direct and indirect fractures

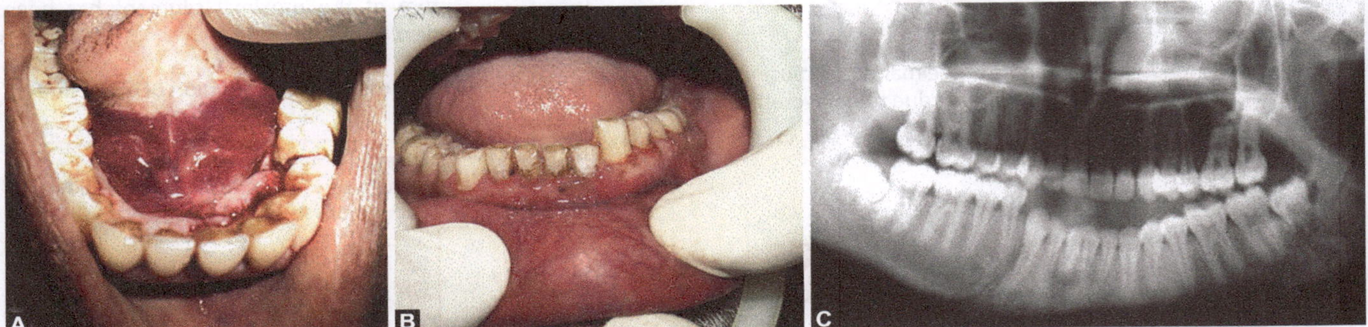

Figs 20.12A to C: (A) Sublingual hematoma (Colman's sign); (B and C) Step deformity

- Facial asymmetry due to edema and hematoma.
- Bleeding per orally from the fracture site.
- The skin may show contusion, abrasion or laceration with discoloration due to injury. In case of symphyseal fracture or subcondylar fracture, laceration is usually present on the chin.
- Trismus and limited excursions of the mandible. The trismus is produced as a result of protective myospasm secondary to pain. The movements increase the pain. When the there is swelling and hematoma, the affected part becomes heavy and the fractured jaw is unable to offer support to the part. Normal movements while speaking, chewing and even the jerks during walking precipitate pain. Thus, the body induces its protective mechanism by inducing myospasm to restrict the movements. The protrusive and lateral excursions are lost when there is a subcondylar fracture, owing to the lack of function of the lateral pterygoid muscle. In case of unilateral subcondylar fracture, the opposite sided lateral excursion is lost.
- Tenderness over the fracture site.
- Crepitus over the fracture site due to grating of the segments over each during the palpation.
- Abnormal mobility across the fracture site.
- Step deformity palpable at the site due to the displacement of the fracture segments.
- Injury to the inferior alveolar nerve in the bony canal during the fracture may lead to neurological deficit in the distribution of the mental nerve.
- In case of bilateral subcondylar fracture, when the proximal segment gets displaced medially due to the pull of lateral pterygoid and the distal segment is pulled superiorly, shortening of the ramus takes place. This phenomenon is called 'telescoping of the fracture' which results in the anterior open bite with gagging of the last molars.
- Derangement of occlusion due to displacement of the fracture segments.
- Step deformity in the arch (Figs 20.12B and C).
- Sublingual hematoma, especially during the fracture involving the denture bearing area. This sign is called '*Colman's sign*'. It should be taken as a pathognomonic sign of fracture, as the sublingual hematoma cannot be formed unless the lingual cortex is fractured and it is unlikely that direct injury to the lingual cortex will occur to the lingual tissue by an external object (Fig. 20.12A).
- The teeth may show luxation, displacement, avulsion with laceration of the gingiva. There may be laceration, ecchymosis in the buccal vestibule. The teeth are sometimes involved in fracture line. When the fracture line passes through the dentate area of the dentulous patient; the teeth are always involved in the fracture line. This fracture is essentially a compound fracture as the intraoral compounding, if the fracture

takes place intraorally, through the periodontal ligament or the pulp of the fractured tooth. The injury to the teeth should be carefully evaluated as such teeth may infect the fracture and delay the healing. All the teeth involved in the fracture line need not be extracted, especially when they are firm, intact, unerupted and do not interfere with the proper reduction or are required to be preserved for esthetic reasons, especially in case of young patients with involvement of the anterior teeth. The teeth, which are grossly luxated, fractured beyond conservation, badly carious or obstruct proper reduction should be extracted (Fig. 20.13).

- When the mandible is held bimanually, keeping index fingers on the occlusal surface on the teeth across the suspected fracture line and the mandible is moved superoinferiorly and anteroposteriorly, abnormal movements are elicited.
- The bilateral parasymphyseal fractures make the genioglossus muscle loose its anchorage onto the bone and the fractured segment tends to collapse lingually, making the tongue to fall back. This is very dangerous in an unconscious patient as it can lead to respiratory embarrassment.
- During the injuries to the chin, which may result in the symphyseal or subcondylar fracture, the mandible gets pushed backwards and superiorly. The cartilage of the external auditory canal gets traumatized between the condyle and the posterior wall of the bony canal and leads to its laceration, resulting into bleeding from the ear. It should be carefully examined and the laceration should be visualized by mopping the blood. The laceration is largely present over the anterior wall. In absence of such laceration, the other causes for bleeding per ear, like fracture of base of the skull, which are more grievous, should be ruled out.

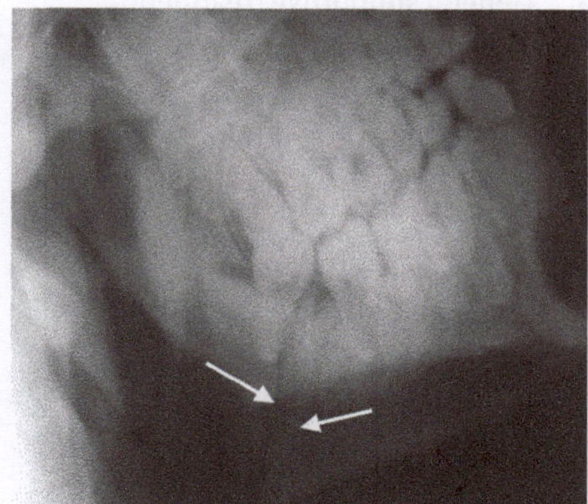

Fig. 20.13: Fracture line passing through the tooth which is also fractured, necessitating its extraction

EXAMINATION OF THE PATIENT

The examination of the patient with suspected fracture of the mandible is done in a methodical ways as follows:

- *General examination* comprising of examination of vital signs, and for ruling out other injuries, visceral injuries, other bone fractures, head injury, spine injury, fractures of ribs, flail chest, etc. to decide priorities in the management as the life-saving measures are undoubtedly the first priority.
- *Local examination* comprises of:
  - **Inspection:** To note swelling, deformity, soft-tissue injuries, limitation of mandibular excursions, derangement of occlusion, step deformity in the arch, Colman's sign, bleeding per orally, bleeding per ear, etc.
  - **Palpation:** The palpation of the mandible starts with the condyles. Even though there is no fracture of the condyle, contusion of the condyle will also produce tenderness over the condyle. The condyle is palpated by placing the fingers over them anterior to the tragus. If there is excessive of edema, the condyles and their movements will be poorly felt in such cases thus, the little fingers are hooked in the external auditory meatus with their pulp placed towards the anterior wall. This will allow the operator to feel the posterosuperior aspect of the condyle. The patient is asked to perform various excursions of the mandible and the condylar movements are felt, which are diminished when the mandible is fractured. They are move severely hampered when the subcondylar fractures are present. If there is a fracture dislocation of the condyle, the glenoid fossa appears empty. Then the palpating finger is passed over the posterior border of the mandible, angle, inferior border up to the midline, bilaterally to note any tenderness, crepitus, step deformity or abnormal mobility (Figs 20.14A to D). Bimanual examination should also be carried out to reach a clinical diagnosis. A clinician must follow certain basic rules as a rule of thumb that:
    - When a fracture or even a laceration is detected in the symphyseal area, bilateral subcondylar area must be thoroughly examined to rule out any indirect fracture.
    - Whenever a parasymphyseal fracture is detected, contralateral subcondylar area must be examined to rule out indirect fracture.
    - Whenever a fracture is detected at the canine area an indirect fracture must be ruled out at the opposite angle of the mandible. The teeth involved in the fracture line must be carefully examined.
  - **Bimanual palpation:** The bimanual palpation is done to elicit abnormal mobility across the fracture line in cases of the fractures involving denture bearing areas, i.e. the symphysis, parasymphysis and the body. The mandible is grasped on either side of the suspected fracture line in such a way that the index finger is on the occlusal surface of the teeth and the thumbs are on the inferior border. The proximal and distal segments are moved in superoinferior and anteroposterior direction, to elicit abnormal mobility (Fig. 20.15). This examination is useful in detecting the fractures which are undisplaced

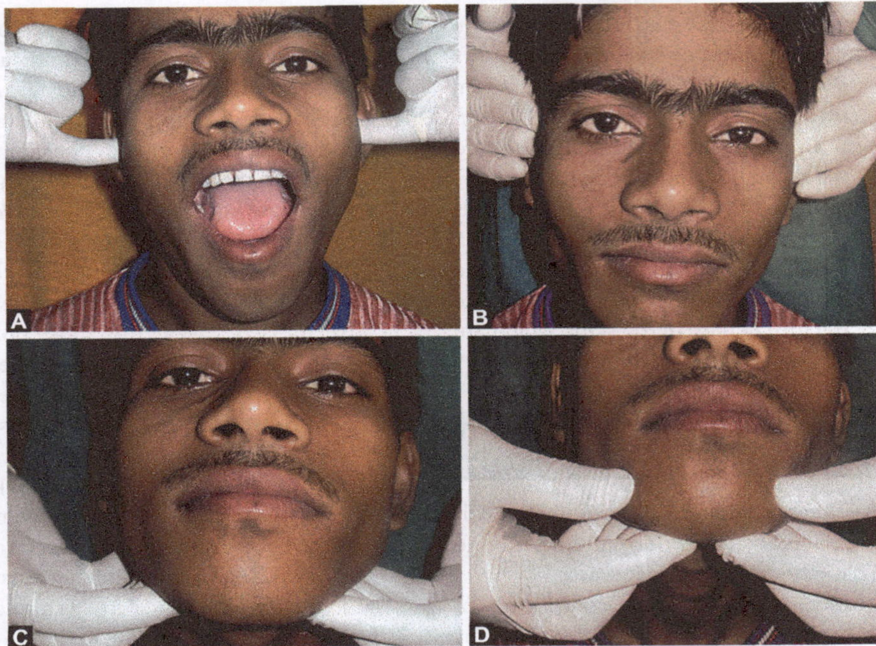

Figs 20.14A to D: Palpatory examination of patient. Start from the condyles and follow through posteriors borders and inferior border

and the fractures of the symphysis/parasymphysis which are not properly visualized on routine radiographs due to superimposition of the shadow of the spine.

- **Compression test:** When there is a hairline, undisplaced fracture of the mandible especially at the symphysis, angle or in the subcondylar areas and it is not conspicuous clinically and radiologically, a compression of the mandible at the symphysis area and over both the sides over the body, using both the palms by the operator, elicits tenderness, which may suggest the fracture (Figs 20.16A and B).

- *Radiographic examination* is the most conclusive evidence of the fracture, however it must be remembered that it is not the substitute for the clinical examination. Even for advising proper radiographic views, the clinical diagnosis of the fracture is essential. The X-rays are the concrete evidence of the fracture and thus, mandatory to be taken and preserved in medicolegal cases. The PA view of mandible and the panoramic X-ray are the screening X-rays of the mandible as they show the complete mandible. The specific views can be advised on the basis of the findings of these screening radiographs to visualize the fracture line properly and to obtain further details. As a rule in orthopedics, the X-ray must be taken in two planes perpendicular to each other, i.e. in the anteroposterior and mediolateral. Thus, apart from the PA view, lateral oblique view is taken for body, angle, ramus and subcondylar fractures. The symphyseal area is poorly seen on PA or panoramic view due to the spinal super imposition (Figs 20.17A to D). In such cases IOPA X-ray or an occlusal film should be taken for better visualization. The condylar head is seen well on transcranial view for intracapsular fractures and the high subcondylar fractures are visualized on the transpharyngeal view. When the fracture line runs obliquely on the bone or due to angulation of the X-rays, two images of buccal and lingual cortical plates fracture are seen giving a false picture of a comminuted fracture. The computed tomography (CT) scans are very helpful and give excellent information (Figs 20.18A to G).

MANAGEMENT OF THE FRACTURE

The management of the fracture of mandible can be discussed under following heads:

- General supportive treatment.

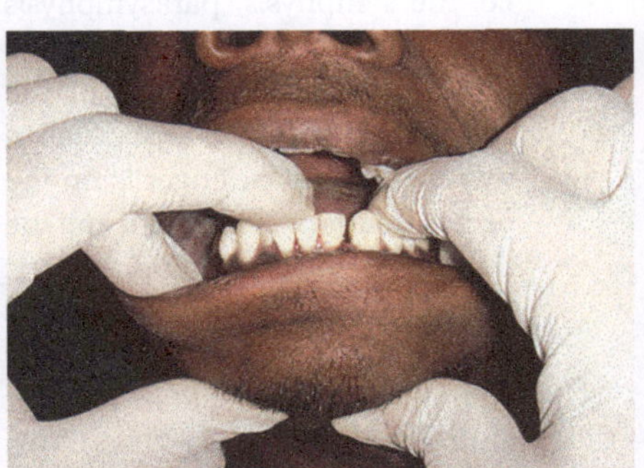

Fig. 20.15: Bimanual palpation of the mandible to elicit abnormal mobility

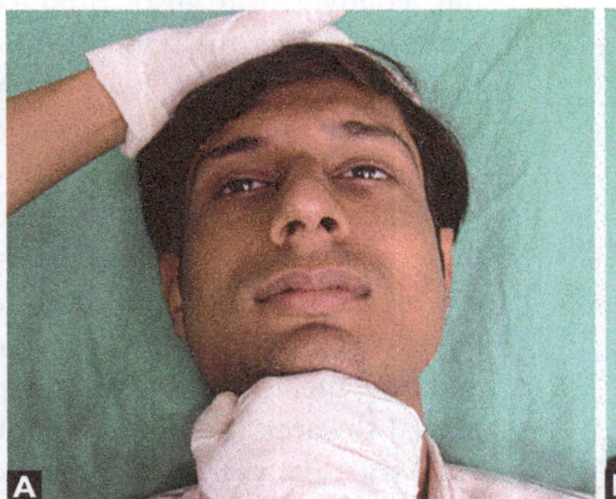

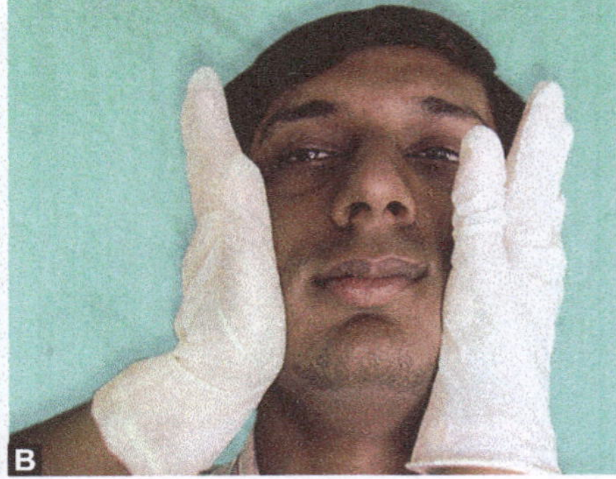

Figs 20.16A and B: Compression test for the undisplaced mandibular fractures at subcondylar, symphyseal (A) and angle region (B)

- First aid management.
- Definitive management.
- Special consideration for management of pediatric, geriatric edentulous fractures and condylar fractures.

GENERAL SUPPORTIVE TREATMENT

The fractures of the mandible do not always occur in isolation, but can be associated with other injuries. The polytrauma patients require priority wise treatment, i.e. the life-saving treatment must be done on priority basis and the management of minor injuries and fractures can be delayed until the patient is stabilized. The priorities in the management are as follows:

- The vital parameters should be critically monitored and airway patency and respiratory support must be given whenever required, to prevent the hypoxia. The circulatory efficiency must be assessed by monitoring pulse, blood pressure (BP) and organ perfusion must be monitored. When there is blood loss, the pulse becomes rapid and thready depending upon the amount of blood loss. When the patient is in hypotension, the peripheral pulse is lost. When the BP is around 60 mm Hg the radial pulse is absent and only carotid pulse is felt. If the BP is around 70 mm Hg, the femoral pulse is palpable and when the BP is around 80 mm Hg, the radial pulse is palpable. The hypotension results in inadequate organ perfusion due to selective peripheral vasoconstriction and fall in mean arterial pressure. The measurement of the urinary output is reliable marker for assessing the organ perfusion. It should be more than 0.5 mL/kg of body weight

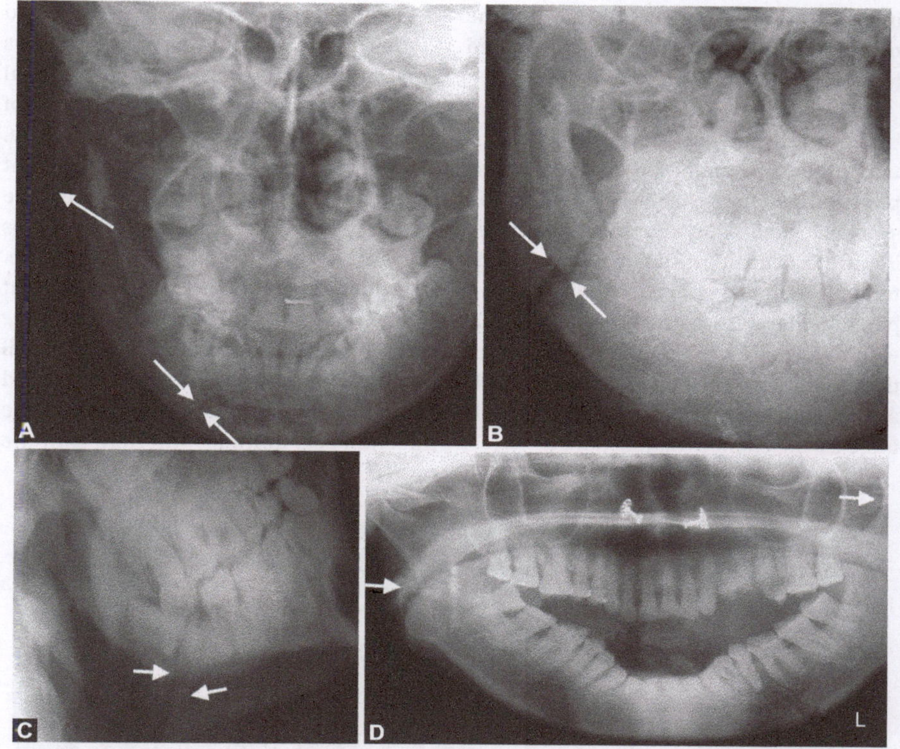

Figs 20.17A to D: PA view, lateral oblique view and panoramic view of the mandible showing fracture

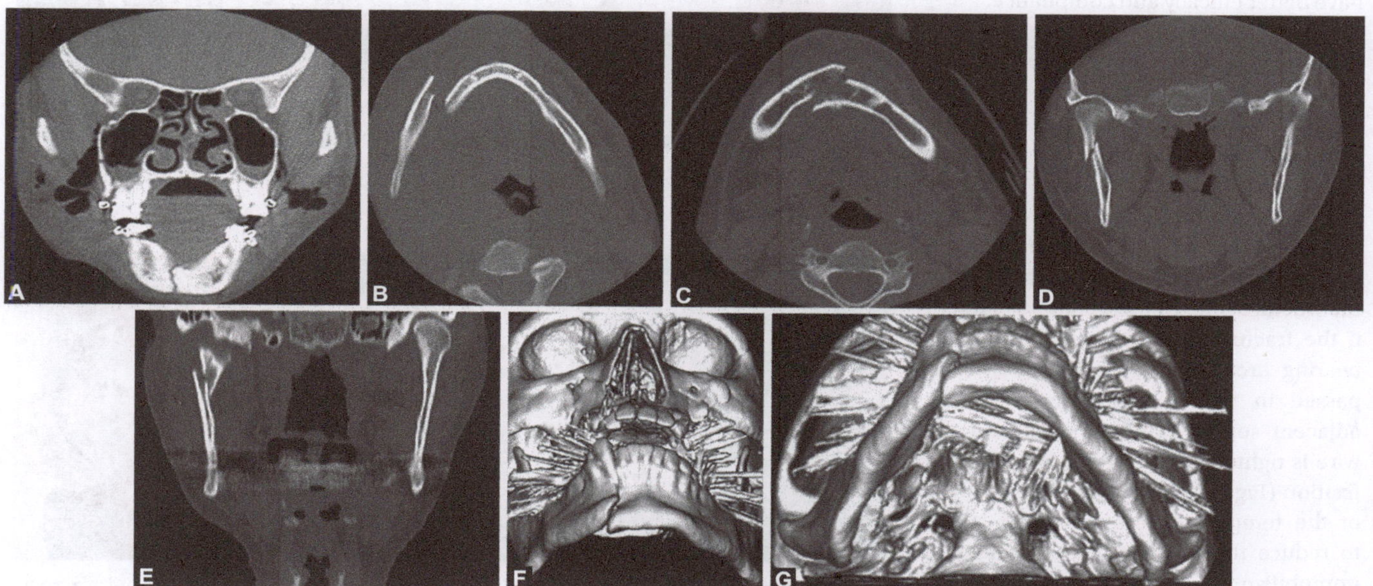

Figs 20.18A to G: CT scans on axial (B, C) and coronal (A, D, E) sections along with 3D reconstruction (F, G) showing fracture of mandible

per minute in adults, 1 mL/kg of body weight/hour in children and 1.5 mL/kg/hour in infants (around 20 mL/hour). If it is less, then replacement of blood volume by parenteral administration of crystalloid solution should be done.

The further bleeding should be arrested by sutures, ligatures, pressure packs or surgical exploration, before blood transfusion is started. Due consideration should be given to the head injury and periodical neurological examination should be carried out to assess the level of consciousness, posture, neurological deterioration and alteration in vital signs. The Glasgow coma scale[2] is assessed periodically to assess the head injury. In the suspected cases, CT scan should be taken and relevant treatment should be started immediately. The neck splinting should be done in case of spinal injuries as the movements may aggravate the injury.

The patient is given prophylaxis against tetanus by administering tetanus toxoid. In severe trauma, where the wounds are badly soiled or there is crushed or devitalized tissue, antitetanus serum (ATS) was administered in the past. If the horse's serum is used, then 1,500 to 3,000 IU of ATS is given IM after the test dose of 200 IU intradermally. The human diploid cell vaccines are available, which have better efficacy and compliance.

The long bone fracture is temporarily immobilized by giving plaster of Paris (POP) casts. The mandibular fractures are also temporarily splinted using the extraoral barrel bandage or the 'four tailed bandage using a crape bandage' (Figs 20.19A and B). Alternatively, intermaxillary fixation may be done by inserting at least one Ivy loop on either side of the fracture line. In the dentulous patient if the fracture is present in the denture bearing area, then a horizontal wire is passed in the embrasure between the adjacent sound, standing teeth and the wire is tightened, this is called horizontal fixation (Figs 20.20A and B). The purpose of the temporary immobilization is not to reduce the fracture but to splint and immobilize the part to provide rest to the part, prevent movement to prevent further bleeding, hematoma, pain and inflammatory edema. The fractured part lacks support and becomes heavy due to edema and hematoma. The movement aggravates pain, inflammation, bleeding and in case of compound fractures, the infection gets pumped in due to the movement, all these things are prevented by temporary splinting.

The patient is given nutritional support by administering parenteral fluids, if he is unconscious or unable to take orally. The patients often have trismus and difficulty in swallowing who they should be prescribed liquid diet or are fed through the nasogastric tube if there is no contraindication for passing the nasogastric tube. The local wound hygiene is maintained. The definitive treatment is under taken as early as possible because the delay will only increase the chances of infection.

Management of Soft-tissue Injuries

The fractures of the mandible are associated with soft-tissue injuries such as abrasions, lacerations of skin, intraoral degloving lacerations (Figs 20.21 and 20.22). The fracture line sometimes gets compounded to intraoral or extraoral environments increasing the chances of contamination/infection of the fracture. An adequate and timely management of the soft-tissue injuries around the fracture line is very important as it helps preventing the infection of the fracture. It is famous quote in orthopedics that '*The bone is like a plant, which has the roots in the soft-tissue*'. The endosteal blood supply of the bone gets disrupted when it is fractured and if the soft-tissue infection sets in it may interfere with the

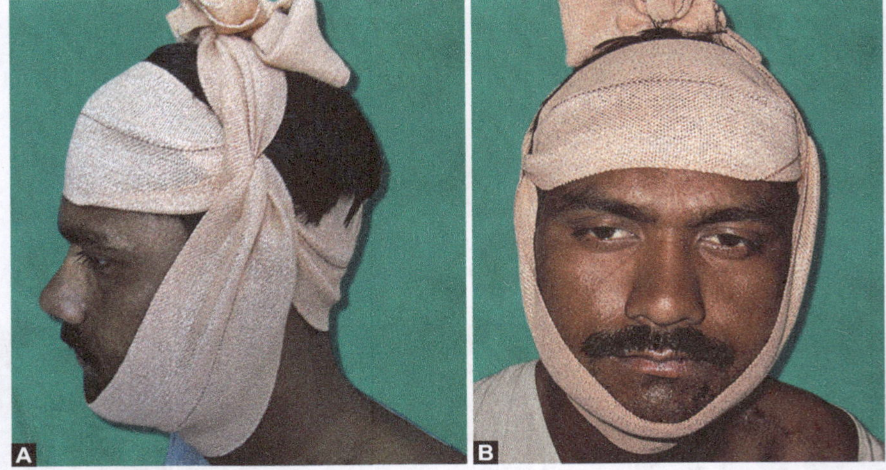

Figs 20.19A and B: Support to the fractured lower jaw using the four tailed bandage

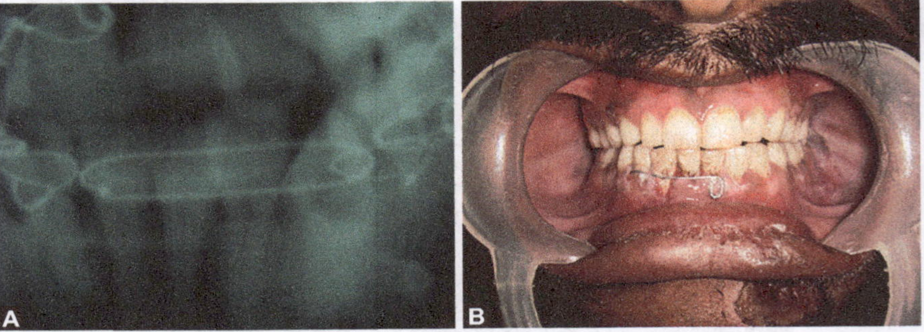

Figs 20.20A and B: Temporary fixation of the fracture with horizontal stay wire across the fracture line

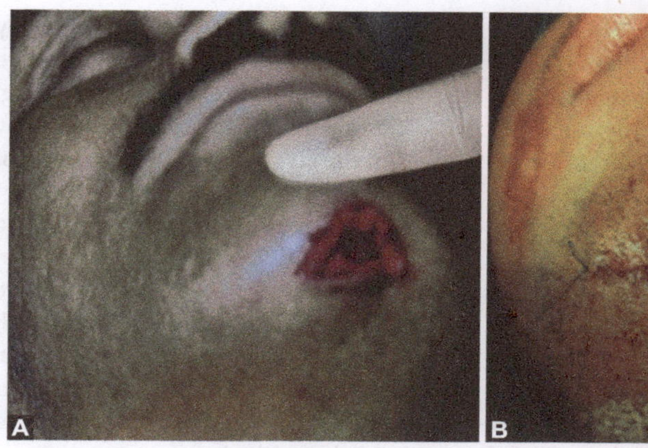
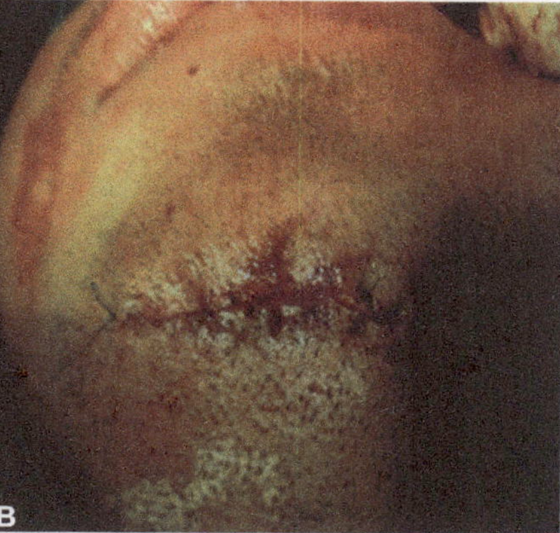

Figs 20.21A and B: Laceration on the chin

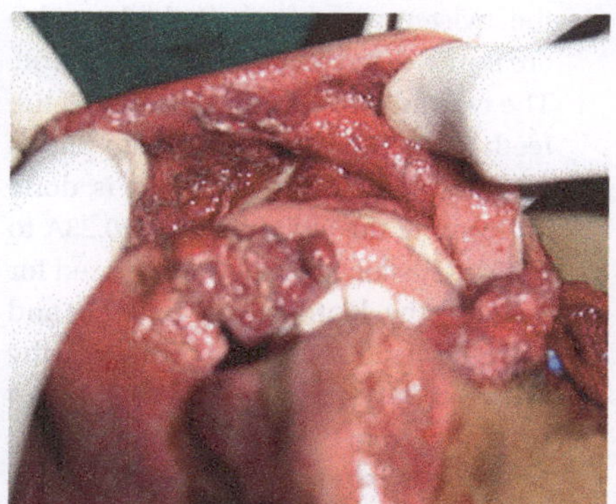

Fig. 20.22: Degloving injury

periosteal blood supply as well, leading to devitalization. And hence, proper management of the soft-tissue injuries is warranted.

The other importance of the lacerated wounds pertaining to fractures of the mandible is that a laceration on the chin is usually associated with fracture at the symphysis and/or the indirect fracture at the subcondylar area (*see* Figs 20.21A and B). Even if there is no symphyseal fracture, the subcondylar fracture could be seen in some patients. Whenever there is an injury to chin, an indirect injury to the temporomandibular joint (TMJ) may be present due to pushing back of condyles against the glenoid fossa and if fracture is not present other injuries such as the contusion, effusion or hemarthrosis may be present, which warrants careful evaluation and management to prevent further complications like ankylosis.

DEFINITIVE TREATMENT

The definitive treatment comprises of following steps:

- Reduction—closed reduction and open reduction
- Immobilization
- Fixation (usually applied to the open reduction when the fracture fragments are fixed with implant).

The reduction is done to bring the fractured segments together in approximation close to their previous anatomical position so that the healing is proper and rapid. This can be done with:

- Manual reduction
- By elastic traction
- During open reduction with bone holding forceps or the bone levers.

The indications for closed reduction are summarized in Box 20.2:

Box 20.2: Indications for closed reduction

1. Undisplaced fractures.
2. Where skill and facilities for open reduction are not available.
3. Medically compromised patients where conservative line of treatment is required.
4. Poor financial status where patient does not afford the cost of treatment.
5. Grossly infected fractures where the implants are likely to be infected.
6. Pediatric fractures with mixed dentition phase.
7. Geriatric fracture with edentulous jaws.

Advantages of the Closed Reduction (Box 20.3)

Box 20.3: Advantages of closed reduction

1. Non-invasive, simple, easy to master.
2. Does not require exposure to general anesthesia.
3. Economical.
4. Less chances of infection.

Disadvantages of Closed Reduction

- The reduction is not 100% perfect, as only superior segment alignment is done by achieving good occlusal relationship. The inferior border may not be adequately reduced.
- The immobilization may not be adequate which delays the healing. It is especially true in case of fractures involving the angle and subcondylar area where the control over the proximal segment is not established and can get displaced with unfavorable muscle pull.
- The healing of bone is by secondary intention, i.e. callous formation. The hyperplastic callous may not be esthetically or functionally acceptable.
- The treatment induces lot of morbidity to the patient as the intermaxillary fixation is kept for long period affecting feeding, speech of the patient.
- The closed reduction is especially problematic when the fracture of mandible is associated with the condylar injuries. For the management of fractures at other sites than the condylar areas, the immobilization is required for a longer period of time. If the associated condylar injury is present, a long-term immobilization increases the risk of fibrous adhesions and ankylosis. If the inadequate immobilization is done, the healing of the other fracture is compromised. The rigid internal fixation has over come this draw back to a large extent.
- Closed reduction is not safe in epileptic patients as during the epileptic seizures the wired teeth can be avulsed or the patient may aspirate during the post convulsive phase.

Modalities of Immobilization

Once the fracture segments are reduced in acceptable position, the segments are held and immobilized in the same position by means of wiring or splints. The reduction is done either by manipulation or the elastic traction. The best example of the use of elastic traction is the subcondylar fracture with telescoping of the fracture segments. In this case, the patient will have anterior open bite and gagging of the last molars. The fracture is not reducible due to muscle spasm. This unfavorable muscle pull can be countered by gradual elastic traction by placing heavy intermaxillary elastics, anteriorly. In closed reduction, the guidance to the proper reduction is achievement of good occlusal relationship, thus, only superior segment alignment is given important. The upper and the lower jaws are immobilized by fixing them together in occlusal relationship (intermaxillary fixation or maxillo-mandibular fixation) using wires or splints. The wires, which are passed between the teeth of the same jaw through the embrasure spaces are called interdental wires which are the means for doing the intermaxillary wiring.

The various modalities used for intermaxillary fixation are:

i. Wiring

- Figure-of-eight wiring
- Essig's wiring
- Continuous wiring
- Risdon's wiring
- Ivy loop wiring
- Continuous Ivy loop wiring
- Gilmour's wiring

ii. Arch bars

iii. Splints

- Cap splints in pediatric patients
- Gunning splints in edentulous patients
- External fixators.

Dental Wiring

Usually the high quality stainless steel wires are used for this purpose. They have good elasticity and do not break readily. The number 26 and number 24 wires are commonly used. The wires are sterilized by autoclaving. The wires are stretched to 10 percent of its original length before use this is called hardening or temporization of the wire, which makes the wire stiff.

- **Figure-of-eight wiring:** This is the simple wiring technique often used to temporarily splint the luxated teeth. It is not used for doing the intermaxillary fixation. It has got inherent draw back that it does not offer good three-dimensional stability.
- **Essig's wiring:** This wiring technique is also used in the management of dentoalveolar fractures and for splinting the luxated teeth. This is a better technique as compared to the figure-of-eight wiring as it gives better stability. In this technique, a piece of 24 gauge stainless steel wire is taken and passed through the distal embrasure between the adjacent healthy teeth to the site of dentoalveolar fracture, i.e. if the incisors are traumatized then the stay wire is passed through the embrasure between the healthy canine and the first premolar tooth. The wire is passed from buccal side and is drawn from the lingual side. The lingual end is passed through the embrasure between the distal embrasures of the sound adjacent tooth present on the other side of the traumatized segment from the lingual to the buccal side and then both the ends are tightened by twisting over each other using a wire twister or heavy straight artery forceps. The wires are always tightened by twisting in a clockwise direction and loosened by twisting in anticlockwise direction. The wire ends are not tightened fully. This wire is called a stay wire. Then pieces of (about 4″ long) number 26 tie wire are taken, which are passed through the embrasure, between the traumatized teeth from the labial to the lingual side, first superior to the labial and lingual stay wire and then drawn lingual to labial side through the same embrasure, but inferior to the stay wires, thus the stay wires are encircled by the tie wire. The tie wire ends are now tightened by twisting fully. The twisting adapts the labial and lingual stay wires to the contour of the traumatized teeth. This procedure is repeated in all the adjacent embrasures in the traumatized segment, thus the stay wire gets nicely adapted to all the teeth. Finally, the incompletely tightened ends of the stay wire are tightened fully, to complete the wiring. The cut ends of the wires are bent away from the soft tissue so that they do not irritate the soft tissue.
- **Risdon's wiring:** In this technique, a long piece of 24 gauge stay wire is taken and passed through the embrasure between the last two standing teeth in the arch from buccal to the lingual side. The lingual end is now taken circumferentially around the last tooth in the arch and both the ends are firmly twisted over each other. The same exercise is done on the other side also the twister wires from both the sides are now twisted together in the midline. The twisted stay wire is ligated to all the teeth in the arch using separate pieces of number 26 tie wires like it is done for legating the arch bar (Figs 20.23A to C). The Risdon's wiring can be used for splinting the dentoalveolar fractures and for intermaxillary fixation by passing the intermaxillary wires inferior to the stay wires placed in both the arches.
- **Ivy loop wiring:** It is the most commonly used by practiced wiring technique. The Ivy loops are prepared from number 24 to 26 SS wire, depending upon the size of the interdental embrasure. To prepare the Ivy loop a 4″ piece of the temporized wire is taken and the loops are prepared as shown in Figures 20.24A to C. The free ends of the loop should be of equal length.

Adaptation of the Ivy Loop

The Ivy loop is adapted to teeth in the arch as follows:

- Both the ends of the Ivy loop are passed buccolingually through the gingival embrasure and drawn lingually. One end is taken circumferentially around the distal tooth and drawn to the buccal side through the distal embrasure. The other end is taken circumferentially around the mesial tooth and drawn buccally through the mesial embrasure. The distal end is now passed through the loop and both the ends are tied by twisting on the mesial/anterior side. The wires are

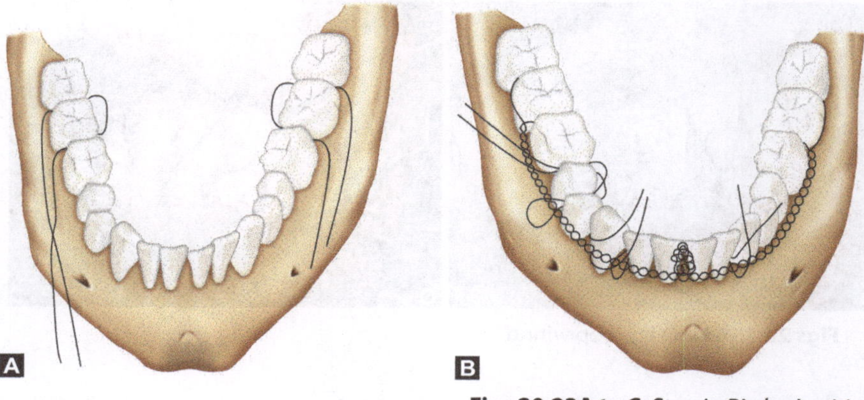
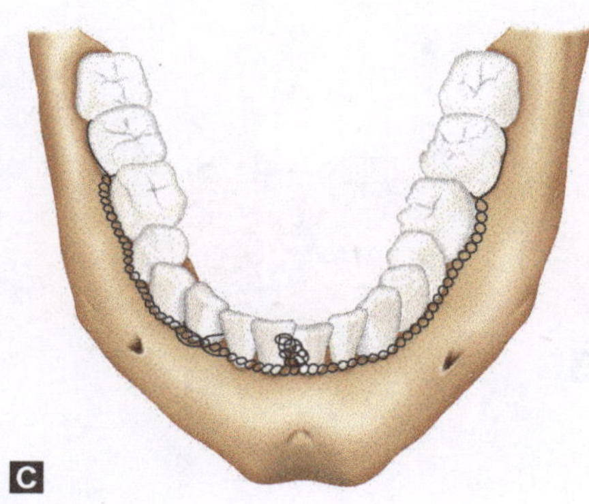

Figs 20.23A to C: Step in Risdon's wiring

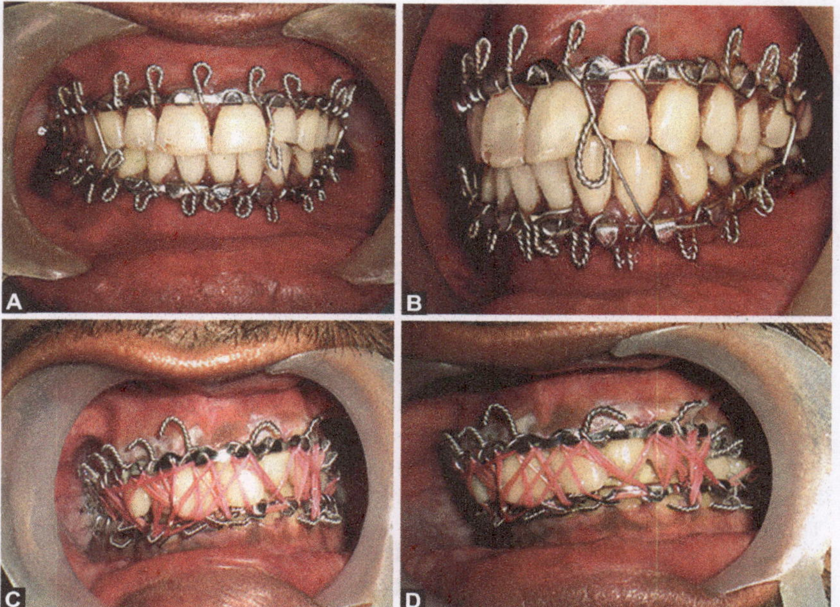

Figs 20.24A to D: Ligation of the Erich's arch bars along with IMF with wires and elastics, note the brackets are facing gingivally

never tied distally as it is difficult to do so. The loop should be tight enough to prevent its slipping or loosening. The twisted ends are cut and bent away from the gingiva to prevent irritation. The Ivy loops are evenly distributed along the arch to give adequate anchorage. If the fracture is present in the denture bearing area then the distribution of the Ivy loops should be adequate on either side of the fracture line. The Ivy loops are placed in both the arches. The intermaxillary wires are passed through the loops in the upper and lower jaws and are tightened to achieve the intermaxillary fixation (Figs 20.25A to C).

Limitation of Ivy Loop Wiring

- It cannot be done in partially edentulous patients.
- It cannot be done if the teeth are periodontally compromised.
- It is not possible to adapt the loop if the adjacent tooth is absent.
- It cannot be done in mixed dentition phase or when the teeth are partially erupted.
- It does not have proper stability when the teeth have wide diastema or when the teeth have unfavorable conical shape.
- **Continuous Ivy loop wiring:** The Ivy loops are similar to that of the interrupted Ivy loop wiring only difference being that they are prepared in the oral cavity, while doing the wiring. Like in case of the continuous wiring one long 26 number wire is taken and passed through the last interdental embrasure in the arch, from buccal to lingual side. The buccal sided wire stays as a stay wire. The lingual wire is drawn through the adjacent embrasure above the buccal stay wire and passed again to the lingual side through the same embrasure below the stay wire, keeping the mirror top handle or a probe in between. The handle is now rotated to twist the wire and an Ivy loop is prepared. The mirror top/probe is removed. The same exercise is repeated in all the adjacent embrasures to prepare multiple Ivy loops. The disadvantage of this technique is that if the wire breaks at one point the whole wiring becomes loose.
- **Gilmour's wiring:**[3] It is also called single tooth wiring. It is very useful when the adjacent tooth is missing and the Ivy loop wiring is not possible. In this technique, a piece of 26 stainless steel wire is taken and passed around a tooth circumferentially mesiodistally and the two ends are twisted till it gets tightly adapted to the tooth near its cervical line, below the height of contour. The wires are ligated to all the teeth in both the arches and then the maxillary wires are tied with the

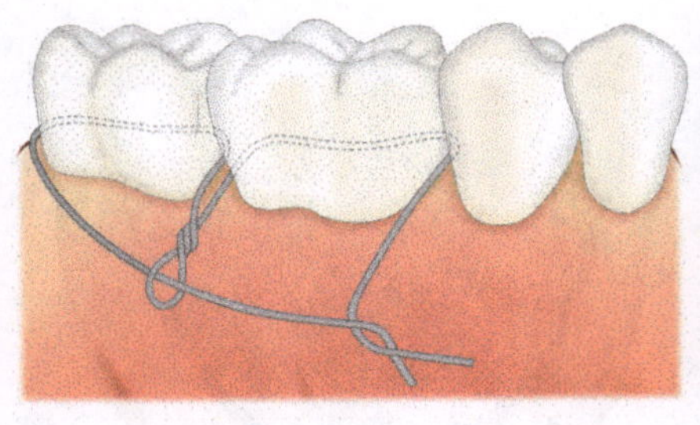
A

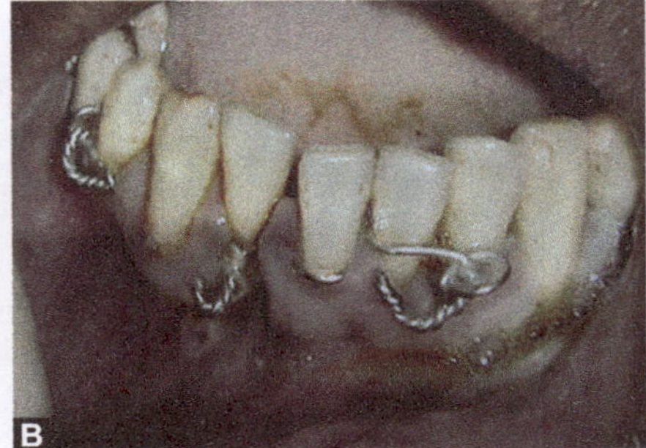
B

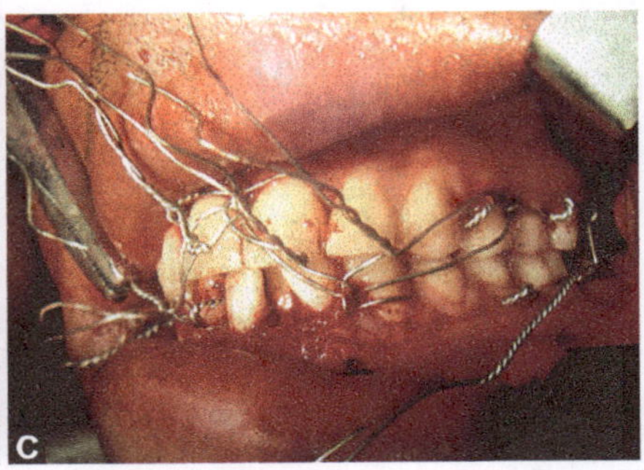
C

Figs 20.25A to C: Ivy loop wiring

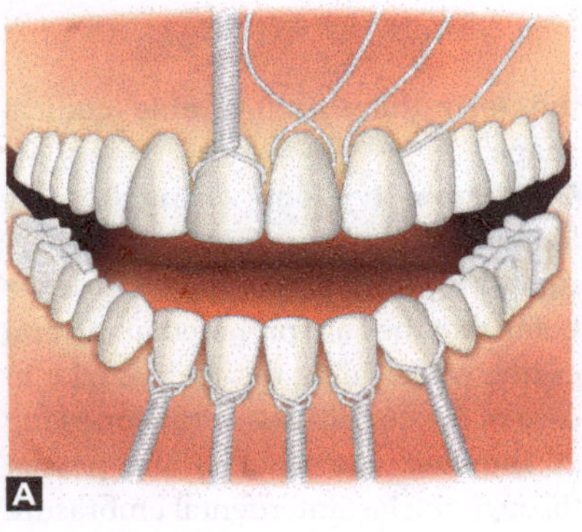
A

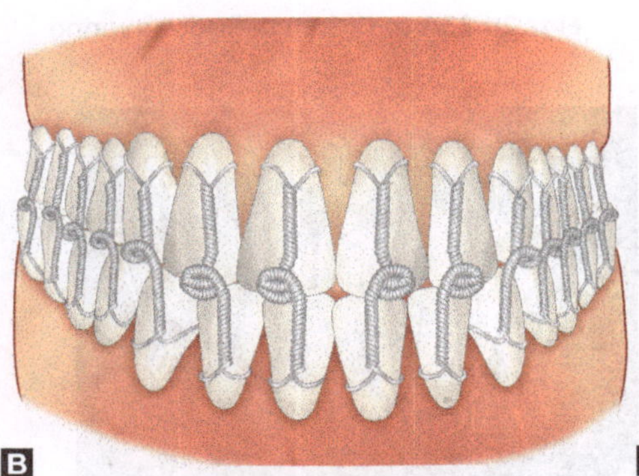
B

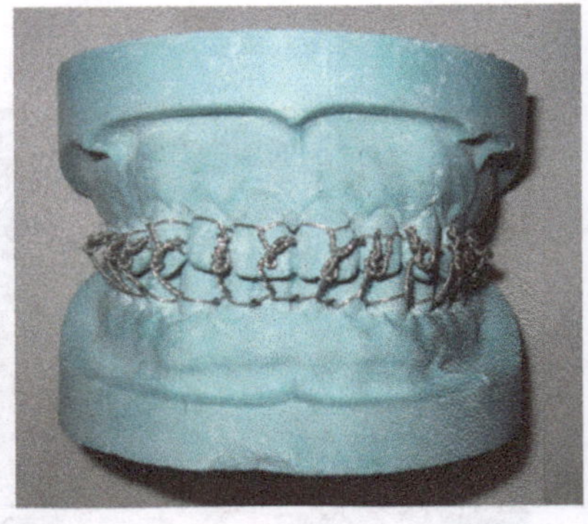
C

Figs 20.26A to C: Gilmour's wiring

mandibular wires to achieve the intermaxillary fixation (Figs 20.26A to C).

Arch Bars

The arch bars are more effective means for the intermaxillary fixation. The wires tend to get loose over a period of time, while the arch bars provide more stable fixation. The arch bars are of two basic types:

- **Rigid arch bars:** They are not commonly used. These arch bars are adapted to the patients cast in the laboratory and then transferred to the patient's mouth for ligation to the dental arch.
- **Soft of flexible arch bars:** They are commonly used. They can be adapted and contoured to the patient's dental arch directly due to their flexibility, e.g. Erich's arch bar (*see* Figs 20.24A to D).

Advantages of the Arch Bar

- They can be used in a patient who is partially edentulous or has uneven distribution of the teeth in upper and lower arches, where wiring is difficult to be done.
- They can be used in presence of teeth having diastema or unfavorable forms. The wires tend to slip when the diastema are present and the contacts between the teeth are absent.
- They can be used when the teeth are periodontally compromised and loose. The arch bar splints the teeth and provides stable anchorage.
- The arch bar has brackets and these brackets are very useful for applying intermaxillary elastics.
- The arch bar while providing assistance in achieving the intermaxillary fixation simultaneously helps in reducing and splinting the associated dentoalveolar injury.

While ligating the arch bar it must be ensured that the brackets of the arch bar face gingivally to facilitate the application of the intermaxillary wires or elastics (*see* Figs 20.24A to D). Similarly, the arch bar should never be ligated across the fracture line, i.e. if the fracture of mandible is in the symphysis area, rather than ligating a single arch bar to entire mandibular arch, two separate arch bars should be ligated on right and the left side leaving the gap at the fracture site. If a single arch bar is ligated, it will splint the fractured segments and hamper proper reduction.

Intermaxillary Fixation Using Screws

The wiring and the arch bar fixation is time consuming and painful procedure for the patient inspite of local anesthesia. Ligation of the arch bar or interdental wiring in the operating room, while the patient is under general anesthesia prolongs the duration of surgery and anesthesia. Moreover, these techniques are uncomfortable for the patient due to excess of hardware in the oral cavity and it is often difficult to maintain proper oral hygiene. The intermaxillary screws are another option for achieving the intermaxillary fixation (IMF). These screws are directly fixed into the alveolar bone through the stab incision in the region of the labial vestibule avoiding injury to the apices of the teeth (Fig. 20.27). If the IMF is planned for long-term then screws are not a suitable option as the fixation is

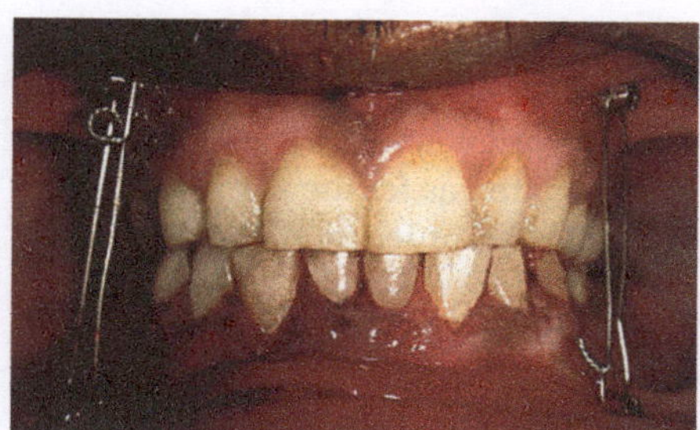

Fig. 20.27: Intermaxillary screws used for IMF

not adequate. The intermaxillary screws should only be used in cases, where only short-term immobilization is required, e.g. while doing open reduction or during the orthognathic surgical procedure.

All the wiring techniques can be done under local anesthesia. The indications for general anesthesia (GA) are uncooperative patients, limited access due to trismus or multiple injuries, severe pain or when the unfavorable muscle spasm or pain prevents adequate reduction of the fracture. Administration of the GA brings about the muscle relaxation and facilitates proper reduction. When the patient is operated under GA and IMF is done, there is always a risk of aspiration of vomitus in the respiratory passage, if the patient vomits during the postoperative recovery period. Hence, the patient should be kept in the head low position with head turned to one side. A wire cutter should be kept readily available bed side to cut open the intermaxillary wires in the event of vomiting to prevent the aspiration.

The intermaxillary wiring is maintained for a period of 6 to 8 weeks as this is a period required for healing of the fracture. In the younger patients, it is kept for shorter time as the healing occurs fast due to excellent healing potential. In the geriatric patients it is kept longer as the healing potential is reduced. Similarly when the jaws are sclerosed, irradiated, having osteodystrophies-like osteogenesis imperfecta, are present the immobilization may be required for longer period.

In case of condylar fractures, the immobilization is done only during acute phase of injury when pain is severe and the part requires rest for resolution of acute symptoms. Hence, the IMF is kept for a short period of 10 to 15 days and an early mobilization of the jaw is ensured to prevent fibrous adhesions and subsequently, ankylosis. The preferred way of IMF is application of the intermaxillary elastics. Even if the proximal segment of the fracture in subcondylar fracture is medially displaced and the fracture is high subcondylar, conservative line of treatment in form of short-term immobilization followed by physiotherapy is advocated. The fracture segments are not reduced and the healing occurs as '*pseudoarthrosis*' (false joint).

Splints

The splints are effective modalities of treating the fracture of mandible in edentulous patients and the pediatric patients with deciduous dentition or mixed dentition.

Cap Splints

The pediatric jaw fractures are treated with specially fabricated cap splints. The deciduous teeth have unfavorable size shape and which does not facilitate the wiring. The teeth are sometimes mobile due to the root resorption or during the mixed dentition some teeth are partially erupted and are not favorable for wiring. In such circumstances, the splint becomes the obvious choice. The open reduction with rigid internal fixation is also not possible as the jaw is occupied with developing teeth buds, which can get traumatized due to the placement of screws or wires. The splint is fabricated by making an impression of the fractured jaw and preparation of the cast. The cast of the upper jaw is also made. The cast of the lower arch is split across the fracture line, where the step is present. The split halves of the lower cast are articulated with the upper cast in pre-existing occlusal relationship, thus the fracture gets reduced *in vitro*. Now the base is poured so that the cast is obtained in the reduced position. The acrylic cap splint is fabricated on this cast, which is finished and sterilized by chemical sterilization. The patient is operated under general anesthesia, the splint is adapted to the lower jaw thus, the fracture gets automatically reduced as the splint is fabricated in reduced position and guides the fractured segments in same position as established in the laboratory. The

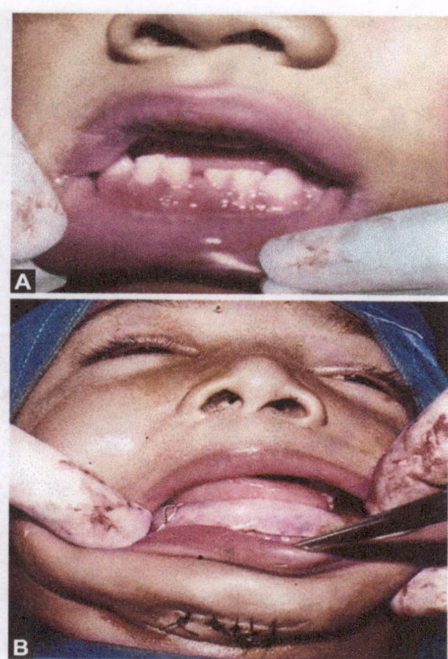

Figs 20.28A and B: Cap splint along with circum-mandibular wiring used to reduce pediatric mandibular fracture

splint is secured to the mandible with the help of circum-mandibular wiring, using a bone awl or long hypodermic needle (Figs 20.28A and B).

Procedure for Circum-mandibular Wiring

Under all aseptic precautions, a stab incision is placed below the inferior border of the mandible up to the bone. The incision should be taken at the site avoiding the facial vessels at the anterior border of the masseter and avoiding the mental nerve in the deciduous molar area. The bone awl (Kelsy Fry) is introduced through the incision along the bone and drawn in the buccal vestibule. A 26 gauge stainless steel wire is passed through the eye of the awl and then the awl is withdrawn and without withdrawing completely from the skin incision passed along the inferior border to the lingual side along the lingual cortical plate and drawn in the lingual vestibule. The wire is detached from the awl and the awl is withdrawn (Figs 20.29A to D). The same procedure is carried out on the opposite side also. The splint is placed in place and the buccal and lingual ends of the wire

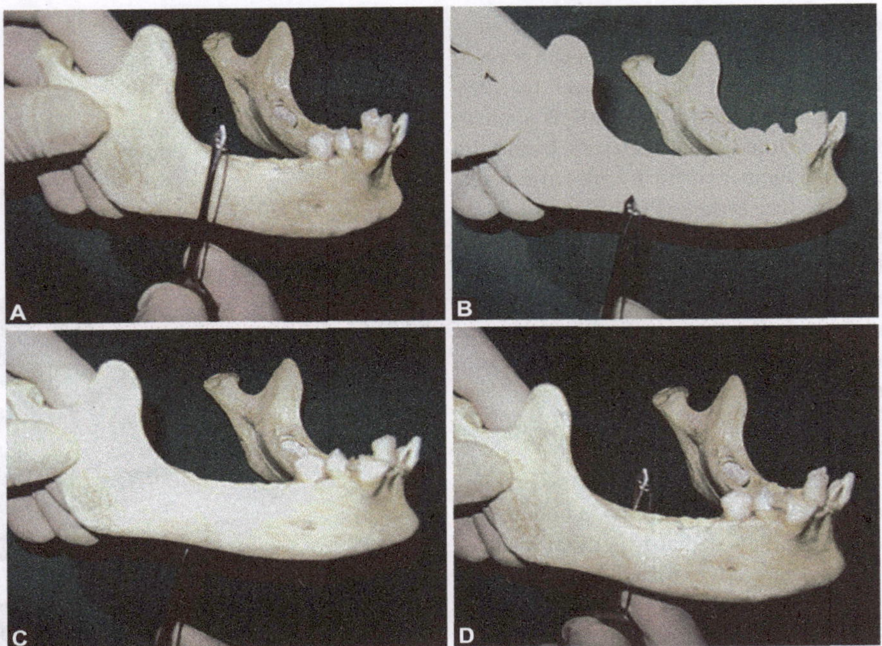

Figs 20.29A to D: Steps in the circum-mandibular wiring

and tightened over it, securing the splint to the mandible (*see* Figs 20.28A and B). The extraoral incision is closed with loose single suture. The splint is kept for 3 to 4 weeks and proper hygiene is maintained around it to prevent infection.

If the bone awl is not available then long (2") hypodermic needle is used for this procedure. Instead of bone awl the needle is passed through the submandibular incision and drawn in the buccal vestibule. A piece of 26 gauge stainless steel wire is taken and passed through the lumen of the needle. The wire is drawn in the buccal vestibule and the needle is withdrawn completely over the wire, leaving the wire in place. The needle is now passed in the lingual vestibule and passed along the bone, to draw it through the submandibular stab incision. The wire end projecting extraorally is passed through the lumen of the needle and is passed in the oral cavity and drawn in the lingual vestibule and the needle is now withdrawn over the wire. The wire is thus passed circumferentially to the mandible. Rest of the procedure is same. It must be remembered that the wire must be along the bone and no soft tissue should be trapped between the wire and the bone as such tissue can under go ischemic necrosis and cause discomfort to the patient and the necrotic tissue can serve as a nidus of infection.

The wires are removed under aseptic care. The oral cavity is disinfected with antiseptic solution. Like in suture removal, the wire is gently pulled up after loosening, so that the portion of the wire, which was buried in the tissue is drawn up and the wire is cut at this point. The wire is pulled out catching the portion, which is projecting in the oral cavity. Thus, the portion of the wire, which was projecting the oral cavity never passes through the tissue. The portion of the wire, which projects in the oral cavity is contaminated and if allowed to pass through the tissue will carry the infection along with it in the deeper tissue planes.

Gunning Splint[4]

It is used for treating the edentulous jaw fractures. If the patient is complete denture wearer, the same denture can be used as the splint, as it was fabricated when the jaw was intact. If the patient is not denture wearer, an impression of the upper and lower fractured jaws are made. The lower cast is split at the fracture site along the step in the ridge. The step is abolished by approximating the two halves in reduced position arbitrarily. The shellac bases are prepared as in case of complete denture, wax rims are also prepared as for the jaw relation (JR). The JR is recorded and the upper and lower rims are sealed. The rims are made discontinuous by removing block of wax intermittently keeping only three blocks of wax, i.e. two in the posterior areas and one anteriorly. The gaps in the rim are useful for feeding the patient. Wire loops or segment of arch bar are incorporated in the splints in each block of wax. The splint is acrylized, finished and sterilized by chemical sterilization. The lower splint is secured to the mandible with circum-mandibular wiring and the upper one is fixed to the maxilla by per alveolar wiring. The IMF is done with the help of wires passing through the loops of wire incorporated in the upper and lower splints during the fabrication (Fig. 20.30).

External Fixators

The fractures can also be treated by introducing the Steinman's pins in the bone percutaneously, on the either side of fracture line. The projecting pins are attached to each other with the help of universal rod and joints, while the fractured fragments are reduced in proper approximation. The disadvantage of the external fixator is that pins and the device project out through the skin for a long period causing lot of morbidity and discomfort to the patient. They produce unesthetic scars on the face. The chances of infection in the fracture line are more as the pins are projecting out through the skin.

Open Reduction

When the fracture line is exposed surgically and the fracture is reduced

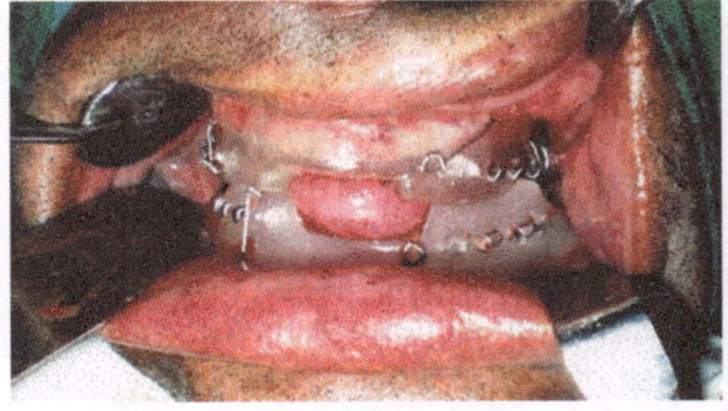

Fig. 20.30: A gunning splint used to achieve IMF in an edentulous jaw fracture

under direct visual supervision, it is called as open reduction. The indications for the open reduction are (Box 20.4):

The modalities for open reduction are as follows:

- Intraosseous wiring—non-rigid fixation.
- Krishener's wire—non-rigid fixation
- Compression bone staples—rigid fixation
- Lag screws—rigid fixation
- Champhy's miniplates—semirigid fixation.

Intraosseous wiring: It was the most common technique of open reduction practiced in the past, before the advent of the bone plates. In this method, the fracture line is exposed surgically and the fracture segments were reduced with the help of bone holding forceps and the bone levers. The intervening granulation tissue, clot, fibrous tissue, loose bone fragments were removed and curetted.

The mandible is first immobilized with intermaxillary fixation in occlusal relationship because that is the primary aim of the surgery. Once the occlusion is established, i.e. the superior border is aligned, then the inferior border is reduced by proper approximation. Holes are then drilled on either side of the fracture line with the help of dental engine and bur preventing damage to inferior alveolar nerve and the roots of the teeth. A 24 number stainless steel wire is passed through the holes across the fracture line and the wire ends are tightened together, holding the fragments in a reduced position. The wire is cut and the ends turned towards the bone to prevent soft-tissue irritation (Fig. 20.31).

Box 20.4: Indications for open reduction

1. Grossly displaced fractures with gross displacement or over riding (telescoping) of the fractured segments.
2. Unfavorable fractures at the angle.
3. Old fractures which do not get reduced due to the fibrous adhesions.
4. Malunited fractures at the condylar neck where the proximal segment gets displaced medially.
5. Fractures in epileptic patients where intermaxillary fixation is contra-indicated.
6. Where the morbidity to the patient due to the intermaxillary fixation is to be avoided.

Krishner's wire: The Krishner's wire (*K wire*) was popularly used in the past not only for stabilization of the fractures, but also for the reconstruction of the mandible after segmental resection of the mandible. It is introduced in the medullary portion of the bone on either side of the fracture line. It is used for fixing the subcondylar fractures. The main disadvantage of the K wire is loosening of the wire and its dehiscence as the wire comes out by perforating the skin. The K wire offers non-rigid fixation (Fig. 20.32). They are no longer used for treating fractures in maxillofacial surgery due to advent of better modalities.

Rigid internal fixation (RIF): The Swiss organization *Arbeitsgemeinschaft für Osteosynthesefragen* (AO) or Swiss Association for the Study of Internal Fixation (AISF) noticed that when the fracture fragments are approximated and compressed together rigidly, with the help of an implant, the healing of the bone is faster and without formation of the callus. The healing occurs by direct proliferation of the osteoblastic cells across the fracture line and they called it as *primary bone healing.* When the fragments are not compressed together rigidly, callus formation takes place, which gets ossified and the bone is formed. They designated it as *secondary bone healing.* Hence, in the former event there is osteosynthesis by way of almost

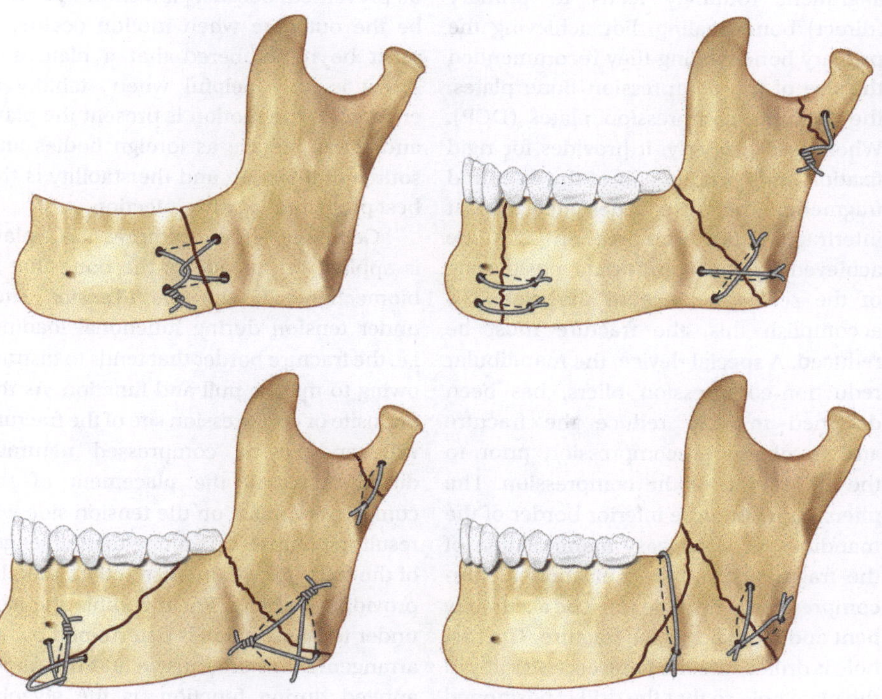

Fig. 20.31: Various techniques for intraosseous wiring

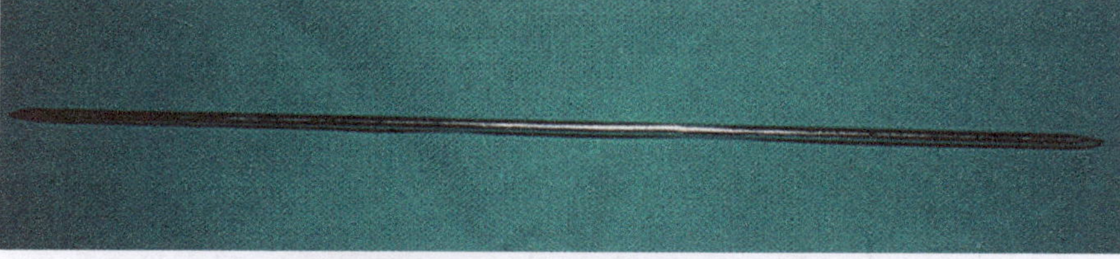

Fig. 20.32: Krishner's wire (K wire)

a regenerative procedure and thus, the quality of healing is better than the latter. In order for this to occur, the stability of the fixed fracture fragments must be enough to neutralize all bending, torsional and shearing forces to which the mandible is subjected to particularly during function. Interfragmental compression increases the friction between fragments and also increases the surface area of the fragments that are actually in contact. This study was first done on the long bones and then applied to the flat bones like the mandible. When the concept of interfragmentary compression was first developed, there was great concern that the pressure against the ends of the fragments would lead to bony necrosis, however, it does not occur. In fact the compression fixation in good alignment routinely leads to primary (direct) bone healing. For achieving the primary bone healing they recommended the use of the compression bone plates, the dynamic compression plates (DCP). When used properly, it provides for rigid fixation and compression of the fractured fragments. The plate is designed so that interfragmentary compression can be achieved by the appropriate positioning of the screws relative to the plate. To accomplish this, the fracture must be reduced. A special device, the mandibular reduction-compression pliers, has been designed to help reduce the fracture and to obtain precompression prior to the application of the compression. The pliers screw into the inferior border of the mandible, allowing easy manipulation of the fragments and their fixation in pre-compression. The plate must be accurately bent and seated over the fracture. The first hole is drilled into the bone eccentrically in the plate hole so that the drill is positioned away from the fracture in the edge of the plate hole. After measuring the depth and tapping the hole, the screw is inserted only until the head of the screw reaches the plate. The first hole in the opposing fragment is then drilled, again positioning the drill in the plate hole so that it is away from the fracture. After measuring and tapping the hole the screw is now placed and tightened alternately with the first screw. As the head of the screw encounters the plate, there will be relative motion between the screw head and the plate until the screws are fully tightened and the screw heads sit flushed within the plate holes. This relative motion will force the screws and therefore the bone fragments, to move towards the fracture site. The fragments are similarly forced to move towards the fracture site, thereby resulting in interfragmentary compression. Additional screws are usually placed neutrally after the interfragmentary compression (Fig. 20.33A). Rest of all additional screws are usually placed neutrally. A minimum of two screws are placed on each side of the fracture line, mandatorily to prevent rotational movement. Any movement between the fragments or gliding between the metal implant and bone surface must be prevented, because, infection will often be the outcome when motion occurs. It must be remembered that a plate and screw is only helpful when stability is ensured. If the motion is present the plate and screw behave as foreign bodies and source of infection and the stability is the best protection against infection.

Generally, the compression plate is applied to the side of the bone that is biomechanically the site (Tension site) under tension during functional loading, i.e. the fracture border that tends to distract owing to muscle pull and function. As the opposite or compression site of the fracture will tend to be compressed naturally during function, the placement of the compression plate on the tension side will result in compression along the full length of the fracture without distraction, thereby providing stability. For mandible the side under tension, which is determined by the arrangement of the muscle and the forces applied during function, is the alveolar side, while the compression side is the inferior border (Fig. 20.33B). Therefore, in order to achieve absolute stability, i.e. the fracture segments are kept in contact during the function without movement, a compression plate used for treating the mandibular fracture should be placed near the alveolar border, if the biomechanical principles are observed. However, due to the anatomical constrains like presence of roots of the teeth, the neurovascular bundle, it is not always possible to place the plate along the alveolar border and have to be placed along the inferior border (compression site). This violates the principle of compression plating. However, the application of the compression plate along the inferior border of the mandible would not only be insufficient to stabilize the fragments, but also cause the flaring of the alveolar side (Fig. 20.34). Function would then cause movement of the fragments, which would result in danger of infection, pseudoarthrosis and malocclusion.

In order to prevent this problem, a tension band or tension plate is applied to the alveolar side. The tension band means the anatomic alignment of the tension site (alveolar) of the fracture via a device that prevents distraction. If the patient has sound teeth then tension band is applied on the teeth, which binds the alveolar segment and prevents the distraction. The alternative to this band is the application of tension plate, which neutralizes the tension forces and the compression plate at the inferior border is called the stabilizing plate (Figs 20.35A and B). The

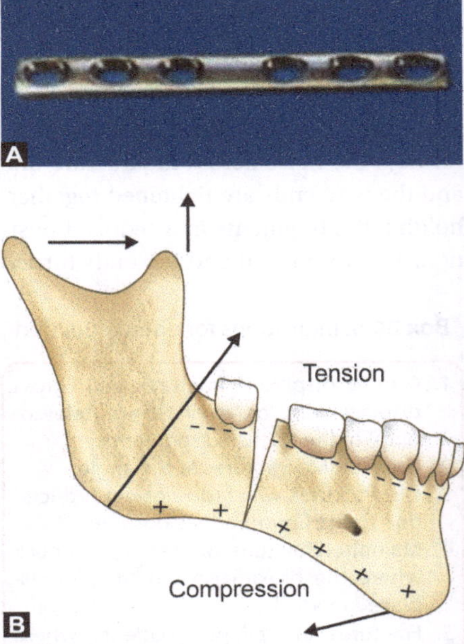

Figs 20.33A and B: (A) Dynamic compression plate causing interfragmentary compression; (B) The alveolar border of the mandible tension site and the inferior border is the compression site

eccentric dynamic compression plates (EDCP) overcome the above difficulty and there is no need to use the tension band or tension plate if the EDCP is used. As the EDCP not only compresses the fracture fragments but also rotates the fracture fragments at the tension site in such a way that the fragments do not flare up at the tension site during the function (Fig. 20.35C).

Before any internal fixation is applied it is mandatory to approximate the superior border, i.e. the alveolar border by achieving the intermaxillary fixation in the occlusal relationship.

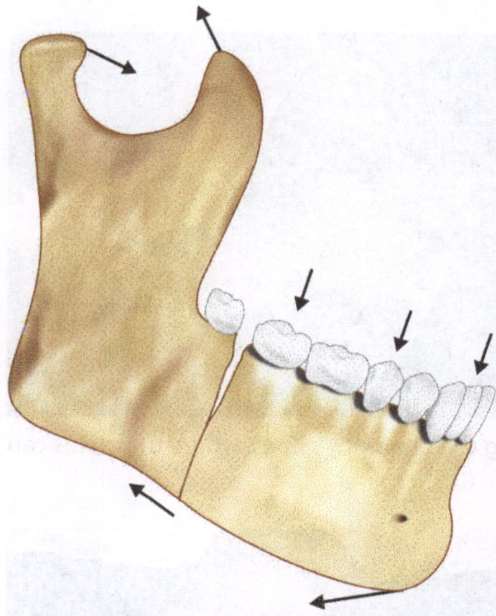

Fig. 20.34: The compression plate fixed at compression site creating opening of the alveolar border

The disadvantage with the compression plate is that the plates are very bulky and may be detectable subcutaneously in certain locations. The technique is complicated and requires lot of precision. The stress shielding effect on the bone below the compression has also been described. **Stress shielding** refers to the reduction in bone density (osteopenia) as a result of removal of normal stress from the bone by an implant (for instance, the compression plates). This is because by Wolff's law, bone in a healthy person or animal will remodel in response to the loads it is placed under. Therefore, if the loading on a bone decreases, the bone will become less dense and weaker because there is no stimulus for continued remodeling that is required to maintain bone mass. The osteoporotic changes have been demonstrated under the compression plate due to the stress shielding effect.

It was observed by Champy[5] that the healing of the mandibular fractures is adequate even in absence of compression and with monocortical screws and non-compression plates also stabilize the fragments sufficiently. The need for bulky plates is also not felt and thinner plates as recommended by him offer reasonable stability. The kind of fixation offered by the Champhy's monocortical plates is semirigid. Champy observed that the osteosynthetic activity is optimum along certain areas during the healing of the fracture and he recommend the application of the plates along these osteosynthetic lines to facilitate good and early healing. In this technique only one cortex comes in full contact while the other opens up to a minor extent. The Champy's osteosynthetic lines are as shown in the diagrams (Figs 20.36 to 20.39).

In the interior region the line is double, i.e. one at the inferior border and the other below the apices of teeth. The line gradually climbs upwards towards the external oblique ridge. The placement of the plates along this line on the buccal cortical plate is recommended. The basic advantage of this technique is the plates are less bulky and all the sites are readily accessible intraorally, thus avoiding a scar on the face. In the mandibular anterior area as the torsional forces are optimum two plates are used, one along each Champhy's lines. In the canine and premolar area while placing the plates intraorally, care should be taken to prevent damage to the branches of the mental nerve. The mandibular angle fractures are treated by placing the plate along the external oblique ridge through an intraoral incision. The subcondylar fractures are fixed through preauricular or Risdon's submandibular incision with retromandibular extension or by Hind's post ramal approach. The low subcondylar fractures are easy to plate, but the high subcondylar fractures are very difficult to manage as the proximal fragment is usually displaced severely and difficult to control.

When the miniplates are used, they should be properly adapted and contoured to the buccal surface of the bone. The gap

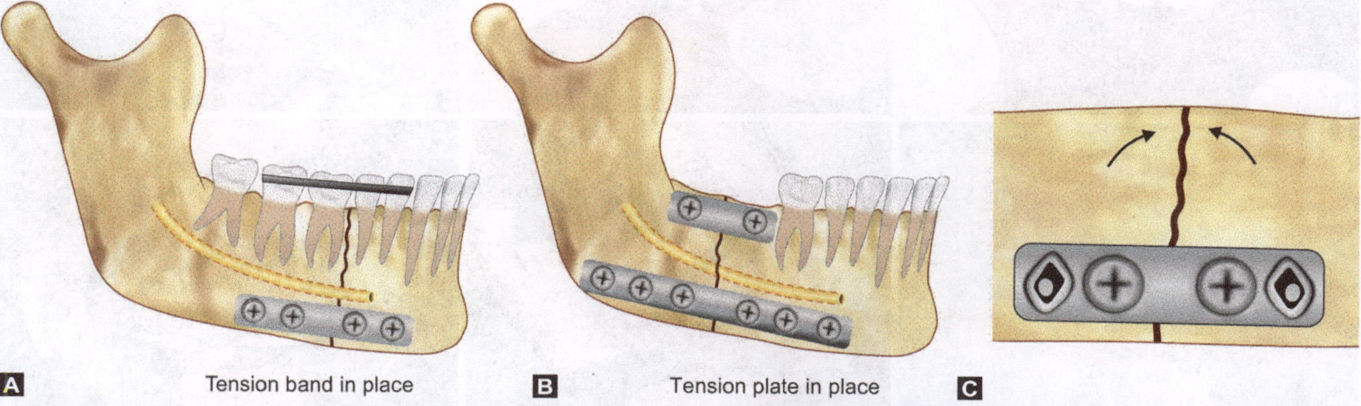

Figs 20.35A to C: (A) DCP with tension band; (B) DCP with tension plate; (C) EDCP eccentric holes at 45 degree angle producing compression and rotation

between the plate and the bone should be minimal. The screws should be secured firmly and tightened until no more turning of the screw is possible with moderate force. Excess of force may lead to micro-fractures around the shaft of the screw leading to loosening of the screw and micro-mobility, which may result into the failure of implant and increased chances of infection. As the Mini plates are applied onto the outer cortex of the bone and the monocortical screws are used to fix them, a good contact between the buccal cortical plate is achieved. However, the lingual cortex flares up slightly. To avoid the flaring of the lingual cortex the slight over contouring of the plate is recommended.

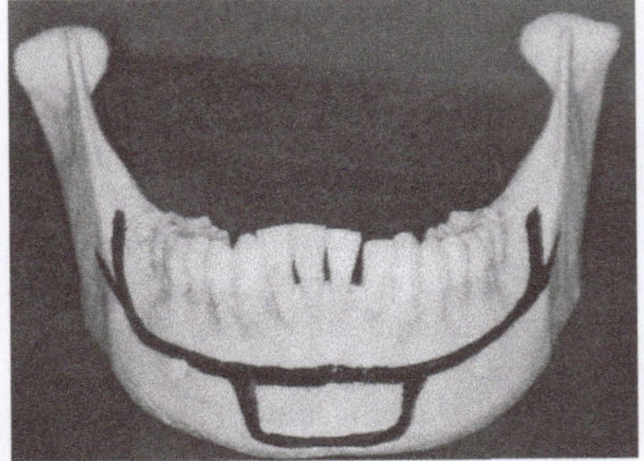

Fig. 20.36: Champhy's lines

The screws that are used for fixing the plate at the fracture site are of 2 types self, tapping and non-self tapping. Self-tapping is the ability of a screw to advance when turned, while creating its own thread. Self-tapping screws come with a sharp, piercing tip or a flat, blunt tip. The sharp-tipped screws are designed for drilling their own hole into bone and do not need a pilot hole. The pilot drill used for creating the tunnel for fixation of the screw should be smaller in diameter than the screw shaft to have better purchase of the screw onto the bone.

In extremely thin layer of cortical bone, such as facial bones, self tapping screws appear to have better holding power than the non-self tapping screws of corresponding size.

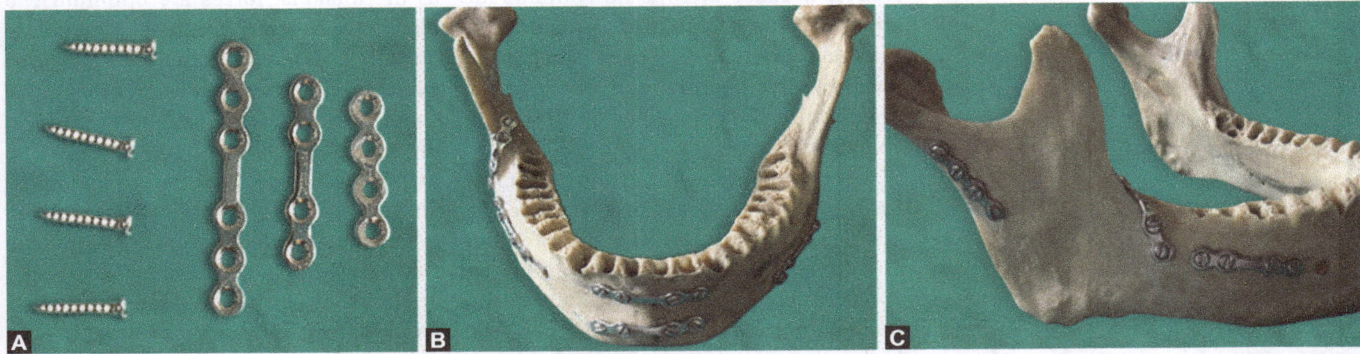

Figs 20.37A to C: Champhy's plates and screws and various locations on the mandible along the Champhy's lines, where the plates can be fixed

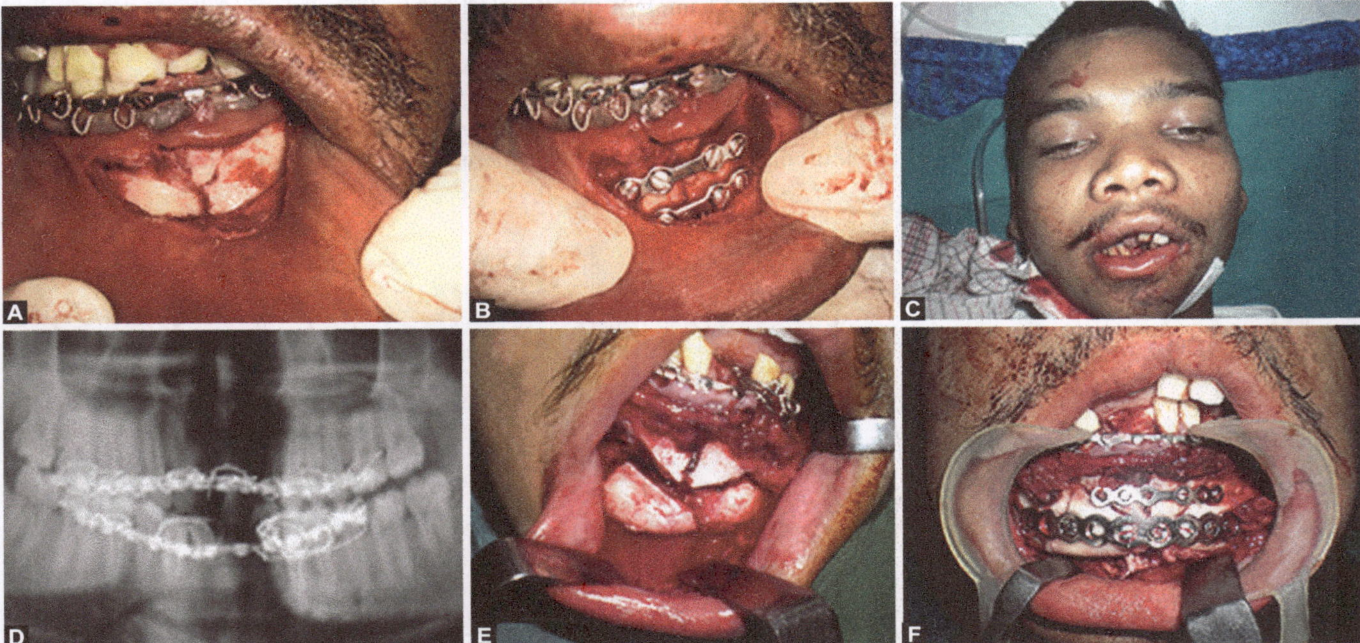

Figs 20.38A to F: Management of the comminuted fracture of the symphysis with a reconstruction plate and mini plate

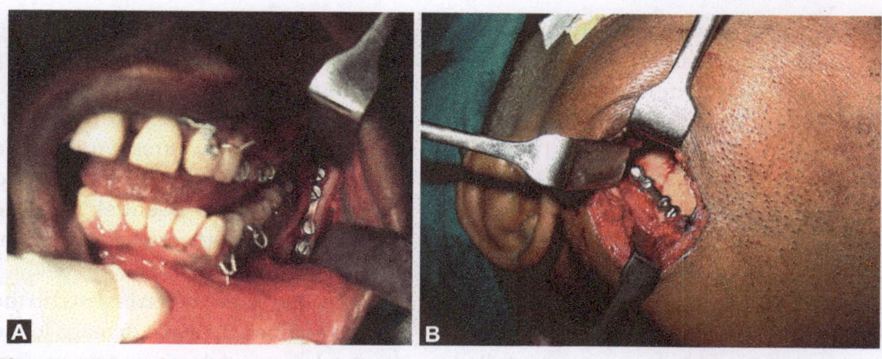

Figs 20.39A and B: Fixation of the Champhy's miniplates at angle and subcondylar areas

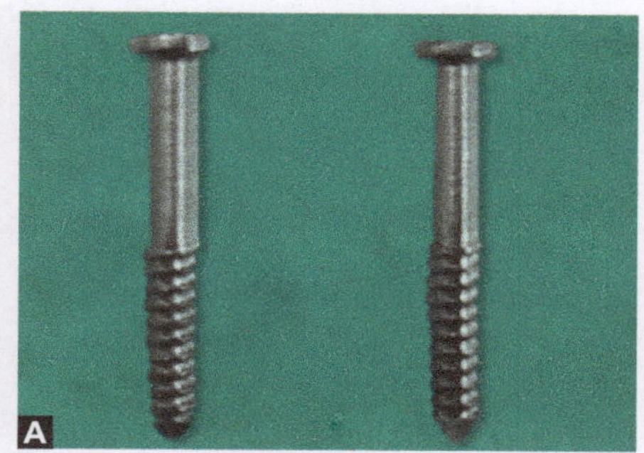

Fig. 20.40A: Lag screws

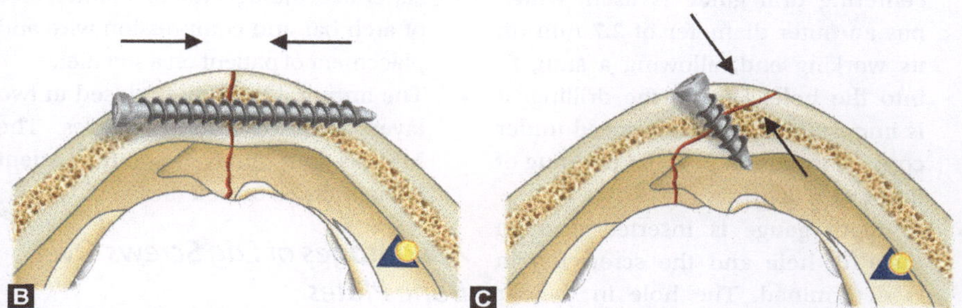

Figs 20.40B and C: Fixation of lag screw at the anterior mandible: (B) Sagittal fractures where two lag screws extending from one buccal plate to other buccal cortical plate are fixed; (C) Oblique fractures where two lag screws can be placed from the buccal to the lingual cortices

Lag Screws

A useful method of providing rigid fixation in the anterior mandible is by using lag screws. The term lag screw is used both, to describe a type of screw as well as a technique of screw placement. A true lag screw has threads only on its terminal end. When used, the threads engage the far cortex, while the head seats against the near cortex, providing compression upon tightening (Fig. 20.40A). A lag screw technique is achieved with a cortical screw, which has threads along its entire length by over enlarging holes in the near cortex. This later procedure has been more commonly used in maxillofacial surgery than true lag screws.

Brons and Boering[6] (1970) first introduced the lag screw technique to maxillofacial surgery who cautioned that at least two screws are necessary to prevent rotational movements of the fragments in oblique fractures of the mandible.

Anatomy and Biomechanics of Anterior Mandible

The anterior mandible from *mental foramen to mental foramen* is uniquely suited to application of lag screw fixations for three reasons:

1. Curvature of the anterior mandible allows the placement of lag screws across the symphysis from one side to other, for sagittal fractures and from anterior to posterior for oblique fractures and those of anterior body region (Figs 20.40B and C).
2. Thickness of bony cortices provide extremely secure fixation when the screws are properly inserted.
3. There are no anatomic hazards below the apices of teeth until the mental foramina are encountered. This makes lag screw placement extremely simple.

The directions of forces that are distributed through anterior mandible vary with the activity of the mandible. The anterior mandible undergoes shearing and torsional forces during functional activities.[7] Therefore, Champy who advocated only one small bone plate in most of the regions of the mandible always placed two bone plates in the symphysis.

One bone screw may not provide adequate stability, since the shear forces may allow rotation of the mandibular fragments around the screw.[3] The only resistance to rotation about one screw is the compaction of one fragment into other by virtue of compression imparted from the lag screw. Application of an arch bar to the teeth may prohibit the rotational force; however, application of a second lag screw is the best insurance for providing rigidity.

Technique

Lag screw technique for anterior mandible can require 2.7 mm screws up to 15 to 40 mm in length. Hence, every screw length up to 40 mm should be available before attempting. Following the ligation of maxillary and mandibular arch bars, a vestibular incision are made from just posterior to one mental foramen to other. The fracture site is exposed and examined following slight distraction to note the obliquity and the relationship of the cortices. If there are extensive areas of communition, the lag screw technique should be abandoned as it has little chance of success in cases, where the continuity of the cortices is disturbed. The IMF is done while simultaneously reducing the fracture. A small bur is used to drill holes approximately 10 mm away from each side of the fracture to provide a purchase for the modified towel clip, which is engaged in these holes and tightened to firmly reduce the fracture fragments. It is helpful to dissect below the inferior border of mandible in the area of the fracture to directly expose the lingual cortex and assure its proper reduction.

Selecting the point of entry into bone and alignment of the drill is crucial since it will determine the success of the procedure and when improperly executed may cause undesirable complications. Lag screw technique in other bones usually involves drilling the screw hole at an angle that is the bisection of angle between line of fracture and outer cortex. Due to its curvature, the path of screw insertion in anterior mandible traverses the fracture in as perpendicular manner as possible. This helps in enhancing the effectiveness of rigid stabilization of the fragments due to compressive force imparted by the lag screws. Lag screws applied obliquely to fracture cause displacement of the fracture. Bony cortex must be engaged with the terminal thread of the screws for anterior mandibular fractures.

Selection of proper point of entry of the drill in buccal cortex is based on:

- Placing it sufficiently away from fracture so that an ample amount of bone is present between the head of the screws and the fracture after drilling and countersinking. This is especially important when drilling along the curved surface of the anterior mandible.
- Providing sufficient space for second screw, thus the first screw must be placed just above the inferior border.
- The 2.7 mm drill is initially placed perpendicular to the buccal cortex at selected point of entry to prevent skidding of drill bit and hole is begun in cortex. The drill is then redirected to previously selected angulation and drilling completed till the medullary bone of first fragment. The drill and drill guide are withdrawn from the hole and counter sinking tool is used at slow speed to provide a smooth platform for screw head seating. While counter sinking the hole, the same angulation should be established by initial 2.7 mm drill hole for which an adjustable guide pin extending beyond the countersinking flutes can be used. Countersinking must be adequate to allow complete seating of screw head. One must avoid countersinking deeper and deeper into the bone to the point, where the screw head rests on medullary instead of cortical bone.
- Drilling through the second fragment with 2 mm drill is next step. To ensure that 2 mm drill is perfectly centered in the 2.7 mm hole previously drilled through the near cortex, a special centering drill guide is used, which has an outer diameter of 2.7 mm on its working end, allowing a snug fit into the hole. During the drilling, it is important to use slow speed under copious irrigation to avoid clogging of flutes with debris.
- A depth gauge is inserted through the drill hole and the screw length is determined. The hole in the far segment is then tapped using a long tap. To prevent tissue engagement and avoid wobble, the same drill guide, which is used in drilling 2.7 mm hole should be used as a tap guide. The hole should be thoroughly irrigated before placing the screws.
- Screw is inserted on a screwdriver into the screw hole. The outer hole is free of threads and screw should slip through until it contacts the thread in the far segment. When tightened, the screw will compress the two segments of bone together. Frequently the screw is over tightened to the point of creating microfractures around the screw head. This should be avoided if possible. It is essential that the screw exits the far cortex for maximal strength (Figs 20.40D to F).
- The second screw is then inserted in the same manner. To avoid damage to the mental nerve while placing the second screw, a bone plate can be placed superior to the lag screw or maintenance of arch bar and compression wire and placement of patient on a soft diet.
- The intraoral incision is closed in two layers with resorbable sutures. The MMF is then removed and the patient is maintained on soft diet.

Advantages of Lag Screws Over Bone Plates

- Lag screws can be applied more rapidly since the time consuming task of adapting the bone plates is obviated and allows more anatomically accurate reduction.
- Displacement of bone fragments is much more common during placement of bone plates, which never occurs while applying lag screw fixation.
- Lag screw also permits the rapid application of fixation without decrease

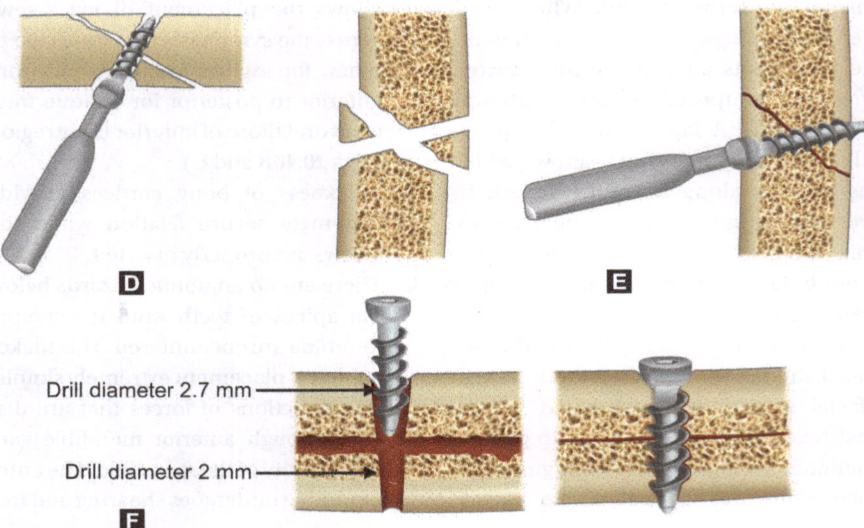

Figs 20.40D to F: Different diameter of drill used to secure the lag screw in the rigid manner

in rigidity of fracture reduction. The fracture gap frequently completely disappears from site due to the great amount of compression that can be imparted with the screw.

- Costs incurred are greatly diminished because the screw cost much less than the bone plate.

Lag screws are however contraindicated when there is a communition and/or bone loss in the fracture gap. If the intervening bone is unstable, due to communition or is missing, compressing across this region will cause displacement of intervening bone fragment, over-riding of segments and/or shortening of the fracture gap, resulting in problems with the occlusion.

Special Considerations

While treating the fractures of the mandible certain special conditions warrant special attention and suitable alterations in the treatment. These areas are pediatric fractures, condylar injuries and the geriatric fractures.

PEDIATRIC FRACTURES

The fractures of the pediatric mandible are usually undisplaced and although the classical green stick fractures like long bones are not seen, due to the elasticity in the bone fragments are not grossly displaced like the fractures in the older patients. The condyles are covered by a fibrocartilaginous cap and have more vascularity and thus, eventhough there is no fracture the contusions of the condyle leads to hemarthrosis and if the mandible is immobilized for longer period, the chances of fibrous and subsequently the bony ankylosis are high. This is partly due to the excellent reparative capacity in the childhood. As the healing potential is excellent in the children the fractures heal faster and do not require the immobilization for the period of 6 to 8 weeks, but 3 to 4 weeks are enough for the healing of pediatric fractures of the mandible.

The pediatric (deciduous) teeth in the jaws are wider at the base (*gingivally*) and thus, the gingival embrasures are very narrow, the interdental wiring is not possible. Secondly, the presence of the mixed dentition poses a great problem in fixing the interdental wires or devices as some teeth might have resorbed roots and are mobile and when the wiring is attempted may get avulsed. The permanent teeth, which are partially erupted, their roots are not fully formed, there are wide open primate spaces between them and the teeth may be in different stages of eruption and at different occlusal levels. Due to all these factors the IMF using the wires may not be possible. In case of minimally displaced fractures requiring short-term immobilization for 3 weeks, bonding the orthodontic brackets and using them for the IMF may be a practical solution however it cannot be useful in all the patients.

The pediatric jaws are small in size and at the age of 7 to 8 years may contain about 42 teeth, including both the erupted and developing. Thus, a large area of the small bone is occupied by the developing teeth buds (Figs 20.41A and B). Open reduction and fixing the fracture with bone plates is not practical as:

- The space to fix the plate is not adequate as the jaw bones are small.
- The chances of injuries to the developing teeth buds are high due to the screws.
- The implant may affect the growth of the mandible or will be required to be removed by second surgery after the fracture healing to prevent the growth retardation.

Thus, the most practical way of treating the pediatric mandibular fractures at the denture bearing area is by fabrication and fixing of the cap splint with a circummandibular wiring. The IMF is not required and thus the mobilization of the jaw prevents the chances of fibrous adhesions in the TMJ. Ideally the fractures need to be reduced accurately, however in pediatric fractures minor discrepancies in alignment and occlusion are acceptable as the erupting teeth compensate the same and the remodeling of the bone also overcomes these discrepancies. In case, the fracture in the body is grossly displaced and warrants management with the open reduction, in such cases the plates may be fixed at the inferior border and small screws (4 to 5 mm) may be used. Such plates should be removed once the fracture heals.

The fractures of the condylar head, subcondylar area can in most of the cases be treated conservatively. Short-term immobilization in the acute stage followed by early mobilization is the key in the treatment. Postoperative physiotherapy may also be useful in preventing the development of ankylosis. In case, the fracture in the subcondylar area is grossly displaced and is indicated for the open reduction, it can be done with bioresorbable plates and screws than the titanium or stainless steel implants as the later two may require their removal.

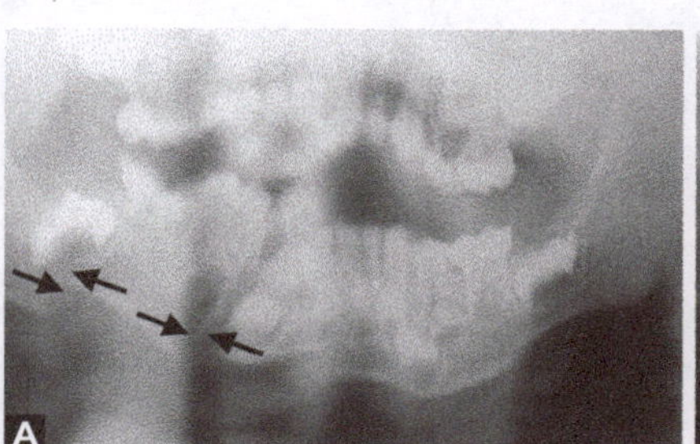
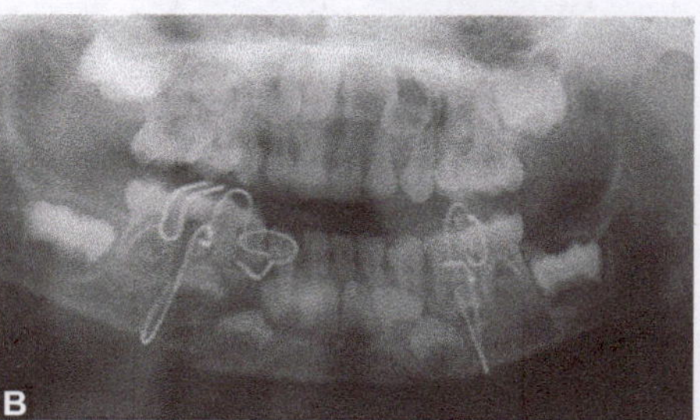

Figs 20.41A and B: Pediatric mandibular fracture treated with cap splin and circumferential wiring

GERIATRIC FRACTURES

The fractures of the mandible in geriatric age group are often difficult to treat. In the elderly patients due to the loss of teeth the alveolar process undergoes severe resorption and the mandible becomes atrophic and thin. The bones become osteoporotic and fragile and fracture readily. In the younger individuals, the blood supply to the bone is said to be centrifugal due to plenty of bone marrow, but in the older patients, it is centripetal, i.e. from periosteum to the center, due to the bone marrow undergoing myelofibrosis and the endosteal blood supply of the mandible is diminished. The periosteum also undergoes fibrosis and thus, the periosteal blood supply also gets reduced. The osteoblastic and healing potential of the bone goes down and the healing of the fracture is a slow process and the complications such as nonunion are more likely to occur. The dentition serves as a good guide for the closed reduction of the mandibular fracture and due to the loss of the teeth the accurate reduction cannot be assessed, nor are the teeth available for fixing interdental wires or devices for IMF in the geriatric patients.

The edentulous geriatric fractures can be treated by closed reduction using the gunning splints or if the patient is a denture wearer, the dentures can be modified by inserting hooks or arch bars in it for doing IMF, which can be used as a splint. The gunning splints can reduce the fractures of the denture bearing area, but the fractures of the ramus, angle and the subconylar area cannot be effectively managed with the gunning splints as the proximal fragment cannot be controlled, especially if it is an unfavorable fracture. Secondly, if the fracture is not grossly displaced, minor discrepancies can be subsequently taken care of while fabricating the denture. But, if the fracture is grossly displaced due to the muscle pull the chances of non-healing are increased further.

The open reduction of the geriatric fractures is often associated with chances of non-union. The bone is already having diminished blood supply as discussed earlier. The endosteal blood supply is disrupted with the fracture. If the open reduction is done by stripping the periosteum excessively the chances of avascular necrosis at the end of the fractured fragments can occur leading to non-union. Thus, the open reduction of the geriatric mandibular fractures should preferably avoided. If the situation necessitates the open reduction, judicious periosteal stripping should be done and the modalities requiring lesser periosteal dissection should be chosen, i.e. lag screws in place of bone plates. Some authors have brought forwards a concept of supraperiosteal plating to avoid the periosteal dissection.

CONDYLAR FRACTURES

The condyles not only facilitate the mandibular excursions, but play a great role in the mandibular growth. The condyle has a head, which rests in the glenoid fossa of the temporal bone. The neck, which is thin and slender connects the head to the rest of the mandible. The glenoid fossa is located at the base of the middle cranial fossa and to avoid its fractures, which may have serious implications, the nature has made the neck of the condyle thin and weak so that whenever there is a force applied on the chin, it gets transmitted along the condyles to the glenoid fossa. The neck is weak and thus, it fractures absorbing the shock and prevent the more grievous injury. However, in growing children, condylar neck is short, stout and broad. It is covered with thick cap of fibrocartilage and the ratio of cancellous to cortical bone is high. Owing to these two factors when vertical forces act, the condyle fractures like cap of mushroom. This phenomenon is intracapsular and is the cause of post-traumatic ankylosis.

The condylar fractures can be classified as:

- Intracapsular fractures (condylar head fractures)
  - Undisplaced.
  - Comminuted.
  - Cortical injuries/cortical chipping usually the medial portion (Figs 20.42A and B).
- Extracapsular fractures (condylar neck fractures)
  - High subcondylar (Fig. 20.43).
  - Low subcondylar (Figs 20.44A and B).

The subcondylar fractures can also be classified as:

- Undisplaced
- Medially displaced (due to pull of lateral pterygoid)
- Laterally displaced (less common)
- Fracture dislocation (the condyle gets dislocated from the glenoid fossa and gets dislocated medially in the infratemporal fossa due to pull of lateral pterygoid muscle) (Figs 20.45A to E).

The intracapsular fractures are essentially treated with closed reduction. There are two schools of thought for the treatment of the high subcondylar fractures. Some people believe in closed reduction, while others believe in the open reduction. The open reduction of the high subcondylar fracture, which is medially displaced or dislocated is often technically difficult. The high subcondylar fractures are approached by the preauricular incision. The fixation is done using a miniplate or lag screws. The use of the K wire for fixation of the subcondylar fracture,[8] as described in the literature is not commonly practiced nowaday due to the availability of better modalities.

The low subcondylar fractures are easily treated with the open reduction. The

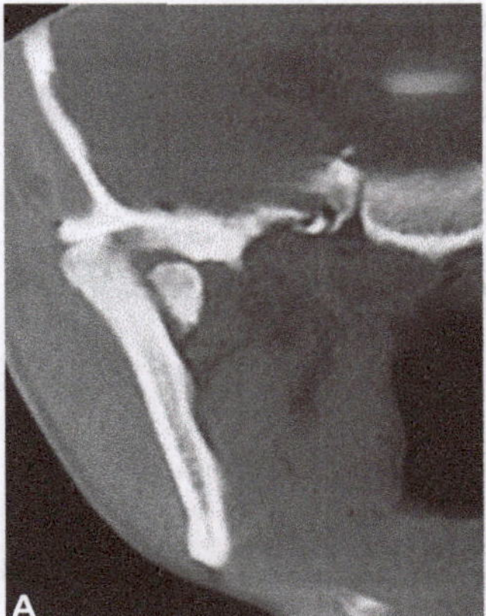

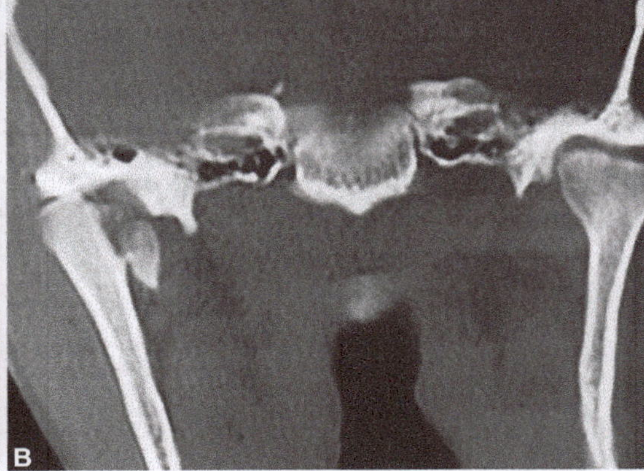

Figs 20.42A and B: Cortical chipping of the medial pole of the condyle

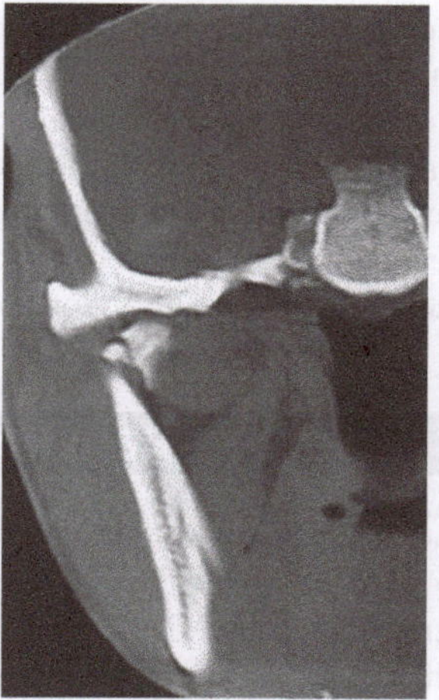

Fig. 20.43: High subcondylar fracture

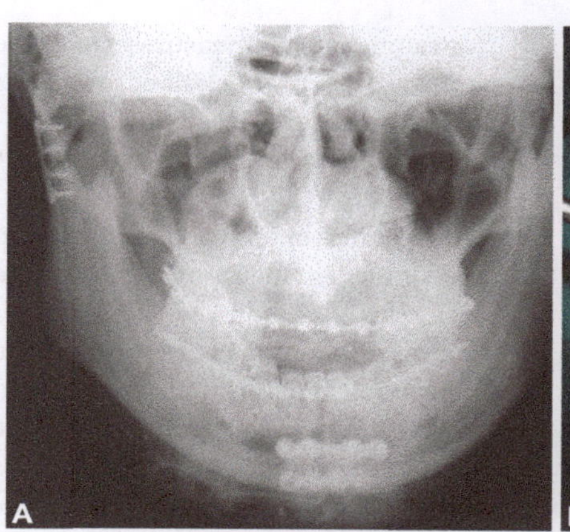

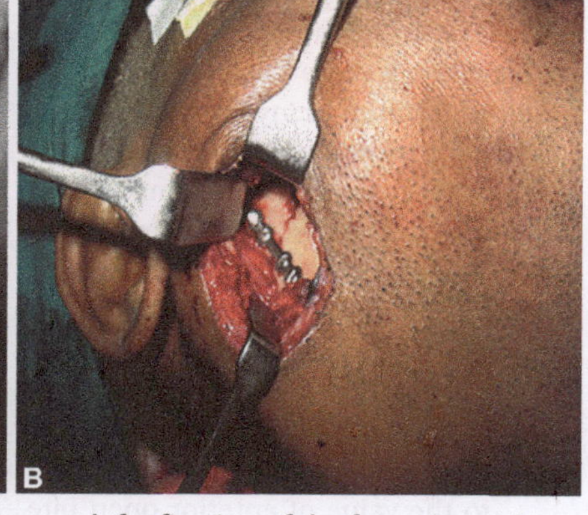

Figs 20.46A and B: Postramal Hind's approach for fixation of the fractures with miniplates

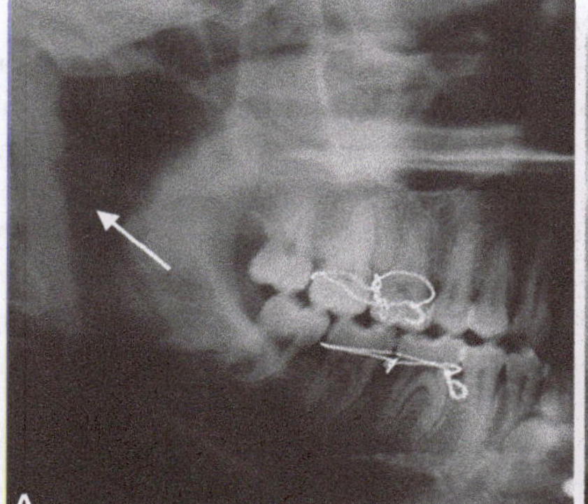

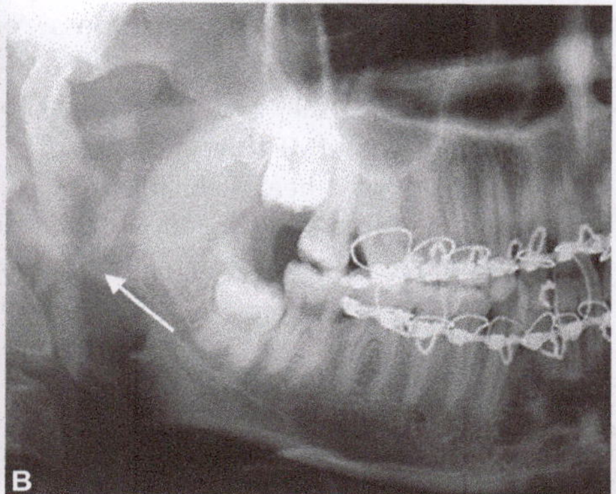

Figs 20.44A and B: Low subcondylar fracture

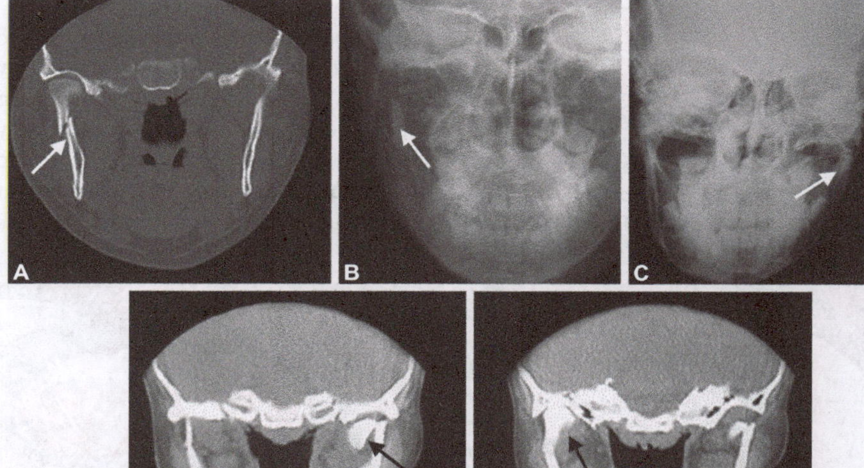

Figs 20.45A to E: (A) Minimally displaced/undisplaced; (B) Laterally displaced; (C and D) Fracture dislocation; (E) Right side medially angulated left side fracture dislocation

site is approached through transbuccal approach or by Risdon's or postramal approach and can easily be fixed with miniplates and screws (Figs 20.46A and B).

The problems with proper reduction and fixation of condylar fractures using a single mini plate have been evaluated by Hammer et al. and they found that the displacement of condylar segment due to the adverse muscle pull of lateral pterygoid muscle and the functional forces acting on the proximal segment exceed the rigidity of one mini plate, plate failure and screw loosening. Hence, they recommended application of two mini plates, i.e. one at the posterior border and one at the anterior border and found the beneficial effect of restoring tension and compression trajectories and providing stability against the muscle pull[9] (Figs 20.47A and B).

The condylar fractures are always associated with injuries to the internal soft tissues of the joint producing joint effusions. If the condylar injuries are treated with long-term immobilization of the jaw, the chances of fibrous adhesions and ankylosis are increased. Hence, while treating them with closed reduction the following protocol should be followed:

- Achieve the occlusion either by reduction manually or under general anesthesia after giving muscle relaxants to overcome the unfavorable muscle pull. The fractures can also be reduced by gradual traction using heavy intermaxillary elastics. In case of telescoping of the fracture fragments, radiographical assessment of the overlap of fracture segments is ascertained and a bite block (fulcrum or hypomochlion[10]) is placed between the posterior teeth, which are gagging or meeting in premature contact, creating anterior open bite (Figs 20.48A to C). The height of hypomochlion should be determined by any of the following two methods:

- **Clinical method:** In which the amount of anterior open bite is recorded (×) and 2 mm is added to the value of anterior open bite (× + 2) + 2 mm signifies the normal overbite value.
- **Radiographic method:** The loss of mandibular ramal height is calculated based upon the measurements taken on a standardized radiograph. The length of the fractured condylar segment is measured on the X-ray (X). The angle of the fractured condylar segment with the distal segment of the ramus is also measured (A°). The loss of vertical height of the ramus (X') due to telescoping is calculated by the following formula:

$$X' = X\,(1 - \cos A°)$$

- The hypomochlion works as a fulcrum and provides mechanical advantage of a class I lever. As the anterior intermaxillary elastics are applied the unfavorable muscle pull is countered and as the mandible rotates over the fulcrum the anterior open bite reduces and proportional lengthening of the ramus occurs due to its downward displacement. The size of the hypomochlion is reduced gradually at the rate of 1 mm per week till satisfactory occlusal relationship of the molars is established, which suggests that the loss of ramal height is corrected.
- After the occlusal relationship is established, the IMF for short-term (2–3 weeks) with heavy elastics may given to maintain and consolidate the established result and do not prefer the IMF for the fear of precipitating ankylosis.
- The patients are advised physiotherapy for long-term to prevent fibrous adhesions and functional adaptation to the new situation generated by this treatment modality, i.e. pseudarthrosis.

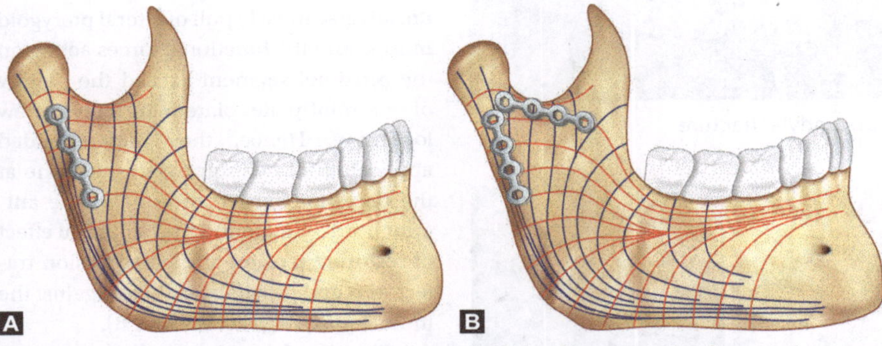

Figs 20.47A and B: Showing the distribution of the forces on the fractured segment and stabilization of the fracture segments using one miniplate (A) and two miniplates (B) (Courtesy: Meyer et al. Journal of Craniomaxillofacial Surgery 2006;34:173-181)

FRACTURE HEALING

In general, fracture results in a well-defined progression of tissue responses that are designed to remove tissue debris, to re-establish vascular supply and to produce a new skeletal matrix. The processes that occur to accomplish healing are dependent on the location of the injured bone and on local and systemic factors.

Like the soft tissue, bone can also heal by primary or secondary intention. Spontaneous bone healing without surgical intervention and healing that occurs after semirigid fixation progress by *secondary intention.* Healing by *primary intention* occurs only when the following conditions are met:

- Excellent anatomic reduction.
- Minimal or no mobility.
- Good vascular supply at the fracture site.
- Rigid fixation and compression of the fracture fragments to abolish micro-movements.

Although similar terminology is also applied to soft-tissue wounds, an analogy between the two should be avoided. In soft-tissue injury, healing by secondary intention involves the filling of a gap by granulation tissue with subsequent replacement by a scar, which is less

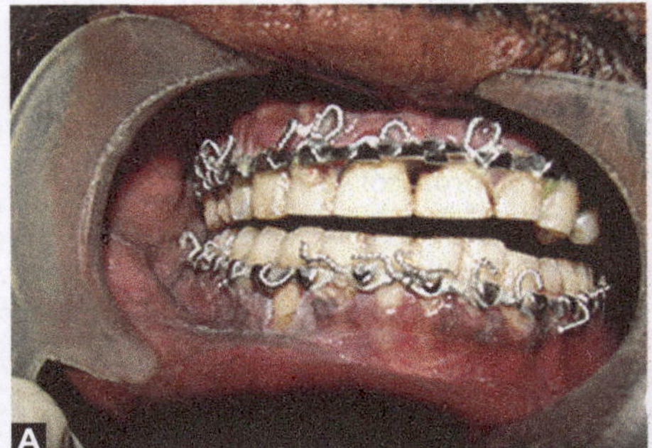

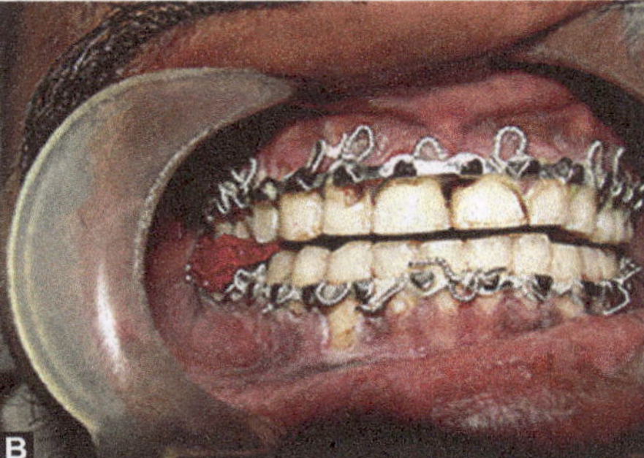

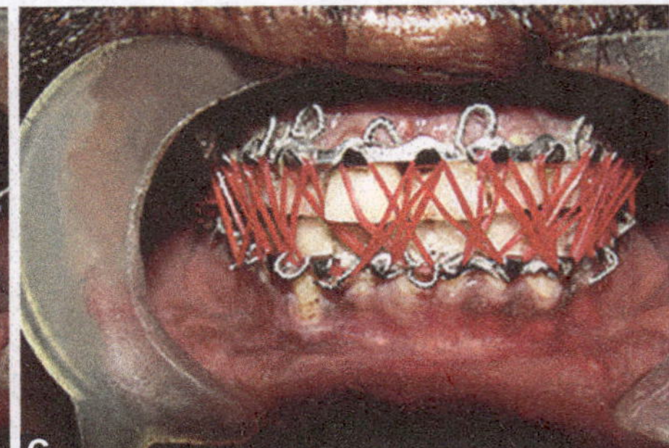

Figs 20.48A to C: A case of subcondylar fracture causing open bite, treated with hypomochlion and anterior elastic traction

functional. Secondary bone healing is so termed because initially an intermediate fibrous tissue (callus) is formed within the fracture gap and is only subsequently replaced by bone, as opposed to primary bone healing, in which no intermediate fibrous tissue (callus) is formed and the bone heals by direct proliferation of the osteoprogenitor cells from either side, which forms bone, osteosynthesis. However, unlike the scar formed by secondary intention healing of the soft-tissue wounds, bones that have healed by secondary intention continue, through adaptation and remodeling process, toward a form and function similar to what was present before the injury.

Secondary Bone Repair

Fractures undergoing spontaneous healing and those treated with a majority of the currently used treatment modalities undergo secondary bone healing. Secondary bone involves a well-defined sequence of steps:[11]

- Initial stage.
- Cartilaginous callus.
- Bony callus.
- Remodeling.

During the initial stage, hematoma formation occurs concurrent with an inflammatory response, which brings new vascularity and the undifferentiated mesenchymal cells differentiate to form a fibrocartilaginous callus. This fibrocartilage then ossifies to form the bony callus, which subsequently undergoes remodeling and functional adaptation in much same way as the preinjured bone.

Initial Stage/Reaction

The disruption of blood vessels and generation of heat from the energy necessary for inducing fractures, lead to hypoxia and cellular death at the fracture site. This situation produces necrosis at the bone ends of the fracture for a variable distance. This aseptic (non-infected) necrosis leads to inflammation and edema. The inflammatory response induces release of numerous vasoactive angiogenic pyrogen, which produce vasodilation within a few hour of injury. Hemorrhage from the dilated, damaged vessel, from the endosteum, periosteum and Haversian system leads to hematoma formation. A great deal of emphasis has been placed on the importance of the hematoma in healing. The clot is invaded by a variety of blood-borne elements, which can contribute to healing. In addition to granulation tissue within the hematoma, fragments of bone and muscle may be found. The small, non-vital muscle undergoes autolysis within 5 to 10 days, and the pedicled, vascularized muscle undergoes fibrosis and does not interfere with healing unless it is trapped between the ends of the fractured bone. Small bone fragments may undergo surface deposition of bone by migrating periosteal cells and associated devitalized marrow undergoes fatty degeneration. Somewhat overlapping this inflammatory hematoma formation is the initiation of cellular proliferation. Within 8 to 12 hours, DNA synthesis and proliferation by the periosteal cells of the cambium layer (inner layer which is close to the bone) begin. This process initially involves the periostium of the entire injured bone, but decreases over a few days to remain only in the area of the fracture.

The basic work of Urist[12] and others has established that these cells are pluripotent and give rise to osteoblasts, fibroblasts and cells with chondrogenic potential. As these cells start to proliferate, capillary in growth begins. The fibroblasts formed during the proliferative stage migrate into the wound and begin to lay down collagen. This combination of collagen and a rich capillary network forms granulation tissue. In this stage, a low oxygen tension and a low pH are noted in the early granulation tissue. It is thought that these conditions of lower pH and relative hypoxia trigger a response within the hematoma toward the formation of hyaline cartilage. In addition to decreased oxygen tension and decreased pH, it is thought that the movement that occurs when bone fragments are not immobilized with rigid internal fixation causes continued compression and tension at the site of the fracture and also directs cells toward the formation of cartilage (Figs 20.49A and B).

Cartilaginous Callus (Soft Callus) Formation

Callus is derived from latin word callum or callus means hard integument. It has been defined as collagenous, revascularizing, osteogenic blastema, which unites the bone fragments and from which the bone regenerates. The term soft callus appears to be contradictory in that the callus implies hardness. Callus formation begins externally and internally. Externally, nodules of cartilage are separated by fibrous septa. As the blood vessels within the septa increase, the tendency toward hypoxemia is reversed and two changes occur simultaneously. First, further calcification of the cartilage takes place, with the trapping of chondroblasts and their conversion to chondrocytes. (Late cartilaginous stage) (Fig. 20.50). Second, osteoblasts increase in number and osteoclasts become apparent for the first time. As this external callus is forming, an internal callus between the bone ends also forms. This area has a better blood supply and therefore less necrosis takes place. No intermediate fibrocartilage is formed instead osteoblasts from the endosteum form an internal bony callus directly. When bone begins to heal after fracture, a cuff or callus, forms around the fracture site to stabilize the involved area. (Bony callus formation) (Fig. 20.49C and D and Fig. 20.51). The callus greatly increases the area of inertia, thereby increasing the strength and stiffness of the bone, especially resistance against bending and torsion, during the healing period. If the fracture is not reduced properly during the healing then the hyperplastic callus is formed (callus adaptation), which undergoes steady remodeling process until the functional adaption to the stresses takes place (Fig 20.52).

Hard Callus (Bony Callus) Formation

In a fashion similar to the endochondral formation of bone that occurs during growth and development, the cartilagenous callus undergoes calcification into woven bone. The spaces within the cartilaginous callus allow for further vascular ingrowth, which

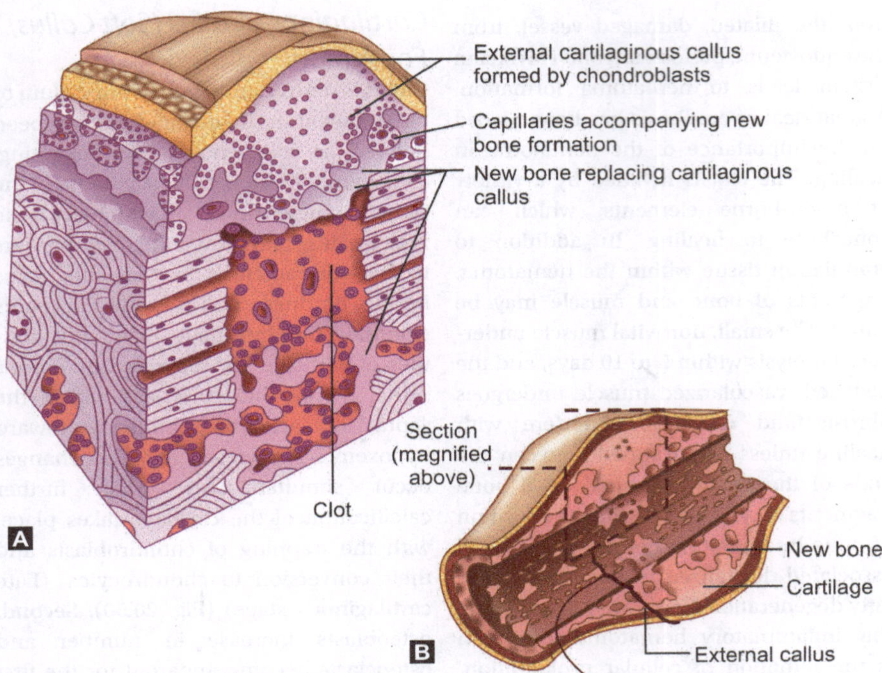

Figs 20.49A and B: Late fibroblastic stage. Osteoblast lay down new bone, in case of low oxygen tension cartilage is laid down by chondroblast

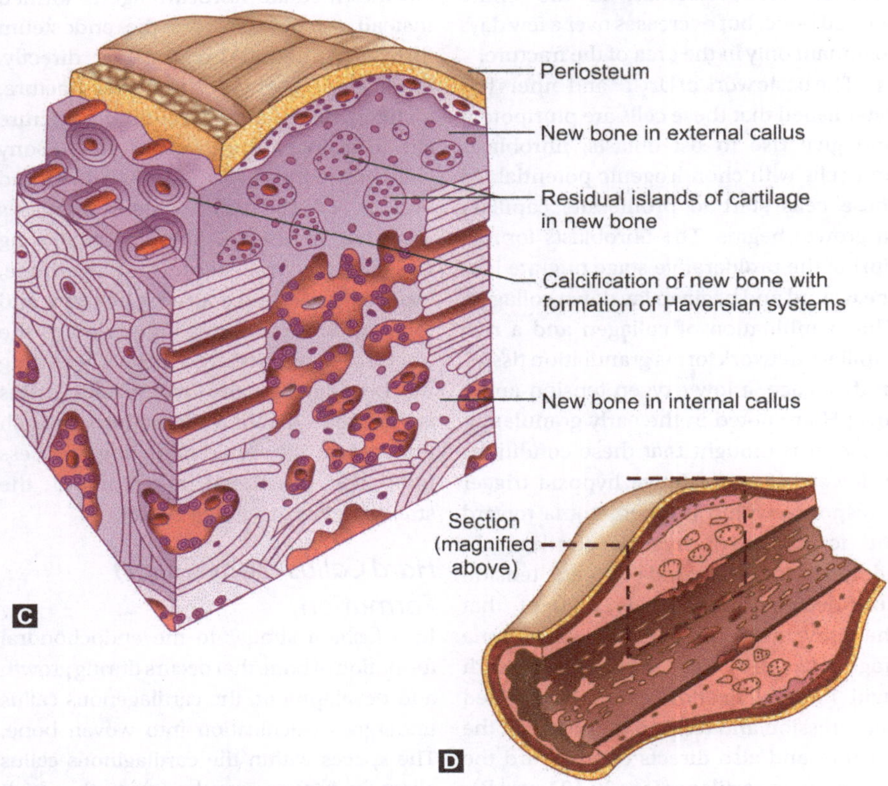

Figs 20.49C and D: Calcification bone with formation of Haversian system

brings with it a change in the environment. The increase in oxygen tension, aided by the transportation of nutrients to the site is conducive to the formation of osteoblasts. These osteoblasts pre-existed at the fracture site and that there was some stimulus that caused them to begin activity. McLean and Urist believed that the cells were derived from connective tissue precursors. Probably both factors contribute somewhat because abundant osteoblasts are present within the endosteum and numerous precursors are available within the connective tissue surrounding the wound. It is well known that these precursor cells can be induced into bone-forming cells both *in vivo* and *in vitro*. The osteoblasts deposit osteoid on the spicules of calcified cartilage and the osteoid then undergoes a calcification process, forming bone. The process begins peripherally and progress as a homogeneous calcification of the cartilaginous callus. Initially the bone that is formed is randomly arranged (*woven bone*); it is then undergoes organization and changes to lamellar bone during the final stage of healing, which is the remodeling stage.

Remodeling

The newly formed woven bone, which is somewhat random in organization, undergoes remodeling into the more familiar pattern of lamellar bone. This slow process progresses in accordance with *Wolff's law*,[13] which states that a change in the functional state of bone causes structural or architectural changes in the tissue through bioelectric field production. As osteoclasts participate in remodeling by resorption of bone, factors are released that help drive and direct the remodeling process further. The bone morphogenic protein (BMP) is a collagenase-resistant glycoprotein, isolated by Urist et al. and is one of these factors. Acting as a mitogenic and tissue growth factor (TGF), the BMP induces differentiation of mesenchymal cells toward bone formation. The preceding overview applies to fractures for which the fixation is such that the movement can occur at the fracture site. Two other situations also exist. The first of these is that of linear fractures of flat bones of the skull and some facial bones. In this case, there is limited

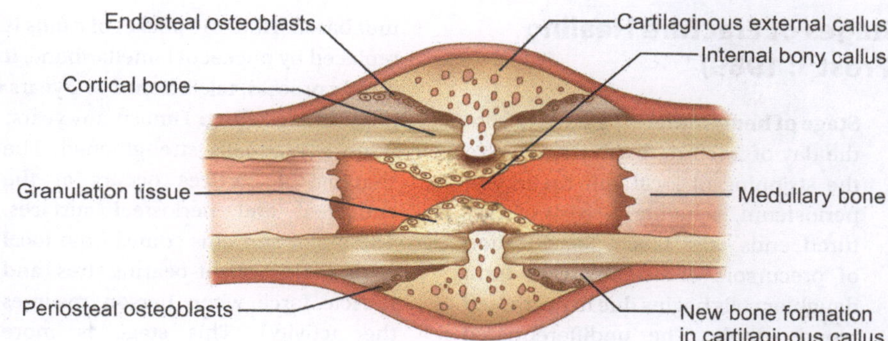

Fig. 20.50: Late cartilaginous stage

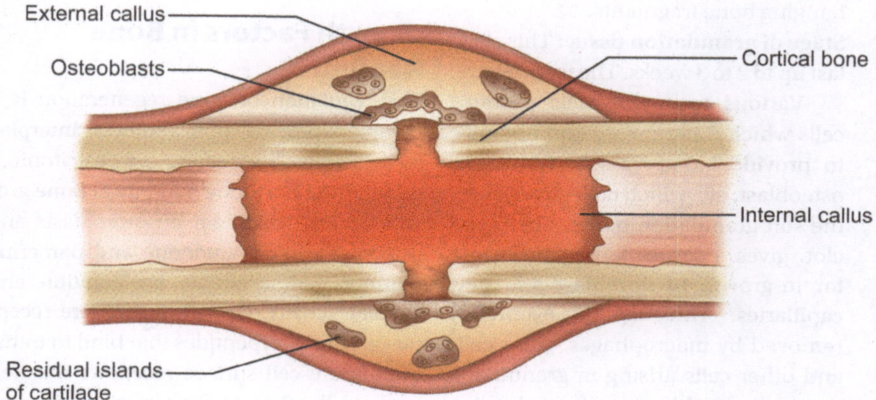

Fig. 20.51: Bony callus formation

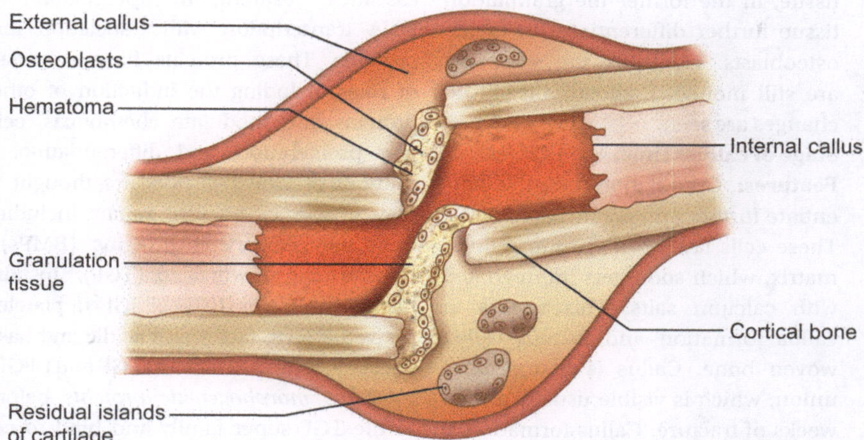

Fig. 20.52: Bony callus stage, fracture with displacement illustrating callus adaptation

movement and the surrounding tissue is very vascular. Periosteal osteoprogenitor cells differentiate into osteoblasts and bone is laid down directly without a cartilaginous phase. The second condition is that which exists when rigid internal fixation is used, so that the effective strain that normally induces callus formation is negated and nearly perfect anatomic reduction is achieved. In this instance healing occurs primarily.

Primary Bone Healing

Primary bone healing occurs when enough rigidity and anatomic reduction exist to preclude the necessity for the mechanical stability afforded by a callus. Primary healing probably occurs in cancellous bone even without this rigid mechanical stabilization if there is no gross mobility. Osteogenic cells and capillaries proliferate in the medullary bone on both sides of the fracture, forming new bone along the fracture site. In cortical bone, union without callus formation was reported as early as 1949 when it was observed that radiographs of long bone fractures that had been plated failed to show callus formation. Schenk and Willenegger[14] were the first to observe the histologic features of primary bone healing. The healing that occurs in cortical bone fractures in which rigid fixation has been accomplished occurs in two different ways:

1. Gap healing
2. Contact healing.

Gap Healing

Even with rigid fixation by means of a device that produces a stable relationship between the fracture ends under the deforming forces produced by muscle pull and function, a perfect anatomic reduction seldom exists. In some areas of the fracture, small gaps occur between the bone segments within a few days after fracture gap healing begins at these points. Blood vessels from the periosteum, endosteum, or Haversian canals invade the gaps, bringing mesenchymal osteoblastic precursors. Bone is deposited directly on the surfaces of the fracture fragments without resorption and without intermediate cartilage formation. If the gaps are less 0.3 mm, lamellar bone forms directly. Gaps from 0.3 mm up to a critical value, 0.5 to 1.0 mm, fill with woven bone and lamellar bone is subsequently laid down within the trabecular spaces.

The formation of lamellar bone occurs over 6 weeks. At the end of this time, the lamellar bundles are oriented at right angles to the longitudinal axis of the remaining bone. Fractures repaired by healing have been shown to be considerably stronger than similar fractures healed by secondary repair in the same time, despite the often large quantity periosteal bone present within the bony callus of secondarily healing bone.

Contact Healing

In areas in which contact is achieved, the interfragmentary gap is essentially zero. Since vascular and cellular ingrowth cannot proceed as it does in fractures in which a gap exists, a special process of bone formation occurs. This process has been termed '*contact healing*'. Contact healing occurs through the formation of a bone metabolizing unit (BMU), a bone remodeling unit (BRU) or a bone repair unit (BRU), all synonyms for the newly forming (or regenerating) osteon. Osteoblasts differentiate and form new bone. The osteoclasts begin to cut away cones on either side of the fracture, progressing toward the fracture site through necrotic bone and into the opposing bone end. The osteoclastic cutting cone proceeds at a rate of 50 to 80 μm per day.[15] The resultant cone which is 200 μm in diameter, provides a pathway for vessel ingrowth and osteoblastic proliferation, with formation of new bone. This process has been likened to a '*pegging together*' of the fracture ends by newly formed bone. The osteon forms at a rate of 1 to 2 μm per day. This lag between resorption and osteon ingrowth produces a transient porosity in the compact bone visible radiographically up to 3 months after fracture in humans, with complete reconstruction of the cortex requiring up to 6 months. During this period, the fixation device must maintain the stability of the fractured segments.

Direct fracture healing consists of direct bone formation without the classical multistage differentiation of connective tissue and cartilage (*callus formation*). The direct union of the fragments in contact and under compression occurs by the remodeling of the Haversian canals by *cutting cones*. These cutting cones contain osteoclasts and a conical surface of osteoblasts, which produce new osteons with incorporated new living osteocytes. These osteocytes are connected among themselves and to the vascular supply in the Haversian canal by a network of canaliculi. The contact in this type of healing is few micrometer.

Stages of Fracture Healing (Frost[16]: 1989)

- **Stage of hematoma:** This stage is from the day of fracture to 7th day. Due to the stripping of local soft tissue and periosteum, ischemic necrosis of fractured ends take place. Sensitization of precursors of osteoblast to form daughter cells begins due to decreased blood supply. The undifferentiated mesenchymal cells also differentiate into the osteoclasts to resorb the overhanging bone fragmants.
- **Stage of granulation tissue:** This stage last up to 2 to 3 weeks. The features are:

  Various precursor cells produce cells which differentiate and organize to provide blood vessels, fibroblast, osteoblast, etc. which collectively form the soft granulation tissue. The blood clot gives rise to loose meshwork for in-growth of fibroblast and new capillaries. The clot is eventually removed by macrophages, giant cells and other cells arising in granulation tissue. From this stage bone healing differs from soft healing in which granulation tissue is replaced fibrous tissue, in the former the granulation tissue further differentiates to create osteoblasts. Clinically the segments are still mobile. Radiographically no changes are seen.
- **Stage of callus:** Time: 4 to 12 weeks.

  Features: Granulation tissue differentiate further and create osteoblasts. These cells lay down an intercellular matrix, which soon gets impregnated with calcium salts. This results in callus formation and is also called woven bone. Callus is first sign of union, which is visible usually after 3 weeks of fracture. Callus formation is slower in adults than in children and in cortical bone than in cancellous bone.
- **Stage of remodeling:** Time: 1 to 2 years. This stage is also called the stage of consolidation. Woven bone is replaced by lamellar structure this process of change is multicellular and unit based. Here the pocket of callus is replaced by pocket of lamellar bone, it is slow process, takes from 1 to 2 years.
- **Stage of modeling:** Time: many years. Bone is gradually strengthened. The shaping of cortices occurs at the endosteal and periosteal surfaces. The major stimulus comes from local bone strain (weight-bearing stress and muscle force when person resumes the activity). This stage is more conspicuous in children and limited in adults.

Growth Factors in Bone Healing

The regulation of bone regeneration is a complex process that requires interplay by systemic hormones, e.g. calcitonin,[17] parathyroid hormone[18] and local bone growth factors, which act on osteoblasts and osteoclasts in an autocrine and paracrine manner and modulate proliferation and cellular activity. Growth factors are receptor-specific polypeptides that bind to transmembrane cell surface receptors on their target cells. Extracellular receptor binding is followed by intracellular changes that lead to activation of second messenger cascades, resulting in upregulation of DNA transcription with translation into proteins. These proteins have a variety of roles including the induction of other proteins and modulate chemotaxis, cellular proliferation, and differentiation. A number of growth factors are thought to play a role in fracture repair including bone morphogenetic proteins (BMPs),[19] transforming growth factor (TGF),[20] insulin-like growth factor (IGF-I),[21] IGF-II, platelet-derived growth factor and acidic and basic fibroblastic growth factor (aFGF and bFGF).

Bone morphogenetic proteins belong to the TGF super family and bind to cell surface receptors that play a crucial role in osteoblast stimulation and recruitment, resulting in bone formation. This group of proteins were first isolated by Urist from rabbit demineralized bone in 1979.[22] With the use of molecular genetics, a number of BMPs have been recombinantly produced and studied. In one of many similar studies, Seto[23] reported the use of BMP-2 in conjunction with small amounts of autologous bone in the reconstruction of continuity defects of primates. In additional research using immunolocalization has demonstrated BMP-2 and BMP-4 in rat callus. In the future, this group of proteins may play a significant role in the management of traumatic and non-traumatic injuries of the facial skeleton.

BMP 2-4 and BMP-7, also known as osteogenic protein-1 (OP-1), are expressed by osteoblasts, osteoclasts and other more primitive mesenchymal cells within the fracture callus during the early stages of membranous fracture healing. These proteins continue to be expressed during the process of bone remodeling, but less prominently. The return of BMP 2-4 and OP-1 immunostaining to baseline intensity coincides with the histological appearance of mature lamellar bone.[3]

Transforming growth factor-beta (TGFs-β) induce normal cells to exhibit neoplastic characteristics through the stimulation of transmembrane receptors and second messengers. A significant amount of data exists to support the role of TGF-β in bone formation and repair. The osteoinductive capacity of TGF-β alone is far less than that of BMP, but studies suggest that this protein may in fact have a role in the potentiation of BMP. TGF-β is synthesized by a number of cells including PMNs, monocytes, platelets, T-lymphocytes and macrophages. It enhances angiogenesis, stimulates collagen synthesis and inhibits its degradation and is chemotactic for fibroblasts and macrophages. Orthopedic animal models of fracture repair in association with exogenous TGF-β have shown augmented healing.

Platelet-derived growth factors (PDGF) and platelet-rich plasma (PRP). PDGF is primarily stored in platelets and released during the clotting cascade. It is angiogenic, a mitogen for fibroblasts and smooth muscle cells and a chemoattractant for PMNs and macrophages. It is composed of two polypeptide chains (A and B), which have been synthesized using recombinant technology. Localization studies demonstrate increased concentrations of PDGF at fracture repair sites, where it is thought to play a role in both osteoblast and osteoclast induction. Although a number of clinical studies have demonstrated a role for PDGF in soft-tissue wound repair, but no definitive evidence exists in regard to fracture repair.[24] The findings related to PDGF and other growth factors released by platelets have stimulated an interest in the role of PRP in fracture repair and reconstruction.

At the present time, basic science in support of the effects of PRP is lacking. Aghaloo et al.[25] studied the effects of PRP on non-critical cranial bone defects in 15 rabbits. The sites were then evaluated with digital subtraction radiography, histologically, and histomorphometry at 1, 2 and 4 months. Their results showed no notable difference with the addition of PRP.

Other Growth Factors

A variety of other growth factors are under investigation in regard to their role in fracture repair (e.g. IGF-I[26] and IGF-II and acidic and basic aFGF and bFGF).[27] It is likely that as technology advances many other similar factors will be identified and their roles delineated in the fracture repair process. All of the growth factors provide exciting possibilities for future applications to traumatic repair of the oral and maxillofacial complex. Recombinant technology allows for the production of large quantities of these proteins, which could potentially be put to clinical use.

Complications of Fracture Healing

The healing of the fracture is sometimes associated with complications like:

- Infection
- Osteomyelitis
- Malunion
- Delayed union
- Non-union.

Infection

The fracture line can get infected due to the following reasons:

- Compound fractures with gross contamination
- Inadequate immobilization
- Loose implants
- Immunocompromised patients, diabetics.

The infection may resolve with the medicinal treatment or get localized to form a localized abscess. The infection can also spread to adjoining tissue planes. Severe bone infections can lead to osteomyelitis. The infection should be prevented by good antibiotic prophylaxis, maintenance of wound hygiene, adequate immobilization, effective management of the teeth involved in the fracture line and ensuring that the implants are not loose. The infection will invariably interfere with the healing of the fracture.

Osteomyelitis

Osteomyelitis is the complication secondary to the infection. If the fracture is comminuted and small fragments of bone are present, which are devoid of the soft tissue attachment, such fragments are likely to turn non-vital and serve as nidus for infection. The fractures of mandible, which are associated with soft tissue laceration, warrant an effective management of the soft tissue trauma. It is being said that the bone is like a plant which has roots in the soft tissue. The bone derives its blood supply from endosteal and periosteal source. The former is disrupted when the fracture occurs. If the periosteum is also separated from it, the bone can undergo avascular necrosis. It is especially true in case of mandible, which is denser and has less collateral circulation than other facial bones. If injudicious stripping of the periosteum is done, while doing the open reduction and in cases of geriatric fractures, the chances of avascular necrosis of the bone are optimized.

The teeth involved in the fracture line always lead to compounding of the fracture intraorally and can lead to contamination and subsequently infection in the fracture line. It is not necessary to extract all the teeth that are involved in the fracture line but there are distinct indications for doing so. The indications for extracting the teeth in the fracture line are:

- Grossly luxated teeth.
- Teeth obstructing the reduction of the fracture.

- Fractured teeth, which are beyond conservation.
- Carious teeth with infective pathologies.

In case the teeth are firm and for cosmetic consideration are decided to be retained, then conservative management like endodontic therapy, splinting, proper local care should be taken to prevent the infection. The teeth which are in the fracture line, but not erupted in oral cavity should not be removed as they do not cause compounding of the fracture.

If the osteomyelitis sets in it should be treated like any other osteomyelitis, immobilization of the jaws with IMF is helpful in healing. During the acute phase of osteomyelitis or when the infection is present the placement of implants like plates, screws should not be attempted. Similarly, the bone grafts should not be used to mend the bony defects subsequent to osteomyelitis when infection is present. Rather it should be done as a second stage surgery after the infection is controlled and adequate soft tissue cover is ensured.

Malunion

The healing of the fracture is an abnormal position is called malunion. It can occur as a result of inadequate reduction, inadequate immobilization or if no treatment is done.[28] The patient often presents with the complaints of inability to masticate, improper occlusion and sometimes poor esthetics. The clinical findings are step deformity in the mandibular arch, extraoral deformity due to hyperplastic callus and derangement of occlusion. The management comprises of surgical exposure of the site, creating a refracture by osteotomising the mandible at the previously fractured site, reduction and recontouring the hyperplastic callus and then reducing the fragments in such a way that satisfactory occlusion is achieved. The fragments are then fixed with internal fixation like miniplates and screws.

Delayed Union and Nonunion

Both these conditions are considered under the same heading because, their etiology is similar. The healing may get delayed due to the following factors.

Local Factors

- Excessive gap or over-riding of the fracture segments.
- Entrapment of soft tissue between the fracture fragments.
- Infection.
- **Inadequate immobilization:** The movement across the fragments does not allow the callus to get stabilized and pseudoarthrosis results rather than bony union.
- Irradiated jaw.
- **Sclerosed bone:** Poor vascularity to the bone delays healing.

Systemic Factors

- Poor general condition, malnourishment.
- Diabetes—where the resistance of the patient against infection is low and the microangiopathy reduces the vascularity.
- Hyperparathyroidism.
- **Old age:** The bones are osteoporotic, vascularity is reduced and the healing potential is low.
- Vitamin D and calcium deficiency.
- Immunosuppression.

The healing is delayed due to any of the above mentioned reasons, the immobilization period is increased to about 8 weeks. If the fracture is treated with RIF, additional IMF may be required to provide rest to the part and avoid stresses on the healing bone. The cause whenever possible must be treated simultaneously. If the infection is present drainage, curettage, extraction of the offending tooth, etc. should be done. If the immobilization is inadequate, it should be corrected. Nutritional deficiencies should be corrected. If there is entrapment of the soft tissue then surgical exploration and removal of intervening tissue may be required.

In case of nonunion, the fragments are united by fibrous tissue rather than the bone and *pseudarthrosis* (false joint) results. The ends of the fragments get covered with cortical bone and the cortical barrier does not allow the fragments to unite. Such ends are called '*eburnated ends*'. The treatment is essentially surgical comprising of surgical exploration of the site, excision of all the fibrous adhesions, freshening of the eburnated ends and fixation of the fragments by rigid means. If the gap between the fragments is wide, to hasten the healing, cancellous bone graft harvested from iliac crest should be placed in the gap. The supportive systemic therapy, additional immobilization with IMF may be given as required in particular case. The hyperbaric oxygen therapy facilitates the healing.

REFERENCES

1. Fridrich KL, Pena-Velasco G, Olson RA. Changing trends with mandibular fractures. A review of 1067 cases. J Oral Maxillofac Surg. 1992; 50:586-9..
2. Teasdale G, Jennett B. Assessment of coma and impaired consciousness. A practical scale. Lancet. 1974;2:81-4..
3. Gilmer TL. A Case of Fracture of the Lower Jaw With Remarks on Treatment, Arch. Dent. 1887;4:388..
4. Gunning TB. Treatment of fractures of the lower jaw by interdental splints. Br J Dent Sci. 1866;9:481..
5. Champy M, Lodde JP, Muster D, et al. Osteosynthesis using miniaturized screwon plates in facial and cranial surgery. Ann Chir Plast Esthet. 1977;22:261-4..
6. Brons R, Boering G. Fracture of the mandibular body treated by stable internal fixation. J Oral Surg. 1970;28:407.
7. Ellis E III, Ghali GE. Lag screw fixation of anterior mandibular fractures. J Oral Maxillofac Surg. 1991;49:13-21.
8. Franc C, Braye F, Ngotene R, et al. Osteosynthesis using intrafocal nailing of low subcondylar fractures in adults. Surgical technics and initial results. Rev Stomatol Chir Maxillofac. 1997;98(1):35-9.
9. Hammer et al. Osteosynthesis of condylar neck fractures: Review of 30 patients.Br J Oral Maxillofac Surg. 1997;35:288.
10. Ulrich Joos, Johannes Kleinheinz. Therapy of condylar neck fractures. International Journal of Oral and Maxillofacial Surgery. 1998;27(4):247-54.
11. Schindeler A, McDonald MM, Bokko P, et al. Bone remodeling during fracture repair: The cellular picture. Semin Cell Dev Biol. 2008;19(5):459-66.
12. Urist MR. Bone: formation by autoinduction. Science. 1965;150(698):893-9.

13. Wolff J, Das Gesetz der. Transformation der Knochen , Hirschwald, Berlin, 1892.
14. Schenk R, Müller J, Willenegger H. Morphological findings in primary fracture healing. Symp Biol Hung. 1967;7:75.
15. Bruce Doll, Matthew Aleef, Jeffrey O. Hollinger. Overview of fracture repair. Musculoskeletal tissue regeneration. Humana Press. 2008:pp. 39-61.
16. Frost HM. The biology of fracture healing: an overview for clinicians. Part I. Clin Orthop Relat Res. 1989;248:283-93.
17. Stanley Wallach. Effects of calcitonin on bone quality and osteoblastic function. Calcified Tissue International. 1993;52(5):335-39.
18. Michael J Gardner. Role of parathyroid hormone in the mechanosensitivity of fracture healing. Journal of Orthopaedic Research. 2007;25(11):1474-80.
19. Wang EA. Bone morphogenetic proteins (BMPs): therapeutic potential in healing bony defects. Trends Biotechnol. 1993; 11(9):379-83.
20. Park SH. O'Connor K, Lin WS. Effect of TGF-[beta]1 and active motion on fracture healing. Journal of Orthopaedic Trauma. 1999;13(4):317.
21. Karachaliou FH, Stamogiannou L. Long bone fracture healing: IGF-I concentrations and specific binding to erythrocytes. J Pediater Endocrinol Metab. 1996; 9(4):491-5.
22. Urist MR, Mikulski A, Lietze A. Solubilized and insolubilized bone morphogenetic protein. Proc Natl Acad Sci USA. 1979;76: 1828-32.
23. Seto I, Asabina I, Oda M, et al. Reconstruction of the primate mandible with a combination graft of recombinant human bone morphogenetic protein-2 and bone marrow. J Oral Maxillofac Surg. 2001;59(1):53-61; discussion 62-3.
24. Andrew JG, Hoyland JA, Freemont AJ, et al. Platelet-derived growth factor expression in normally healing human fractures. Bone. 1995;16(4):455-60.
25. Aghaloo TL, Moy PK, Freymiller EG. Investigation of platelet-rich plasma in rabbit cranial defects: A pilot study. J Oral Maxillofac Surg. 2002;60(10):1176-81.
26. Schmidmaier G, Wildemann B, Gäbelein T, et al. Synergistic effect of IGF-I and TGF-beta1 on fracture healing in rats: single versus combined application of IGF-I and TGF-beta1. Acta Orthop Scand. 2003;74(5):604-10.
27. Simpson AH, et al. The role of growth factors and related agents in accelerating fracture healing. J Bone Joint Surg Br. 2006; 88-B: 701-5.
28. Li Z, Zhang W, Li Z, Li J. Abnormal union of mandibular fractures: A Review of 84 Cases. Journal of Oral and Maxillofacial Surgery. 2006;64(8):1225-31.

21 Fractures of Middle Third of Facial Skeleton

Borle Rajiv M, Arora Aakash, Bhola Nitin, Yadav Abhilasha

The middle third of the facial skeleton is the area between the imaginary lines passing superiorly through the supraorbital ridges and inferiorly through the tip of the maxillary alveolar bone, when the patient is edentulous and through the incisal edges of the teeth when the patient is dentulous (Fig. 21.1).

The middle third of facial skeleton is formed by many small, fragile bones, which articulate with each other in immobile sutural joints. The bones taking part in the formation of the middle third of face are (Fig. 21.2):

- Two maxillae
- Paired nasal bones
- Paired zygomatic bones
- Two ethmoidal bones
- Two lacrimal bones
- A vomer
- Paired palatine bones
- Sphenoid bone.

These bones are further undermined due to presence of anatomical cavities like the air sinuses nasal cavity and orbital cavities. But, in certain areas like the orbital rims the bone is buttressed to protect the vital structure like eye. The bones articulate at the base of the cranial cavity with the cranial bones and thus, the cranial involvement commonly occurs when middle third of facial skeleton fractures occur in severe facial injuries. The middle third of the facial skeleton articulates with the cranial base at three sites, i.e. the frontonasal buttress, the pterygoid plates and the frontozygomatic suture/buttress. These three buttresses are designated as the pillars (like pillars of a building) of the facial skeleton (Figs 21.3A and B). The bone grains are oriented along these buttressing areas and thus, the facial skeleton withstands force/trauma better from the inferior direction than the horizontal direction.

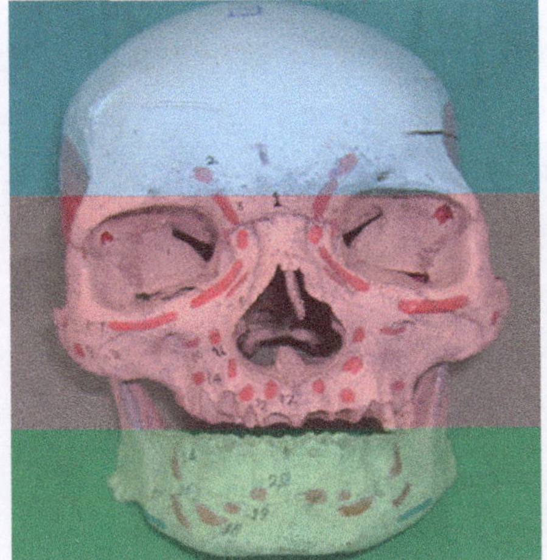

Fig. 21.1: Division of facial skeleton in three parts

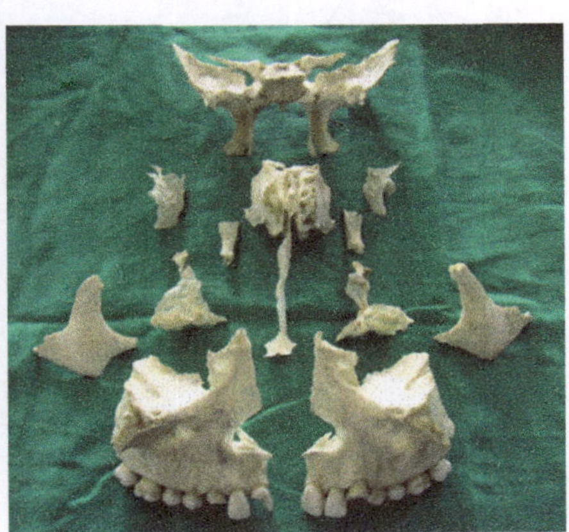

Fig. 21.2: Disarticulated facial bones

PATHOPHYSIOLOGY OF MAXILLOFACIAL INJURIES

The fractures of this area are commonly seen in clinical practice due to increasing

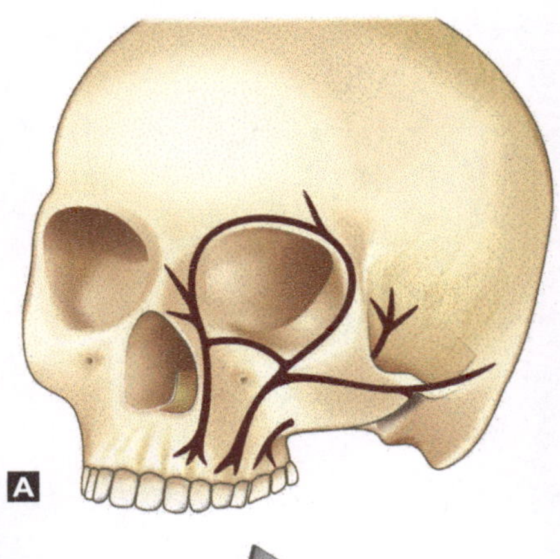

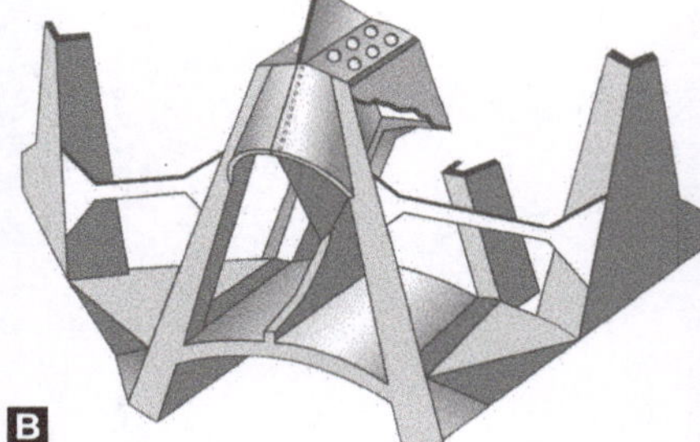

Figs 21.3A and B: The frontonasal buttress, the pterygoid plates and the frontozygomatic suture/buttress

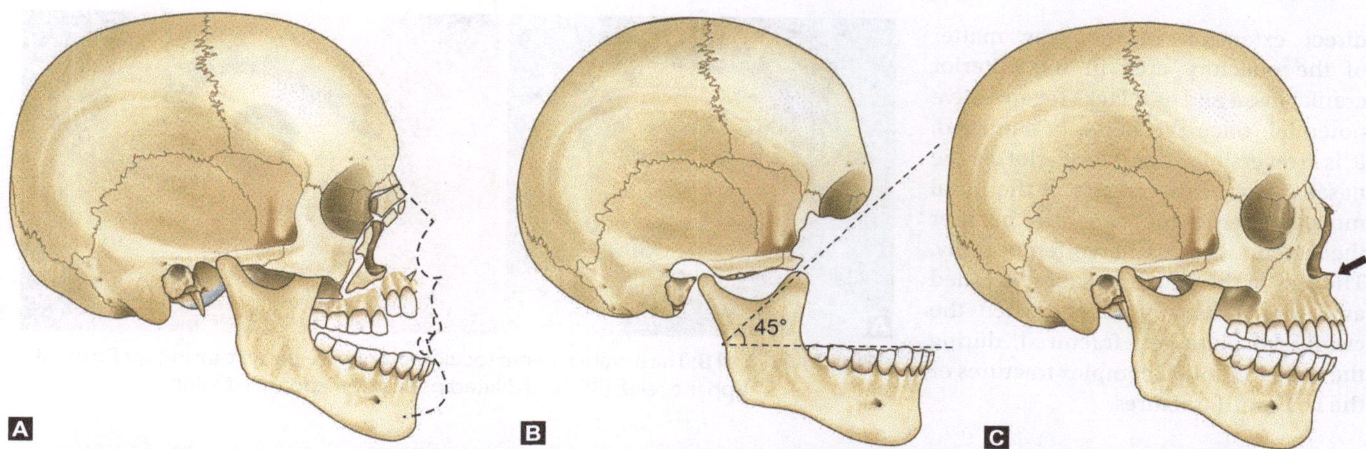

Figs 21.4A to C: (A) Displacement of mid third of facial skeleton posteriorly and downwards, along the slope of the sphenoid; (B) Leading to facial elongation and open bite due to gagging of molars; (C) Showing direction of the force

number of road traffic accidents (RTAs) and interpersonal violence. The face is a precious possession of every individual and everybody cares for it and wants to look good. Thus, inflicting damage to it leaves a psychological dent on the individual and this is the reason that during the assault it becomes a favorite and tempting site to be hit. If the facial fractures are common then the incidence of grievous head injuries should also be high considering their anatomical proximity. But, the nature has given us a protection against it by way of making the facial skeleton weak and fragile. In the event of trauma, the fragile facial bones fracture and absorb the shock and prevent it from being transmitted to the cranium and thus, prevent injury to it. Secondly, if a line is drawn from the nasion to the tip of the mastoid process, it forms an angle of 45 degree with the occlusal plane. It is called the slope of the sphenoid (Figs 21.4A to C). When the facial bones fracture and get displaced along this slope of the sphenoid, posteriorly and downward rather than only posteriorly. Thus, the bones are displaced away from the cranium and injury to the cranium and its contents is prevented. Due to its fragile character the facial skeleton is compared with match box (Fig. 21.5).

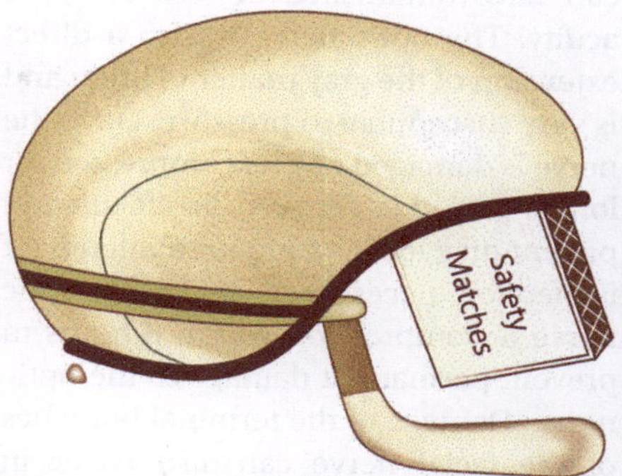

Fig. 21.5: Fragile mid third facial skeleton compared with 'Matchbox'

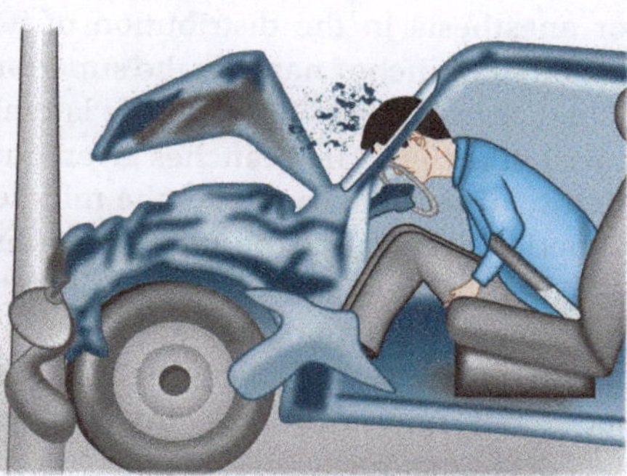

Fig. 21.6: Dashboard injury causing impact on the mid third of facial skeleton

The maxillofacial injuries usually result from what is conventionally called dash board injuries. When a person is traveling in a vehicle at a high velocity and suddenly the vehicle comes to stand still, due to the gathered momentum (inertia) the driver is thrown forward and his head strikes against the dash board and the middle third of the face gets traumatized. Similarly the chest gets traumatized against the steering wheel resulting in injuries to the rib cage (Fig. 21.6). This is called *coup-counter-coup* injury or acceleration declaration injury. The arrangement of the facial bones and the bone grains are such that the middle third of the face tolerates the forces better from the inferior direction than the anteroposterior direction. The masticatory forces are transmitted along the bone grains around the anatomical cavities to the base of the skull and are disturbed over a large area, due to the peculiar orientation of the bone grains.

INVOLVEMENT OF VARIOUS STRUCTURES DURING MIDDLE THIRD FRACTURES

During the middle third facial fractures various anatomical structures in this area are traumatized. They are as follows.

Involvement of the Nerves

Various nerves pass through the facial bones which are involved during the fractures of the middle third of facial skeleton.

Olfactory Nerve

The olfactory nerves are multiple, small nerves that pass through the cribriform plate of the ethmoid bone and supply the olfactory perception area situated at the roof of the nasal cavity. They are responsible for carrying the smell sensation. The olfactory nerve is the direct extension of the gray matter of the olfactory area in the anterior cranial fossa and as it lacks regenerative potential, once the nerve is damaged, it is irreversible. The blood clot in the nasal cavity or the edema of the nasal mucous membrane can also hamper the function of this nerve temporarily. The loss of the smell sensation is called anosmia. It usually occurs when the cribriform plate gets fractured, during the nasoethmoidal complex fractures or the Le Fort III fractures.

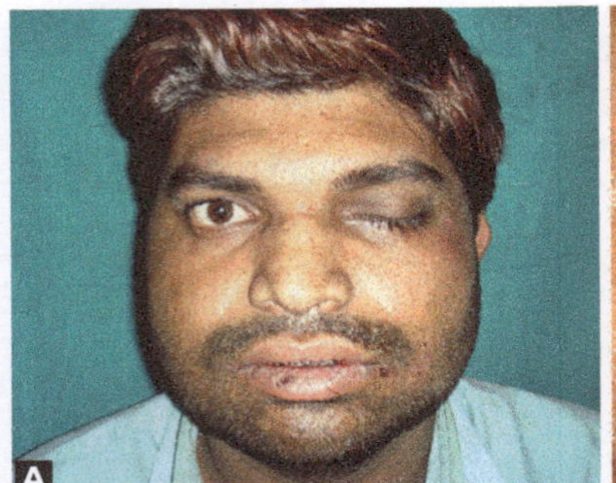
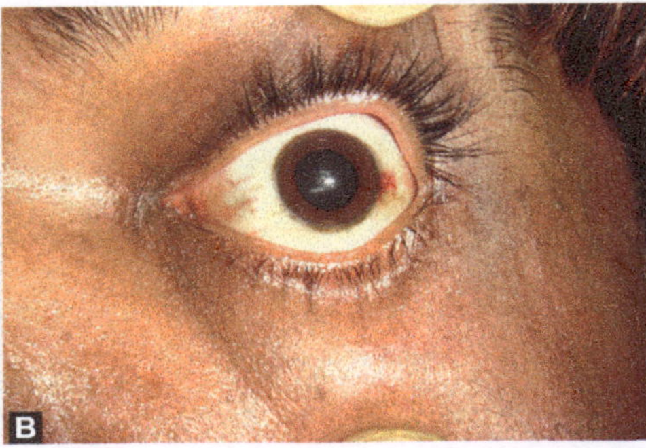

Figs 21.7A and B: Third cranial nerve (oculomotor nerve palsy) causing (A) Ptosis of upper eyelid; (B) Fixed dilated pupil nonresponsive to light

Infraorbital Nerve

The infraorbital nerve is involved in the Le Fort II fractures, zygomatic fractures and the orbital floor fractures. It is manifested in the form of hypoesthesia or anesthesia in the distribution of its terminal branches namely, the superior labial, inferior palpebral and the lateral nasal branches. The branches given out in the infraorbital canal, i.e. the middle superior alveolar and the anterosuperior alveolar are also involved producing numbness in the maxillary anterior and premolar teeth and the gingiva. The latter two nerves are also involved in Le Fort I fracture.

The III (Oculomotor), IV (Trochlear), VI (Abduscent) Cranial Nerves

These three nerves are collectively called oculomotor nerves. These nerves are involved when the fractures of the orbital walls take place and the nerves get compressed in the superior orbital fissure due to hematoma, bony fragments or as a result of direct injury to them. It produces paresis of the extraocular muscles producing 'external ophthalmoplegia' (loss of movements of the eyeball) and diplopia. The blockade of the parasympathetic supply to the eye, which comes from the Edinger-Westphal nucleus, via the IIIrd cranial nerve is disrupted and results into a fixed dilated pupil, not responding to light, ptosis of upper eyelid (Figs 21.7A and B). The fixed dilated pupil, not responding to light leads to paralysis of accommodation (internal ophthalmoplagia). The second cranial nerve (optic nerve) is well guarded by the thick cortication of the optic foramen and is not usually traumatized. However, if there is retrobulbar bleed or the fractured segments get displaced and impinge upon the nerve, the patient can have diminished or loss of visual acuity. The optic nerve is also a direct extension of the gray matter of brain and is very susceptible to pressure. Once the nerve is damaged or gets compressed for longer period its recovery is difficult and patient may loose vision permanently. It is therefore necessary to undertake optic nerve decompression within 6 hours to prevent permanent damage to the optic nerve. Damage to the terminal branches of the facial nerve can also occur in compound zygomatic fractures.

Cranial Involvement

The involvement of the cranial cavity in the middle third fractures is not an uncommon phenomenon. In severe mid facial trauma the fracture of the cribriform plate results in cerebrospinal fluid leakage in the nose producing CSF rhinorrhea (Fig. 21.8). The anterior fossa injury produces bilateral circumorbital ecchymosis (Raccoon's eye) (Figs 21.9A and B). The fracture of the base of the skull produces bleeding per ear, hematotympanum (blood behind tympanic membrane), CSF otorrhea and the *Battle's sign* (ecchymosis over the mastoid process in absence of evidence of direct trauma to it). Battle's sign, is also an indication of fracture of the base of the middle cranial fossa and may suggest underlying brain trauma. Battle's sign consists of bruising over

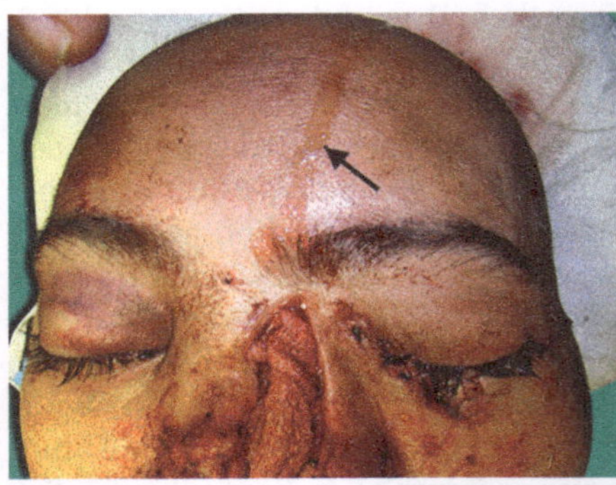

Fig. 21.8: Cerebrospinal fluid rhinorrhea. Arrow showing clear CSF flowing out of the fracture site

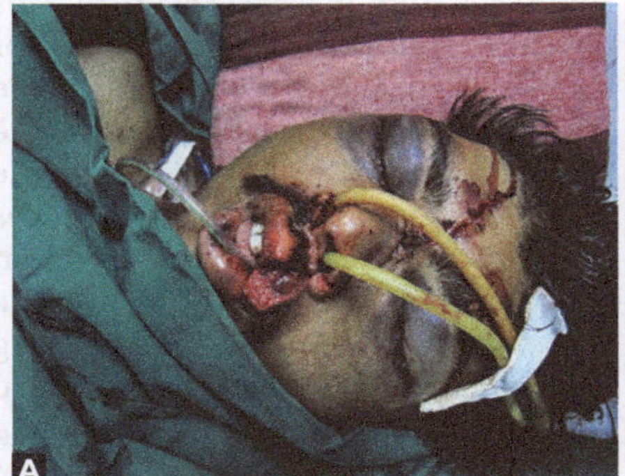
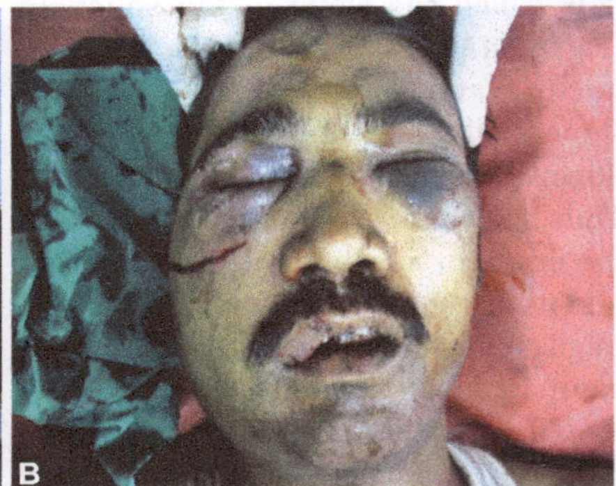

Figs 21.9A and B: Bilateral black eye (Raccoon's eye)

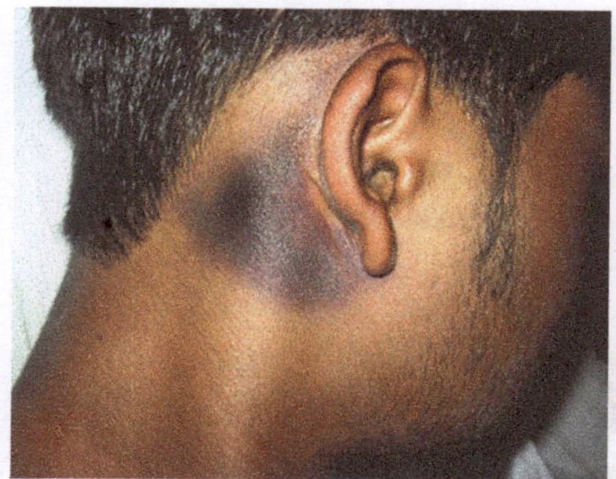

Fig. 21.10: Ecchymosis over the mastoid area (Battle's sign)

the mastoid process, as a result of extravasation of blood along the path of the posterior auricular artery.[1] The sign is named after William Henry Battle (Fig. 21.10). The danger associated with such cranial involvement is spread of the infection in the cranial cavity, producing meningitis to brain abscess. The other types of the head injuries like intercranial bleeding, cerebral concussion, cerebral contusion or laceration produces cerebral edema and compression may be present, which deserves treatment on priority as they can be life-threatening. In a polytrauma patient the treatment needs to be prioritized. The life saving treatment should be undertaken first and the management of facial fractures can be delayed until the patient is stable.

Involvement of the Blood Vessels

The major blood vessels are not involved, but the branches of the internal maxillary artery are involved producing hemorrhage from the injury sites and the epistaxis.

Involvement of the Paranasal Air Sinuses

The involvement of the maxillary sinus occurs in Le Fort I and II fractures, zygomatic fractures, blow out orbital fractures, producing epistaxis due to bleeding in the sinus, which escapes in the nose through the osteum maxillary. The surgical emphysema is produced due to leakage of the air in the soft tissue planes. In case of Le Fort II, III fractures, nasoethmoidal fractures, blow out fractures of the orbit involving in the medial wall, ethmoidal air cells get exposed and the infection occur, which can extend intracranially, through the emissary veins producing intracranial infections.

Involvement of the Orbit

During the Le Fort II, III fractures, zygomatic fractures and the orbital wall fractures, the orbit and its contents are involved. The bleeding that occurs due to the fractured bone travels in the subperiosteal plane and escapes in the subconjuctival plane to manifest as subconjuctival hemorrahage which is bright red in color and as the source of bleeding is subperiosteal its posterior extent is not seen (Figs 21.11A and B). If the blood escapes in the subcutaneous plane it produces circumorbital ecchymosis (Black eye) (Fig 21.12). When the orbital walls are displaced outwards, the orbital volume increases. The retracting action of the extraocular muscles draws the eyeball inside and enophthalmos is produced. When the orbital walls are displaced inward, the orbital size decreases and the eyeball is pushed out leading to proptosis. The entrapment of the extraocular muscles in the fracture fragments hampers their action and the eyeball fails to move in a particular direction depending on which muscle is involved. The eyeball on the unaffected side moves freely and the eyeball on the affected side fails to reciprocate leading to disruption of the focal axis, producing parallax between the images, resulting in double image perception of the single object (*double vision or diplopia*). The binocular diplopia occurs due to the vertical imbalance of the globe whereas the monocular diplopia results because of hemorrhage in the anterior chamber of the eye, mostly due to the detachment of the lens which requires immediate intervention unlike the binocular diplopia, which results due to either muscle entrapment or retrobular hemorrhage, which resolves with time and the diplopia could be reversed.

A similar kind of phenomena occurs when the III, IV or VI cranial nerves are involved. The paresis of the nerve leads to paralysis of the corresponding extraocular muscle and eyeball fails to move in that direction producing diplopia. The orbital walls, especially the inferior and the medial, are thin and fragile. The eyeball is non-compressible structure and thus, when the intraorbital pressure increases as a result of trauma, these fragile walls give way and blow out fracture of orbit results. As a result of this fracture the orbital size increases and the orbital contents herniate outside, causing retraction of the eyeball resulting in enophthalmos.

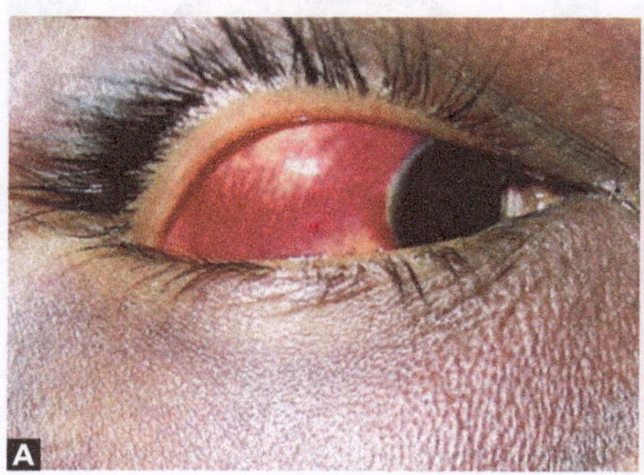

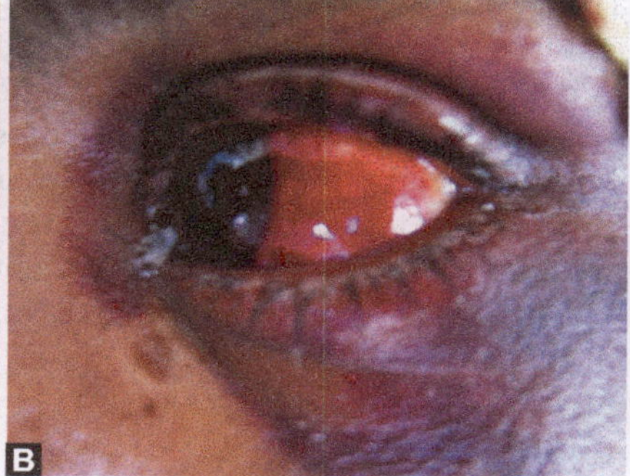

Figs 21.11A and B: Subconjunctival hemorrhage, note the flame shape, posterior boundary not seen and bright-red color

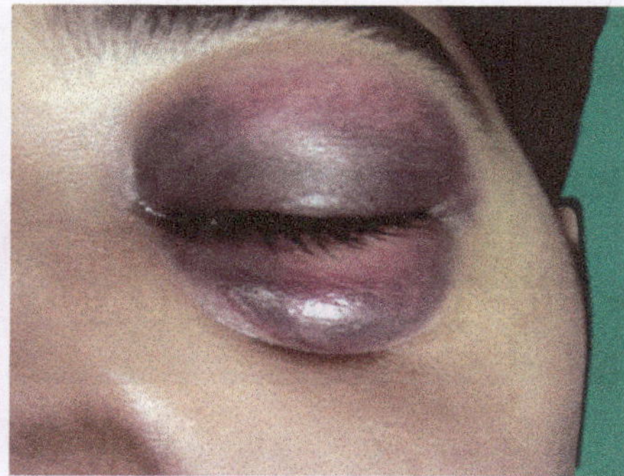

Fig. 21.12: Black eye (circumorbital ecchymosis) blackish-red in color

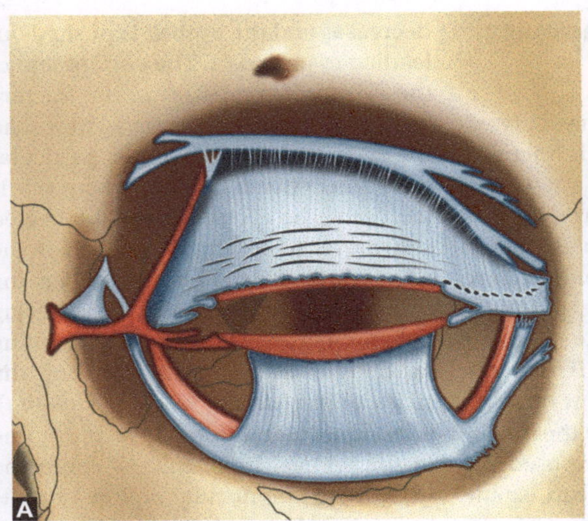

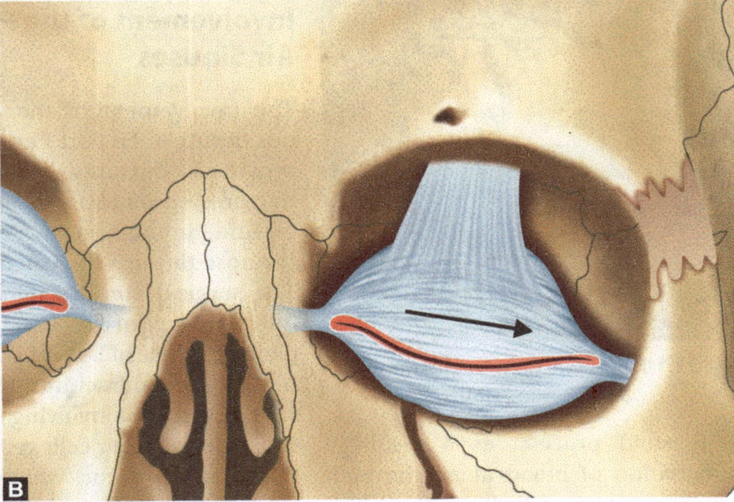

Figs 21.13A and B: (A) Suspensory ligament of lockwood; (B) Its displacement inferiorly produces hypoglobus and hooding of the globe

The eyeball is supported from the inferior side by the suspensory ligament of Lockwood, which is attached medially to the frontal process of maxillary bone and laterally to the Whitnall's tubercle present on the orbital process of the zygomatic bone. Whenever, the fracture occurs superior to the Whitnall's tubercle and the zygoma is displaced inferiorly, the eyeball also sinks down producing alteration in the level of globe (hypoglobus). The lateral canthal ligament moves inferiorly along with the fracture fragment and the upper lid also follows it and produces a characteristic 'Hooding of the globe' (Figs 21.13A and B), which becomes obvious after the initial edema subsides.

More severe orbital injuries are superior orbital fissure syndrome (involvement of III, IV, V, VI cranial nerves in the superior orbital fissure) and orbital apex syndrome (all the nerves in the superior orbital fissure syndrome plus the involvement of the optic nerve).

CLASSIFICATION OF THE FRACTURES OF THE MIDDLE THIRD (ROWE AND WILLIAMS[2])

The fractures are classified as given in Table 21.1.

Table 21.1: Rowe and Williams' classification of midface fractures

1. Central area fractures
   A. Those involving occlusion:
      i. Dentoalveolar fractures
      ii. Le Fort I fracture
      iii. Le Fort II fracture
      iv. Le Fort III fracture
   B. Those not involving occlusion:
      i. Fracture of the nasal bones
      ii. Fracture of the frontal process of the maxilla
      iii. Fracture of the lacrimal bone
      iv. Fracture of the ethmoidal bone
      v. Combination of I, II, III, IV
2. Lateral area fractures
   A. Zygomatic bone fractures
   B. Zygomatic arch fractures
   C. Orbital fractures:
      i. Blow out fractures—pure, impure
      ii. Blow in fracture

DENTOALVEOLAR FRACTURE

The fracture of the alveolar bone along with the injuries to the teeth is termed as dentoalveolar fracture. There can be a simple linear fracture of the alveolus or a severe comminution of the alveolar bone. The teeth are also injured leading to their fracture, luxation, displacement or avulsion. The injuries to the teeth can be classified as:

- Luxation—instrusive, extrusive
- Proclination
- Retroclination
- Traumatic exfoliation or avulsion (Fig. 21.14).

The fractures of the teeth can be further classified as:

- Class I—those involving only enamel.
- Class II—those involving the enamel and dentine.
- Class III—those involving enamel, dentine and pulp
- Class IV—fracture at the cervical level.
- Class V—fracture of the root below the cervical level.

The dentoalveolar injuries are caused by RTA, assault, fall, sports injuries and are commonly seen in the clinical practice. In the anterior region these are caused by a hard and blunt object when

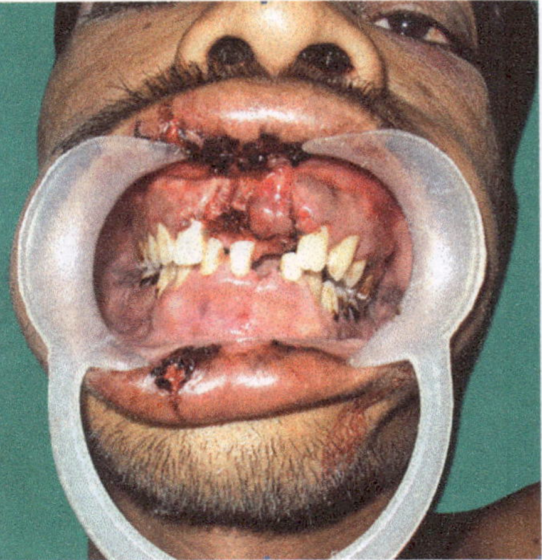

Fig. 21.14: Dentoalveolar fracture with traumatic avulsion of the incisors

it strikes the maxilla at lower level. In the posterior area they are caused by similar cause, but are rare. The posterior area can also be traumatized by accidental fracture of the dentoalveolar segment during the extraction of the maxillary posterior teeth. The clinical features are:

- Bleeding per orally
- The upper lip is traumatized between the object and the teeth, alveolus and hence there is abrasion/contusion or laceration of the lip. The lip is edematous and the mucosal aspect of the lip shows laceration or ecchymosis.
- The gingivae are lacerated and bleeding is seen from its margins.
- The teeth are traumatized and may show fracture/displacement/mobility and the occlusion is deranged.
- The luxated teeth come in the way of occlusion, especially when they are retroclined and the patient is unable to close the jaw.
- The intraoral periapical X-ray shows widening of the lamina dura and fracture line on the alveolar bone.
- In severe intrusive displacement, the root may perforate the nasal floor and is seen in the nasal cavity.
- The patient complains of pain and sensitivity especially when the teeth are fractured.
- The teeth turn nonvital due to the damage to the periapical vessels.

Management

The management of the dentoalveolar fracture comprises of two steps:

1. Reduction and splinting of the luxated teeth.
2. Conservation of the traumatized teeth.

Reduction and Splinting of the Luxated Teeth

The teeth, which are displaced are reduced in their normal position and to facilitate the healing, they are splinted till the healing takes place. The soft tissue injuries are also managed simultaneously. The lacerations of the lip are sutured. If the tooth is fractured and the fragment is lost and if the patient has lacerated wound (LW) on the inner side of the lip, then *before closing the laceration, the lip must be carefully inspected and palpated as the tooth fragments may be embedded in the lip laceration.* The lacerated gingiva should be sutured. The teeth are splinted after reduction by any of the following methods:

- Figure of 8 wiring
- Essig's wiring
- Ligation of arch bar
- Using splints—lateral compression splint
- Composite resin splints
- Lead foil splinting (not practical).

Conservation of the Fractured Teeth

The traumatized teeth are examined for vitality as the nonvital teeth can serve as nidus for infection, elective endodontic therapy should be undertaken. The restoration of the teeth is done subsequently.

FRACTURES OF MAXILLA

Rene Le Fort[1] (1902), studied the fractures produced on the cadaver after hitting it with heavy stones and upon autopsy that a typical pattern of injuries were produced, depending upon the level of the impact. He described three types of fracture lines and they are eponymously named as Le Fort I, II or III fracture lines. One must remember that these fracture lines which are described are standard patterns but, no injury is ideal, or no two injuries are identical or no two individuals can have similar bony configurations. The severity of the trauma, strength of bone, nature of object causing injury and its velocity vary and thus, in the clinical practice some deviations from what is classically described in the textbooks is observed. However, for understanding the deviations from the normal, the normal pattern must be known.

Le Fort I Fracture

The Le Fort I fracture is also called Guérin fracture or a low level horizontal fracture. As the fracture line runs below the zygomatic bone it is also called subzygomatic fracture. This type of fracture is produced due to the maxillary trauma at a lower level from the anterior or anterolateral direction (Fig. 21.15). The fracture could be unilateral or bilateral. The bilateral Le Fort I fracture is also called *'Floating maxilla'*.

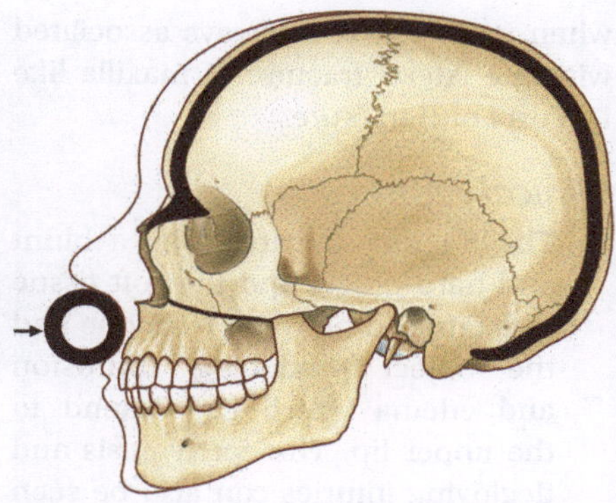

Fig. 21.15: Lower level of impact causing Le Fort I fracture line

The classical Le Fort I line starts from the lateral margin of the pyriform aperture, at the junction of the superior thin portion and the inferior thick portion, which forms the line of weakness. The fracture line then runs laterally on the anterior surface of the maxilla, above the apices of the teeth, crosses the canine fossa superior to it to reach the zygomaticomaxillary buttress. The buttress is a thick, condensed area and thus, the fracture line curls around it and continues over the posterolateral wall of the maxillary sinus, then it crosses the pterygomaxillary fissure and fractures the pterygoid plates at the junction of the lower one-third with the upper two-third (Figs 21.16A to D). This is the fracture line on the lateral side. The fracture line also runs on the medial side, i.e. on the lateral nasal wall and runs posteriorly on it to reach the lateral fracture line at the pterygoid plates. When a bilateral fracture line is produced, the whole lower maxilla gets detached from rest of the facial skeleton and moves freely, thus the name, floating maxilla. It may be associated with the mid palatine split. The mid palatine split cannot occur in an isolated way and when it is seen it is always associated with the lateral fracture of maxilla like Le Fort I or II fracture.

Clinical Features

- The fracture is caused by a blunt and hard object and the soft tissue gets crushed between the bone and the object producing contusion and edema which can extend to the upper lip. The ecchymosis and degloving injuries can also be seen in the gingivolabial sulcus.
- There is tenderness, step and crepitus in the gingivolabial sulcus on lateral margin of the pyriform aperture and anterior surface of maxilla.
- As the fracture line passes over the walls of the maxillary sinus, there is bleeding in the maxillary sinus, which escapes in the nasal cavity through the osteum maxillary, producing epistaxis.
- The anterior and middle superior alveolar nerves are traumatized, which results in heaviness in the anterior teeth and gingiva.
- There is an ecchymosis on the zygomaticomaxillary buttress area, step formation and tenderness.
- An ecchymosis over the junction of hard and soft palate may be seen which is called Guérin sign[3] (Alphonse François Marie Guérin) (Figs 21.17A and B).
- The maxilla gets displaced posteriorly and downwards causing derangement of occlusion.
- When the maxilla is palpated bimanually, keeping the thumb and index finger of the left hand on the lower one-third of the maxilla on either side and the anterior teeth and alveolus are grasped with the thumb and the index finger of the right hand and the jaw is moved anteroposteriorly, the movements are felt by the fingers of the left hand kept on the anterior surface of the maxilla (Fig. 21.18). In cases of bilateral fracture the movements are felt bilaterally and are free, giving the maxilla floating appearance.

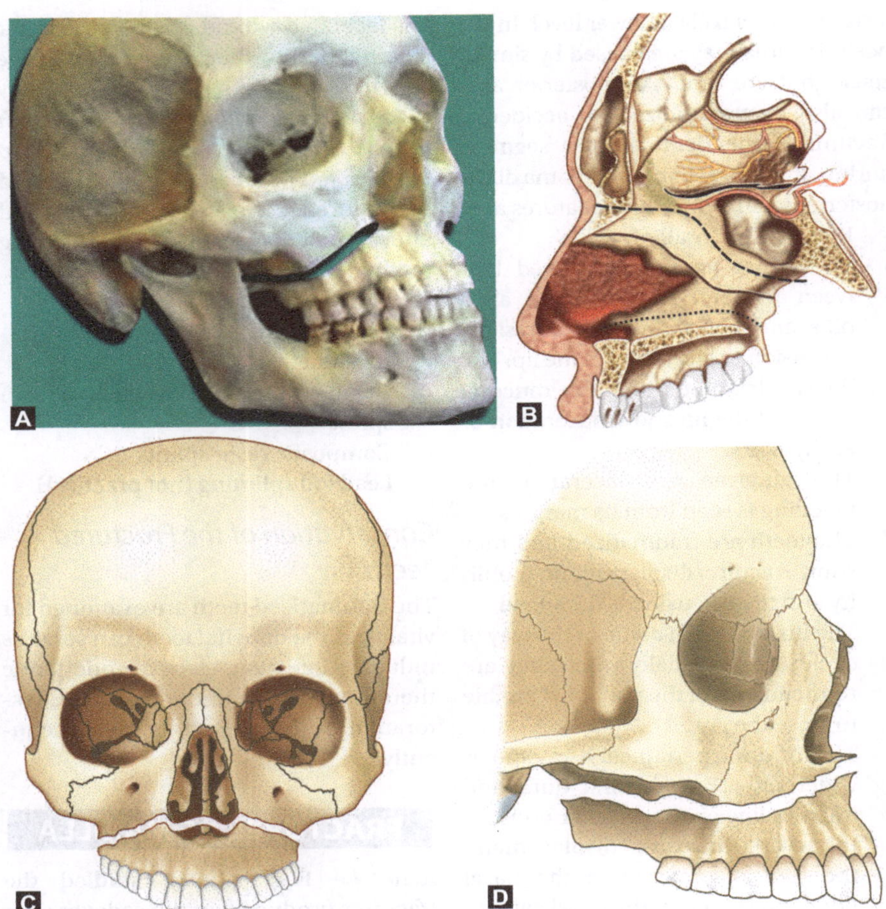

Figs 21.16A to D: Le Fort I fracture line

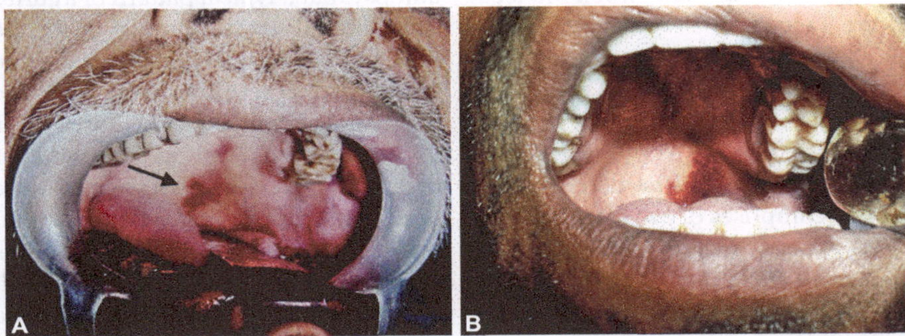

Figs 21.17A and B: Ecchymosis at the junction of hard and soft palate 'Guérin sign'

- When the maxillary teeth are percussed a typical crack pot sound is produced.

The Le Fort fractures are not properly seen on the X-ray. The X-ray paranasal sinus (PNS) shows break in continuity in the lateral wall of the nasal aperture, haziness in the maxillary sinus, step or broken cortication in the zygomatic buttress area. The fracture line over the anterior maxillary wall is not clearly seen due to super imposition of various cranial and spinal shadows. The true lateral view also shows the fracture line, but again not very clearly. The CT scans in both, the axial and coronal sections

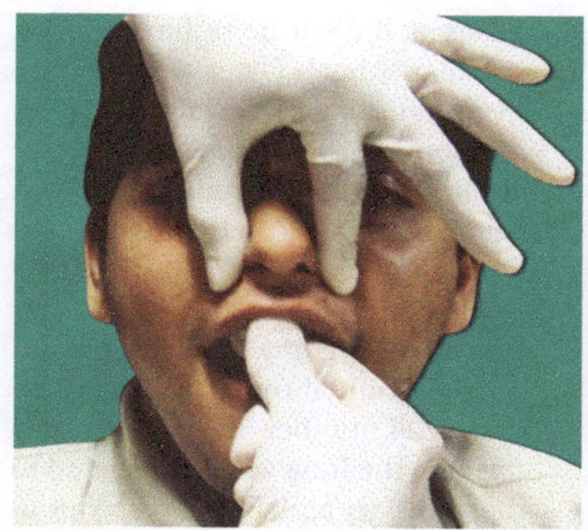

Fig. 21.18: Bimanual palpation for Le Fort I fracture, one hand grasps the maxilla and elicits the mobility, while the fingers of the other hand kept lateral to the pyriform fossa feel the abnormal mobility

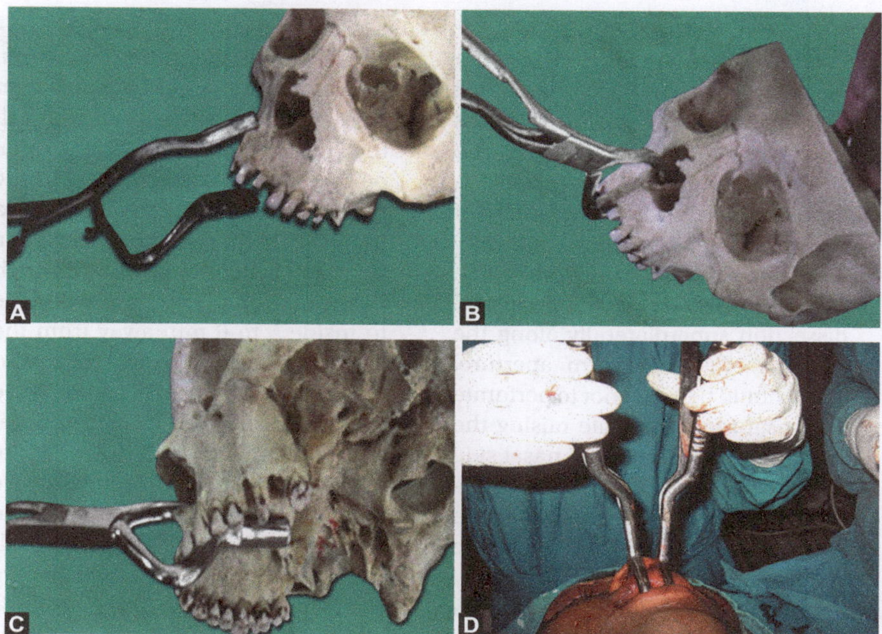

Figs 21.19A to D: Application of the Rowe's disimpaction forceps

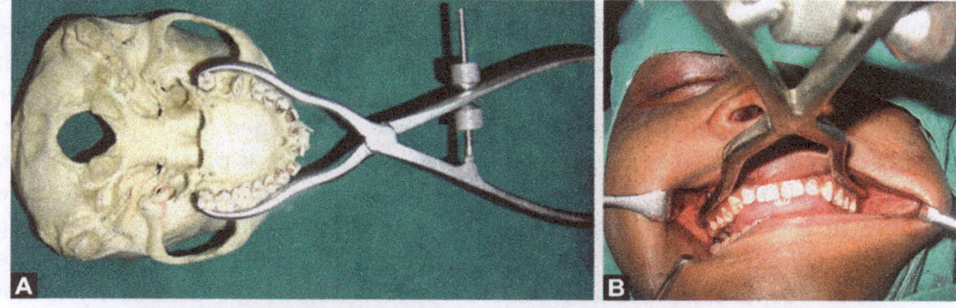

Figs 21.20 A and B: (A) Application of the Hayton-William's disimpaction forceps; (B) Application of the Hayton-William's forceps

are very helpful and show the fracture lines clearly. The 3D reconstruction of the CT scans can be very informative.

Management of the Le Fort I Fracture

The Le Fort I fractures are managed by:

- Closed reduction and immobilization by:
  - Internal suspension
  - External suspension
- Open reduction and fixation with plates and screws.

Proper disimpaction of the fracture and its reduction is very important to achieve proper occlusal relationship and for restoring the facial symmetry, prior to fixation. The reduction is done using a pair of Row's maxillary disimpaction forceps (Figs 21.19A to D). The operator stands behind the head of the patient and the Row's disimpaction forceps are applied to hold the maxillae bilaterally by placing its beaks on the nasal floor and the curved beak goes over the maxillary anterior teeth and rests on the hard palate. The beaks are padded to prevent trauma to the mucosa. The maxillae are disimpacted by applying forceps which are directed backwards towards the operator, giving downwards and side to side rocking movements and then reduced by applying traction in the anterosuperior direction. The Hayton-William's maxilla holding forceps can also be used for reduction of the fractured maxilla but, it can move the fractured segment only in anteroposterior plane and proper disimpaction cannot be achieved. It is not suitable in case of maxillary fractures with mid palatine splits as the maxillae tend to get collapsed due to the lateral pressure applied by these forces (Figs 21.20A and B). The Hayton-William's forceps are more suitable for the manipulation of maxilla during the Le Fort osteotomies. The guidance for proper reduction is achievement of satisfactory occlusion.

When there is unilateral Le Fort I fracture, the fractured maxilla is reduced and then sandwiched between the mandible and the contralateral intact maxilla with intermaxillary fixation (IMF). The contralateral, intact maxilla prevents pulling down of the fractured maxilla when the mandible is depressed. This is called '*Sandwich technique*'.

When the fracture is bilateral, only IMF is not adequate as the depression of the mandible will pull dawn the fractured maxilla. Hence, the fractured maxilla needs to be fixed against the intact facial bones superior to the fracture line. This is achieved by either internal suspension or external suspension.

Internal suspension

- **Pyriform fossa wiring:** A degloving incision is placed in the labial vestibule anteriorly and full thickness mucoperiosteal flap is raised. The anterior surface of the maxilla is exposed and the lateral boundary of the pyriform aperture is identified by identifying the anterior nasal spine and then carrying the subperiosteal dissection superolaterally along the margins of the pyriform aperture. Care should be taken not to perforate the nasal mucosa, while raising the *mucoperiosteum* from the nasal side of the aperture. The nasal mucous membrane is reflected and the lateral wall of the pyriform aperture is exposed. Keeping a guard medially to protect the nasal mucosa a hole is drilled from lateral side, 5 to 6 mm apart from the lateral boundary of pyriform aperture to prevent fracture of the bony margin. A piece of 24 gauge stainless steel wire is passed through the hole and both the ends of the wire are drawn in the oral cavity, through the vestibular incision. The wire ends are legated to the arch bar or Ivy loop in the maxillary arch, after the IMF is achieved in the desired position (Fig. 21.21).

  This suspension prevents the downward displacement of the maxilla when the mandible is depressed. The incision is closed and the wires project through the incision line in the oral cavity.

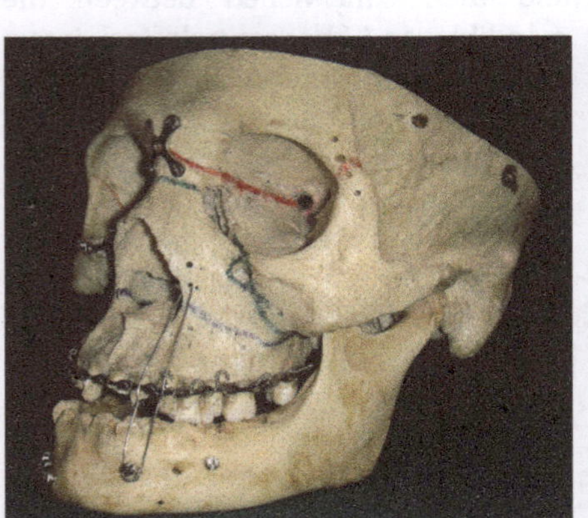

Fig. 21.21: Pyriform fossa wiring

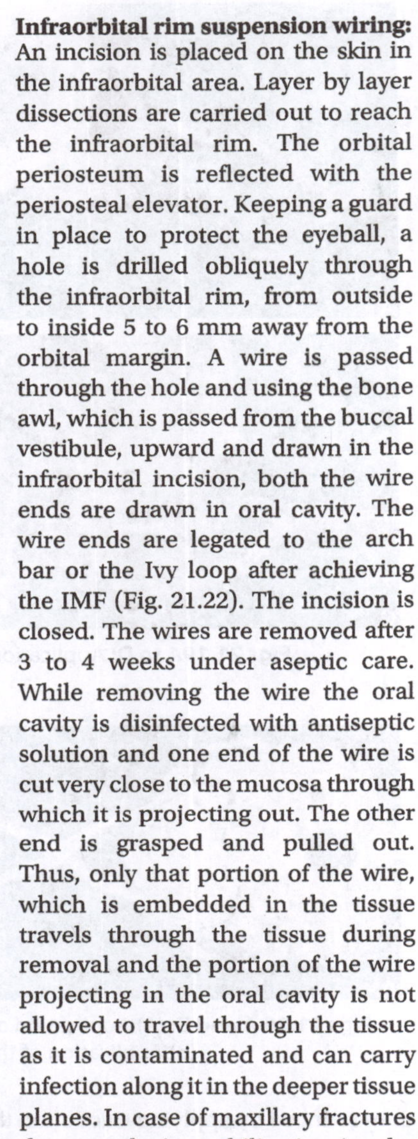

- **Infraorbital rim suspension wiring:** An incision is placed on the skin in the infraorbital area. Layer by layer dissections are carried out to reach the infraorbital rim. The orbital periosteum is reflected with the periosteal elevator. Keeping a guard in place to protect the eyeball, a hole is drilled obliquely through the infraorbital rim, from outside to inside 5 to 6 mm away from the orbital margin. A wire is passed through the hole and using the bone awl, which is passed from the buccal vestibule, upward and drawn in the infraorbital incision, both the wire ends are drawn in oral cavity. The wire ends are legated to the arch bar or the Ivy loop after achieving the IMF (Fig. 21.22). The incision is closed. The wires are removed after 3 to 4 weeks under aseptic care. While removing the wire the oral cavity is disinfected with antiseptic solution and one end of the wire is cut very close to the mucosa through which it is projecting out. The other end is grasped and pulled out. Thus, only that portion of the wire, which is embedded in the tissue travels through the tissue during removal and the portion of the wire projecting in the oral cavity is not allowed to travel through the tissue as it is contaminated and can carry infection along it in the deeper tissue planes. In case of maxillary fractures three weeks immobilization is adequate as the flat bone having good vascularity heals faster.

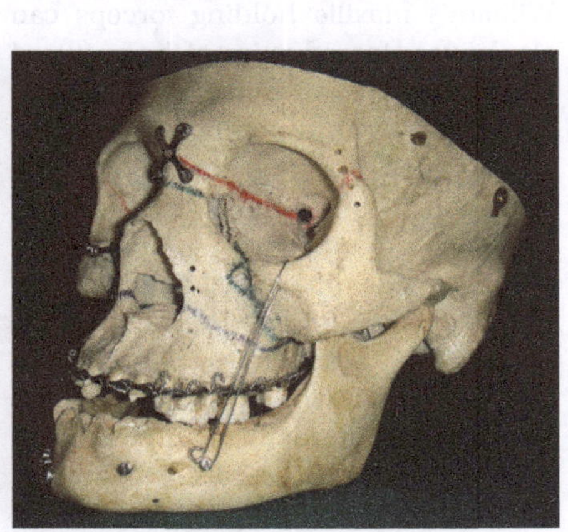

Fig. 21.22: Infraorbital rim suspension wiring

- **Zygomatic suspension wiring:** An incision is placed in the buccal vestibule in the molar area. A subperiosteal dissection is carried out along the bone to expose the zygomatic buttress. The maxillary process of zygoma is identified and a through and through hole is drilled in it. A 24 number SS wire is passed through the hole which is legated to the maxillary arch bar or Ivy loops to achieve the zygomatic suspension. This suspension wiring is very useful in firmly stabilizing the maxilla along with the pyriform aperture wiring or plating, not only in cases of Le Fort I fracture, but also in cases of Le Fort I osteotomies.
- **Circumzygomatic wiring:** The wire is passed around the zygomatic arch to suspend the fractured maxilla. It is mandatory to rule out fracture of the zygomatic arch before the wiring is done, by good clinical examination and the submentovertex radiographs. The fracture of the arch is contraindication for this wiring. In this technique a small 0.5 cm incision is taken superior to the zygomatic arch and the tissues are dissected up to the superior border of the arch. An Obwegeser bone awl is passed through the incision lateral to the arch, directing it inferiorly and slightly anteriorly until it is drawn intraorally in the buccal vestibule. A 24-gauge stainless steel wire is fed in the eye of the awl and secured by giving few twists. The awl is retracted back slowly without withdrawing it fully through incision. As the tip of the awl reaches the superior border of the arch, the awl is reinserted in the same direction, medially to the arch and drawn through the same site intraorally. Both the ends of the wire are ligated to the arch bar or the Ivy loop in the maxillary arch (Figs 21.23A to D). While doing the circumferential wiring it must be remembered that the wire must pass very closely to the bone and no soft

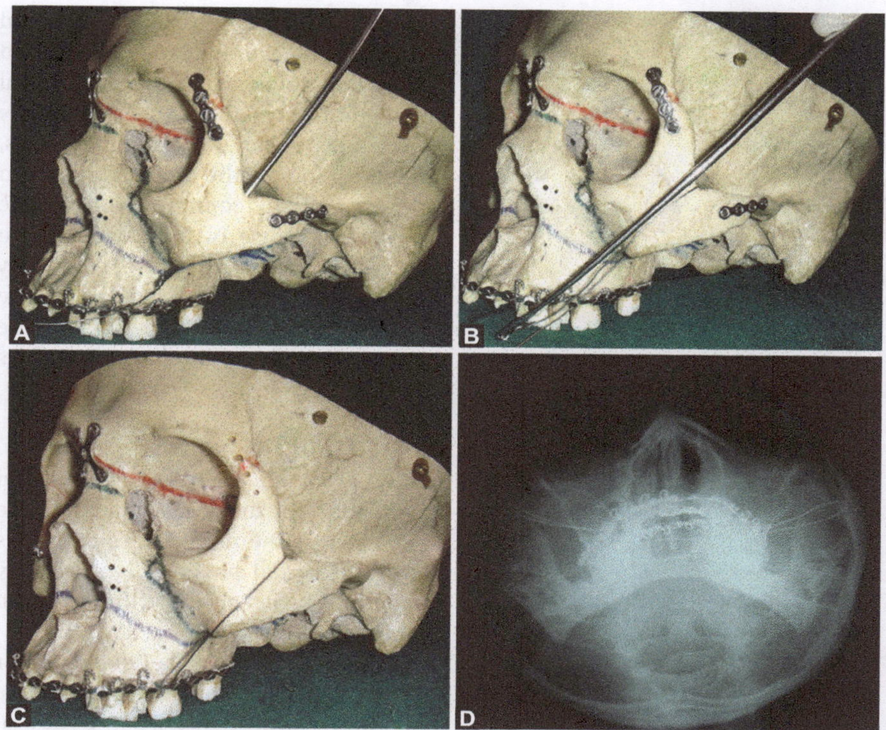

Figs 21.23A to D: Circumzygomatic wiring using *Obwegeser bone* awl

tissue should be trapped between the wire and the bone, as the pressure necrosis can occur and the patient may experience pain. Proper hygiene must be maintained around the wire to prevent infection and the wires are removed under aseptic care after 3 to 4 weeks.

- **Supraorbital rim suspension wiring:** In this technique a lateral eyebrow incision is taken. The tissues are dissected layer by layer till the bone is reached. The orbital periosteum is reflected and keeping a guard in place, a through and through hole is drilled in the supraorbital rim. A wire is passed through the hole. A long bone awl is taken and passed percutaneously through the incision inferiorly and it is drawn intraorally in the buccal vestibule. Rest of the procedure is same as in case of any other suspension wiring (Fig. 21.24).

External suspension

The external suspension wiring is done by using the plaster of Paris (POP) head

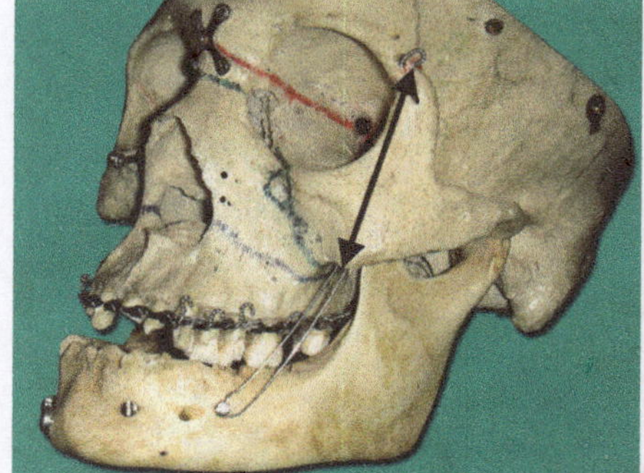

Fig. 21.24: Supraorbital rim wiring

frames or hallows and cheek wiring. The prefabricated frames are fixed to the shaved head using a POP roll. The head frame has a cap like projection. A bone awl is passed from the buccal vestibule to the skin surface 1′ below the outer canthus of the eye. A stainless steel wire (24–26 number) is passed in the oral cavity, using the awl. The extraoral end of the wire is legated to the head frame and the intraoral end is legated to the arch bar or Ivy loop in the maxillary arch (Fig. 21.25). The wire is used to give anterior and superior traction to the

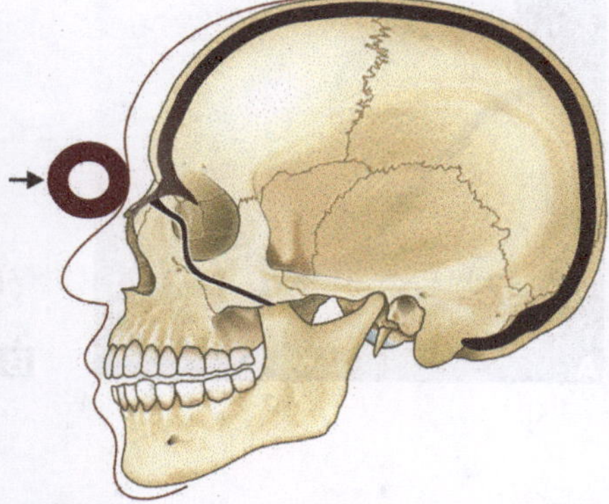

Fig. 21.25: Impact at the level of base of nose causing Le Fort II fracture

maxilla. The head frame can also be used for anchoring the universal rods with the help of the universal joints (Figs 21.26A to E). A rod suspended from the frame anteriorly can also be used for giving anterior traction to the maxilla when it is displaced posteriorly and is impacted. The external suspension wirings are basically indicated for the Le Fort III fractures or other Le Fort fractures where there is poly trauma and facial skeleton is fractured at multiple sites or when there is gross comminution, which prevents/contradicts the internal suspension wirings.

Open reduction

The Le Fort I fracture can be treated by open reduction. This is very effective modality and avoids morbidity to the patient, which occurs as a result of the IMF and suspension wiring. The internal suspension is better tolerated than the external suspension as the projecting wires, POP head cap, head frame are very uncomfortable to the patient. The head frame and the POP head cap tend to get loose, impinge upon the skin, cause pressure sores and do not allow the patient to sleep in lateral position. The open reduction ensures proper reduction and more rigid immobilization and faster healing. In addition to this the miniplates can be fixed transorally and thus, cosmetically more acceptable to the patient. The fracture line is accessible at lateral to pyriform fossa and the zygomatico-maxillary buttress area, intraorally.

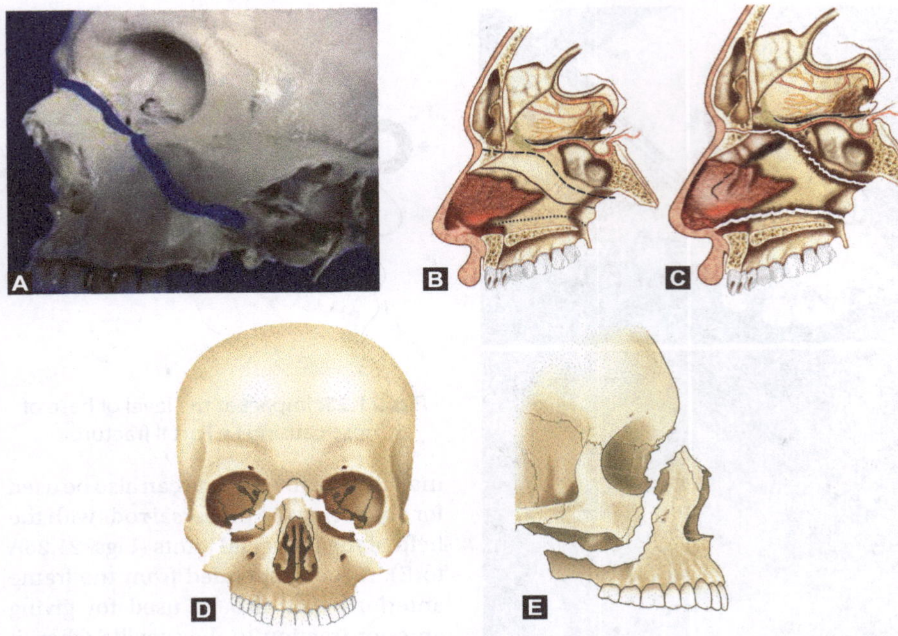

Figs 21.26A to E: Le Fort II fracture line

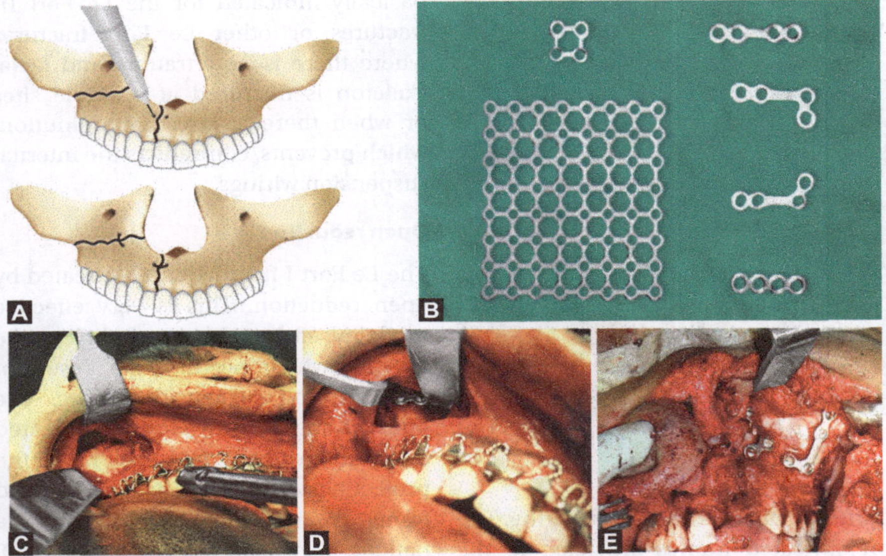

Figs 21.27A to E: (A) Intraosseous wiring; (B) Various implants used for the RIF; (C and D) Exposure of fracture line at the buttress through a degloving incision and plating; (E) Plating at the buttress and lateral to pyriform fossa

A degloving incision is placed in the buccal vestibule in the anterior and the premolar-molar area to expose the fracture line. The fracture is reduced by using a pair or Row's maxillary disimpaction forceps, as described previously. A 4 holed 'L' shaped plate is used for fixing the fracture, lateral to the pyriform aperture. The L shaped plate with 135 degree angulation is better suited for application lateral to the pyriform aperture than the regular L shaped plate with 90° angulation. The plate is adapted to the bone and fixed across the fracture line with 5 mm long screws as the bone is very thin. The plate that is fixed at the buttress is a four holed straight plate without gap or a L shaped plate, depending upon the anatomical configuration of the bone, availability of sound bone for anchoring the screws, the direction of the fracture line and presence of any comminution of bone may warrant use of a particular form and size of bone plate. The plate is nicely adapted to the bone and fixed across the fracture line using 5 mm screws. The 2 mm plates are commonly used (Figs 21.27A to E).

Le Fort II Fracture

The Le Fort II fracture is also called pyramidal fracture. The fracture line originates at the nasal bones and ends at the pterygoid plates. It is caused by trauma at the higher level of the face, from the anterior direction (*See* Fig. 21.25).

The fracture can be unilateral or bilateral. The nasal bones articulate superiorly with the frontal bones at frontonasal suture and with each other in the midline at internasal suture. The nasal bones are thicker at the frontonasal suture and as the inferior border is reached they become thin. The junction between this thick and the thin part of the nasal bone constitutes a line of weaknesses. In the event of trauma the Le Fort II fracture line originates at this point and runs laterally on the frontal process of maxilla and then extends on to the lacrimal bone. Then it crosses the inferior part of the lamina papyracea of the ethmoidal bone, exposing the ethmoidal air cells. The fracture line runs on the floor of the orbit towards the infraorbital rim and crosses the same at the level of zygomaticomaxillary suture. It then runs on the anterior surface of the maxilla, runs inferiorly towards the zygomatic buttress, during this course it runs around the infraorbital foramen and does not involve the foramen as its walls are corticated. It then runs inferiorly around the buttress and runs on the posterolateral wall of the maxillary sinus, crosses the pterygomaxillary fissure to the fracture the pterygoid lamellae half way (*See* Figs 21.26A to E). The fracture also continues medially, from its origin over the lateral nasal wall, runs posteriorly to meet the lateral fracture line behind the pterygoid plates. When the bilateral fracture occurs it assumes the shape of a pyramid and thus the name 'pyramidal fracture'.

Clinical Features

The clinical features of the Le Fort II fracture are as follows:

- Due to the fracture of the nasal bones there is edema over the nasal bridge and epistaxis. Bilateral circumorbital edema and/or ecchymosis may be present. There is tenderness over the nasal bridge.
- As the fracture passes over the medial orbital wall, there may be subconjunctival bleeding, which is more pronounced medially. The subconjunctival hemorrhage and then circumorbital ecchymosis are a result of the bleeding at the site of fracture, which through the subperiosteal plane escapes in different tissue planes. If it goes in the subcutaneous plane, it will present as a circumorbital ecchymosis and if it goes in the subconjunctival plane, subconjunctival hemorrhage is the presentation.
- There is a step defect in the infraorbital rim. It also contributes to the circumorbital edema and ecchymosis.
- As the fracture line passes on the floor of the orbit, the infraorbital nerve gets traumatized in the infraorbital canal and it results in the neurological deficit in the area of distribution of the infraorbital nerve. The infraorbital nerve seldom gets traumatized due to the fracture passing through the foramen as the line gets deflected around the foramen due to its cortication. The lateral nasal, inferior palpebral, and superior labial branches are involved along with the anterior and middle superior alveolar branches.
- There could be tenderness and step over the buttress intraorally.
- The maxilla gets displaced posteriorly and downward resulting in anterior cross bite, gagging of molars and anterior open bite.
- On bimanual palpation, keeping thumb and index finger of the left hand on the nasal bones and grasping the anterior maxillary teeth with the thumb and index fingers of the other hand if the maxilla is moved, the movements are felt at the nasal bone suggesting fracture at the site. Similar bimanual palpation also elicits the abnormal mobility over the infraorbital rims (Figs 21.28A and B).
- The face becomes flat or concave due to the posterior displacement of the mid third of facial skeleton resulting in classical '*dish face deformity*' (Fig. 21.29A).
- In a classical Le Fort II fracture, the injury to the cribriform plate of ethmoid is not present and thus CSF rhinorrhea does not take place, unless there is associated fracture of cribriform plate of ethmoid.
- As the walls of the maxillary sinus get involved there could be leakage of the air in the soft tissue producing crepitus on palpation (surgical emphysema) and the maxillary sinus appears hazy on X-ray due to bleeding in the sinus.

Investigations

The X-ray paranasal sinus (PNS) is usually adequate. The maxillary sinus appears hazy due to bleeding in it. Step deformity is also seen in the infraorbital rim (Figs 21.29B and C). The fracture line is also seen at the level of the nasal bones. The Campbell-Trapnell lines are useful in reading the X-ray properly (Fig. 21.30).

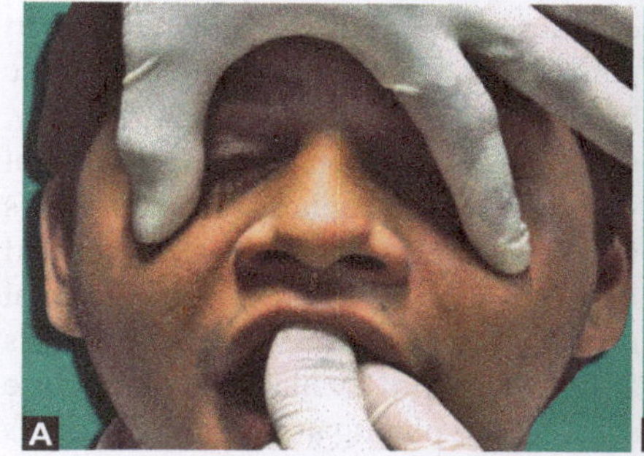
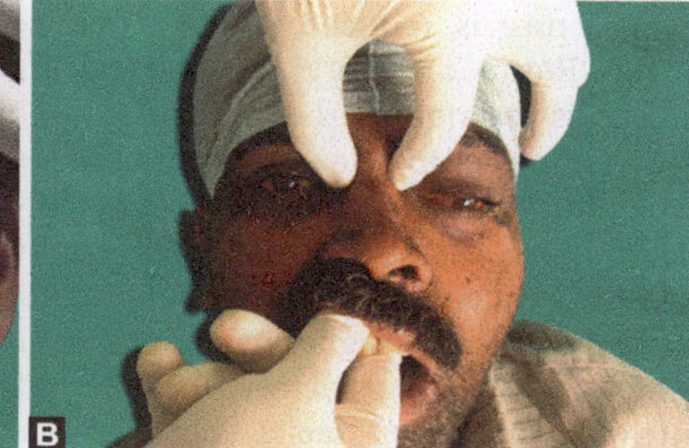

Figs 21.28A and B: Bimanual palpation in a case of Le Fort II fracture, one hand grasps the maxilla and elicits the mobility, while the fingers of the other hand kept over the infraorbital area feel the abnormal mobility

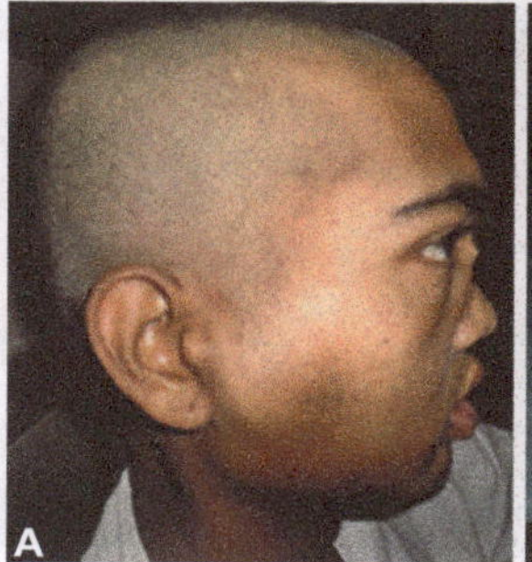
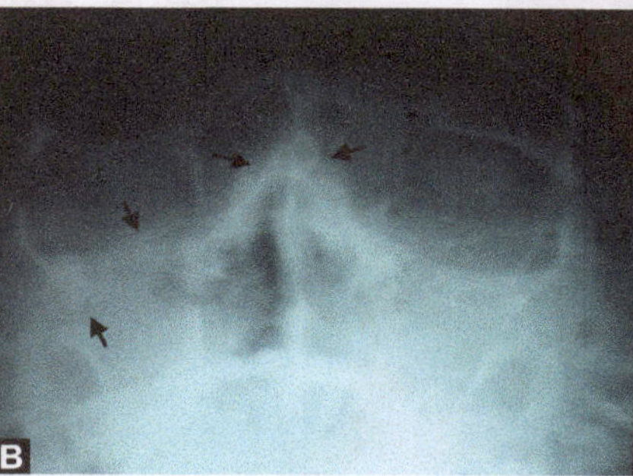
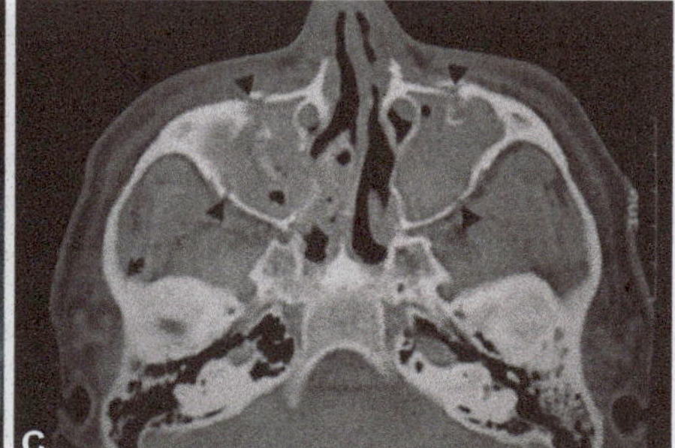

Figs 21.29A to C: (A) Dish face deformity; (B and C) X-ray and CT scan showing Le Fort II fracture

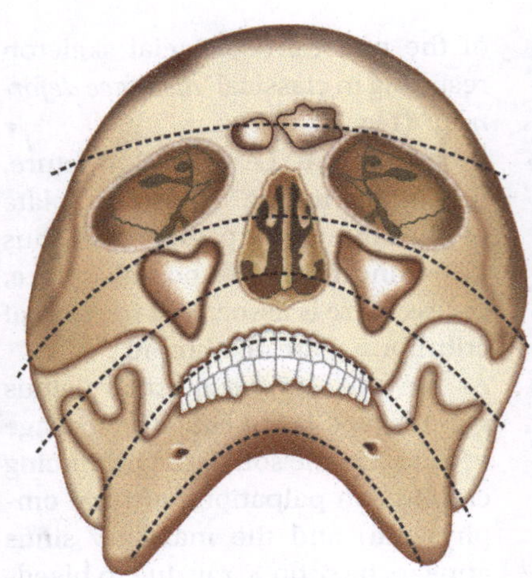

Fig. 21.30: Campbell-Trapnell lines

The fracture lines are appreciated on a CT scans in a better way than the conventional X-rays.

Management

The management of the Le Fort II fracture is by:

- Closed reduction
- Open reduction

Closed reduction

The fracture is reduced using a pair of the Row's maxillary disimpaction forceps as described earlier. The maxilla is disimpacted in the anterosuperior direction. When the fracture is old or the fracture segments are impacted, traction with the help of extraoral device using pulley and weights or elastics is done. Achieving satisfactory occlusion and correction of facial deformity are the markers of proper reduction. Intermaxillary fixation is done and the fractured middle third is secured with the intact superior skeleton with the help of either:

A. Internal suspension
B. External suspension.

The internal suspension is similar to the Le Fort I fracture except, the pyriform fossa wiring suspension and infraorbital rim wirings are not used for treating the Le Fort II fracture as the fracture line passes above these points. The circumzygomatic suspension wiring or supraorbital rim wiring can be done. External suspension with the help of POP head frame can be done.

Open reduction

The fracture line can be accessed at the infraorbital rim and the zygomatic buttress area. Through the infraorbital or subcilliary incision; the infraorbital rim is exposed and after carefully reflecting the orbital periosteum holes are drilled on either side of the fracture line and intraosseous wiring is done. If the plates are used, orbital plates with gap having 4 to 6 holes is carefully adapted and contoured to the bone and secured in place using 5 mm screws. The zygomatic buttress area is accessible intraorally, through an incision placed in buccal vestibule in the molar area. The plates are fixed in a similar way as described in the Le Fort I fracture. The infraorbital rim is grossly comminuted sometimes and bone is not available for fixing the screws. The plating at the nasal bones is usually not required and the nasal bone fractures can be managed conservatively by simple reduction and stabilization by nasal packing and external POP splints. The two point fixation at the infraorbital rim and the zygomatic buttress is usually adequate (Figs 21.31A to C). It is also observed that the infraorbital rim area is comminuted in high velocity trauma and sound bone for anchoring the screws is not available, in such cases or in the cases where the fracture is minimally displaced single point plating at the buttress area may be opted. If the stability of the fracture fragments is doubtful with one point fixation then additional measures such as IMF for ten days may be resorted to facilitate uneventful healing.

Le Fort III Fracture

The Le Fort III fracture is also called craniofacial disjunction, as the mid third of facial skeleton gets disarticulated from the cranial base. This fracture is a suprazygomatic fracture. It results from an impact that occurs at a high velocity at the level of frontonasal suture (Fig. 21.32).

The fracture line starts at the frontonasal suture, runs horizontally to separate the frontomaxillary suture, runs over the lacrimal bone, the lamina papyracea of the ethomoid bone and runs towards the optic foramen. As the optic foramen is guarded by thick cortication, to protect the optic nerve, the fracture line goes around it to reach the medial boundary of the inferior orbital fissure, which provides a readymade passage for the fracture line. At the medial

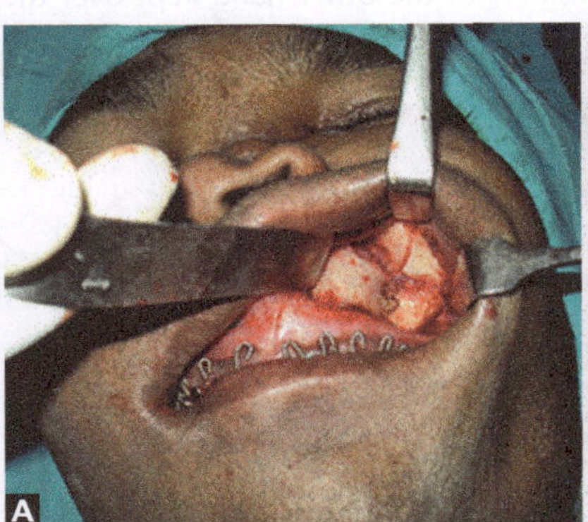

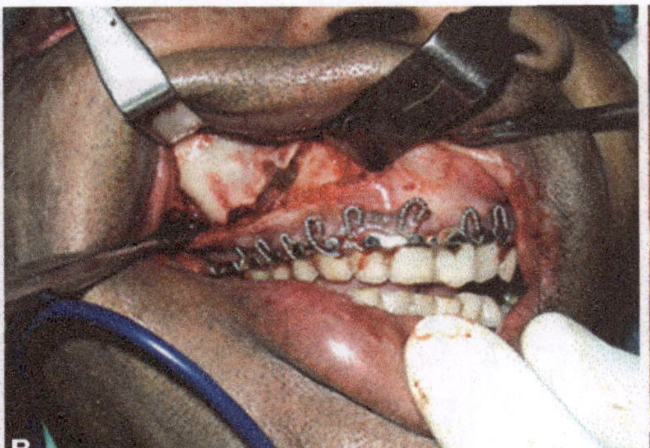

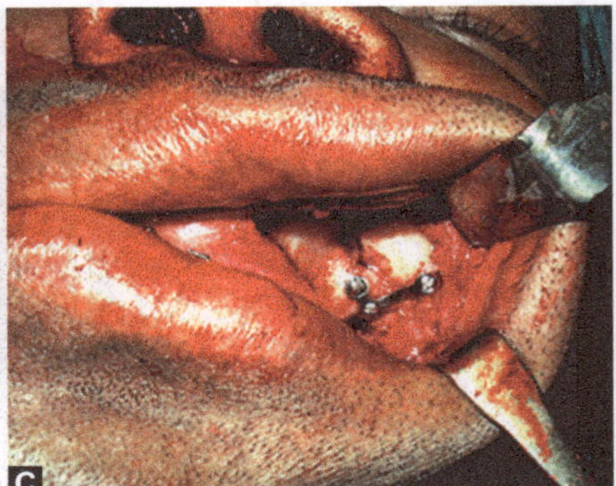

Figs 21.31A to C: Management of bilateral Le Fort II fracture by fixation at the buttress area

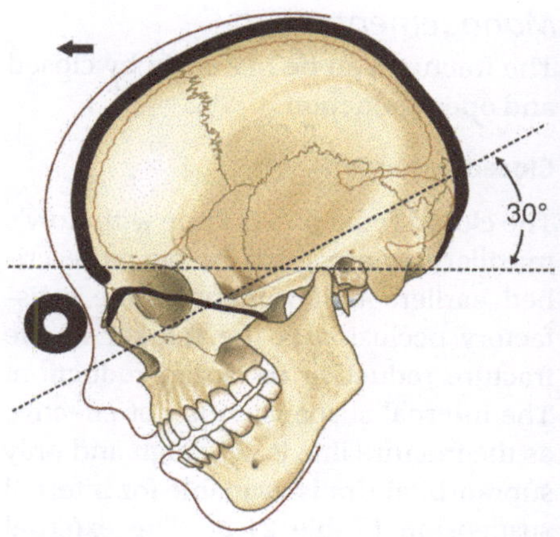

Fig. 21.32: High velocity impact at the level of frontonasal suture

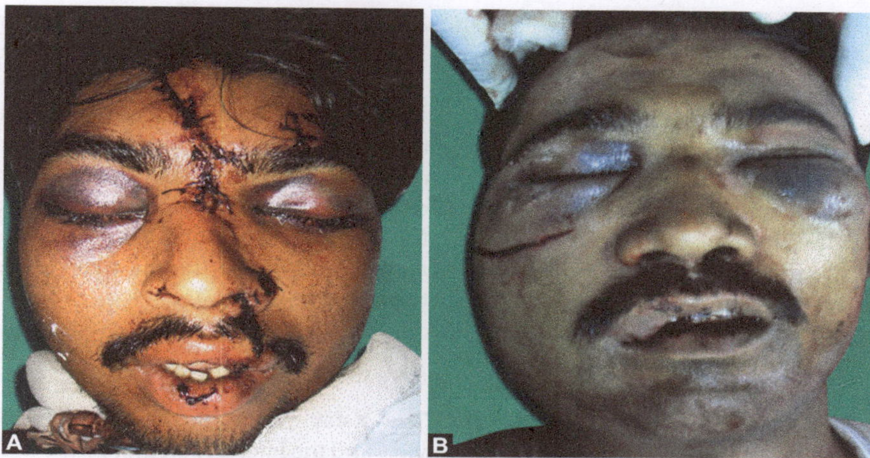

Figs 21.34A and B: Clinical cases of Le Fort III fracture, note gross edema of face in figure B

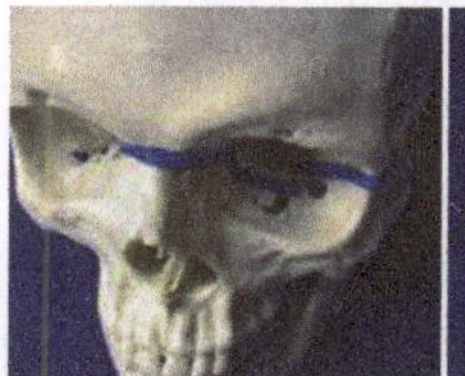
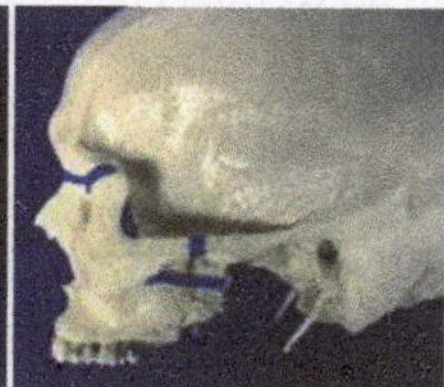

Fig. 21.33: Le Fort III fracture line

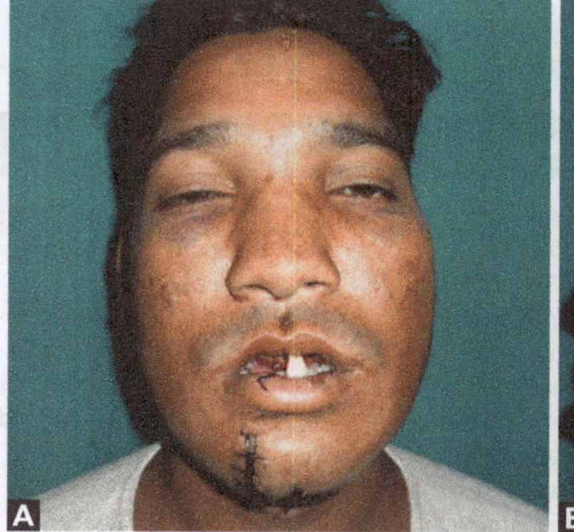

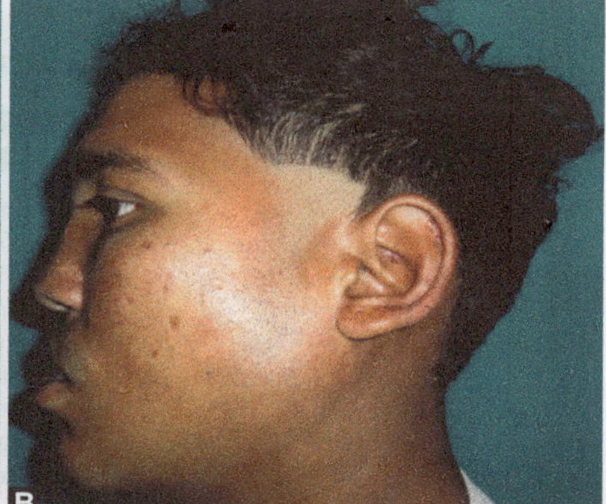

Figs 21.35A and B: Clinical case of Le Fort III fracture showing elongation of the face

boundary of the inferior orbital fissure the fracture line divides/bifurcates in two lines. One line passes around the frontozygomatic suture to separate the zygomatic bone from the frontal bone. The other line passes posteriorly to fracture the pterygoid plates at the root, thus separating them from the cranial base. Hence, in this fracture the facial skeleton is separated from the cranium at frontonasal suture, frontozygomatic suture and the pterygoid plates thus, total craniofacial disarticulation takes place and hence the name, craniofacial disjunction. The fracture line also runs medially from its point of origin runs over the lateral nasal wall to meet the lateral fracture line behind the pterygoid plates (Fig. 21.33).

Clinical Features

- There is massive edema of the face.
- Bilateral circumorbital edema/ecchymosis is present (Figs 21.34A and B).
- Subconjunctival hemorrhage is also present.
- There is flattening of the nasal bridge.
- Profuse epistaxis is present.
- As the facial bones are disarticulated from the cranial base the elongation of the face takes place leading to long face syndrome (Figs 21.35A and B). The facial bones not only get displaced inferiorly, but also posteriorly along the slope of the sphenoid leading to concavity, which gives a classical '*dish face deformity*'.
- The posteroinferior displacement of the facial bones leads to derangement of occlusion, anterior open bite and cross bite deformity.
- There may be fracture of the cribriform plate of the ethmoid, which may lead to dural injury leading to the leakage of the CSF in the nasal cavity, which is called CSF rhinorrhea. If the patient is in upright position the CSF leads in the nasal cavity and flows out. It appears as a glistening, clear fluid. It is often difficult to detect the CSF as it is admixed with the blood. The blood clots and dries earlier and the flowing CSF washes the dried blood on the face as it flows dawn producing classical rail tracts. It also forms classical ring around the clotted blood on the pillow. If the patient is in supine position it passes in the pharynx giving salty taste.
- The damage to the branches of the olfactory nerve or even edema or clot in the region of superior meatus leads to hampering of sense of smell

thus, causing anosmia. In case of former it is irreversible but in case of latter it is transient.

- The exposure of the ethmoidal air cells can lead to infection, which can pass intracranially and cause intracranial infections.
- The size of the orbit increases and as the fracture occurs at the frontozygomatic suture area the Whitnall's tubercle along with the Lockwood's suspensary ligament attached to it migrates inferiorly to produce hypoglobus and hooding of the eye.
- Bimanual palpation as described earlier, depicts abnormal mobility at the fronto-nasal and frontozygomatic sutures.
- Step deformity is present at the frontonasal and frontozygomatic sutures.

The Le Fort III fracture may be associated with head injury more frequently than any other facial fracture due to the anatomical proximity of the fracture to the cranial base and the higher level of the trauma that causes the fracture.

Investigations

The X-ray PNS, posteroanterior (PA) view and the lateral radiographs are useful in assessing the fracture. CT scans are the best method to visualize the fracture, as in normal radiographs the superimposition obscures the fracture line.

Management

The fracture can be managed by closed and open reduction.

Closed reduction

The closed reduction is done with Row's maxillary disimpaction forceps as described earlier. Achievement of the satisfactory occlusion is the marker of the fracture reduction in closed reduction. The internal suspension is not effective as the fracture line is very high and only supraorbital rim is available for internal suspension (Table 21.2). The external suspension with POP head frame or halo frame is possible, through the cheek wires with the anterior traction, through the vertical suspended rods from the head frame (Figs 21.36 and 21.37).

Table 21.2: Methods of closed reduction in mid-face fractures

	Le Fort I fracture	Le Fort II fracture	Le Fort III fracture
Closed reduction (for internal suspension, point from which the suspension is done is superior to the fracture line)	***Internal suspension*** Pyriform fossa Infraorbital rim Circumzygomatic Supraorbital rim ***External suspension*** Craniomaxillary suspension using halo frame and cheek wires or universal rods and joints ***Sandwich technique*** In case of unilateral Le Fort I fracture	***Internal suspension*** Circumzygomatic Supraorbital rim ***External suspension*** Craniomaxillary suspension using halo frame and cheek wires or universal rods and joints	***Internal suspension*** Not desirable as the fracture is at a higher level and all the suspension points are below the fracture line ***External suspension*** Craniomaxillary suspension using halo frame and cheek wires or universal rods and joints
Open reduction	Plating at lateral margin of pyriform fossa and the zygomaticomaxillary buttress area	Plating at the zygomatico-maxillary buttress areas, if the fracture is unstable then plating at infraorbital rim and at the frontonasal area, which is seldom required	Plating at the frontozygomatic sutures and if the fracture is still unstable then at the frontonasal area

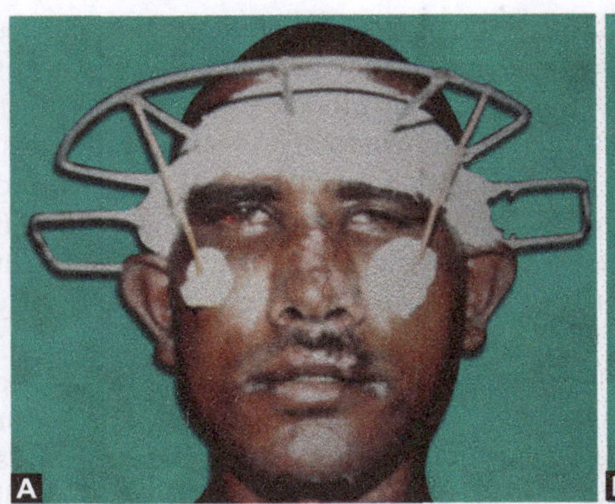

A

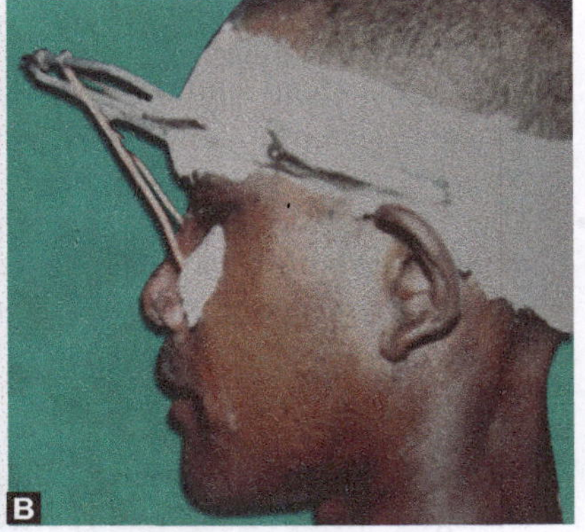

B

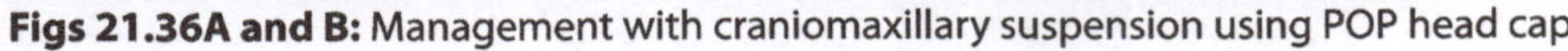

Figs 21.36A and B: Management with craniomaxillary suspension using POP head cap

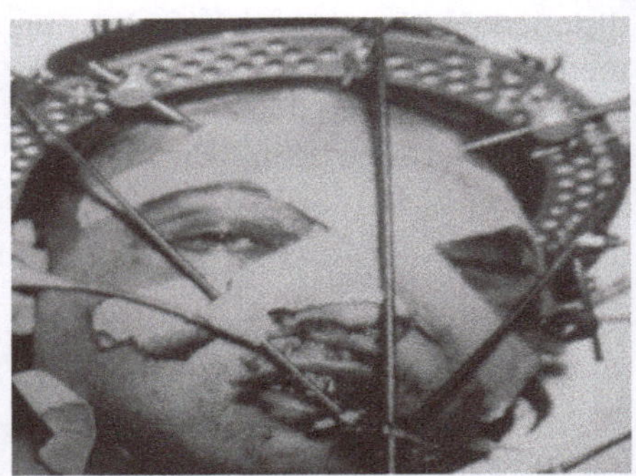

Fig. 21.37: Management with craniomaxillary halo frame

Open reduction

The open reduction is done with the help of intraosseous wires or bone plates placed at the frontozygomatic suture and frontonasal sutures. In case of pan facial trauma when there are multiple facial fractures, the outer most fractures are first reduced and the inner fractures are treated later, i.e. the fracture at the zygoma and mandible will be reduced first and the nasal bone fracture at the end to avoid facial widening (Fig. 21.38). The advantage of open reduction in the treatment of mid third fractures is that it causes least morbidity to the patient and not only the occlusion, but the facial deformities are also corrected more accurately.

If the Le Fort III fracture is associated with the head injury then the management of the fracture is always the second priority. The head injury and other life threatening, grievous injuries must be attended to first. If the CSF leakage is present then neurosurgical opinion must be sought, antibiotics that cross the blood brain-barrier (BBB) like chloromycetin, third generation celephalosporins should be started to prevent the intracranial infections. The ethmoidal air cell exposure must also be covered with the similar antibiotic therapy.

While studying the mid facial fractures certain associated conditions must be elaborated, which matter a lot in the management and the clinician must be aware of. The CSF rhinorrhea is one such condition.

CSF Rhinorrhea

The leakage of the CSF through the nose following the fracture of the cribriform plate of the ethmoid bone results in CSF rhinorrhea as the dural attachment at this site gets torn and the leak results. This can occur commonly in Le Fort III fracture and the nasoethmoidal fracture and occasionally Le Fort II fracture, if the associated injury to the ethmoid is present. The CSF leaks in the nasal cavity and trickles out through the nose. It is glistening, clear fluid. When the patient is in supine position, the CSF instead of flowing out, trickles in the throat, giving salty taste in a conscious patient. Immediately following the trauma the CSF is mixed with blood and is difficult to detect. The blood flows dawn the face and clots and dries but the CSF does not clot and flows dawn the face washing out the dried blood on the face along the path of its flow and creates classical rail tracks. The blood mixed with the CSF collects on the pillow of the patient. The blood clots earlier and forms the central area of clotted blood around which the CSF forms a ring of clear fluid. This is the ring test. Similarly, a drop of blood with CSF is taken on the blotting paper the blood clots and forms the central area around which clear CSF forms a ring. The CSF must be differentiated from the serum which is expressed out when the blood clots and from the mucous secreted by the nasal mucous membrane. Both of them have lower glucose content than the CSF (Identification of CSF rhinorrhea: clear CSF should be collected in a vial and a glucose level of 45 mg/dL or more confirms its presence, as does the absence of it's sedimentation. CSF will not stiffen the handkerchief, whereas nasal secretions will. CSF also produces concentric rings when poured on linen).

The leakage of the CSF can lead to progress of retrograde infection in the cranial cavity which can result in meningitis, venous thrombosis to more severe intracranial sepsis, which could prove fatal. Thus, every attempt must be made to prevent the infection, the antibiotics that cross the BBB should be prescribed. The minor CSF leakage is managed conservatively with antibiotic prophylaxis, propped-up position formation of blood clot and organization of the same may lead to spontaneous arrest of the CSF leak. Nasal packing, nasotracheal intubation, passing of the nasogastric tube (Ryle's tube) is strictly contraindicated in presence of the CSF rhinorrhea. If the leak is profuse and does not get arrested spontaneously, then the neurosurgical intervention is required and cranioplasty is done to repair the dural tear.

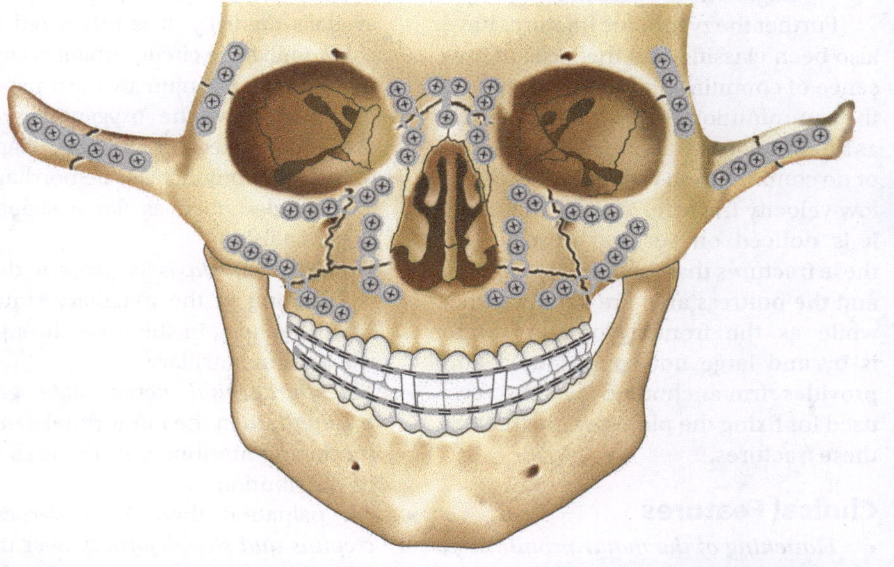

Fig. 21.38: Various sites on facial skeleton where plates can be fixed during internal fixation

FRACTURES OF THE ZYGOMATIC BONE

The zygomatic bone is also called malar bone; it forms the prominence of the cheek and thus, also referred as cheek bone. It is a flat bone and has four processes, the frontal process which articulates with the frontal bone, superiorly at the frontozygomatic (F-Z) suture. The maxillary process articulates with the zygomatic process of the maxillary bone to form the zygomaticomaxillary suture, near the zygomaticomaxillary buttress.

The temporal process articulates with the zygomatic process of temporal bone to form the zygomaticotemporal suture and both these processes form the zygomatic arch. The orbital processes of the zygoma forms the lateral orbital wall. Because of the three processes of the zygomatic bone are involved in the fracture these fractures are often described as tripoid fractures. As the forth process, the orbital process is also involved some clinicians describe it as quadripoid fracture. All the joints with adjacent bones are sutural joints.[4] Below the F-Z suture, on the lateral orbital margin a small bony projection is seen, which is called Whitnall's tubercle which gives attachment to the suspensary ligament of Lockwood, which is a Hammock like ligament and supports the eyeball.[5] The masseter muscle originates from the inferior border of the zygomatic arch and the deep temporal fascia is attached to it superiorly. Due to these attachments the displacement of the zygoma is prevented in superoinferior direction in the event of the fracture.[6] The sutural joints existing between the zygoma and adjacent bone leads to separation of these sutures and if reduced properly the interlocking of the sutures makes the fracture self-retaining.

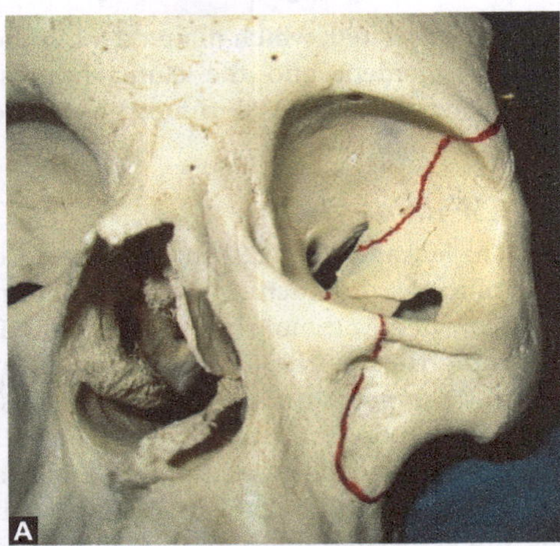
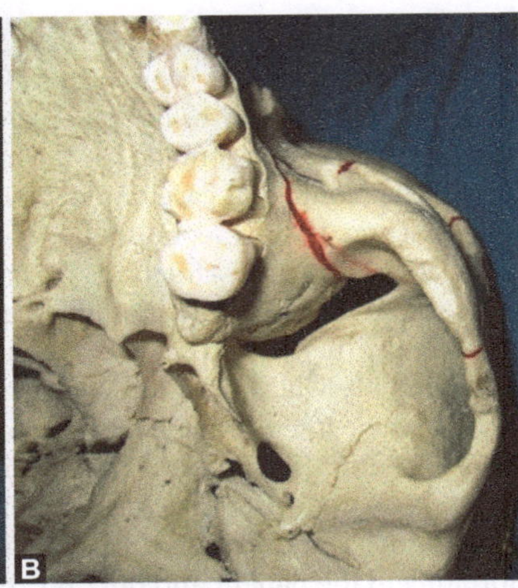

Figs 21.39A and B: Fracture of the zygomaticomaxillary complex

The fractures of the zygoma are divided into two categories, which produce distinct clinical signs and symptoms. They are:

- Fractures of the body of zygoma (malar bone fractures).
- Fractures of the zygomatic arch.

The fractures of the zygoma were previously called as the zygomaticomaxillary complex fractures as the zygomaticomaxillary suture is involved. However, presently they are referred to as zygomatico-orbital complex fractures as the involvement of the orbital rim is inevitable (Figs 21.39A and B).

Many authors have devised classification schemes for zygomaticomaxillary complex (ZMC) fractures (Ellis,[7] 1985; Yanagesawa,[8] 1973; Knight,1961).[9] Zingg[10] (1992), Yamashiro M[11], 1983.

The zygomatic fractures can be classified as:[9]

- As per the conspicuous presentation of step:
  - 3 o'clock position
  - 6 o'clock position
  - 9 o'clock position
  - 12 o'clock position
- According to the displacement along the vertical and the horizontal axis (Figs 21.40A to E):
  - Undisplaced fractures—only the sutures are widened without gross displacement of the bone
  - Upward and inward displacement—the zygoma encroaches upon the orbital cavity
  - Downward and outward displacement—size of the orbit gets expanded
  - Comminuted fracture—multiple fragments are present.

Further the zygomatic fractures have also been classified on the basis of presence of comminution at the sutures. If the comminution is present it is referred as a high velocity fracture and if minimal or no comminution is present it is called low velocity fracture. Most of the times it is noticed on surgical exposure of these fractures that the infraorbital area and the buttress area are communited, while as the frontozygomatic suture is by and large not comminuted and provides firm anchorage for the screws used for fixing the plates, while treating these fractures.

Clinical Features

- *Flattening of the malar prominence,* in case of the depressed fractures. The depression is seen immediately following the trauma and later it is masked by the edema. It can be seen again when the edema subsides. In case of outward displacement the malar prominence is accentuated (Fig. 21.41).
- *Circumorbital edema* is present. Bleeding below the periosteum escapes below the subcutaneous plane to produce circumorbital ecchymosis (Fig. 21.42A).
- *Subconjunctival hemorrhage* is present laterally. As it is produced as a result of bleeding in the subperiosteal plane due to fracture which escapes in the subconjunctival plane, its posterior boundary is not seen when the patient is asked to look medially, rotating the eyeballs medially. It is bright red in color, unlike the circumorbital ecchymosis, as the conjunctiva are paper thin and allow the oxygenation of the extravasated RBCs. The shape of the subconjunctival hemorrhage is often described as flame shaped (Fig. 21.42B).
- *Unilateral epistaxis* is present due to bleeding in the maxillary sinus, which escapes in the nose through the osteum maxillary.
- The *infraorbital nerve often gets traumatized* in the infraorbital canal producing numbness in the area of its distribution.
- On palpation there is *tenderness, crepitus and step deformity* over the frontozygomatic suture. Similar findings are also present over the

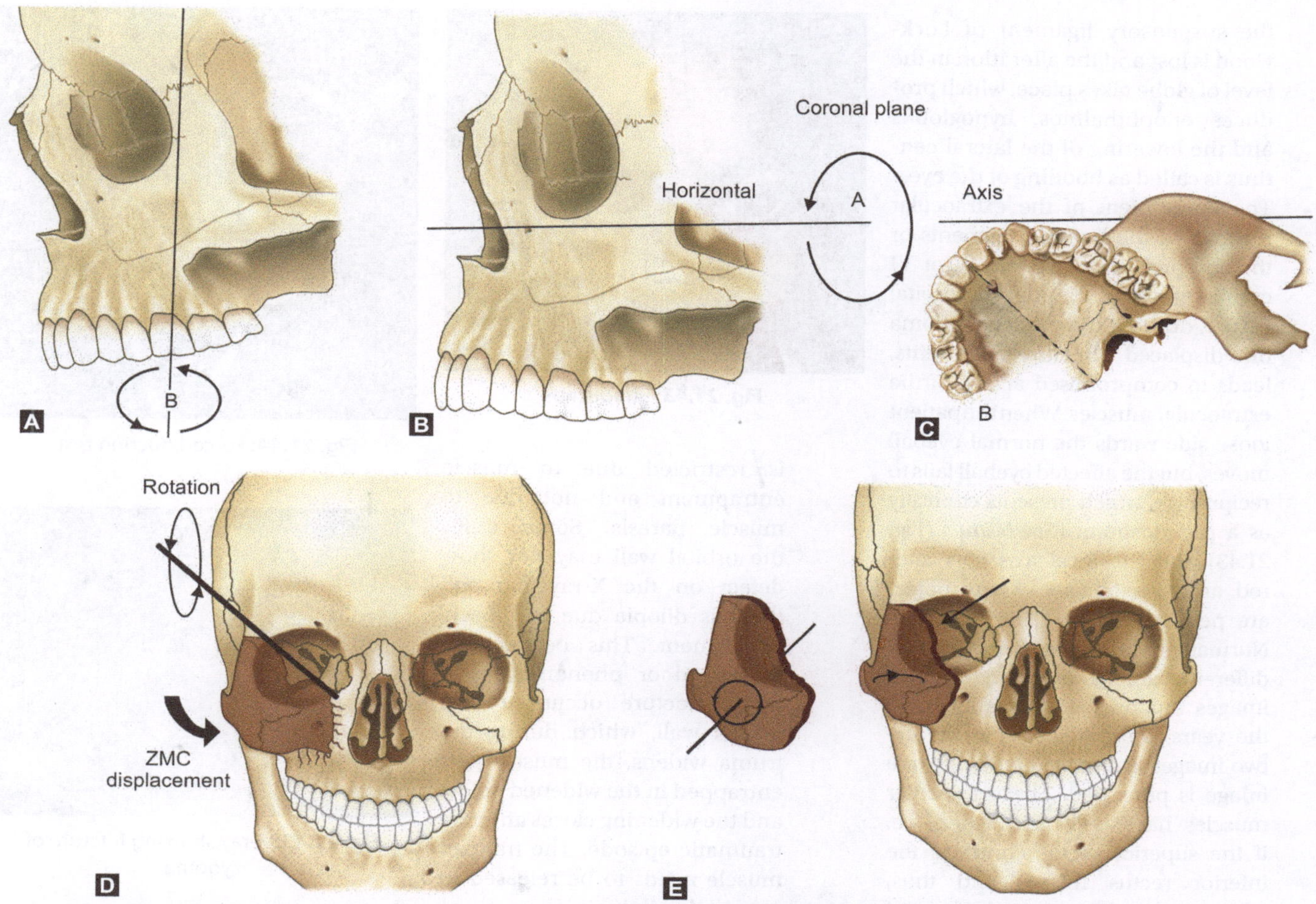

Figs 21.40A to E: Classification of ZMC according to the displacement along the vertical and the horizontal axis (Adopted from Rowe and William's maxillofacial injuries. Churchill Livingstone 1994)

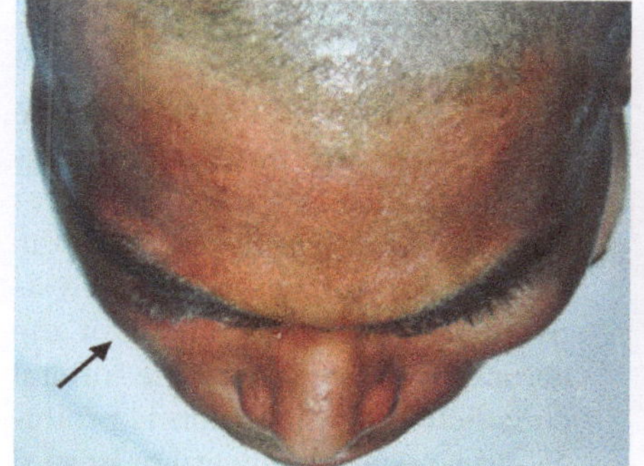

Fig. 21.41: Flattening of malar prominence

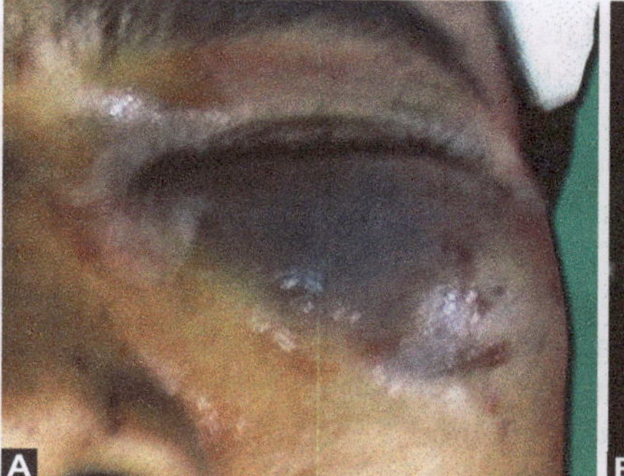

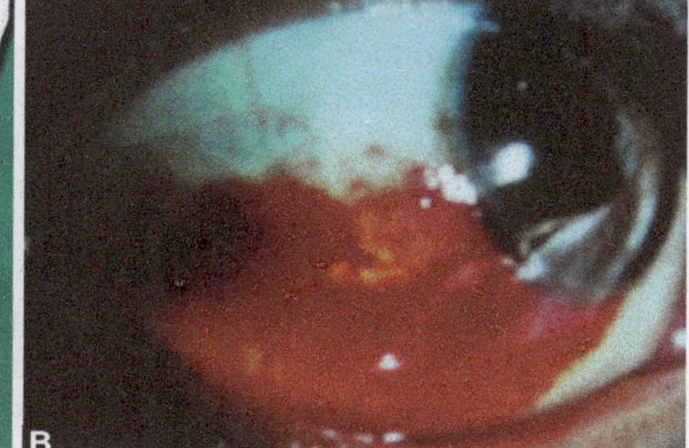

Figs 21.42A and B: (A) Circumorbital ecchymosis; (B) Subconjunctival hemorrhage (note the bright-red color)

zygomatic arch, infraorbital rim and the zygomaticomaxillary buttress area. In high velocity accidents the infraorbital area is usually comminuted and so is the area of zygomaticomaxillary buttress. The frontozygomatic suture is usually not comminuted and offers a stable point for internal fixation during the management.

- When the fracture is inwardly displaced, i.e. depressed fracture, the orbital size gets reduced and the eyeball is pushed out causing proptosis. When the fracture is displaced outwards the orbital size increases and the retracting action of the extraocular muscles pull the eyeball in, causing enophthalmos.
- When the fracture is severely displaced downwards, the support of

the suspensory ligament of Lockwood is lost and the alteration in the level of globe takes place, which produces enophthalmos, hypoglobus and the lowering of the lateral canthus is called as hooding of the eye.

- The entrapment of the extraocular muscles in the fracture segments or the compression of the III, IV or VI cranial nerves in the superior orbital fissure, due to intraorbital hematoma or displaced fracture segments, leads to compromised action of the extraocular muscles. When the patient looks side wards the normal eyeball moves, but the affected eyeball fails to reciprocate, which presents clinically as a pseudosquint (*Strabismus* (Fig. 21.43) and the focal axis gets altered and two images of one object are perceived. It is called diplopia. Normally the two eyes work like two different cameras and produce two images but due to adaptation over the years, the parallax between the two images is removed and only one image is perceived. The extraocular muscles have pully like action, i.e. if the superior rectus contracts the inferior rectus relaxes and thus, the eyeball moves upwards. If any of the extraocular muscles is entrapped or is paralyzed, it fails to complement the action of its antagonist muscle and the movements of the eyeball are hampered producing diplopia. The Hess chart shows directions or gazes of the diplopia which is produced due to involvement of the particular extraocular muscle.
- The soft tissue around the eye ball is anesthetized using 4 to 5 percent sterile ledocaine solution and forcibly moved with forceps as indicated in Fig. 21.44.
  - If the eye moves freely to forced movement, then this indicates that any restriction in eye movement in that direction is caused by a muscle paresis.
  - If the eye cannot be moved, even with this forced duction in a particular gaze direction, then it suggests that the eye movement is restricted due to muscle entrapment and not due to muscle paresis. Some times the orbital wall may not show defect on the X-ray but still there is dilopia due to muscle entrapment. This occurs due to trap door phenomenon. A linear fracture occurs in the orbital wall, which during the truma widens, the muscle gets entrapped in the widened defect and the widening closes after the traumatic episode. The trapped muscle needs to be released to correct the diplopia.

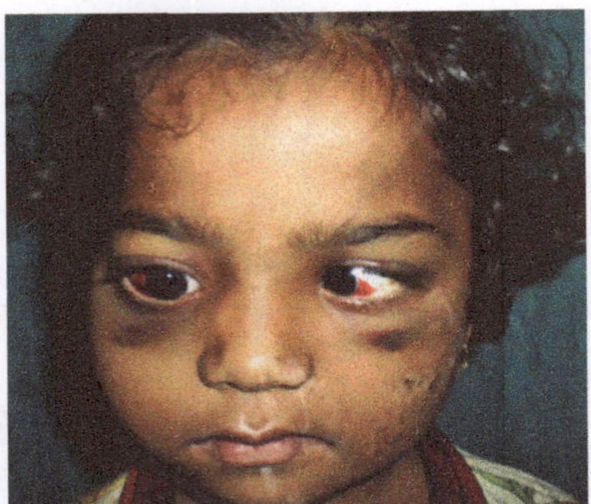

Fig. 21.43: Strabismus

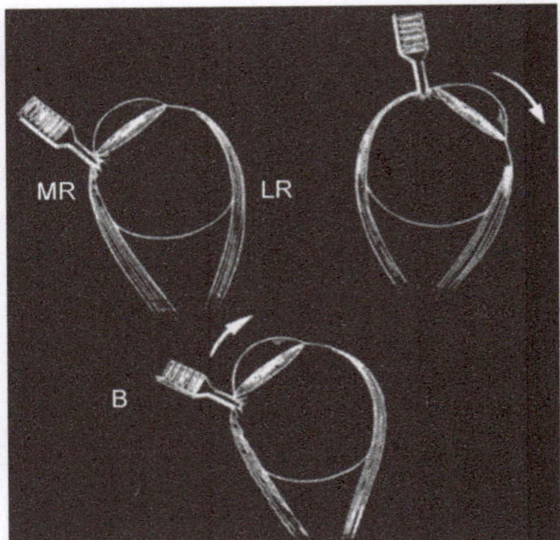

Fig. 21.44: Forced duction test

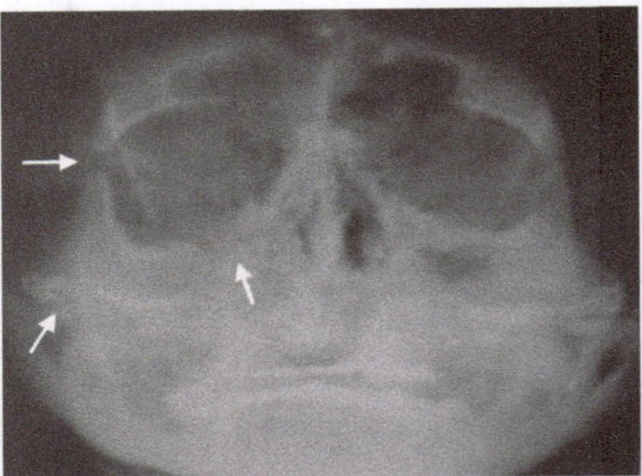

Fig. 21.45: X-ray showing fracture of zygoma

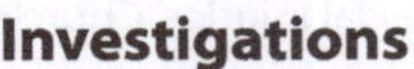

Investigations

X-ray PNS shows the zygomatic bone and all its sutures very well. This X-ray is not good to visualize the arch. The undisplaced fracture is seen as widening of the sutures.[12] The displaced fractures result in break in continuity of the orbital rims. The maxillary sinus appears hazy due to bleeding in the sinus (Fig. 21.45). Due to superimpositions of adjacent anatomical structures the visualization of the fracture line and the displacement therfeof is not properly visualized. However, the CT scan often provide more precise information about the fracture line and the displacement (Figs 21.46A to C).

Management of the Zygomatic Bone Fracture

The zygomatic bone fractures can be managed by either closed reduction or by open reduction. All the fractures do not require treatment, but there are distinct indications where the fractures are treated surgically. The indications are:

- For cosmetic consideration—where the displacement causes facial disfigurement.
- For considerations of function—the mandibular movements are restricted due to impingement of the coronoid process and the orbital constriction or expansion is produced as a result of outward or inward displacement of the fractured segment. The orbital size changes produce inophthalmos or proptosis. The entrapment of the muscles causes diplopia. In such cases the fracture needs to be treated.

The undisplaced fractures without any cosmetic or functional problems may be treated conservatively.

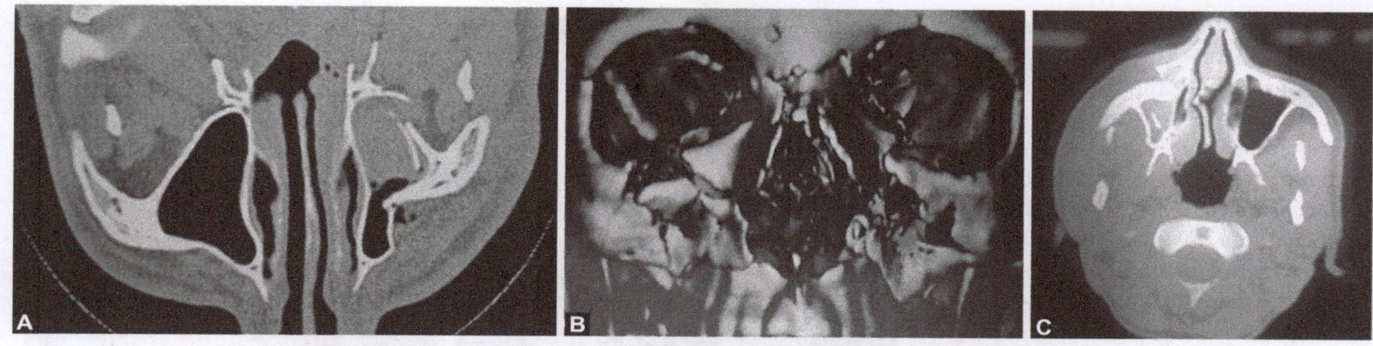

Figs 21.46A to C: CT scans showing fracture of zygomatic bone and bleeding in the sinus

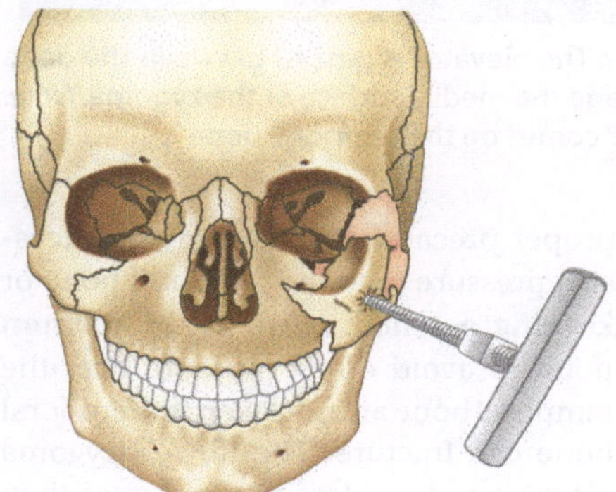

Fig. 21.47: Girard-Carroll screw

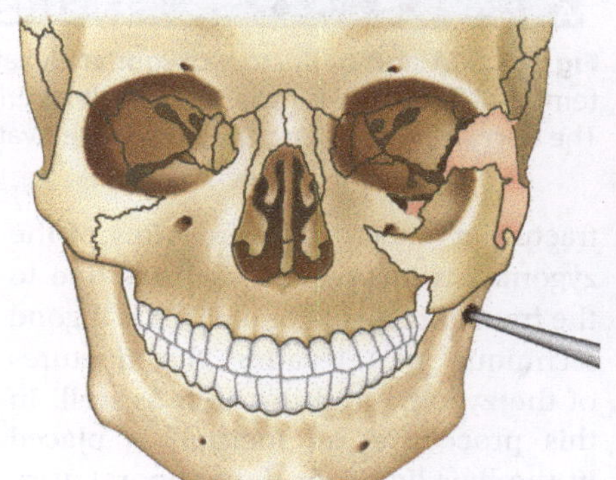

Fig. 21.48: Poswillow's hook

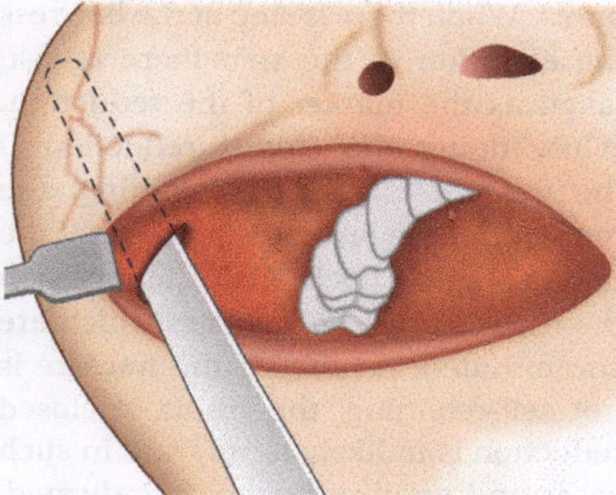

Fig. 21.49: Bristow's elevator through the modified Keen's approach

Closed Reduction

The closed reduction of the fracture is based on the assumption of the self-retaining nature of the fracture. The zygomatic fractures are self-retaining due to its sutural joints with the adjacent bones and as the fractures results in the separation of the sutures and when the fracture is reduced properly there is interlocking of the sutures, which makes the fracture self-retaining. However, most of the fractures show communition of edges and this philosophy does not work. Secondly, the masseter is attached to the inferior border of the zygomatic arch and the deep temporal fascia is attached to its superior border, both these anatomical structures splint the bone and prevent its superoinferior movement. For doing the closed reduction the fracture should be treated within 72 hours as more the time lapse more are the chances of the resorptive and remodeling activity at the sutural border and rounding of the sutures, which makes the fracture less self-retaining. Hence, older fractures are treated with the open reduction. As the time lapses the adhesions may develop around the fracture ends which also prevents the reduction of the fracture. The comminuted fractures are treated with open reduction as the self-retaining phenomenon is absent due to multiple fragments.[13]

In the past, the concept of the percutaneous elevation of the zygomatic fracture was in place which was accomplished using either the Girard-Carroll screw or Poswillow's hook, but it did not last longer as it lacked precision and was not esthetically viable as it involved scar on face due to small access incision (Figs 21.47 and 21.48).

For doing the closed reduction the approaches are:

- Keen's intraoral approach[14]
- Gillies temporal approach[15]
- Transantral approach[16]
- Other approaches mentioned in the literature like transnasal approach,[17] direct approach are impractical and are seldom practiced.

Keen's intraoral approach

Keen in 1932[14] described this method of reducing the fractured zygomatic bone (Fig. 21.49). In this approach an incision is placed in the buccal vestibule, over the zygomaticomaxillary buttress area. The tissues are dissected carefully by sharp and blunt dissection and along the medical surface of the zygomatic bone. A bone lever or the periosteal elevator is passed behind the body of the zygoma. The key is to stay in the subperiosteal plane and dissect along the bone as one may enter in the infratemporal fossa if this plane is missed and encounter bleeding due to the damage to the pterygoid plexus of the veins. Using the buccal alveolar bone as fulcrum the zygoma is gently elevated. Simultaneously, the orbital rims are palated with the finger of the other hand at the frontozygomatic suture and over the infraorbital rim to feel the step deformity, which gets abolished as the fracture is elevated and reduced. The comparison of the malar prominence on both the sides is also done to assess the correction of the malar prominence flattening. When the edema is conspicuous, the malar prominence is masked and it is not possible to assess, it and one has to rely on the palpation of the orbital rims only.[18] When there is step at the buttress the abolition of the step there is also taken as the marker of the reduction. While doing the closed reduction if the fracture is not self-retaining, the moment of the leverage is released, the zygoma sinks back. This happens in the old fractures or fractures which are comminuted. As such if the fracture is not self-retaining, the result of closed reduction is unlikely to stay and in such cases and open reduction is indicated. In the literature it is mentioned that the Bristow's zygoma elevator is used to elevate the fractured zygoma, but it is too bulky to be used intraorally.[19] The Keen's approach is suited for the reduction of the zygomatic bone, but it is cumbersome for reducing the fractures of the arch. The wound is closed primarily. During the postoperative period the assistants are instructed not to handle the area of the fracture as the fracture may sink back due to the pressure. The zygomatic area is marked with red ink cross indicating that the area should not be handled, while turning the head of the patient or while shifting the patient. The patient is not allowed to sleep on that side and sand bag support is given to prevent so. The supportive treatment in form of anti-inflammatory/analgesics is prescribed. Antibiotics are also prescribed as prophylaxis.

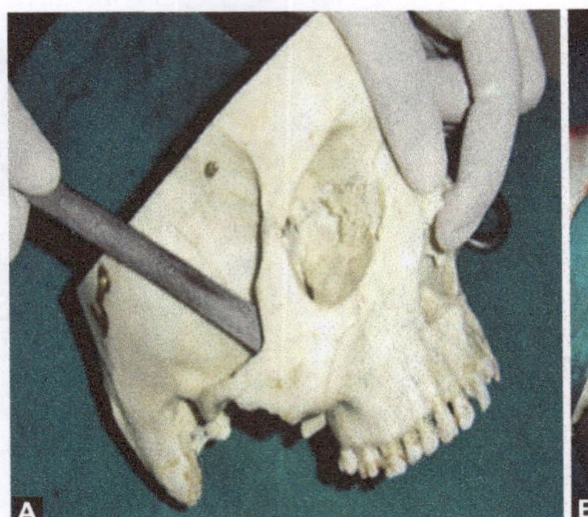

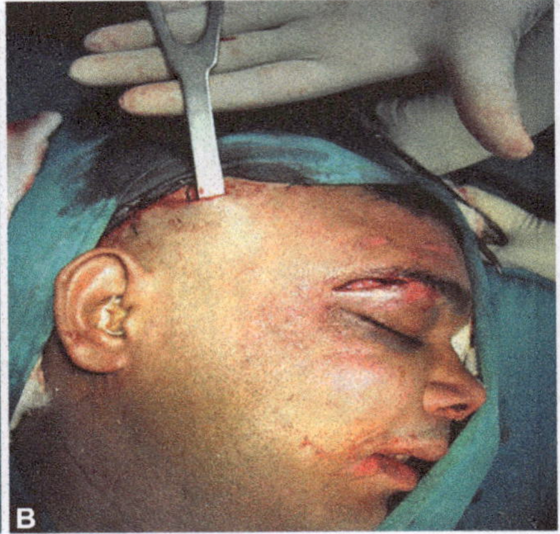

Figs 21.50A and B: Bristow's zygoma elevator. The elevator is passed between the deep temporal fascia and temporalis muscle to engage the medial surface of the zygoma. *Note:* The fulcrum, while using the Bristow's elevator comes on the temporal bone

Gillies temporal approach[15]

Gillies temporal approach is a popular approach for elevating the fractures of the zygoma. The word elevation is commonly used to describe the reduction of the fracture as most of the fractures of the zygoma are depressed fractures due to the inward displacement. This is a good technique for elevating the fractures of the zygoma and the arch as well. In this procedure, an incision is placed in the hair line over the temporal area, 45 degree to the vertical line in preauricular fold. This incision goes between the bifurcation of the superficial temporal vessels and avoids trauma to them and the scar is also hidden in the hair line. The skin, superfacial facia are dissected in layers to expose the deep temporal fascia, which looks as a white tenacious structure. The deep temporal facia is divided and plane is created between it and the temporalis muscle. The Bristow's zygoma elevator is passed between these two structures to engage the medial surface of the zygoma (Figs 21.50A and B). The leverage is given to elevate the zygoma in its proper reduced position. The marker of the reduction is the correction of malar flattening and the abolition of the step in the orbital rim. The postoperative check X-rays help in ascertaining the adequacy of reduction of the fracture. Rest of the postoperative precautions and management is similar to that described in the Keen's approach. The disadvantage with the Bristow's elevator is that the fulcrum point comes in the region of the squama of the temporal bone, which is thin and delicate. If proper precautions like avoiding excessive pressure over the temporal bone or keeping a rolled gauze at the fulcrum point to avoid direct pressure over the temporal bone are not taken the temporal bone can fracture. The Rowe's zygoma elevator is considered to be better than the Bristow's elevator as it avoids the fulcrum point on the temporal bone and the fulcrum lies at the junction of the two blades of the elevator. The position of the handle (outer blade) corresponds to the position of the inner (lever) blade as their length is same and gives the operator an idea regarding the position of the lever blade, which goes in the tissue plane and elevates the zygoma (Figs 21.51A to D).

Transantral approach[11]

The apex of the maxillary sinus extends into the zygoma and the later also constitutes a part of the anterolateral wall of the maxillary sinus. Thus, the sinus gets involved in the fractures of the zygoma. The inwardly displaced fractures encroach upon the maxillary sinus and hence for reducing (elevating) such fractures transantral approach is useful. In this technique a Caldwell-LuC opening is created and the antrum is opened the fracture is manipulated by inserting a finger in the sinus. After the fracture is reduced satisfactorily, the sinus is packed with a roll guaze soaked in White head's varnish or petroleum

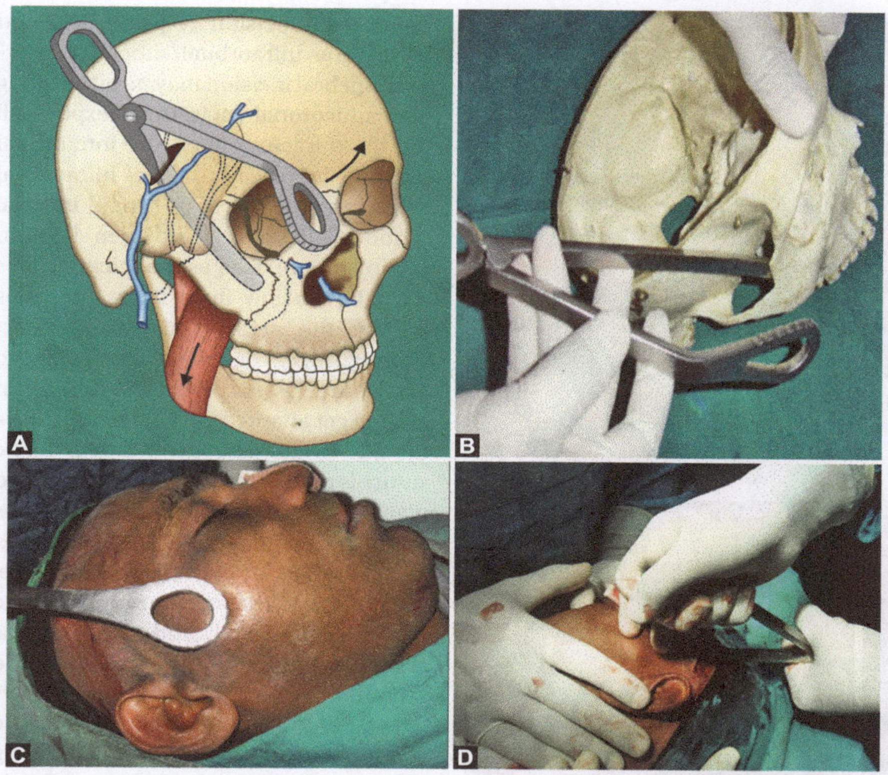

Figs 21.51A to D: Application of Row's zygoma elevator, note the similar lengths of both the blades and avoiding the fulcrum on the temporal bone

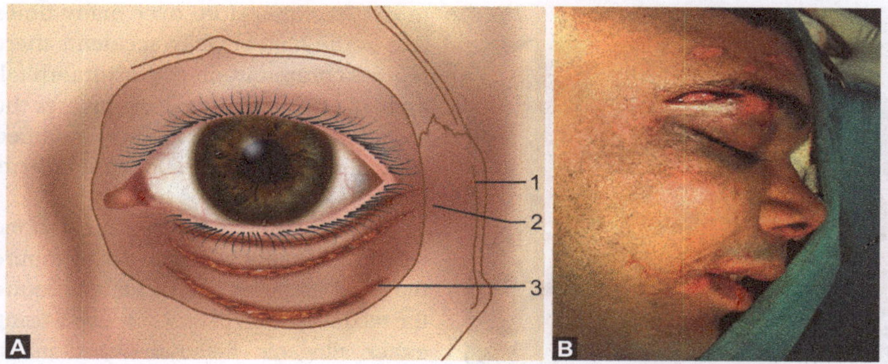

Figs 21.52A and B: (A) 1–Inferior palpebral, 2–Subcilliary, 3–Infraorbital incisions; (B) Lateral eyebrow incision

gelly created separately in the inferior meatus.[20] The pack supports the fracture from within. The intraoral incision, which is taken for Caldwell-Luc's operation is closed primarily. The pack is left *in situ* and removed after 3 to 4 days.

Open Reduction

The open reduction of the fracture of the zygoma is indicated in:

- Severely displaced and impacted, fractures which do not yield to the closed reduction
- Old fractures, which are not self-retaining
- Malunited fractures
- Comminuted fractures
- Fractures where functional loss is like diplopia, inophthalmos, proptosis, restriction of the mandibular excursions are present due to displacement of the fracture.

The open reduction is followed by fixation of the fracture segments with the help of either intraosseous wires[21,22] or miniplates.[23] The wires or plates can be fixed at frontozygomatic suture, infraorbital rim, the buttress and rarely at the zygomaticotemporal suture. The fractures should be fixed at minimum two points. For exposing the fracture line at frontozygomatic suture, a lateral eyebrow incision is taken. While taking the incision precaution must be taken that the direction of the blade is parallel to the hair follicles and not through them, as it leaves unsightly alopecia in the region of the eyebrow. The incision is masked in the hair as they grow. The orbital rim is exposed and the orbital periosteum is reflected carefully taking care not to injure the eyeball or other intraorbital structures. A malleable copper retractor is kept as a guard and after reducing the fracture, through and through holes is drilled on the either side of the fracture line on the lateral orbital rim. A piece of 26 number stainless steel wire is passed and intraosseous wire is tied across the fracture line.

The infraorbital rim is exposed through inferior palpebral, subcilliary or infraorbital incisions (Figs 21.52A and B).[24] All the incisions are intended to be cosmetically acceptable. Through the layer by layer dissection the infraorbital rim is exposed and the orbital periosteum is reflected. If the orbital contents are herniated through the fracture they are carefully separated and the fracture is reduced by elevation. Two holes are drilled on either side of the fracture line, keeping a guard for protecting the eyeball, using a 26 number stainless steel wire, intraossesous wiring is done. The zygomaticotemporal suture is exposed by placing a direct incision on the arch. But this incision is not cosmetically acceptable and the chances of injuring the branches of facial nerve are optimum.

The best incision of approaching the frontozygomatic suture and the zygomaticotemporal sutures is the

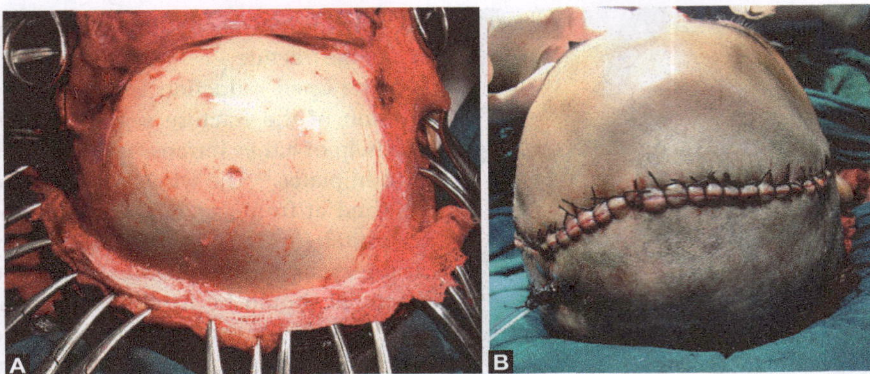

Figs 21.53A and B: Bicoronal incision

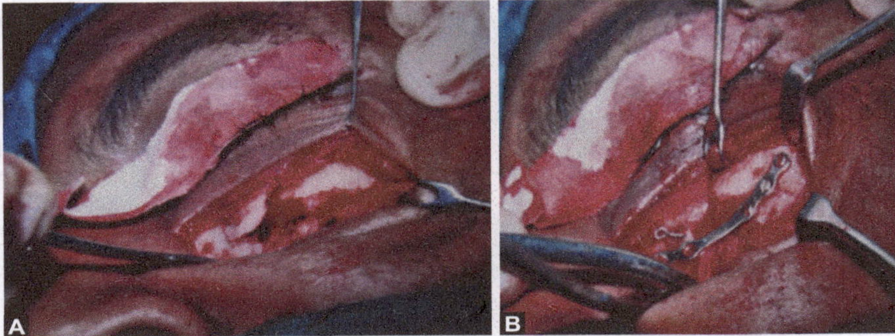

Figs 21.54A and B: Comminuted infraorbital rim plated with orbital plate

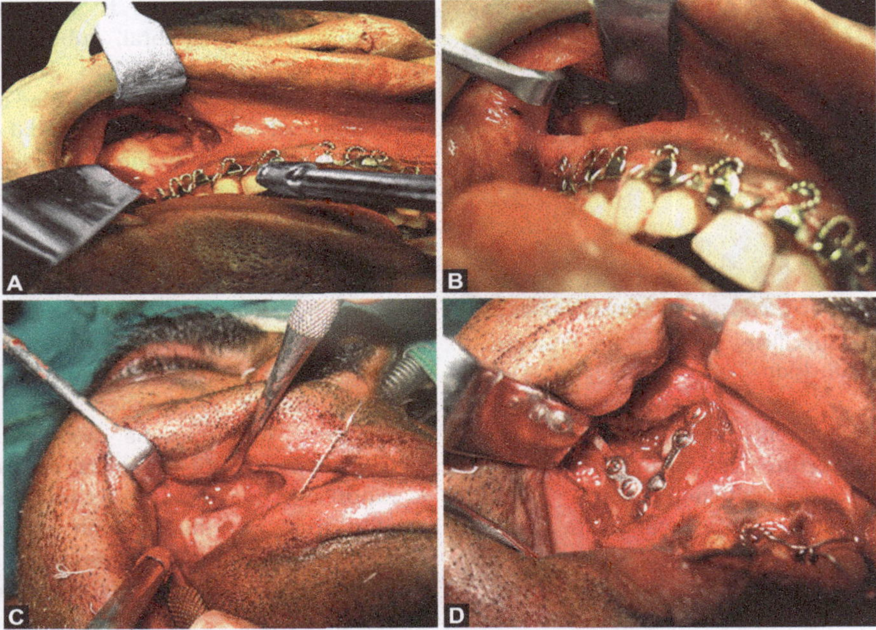

Figs 21.55A to D: Plating at zygomatic buttress

unicoronal incision (Figs 21.53A and B).[25,26] The infraorbital/subcillary/inferior palpebral incision may be taken along with unicoronal incision to expose all the three fracture lines, the infraorbital incision is placed in the infraorbital groove to hide the scar. If rigid internal fixation (RIF) is planned then 1.5 mm miniplates are used as the thicker plates may show below the skin as the plates are on the areas, which are almost subperiosteal. The orbital plates with 4 to 6 holes are best for plating the orbital rim as they get adapted well to the curvature of the orbit. The temporozygomatic suture is plated using straight 4 to 6 holed plate. The screws used at these locations are 4 to 5 mm long as the bones are thin.

Although all the four areas, i.e. the frontozygomatic, temporozygomatic (arch), infraorbital and the buttress areas can be used for the fixation of the zygomatic bone fractures, it is not always necessary to fix all the four points. The two point fixation, one point each along the vertical axis, i.e. frontozygomatic suture and the horizontal axis, i.e. at the buttress area, is usually adequate to give adequate fixation and the stability to the fracture. More over many times due to the high velocity accidents there is gross comminution at the infraorbital, arch and buttress area in such cases the technique needs to be suitably modified as per the presentation and requirements in each case (Figs 21.54 to 21.59).

The fractures of the zygomatic bone with involvement of orbital floor (Impure blow-out fractures of orbit) often require the reconstruction of the orbital wall using either allogenic material like titanium mesh, silastic, etc. or autogenous grafts like iliac crest or calvarial grafts, along with the fixation of the fracture of the zygomatic bone (Figs 21.60A to F).

Complications

- Infection
- Osteomyelitis
- Dehiscence of the plates
- Damage to the branches of the facial nerve

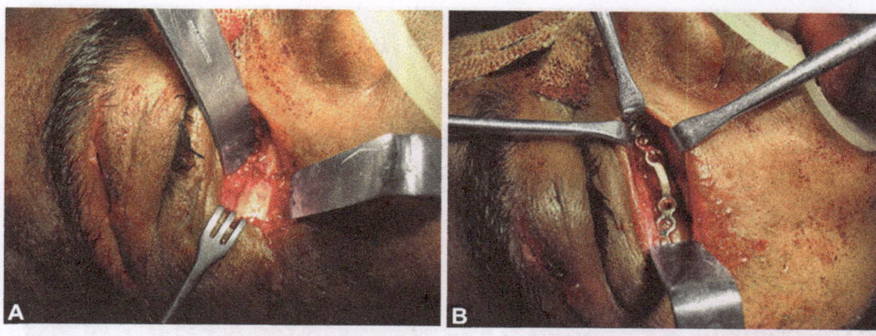

Figs 21.56A and B: Plating at the infraorbital area

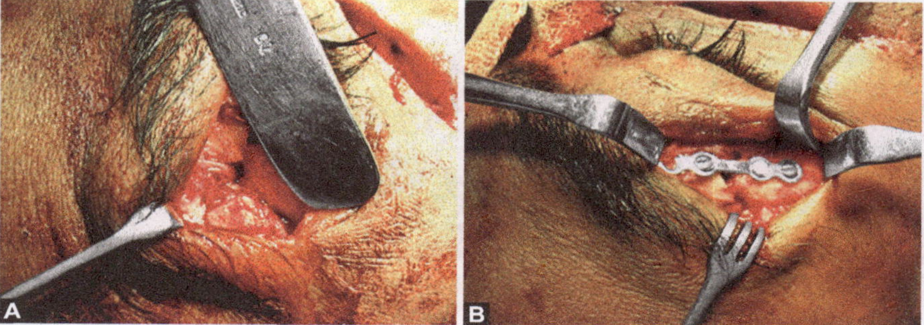

Figs 21.57A and B: Plating at the frontozygomatic suture

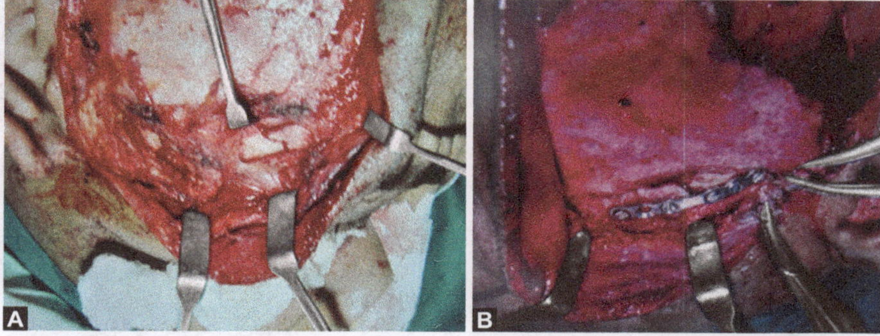

Figs 21.58A and B: Plating of the zygomatic arch through coronal exposure

- Ophthalmic complications like diplopia, proptosis, inophthalmos, superior orbital fissure syndrome, orbital apex syndrome.
- Showing of the plates below the skin.

SUPERIOR ORBITAL FISSURE SYNDROME

Superior orbital fissure syndrome, also known as Rochon-Duvigneaud syndrome.[27] Hirschfeld[28] first described superior orbital fissure syndrome in 1858. The superior orbital syndrome results secondary to the compression of the contents of the superior orbital fissure as a result of raised intraorbital pressure due to hermatoma or the displaced fracture segments.[29] The structures that pass through the superior orbital fissure are the 3rd, 4th, 6th cranial nerve, the ophthalmic division of the 5th cranial nerve, ophthalmic artery, and ophthalmic vein (Fig. 21.61). Owing to the raised intraorbital pressure these structures are compressed resulting in the paresis of the nerves and neurological deficit in their distribution. The 3rd (oculomotor) nerve supplies the superior rectus, medial rectus, inferior rectus and inferior oblicus muscles of the eye. The lateral rectus is supplied by the 6th (abduscent) nerve. The 4th (trochlear) nerve supplies the superior oblicus muscle of the eye. Due to the involvement of the nerves all these extraocular muscles undergo paralysis and the eyeball fails to move, which is called 'external ophthalmoplegia'. As the affected eye does not move while the contralateral normal eyeball moves the focal axis gets distributed and two images of one object are perceived producing diplopia. The IIIrd cranial nerve relays the preganglionic parasympathetic fibers from the Edinger-Westphal nucleus in the mid brain, which are relayed in the ciliary ganglion situated on the lateral rectus muscle. The postganglionic fibers are distributed the papillary and ciliary muscles of the pupil through the short ciliary nerve. Normally the parasympathetic stimulation leads to constriction of the pupil. As the IIIrd carnial nerve gets paralyzed, the parasympathetic supply is cut off and it results in sympathetic predominance, leading to fixed dilated pupil not responding to light. This is called '*internal ophthalmoplegia*' (Figs 21.62A and B). The parasympathetic fibers also go to the upper eyelid and they help in maintaining the tonus of the upper lid. Due to the interruption of the parasympathetic supply to the lid it drops dawn like a curtain and it is called ptosis of the eye, characterized by obliteration of the supratarsal fold. The optic nerve is not involved in this syndrome. But when in addition to this if the optic nerve is also involved it is called the 'orbital apex syndrome'.

Management

The management comprises of conservative and surgical. The conservative management is resorted to when the symptoms are mild. The CT scan or MRI of the orbit is done to find the cause. If a large hematoma is present retrobulbar or in the muscle cone or a fracture is severely displaced or some fragment is impinging upon the superior orbital fissure then surgical decompression is indicated.

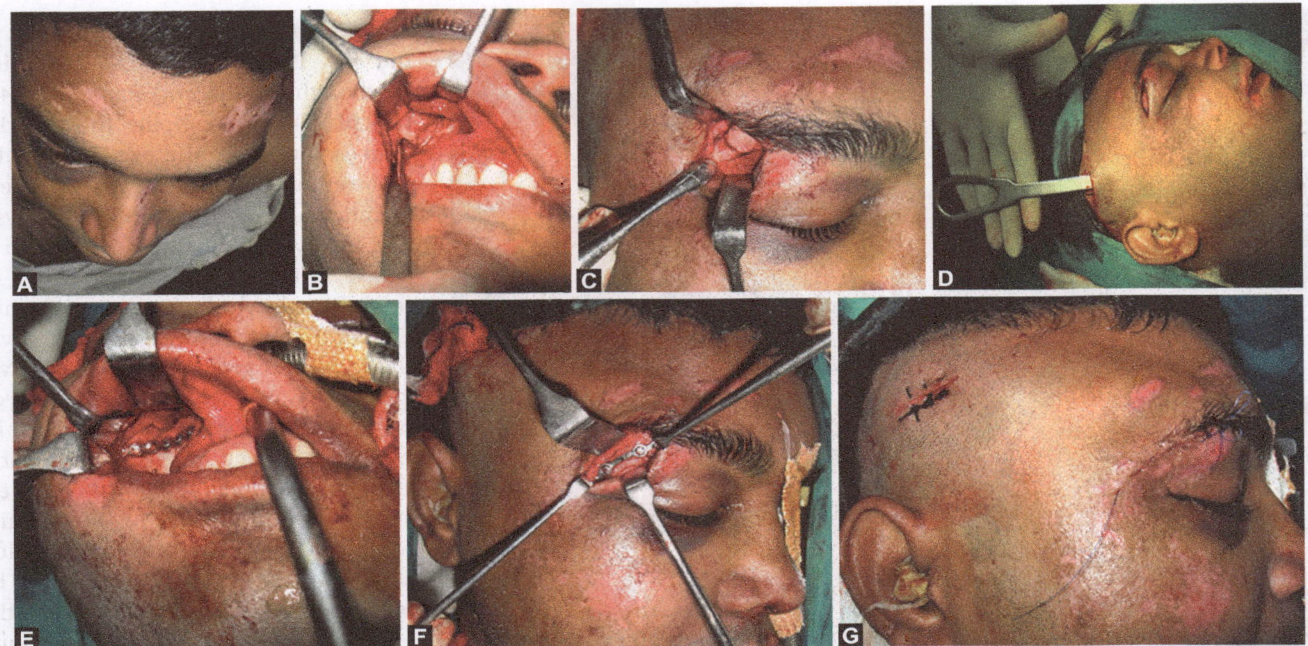

Figs 21.59A to G: Management of zygomatic fracture by two point fixation at the frontozygomatic suture and buttress

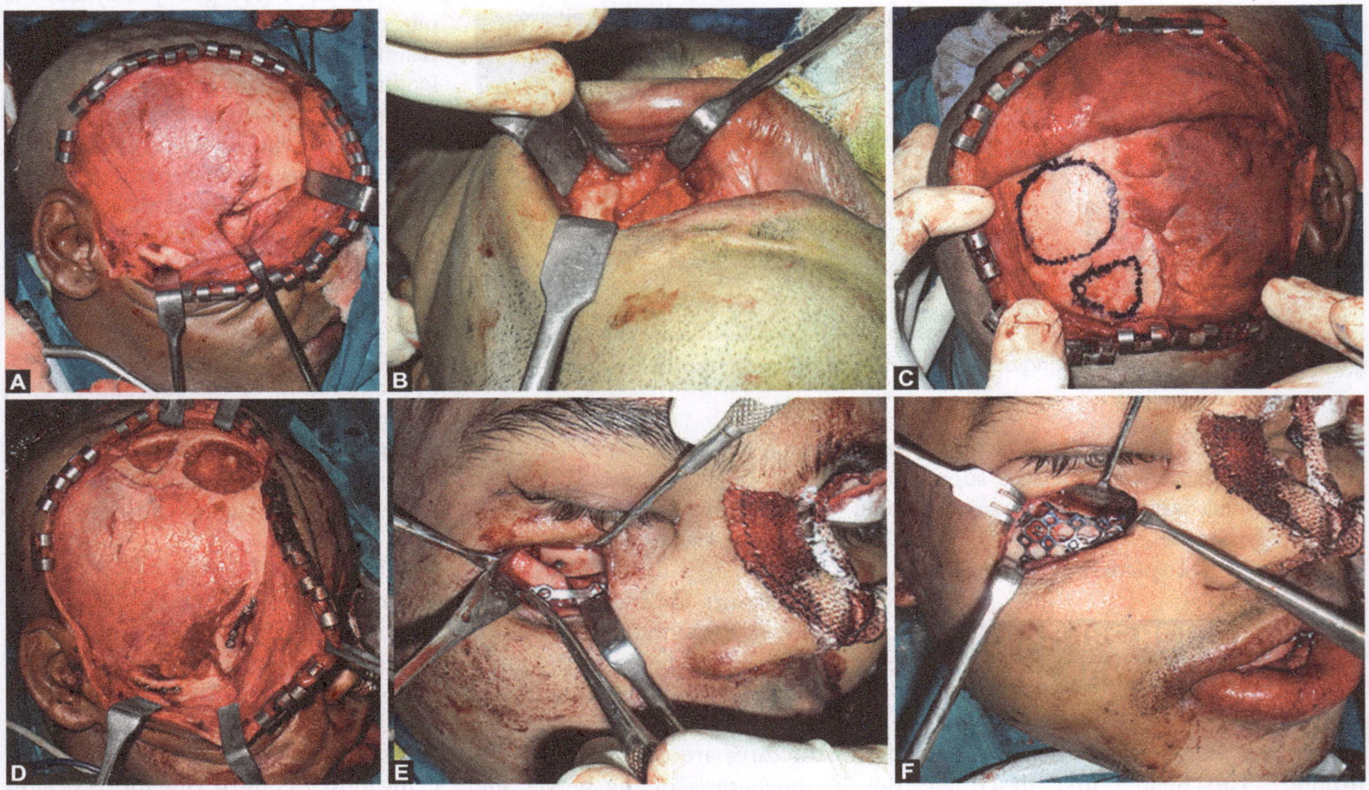

Figs 21.60A to F: Impure blow out fracture treated with reduction of zygomatic fracture and reconstruction of orbital floor with a calvarial graft

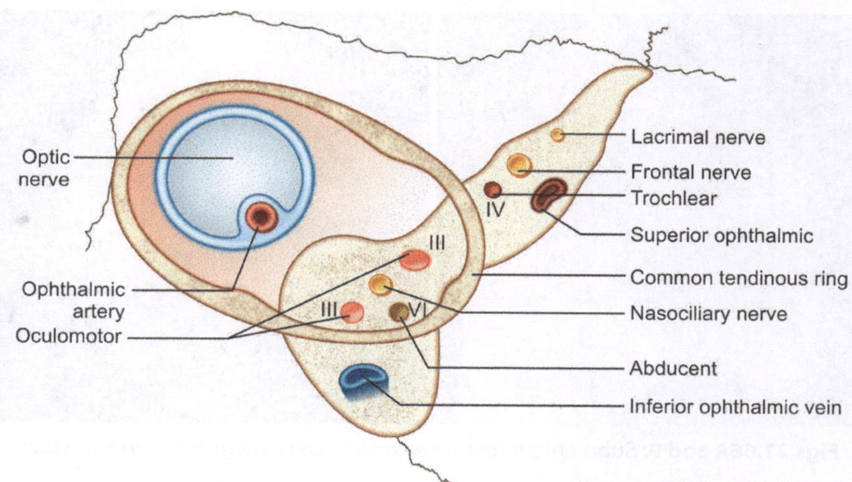

Fig. 21.61: Structures involved in superior orbital fissure syndrome

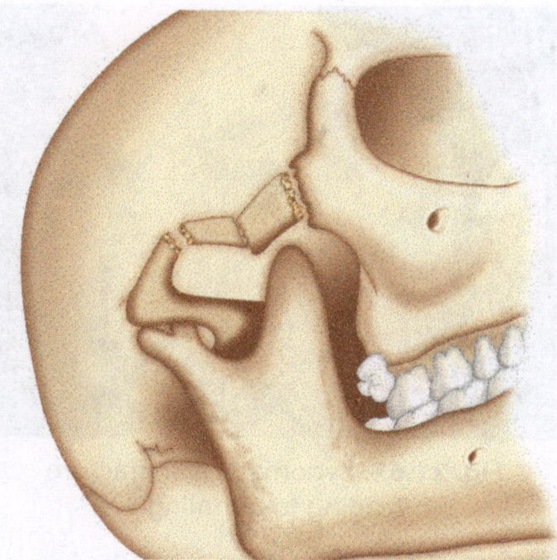

Fig. 21.63: Diagrammatic representation of V in zygomatic arch fracture

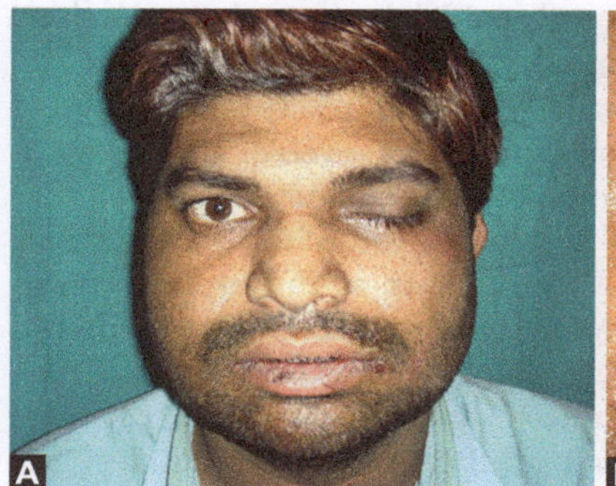

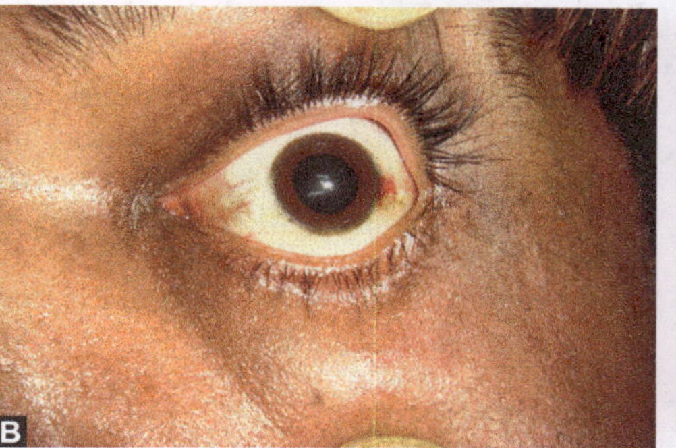

Figs 21.62A and B: Superior orbital fissure syndrome note the ptosis of eyelid, fixed dilated pupil and lack of extraocular movements (external ophthalmoplegia)

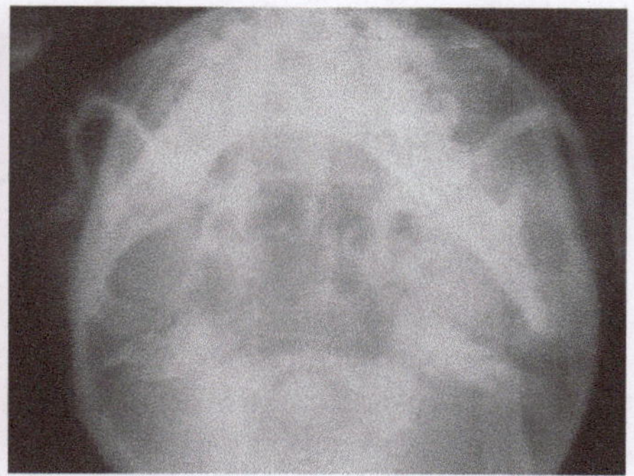

Fig. 21.64: Submentovertex view showing V in type of zygomatic arch fracture

Supportive treatment in the form of corticosteroid therapy, ocular physiotherapy should be prescribed to the patient.

FRACTURES OF THE ZYGOMATIC ARCH

Although the arch is anatomically very close to the zygoma, the isolated fracture of the arch can take place and they produce distinct clinical features. The arch is formed by the temporal process of the zygoma and the zygomatic process of the temporal bone. The masseter originates from the inferomedial border of the arch and the deep temporal fascia is attached to it superiorly. Both these structures prevent the superoinferior displacement of the arch in the event of the fracture. The coronoid process of the mandible lies deep to the arch and when there is severe medial displacement of the fracture the coronoid process gets obstructed mechanically and the mandibular movements are restricted.

The fractures of the arch can be classified as:

- Undisplaced fractures
- 'V' in type of the fractures (Figs 21.63 and 21.64)
- A 'V' in fracture results when the zygomatic arch fractures at 3 points, thus, there are more than two fracture fragments and the V in fracture in true sense is a comminuted fracture.

Clinical Features

- Dimpling over the arch—the dimpling is seen immediately following trauma (Fig. 21.65) and it is masked by the edema in short period of time. It is seen cases of depressed (V-in) fractures.
- Edema over the temporal and the preauricular area. The edema may extend to the adjacent structures.
- Trismus and restricted mandibular excursions. When the fracture is a V-in type in trismus can be produced due to the spasm of the masseter and the mechanical obstruction of the coronoid process.
- Pain or mastication as a result of contraction of the masseter during function, which brings about the movement across the fragments and produces pain.
- Tenderness, crepitus and step deformity over the arch.

Investigations

The submentovertex view of the skull (Jug handle view) is taken to visualize the arch. The medicolateral displacement is better assessed on the X-ray. The

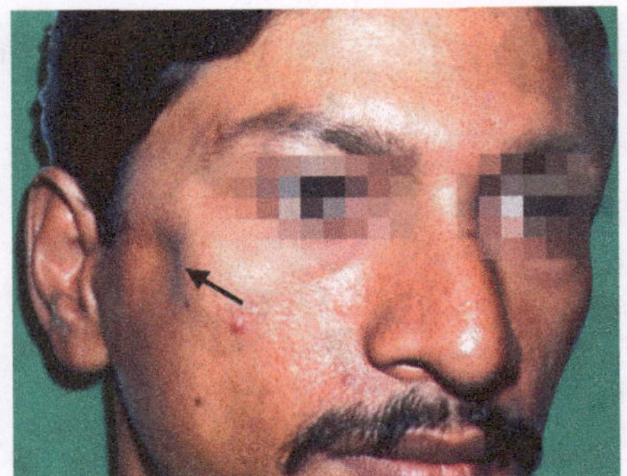

Fig. 21.65: Zygomatic arch fracture leading to dimpling

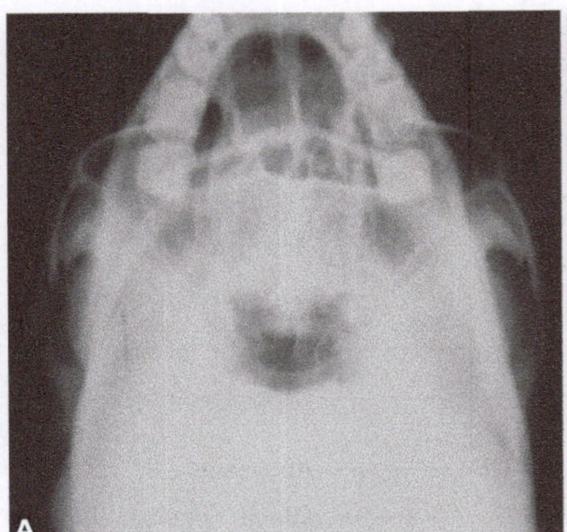

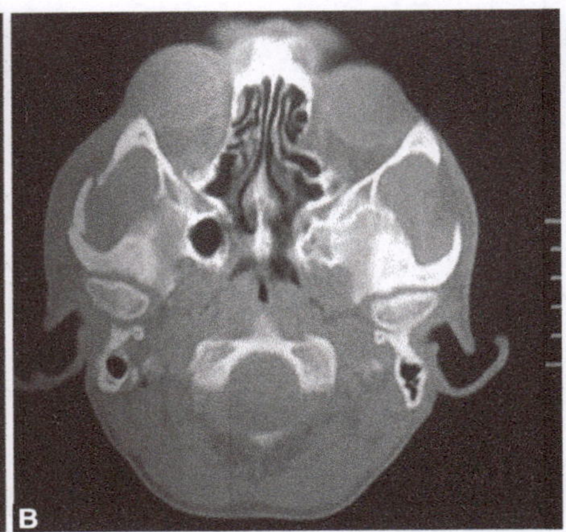

Figs 21.66A and B: Submentovertex view and CT scan of zygomatic arch fracture

X-ray PNS also shows the arch, but not very clearly. The submentovertex view of skull is often adequate to properly visualize the zygomatic arch fracture but the CT scan provides better details (Figs 21.66A and B).

Management

The management comprises of closed and open reduction. The closed reduction is done by the intraoral Keen's approach[14] or by extraoral Gillies temporal approach.[15] The Bristow's zygoma elevator is used for the same. The procedure is the same as described for the zygomatic bone reduction, only difference being the direction of the elevator is little posteriorly towards the arch. The indicator of the adequate reduction is correction of the dimpling and abolition of the step over the arch. To prevent the collapse of the reduced arch, an external splint is applied on the reduced arch and is secured in place with the help of thick suture thread passed circumferential to the arch and tying a knot above the splint. Postoperative radiographs are often helpful in ascertaining the proper reduction. The comminuted old fractures are treated by open reduction as they are not self-retaining and tend to collapse after elevation. The open reduction of the arch is done either through direct approach, taking incision over the arch and exposing the arch by layer by layer dissection, the fracture is reduced using a bone lever and intraosseous wiring or miniplates can be used to plate to stabilize the segments. While dissecting the soft tissue care must be taken not to dissect the periosteum injudiciously as there can be a vascular necrosis due to excessive periosteal stripping. The disadvantages of the direct approach are poor esthetic results due to scar, chances of damage to the zygomatico- temporal branch of the facial nerve. To avoid such complications hemicoronal exposure is preferred (Figs 21.58A and B).

Complications

- Osteomyelitis
- Malunion
- Fusion of the arch with the coronoid process leading to false ankylosis.

ORBITAL FRACTURES

The orbit is conical cavity with its base anteriorly and the apex directed at the optic foramen. It has four walls composed of seven bones; ethmoid, frontal, lacrimal, maxillary, palatine, sphenoid and zygomatic. The walls (roof, lateral, medial, floor) taper posteriorly to the apex and optic canal. The medial orbital walls are approximately 1 cm apart and parallel and the adult orbit volume is 30 cc. The orbital boundries are called the rims of the orbit, which are dense, corticated to protect the eyeball. The medial wall and the floor of the orbital are thin and fragile, while the roof and the lateral walls are stronger. The floor is weakened due to the infraorbital canal passing through it and the medial wall is formed by lamina papyracea of the ethmoidal bone and the lacrimal bones, which themselves are thin and fragile (Fig. 21.67).[30] The vital content of the orbit is the eyeball and it is noncompressible structure. The eye has six extraocular muscles, which control the movements of the eyeball, which originate from the common tendinous fibrous ring. The Annulus of Zinn is a fibrous ring formed by the common origin of the four rectus muscles. The eyeball and the muscles are cushioned in the orbit with the periorbital fat. The optic foramen is guarded by thick, corticated rim, which protects the optic nerve. The optic nerve is a direct extension of the gray matter. It is very sensitive to compression and once damaged fails to regenerate. The superior orbital fissure transmits the 3rd, 4th, 6th ophthalmic division of the 5th cranial nerve in addition to the ophthalmic vein and the artery. These cranial nerves innervate the extraocular muscles and the 3rd cranial nerve also relays the preganglionic parasympathetic fibers. The eyelids contain cartilaginous plates called tarsal plates. In the event of the trauma the thick rims protect the eyeballs and absorb shock by way of fracturing themselves. The orbital walls especially the medial and the floor can also fracture in an isolated way and get the displaced inwards or outwards and such fractures are called blow in and blow out fractures, respectively. When

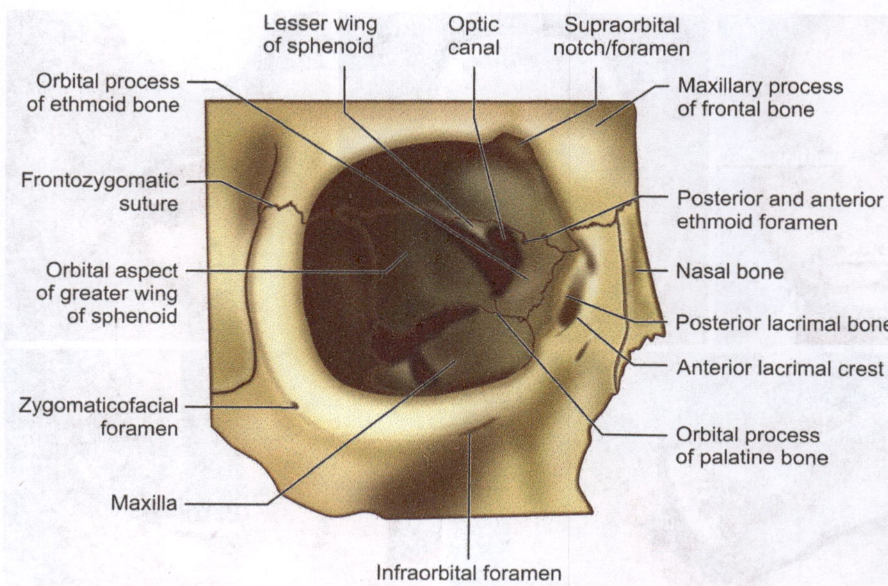

Fig. 21.67: Anatomy of the bony orbit

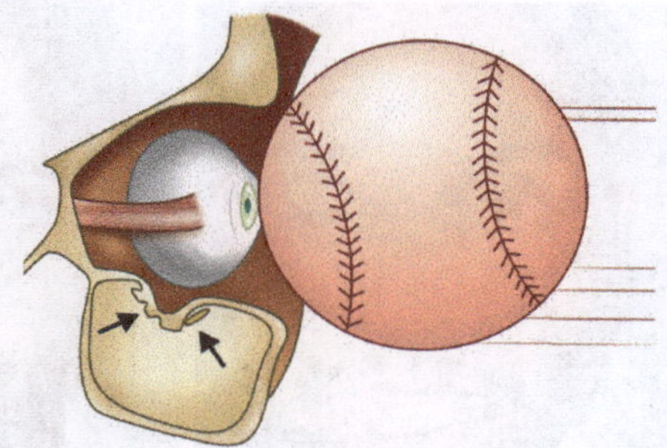

Fig. 21.68: Pathophysiology of blow out fracture of the orbit

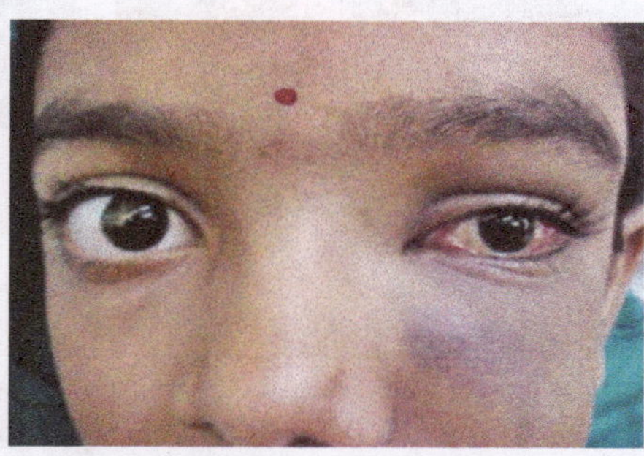

Fig. 21.69: Enophthalmos following the blow out fracture

the orbital walls fracture in isolation they are called pure blow out or blow in fractures. When the walls fracture along with the rim it is called impure blow out or blow in fracture depending upon the direction of the displacement of the wall.

Blow Out Fracture of Orbit

The term 'blow out fracture' was coined in 1957 by Smith and Regan[31] who were investigating injuries to the orbit by placing a hurling ball on cadaverous orbits and striking it with a mallet. According to Ng P et al., orbital floor fractures first were described by MacKenzie in Paris in 1844.[32] The pathophysiology of the blow out fracture is that the eyeball is a noncompressible structure. When an object which is larger in size than the orbit strikes the orbit, the eyeball is compressed, but as it is incompressible the intraorbital pressure increases and the pressure is exerted indirectly on the walls of the orbit. As the walls are thin and fragile they give way and fracture and are blown outward, this produces the blow out fracture (Fig. 21.68) thus, the thin and fragile nature of the medial wall and the floor is a natural protection offered by the nature. As they fracture readily and the orbital size expands and the raised intraorbital pressure is compensated. This fragility of walls prevents the rupture of the eyeball which is vital. The blowing out of the walls results in herniation of the periorbital fat and thus, the orbital contents are also reduced and due to the retracting action of the extraocular muscles the eyeball sinks in, resulting in inophthalmos. The extraocular muscles especially the inferior rectus and the inferior oblicus get entrapped in the fracture fragments and diplopia results in vertical gage.

Clinical Features

- Due to the trauma there is circum orbital edema, which sometimes is so severe that the examination of the eye may not be possible until it recedes.
- Due to the fracture of the wall there is subperiosteal bleeding, which escapes in the subconjunctival plane to produce subconjunctival bleeding.
- As the walls are blown out the orbital size expands and the eyeball sinks in resulting in inophthalmos (Figs 21.69 and 21.70A).
- Due to the fracture of the wall the periorbital fat herinates through it producing further increase in the size of the orbit (Fig. 21.70C).
- If the floor is fractured the periorbital fat herniates in the maxillary sinus and on X-ray PNS produces a classical 'hanging drop' appearance.
- The fracture and herination of the orbital contents also leads to bleeding in the antrum producing unilateral epistaxis.
- The infraorbital nerve gets traumatized producing numbness in its area of distribution.
- The inferior rectus and the inferior oblicus get entrapped in the fracture producing inability of the eyeball to move in vertical direction producing diplopia on vertical gage.
- When the medial wall is blown out in addition to inophthalmos, epistaxis, the diplopia will be produced on medial gage.

Management

The orbital fractures are assessed by X-ray PNS, which shows haziness of the maxillary sinus and a classical hanging drop appearance. In case the medial

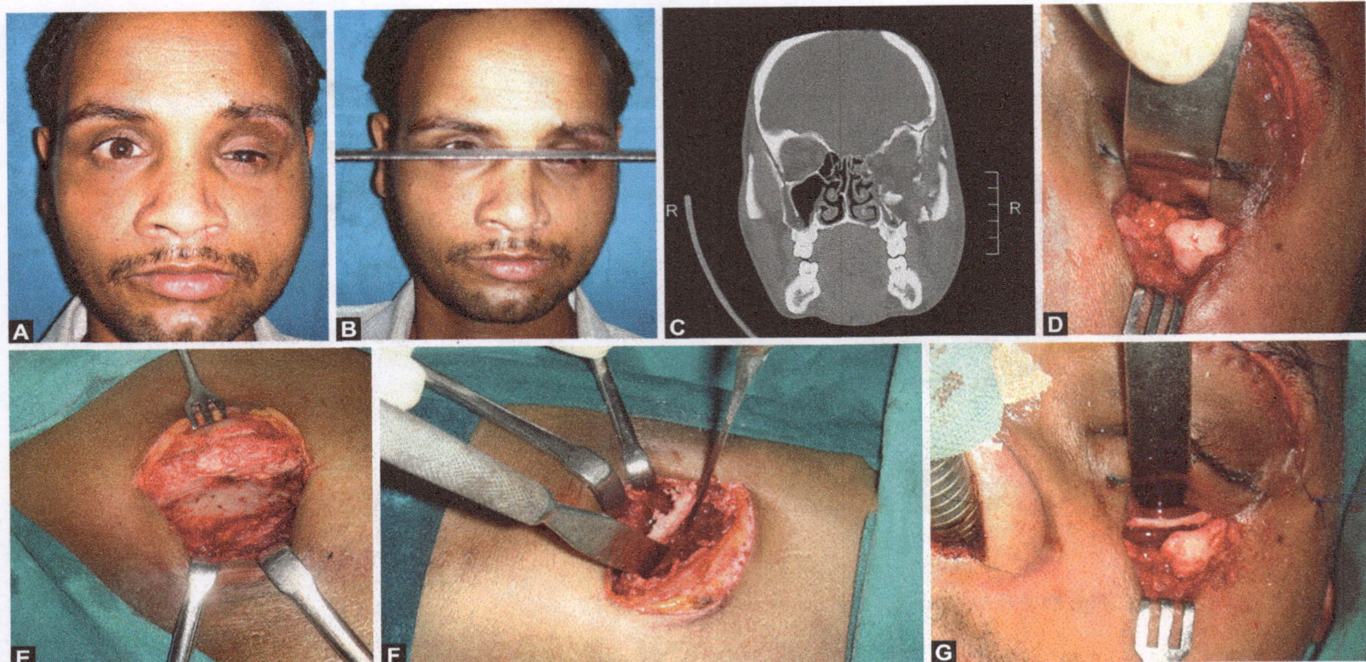

Figs 21.70A to G: A case of blow out fracture managed by bone graft, (A and B) Change in the level of the globe (enophthalmos); (C) Fracture of the floor of the orbit; (D) Exposure of the floor of the orbit through infraorbital incision and lateral wall of orbit through eyebrow approach; (E and F) Harvesting of bone graft from iliac crest; (G) Placement of iliac crest bone graft to reconstruct the floor of the orbit

wall fracture the nasal passage locks obliterated on the affected side. The better evaluation is by the CT scan[33] (Fig. 21.70B) and the assessment of the periorbital structures is done with MRI, which gives fair idea of the injury to the extraocular muscles.

The floor of the orbit fractures can be managed by closed reduction or by open reduction.[34]

Closed Reduction

The closed reduction is done by:

- **Transantrally**: Caldwell-Luc operation is performed and the herniated orbital contents are carefully elevated with digital pressure then the maxillary sinus is packed with a guaze soaked in petroleum jelly to support the fractured floor and the end of the roll guaze is drawn out through the nasal antrostomy opening in the cavity. The intraoral incision is closed primarily. The pack is removed on 5th to 6th postoperative day.
- **Transnasally:**[35] A nasal antrostomy is performed through the inferior turbinate approach, using a trochar and cannula. A balloon catheter (Foley's catheter) is passed through the antrostomy site in the maxillary antrum and the ballon is inflated (Fig. 21.71). As the balloon gets inflated the herniated orbital contents get lifted. The catheter is left *in situ* in inflated condition for support 5 to 6 days.

Disadvantage: The disadvantage of the closed reduction is that the reduction is arbitrary. The sharp bony fragments may injure the eyeball and the entrapped muscle is not released and thus the diplopia may persist.

Open Reduction

The open reduction is the more accurate method of reducing the blow out fracture as this is not only reduces the fracture, but also released the entrapped muscles and the help in correcting the diplopia. The orbital floor invariably fractures in small fragments and often needs reconstruction and thus, the open reduction is not only reduction but processes of the reconstruction of the fractured floor. The inferior orbital rim is exposed through the infraorbital/subcilliary/inferior palpebral incision. The orbital periosteum is identified and carefully raised by subperiosteal dissection. The entrapped muscles are released. The herniated structures are present above the periosteum and hence, if the periosteum is lifted the herination is automatically corrected. Sometimes, the wall is severely damaged

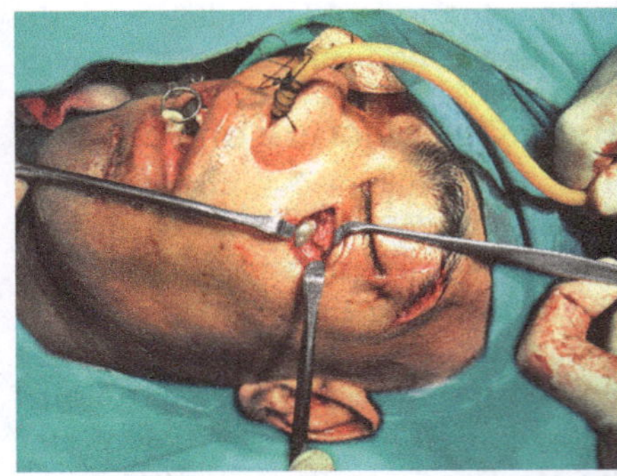

Fig. 21.71: Impure blow out fracture, the herniated floor of orbit elevated by a Foley's catheter introduced in the sinus through transnasal antrostomy and the infraorbital rim exposed for plating

and the periosteum is also lacerated in such cases the herniated contents are lifted and the eyeball is retracted upward using an eyeball retractor. The fractured floor is examined and the modality of reconstruction is decided. The average depth of the orbit is 40 to 45 mm and the graft/implant/mesh should cover 2/3rd the depth of the orbit (25 mm) for proper and adequate reconstruction of the floor of orbit defects during the management of the blow out fractures of the orbit. The extension of the dissection should not be extended beyond the 25 mm as the anterior ethmoid artery or optic nerve can be injured.

The orbital floor can be reconstructed with[36]

- Alloplastic material[37-39] like proline mesh, titanium mesh,[40] silastic, stainless steel (SS) mesh, etc. (Figs 21.72 and 21.73).
- Autogenous material[41] like cartilage, iliac crest cortico cancellous bone graft (*See* Figs 21.70A to G) (*See* Figs 21.65 and 21.74), Calvarial bone graft (*See* Fig. 21.60 A to F), split rib graft, nasal septal cartilage, etc. The calvarial graft are best suited for this purpose as they are thin, provide natural favorable curvature and most importantly show least resorption. After the surgery ocular physiotherapy is prescribed to correct the diplopia.

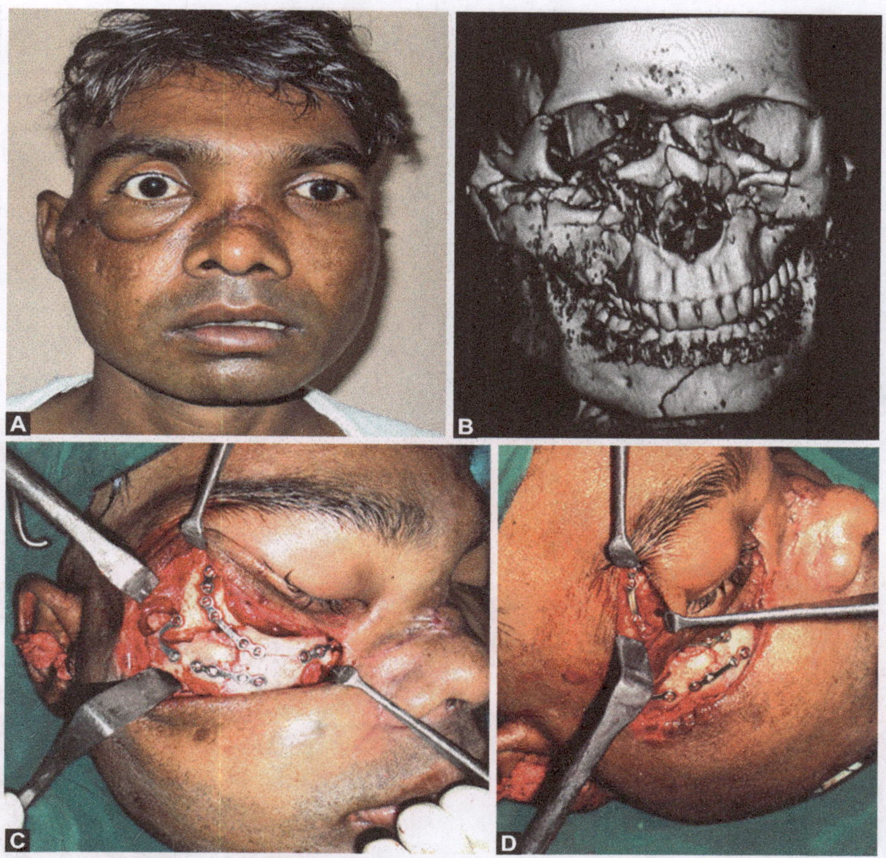

Figs 21.72A to D: (A and B) Clinical and CT scan view showing comminuted fracture of the orbit; (C and D) Exposure of the fracture through pre-existing laceration/scar

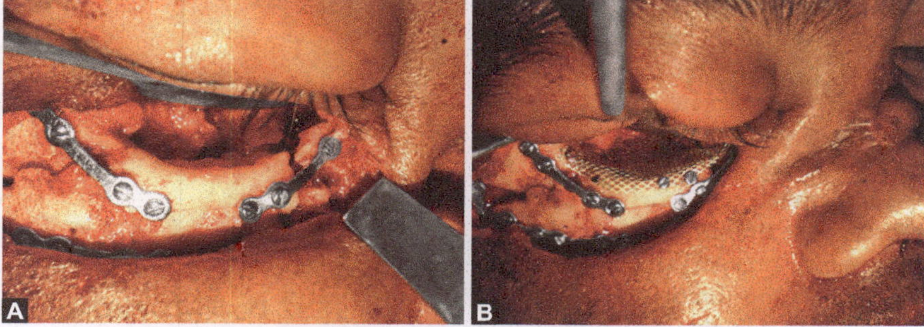

Figs 21.73A and B: Reconstruction of the orbit and its floor using the titanium mesh and fixation of the fracture using miniplates

NASAL BONE FRACTURES

The nasal bone is the most commonly fractured bone due to its prominent position on the face, little protection and support and minimal force required for it to fracture. It most commonly occurs in males than females. Highest incidence is between ages of 15 to 25 years in males and more than 60 years old females. The most common causes are road traffic accident in 70 percent of cases other causes are assault, sports injuries, industrial injuries.

Applied Anatomy

The nasal bones are small, paired bones, which constitute the nasal bridge. Superiorly the nasal bones articulate with the frontal bone at the frontonasal suture and laterally they articulate with the frontal process of the maxilla while they articulate with each other in the midline at the internasal suture. The perpendicular plate of the ethmoid lies below the internasal suture. The nasal bones can fracture in isolated way, but with a trauma of greater velocity, the fractures of adjacent bones like the frontal process of maxilla, the ethmoid bone and the lacrimal bone can also occur and in such cases the fractures are termed the nasoethmoidal complex fracture. The nasal bone fractures lead to the deformities of the nasal bridge and are comparatively easier to treat, but the nasoethmoidal fractures are complicated and may have anterior cranial fossa involvement and are

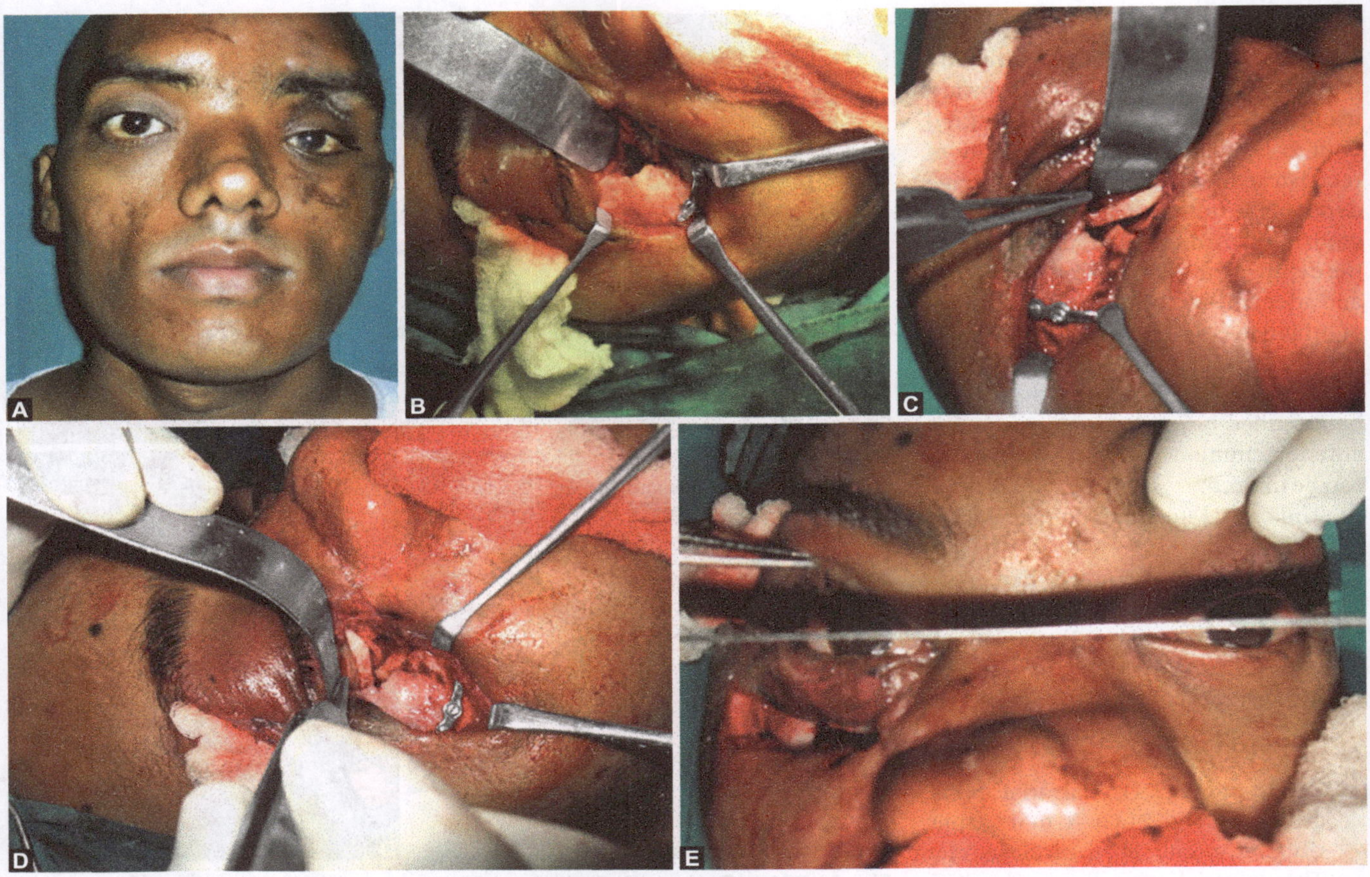

Figs 21.74A to E: A case of blow out fracture managed by bone graft

difficult to treat. The nasoethmoidal complex fracture may be associated with the detachment of the medial canthal ligament and injury to the nasolacrimal duct.

Kiesselbach's plexus or Little's area: It is the important area of arterial anastomosis present at anterior nasal septum, linking branches of greater palatine, superior labial, sphenopalatine and anterior ethmoid arteries. This area is most common source of epistaxis when fracture line or trauma effects this area. The nasal mucosa is highly vascular and is lined by pseudostratified columnar ciliated epithelium.

Classification

The isolated nasal bone fractures can be classified as:

- Undisplaced

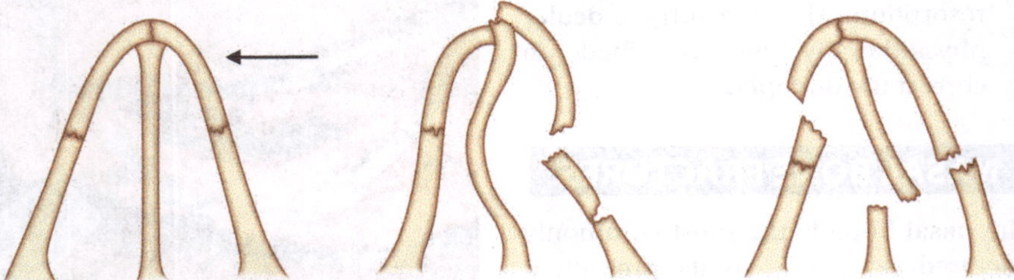

Fig. 21.75: Mechanism of fracture of nasal bone due to injury from lateral aspect

- Laterally displaced
- Comminuted.

Rowe and Killey Classification (1968)

Described lateral and anterior nasal injuries resulting from impact either from lateral or anterior direction.

- **Injuries from lateral aspect (Fig. 21.75):**
  - Moderate force result in depression of nasal bones and associated anterior edge of the frontal process of maxillary bone and buckling of nasal septum.
  - Severe force results in displacement of nasal pyramid to opposite

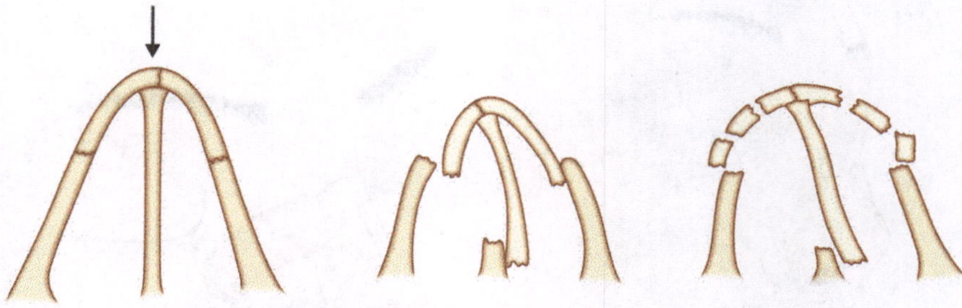

Fig. 21.76: Mechanism of fracture of nasal bone due to injury from anterior aspect

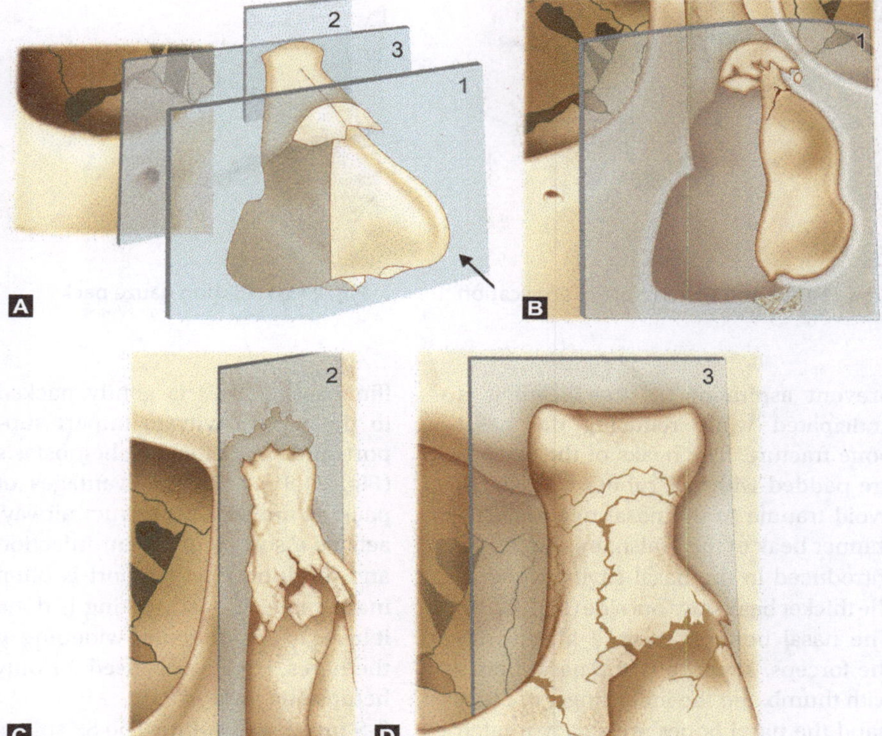

Figs 21.77A to D: (A) Stranc and Robertson classification (plane 1, 2 and 3); (B) Stranc and Robertson classification (plane 2); (C) Stranc and Robertson classification (plane 2); (D) Stranc and Robertson classification (plane 3)

side and fracture of nasal septum.

- **Nasal injuries from anterior impact (Fig. 21.76):**
  - Moderate force frequently results in fracture of nasal pyramid.
  - Severe impact results in fracture of the septum and comminution of nasal pyramid resulting in so called 'open book' nasal fracture.

Stranc and Robertson Classification (1979) (Fig. 21.77A)

Plane 1: Injuries do not extend beyond a line joining the lower end of nasal bones to anterior nasal spine (Fig. 21.77B).

Plane 2: Injuries are limited to the external nose and do not transgress the orbital rims (Fig. 21.77C).

Plane 3: Injuries are more serious and they involve orbital and possibly intracranial structures (Fig. 21.77D).

Clinical Features

The clinical features of the isolated nasal bone fractures are:

- Edema over the nasal bridge.
- Bilateral circumorbital edema and ecchymosis.
- Depression/flattening of the nasal bridge in the cases of anterior impact leading to open book deformity and deviation of the nasal bridge due to lateral impact leading to lateral displacement of the nasal bones.
- Epistaxis due to injury to nasal mucosa and the Little's zone.
- Septal dislocation from the groove of the vomer and deviation or buckling on one side (traumatic DNS). The presence of blood clot, edema of nasal mucous membrane and the deviated nasal septum (DNS) leads to nasal stuffiness or obstruction.
- Fracture and disruption of the nasal cartilage leads to deformities of the cartilaginous part of the nose.

Treatment of Nasal Injuries

- Careful preoperative clinical and radiological diagnosis is made.
- Radiographs are taken in two directions, PA and lateral.
- Nasal bone fractures are usually visualized on soft tissue radiographs of nose, lateral nasal radiograph and CT scans.
- The septal deviations are visualized on the X-ray PA Water's view (PNS).

Soft tissue injuries of the distal portion of the nose or injuries overlying the cartilaginous portion supported internally with packing or internal stabilization for 24 to 48 hours.

Closed Reduction

Timing of treatment

- Isolated nasal fracture can be reduced in first 24 hours.
- Treatment can be delayed until the 10th to 12th day.
- Nasal fractures associated with other fractures should be treated at the same time.

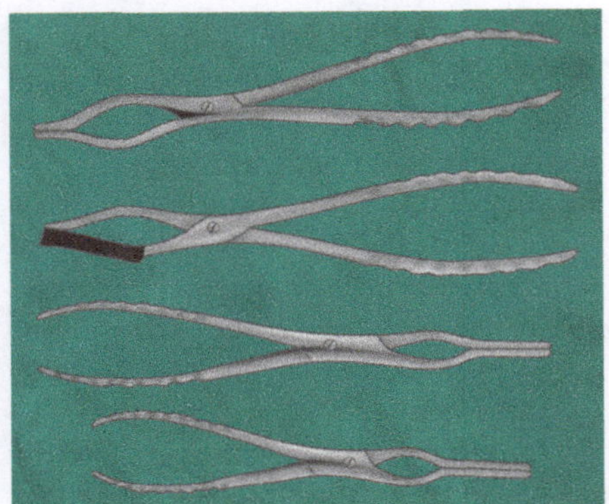

Fig. 21.78: Instruments—Walsham's forceps and Asch septum forceps

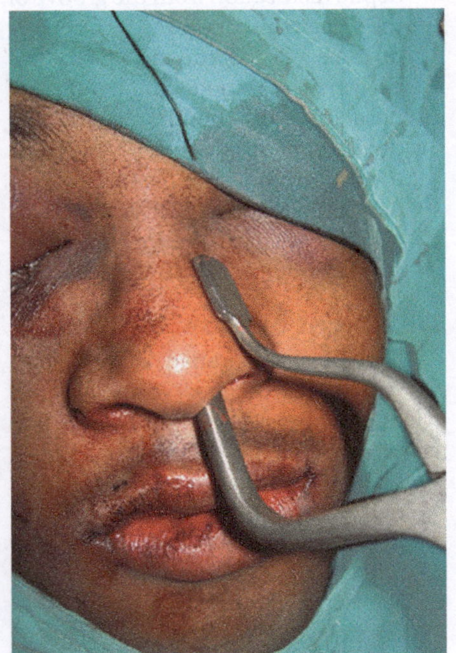

Fig. 21.79: Application of Walsham's forceps

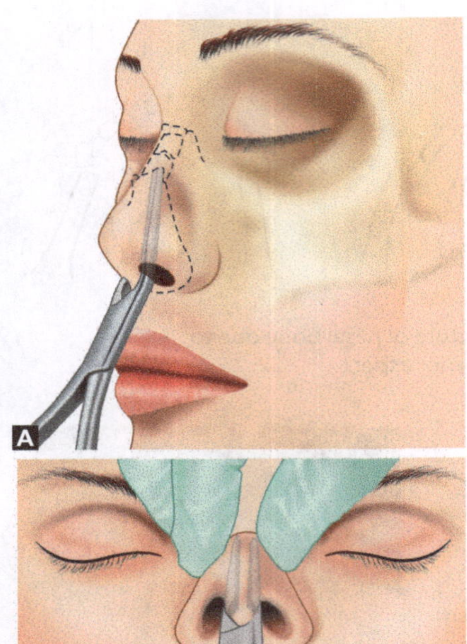

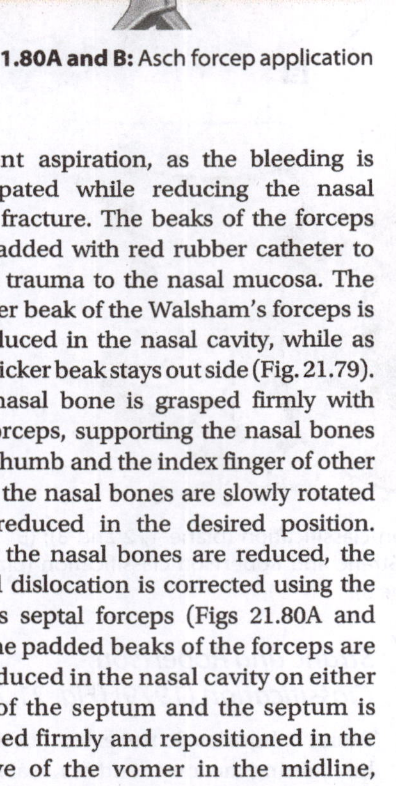

Figs 21.80A and B: Asch forcep application

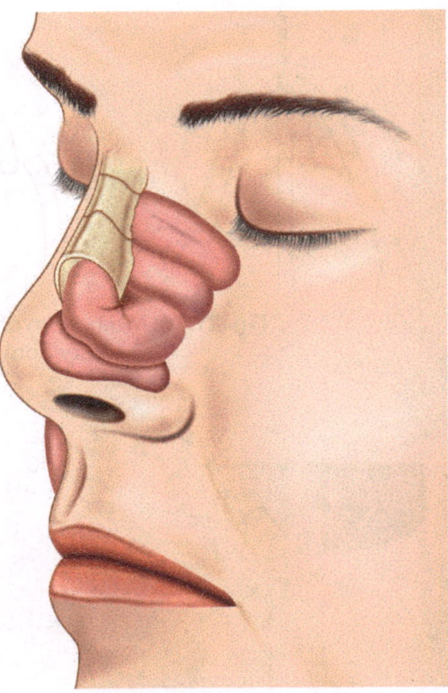

Fig. 21.81: Ribbon gauze pack

The closed reduction comprises of reducing the nasal bone fractures using the Walsham's nasal bone forceps and reducing the dislocated septum using Asch septum forceps (Fig. 21.78). The patient is operated preferably under general anesthesia. As the nasal bones are required to be handled nasal intubation is not done, but oral intubation is preferred with a cuffed endotracheal tube and meticulous pharyngeal packing to prevent aspiration, as the bleeding is anticipated while reducing the nasal bone fracture. The beaks of the forceps are padded with red rubber catheter to avoid trauma to the nasal mucosa. The thinner beak of the Walsham's forceps is introduced in the nasal cavity, while as the thicker beak stays out side (Fig. 21.79). The nasal bone is grasped firmly with the forceps, supporting the nasal bones with thumb and the index finger of other hand the nasal bones are slowly rotated and reduced in the desired position. Once the nasal bones are reduced, the septal dislocation is corrected using the Asch's septal forceps (Figs 21.80A and B). The padded beaks of the forceps are introduced in the nasal cavity on either side of the septum and the septum is grasped firmly and repositioned in the groove of the vomer in the midline, abolishing the septal deviation. The achieved result needs to be maintained by using the following methods:

Methods of immobilization

- **Ribbon gauze packs:** A 2.5 cm ribbon gauze in paraffin/flavine emulsion or bismuth iodoform paraffin paste (BIPP) is gently packed in the nasal cavity to impart support and for achieving hemostasis (Fig. 21.81). The disadvantages of packing are that it obstruct airway, acts as a source of potent infection and the intranasal support is often inadequate. If over packing is done it leads to postoperative widening of the nares. Hence, it is used for only hemostatic purpose.
- **S-S intranasal splint:** The SS splints were described by Sear in 1977. They provide better support when anteroposterior collapse is present. They are fixed using a transnasal wiring. Instead of the SS splints, custom made acrylic splints can be fabricated and used as per the need of the case. The splints are useful and rapid method when treating patients of multiple trauma.
- **POP splint:** The 'Butterfly shaped' are prepared by cutting 4 to 5 layers of 10 cm POP bandage and is moistened in water. The splint is applied to the nasal bone contour and held in place till the plaster of Paris sets. The set splint is lined by thin layer of cotton

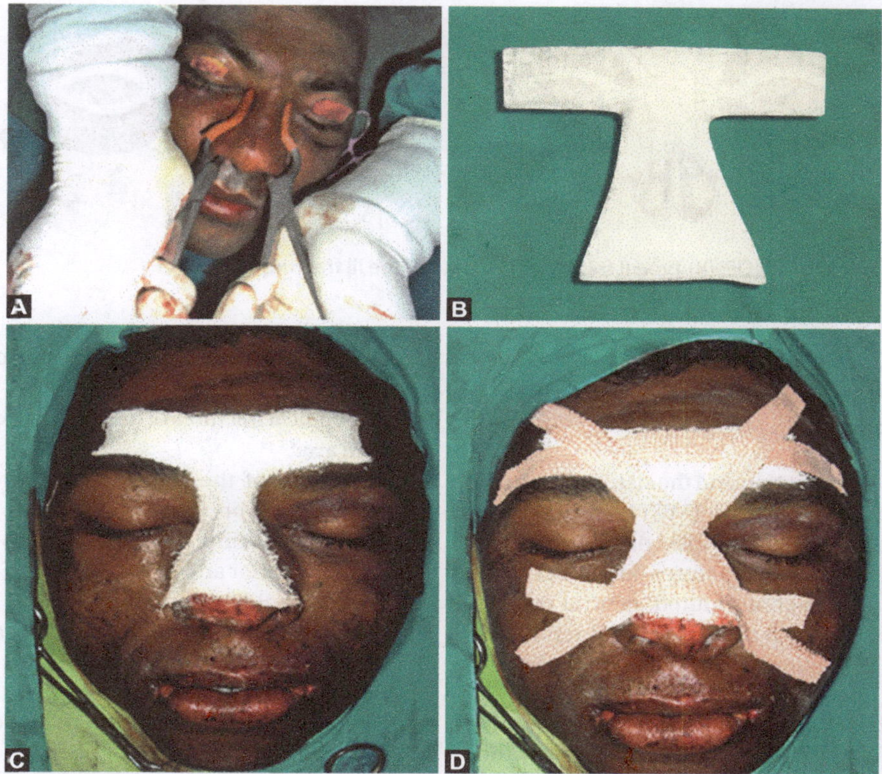
Figs 21.82A to D: POP splint and nasal packing for splinting the nasal bone fracture

wool to prevent pressure injuries to skin. Care should be taken to ensure that the splint margins are medial to the inner canthus of each eye. The splint is fixed in place using adhesive plaster strips (Figs 21.82A to D).

- **Collodion gauze and soft metal sheet (*Asch soft-metal sheet—tin/lead alloy*):** Several layers of cotton gauze are cut to size and soaked in collodion solution. A piece of soft-metal sheet is cut to shape, applied and contoured.

Open Reduction

The indications for the open reduction of the nasal bone fractures are:

- Malunited Nasal bone fractures.
- The grossly displaced fragments where stable reduction is not possible without opening.
- Comminuted fractures.
- Visibly displaced nasal bone and disruption of septal cartilage.

(details of the procedure are given under the nasoethmoidal complex fractures).

Complications

Hemorrhage—the posterior nasal bleed can be controlled by pressure applied through the postnasal packing.

Anterior nasal bleeding can be effectively controlled by pressure applied through the anterior packing using the ribbon gauze soaked in petroleum gelly or by cauterizing the bleeding points.

- Scarring or mucosal adhesions.
- Septal hematoma.
- Incomplete reduction leads to airway (nasal) obstruction.
- Traumatic deviated nasal septum (DNS).

NASOETHMOIDAL FRACTURES

Nasoethmoid fractures typically result from a forceful blow to the central area of the midface.[42] The fractures of the nasal bones can occur in isolation or they may be accompanied with the fractures of the ethmoidal bone, frontal process of the maxilla and the lacrimal bone (Figs 21.83A to C). The complex injuries involving these bones are often termed nasoethmoidal complex injuries.

The ethmoidal bone has various processes. The lamina papyracea forms the medial wall of the orbit and behind it the ethmoidal air cells are present. The cribriform plate forms the floor of the anterior cranial fossa and the perpendicular plate forms the superior part of the nasal septum and superiorly projects in the anterior cranial fossa (*crista galli*) to which the dura is attached. The cribriform plate transmits the

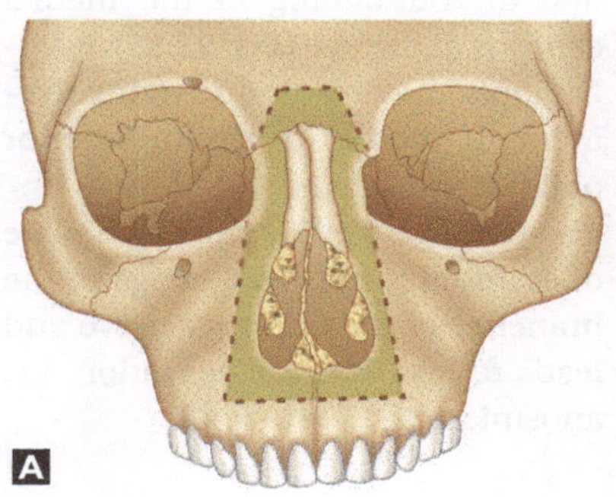

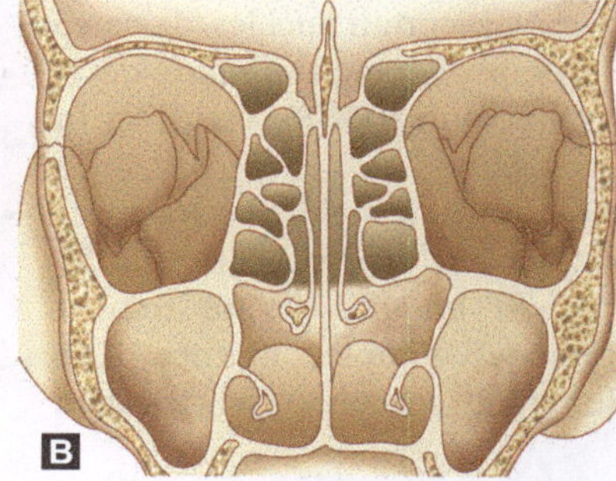

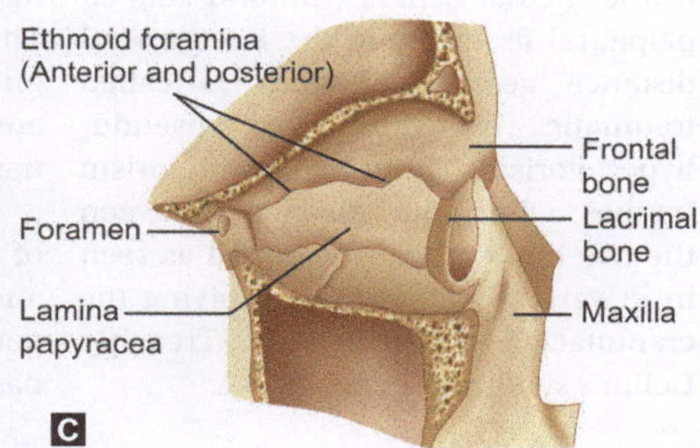

Figs 21.83A to C: Anatomy of the nasoethmoidal region

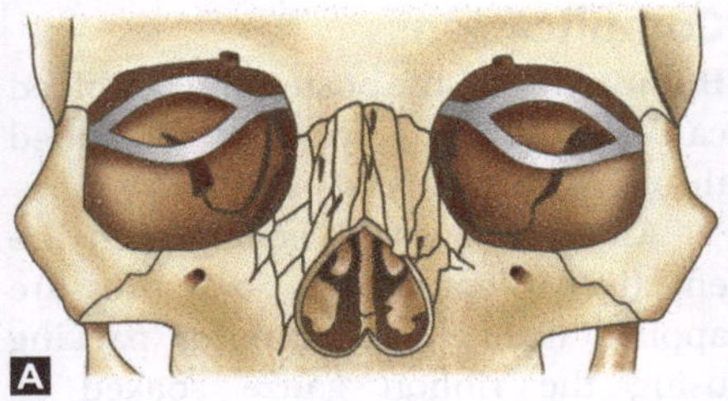
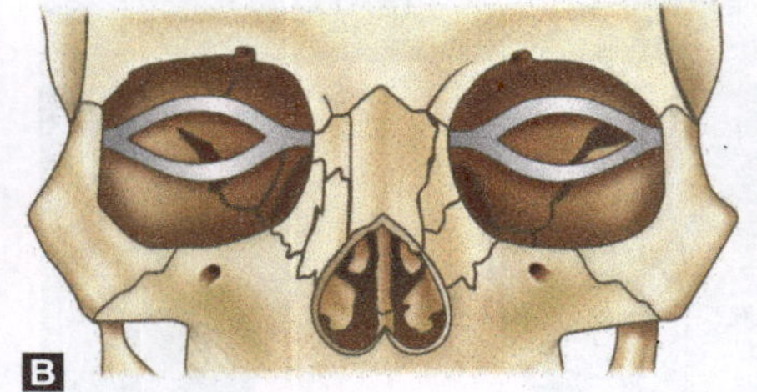
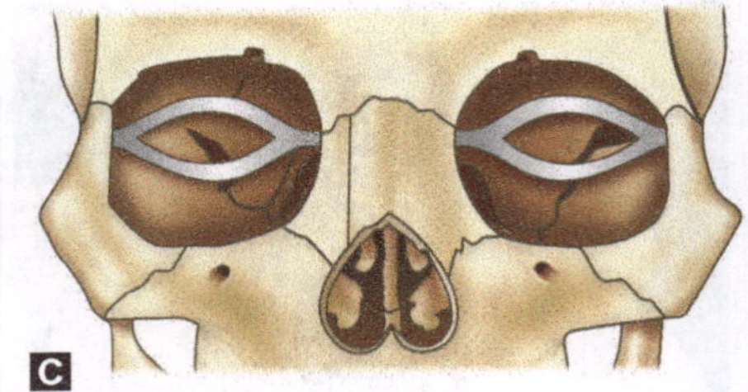

Figs 21.84A to C: (A) Type I fracture of NOE; (B) Type II fracture of NOE; (C) Type III fracture of NOE

emissary veins and the olfactory nerves. The ethmoidal air cells are normally not exposed to the external environments and in the event of the fracture they get exposed and infected and the infection can pass in a retrograde manner in the cranial cavity through the veins resulting in the intracranial infections like meningitis. The olfactory nerves are in the direct extension of the gray matter and lacks regenerative potential, which results in permanent loss of the smell sensation (anosmia) once it is traumatized. The crista galli provides attachment to the dura in the anterior cranial fossa, in the event of fracture of the cribriform plate the dural attachment may get torn and result in CSF rhinorrhea.

The nasal bones are paired and articulate with each other in the midline at the internasal suture. Laterally they articulate with the frontal process of the maxilla and superiorly with the frontal bone by frontonasal suture. The medial canthal ligament is attached to the frontal process of the maxilla and is responsible for the shape of the medial canthus of the eye. The fracture of the frontal process of the maxillary bone leads to detachment of the medial canthal ligament leading to rounding of the medial cantus (Almond shaped palpabral fissure) and the intercanthal distance gets widened, it is called traumatic telecanthus or pseudo-hypertelorism. The term hypertelorism implies when the distance between the two bony orbits is widened as seen in in various deformities involving the craniofacial skeleton (e.g. Treacher Collin's syndrome).

Classification of Nasoethmoidal Complex Fractures[43]

Comminution and the status of the medial canthal tendon (MCT) separate NOE fractures into the following three groups:[44]

1. **Type I:** Fractures involve a single, non-comminuted, central fragment without medial canthal tendon disruption (left-unilateral, right-bilateral) (Fig. 21.84A).
2. **Type II:** Fractures involve comminution of the central fragment without medial canthal tendon disruption (Fig. 21.84B).
3. **Type III:** Fractures result in severe central fragment comminution with medial canthal tendon disruption (Fig. 21.84C).

The nasal bones are articulate with each other at an angle of about 45 degrees and form the nasal bridge. The septum is formed by the vomer, septal processes of the palatine bone and the perpendicular plate of the ethmoid superiorly. The vomer has a groove anteriorly in which the septal cartilage articulates. The septum is located behind the internasal suture and is traumatized during the nasal bone injuries and gets dislocated from the groove of the vomer. The dislocated septum buckles/deviates on one side producing traumatic deviated nasal sebtum (DNS), resulting in nasal obstruction.

When associated with the fractures of the frontal process of maxilla and ethmoid bone they are termed nasoethmoidal complex injuries. The nasoethmoidal complex injuries can occur in isolation or may be associated with Le Fort II or III fractures.

The clinical fractures of the nasal bone fracture are:[45-49]

- Flattening of the nasal bridge producing open book deformity.
- Epistaxis—Hemorrhage due to rupture of anterior and posterior branches of ethmoidal artery.
- Due to the loose areolar tissue around the eye there is bilateral circumorbital ecchymosis/edema.
- There is tenderness, crepitus over the nasal bones.
- Subconjunctival hemorrhage medially.
- The nasal septum gets dislocated from the groove of the vomer and may lead to deviated nasal septum (DNS).
- The fracture of the frontal processes of maxilla can result in the detachment of the medial canthal ligament and the canthal angle becomes rounded. This apparently increases the distance between the medial canthi of both the eyes. The normal distance is about 36 mm and this increases beyond the normal value and the condition is called telecanthus. Thus, the traumatic telecanthus results.[50]
- *Almond shaped* palpabral fissure due to roundening of the medial canthus of the eye (Fig. 21.85).
- Diplopia may result due to involvement of medial rectus or inferior obliques muscle.
- The damage to the cribriform plate of ethmoid results in damage to the branches of the olfactory nerve and leads to loss of smell sensation, i.e. anosmia.

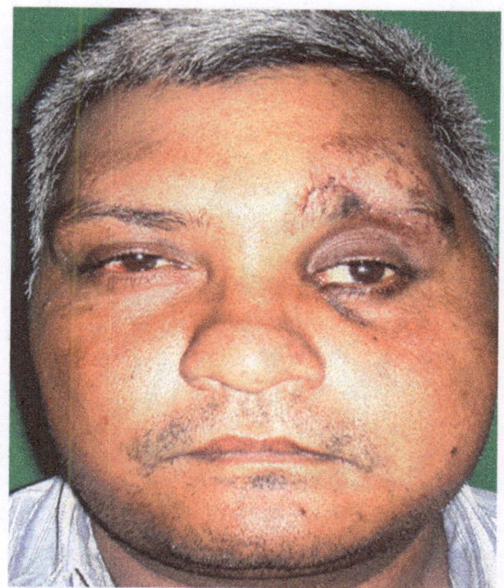

Fig. 21.85: Almond shaped palpebral fissure on left side due to detachment of medial canthal ligament

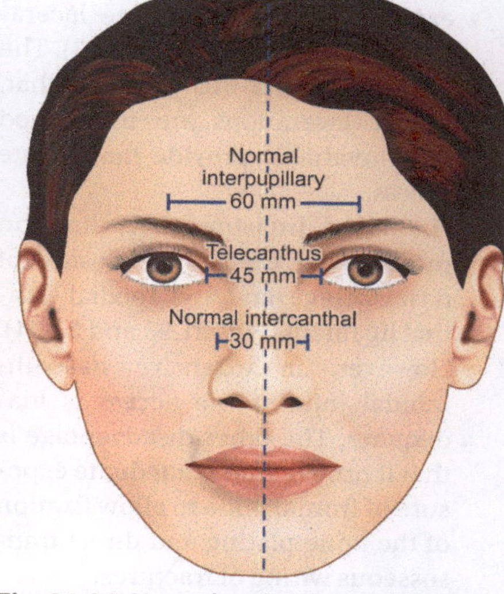

Fig. 21.86: Normal and abnormal intercanthal distance and interpupillary distance

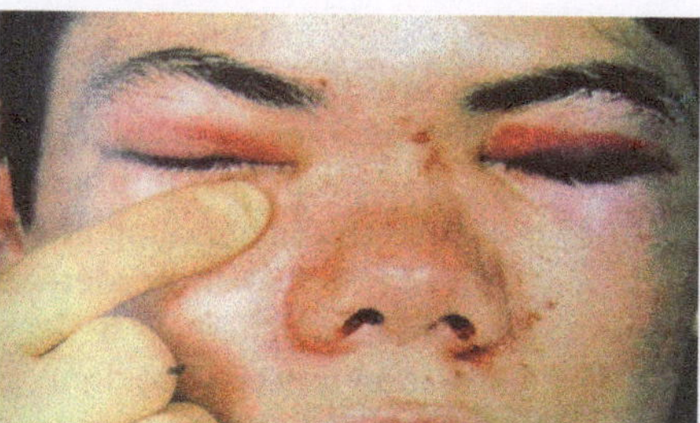

Fig. 21.87: Lateral tension test

- The fracture of the cribriform plate of ethmoid also results in detachment and tear of the dura and CSF rhinorrhea results.
- The ethmoidal air cells get exposed due to the fracture of the lamina papyracea of the ethmoid. Both the later condition facilitate the spread of infection in the cranial cavity resulting in meningitis.

Criteria for Making Diagnosis

- High index of suspicion and possibility of canthal spread should be considered with all severe nasal and midfacial injuries.
- **Measurement:** Normal intercanthal distance—the intercanthal distance is 32 to 33 mm in females and 33 to 34 mm in males. The intercanthal distance of more than 35 mm is indicative of canthal spread (telecanthus) (Fig. 21.86).
- **Palpabral fissure:** It becomes narrowed and almond shaped. The medial canthal angle becomes blunted with obliteration of caruncle and may be displaced down and laterally, due to the disruption of the medial canthal ligament tendon.
- **Eyelids:** Becomes lax and epicanthal fold becomes prominent
- **Canthal ligament:** The medial canthal ligament is assessed by lateral tension test (Fig. 21.87). On palpation there is diminished tension of the canthal ligament, which normally is firm and tensed and this sign is frequently visible clinically in cases where the canthal ligament is disrupted.
- **Examination of the nasal cavity:** A complete intranasal examination for nasal septum deviation, bleeding, concha, nasal mucosa, position of osseous structures and the presence of the CSF rhinorrhea (Figs 21.88A to C).

Investigations

The nasal bone fractures are seen on the true lateral view of the skull. The X-ray PNS shows the nasal septum and its deviation. Proper assessment of the nasoethmoidal complex is possible CT scan (Fig. 21.89).

Management[51-55]

The management of the nasoethmoidal complex fractures is more complex as compared to the isolated nasal bone fractures. Due to the involvement of many tiny bones, presence of comminution, gross displacement, detachment of the canthal ligaments and severe deformity, most of the nasoethmoidal complex fractures are treated with open reduction. The presence of cranial involvement in

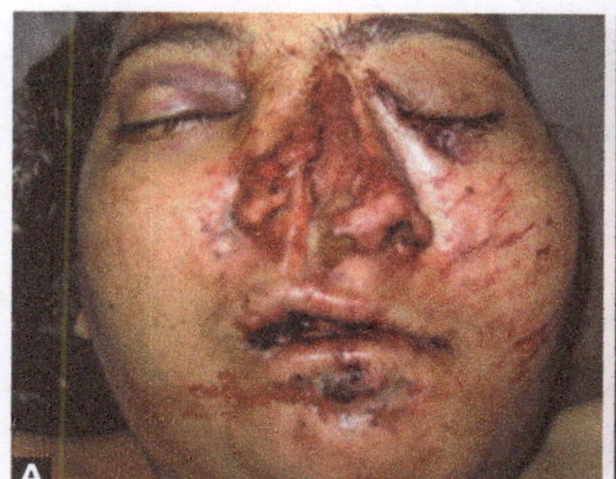
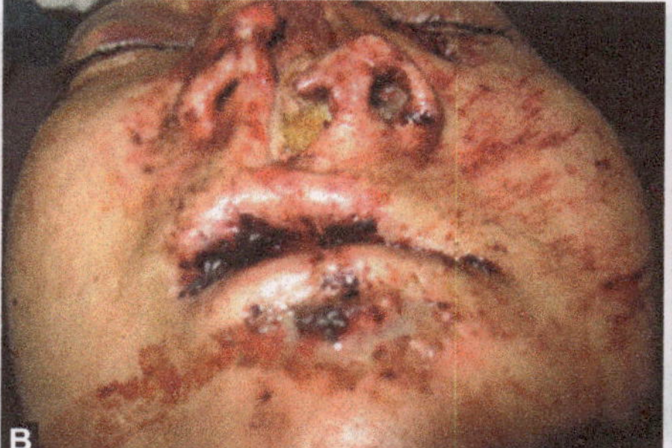
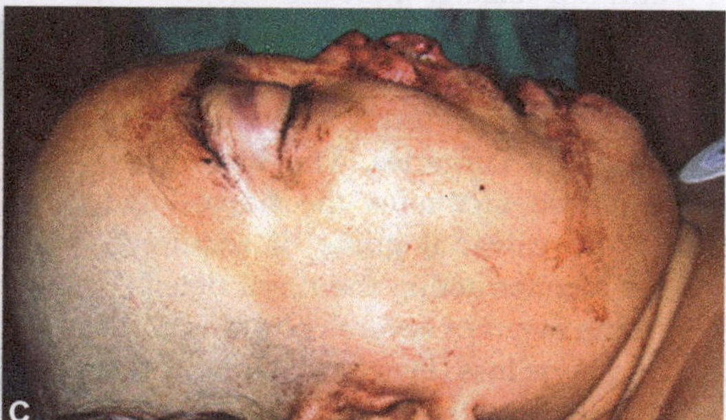

Figs 21.88A to C: Severe nasoethmoidal injury

the form of presence of CSF rhinorrhea further complicates the management.

In the presence of severe nasoethmoidal injuries the nasotracheal intubation is contraindicated as the handling of the area may lead to CSF leak in borderline cases. In the presence of active CSF leak the nasal intubation must not be done as it can widen the dural defect and can lead to infection and meningitis. In such cases the oral intubation is best suited as the nasoethmoidal complex fractures do not involve occlusion and IMF is not required. However, in polytrauma patients when the nasoethmoidal fracture is associated with a Le Fort II or III fracture and if the IMF is required during the reduction and the fixation of these fractures then oral intubation is not suitable and either a *transmyelohyoid* (Fig. 21.90) or if that is not possible tracheostomy should be done. The airway must be guarded using cuffed endotracheal tubes of by meticulous pharyngeal packing to prevent aspiration of the blood in the lower respiratory passage, as the bleeding is anticipated during the management of nasoethmoidal fractures. The packing of the nasal cavity is contraindicated in presence of CSF rhinorrhea as it increases chances of the intracranial infections.

For accomplishing the open reduction of the nasoethmoidal fractures different surgical approaches are described.

- **Bicoronal approach** is commonly used. It provides excellent exposure of the nasoethmoidal area and the glabella. It is useful if the frontal sinus fractures or frontal bone fractures are also present and facilitates the fixation of the plates. In case of anterior cranial fossa involvement and CSF leakage if the dural repair is also planned simultaneously, using a galial flap, the bicoronal incision provides opportunity to accomplish both the surgeries. The bicoronal flap also facilitates the harvesting of the calvarial grafts, if required for reconstructing the nasal defects in the event of severe comminution and bone loss (Figs 21.91A and B).
- **Through exsisting laceration:** If the compound nasoethmoidal injuries are present the fracture site can be exposed through the same laceration or scar (Figs 21.92A and B). The disadvantage of this access is that, as the lacerations are unplanned they invariably provide inadequate access.
- **H-shaped incision:** This incision provides an excellent exposure of nasal bridge and the medial canthal ligament (Figs 21.93 and 21.94). However, in extensive nasoethmoidal injuries the access is inadequate. The other disadvantage is that it provides an inadequate exposure of frontal bone to allow fixation of the bone plating and direct transosseous wiring of fractures.
- **Bilateral Z approach** described by Digman et al. the two Z incisions can be joined by a horizontal incision at base of nose to enhance the exposure of the fracture site (Fig. 21.95). This access also has the same merits and demerit as the 'H' incision.
- **Midline vertical approach:** It was described by Stranc. In this technique a 2 to 3 mm incision

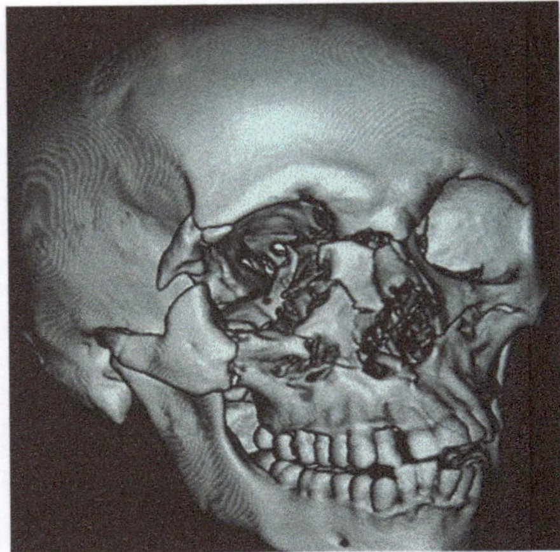

Fig. 21.89: CT scan of NOE fracture

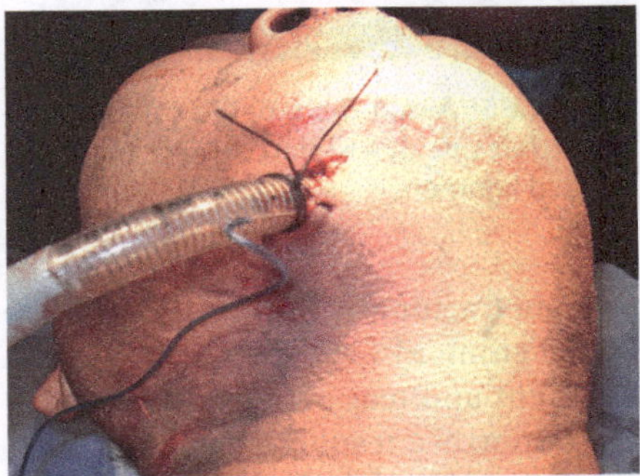

Fig. 21.90: Transmyelohyoid intubation

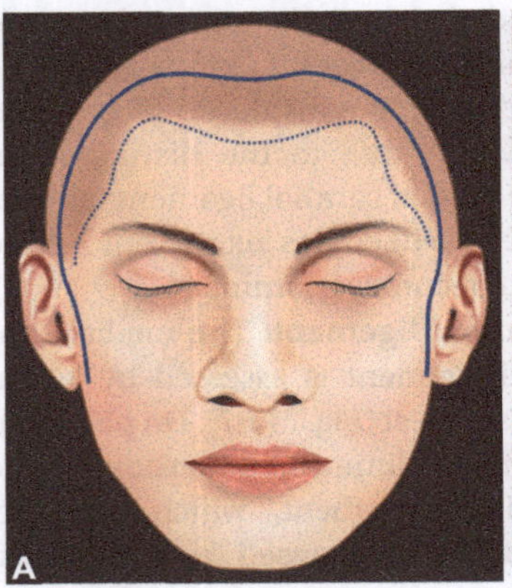

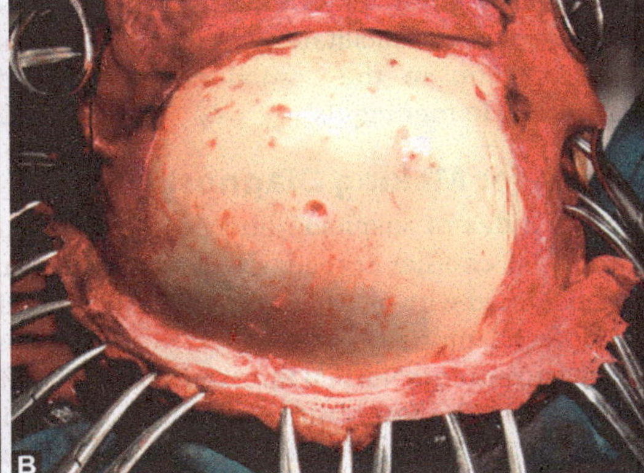

Figs 21.91A and B: Bicoronal incision

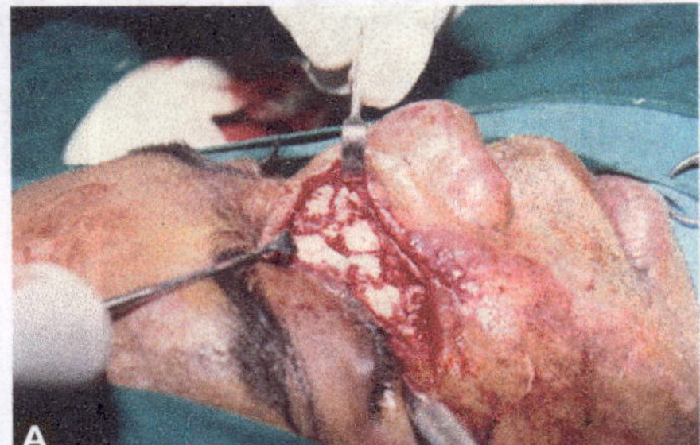

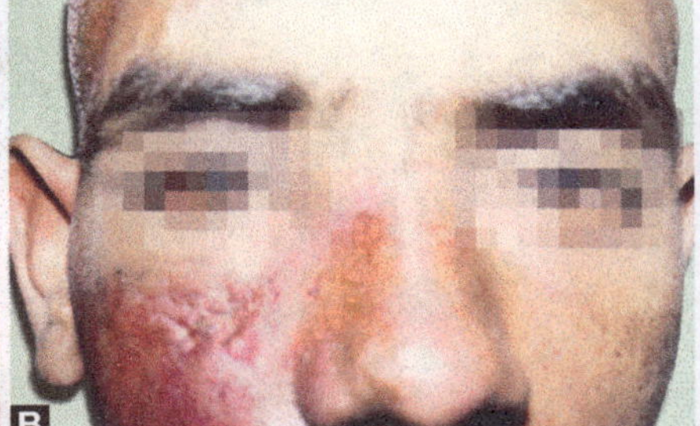

Figs 21.92A and B: Exposure of NOE fracture through existing laceration

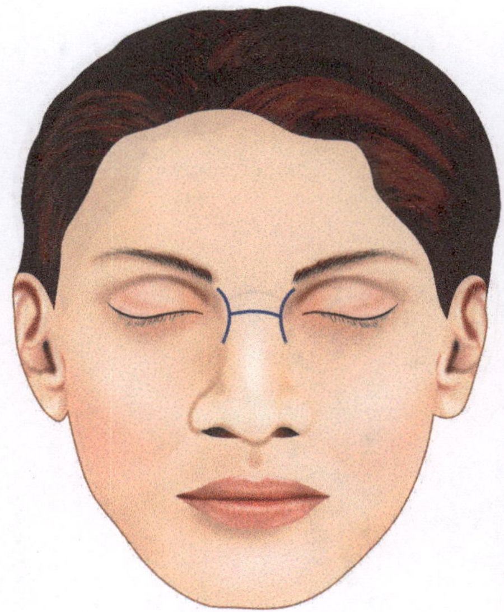

Fig. 21.93: H-shaped incision

made from forehead to base of nose (Fig. 21.96). Although it gives an excellent visibility, but difficulty in wiring or plate fixation. The ensuing scar is unesthetic and unacceptable hence not commonly practiced.

- **W-shaped approach described by Bowseman**: The incision is made across: the base of nose within the skin crease (Fig. 21.97). Provides excellent access and visibility, but produces an unacceptable scar on the base of nose.

Edward Ellis in 1993 suggested a 8-step protocol for the management of Nasoethmoidal complex fractures, which gives priorities in the management (Table 21.3).

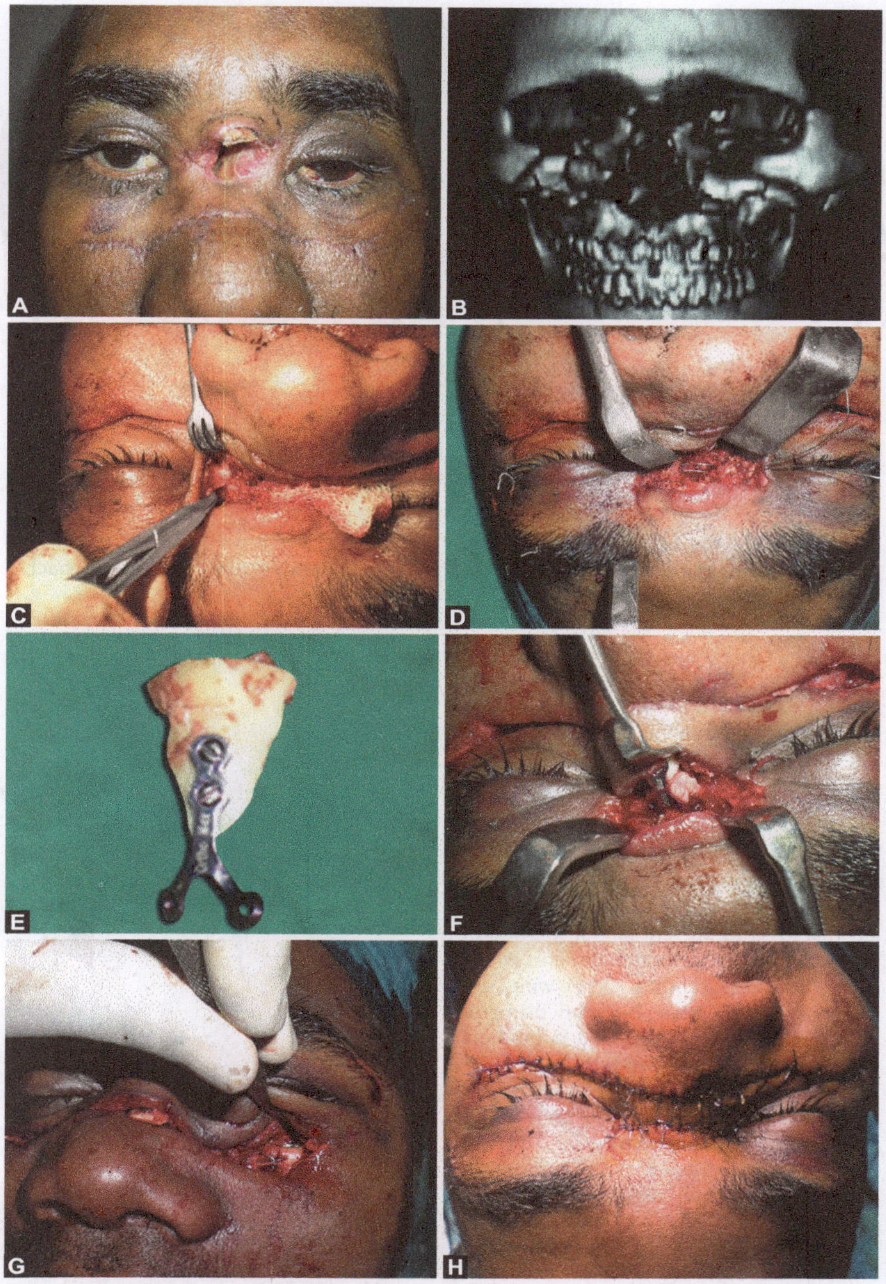

CANTHOPLASTY

Medial Canthal Anatomy

Medial canthus is formed by medial aspect of upper and lower eyelid, which converges into an acute angle. It has two limbs. Between anterior and posterior limb lies the lacrimal punctum, superior and inferior canaliculi and superior 1/3 of lacrimal sac.

As the tendon serves as the insertion for orbicularis occuli muscle, loss of anchorage allows the muscle to contract unopposed, producing a rounded canthal ligament.

Figs 21.94A to H: Management of NOE fracture with bone graft: (A) Clinical; (B) Radiological presentation of NOE fracture; (C and D) Exposure of the fracture through pre-exisiting laceration; (E) Bone graft harvested from anterior wall of maxillary sinus; (F) Fixation of the bone graft to reconstruct the base of the nose; (G) Fixation at infraorbital rim with miniplate based on Champy's principle; (H) Closure of the incision with prolene sutures

Most important part of medial canthal ligament to be secured at the repair is the anterior limb. When it is correctly and securely repositioned, fixed and splinted the complications like dacryocystitis, post-traumatic hypertelorisim, epiphoria and widening of nasal bridge are uncommon.

Method of Securing Tendon (Figs 21.98A and B)

Direct suturing of the tendon to the loop of the wire with a braided non-resorbable suture.

Passing the free end of the wire through the tendon in a continous fashion

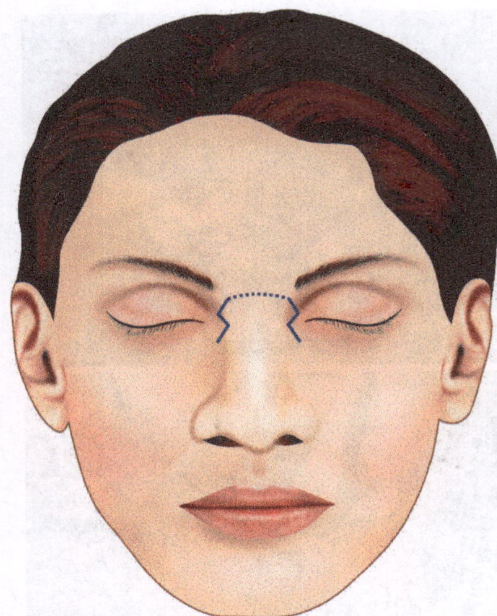
Fig. 21.95: Bilateral Z approach

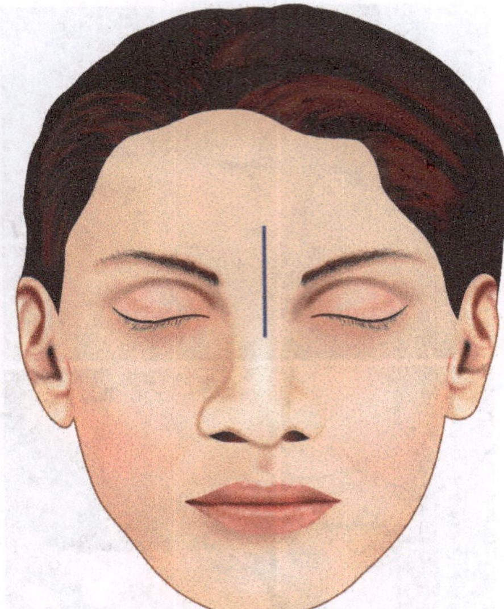
Fig. 21.96: Midline vertical approach

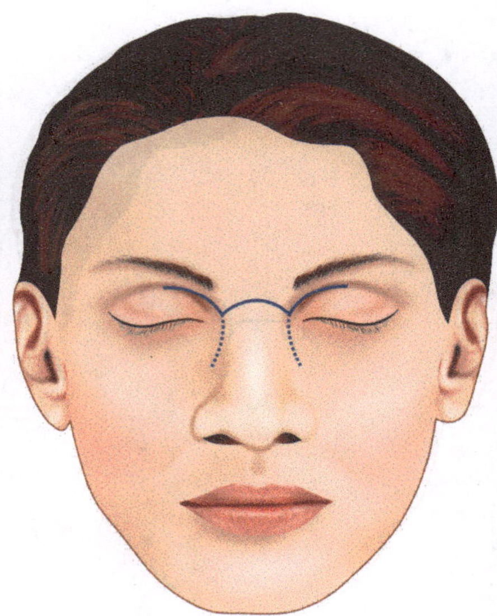
Fig. 21.97: W-shaped approach

Table 21.3: Sequencing naso-orbito-ethmoidal fractures Edward Ellis 1993

Eight steps in treatment:
Step I—exposure through existing laceration, open sky and/or W incision, coronal + lower eyelid.
Step II—identify the medial canthal tendon/tendon bearing bone
Step III- reduce/reconstruct the medial orbital rim. Atleast one hole is drilled posterior to lacrimal fossa to prevent lateral splaying of posterior portion of bonefragment, which can result in telecanthus. Other wire superior to lacrimal fossa. 2–4 mm diameter hole so that ligament is pulled in the hole canthal bearing bone fixed first.
Step IV—reconstruction of medial orbital wall with bone graft (rib, cranial bone)
Step V—transnasal canthopexy
Step VI—reduce septal fracture/displacement (upwards, anteriorly)
Step VII—nasal dorsum reconstruction/augmentation
Step VIII—soft tissue readaptation, nasal split, transnasal bistress silicone sheeting

before directing the wire through the second transnasal channel. If both canthal tendons are detached and separated wire loop is used for each attachment.

When contralateral stabilization of wire is compromised by insufficiency of bone a '*toggle bone*' graft may be used to anchor the wire or a screw can be placed into solid bone and the wire secured to the screw.

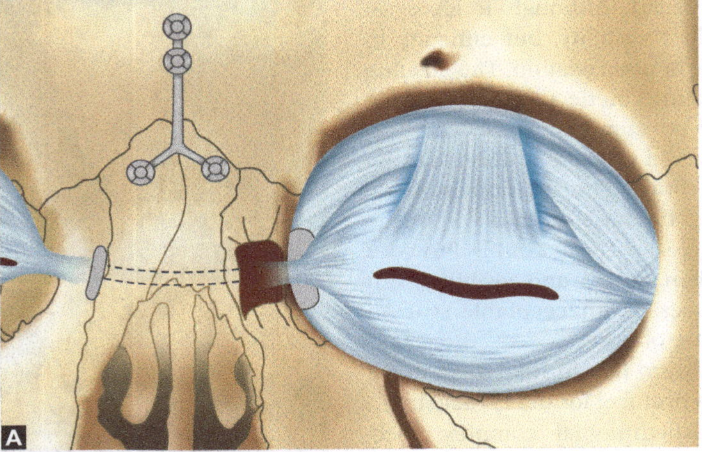

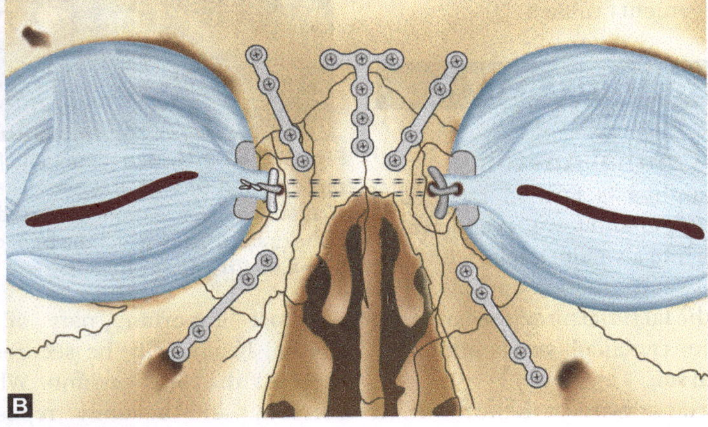

Figs 21.98A and B: Method of securing medial canthal tendon

Table 21.4: Complications of the NOE fractures

Complications of NOE fractures	
Immediate	Delayed
Anosmia	Meningitis, epiphorea
Enophthalmos,	Uncorrected deformity,
Diplopia	soft tissue thickening and contracture
	Prominent plate and
Nasal obstruction	screws.

The complications of the nasoethmoidal complex fractures can be either of immediate or delayed nature and are summarized in the Table 21.4.

PRIORITIES IN THE MANAGEMENT OF A POLYTRAUMA PATIENT (BOX 21.1)

Box 21.1: Priorities in the management of polytrauma patient

1. Lifesaving treatment first
2. Management of fractures later
   a. Airway/breathing
   b. Shock/circulation
   c. Head injury
   d. Cervical spine fracture

a. Air way
- Clean the oral cavity of blood, clot, secretions, foreign bodies
- Prevent tongue fall-air way, tongue stitch, oropharyngeal or nasopharyngeal airway
- Intubate
- Tracheostomy
- Cricothyroidectomy
- Assisted ventilation if indicated

b. Circulation/Hemorrhagic shock
- Fluid resuscitation—crystalloids, colloids
- Control bleeding
- Vasopressors, steroids, O_2, correction of acidosis
- Blood transfusion.

c. Head injury
- History of unconciousness, convulsions, vomiting
- Orientation
- Amnesia
- Level of consciousness
- ENT bleeding
- Posture
- Neurological examination.

Establish the Glasgow coma scale score and necessary neurosurgical intervention to be done immediately.

d. Cervical spine fracture
- Tenderness
- Splinting
- Neurological deficit
- Careful shifting
- Avoid ET intubation/tracheostomy, cricothyroidectomy best suited.

Most of the maxillofacial injuries are as a part of poly trauma. The high velocity RTA results in the injuries at multiple areas of the body and some of them are more critical and warrant urgent attention due to their fatal consequences. The maxillofacial injuries may be associated with the head injury, spinal injuries, fractures of the long bones, injuries to the ribs, flail chest, blunt injuries to the abdomen with visceral lacerations/ruptures. Thus, the management is usually a teamwork and priority wise that means the lifesaving treatment must be done first and then the management of the fractures. The patient who has head injury must be evaluated and get neurosurgical attention first. In view of cervical spine injuries, need to be handled carefully, while shifting the patient. The neck should be supported with sand bags, rigid collar or pneumatic splints as the movements may aggravate the spinal damage. The endotracheal intubation and tracheostomy is contraindicated in the patients with cervical spine fractures as it requires extension of the neck. A cricothyroidotomy should be resorted to in case access to the air way is required. The other injuries like rupture viscera, fractures of long bones lead to massive blood loss and the patient may land in a state of hypovolmic shock and thus, restoration of the circulatory efficiency must be the priority by appropriate measures. The traumatized brain has diminished tolerance to hypoxia and thus it becomes imperative to restore circulatory efficiency and maintain adequate perfusion of vital organs.

Careful neurological examination comprising history of the event, unconsciousness, convulsions, vomiting should be obtained as these signs may suggest cerebral concussion. The level of consciousness should be ascertained periodically and presence of any amnesia should be noted. The retrograde amnesia is more significant finding than the anterograde amnesia. The posture of the patient should be observed as abnormal posturing like decerebrate or decorticate could be present in patients with head injury. The Glasgow coma scale score should be recorded and should be periodically monitored as a prognostic index in the patients with head injury. The presence of rigidity/flaccidity, tendon reflex, planter reflex should be done. The papillary signs such as size, light reflex (3rd cranial nerve evaluation) is an important examination in presence of raised intracranial pressure and coning of the brain (transtentorial herniation). The evaluation of individual cranial nerve examinations should be done to complete the neurological examination. The cases with head injury be further evaluated by CT scans or MRI scans and appropriate neurosurgical interventions should be undertaken along with attempts to reduce raised intracranial therapy like use of steroids, mannitol, etc. The use of sedatives and narcotic analgesics should be avoided in patients with head injury as they may interfere with level of consciousness, pupillary signs and the subsequent neurological evaluation may be difficult.

The circulatory efficiency should be monitored by detecting the signs of hypovolumia such as thready pulse, hypotension, oliguria, collapsed peripheral veins, pallor, tachypnea, cyanosis, etc. the blood loss should be ascertained and signs of intraperitoneal bleed should be elicited. The fracture of the femur can sequestrate about 750 mL of blood in the muscle compartment and the intraperitoneal bleed can loose about 1,500 to 2,000 mL blood. The signs of intraperitoneal bleed such as guarding, rigidity, distension, Turner's hematoma should be elicited. Some of these signs may be masked in a patient with head or spinal cord injuries especially in presence of generalized rigidity and flaccidity. The scalp lacerations may appear small, but are known to bleed disproportionately, as the open blood vessels fail to collapse due to the presence of dense aponeurosis. The replacement of the lost blood volume with crystalloids, colloids or blood transfusion be undertaken along with the measures to arrest the bleeding.

The chest should be evaluated for the presence of contusions, fractures of the ribs, presence of flail chest (fracture of more than 2 ribs at more than one point), presence of pnemothorax, hemothorax and necessary drainage using the intercostals drain should be undertaken. All such injuries may lead to compromised chest expansion, collapse of lung and compromise respiratory efficiency. The patients who have compromised respiratory efficiency due to either central or peripheral cause may be provided with assisted ventilation, nasal O_2 suppliments as indicated in a given case.

An oral and maxillofacial surgeon is expected to consider all these things, be able to provide basic lifesaving and supportive treatment and summon help in time from concerned specialists, if he happens to be the first person to handle the case. The patients with grievous injuries are monitored critically and should be provided critical care.

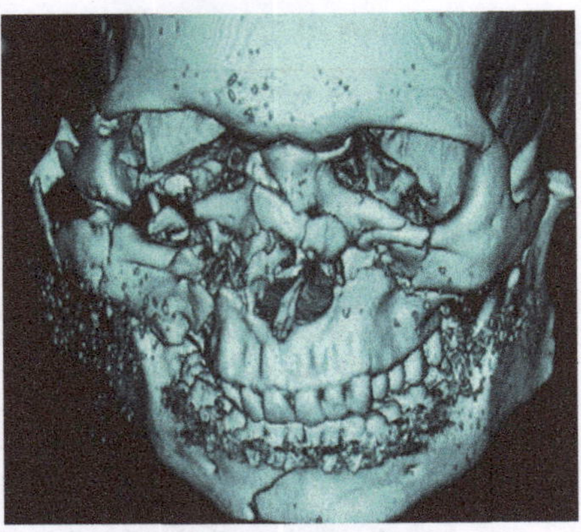

Fig. 21.99: CT scan with 3D reconstruction for a facial polytrauma patient

The patients are given good prophylaxis against the infections with appropriate antibiotics and immunization against tetanus. In the patients with clean contaminated wounds routine antibiotics with immunization with tetanus toxoid will be enough, but in cases where the wounds are badly contaminated, soiled, plenty of crushed, devitalized tissue is present then the antibiotics should be broad spectrum. In the presence of cranial involvement such as CSF rhinorrhea the antibiotics that can cross BBB should be opted to prevent the intracranial sepsis. The prophylaxis against tetanus should be with injection of tetanus toxoid 1 mL, intramuscularly, if the patient is previously immunized against tetanus. The tetanus toxoid is an antigen and it evokes active immunity which takes about 3 weeks to be fully established. However, if the wound is badly soiled and there is crushed, devitalized tissue, which enhances the chances of contracting tetanus, the patient requires immediate protection in such cases passive immunity in the form of human diploid cell vaccines (antibodies) can be given along with the tetanus toxoid. The passive immunity provides immediate cover against the tetanus and lasts for 8 to 10 days only. By the time the passive immunity wanes the active immunity develops and provides longer protection against the tetanus. In the past antitetanic serum (ATS), which was the horse's serum was used in place of human diploid cell vaccines. As it was a foreign protein there was a risk of severe allergic reactions, which is minimized largely due to the advent of diploid cell vaccine. The ATS was administered in a dose of 1,500 to 3,000 IU, after the intradermal test dose of 200 IU to avoid severe allergic reactions.

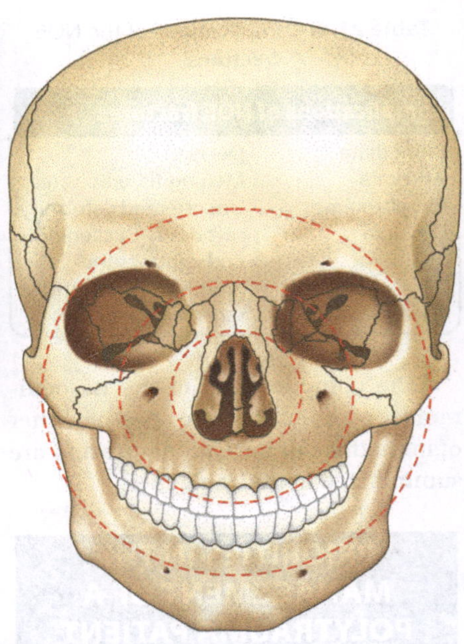

Fig. 21.100: Golden rule to fix the fractures, i.e. fixation of outer ring first and the central area fractures at the end

Once the condition of the patient is stabilized, the treatments of the fractures of the facial skeleton may be undertaken. If the patient has multiple facial fractures (Fig. 21.99) then the golden rule is that treat the injuries or fix the fractures in the outer ring first and the central area fractures are treated at the end, i.e. the zygomatic fracture is treated first then the nasal bone fracture (Figs 21.100 and 21.101).

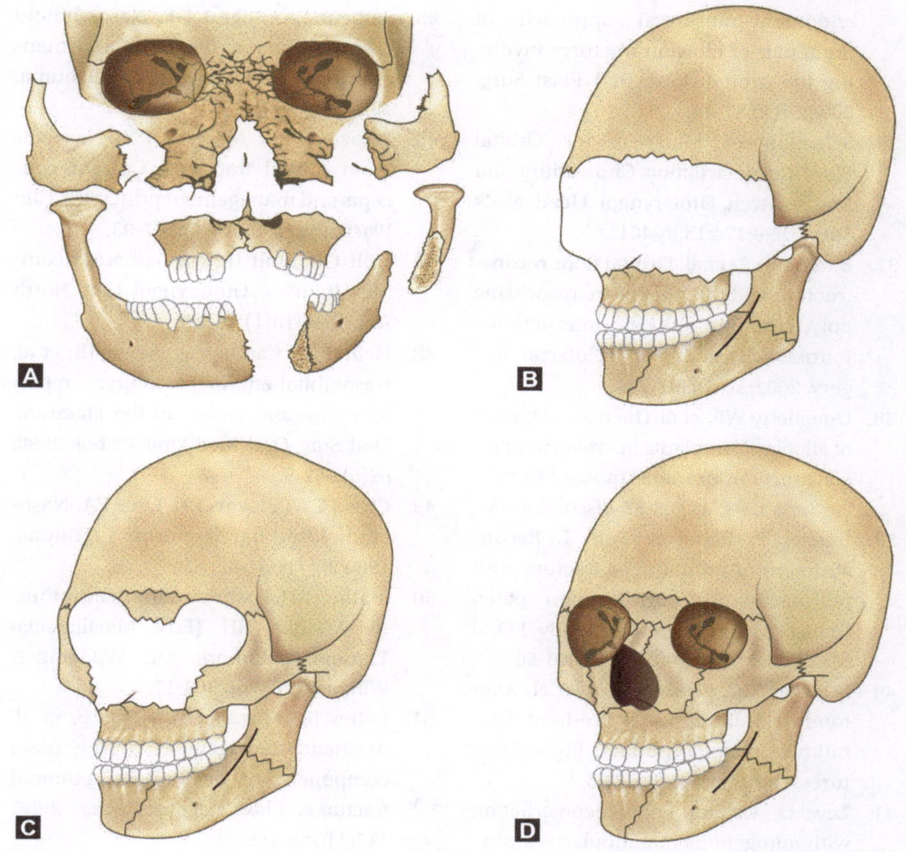

Figs 21.101A to D: Sequence of fixations of fracture in panfacial trauma case lower to upper and outer to inner

REFERENCES

1. Lefort R. Etude experimentale Sur les fractures de le menchoire superieure, Rev Chir. 1901;20:8.
2. Row NL (Ed). William maxillofacial injuries. New York: Churchill Livingston, 1985.pp.538-58.
3. Guérin AF. Des fractures des maxillaires supérieurs. Nouveu moyen de les reconnaitre dans les cas fréquents ou elles ne s'accompagnement pas de déplacement Archives générales de médecine, Paris. 1866; 2:5-13.
4. Strong EB, Sykes JM. Zygoma complex fractures. Facial Plast Surg. 1998;14(1): 105-15.
5. Manson PN, et al. Mechanisms of global support in post-traumatic enophthalmos: the anatomy of the ligament sling and its relation to intramuscular cone orbit fat. Plastic Reconstr Surg. 1986;77:193-8.
6. Frank Dal Santo, Edward Ellis III, Gaylord S Throckmorton. The effects of zygomatic complex fracture on masseteric muscle force. J Oral Maxillofac Surg. 1992;50:791-99.
7. Ellis E 3rd, el-Attar A, Moos KF. An analysis of 2,067 cases of zygomatico-orbital fracture. J Oral Maxillofac Surg. 1985;43(6):417-28.
8. Yanagisawa E. Symposium on maxillofacial trauma. 3. Pitfalls in the management of zygomatic fractures. Laryngoscope. 1973;83(4):527-46.
9. Knight JS, North JF. The classification of malar fractures: an analysis of displacement as a guide to treatment. Br J Plast Surg.1961;13:325-32.
10. Zingg M, Laedrach K, Chen J, et al. Classification and treatment of zygomatic fractures: a review of 1,025 cases. J Oral Maxillofac Surg. 1992;50(8):778-90.
11. Fujii N, Yamashiro M. Classification of malar complex fractures using computed tomography. J Oral Maxillofac Surg. 1983;41(9):562-7.
12. Ardekian L, Kaffe I, Taicher S. Comparative evaluation of different radiographic projections of zygomatic complex fractures. J Craniomaxillofac Surg. 1993;21:120-8.
13. Perino KE, Zide MF, Kinnebrew MC. Late treatment of malunited malar fractures. J Oral Maxillofac Surg. 1984;42(1):20-34.
14. Keen WW. Surgery, its principles and practice. Saunders (Ed). Philadelphia; 1909.
15. Gillies HD, Kilmer TP, Stone D. Fractures of the malar-zygomatic compound with a description of a new X-ray position. Br J Surg. 1927;14: 651.
16. Lothrop HA. Fractures of the superior maxillary bone caused by directs blows over the malar bone. Boston Med Surg J. 1906;154:8.
17. Shea JJ. The management of fractures involving the paranasal sinuses. JAMA. 1931;96:418.
18. Fryer MP. A simple direct method of reducing a fracture-dislocation of zygoma. Surg Clin North Am. 1950; 30:1361.
19. Balasubramanian S. Intraoral approach for reduction of malar fractures. Br J Oral Surg. 1967;4:189-91.
20. Wavak P, Zook EG. Immobilization of fractures of the zygomatic bone with an antral pack. Surg Gynecol Obstet. 1979;149(4):587-89.
21. Adams WM. Internal wiring fixation of facial fractures. Surgery. 1942;12:523.
22. Dingman RO, Alling CC. Open reduction and internal wire fixation of maxillofacial fractures. J Oral Surg. 1954;12:40.
23. Michelet FX, Deymes J, Dessus B. Osteosynthesis with miniaturized screwed plates in maxillofacial surgery. J Maxillofac Surg. 1973; 1: 79-92
24. Holtmann B, Wray CR. Little AG. A randomized comparison of four incisions for orbital fractures. Plast Reconstr Surg. 1981;67:731-7.
25. Abubaker AO, Sotereamos G, Patterson GT, Use of the coronal surgical incision for reconstruction of severe craniomaxillofacial injuries. J Oral Maxillofac Surg. 1990; 48: 579-86.

26. Frodel JL, Marentette LJ. The coronal approach. Anatomic and technical considerations and morbidity. Arch Otolaryngol Head Neck Surgery. 1993; 119: 201-7.
27. Rochon-Duvigneaud. Quelques cas de paralysie de tous les nerfs orbitaires (ophthalmoplegie totale avec amaurosse en anesthésie dans le domaine de l'ophthalmique d'origine syphilitique). Archives d'ophthalmologie, Paris, 1896; 16:746-60.
28. Zachariades N, Vairaktaris E, Papavassiliou D, Papademetriou I, Mezitis M, Triantafyllou D. The superior orbital fissure syndrome. J Maxillofacial Surg 1985; 13:125-8.
29. Bun RJ, Vissink A, Bos RRM. Traumatic superior orbital fissure syndrome: report of two cases. J Oral Maxillofacial Surg 1996; 54:758-61
30. Burm JS, Chung CH, Oh SJ. Pure orbital blowout fracture: new concepts and importance of medial orbital blowout fracture. Plast Reconstr Surg. 1999; 103(7):1839-49.
31. Blowout fracture of the orbit: mechanism and correction of internal orbital fracture. By Byron Smith and William F. Regan, Jr". Adv Ophthalmic Plast Reconstr Surg 1987;6:197-205.
32. Ng P, Chu C, Young N, Soo M. Imaging of orbital floor fractures. Australas Radiol. Aug 1996;40(3):264-8
33. Gilbard SM, Mafee MF, Lagouros PA, et al. Orbital blowout fractures. The prognostic significance of computed tomography. Ophthalmology. 1985;92 (11):1523-8.
34. Hawes MJ, Dortzbach RK. Surgery on orbital floor fractures. Influence of time of repair and fracture size. Ophthalmology. 2183;90(9):1066-70.
35. Kackibushi M, Fukazawa K, Fukada K. Combination of transconjunctival and endonasal-transantral approach in the repair of blowout fractures involving the orbital floor. Br J Plast Surg. 2004;57(1):37-44.
36. Selection of Materials for Orbital Floor Reconstruction Chowdhury and Krause Arch Otolaryngol Head Neck Surg. 1998;124:1398-401.
37. Baumann A, et al. Orbital floor reconstruction with an alloplastic resorbable polydioxanone sheet International Journal of Oral and Maxillofacial Surgery. 2002;31(4):367-73.
38. Dougherty WR, et al The natural history of alloplastic implants in orbital floor reconstruction: an animal model. J Craniofac Surg. 1994;5(1):26-32; discussion 33.
39. Buchel P, Rahal A, Seto I. Reconstruction of orbital floor fracture with polyglactin 910/polydioxanon patch (ethisorb): a retrospective study. J Oral Maxillofac Surg. 2005;63(5):646-50.
40. Metzger MC, Schon R, Weyer N. Anatomical 3-dimensional Pre-bent Titanium Implant for Orbital Floor Fractures. Ophthalmology 2006.
41. Lew D. Orbital floor reconstruction with autogenous mandibular symphyseal bone grafts. J Oral Maxillofac Surg. 1977;55(4):330-32.
42. Sargent LA. Nasoethmoid orbital fractures: diagnosis and treatment. Plast Reconstr Surg. 2007;120(7 Suppl 2):16S-31S.
43. Morgan RF, et al. Management of nasoethmoid-orbital fractures. Am Surg. 1982;48:447.
44. Markowitz BL, Manson PN, Sargent L, et al. Management of the medial canthal tendon in nasoethmoid orbital fractures: the importance of the central fragment in classification and treatment. Plast Reconstr Surg. 1991; 87(5):843-53.
45. Sargent LA, Rogers GF. Nasoethmoid orbital fractures: diagnosis and management. J Craniomaxillofac Trauma. 1999;5(1):19-27.
46. Leipziger LS, Manson PN. Nasoethmoid orbital fractures. Current concepts and management principles. Clin Plast Surg. 1992;19(1):167-93.
47. Holt GR, Holt JE. Nasoethmoid complex injuries. Otolaryngol Clin North Am. 1985;18(1):87-98.
48. Heine RD, Catone GA, Bavitz JB, et al. Nasoorbital-ethmoid injury: report of a case and review of the literature. Oral Surg Oral Med Oral Pathol. 1990; 69(5):542-9.
49. Cruse CW, Blevins PK, Luce EA. Nasoethmoid-orbital fractures. J Trauma. 1980;20(7):551-6.
50. Mathog RH. Posttraumatic telecanthus. In: Mathog RH (Ed). Maxillofacial Trauma. Baltimore, Md: Williams & Wilkins; 1984: pp.303-17.
51. Potter JK, Muzaffar AR, Ellis E, et al. Aesthetic management of the nasal component of naso-orbital ethmoid fractures. Plast Reconstr Surg. 2006; 117(1):10e-18e
52. Crockett DM, Funk GF. Management of complicated fractures involving the orbits and nasoethmoid complex in young children. Otolaryngol Clin North Am. 1991;24(1):119-37.
53. Ellis E. 3rd Sequencing treatment for naso-orbito-ethmoid fractures. J Oral Maxillofac Surg. 1993;51(5):543-58.
54. Fedok FG. Comprehensive management of nasoethmoid-orbital injuries. J Craniomaxillofac Trauma. 1995;1(4):36-48.
55. Sargent LA, Rogers GF. Nasoethmoid orbital fractures: diagnosis and management. J Craniomaxillofac Trauma. 1999;5(1):19-27.

22 Facial Burns

Jajoo Suhas N, Yadav Abhilasha, Garg Rajat

INTRODUCTION

A very few areas of medicine are as challenging medically or surgically as the burn care. It affects mainly young and children and in both sexes equally. It may vary from small minor burn injuries, which can be managed as outpatient to more extensive injuries resulting in multiorgan system failure and subsequent mortality.

Improvement in resuscitation facilities, use of topical antimicrobials and practice of early burn wound excision has contributed to the improved outcome of treatment with probably lesser morbidity.

The facial burns are most challenging to manage, as the esthetic and functional outcome is critical and is intimately related to feelings of self-esteem and social acceptance.

ETIOLOGY

Burn injuries could be caused due to:

- Dry heat- flame burns
- Moist heat
- Electrical
- Radiation
- Flash friction
- Blast or frost bite
- Contact burns due to direct contact of hot object, which are localized but deep.[1]

Moist heat-scald, steam are the most common causes of the burn and the scald being the most common in children. Chemical burn of face is usually which can be accidental or inflicted by someone. The facial burns can be isolated or they may be part of the whole body burn. The burn injuries can be caused due to suicidal, homicidal intent or could be accidental.

EVALUATION

Airway, breathing and circulation are assessed immediately. Associated life-threatening injuries should be excluded. Vital signs like pulse, blood pressure along with the level of consciousness should also be assessed and basic life support be initiated.

Thorough history is mandatory as it affects the management. Location of injury (indoor/outdoor), history of standing or running with flames (respiratory burn due to fumes) type of liquid involved in the scald or chemical burn, duration required to extract the patient out of heat or dilution of chemicals are all important.

Admission is required for large burns, which require resuscitation or full thickness burns, which needs an early surgical intervention. The patients are also susceptible to infection and need to be kept under controlled, aseptic environments. Minor burns can be treated on outpatient basis, if the proper care from the family members is assured.

Determination of the Extent of Burn

When calculating the TBSA (Total Body Surface Area), only those areas having partial and full thickness dermal burn injuries are included. Erythema (superficial burn involving epidermis only) is not included.[2]

Wallace's rule of nine (Fig. 22.1) is good for adults for assessing the burn percentage, but proportion of surface area in infants and children are different.[1] Patient's palm approximately is 1 percent TBSA. Lund and Browder charts are more accurate method of assessing the extent of burn injury[3] (Fig. 22.2).

Depth of the Burn Injury

The depth of burn injury is very important from the management and prognostic point.[1] It is dependent upon:

- Initial temperature of object causing the injury.
- Duration of contact.
- Viscosity of liquid causing injury.

Facial burns are usually associated with inhalational respiratory injury due to inhalation of smoke, gases and irritant chemical fumes. Thus, the most critical issue is airway especially, when it is a closed space fire.

Assessment of depth of injury is important as it is an important marker for the wound management.[1] There are four degrees of burn[2] as given below:

First degree: Erythema (Figs 22.3A and B).

Second degree: Superficial partial thickness (Figs 22.4 and 22.5). Epidermis and superficial dermis is damaged. Generally this condition does not advance to full thickness if proper care is constituted.

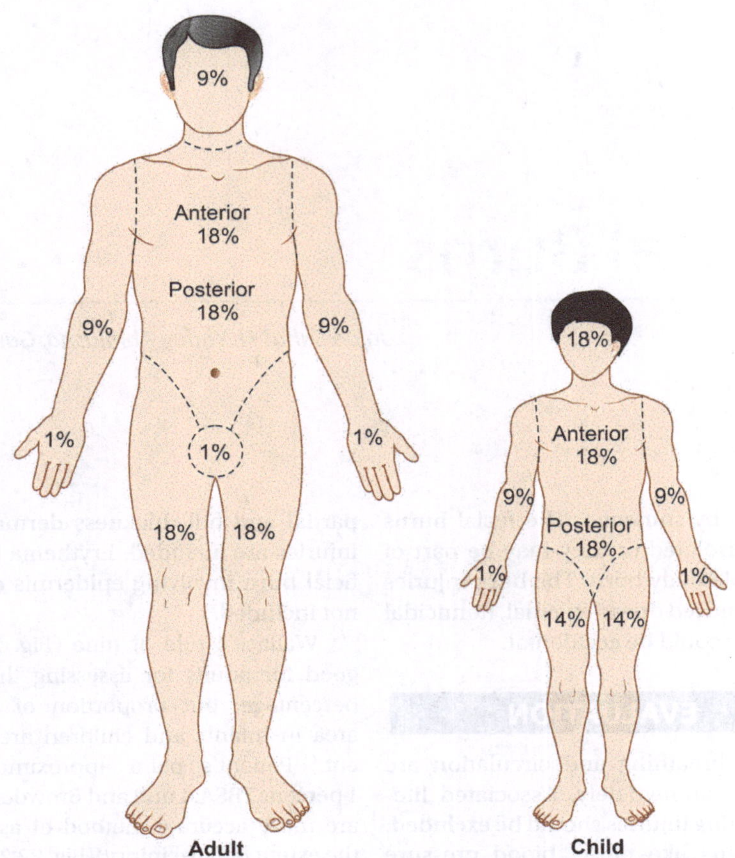

Fig. 22.1: Wallace's rule of nine

a. *Superficial Partial Thickness (second degree A)*
b. *Deep Partial Thickness (second degree B) (Figs 22.6 to 22.8)*: Regeneration progresses very slowly and conversion to full thickness burns is high. These burns are best treated conservatively and sequelae are rare.

Third degree (Full thickness): These injuries cannot heal spontaneously and treatment involves excision of injured tissue followed by skin grafting/Flap (Figs 22.9A and B).

Fourth degree (Full thickness involving deep structures): Thrombosis of subcutaneous venous plexus occurs. Pain involved in these injuries is low as all sensory terminations to skin are destroyed. Potential for infection is high, if not excised (Figs 22.10 to 22.12).

Burnt tissue shows three different zones, zone of necrosis, zone of stasis and zone of hyperemia (Fig. 22.13). The zone of stasis is the area, which needs to be protected, otherwise depth of the burn increases, i.e. conversion of partial thickness into full thickness burn. The most important part of the management is to prevent deep partial thickness burn getting converted into a full thickness burn owing to dryness of tissue due to exposure, secondary infection and use of antiseptic solutions in an inappropriate concentration, thus reducing the morbidity and mortality.

Three epithelial elements, i.e. sebaceous gland, hair follicle and sweat gland help in healing of the wound, being helped by basal layer of epidermis from periphery. After burn, if more the epithelial elements are damaged, poorer will be the healing along with bad scars. The degree of burn and its correlation with the involvement of epithelial elements is given in Table 22.1.

Accurate determination of depth of the burn injuries and their healing potential is challenging. The depth changes with time as there is gradual proximal extension of the vascular thrombosis at the burn site. The assessment of burn which is done initially may not be accurate as it changes according to the duration due to the loss of tissue due to dryness, infection, chemical insult and progressive vascular thrombosis. The wound, which is anticipated to take more than 3 weeks for healing should be managed by excision and skin grafting because it will heal slowly by granulation tissue formation ultimately leading to scarring and increased morbidity.[3] Also the chances of infection to occur will be more in an open wound for such a long period.

Burn depth can be assessed by fluorescein dyes, ultrasound, LASER Doppler and magnetic resonance imaging (MRI), but they are no better than a clinical acumen of experienced burn surgeon.[3]

Classification of Burn Severity

This simplified classification helps the clinician in prioritizing the treatment and thereby rendering the necessary treatment according to the need.

The burn severity can be classified as under (Box 22.1).

First-aid Treatment

Needs to be initiated at the scene of accident to minimize extent of injury and the ensuing complications.

- Try to extinguish the fire.
- Prevent the patient from running as running may flare up the fire.
  - Place the patient in a supine position to avoid inhalation injury.
  - Pour cold water to dissipate the heat and prevent the deeper penetration of the heat to cause more complicated deep burns.
  - Wash/irrigate the chemical burn copiously with water to dilute the chemical to reduce the extent of the injury.

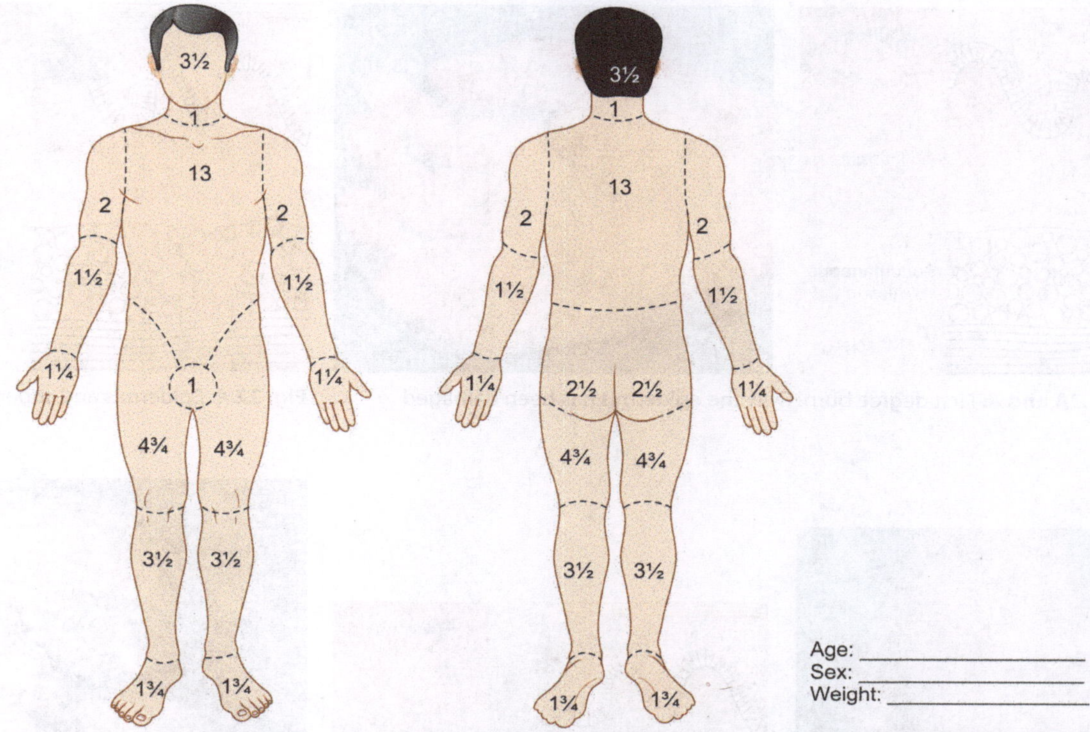

Area	Birth–1 year	1–1 year	5–9 years	10–14 years	15 years	Adult	Partial thickness 2°	Full thickness 3°	Total
Head	19	17	13	11	9	7			
Neck	2	2	2	2	2	2			
Anterior trunk	13	13	13	13	13	13			
Posterior trunk	13	13	13	13	13	13			
Right buttock	2½	2½	2½	2½	2½	2½			
Left buttock	2½	2½	2½	2½	2½	2½			
Genitalia	1	1	1	1	1	1			
Right upper arm	4	4	4	4	4	4			
Left upper arm	4	4	4	4	4	4			
Right lower arm	3	3	3	3	3	3			
Left lower arm	3	3	3	3	3	3			
Right hand	2½	2½	2½	2½	2½	2½			
Left hand	2½	2½	2½	2½	2½	2½			
Right thigh	5½	6½	8	8½	9	9½			
Left thigh	5½	6½	8	8½	9	9½			
Right leg	5	5	5½	6	6½	7			
Left leg	5	5	5½	6	6½	8			
Right foot	3½	3½	3½	3½	3½	3½			
Left foot	3½	3½	3½	3½	3½	3½			
						Total			

Fig. 22.2: The Lund and Browder chart. It provides more accurate estimate of burns TBSA for each body part based on the patient's age (*Source:* Advanced Life Support Burn Manual Chicago, American Burn Association, 2005)

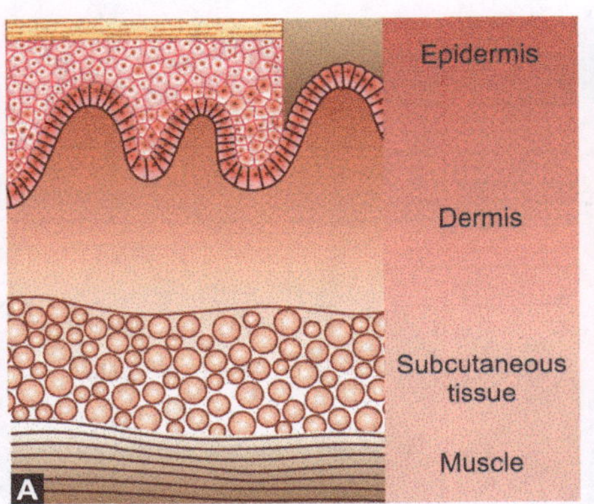

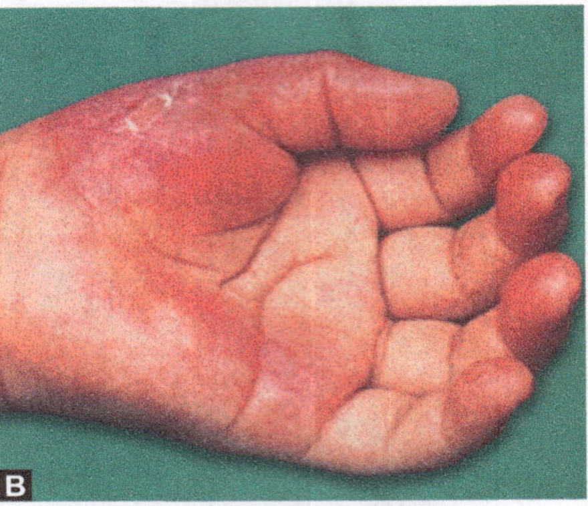

Figs 22.3A and B: First degree burn. Only the epidermis has been damaged

Fig. 22.4: Epidermis and superficial dermis

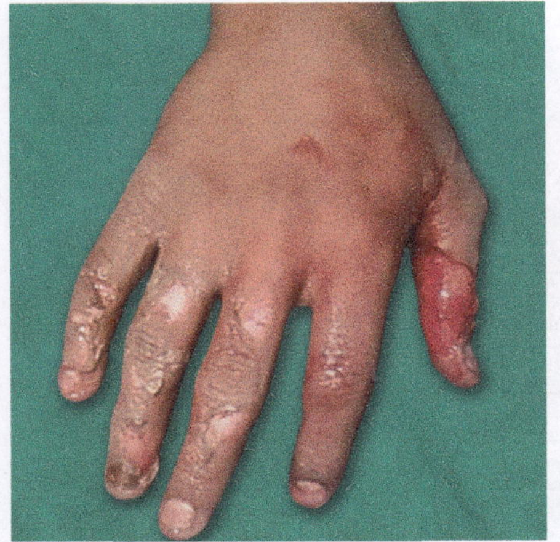

Fig. 22.5: Superficial second-degree burns damaging dorsa of fingers

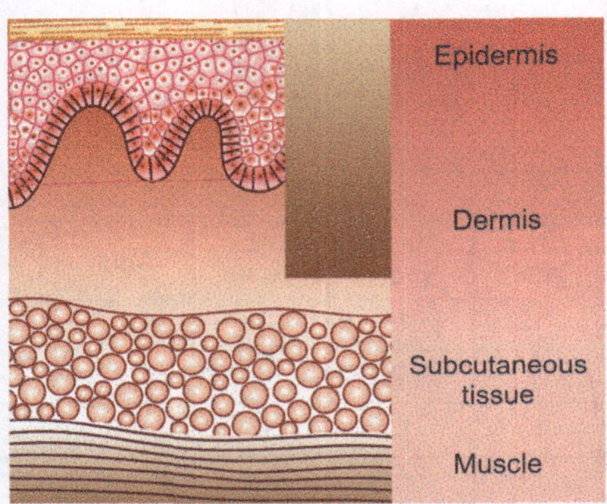

Fig. 26.6: Deep second-degree burn (deep partial thickness burn). Epidermis, papillary dermis, and various depths of reticular (deep) dermis have been damaged

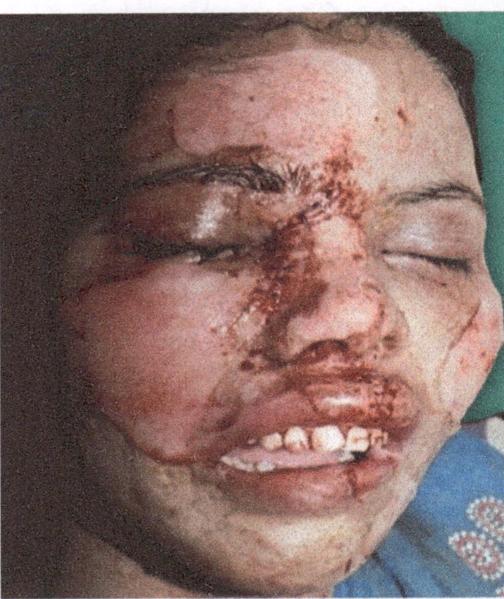

Fig. 22.8: Sutured lacerated wound. Deep partial thickness burn due to steam following pressure cooker blast

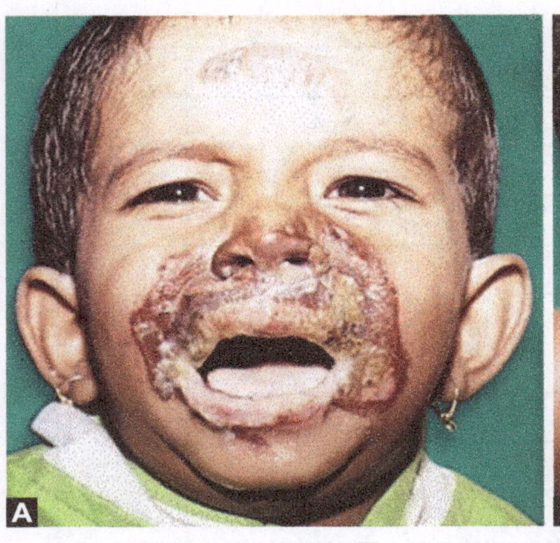

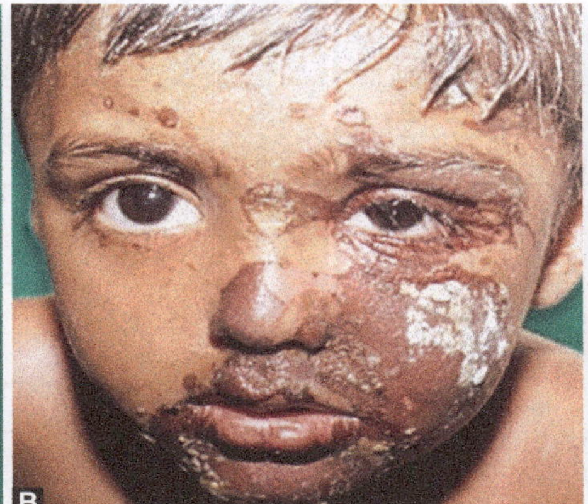

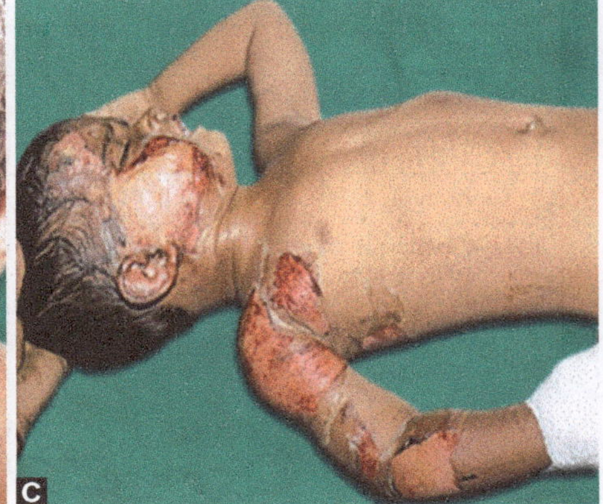

Figs 22.7A to C: Deep partial thickness burn

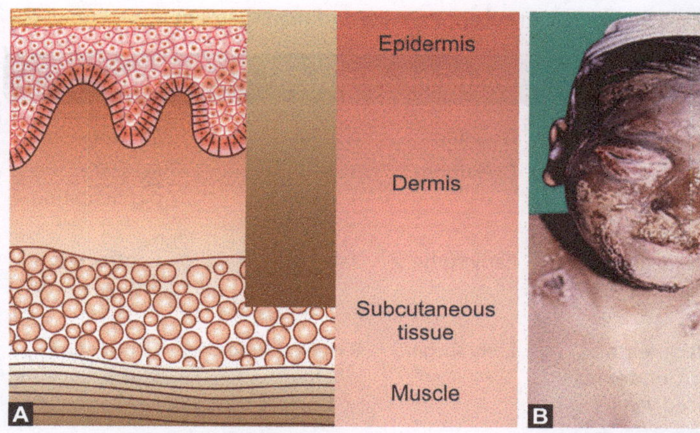

Figs 22.9A and B: Third degree burn (full thickness burn). Epidermis, papillary and reticular dermis, and different depths of subcutaneous tissue have been damaged

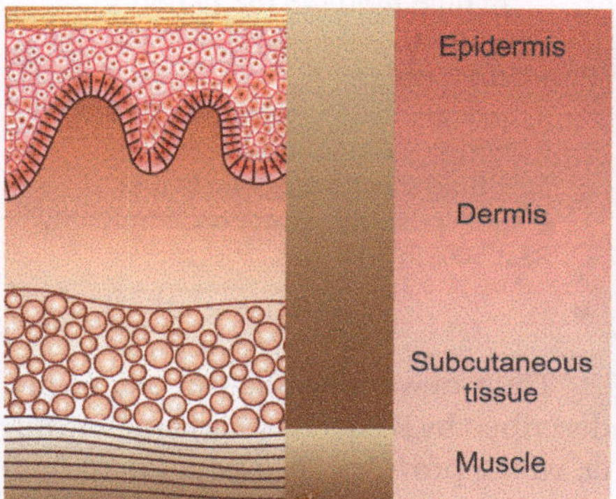

Fig. 22.10: Fourth-degree burns (full thickness burns with involvement of deep structures, like muscle and bone, is present)

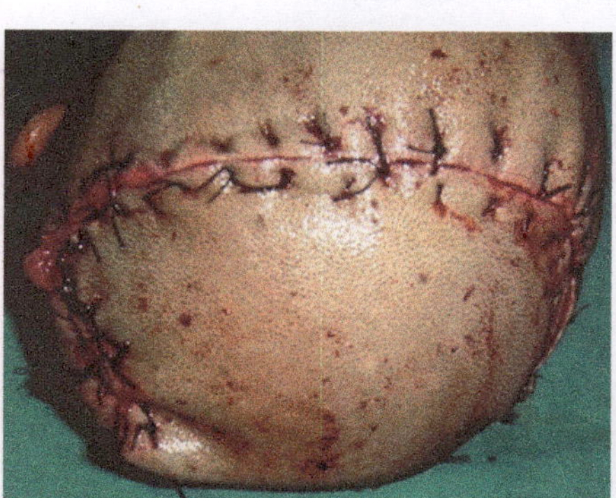

Fig. 22.12: Closure done using scalp rotation flap

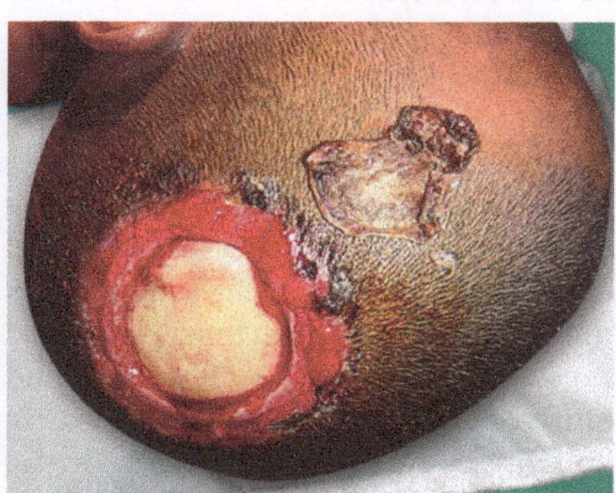

Fig. 22.11: Fourth-degree electrical injury following contact with a high power wire

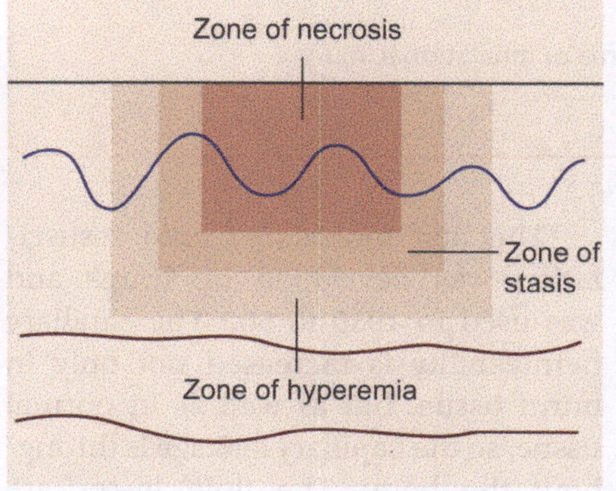

Fig. 22.13: Zones of necrosis, stasis and hyperemia corresponding to a partial thickness burn[5]

- In case of electrical burns switch off the electrical supply before you touch the patient.
- Cover the area of burn injury with clean sheet to prevent contamination and dehydration.
- No household medicament should be applied as they may lead to contamination of the wound.
- Oral feeds are withheld, if the burn injuries are more than 30 percent of surface area.

Acute Complications of Burn

The acute complications of burn are as follows:

- Carbon monoxide poisoning due to inhalation of the smoke and fumes is treated with administration of oxygen through a mask.
- Ventricular fibrillation—the patient needs to be defibrillated.
- Neurogenic shock—the patient is to be treated with necessary resuscitation and basic life support (BLS).

Management of Burns on Outdoor Basis

The following precautions can be taken for burns on outdoor basis[4]:

- Wound protection—topical antibacterial and dressing
- Analgesics
- Antibiotics
- Tetanus prophylaxis
- Scar care and physiotherapy to prevent scar contracture and subsequent morbidity.

Management of Burns in the Inpatient Department

The BLS comprising of airway, breathing, circulation (ABC) should be started immediately.

Airway

Methods of securing the airway like oropharyngeal, nasopharyngeal airway or endotracheal intubation should be carried out to maintain patency. Tracheostomy is done as a last resort and is needed especially, when inhalational injury has occurred.

Breathing

Oxygenation of the patient is carried out through the mask or airway, if the patient's own respiratory effort is adequate, but in the unconscious patients with diminished respiratory drive or effort, assisted ventilation or positive pressure ventilation using a ventilator is provided to prevent hypoxia.

Circulation

Significant burn injury, not only result in local tissue injury, but initiates a generalized inflammatory response that

Table 22.1: Correlation of degree of burn, structures involved, clinical appearance and management

Degree of burn	Involves	Appearance	Treatment	Heals	Result
• Superficial (Erythema)	Only epidermis	Erythematous, painful	Dressings	3–5 days	No scar
• Superficial partial thickness	Superficial dermis, hair follicle, sweat glands not destroyed	Pink, moist, painful	Dressings	2 weeks	No scar, pigmentation +
• Deep partial thickness	Reticular dermis–hair follicle destroyed. Sweat gland not destroyed	Dry, mottled, pink, white variable sensation	Early surgery	3–8 weeks	Contraction + Scar +
• Full thickness	Full dermis reaching fat, hair follicle, sweat gland destroyed	Brown black, leathery, insensate, dry, depressed thrombosed veins seen	Early surgery	8 weeks–6 months	Contraction+ Scar +

Box 22.1: Classification of burn severity

Minor burn
- 15% TBSA or less in adults
- 10% TBSA or less in children and the elderly
- 2% TBSA or less full thickness burn in children or adults without cosmetic or functional risk to eyes, ear, face, hands, feet, or perineum

Moderate burn
- 15–25% TBSA in adults with less than 10% full-thickness burn
- 10–20% TBSA partial-thickness burn in children under 10 and adults over 40 years of age with less than 10% full thickness burn
- 10% TBSA or less full-thickness burn in children or adults without cosmetic or functional risk to eyes, ears, face, hands, feet, or perineum

Major burn
- 25% TBSA or greater
- 20% TBSA or greater in children under 10 and adults over 40 years of age
- 10% TBSA or greater full-thickness burn
- All burns involving eyes, ears, face, hands, feet, or perineum that are likely to result in cosmetic or functional impairment
- All high-voltage electrical burns
- All burn injury complicated by major trauma or inhalational injury
- All poor-risk patients with burn injury
- TBSA, Total Body Surface Area

can affect nearly every organ system. The release of inflammatory mediators [histamine, kinins, prostaglandins, cytokines, interleukins, tumor necrosis factor (TNF)-alpha] can lead to decreased cardiac output, increased vascular permeability and alteration in cell membrane potential (sick cell syndrome) and a state of oligemic shock. Decrease in cardiac function is due to myocardial depressant factor (it is claimed, but not yet identified) and the effect of cytokines.

The purpose of fluid resuscitation is to provide adequate replacement for fluid lost in skin and interstitium to maintain organ perfusion.

The first formula of fluid resuscitation was developed by Evans and was used in 1950 to 60.[4] The capillary permeability is increased not only in burnt tissue, but as well as in normal tissue, so the capillary leakage is throughout the body. The fluid losses are still greater, if the inhalation injury is present. According to Evan's 1.0 mL/kg/percent of burn of crystalloid and equal amount of colloid should be given in first 24 hours, but permeable capillaries are unable to hold colloids as the space between endothelial cells increases. Thus, there is no logic to use colloids in first 24 hours.

Box 22.2: Parkland formula for estimation of fluid required for 24 hours

Parkland formula
- 4 mL/kg/% TBSA = total fluid for first 24 hours—all ringer lactate
- 50% fluid should be given in first 8 hours post burn (not post admission)
- Rest 50% in 16 hours.

Thus, newer formula came in vogue, described by Baxter, i.e. Parkland formula, which provides an estimation of fluid required for 24 hours[4] shown in Box 22.2.

The Parkland formula quantifies the burn trauma and is a guideline only. Monitoring and urine output 50 to 70 mL per hour is maintained, which decides the fluid administration. Fluid administration in children is different.

Monitoring

Urine output is the best monitoring criteria. Good bouncing pulse, good capillary circulation, clear sensorium is the best criteria. Drop in pulse and blood pressure (BP) is late manifestations and aim of fluid replacement is to preserve end organ perfusion and prevent the shock rather than treating it. Hematuria suggest acute tubular necrosis and myoglobinurea is seen with extensive burn injury.

Invasive hemodynamic monitoring

Invasive hemodynamic monitoring is especially useful when associated premorbid conditions, i.e. when cardiac or pulmonary diseases are present. Pulmonary artery catheters pulmonary wedge pressure monitoring help to avoid over infusion.

Analgesics

Analgesics should always be given intravenous (IV) and never intramuscular (IM) as the patient is in circulatory shock and absorption of the drug from muscles would be reduced because of decreased circulation and patient may not get relief. Later when circulation is re-established all this drug in muscles will be absorbed which can lead to increased toxicity of the drug if multiple doses have been given.

Tetanus Prophylaxis

Discussed elsewhere under Chapter 19, Management of Soft Tissue Injuries.

Inhalation Injury Management

Inhalation of products of combustion can lead to devastating pulmonary injury and increases burn mortality significantly. Three clinical aspects are seen:

1. Carbon Monoxide (CO) poisoning.
2. Thermal airway injury.
3. Smoke inhalation.

Diagnosis is based on circumstances surrounding the burn injury and findings on physical examination. History of burns in an enclosed space, while on run, neurologic impairment should suggest it. CO poisoning interferes with oxygen delivery and is toxic to muscles so also causes demyelination of central nervous system (CNS).

Thermal airway injury causes mucosal edema, ulceration and hemorrhage of upper airway. Steam and exploding gases cause lower respiratory injury leading to untractable asphyxiation. Smoke inhalation cause chemical irritation of respiratory tract through 280 carbonaceous toxic products identified. It leads to stridor, wheeze, ronchi and carbonaceous sputum comes out. Loss of alveolar surfactant leads to atelectasis, hypoventilation, hypoxia and acute respiratory distress syndrome (ARDS).

Treatment: Endotracheal intubation is done and oxygen therapy instituted with assisted ventilation. Bronchodilators, nebulization, chest physiotherapy are supportive measures. Blood gas analysis helps deciding treatment. Tracheostomy can also be done as a last resort. Hyperbaric oxygen therapy can be tried. The role of surfactant is doubtful in the overall management of respiratory complications.

Wound Management

Aim of the treatment is prevention of infection, reducing the morbidity and avoiding the complications. Gentle cleansing with antiseptic solution like 0.5 percent savlon is done. Loose burnt tissues are debrided. Blisters should not be broken unless they are more than 6 cm in size. They get absorbed avoiding protein loss, infection and pain.

Escharotomy is indicated for full thickness circumferential burns of extremities or chest wall to improve the vascular supply and overcoming the breathing difficulty.

Fasciotomy is indicated only when the electrical burns are causing compartment syndrome.

Topical wound agents

The wound should be cleaned with 0.5 percent savlon and all the loose tissue is to be debrided. The blisters need not be opened as keratin layer of blister works as biological dressing and avoids pain and infection of raw surfaces. No forceful rubbing should be done, while doing the dressing. Exposure therapy is used only on face and perineum, whereas all other areas should be covered with dressing. Dressings are needed to avoid loss of epithelial cells from drying and dying. It protects from infection, reduces evaporative loss and reduces pain.

Choice of topical wound agents depends on depth of injury and goals of management.

Superficial burn wounds (erythema) requires soothing lotions such as aloevera that can expedite epithelialization process. Superficial partial thickness burn wound need coverage that keeps the wound moist and provide antimicrobial protection. Deep partial thickness wounds need dressings for the same purpose till the wound starts epithelializing. The dressings are changed, which help the epithelium to grow. Full thickness burn needs cover of topical agents to avoid infection until burn excision is contemplated.[5] One percent silver sulfadiazine is the most commonly used topical antibacterial agent[6] with excellent streptococcal and staphylococcal coverage. Principal drawbacks of silver sulfadiazine therapy are:

- Leucopenia, which is self-limiting.
- It does not penetrate eschar, thus less useful in infected burn wounds.
- It may evoke allergic reactions.

It impedes epithelization, hence it should not be used once the necrotic tissue is debrided. It should not be used in pregnant women, nursing mothers and infants less than 2 months of age. Mafenide[7] (sulfamylon) readily penetrates burn eschar and is an excellent drug for burn wound infection. It protects against suppurative chondritis, thus used on nose and ear (as good as silver sulfadiazine).

Drawbacks are:

- It is a potent carbonic anhydrase inhibitor. This can cause metabolic acidosis.
- Application is painful.

Other topical agents are:

- Silver nitrate
- Bacitracin
- Neomycin
- Polymyxin B.

Bacitracin, neomycin and polymyxin B accelerate epithelialization, commonly used for superficial facial burns. Mupirocin is used only when cultured proven MRSA (Methycillin Resistant *Staphylococcus aureus*) is present.

Prophylactic use of systemic antibiotic has no role because they increase the chances of opportunistic infection. Burn eschar has no microcirculation, thus, the systemic antibiotics do not penetrate it. Thus, topical antibacterial agents and subeschar delivery of antibiotics (Subeschar clysis) is useful. Once there is healthy granulation tissue is present, it should be grafted with split thickness graft.

Biologic wound dressings

Allogeneic amnion

Innermost layer of fetal membrane is used as protective dressing on partial thickness burn wound. However, with this the risk of biologic transmission can never be eliminated completely, e.g. Hepatitis, HIV.

Synthetic tissue engineered dressings: The advantages of these dressings are less pain, shorter wound healing time, better scar, e.g. Biobrane, Hydrocolloid dressings, Transcyte.

Human cadaveric allografts and pig xenografts can be used in extensive burns. A variety of proteolytic enzymatic agents have been used to debride the wound, but it causes bacteremia in extensive wounds.

Surgical management

Traditionally burn eschar was allowed to separate by proteolytic enzymes. The underlying granulation tissue was then skin grafted. In extensive burn injury this delay in covering the wound leads to burn wound sepsis due to extensive bacterial colonization, catabolic state, multiorgan failure and death.

The practice of early burn wound excision has significantly decreased the incidence of burn wound sepsis and improved survival.

This should be done between 3rd to 5th post burn days in staged manner spaced 2 to 3 days apart. This spacing helps stabilization and resuscitation of burns. Excised wounds are covered with auto or homografts or synthetic biological dressings.

- Tangential excision—sequential removal of eschar till viable tissue appears. It leads to substantial blood loss.
- Fascia excision—excision down to the layer of muscle fascia. Although blood loss is less, one removes viable tissue also leading to unsightly contour deformity and lymphedema.

Newer device is water jet powered versajet, which is very good for concave surface of hand and feet and for excision at eyelids, ears and nose.

The resultant raw areas are covered with a skin graft. Adequate hemostasis is critical to minimize hematoma to avoid graft loss. Epinephrine, topical pressure, cauterization and use of tissue sealants are the various methods used.

Skin graft used can be either as a sheet or meshed. Sheet graft placed as per esthetic zones of face give best results. In larger burns, there is inadequate skin available thus, grafts are meshed 3 to 6 times, but mostly 2 : 1 is used.

Grafts can be stapled or sutures are placed to fix it to the bed. Hypafix is a elastic adhesive dressing, which can be used with mastisol as adhesive.[8] Vaccum assisted closer device is used along with graft to help closure of wound.

Advances in wound closure

Dermal replacement material such as Integra,[9] Terudermis[10] can be used to reduce chances of contracture. Use of cultured skin (cultured epithelial autografts) although promising have problems of shearing and blistering.

Tissue engineering technology providing skin is expected to deliver spectacular results. Stem cell culture technology is also in offing.

Infections

Infection is a significant risk following burn injury. Colonization of burn eschar, prolonged periods of intubation and mechanical ventilation, respiratory, urinary tract infection and thrombophlebitis also contribute to development of infection (Fig. 22.14).

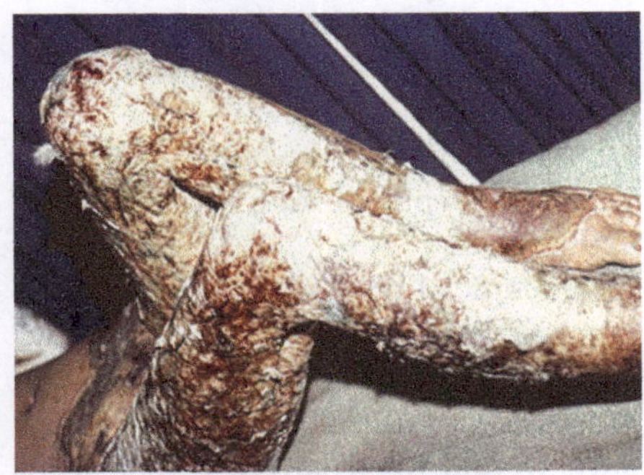

Fig. 22.14: Infection at burn site

These patients are also functionally immunocompromised as cellular and humoral responses are compromised. All these risk factors are further complimented by the risk of cross infection from self, attending personnel and atmosphere.

Colonization of eschar, spreading to normal tissues and then to the blood stream, i.e. burn wound sepsis to septic shock follows.

Best treatment is prevention of burn wound sepsis for which early burn wound excision is propagated.

Diagnosis of infection can be done by regular and repeated culture studies of wound surface, blood, urine and stool. These are evidences, but may not be available at the time of sepsis barring trend of hospital is understood. Surface culture may not match the bacteria causing sepsis.

Best modalities are:

- Burn wound biopsy with more than 10^5 organism/gram of tissue and/or histologic evidence of viable tissue invasion
- Positive burn wound biopsy and blood culture.
- Urinary tract infection (UTI) with more than 10^5 organism/mL of urine
- Pulmonary infection.

Extremely virulent organisms are *Pseudomonas*, *Fusarium* and *Candida* can be isolated from burn wounds.

Nonbacteriologic causes of infection are viruses, e.g. *Cytomegalovirus*, herpes, chicken pox and fungi. Fungi commonly are *Candida, Aspergillus, Fusarium* and anaerobes (*Bacteroides* and *Fusobacterium* species).

Burn associated infections are chondritis, pneumonia, UTI, thrombophlebitis and venous abscesses and suppurative sinusitis. 'Ghosting' of grafts, i.e. disappearance of graft which was already taken up is a clinical problem with obscure etiology.

Clinically fever and leukocytosis may be due to systemic inflammatory response syndrome (SIRS) rather than infection. Periodic culture after 72 hours is useful in making diagnosis of infection. (Urine, sputum, blood, central lines).

In addition to identification of septic source following criteria should be watched for:

- Tachypnea
- Paralytic ileus
- Hyperthermia or hypothermia
- Altered mental status
- Thrombocytopenia
- Leucopenia or leukocytosis
- Metabolic acidosis
- Hyperglycemia.

Local evidence of invasive wound infection includes black or brown patches of wound discoloration, rapid eschar separation, wound conversion to full thickness and ecthyma gangrenosum.

When patient exhibits signs and symptoms of sepsis, immediate institution or broadening of coverage antibiotics is mandatory, while awaiting confirmatory cultures depending on routine hospital flora and its resistance pattern. In addition there should also be a rapid aggressive surgical intervention for the control of infection. In presence of human immune deficiency virus (HIV) (CD_4 and CD_8) immunosuppression adds to the problem and graft survival is compromised.

Antibacterial agents include coverage against gram-positive (streptococci, staphylococci and enterococci), gram-negative (*Pseudomonas aeruginosa, Escherichia coli* and *Klebsiella*) and yeast and fungal infections.

Nutritional Support

Less nutritional intake, hypermetabolism and hypercatabolism persists until complete wound coverage is achieved. Supporting the increased nutritional needs is a cornerstone of burn patient management. If not done, it results in severe weight loss, debility, anemia, hypoproteinemia, immunocompromised state, sepsis and death.[11]

Burns up to 20 percent burn can be managed by total oral and or enteral (TEN) route alone. But more than 20 percent may need total parenteral support (TPN).

There are several equations for estimation of nutritional requirements, i.e. Long's modification of Harris-Benedict's formula[11] and Curreri formula[12] as shown in Table 22.2.

Table 22.2: Harris-Benedict's formula and Curreri formula

Formula	
Harris- Benedict's formula	Basal energy expenditure: Men: 66.5 + (13.8)W + (5)H – (6.76)A Women: 655 + (9.6)W + (1.85)H – (4.68)A Adjust for stress by multiplying BEE by a factor of 1.2 – 2.0.
Curreri formula	Age 16–59: (25)W + (40)TBSA Age ≥ 60: (20)W + (65)TBSA

W–weight in kg, H–height in cm, A–age in years.

Nutritional expert should be available to support and look after supervision and persuasion in TEN as well as ileus and intubated states compelling TPN needs are helped by them. Immunological support is needed, but still is in research phase. Psychological support is mandatory keeping in mind the etiology of burn, its scar deformities and disabilities.

Rehabilitation

It includes:

- Splinting in acute burns.
- Splinting after wound has healed.
- Compression by elastic garments for hypertropic scar and keloid.
- Physiotherapy—active and passive for joint mobilization.
- Pigmentation—hypo- and hyper-pigmentation needs dermatologist's advice.
- Operative correction and reconstruction after scar has matured.

FACIAL BURN

Facial burns are most challenging as esthetic and functional outcomes is critical to the daily life of the patient and is intimately related to feeling of self-esteem. Many patients with facial burns sustain inhalation injury and need intubation. Endotracheal tube should be secured in such a way as to minimize pressure necrosis of lip. Same is true with nasogastric tube, which can cause pressure necrosis of ala and columella.

In periorbital burns, look for injury to eyeball, which is more common with acid splash. Exposure keratitis needs to be cared for, especially with lid contracture. In such cases tarsorrhaphy may be needed. Traditional method was to perform daily wound care until the facial wound has either healed or the eschar got separated so that the raw can be grafted. It is now clear that better outcomes can be achieved if the nonhealing areas are excised (likely to take 3 weeks or more) and then skin grafted. The donor skin needs to be taken from area above the nipple for the best color match. Many surgeons favor the scalp skin but, alopecia and hair growth from transplanted skin is of concern whereas the upper part of back has thick skin.

Facial excision is carried out using Goulian knives or versajet water dissector. Exposed cartilage needs excision with closure of skin.

Sheet of autografts are used as the meshed grafts are cosmetically unacceptable. Epinephrine clysis is essential to limit hemorrhage. A face mask should be placed to help immobilization of skin graft. Graft should be placed in such a fashion as to mimic the esthetic units. Fibrin glue can be used to enhance the graft adherence. Post-operative facial elastic mask compression helps in avoiding hypertrophic scar.

In the cold cases of burn, the burn contractures are common which lead to significant morbidity. In presence of the neck contractions, administering General anesthesia for release of contraction with multiple Z plasties and subsequent

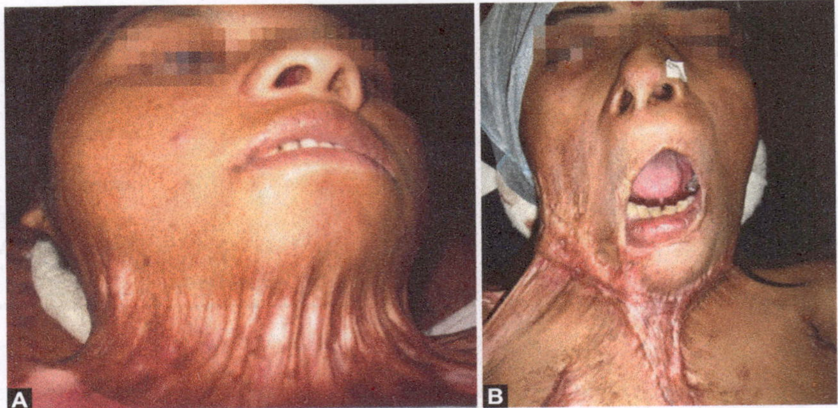

Figs 22.15A and B: Burn contracture of the neck preventing extension of the neck

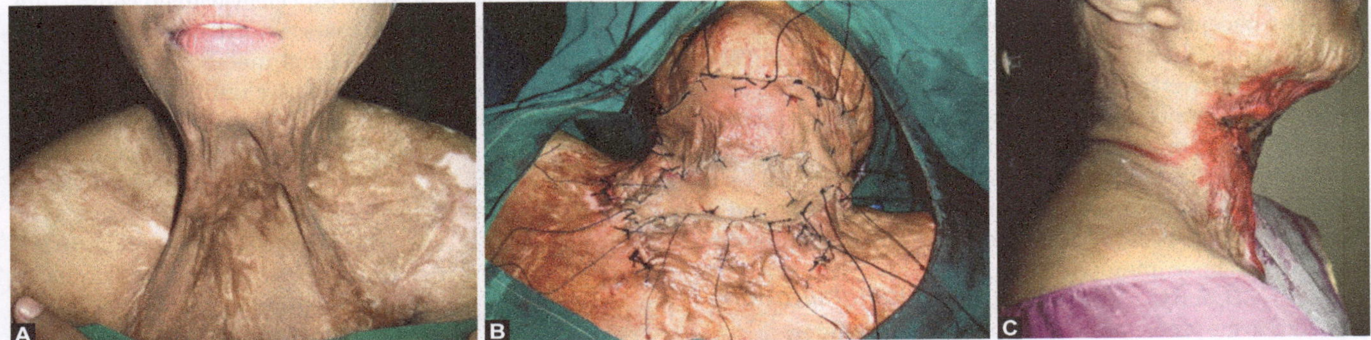

Figs 22.16A to C: (A) Burn contracture of the neck; (B) Contracture released and skin graft placed; (C) Postoperative view

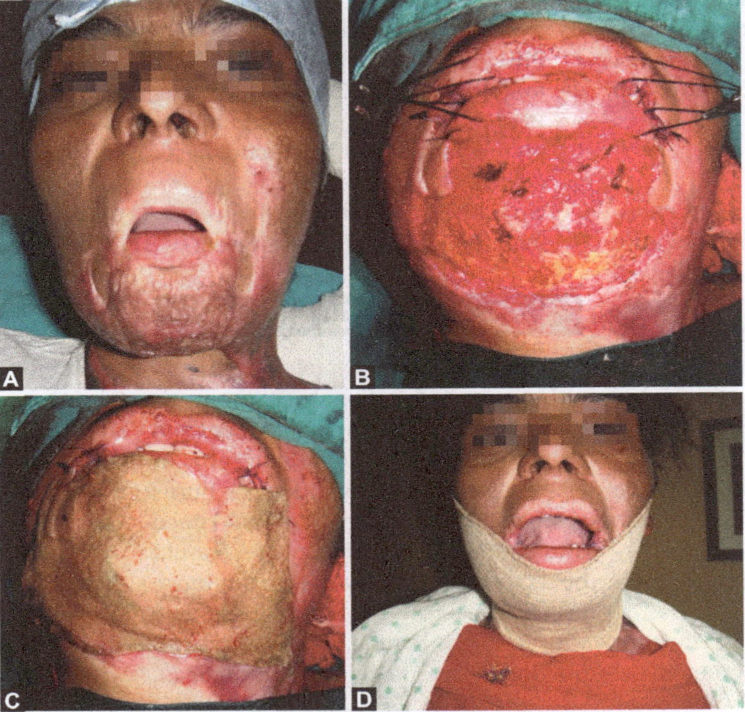

Figs 22.17A to D: (A) Burn contracture of face; (B) Contracture released; (C) Skin graft placed; (D) Elastic bandage applied for better graft uptake

skin grafting is very difficult and sometimes, not possible as laryngoscopy cannot be done and neck angulation is not favorable for intubation (Figs 22.15A and B). In such cases fiber optic guided intubation can be done or else the patient is given ketamine and local anesthesia and the contracture is released. After the release of the contracture, the patient can be safely intubated and administered general anesthesia and split thickness skin grafting can be done. Grafts on the neck should be carefully harvested as long sheets and the defect is covered with skin graft, while the neck is in hyperextension (Figs 22.16A to C). The postoperative spint should be given to keep the neck extended to prevent graft contracture and relapse. Long term physiotherapy with neck extension exercises are advocated to get optimum results and to prevent contractures (Figs 22.17A to D).

REFERENCES

1. David Herndon. Total burn care third edition page no 78-9.
2. Juan P. Barret. Colour atlas of burn care, page 2-7.
3. A. Forage. The history of the classification of burns (diagnosis of depth). British Journal of Plastic Surgery, Volume 16, Issue null, Pages 239-42.
4. Mertens DM, Jenkins ME, Warden GD. "Outpatient burn management". Nurs Clin North Am. 1997;32(2): 343-64.
5. Orgill DP. Excision and skin grafting of thermal burns. N Engl J Med. 2009; 360(9):893-901.
6. Charles L. Fox, jun. Silver sulphadiazine-poly hydroxyethylmethacrylate (PHEMA) dressing. Burns. 1981;7(4). pp. 295-7.
7. Lee JJ, Marvin JA, Heimbach DM, et al. Use of 5% Sulfamylon (mafenide) solution after excision and grafting of burns. J Burn Care Rehabil. 1988;9:602-5.
8. Cassey JG, Davey RB, Wallis KA. Hypafix—a new technique of skin graft fixation. Aust NZJ Surg. 59:479.
9. Jeng JC, Fidler PE, Sokolich JC, et al. Seven years experience with Integra as a reconstructive tool. J Burn Care Res. 2007;28(1):120-6.
10. Terashi Hiroto. Successful Application of Artificial Dermis (Terudermis) for Deep Burn on Big Toe with Bone Necrosis. Nishinihon Journal of Dermatology. 2001;63(5):557-60.
11. Long CL, Schaffel N, Geiger JW, et al. Metabolic response to injury and illness: estimation of energy and protein needs from indirect calorimetry and nitrogen balance. JPEN J Parenter Enteral Nutr. 1979;3(6):452-6.
12. Curreri PW, Luterman A.: Nutritional support of burned patients. Surg Clin North Am. 1978;58:1151-6.

23 Medicolegal Aspects of Injury

Anjankar AJ, Borle Rajiv M, Garg Rajat

Today is a world of the fast and the furious. On one hand newer technological innovations have proved to be a boon for the upliftment of mankind, however, on the other hand they have also led to an increase in the number of accidents and associated injuries. These days due to increased interpersonal violence and the increasing hatred amongst mankind, it is absolutely necessary to rule out any foul play in case of any injury, whether major or trivial. Also, these injuries may be associated with lawsuits and insurance claims. Hence, it becomes mandatory to record the injuries when they are first reported. As a doctor is the first one to see such patients, he is under legal obligation to correctly report them to the concerned police station and is also an important witness in such cases. He might even be one of the first persons to report the incident to the law enforcing authorities. In this chapter we will discuss about the various duties of doctor on duty, preparation of injury report and record keeping. Injury report form must be filled for every patient who is seen in casualty by medical officer on duty to report that case in a police station for medicolegal purpose. To fill up this form (*Annexure-I, page 493*) doctor should examine the patient carefully and should record all the injuries nature, type, number, depth, size, site, edges and line of direction. For all this he/she must have a thorough basic knowledge how various injuries are classified and characteristics of various injuries.

TYPES OF INJURIES

Before proceeding to details of types of injuries we will discuss about the nature of injuries (Table 23.1). It can be as follows:[1]

GRIEVOUS INJURIES

These are the injuries as described under section 320 of the Indian Penal Code (IPC), refers to the following:[2]

- Emasculation—it is castration or loss of power of erection (spinal injury).
- Permanent privation of the sight of either eye.
- Permanent privation of the hearing of either ear.
- Privation of any member or joint.
- Destruction or permanent impairing of the powers of any member or joint.
- Permanent disfiguration of the head or face.
- Fracture or dislocation of a bone or tooth.
- Any hurt, which endangers life or which causes the sufferer to be, during the space of 20 days, in severe bodily pain or unable to follow his ordinary pursuits.

Table 23.1: Types of injuries

- *Simple:* A simple or slight injury is neither extensive nor severe and heals rapidly without leaving permanent deformity or disfigurement.
- *Grievous:* These injuries are serious, severe, deforming and heal slowly.
- *Dangerous:* Grievous injury, which endangers life immediately.

INJURIES CAUSED BY MECHANICAL VIOLENCE

For medicolegal purposes, injuries caused by mechanical violence are divided into:

- Abrasion
- Contusion
- Incised wound
- Laceration
- Stab (penetrating, punctured)
- Ballistic injuries.

Abrasion

Abrasions are injuries involving loss of the superficial epithelial layer of the skin and they do not leave a scar on healing (Fig. 23.1). These blunt impact injuries (usually friction against the hard blunt surface or object) are hardly of any significance from the point of view of loss of life, but medicolegally they are of great importance. Abrasions may also be covered with mud and straw and their shape and pattern may indicate the type of surface on which the victim may have

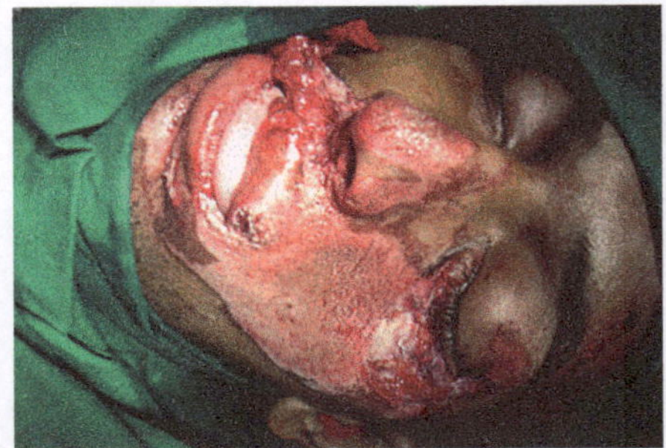

Fig. 23.1: Grazing type of abrasion due to RTA

been impacted or dragged. The direction of the abrasion may be made out by the heaped surface layer (epidermis) or tags at one end. Abrasions caused by finger nails indicate a struggle and an assault are usually seen on the exposed parts of the body.

Types of Abrasions[2]

- **Scratch:** Cause by sharp pointed object. They are linear in shape. Its beginning is clean and end is heaped indicating direction of injury.
- **Grazing/Sliding/Gliding:** As the name suggests it occurs due to sliding between an object and skin. It occurs in road traffic accidents. They are present as multiple, parallel and longitudinal lines.
- **Patterned or Imprint or Impact:** It is caused by tyre marks and radiator grill.
- **Crushing or Pressure:** It occurs in ligature strangulation of hanging and strangulation. Pressure is sustained.[3]

Age of an Abrasive Wound

It can be judged by inspecting the injury. It is also a very important finding in medicolegal cases (Table 23.2).

Postmortem abrasions are pale white in color and usually caused by ant bites and no changes can be seen with days in abrasions as in antemortem abrasion.

Contusion

Hemorrhage into skin, subcutaneous tissue or deep without break in continuity of skin (Fig. 23.2). These are the injuries, which are caused by a blow from a hard and blunt weapon such as lathi, iron bar, stone, fist, boots or by a fall. These are accompanied by a painful swelling and crushing or tearing of the subcutaneous tissues without solution of continuity of the skin. The swelling is due to rupture of small subcutaneous blood vessels producing in the cellular tissues, extravasation of blood, known as ecchymosis. Hematomas are formed when large blood vessels are injured. They appear after sustaining the injury. Sometimes it is delayed by 1 or 2 days. Contusion can be divided as[2]:

- Intradermal
- Subcutaneous
- Deep (may be associated with abrasion)
- Collection may be distant to the site of injury. Blood may gravitate to some other place in the same anatomical plane—'black eye'.

Table 23.2: Age of an abrasive wound

Fresh	No scab or red in color
12–24 hours	Dark red scab
1–2 days	Brownish red scab
3–5 days	Dark brownish red scab
5–7 days	Peripheral healing with shrinkage of the scab and falling off

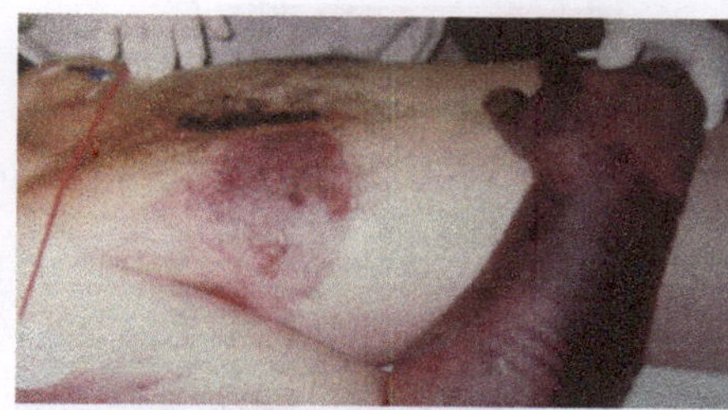

Fig. 23.2: Contusion over right side of chest

The age of a bruise may be ascertained from the color changes, which its ecchymosis undergoes. These changes commence from 18 to 24 hours after its infliction and pass through various stages (Table 23.3).

Color Changes seen in Contusion

Bruises are as a rule, simple injuries. They are seldom fatal unless accompanied by the rupture of an internal organ or by extensive crushing of the tissues and large extravasation of blood, producing sloughing and gangrene of the parts. However, several bruise, though trivial individually, may cause death from shock.

Table 23.3: Color changes in contusion

Fresh	Reddish in color (Hemoglobin)
24 hours	Bluish in color (reduced hemoglobin)
2–4 days	Bluish-black to brownish (hemosiderin)
5–7 days	Greenish – hematoidin
7–12 days	Yellowish (bilirubin)
12–14 days	Fades to normal

Postmortem bruise do not show any color changes, but if the red blood cells have not hemolyzed, and the blood is in a liquid state, then severe trauma, like a forcible blow drive the blood into the issues through ruptured blood vessels and produce a bruise similar to an antemortem bruise.[4] However, it is mostly restricted to bony prominences, while antemortem can be anywhere.

Incised Wound

Incised wounds are sharp with clear cut margins by a sharp object drawn across the skin. Sharp instruments may be like knife, razor, scissors or sword, axe, hatchet. Incised wound is always broader than the edge of the weapon causing it owing to the retraction of the divided tissues (Fig. 23.3). It is somewhat spindle is shaped; its length greater than depth and width. The direction of the injury can be decided as these injuries have deep beginning and superficial end or tails off towards the end called '*tailing*'. When a curved weapon is used it always produces a stab or punctures and than an incised wound.

Age of the wound can be decided by inspecting Table 23.4.

The differences between antemortem and postmortem incised wounds are as that of laceration. The only

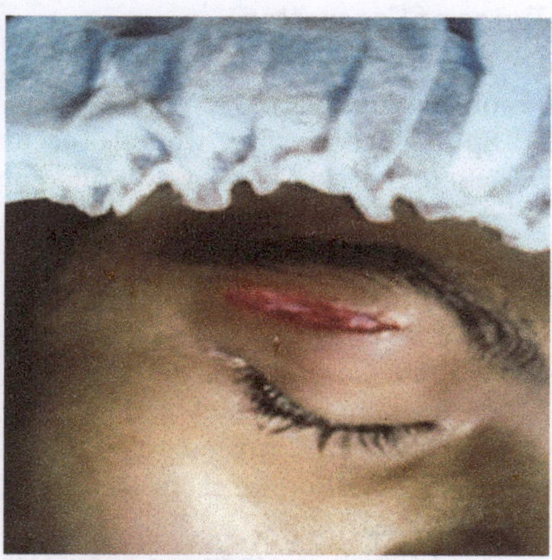

Fig. 23.3: An incised wound over upper eyelid

Table 23.4: Age of an incised and lacerated stab wounds

Age of the wound—lacerated or incised stab wounds	
Unsutured	
Inflamed skin edges	12–24 hours
Appearance of infection	36–48 hours
Sutured	
Inflamed edges	12–24 hours
Edges can be easily separated	1–3 days
Firm union—edges are difficult to separate	3–5 days
Red, linear, tender scar	7–10 days
Pale, firm, nontender scar	> weeks

difference is that when incised wound is made, no gaping (due to loss of elasticity of skin) is formed and it is straight.

Beveling Cuts

When sharp weapon struck obliquely will cause beveling of one edge of the wound and also indicate the direction of the blow, while if the sharp edge struck almost horizontally, it produces a wound with a flap.

Hesitation Cuts

They are usually suicidal or self-inflicted. It is formed when the blade moves in saw like fashion. These are small, multiple, superficial cuts usually parallel.

Laceration

Laceration means the edges are irregular with surrounding abrasion or bruises and the deeper tissues are torn irregularly.

Types of Laceration

- **Tears:** Caused due to projecting object (Fig. 23.4).
- **Split:** Incision like wounds occur when the skin is closely adherent the bone—iliac crest, scalp due to a perpendicular impact (Fig. 23.5). To differentiate it from incised wound, examination with hand lens is a must.
- **Stretch:** Caused in a run over by a motor vehicle. Hanging skin is an indication of a run over producing flap. For example, scalp laceration (Fig. 23.6).
- **Avulsion:** It is otherwise known as degloving of the skin. The skin of the affected limb is separated from the underlying tissues and hangs loosely (Fig. 23.7).
- **Crushing:** Compression of the skin, crushing of the underlying tissues and bones (Figs 23.8 and 23.9).

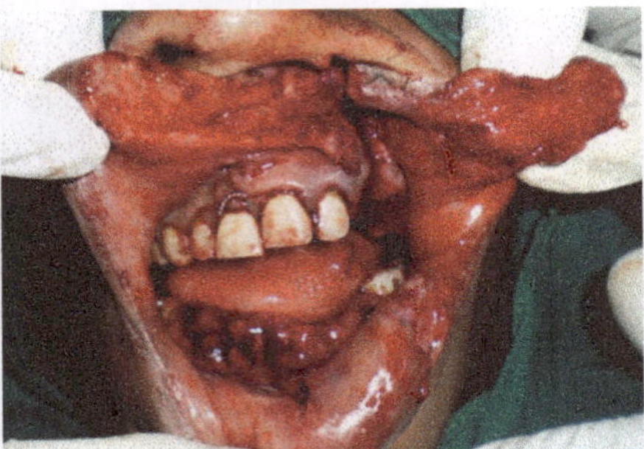

Fig. 23.4: Tear type of laceration over the face

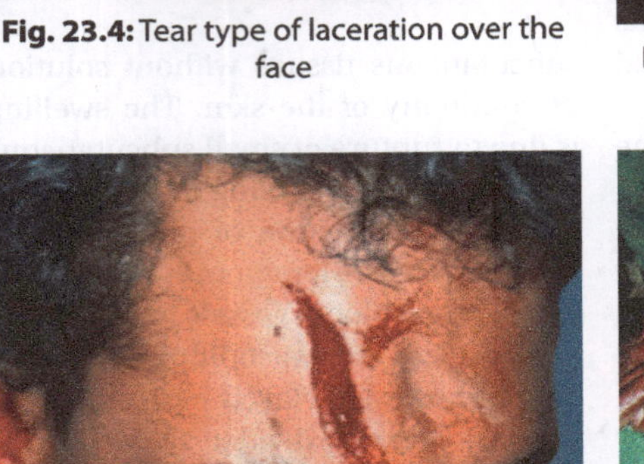

Fig. 23.5: Split laceration over the forehead

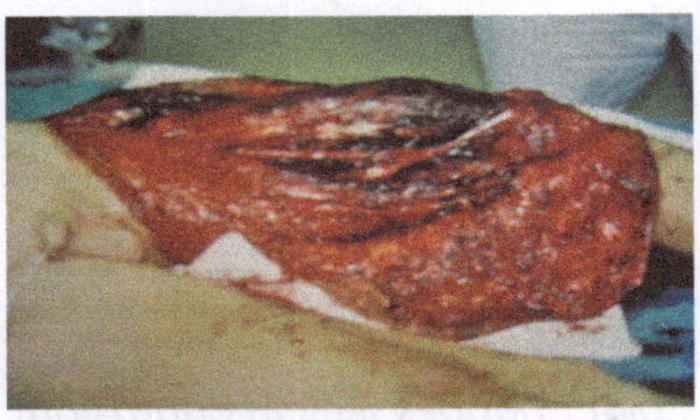

Fig 23.6: Laceration over left thigh with a hanging skin flap

Differences between Antemortem and Postmortem Lacerations

The difference between antemortem and postmortem lacerations is described in Table 23.5.

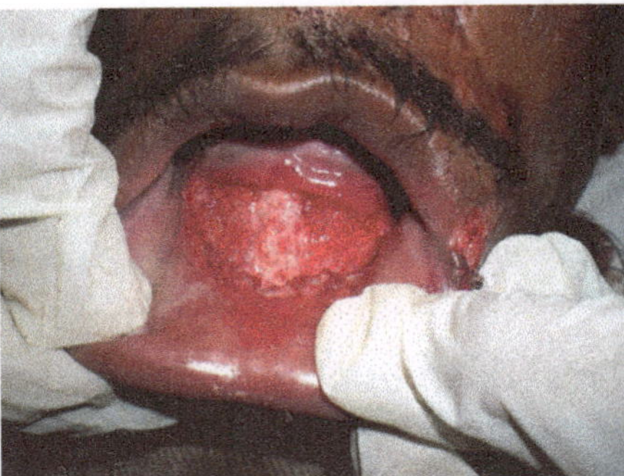

Fig. 23.7: Degloving laceration in lower labial vestibule

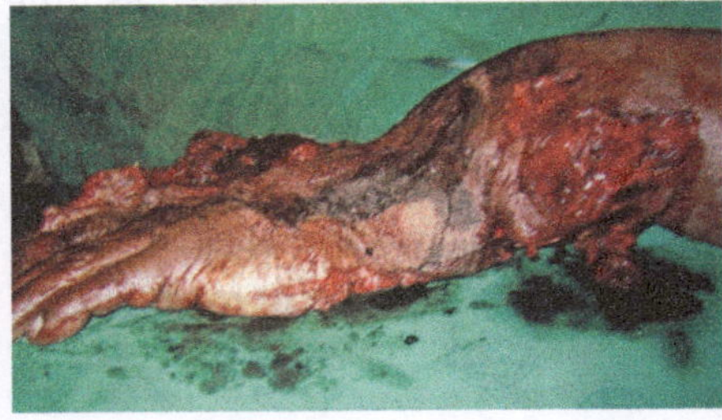

Fig. 23.8: Crush injury of hand

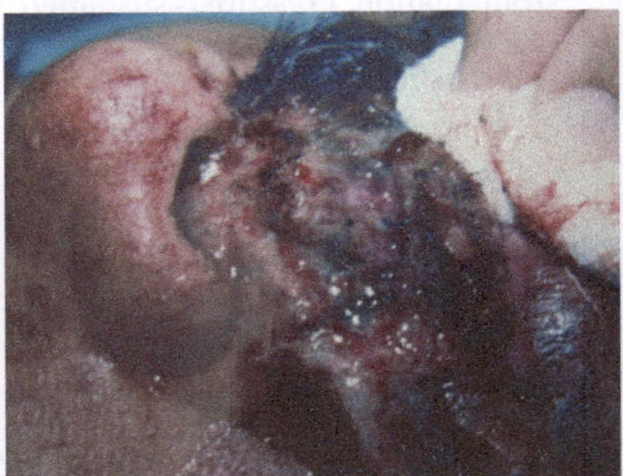

Fig. 23.9: Contused lacerated wound on upper lip

Punctured or Stab Wounds

Punctured or stab wounds are also called penetrating injuries when passing through the tissues, they enter a cavity of the body. It is due to pointed sharp object with greatest dimension at depth. For example, dagger, needle, spear, arrow, scissor, ice pick. The length of stab wound is equal to the breadth of the blade at the point of entry wound. The deeper point of the wound is tapering if tapering knife is used. If the ends are sharp that means knife having both edges sharp where as with one-sided blunt knife wound have ragged margins on blunt side of the knife.[2]

Table 23.5: Differences between antemortem and postmortem laceration

Antemortem	Postmortem
Extravasated blood cannot be wiped out	Extravasated blood can be wiped out
Coagulated blood is seen	Coagulated blood is absent
Increased enzyme activity is seen at the periphery of the wound	No enzyme activity
Signs of healing present	No signs of healing

In case of a punctured wound perforating a part of the body, there are two wounds, one of entry and the other of exit. The wound entry is usually larger with inverted edges and the wound of exit is smaller and has everted edges. The site of wound indicates whether it is suicidal or homicidal. A careful examination of the clothes for cuts may reveal valuable information.

Ballistic Injuries

Ballistic injuries it is essential for a medical person to have some basic knowledge of the common firearms and physical aspects of firearms injuries (forensic ballistics). The term ballistic trauma (generally referred to by the type of weapon, such as gunshot wound, etc.) refers to a form of physical trauma sustained from the various weapons.[5] Gunshot injuries are an increasing problem in many countries, with the continuation of warfare in many parts of the world, together with a very large number of guns in circulation, there has been an increase in the number of gunshot injuries and fatalities since the 1970s. The most common forms of ballistic trauma is from small arms fire, namely semiautomatic pistols, machine guns, submachine guns, and assault rifles used in armed conflicts, civilian sporting and recreational pursuits, and criminal activity.[5]

Gunshot injuries are classified as low velocity if the bullets traveled at less than 1,000 feet per second and high velocity if the bullets traveled at more than 2,000 feet per second. This is an arbitrary definition and varies among different authorities. Clearly the inference is that high-velocity wounds are more serious

Table 23.6: Factors determining severity of bullet injury

Bullet characteristics	Tissue characteristics
Velocity	Distance and path within body
Mass	Biological characteristics of tissues
Shape	Mechanism of tissue disruption
Design and composition	
Range	

and there is no doubt that bullet velocity is an important determinant of wound severity. The kinetic energy transferred to the target is defined as mass multiplied by velocity to the second power ($KE = MV^2$). A number of factors determine the severity of injury (Table 23.6).

The mass, velocity, shape and compositions of the bullet all help determine the degree of injury. Larger bullets traveling at lower velocities may cause more damage than smaller high-velocity bullets. Tissue characteristics are also important. As a bullet passes through the tissues, they offer resistance, which depends on their elasticity, cohesiveness and density. Thus, although liver and muscle absorb about the same amount of energy per centimeter of tissue, their different structural characteristics mean that the liver is more severely traumatized by bullet wounds.

When assessing the likely severity of gunshot wounds, the numerous variables include the following, considered singly or in concert:

- The particular type of weapon used; rifles are generally more destructive than handguns.
- Caliber of the weapon. For example, a wound from a small diameter bullet is generally less severe than a wound inflicted by a larger diameter at the same velocity.
- Design of the bullet and its velocity; expanding bullets are more damaging than nonexpanding. Of the nonexpanding bullets, flat or very blunt-nosed bullets are more damaging than more pointed bullets, as the more pointed bullet may push some tissue aside. Heavier bullets will penetrate more deeply than lighter bullets at the same velocity.
- Range at which the victim was shot; i.e. wounds inflicted from a distance of 5 meters, invariably are more severe than those fired from 500 meters, if all other factors are equal.
- Path of the wound—initial entry is a poor guide, as it is only a single point where as the exit point is more severe in expanding type of bullets.

Bomb Blast Injuries

Civilian bomb blast injuries are often industrial and occur in mining, chemical storage facilities, explosive and fireworks manufacturing plants and stone-crushing industries. Explosions are classified into atomic, mechanical and chemical explosions.

The principal chemical explosives are black powder, nitroglycerine, dynamite and trinitrotoluene (TNT). TNT is a most common conventional military explosive. Chemical explosives can be gaseous, liquid or solid. Chemical explosives are also classified as:

- Low explosives or deflagrating explosives
- High explosives.

Royal demolition explosive (RDX) or cyclotrimethylene trinitramine is a most powerful explosive used in military. When an explosion occurs, the explosive material is suddenly converted into a large volume of gas with the release of a tremendous amount of energy. Pressures of up to 1,000 tons per square inch (psi) can be generated. The temperature of explosive can rise to 3,000°C.

A person can be injured by explosive in many ways:

- If he is near the seat of the explosion, he can be blown to pieces and scattered by the force of the explosion gases.
- If he is near enough for the skin to be in contact with the explosion flame, he can sustain the usual kind of flame burn. This type of burn is also caused by contact with clothing or other material ignited by the explosion.
- The person can be struck by flying missiles propelled by the explosion.
- He can be injured or crushed by debris usually of building demolished by explosion.
- The person can be injured by the wave of pressure, which spreads concentrically from the blast center. This air blast can:
  - Damage the ear by hyperemia or punctate bruising or rupture of the tympanic membrane. Even it can lead to damage to the cochlea.
  - The lung lesion takes the form of alveolar hemorrhage, its severity varying directly with the size of the explosion charge and becoming greater, the nearer the victim is to the explosion.

Clinical effects after air blast injuries can be:

- Pulmonary hemorrhage
- Pulmonary edema
- Circulatory failure
- Systemic air embolism
- When it is extensive, copious bloody froth in the air passage, the victim may suffocate.
- Obstruction of respiratory passages or pulmonary circulation and lethal reflexes initiated in the vagus nerve lead to profound circulatory changes.

The following samples should be collected after blast injuries for forensic examination:

- **For toxicology:** Blood; urine; liver and stomach and their contents if required.
- **For tissue matching:** Hair and blood.
- **Other trace evidence:** Powder traces; paint fragments; oil or grease stains and any foreign material.
- Clothing and footwear.

DIFFERENCES BETWEEN SUICIDAL WOUNDS AND HOMICIDAL WOUNDS

The difference between suicidal and homicidal injuries are given in Table 23.7.

Note: Homicidal wounds are usually produced to support a false charge of assault or attempted murder against an opponent, which one has already received during a quarrel, to prove self-defense.

AGE OF INJURY

It is not possible for a doctor to give exact time of infliction of any injury, but an approximate time can be given with following data:

- The age of a bruise may be ascertained from the color changes, which its ecchymosis undergoes. These changes commence from 18 to 24 hours after its infliction and pass through various stages.
- The age of wound may be ascertained from observing the stages of healing process.
- In the fracture of a bone following data can provide us the approximate age of the fracture (Table 23.8).
- In the dislocation of joint the time can be judged from the color changes of a bruise, when caused by violence.
- When a tooth has been knocked out, bleeding from its socket stops in about 24 hours. The cavity of the socket usually fills up in 7 to 10 days and the alveolar process becomes quite smooth after 14 days.

TYPES OF WEAPON

Kind of weapon used can be inferred by examining the edges, margins, ends, width and shape in case of a wound. Width of the wound is important as by examining width, we can judge actual penetration of knife in wound as width varies of knife from tip onwards. When there is any doubt whether the wound is lacerated by a weapon or contusion by a fall, it is always better to mention both possibility and probability.

Table 23.7: Differences between suicidal and homicidal injuries

Suicidal or self-inflicted	Homicidal
Accessible and elective anatomical sites like wrist or neck	Anywhere in the body
Multiple, linear, parallel cuts	Their position and shape vary
Usually incised stab wound	Usually chop wounds. Stabs and lacerations may also be present
They are superficial at the commencement and end is deeper	They are deeper at the commencement and end is superficial
In right handed persons from left to right and from above downwards	Any direction
Defense or protection cuts absent	Defense or protection cuts present usually over the ulnar border of forearm
Hesitation cuts usually present	Hesitation cuts usually absent
Weapons are usually found grasped due to cadaveric spasm or found near body	Weapons are usually missing
Scene of crime is usually closed room. There are no disturbances of surroundings	Scene of crime is disturbed and signs of struggle may present
Clothes not damaged	Clothes may be damaged

Table 23.8: Criteria for determination of age of fractures

1–3 days	Signs of inflammation and exudation of blood (hematoma) around fracture ends in soft part
3–14 days	Soft provisional callus formation
14th day – 5 weeks	Ossification of callus
6–8 weeks	Fracture ends united entirely by bone

Annexure I: Proforma for Injury Report Form

Place: ________________ Date: ________________ Time:

1. Full Name: ________________ Age: ________________ Sex: ________________
2. Address: Village/Town: ________________ PS: ________________
   Tah. ________________ Dist. ________________
3. Brought by: PC ________________ Buccal No. ________________ Police Station (PS): ________________
4. Consent : I am willing to be examined by Dr. ________________
   Signature or thumb impression ________________
5. Marks of Identification: a. ________________
   b. ________________
6. Brief history: ________________
7. General examination: ________________
8. Local examination of injuries:

S. No. of injury	Type of injury	Size and shape	Situation on body	Simple or grievous	Approx. age of injury	Kind of weapon used
1.						
2.						
3.						

N. B. Separate paper may be used if injuries are much more in number.

9. Healing period required: ________________
10. Exfoliated/extracted teeth; weapon inspected and handed over to PC after sealing: Yes/No
    Signature of PC: ________________ Signature of MO: ________________
    Name of PC: ________________ Name of Dr: ________________
    No: ________________ PS: ________________ Designation: ________________
    Date: ________________ Seal if any:

Left thumb impression of the patient

REFERENCES

1. Parikh CK. Textbook of Medical Jurisprudence, Forensic Medicine and Toxicology. New Delhi. CBS Publishers and Distributors; 6th Ed. 2005.
2. Mathiharan K, Patnaik AK. Modi's Medical Jurisprudence and Toxicology. Eastern book co. Calcutta, 23rd edition, 4th reprint 2005.
3. Keith Mant A. Taylor's Principles and Practice of Medical Jurisprudence. Churchill Livingstone, UK 13th Ed 1984.
4. Bernard Knight, Simpson's Forensic Medicine CRC Press; 11 edition, 1996.
5. Kumar K. Forensic Ballistics in Criminal Justice. Eastern Book Company, 1987.

Section 8

Facial Deformities

- Introduction to Cleft Lip and Palate
- Orthognathic Surgery

24 Introduction to Cleft Lip and Palate

Jajoo Suhas N, Yadav Abhilasha, Garg Rajat

INTRODUCTION

Cleft lip is the second most common embryological (Congenital) deformity, after the clubfoot (Figs 24.1A to D). Although it is localized to a small anatomic area, but being on face it requires more attention and priorities. It is a three-dimensional anomaly involving soft and skeletal tissue that changes in the fourth dimension with growth and function. Successful treatment of these children requires a multidisciplinary team approach including pediatrician, oral and maxillofacial surgeon, plastic surgeon, craniofacial surgeon, orthodontist, pedodontist, ENT surgeon, anesthetist, prosthodontist, speech therapist and psychiatrist with technical skill, in-depth knowledge of the abnormal anatomy and appreciation of three-dimensional facial esthetics.

HISTORICAL ASPECT

In ancient times many congenital deformities, including cleft lip and palate, were considered to be evidence of an evil spirit in an afflicted child. These children were often removed from the tribe or cultural unit and left to die in the surrounding wilderness.

Boo-Chai[1] (1966) reported a case of successful closure of a cleft lip in approximately 390 AD in China. Yperman (1295–1351) was a Flemish surgeon who appears to have written the first fully documented description of cleft lip and its surgical repair.[2] Treatment of protruding premaxilla using a head bandage to achieve external compression of the premaxillary segment, thereby bringing it to more favorable position was introduced by Desault and Bichat (1798) (Figs 24.2A to F). Mirault[3] introduced the modern cross flap technique of lip closure in 1844 and Hagedorn[4] in 1884 modified this technique by rectangular flap technique to prevent linear contracture. Then period of Z-plasties came, which led Tennison[5] (1952) to introduce low triangular flap technique and the high Z-plasty rotation flap of Millard[6] (1958).

However, it was as late as the 16th century that Franco[7] (1561) noted "patients having cleft palate are more difficult to cure". In ancient times around 2,500 BC use of dental prosthesis was introduced for cleft palate mostly made of gold or silver.

Von Graefe[8] in 1816 and Roux[9] in 1819 were the first to perform the successful surgery of soft palate and later Dieffenbach[10] recommended separation of the hard palate mucosa from the bone as a mean of closing the cleft of palate.

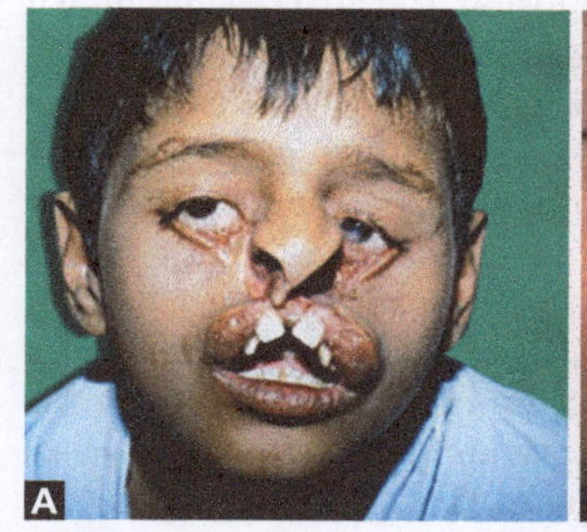

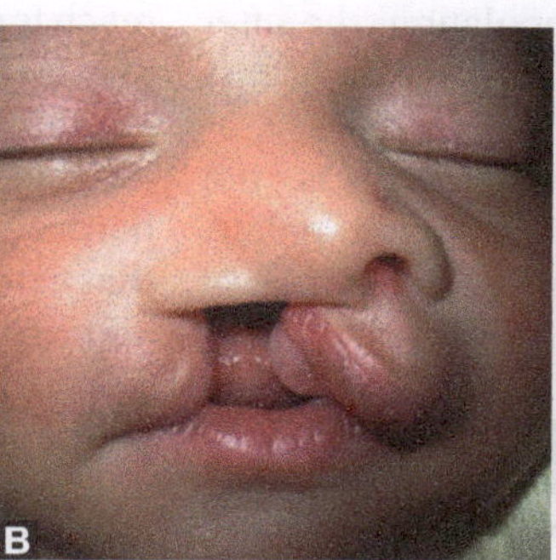

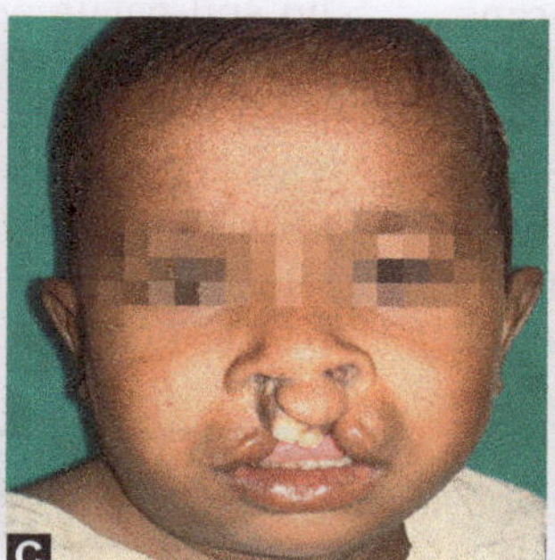

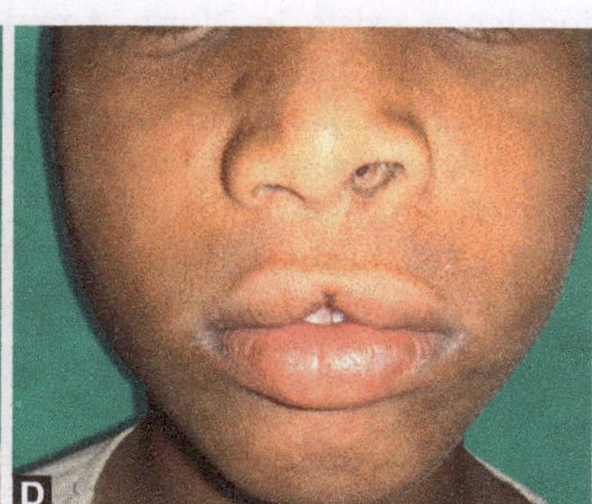

Figs 24.1A to D: Different craniofacial cleft deformities seen among children: (A) Oro-occular cleft; (B) Unilateral cleft; (C) Bilateral cleft; (D) Midline cleft

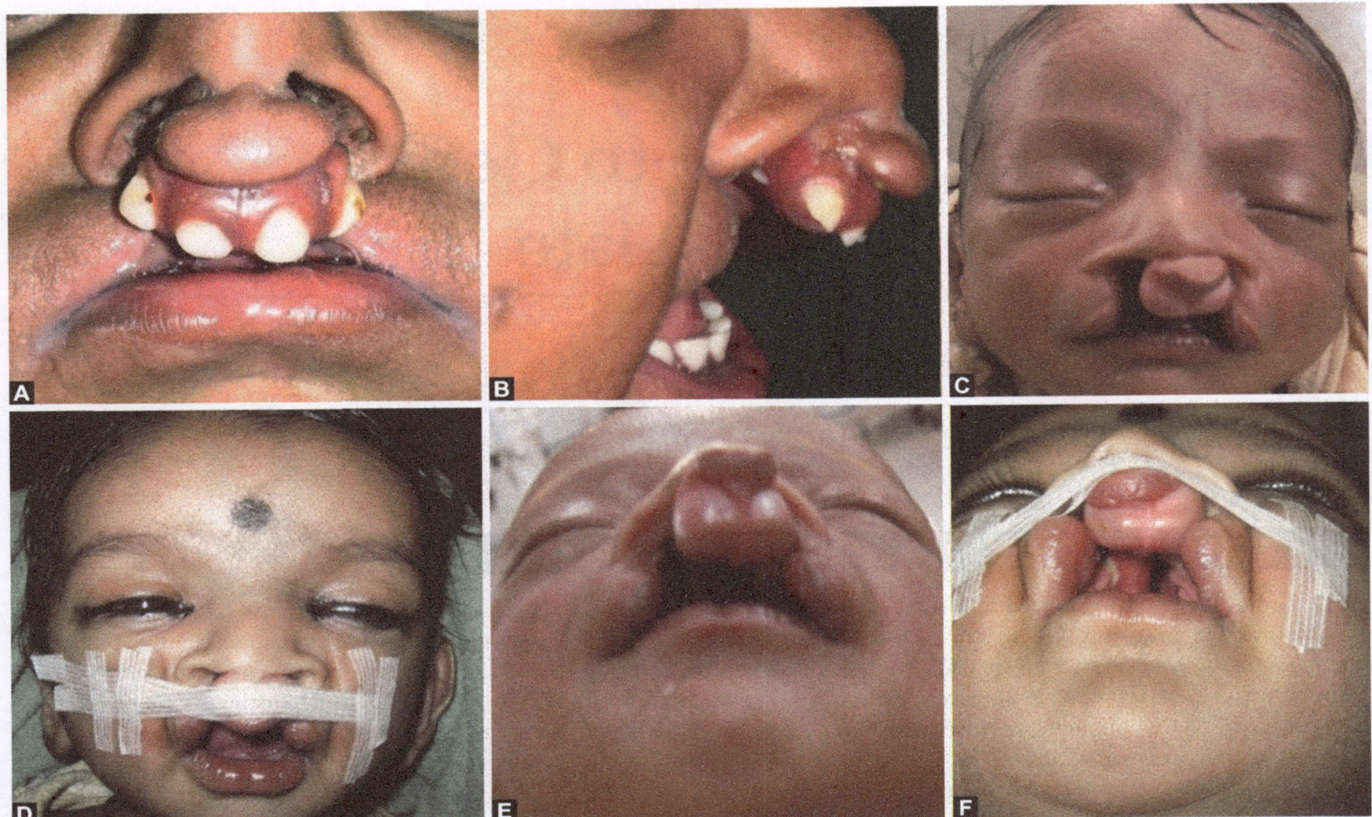

Figs 24.2A to F: Protruding premaxilla treated with external band compression in bilateral cleft lip and palate: (A) Frontal view; (B) Lateral view; (C) Protruding premaxilla-pretreatment; (D) Adhesive tape in place to retract the premaxilla; (E) Pretreatment worms view; (F) Posttreatment worms view

Von Langenbeck[11,12] collaborated these concepts and emphasized on subperiosteal undermining and use of mucoperiosteal flap, which was a major factor in healing of wound.

EPIDEMIOLOGY

Cleft lip occurs in approximately 1 in 750 to 1,000 live births.[13] The highest incidence exists in North Americans, Indians and Japanese (approximately 1 in 350 births). African Americans and Africans represent the lowest incidence of cleft lip deformity (approximately 1 in 1,500 births). There is a higher incidence of cleft in certain populations of Scandinavia and Middle European countries.

Among the cleft lip and palate population, the most common diagnosis is:

- Cleft lip and palate at 46 percent, followed by isolated cleft palate at 33 percent, followed by isolated cleft lip at 21 percent.
- The majority of bilateral cleft lips (86%) and unilateral cleft lips (68%) are associated with a cleft palate.
- Unilateral clefts are nine times as common as bilateral clefts and occur twice as after frequently on the left side than on the right.
- Males are predominant in the cleft lip and palate population, the after whereas isolated cleft palate occurs more commonly in females.
- This racial heterogeneity is not observed for isolated cleft palate, which has an overall incidence of 0.5 per 1,000 live births.

APPLIED SURGICAL ANATOMY

Important structures of the embryo's mouth form at 4 to 7 weeks of gestation. Development during this period entails migration and fusion of mesenchymal cells with facial structures. If this migration and fusion is interrupted, a cleft can develop along the lip and palate. The type of cleft varies with the embryonic stages of development. Important thing to remember is basically abnormality of mesoderm for a cleft to occur, either mesoderm is less or mesoderm does not reach for fusion, if at all it reaches then it may be late.

There are several types of cleft lip, ranging from a small groove on the border of the lip to a larger deformity that extends into the floor of the nostril and part of the maxilla.

Unilateral cleft lip results from failure of the maxillary process on the affected side to fuse with median nasal prominences (Fig. 24.3). The result is called as persistent labial groove. The cells of the lip become stretched and the

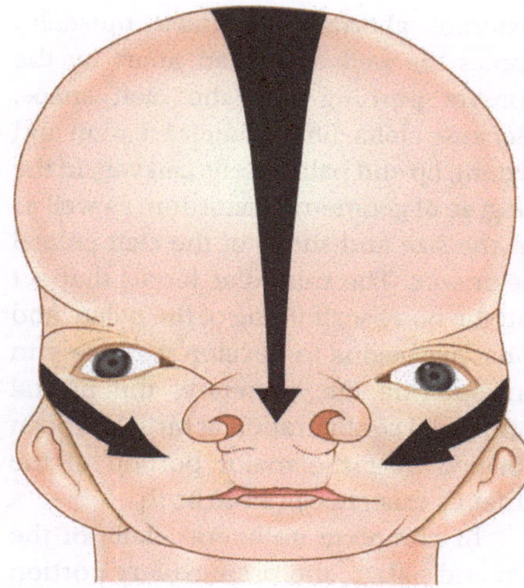

Fig. 24.3: A developing embryo showing fusion of both the maxillary processes on either side with median nasal process in center. Any abnormality in fusion leads to cleft

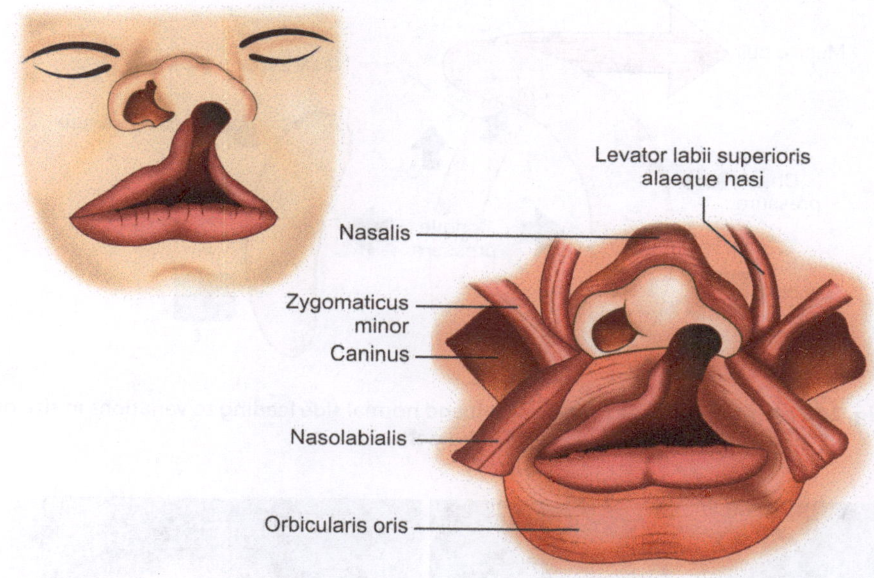

Fig. 24.5: Depiction of the abnormal musculature surrounding a cleft lip

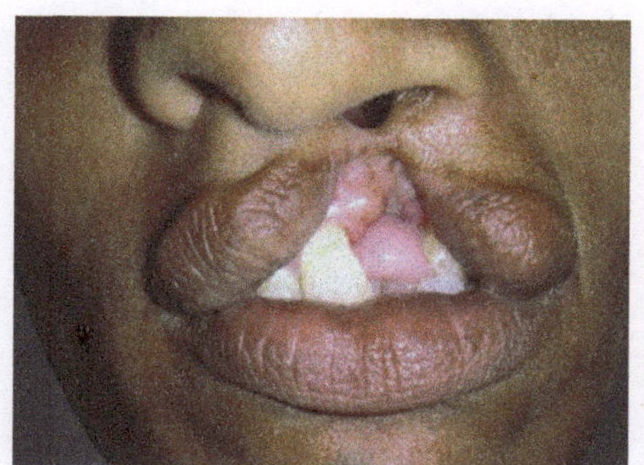

Fig. 24.4: Simonart band joining lip on both the sides of cleft

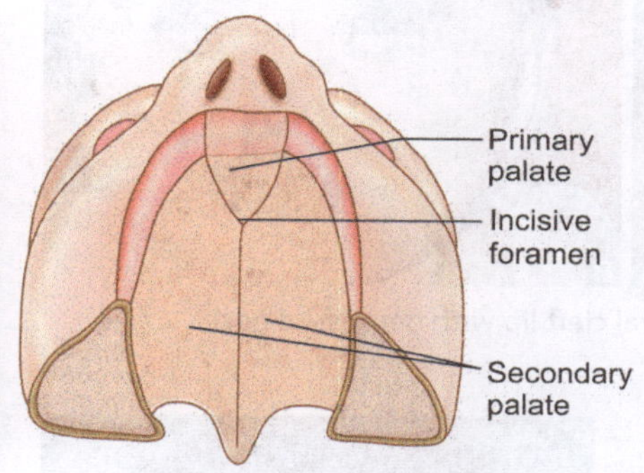

Fig. 24.6: Development of palate

tissues in the persistent groove break down, resulting in a lip that is divided into medial and lateral portions. In some cases, a bridge of tissue (Simonart band) joins together, the two incomplete lip portions shown in Figure 24.4. The orbicularis oris muscle anatomy is abnormal in the cleft lip patients. The orbicularis muscle fibers do not decussate transversely across the midline over the maxilla but tend to run-up parallel to the cleft edges toward the base of the nose (Fig. 24.5).

Bilateral cleft lip occurs in a fashion similar to the unilateral cleft. Patients with bilateral cleft lip may have varying degrees of deformity on each side of the defect. An anatomical structure prolabium projects to the front and hangs unattached. Defects associated with bilateral cleft lip are particularly problematic due to discontinuity of the muscle fibers of the orbicularis oris.

FORMATION OF PALATE

The palate is formed with the fusion of primary palate (median palatine process), which is derived from the frontonasal process and the secondary palate (lateral palatine processes), which are derived from the maxillary prominences on both sides. All these three elements are initially widely separated because of the presence of tongue.[14] During 8th week, the orientation of the lateral palatine processes alters from vertical to horizontal to initiate their fusion. During this process the mandible becomes more prognathic, thereby allowing the tongue to move downwards to avoid any interference for fusion to occur.

Fusion then occurs between the secondary palate and primary palate as shown in Figure 24.6.

Ossification occurs in the primary palate and the anterior portion of the secondary palate to form the hard palate, while the posterior portion of the secondary palate does not undergo ossification and remains as the soft palate.

The embryologic basis of cleft palate is failure of the fusion of these processes with each other. Cleft of either the primary or secondary palate can be complete or incomplete, depending on the degree of fusion that occurred during embryonic development.

A cleft of the lip and palate is the result of the failure of lip elements, and right and left palatal segment, to come together within the first 9 weeks of fetal

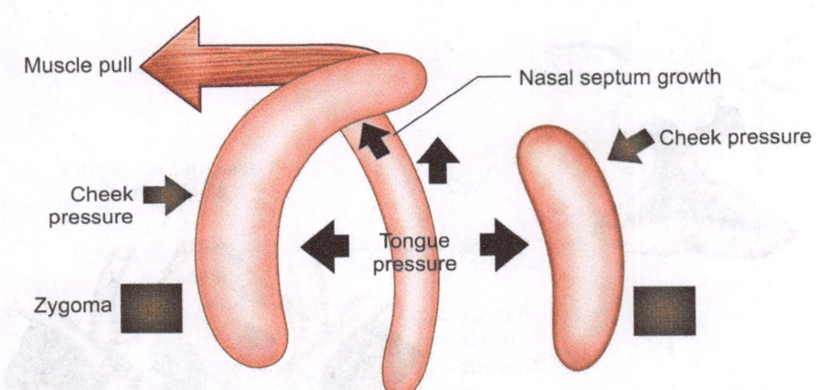

Fig. 24.7: Abnormal forces acting on cleft and normal side leading to variations in size of the cleft

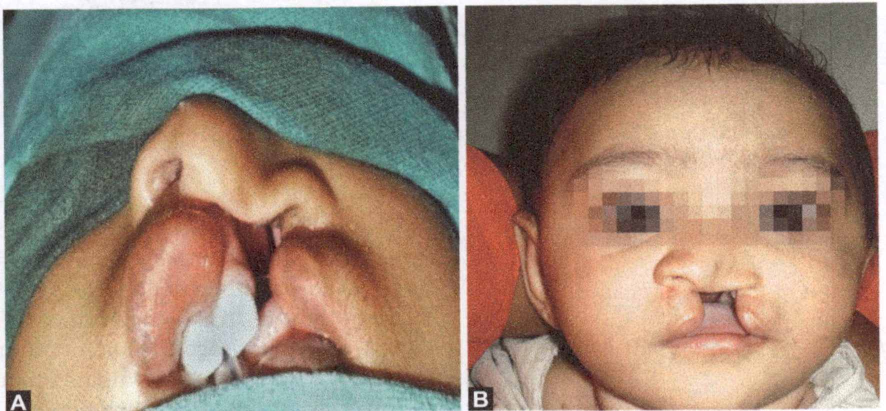

Figs 24.8A and B: Wide unilateral cleft lip with depressed nose

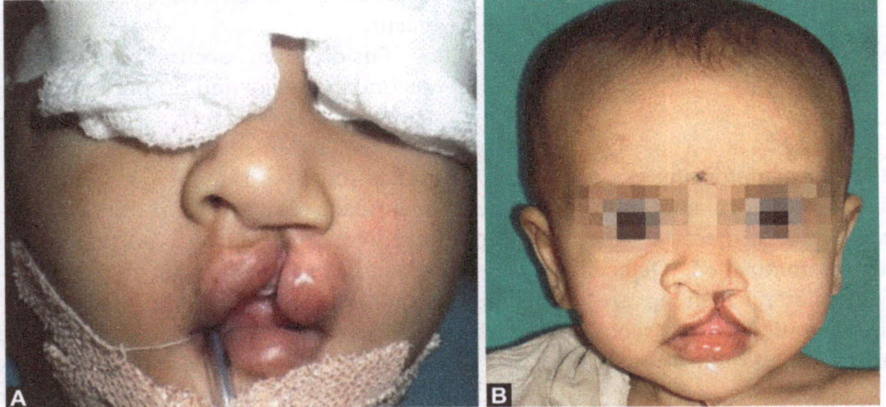

Figs 24.9A and B: Minimally displaced cleft margins due to Simonart band

life. The loss of muscular continuity of the orbicularis oris-buccinator-superior constrictor ring in complete unilateral and bilateral clefts changes the normal muscular force. The aberrant muscular forces act to displace tissue masses (Fig. 24.7). In complete clefts of the lip and palate, if the lateral palatal cleft segments are detached from the vomer, they will be pulled laterally by the external aberrant lip-cheek muscular forces, as well as spread apart by the tongue pushing into the cleft space. Because clefts differ in their location and extent, lip and palate clefts can vary in the degree of geometric distortion, as well as in the size and shape of the cleft palatal segments. The muscular forces that act on the bony scaffolding of the palate and pharynx begins to develop very early in intrauterine life; therefore, the palatal and facial configuration at birth has been formed over the major portion of the infant's existence prior to birth.

In complete unilateral clefts of the lip and palate, the premaxillary portion of the non-cleft segment is pulled anterolaterally. In addition to the lateral displacement of the lateral palatal segments, the premaxilla in the larger segment is carried forward in the facial skeleton. Alveolar bone deficiencies can be seen in related abnormal tooth development or absence, as growth of alveolar bone is based on tooth development. Nose is also deviated to the normal side because of muscle pull except the alar base of cleft side, because of which nose appears to be depressed as shown in Figures 24.8A and B. If a soft tissue, which collectively form Simonart band, bridges the alveolar cleft, the attached palatal segments are limited in their degree of geometric displacement (Figs 24.9A and B).

In complete bilateral cleft lip and palate, there is excessive growth in the premaxillary-vomerine suture is caused by increased tension at this site, precipitated by mechanical force stresses during periods of rapid growth (Figs 24.10A and B). This growth is continuous during early postnatal years and provides a fourth dimension to the deformity, which can alter the cleft palatal segments and their associated parts and either simplify or complicate treatment.

In complete cleft palate cases, there is abnormal muscle attachment seen at the junction of hard palate and soft palate. In the normal palate, complete ring of muscles (tensor veli palatini and levator veli palatini) can be seen, where as in cleft there are abnormal attachment of these muscles on the posterior border of hard palate, instead of intermingling with each other in center as seen in normal palate. This abnormal attachment restricts the normal movement of soft palate, while performing various functions (Figs 24.11A and B).

Maxillary growth occurs on posterior surface of maxilla with the forward push of maxilla against basal bone and deposition of bone at the tuberosity region. In the cleft palate surgery mucoperiosteal flap is raised and sutured leaving denuded bone area on both sides, which heals with scar tissue. This tissue contracts, while healing helps in reducing width of the maxillary arch form although this effect is minimal. At the same time if hamulus is fractured in pterygopalatomaxillary junction scar tissue may form across this sensitive area of growth and inhibits forward movement of maxilla. It also affects eruption of teeth, teeth erupts more palatally than its normal eruption pathway.

In infants with cleft lip and palate, feeding is a major problem as child cannot suck, because of inability to create negative pressure in mouth. Poor feeding also leads to improper growth of the child. Otitis media is also a common problem with cleft palate patients, as ventilation of ear is affected due to abnormal muscle attachment, blockage of eustachian tube and its pull, which leads to accumulation of fluid in ear and leading to inflammation.[15] Children have speech related difficulties as there is no closure of nasopharynx (velopharyngeal incompetence), hence a nasal twang is present, which makes words incomprehensible.

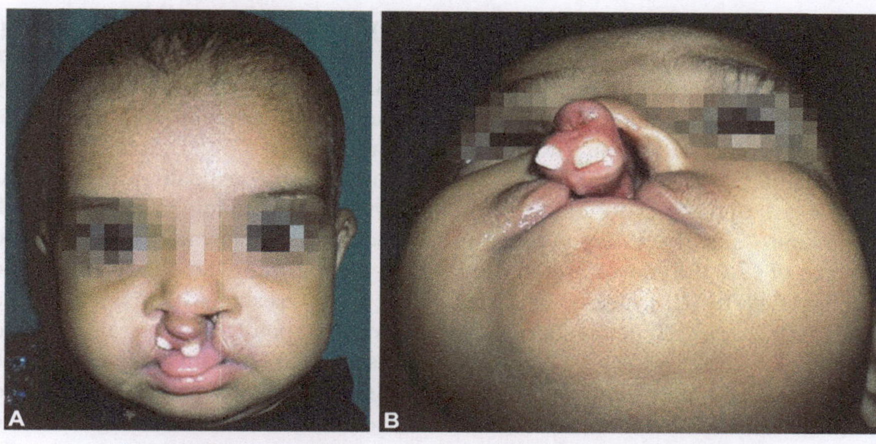

Figs 24.10A and B: Displaced unsupported premaxilla and palate

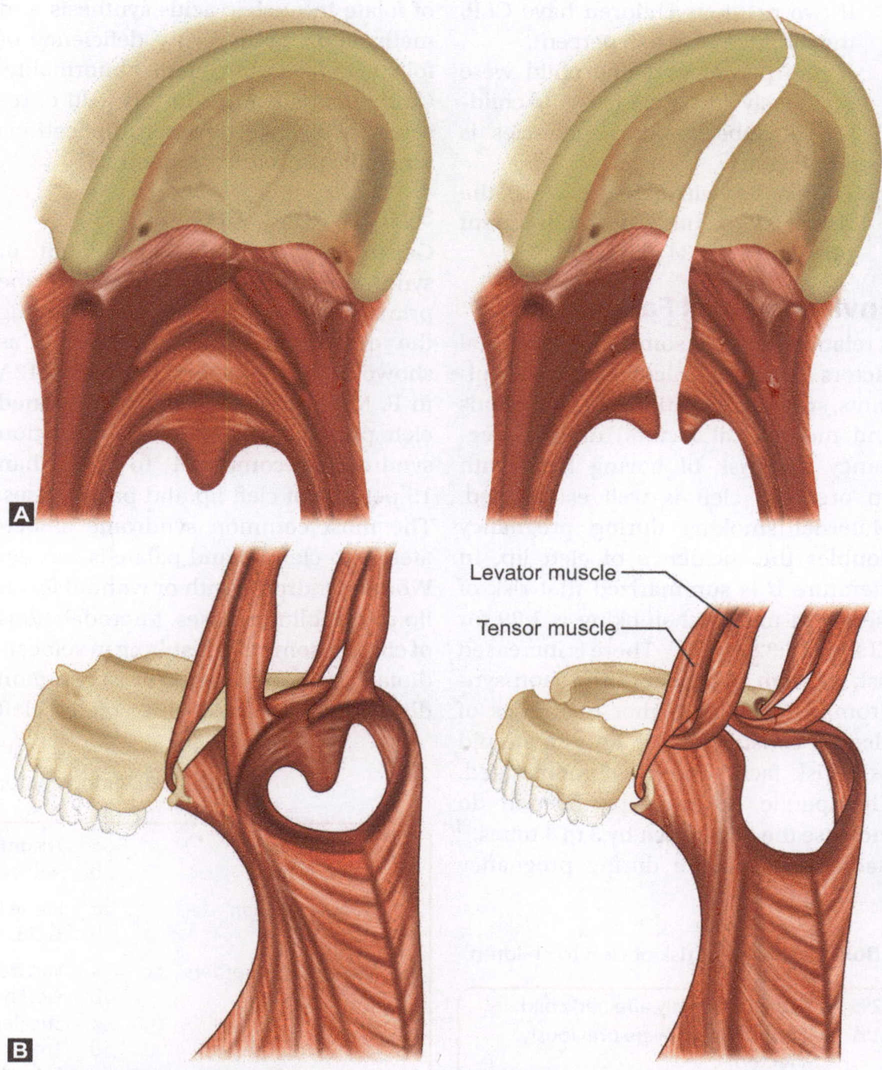

Figs 24.11A and B: Abnormal attachment of palatal musculature in cleft palate (*Courtesy:* Salyer and Bardach's Atlas of Craniofacial and Cleft Surgery: Craniofacial Surgery, Vol. 1 by Kenneth E Salyer, Janusz Bardach)

ETIOLOGY

Both environmental and genetic factors are implicated in the genesis of cleft lip and palate. Facial clefts can occur as part of a syndrome or an isolated clefts. Factors most commonly causing cleft are as follows:

- Genetic factors
- Environmental factors
- Syndromic clefts.

Genetic Factors

Parents with a non-syndromic child having cleft, often have a query whether their subsequent child will also have CLP deformity. However, it should be explained to such parents that the relative risk of having CLP deformity in subsequent offsprings depends upon the type of CLP the previous child had, i.e. cleft lip alone (CL), cleft lip with cleft palate (CLP) or a cleft palate alone (CP) (Box 24.1).

- If the family has one affected child or parent with CLP, the risk of the child of the next pregnancy having CLP is 4 percent.[16]
- If two previous children have CLP, the risk increases to 9 percent.
- If one parent and one child were previously affected, the risk to children of subsequent pregnancies is 17 percent.
- For families with a history of CP, the risk of CP to children of subsequent pregnancies is 34 percent.

Environmental Factors

A relation between some environmental factors (smoking, alcohol, anticonvulsants, steroids, radiation, viral infections and mechanical factors) during pregnancy and risk of having baby with an orofacial cleft is well established. Maternal smoking during pregnancy doubles the incidence of cleft lip. In literature it is summarized that risk of cleft with maternal smoking is 1:29 for CLP and 1:32 for CP.[17] There is increased risk of both syndromic and non-syndromic cleft with higher quantities of alcohol consumption.[18] Role of steroid as a risk factor is well demonstrated. Therapeutic doses of prednisone do increase the risk of cleft by 3 to 4 times.[19] Radiation exposure during pregnancy and viral infections also predisposes to cleft lip and palate. Mechanical factors are like attempt to abort the baby by uterine manipulation and hormonal therapy.

Intrauterine exposure to the anticonvulsant phenytoin,[20] valproic acid, oxazolidine is associated with a 10 fold increase in the incidence of cleft lip. The drug methotrexate which is used as a chemotherapeutic agent is also said to be associated with increase in the risk of clefts.[21] Deficiency of folic acid also causes cleft in human beings but the exact etiopathogenesis for this is still unclear, most accepted being the role of folate in nucleic acids synthesis and methylation cycle.[22] Any deficiency of folic acid leads to genetic abnormality. Continuing advances in this field of research will have obvious implications for global prevention programs.

Syndromic Clefts

Genetic abnormalities can result in syndromes that include clefts of the primary or secondary palate among the developmental fields affected as shown in Box 24.2 and Figures 24.12A to F. More than 40 percent of isolated cleft palates are part of malformation syndromes, compared to less than 15 percent of cleft lip and palate cases. The most common syndrome associated with cleft lip and palate is van der Woude syndrome with or without lower lip pits or blind sinuses. Microdeletions of chromosome 22q resulting in velocardiofacial syndrome is the most common diagnoses associated with isolated cleft palate with congenital heart diseases, hypernasal speech and learning disabilities. Syndromes associated with cleft are many. Some of them commonly seen as given in Box 24.2.

CLASSIFICATION

Many different classification systems of varying complexity have been proposed for cleft lip and palate, but few have found wide clinical acceptance and application.

In 1922, Davis and Ritchie,[23] classified congenital clefts in three groups according to the position of the cleft in relation to the alveolar process (Box 24.3).

In 1931, Veau[24] suggested a classification, which has four categories (Box 24.4).

However, this classification is incomplete because it makes no provision for isolated cleft lip and cleft alveolus. Fogh-Andersen[25] introduced embryological concepts into his simple classification, which he used to describe the epidemiology of cleft lip and palate in Denmark in 1942. Kernahan and Stark[26] further developed this concept in 1958 and Kernahan[27] represented symbolically as a 'striped Y' in 1971 (Fig. 24.13). The involved area is filled in by pen and provides rapid graphic presentation of the site and extent of cleft involvement.

However, it has got few limitations like no differentiation of cleft lip with and without involving nose and clefts of secondary palate cannot be classified into right or left sides. Kernahan later on

Box 24.1: Genetic risk of cleft to children

2%	If one previously affected child
1%	If two children were previously affected
6%	If one parent has CP
15%	If one parent and one previous child have CP.

Box 24.2: Various syndromes associated with cleft

1. Chromosomal	a. Trisomy 13 and 18 b. Velocardiofacial syndrome
2. Non-mendelian	a. Pierre Robin's syndrome b. Goldenhar syndrome
3. Mendelian disorders	a. Van der Woude syndrome b. Gorlin syndrome c. Stickler's syndrome d. Treacher-Collin's syndrome e. Ectrodactyly-ectoderm
4. Unknown	a. Kabuki syndrome b. de Lange syndrome

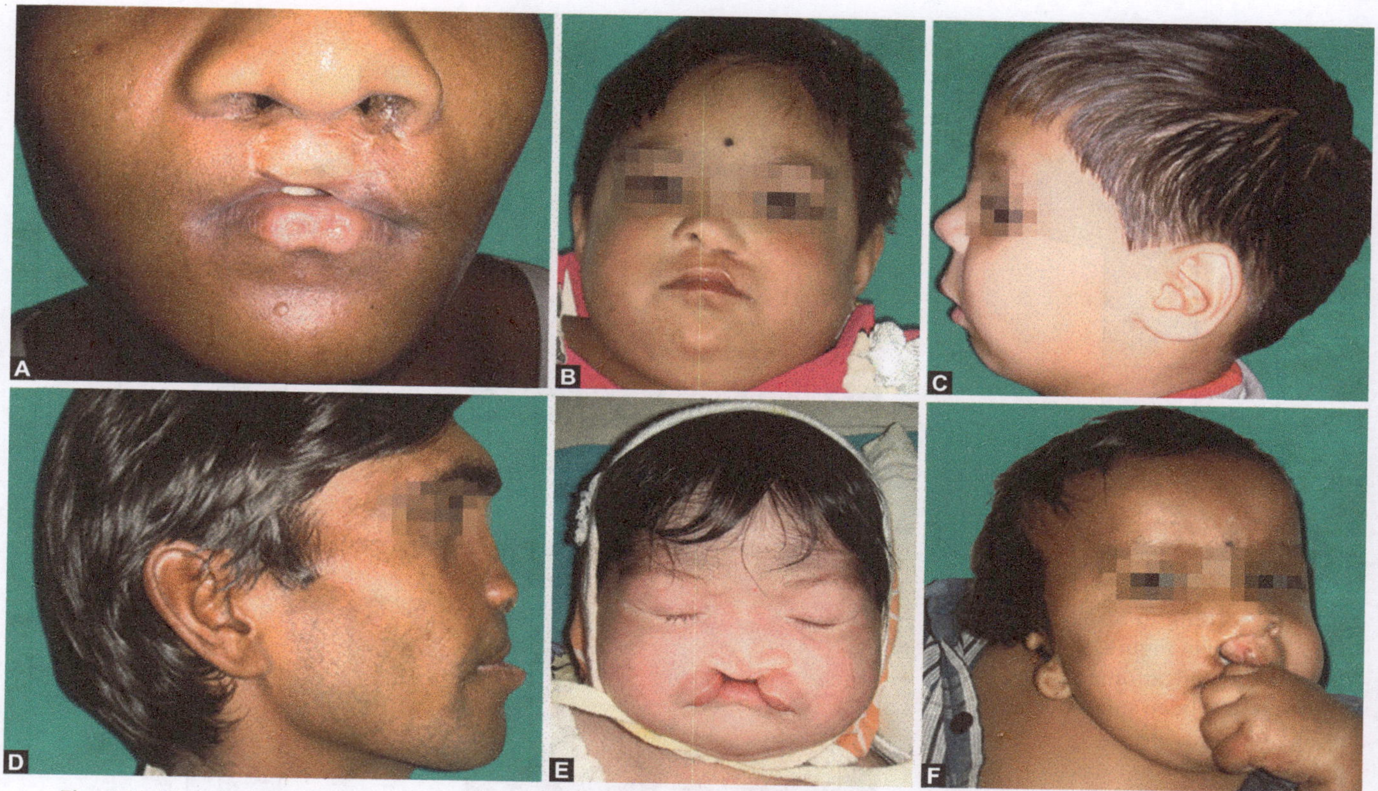

Figs 24.12A to F: (A) Van der Woude syndrome; (B) Down syndrome; (C) Pierre Robin sequence; (D and E) Binder, syndrome; (F) Goldenhar syndrome

Box 24.3: Davis and Ritchie's classification of clefts

Group 1	Prealveolar clefts, unilateral, median or bilateral.
Group 2	Postalveolar clefts involving the soft palate only, the soft and hard palates or a submucous cleft.
Group 3	Alveolar clefts, unilateral, bilateral or median.

Box 24.4: Veau's classification

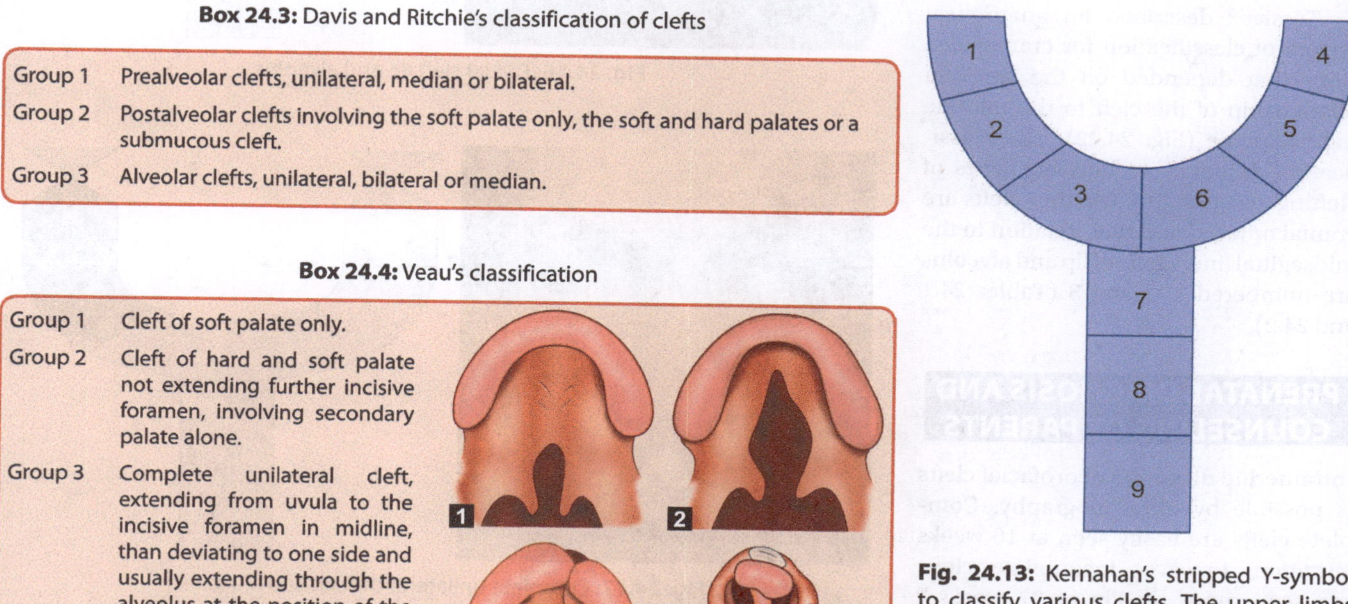

Group 1	Cleft of soft palate only.
Group 2	Cleft of hard and soft palate not extending further incisive foramen, involving secondary palate alone.
Group 3	Complete unilateral cleft, extending from uvula to the incisive foramen in midline, than deviating to one side and usually extending through the alveolus at the position of the future lateral incisor tooth.
Group 4	Complete bilateral cleft, same as group 3 with two clefts extending forward from the incisive foramen through the alveolus.

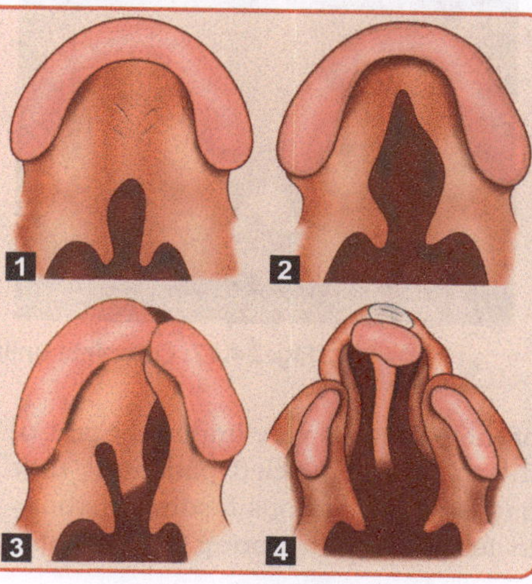

Fig. 24.13: Kernahan's stripped Y-symbol to classify various clefts. The upper limbs represent the right (1, 2, 3) and left sides (4, 5, 6) lip (1 and 4), alveolus (2 and 5), hard palate anterior to the incisive foramen (3 and 6). The lower limb represents the hard palate posterior to the incisive foramen (7 and 8) and soft palate (9)

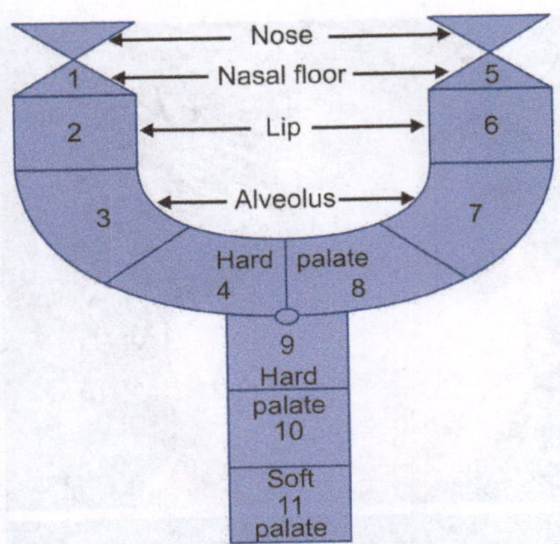

Fig. 24.14: Modified Kernahan classification

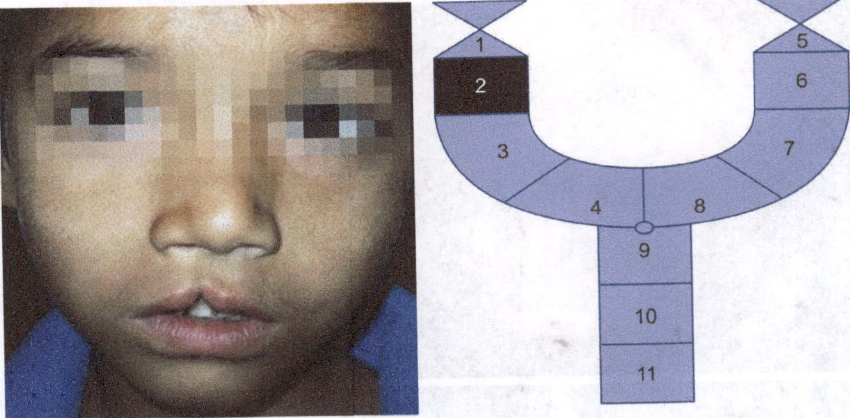

Fig. 24.15: Partial cleft lip

modified his stripped Y to involve nose and nasal floor as shown in Figure 24.14.

Various types of clefts and how to classify according to Kernahan classification is given in Figures 24.15 to 24.21.

A new classification, Nagpur classification has also been suggested as shown in Box 24.5.

Still remaining is a group of rare craniofacial clefts that lie outside the classification systems of the clefts of the lip and palate deformities, described previously.

Tessier[29] described an anatomical system of classification for craniofacial clefts that depended on the site and relationship of the cleft to the midline sagittal plane (Fig. 24.22). The classification describes 14 different types of clefting according to, whether clefts are cranial or facial and their relation to the midsagittal line. Clefts of lip and alveolus are numbered 1, 2 and 3 (Tables 24.1 and 24.2).

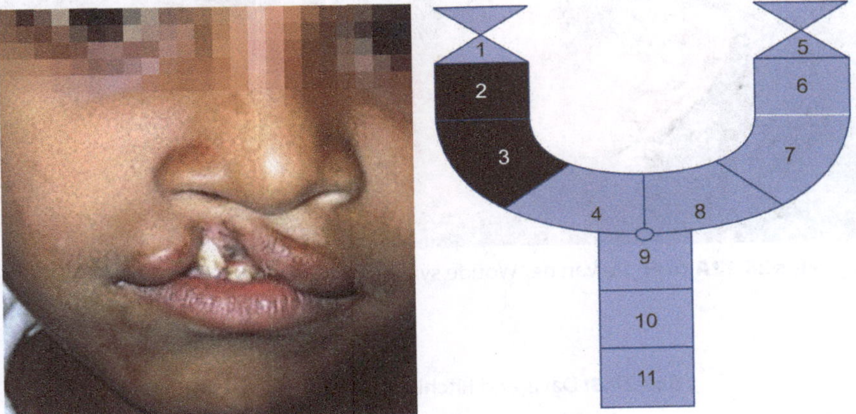

Fig. 24.16: Partial cleft lip and alveolus

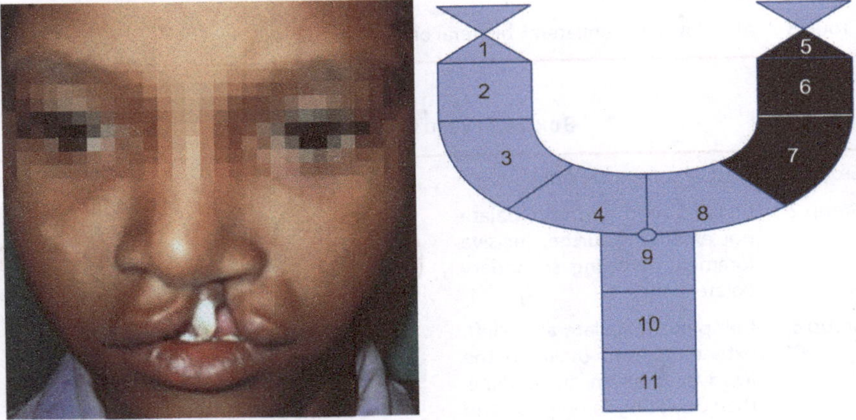

Fig. 24.17: Complete unilateral cleft lip and alveolus

PRENATAL DIAGNOSIS AND COUNSELING OF PARENTS

Intrauterine diagnosis of orofacial clefts is possible by ultrasonography. Complete clefts are easily seen at 16 weeks gestation, however incomplete clefts are seen more readily at 27 weeks.[30] Palatal clefts are difficult to visualize by prenatal ultrasonography (Figs 24.23A to I). Prenatal diagnosis can be done during routine screening and with high resolution ultrasonography. Counseling of the parents is very important part of the treatment for cleft patient as they have to learn various feeding methods to feed the child during infancy, also the parents should be psychologically prepared to be the part of the team for the management of the child. Counseling is also important as sometimes parents

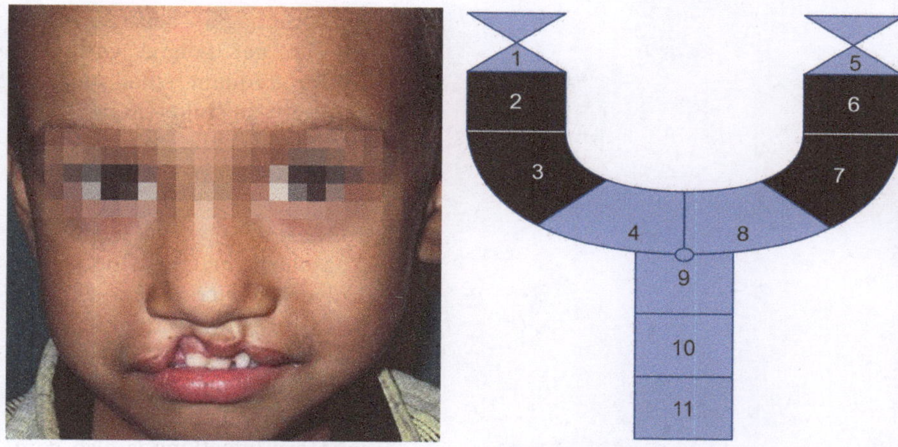

Fig. 24.18: Partial bilateral cleft lip and alveolus

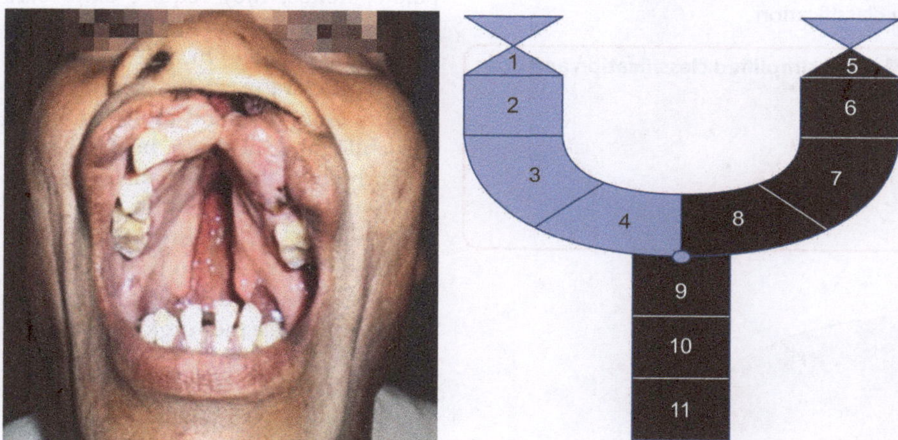

Fig. 24.19: Complete unilateral cleft lip, alveolus and palate

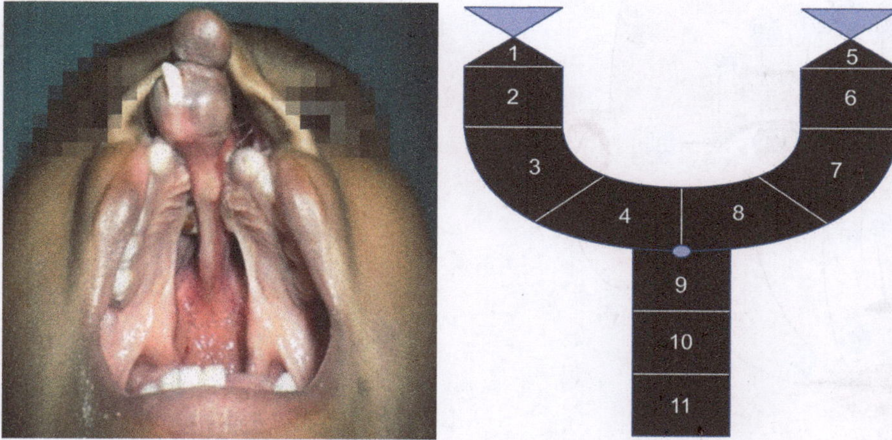

Fig. 24.20: Complete bilateral cleft lip, alveolus and palate

may want to terminate pregnancy, but parents must be explained about the treatment options available for cleft patients, but if the child is syndromic and having other congenital anomalies, then it may be an indication for termination of pregnancy. Intrauterine foetal surgeries are the upcoming modalities to avoid such terminations.

MANAGEMENT PROTOCOLS FOR THE PATIENTS WITH CLEFT LIP AND PALATE

Many treatment protocols have been given in the literature for the management of cleft deformities however, only standardized and widely acclaimed and practiced treatment modalities are discussed in the present chapter. The comprehensive treatment of cleft lip and palate deformities requires thoughtful consideration of the anatomic complexities of the deformity and the delicate balance between intervention and growth. There are many modalities, but all have same aims and objectives to achieve:

- Normal dentofacial growth and development.
- Normalized esthetic appearance of face.
- Intact primary and secondary palate.
- Normal speech, language and hearing.
- Nasal airway patency.
- Class I occlusion with normal masticatory function.
- Good dental and periodontal health.
- Normal psychosocial development.

To achieve all these goals only surgical procedure is not sufficient enough. The line of treatment for the child is as follows:

- Preoperative management.
- Primary operative management.
- Secondary management.

Preoperative Management

During the first day of life the most critical aspect is feeding, as child cannot generate negative intraoral pressure having cleft palate, parents have to feed the child. Otherwise caloric requirements of the child will not be met. There are various devices available to aid in feeding (Figs 24.24 to 24.27).

The child must be fed in sitting up position and frequent burping is required as child ingests air along with

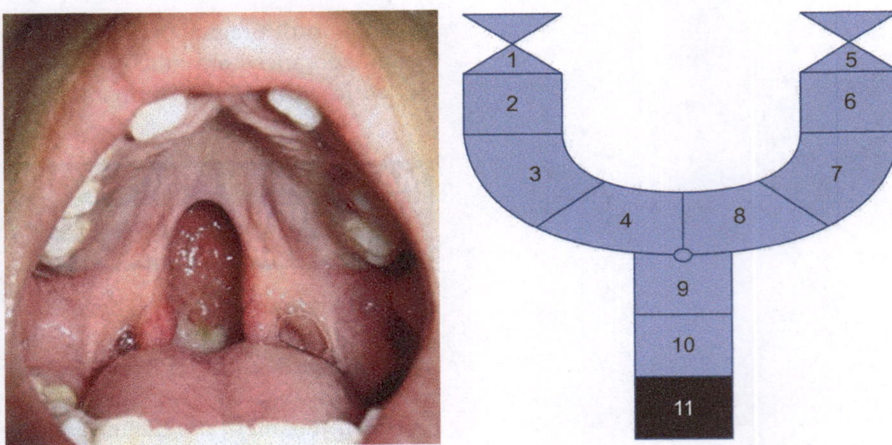

Fig. 24.21: Cleft soft palate and uvula

Box 24.5: Nagpur classification

Nagpur classification for cleft lip and palate[28]: It is a simplified classification and does not tell whether cleft is complete or incomplete.

Group 1—cleft lip.
Group 1A—cleft lip and alveolus.
Group 2—cleft palate.
Group 3—cleft lip and palate.
It could be unilateral or bilateral.

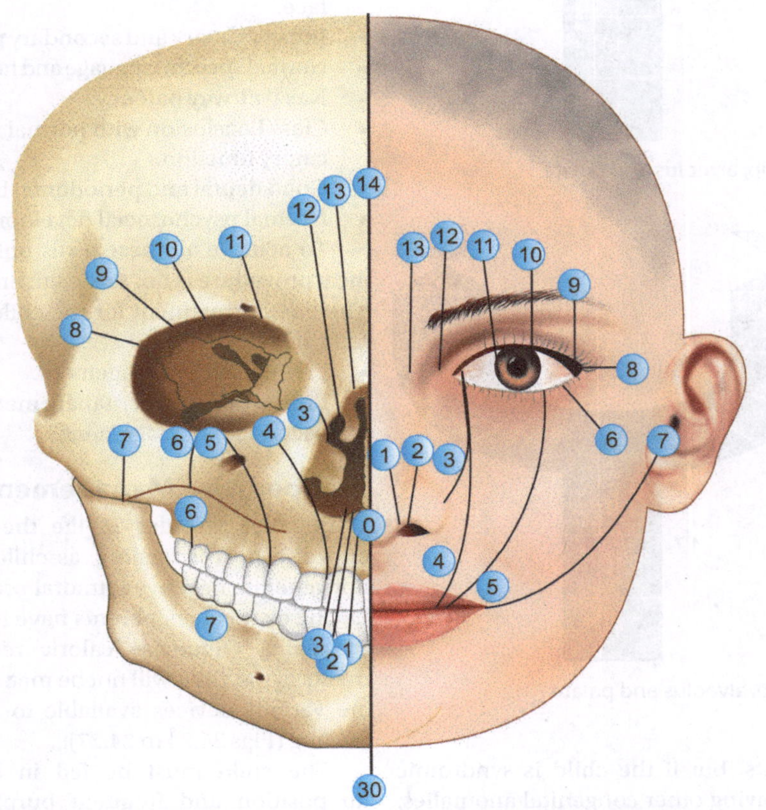

Fig. 24.22: Tessier classification of craniofacial clefts. Right side depicts the osseous clefts while the left side shows soft tissue clefts (Numbers 0 and 30 represent midline clefts)

the food (aerophagia), because of this cleft children get fatigue early and they require frequent small quantity of feeds, otherwise child will be undernourished. If the child cannot be fed with this method, a palatal prosthesis, which spans the defect may be required. The prosthesis helps in feeding as well as nasoalveolar moulding (NAM) preoperatively to decrease the width of the cleft. Despite these attempts, more than 25 percent of CLAP children have feeding difficulties with poor weight gain until palatal repair.

Respiratory infections is also common in children with cleft lip and palate, hence, they require extra care by the parents to prevent any infection and avoid people having respiratory infection coming close to the child. Parents need to spend more time with the child and need to be counseled properly about the importance of regular follow-up for hemoglobin estimation, management of recurrent diarrhea, needful interventions to prevent weight loss, as all these factors delay the surgery and compromise the surgical outcomes.

Presurgical Orthodontics

The goal of presurgical orthodontics is to move the abnormally positioned maxillary arches into a normal relationship prior to the surgery. The soft tissues follow the bony foundation and cleft lip elements move closer to each other narrowing the cleft. There are many devices used for this, such as:

- Extraoral devices
  - Simple surgical tape on lip from cheek to cheek.
  - Head bonnet with elastic strap.
- Intraoral devices
  - Passive devices (palatal obturators).
  - Active devices (pin retained devices 'Latham appliance') (Figs 24.28A and B).

Extraoral devices are economical and simple to apply, but they require cooperation from parents for application of new tapes and adjustment of straps at periodic intervals. The appliance is visible externally and can damage the tender skin of the child.

Table 24.1: Tessier's classification showing bony clefts

Bony or skeletal clefts	Extent
#14	Midline Cleft
#13	On the cranium comes through frontal bone through olfactory groove between nasal bone and frontal process of maxilla
#12	Through lateral mass of ethmoid
#11	Upper medial orbital cleft, cranial counterpart of #3
#10	It is a central orbit cleft, extends to roof of eye socket and forehead, the cranial extension of #4
#9	Upper lateral orbital cleft, seems to correspond with #5
#8	Frontozygomatic cleft which appears to be the cranial counterpart of #6
#7	Temporozygomatic cleft with absence of zygomatic arch, deformities of mandibular ramus, condyle and coronoid process
#6	Maxillary zygomatic cleft opens into infraorbital fissure travels through back of upper jaw with high palate and choanal atresia (absence of inner ear structure)
#5	It runs through infraorbital rim, orbital floor and maxilla lateral to the infraorbital nerve and maxillary ainus, proceeds to alveolus behind canine tooth in premolar region
#4	It is a central orbito–maxillary cleft through infraorbital rim, orbital floor and medial to infraorbital nerve through maxillary sinus or alveolus
#3	Runs from inside (medial) lower edge of orbit through lacrimal bone, across maxilla and alveolus to lateral incisor
#2	Across premaxilla, 2 appears to split the tooth
#1	From between central and lateral incisor to floor of nasal cavity

Table 24.2: Tessier's classification showing soft tissue clefts

Soft tissue clefts	Extent
#14	Midline facial cleft
#13	Cranial Counterpart of #1, medial to the eyebrow
#12	Cranial cleft between nasal bridge and inner corner of eye, coloboma of the root of the eyebrow
#11	Notch of upper lid and eyebrow
#10	Notch of the upper lid and divides the eyebrow
#9	Upper lateral orbital cleft in the outer third of upper eyelid
#8	True cleft of lateral canthus associated with Goldenhar syndrome
#7	Presents as macrostomia and preauricular tags
#6	Lower lid coloboma with a marked furrow across cheek
#5	Lateral orbito–maxillary cleft through the outer third of lower lid through cheek to lip near outer corner of mouth
#4	Lateral to the tear duct, across the cheek, skirting the nose, to the lip between the cuspid's bow and corner of mouth
#3	Through the lacrimal punctum around the nostril and into the lip at the cuspid's bow
#2	Slightly to the outer curve of the nostril and into the lip
#1	Through the dome of the nostril cartilage, occasionally through the lip

Intraoral devices aid in feeding and presurgical orthodontics. Latham appliance is used most commonly in bilateral cleft patients to expand the dental arch, so that displaced premaxilla can be retropositioned. This device is given at 6 weeks of age and removed by 2 to 3 months of age for definitive lip repair. Their major disadvantage is that they require specialized orthodontic care, they are expensive and frequently need short anesthesia for making necessary adjustments.

Nasoalveolar Molding[31]

Nasoalveolar Molding (NAM) is a non-surgical method of reshaping the alveolar processes, lip and moulding the nasal cartilages in favorable position before the cleft lip and palate surgery, to facilitate the surgical procedure and enhance the outcomes. It is used mainly in children with wide clefts (Figs 24.29 and 24.30). NAM is employed in early management of both unilateral and bilateral cleft anomalies in newborns. The therapy is started as early as 2 weeks postnatally, as the cartilage and the ridges have high elasticity and can be easily molded in the desired way. The delay in initiating the therapy by few months fails to produce the desired results. It gives excellent early results, but, the long-term results are questionable. Surgery is performed after the molding is complete, approximately 3 to 6 months after birth.

Purpose of NAM:

- Minimal tension in soft tissue during surgical repair.
- Preoperative NAM aid in obtaining optimal scar.
- Increases symmetry of nose.
- Reduction in number of revision surgeries.
- Reduction in overall cost of therapy.

Primary Operative Management

Treatment Planning and Timing of Surgery

The timing of cleft lip and palate repair is controversial. Despite several meaningful advancements in the care of patients with cleft lip and palate, a lack

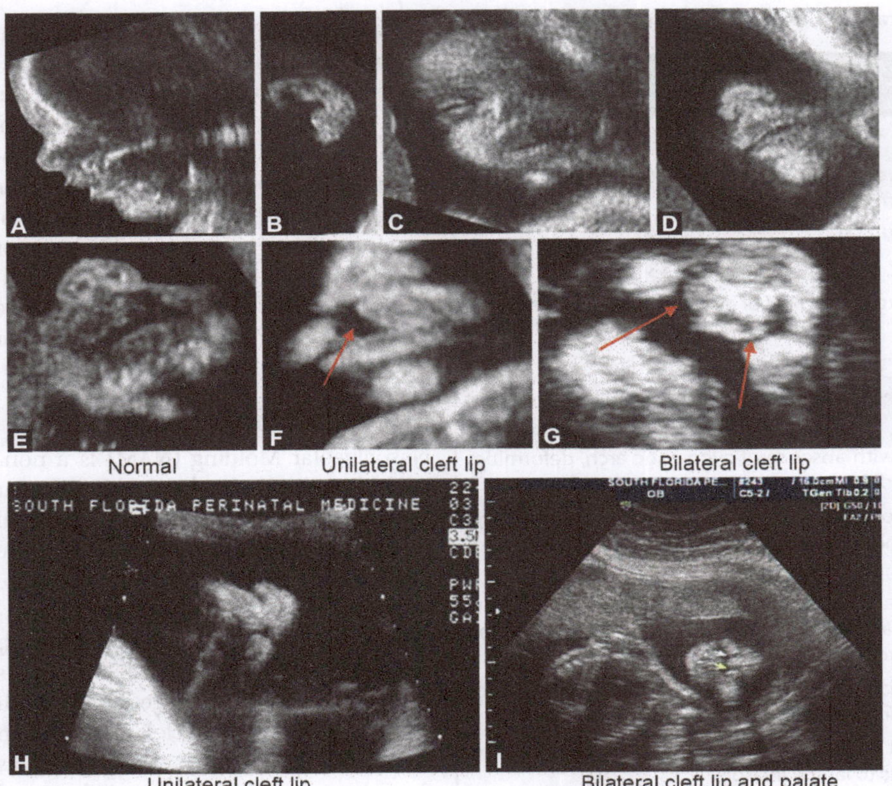

Figs 24.23A to I: Various transvaginal ultrasound images of the fetus with normal lip and cleft lip (*Source:* Cleft Lip and Palate Editor Samuel Berkowitz 2nd Edition, Chapter 2 Prenatal Diagnosis of Oral Clefts pages 23 and 14)

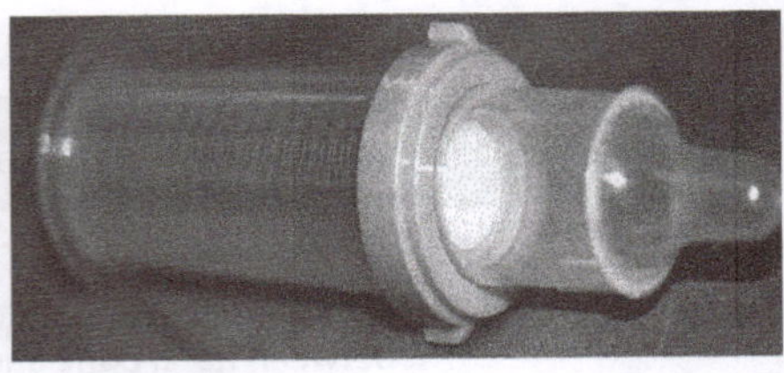

Fig. 24.24: Soft bottle with a large hole, as this fills the palatal defect and requires minimal sucking by the neonate

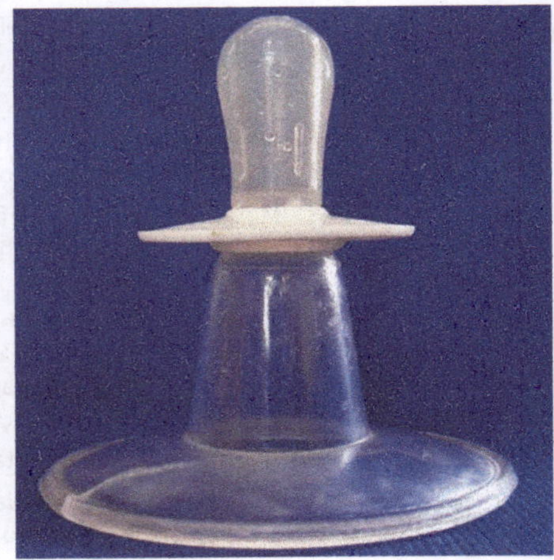

Fig. 24.25: Haberman nipple—it delivers milk under slight pressure, more posteriorly in the oropharynx

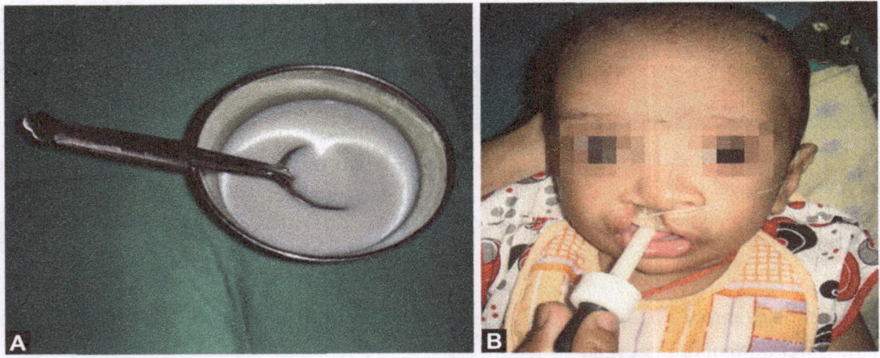

Figs 24.26A and B: (A) Bowl and spoon; (B) Dropper if these nipples are not available

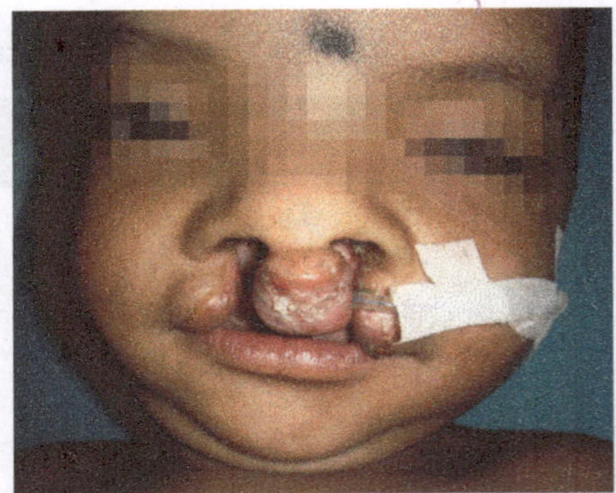

Fig. 24.27: Feeding tube secured to feed the cleft child

of consensus exists regarding the timing and specific techniques used during each stage of cleft reconstruction. Timing of surgery depends on the balance between functional needs, aesthetic concerns, and the issue of ongoing growth of the child. Due to many different treatment philosophies, the timing of treatment interventions is considerably variable amongst cleft centers. Therefore, it is difficult to produce a timing regimen that everyone agrees upon.

The staged reconstruction of cleft lip and palate deformities are shown in Table 24.3.

Cleft lip repair is generally undertaken at some point after 10 weeks of age because:

- It allows a complete medical evaluation of the patient so that any associated congenital defects affecting other organ systems (e.g. cardiac or renal anomalies) may be detected.

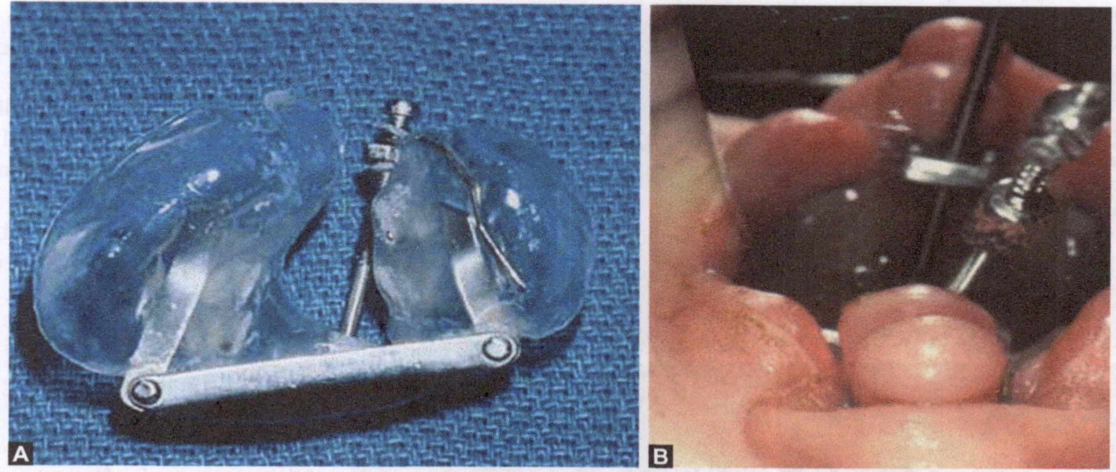

Figs 24.28A and B: Latham's appliance (*Source:* Clefts of the Lip and Palate—Tennessee Craniofacial Center 1(800) 418-3223)

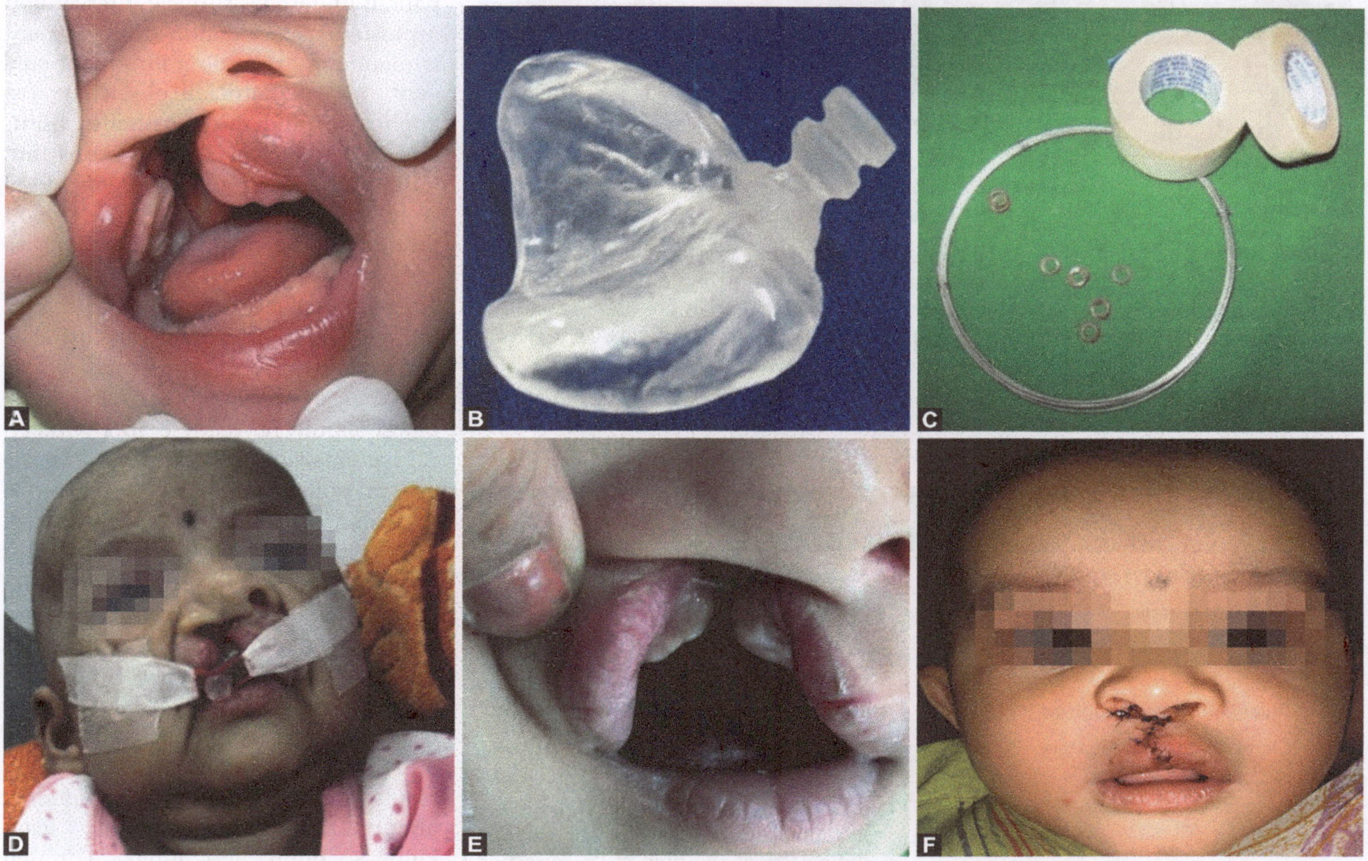

Figs 24.29A to F: Nasoalveolar moulding: (A) Child with a wide unilateral complete cleft lip, alveolus and palate; (B) Custom made tray; (C) Wire, elastics and bandage used to secure the custom made tray; (D) Appliance *in situ*; (E) Reduced size of the defect post therapy; (F) Surgical result post NAM

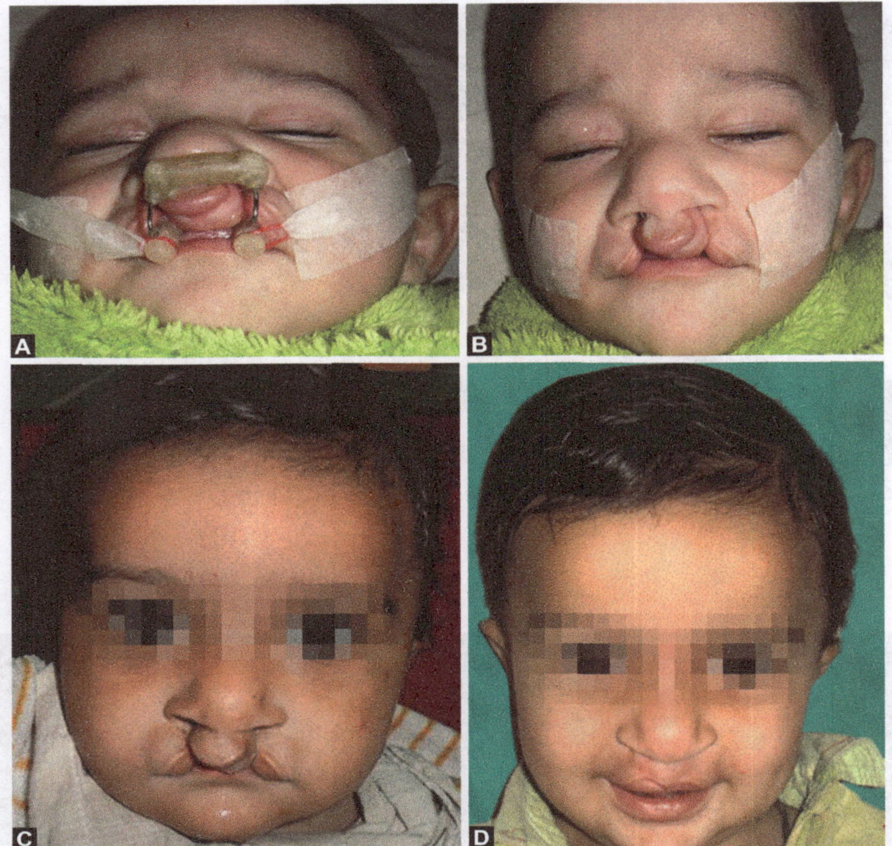

Figs 24.30A to D: Nasoalveolar moulding—Child with bilateral cleft lip, alveolus and palate. To correct the protruding premaxilla a custom made tray is prepared which is secured in mouth using elastic bandages. Retrusion can be seen in pre therapy and post therapy pictures: (A) NAM appliance *in situ*; (B) Retrusion of premaxilla after NAM; (C) Frontal view after NAM; (D) Postsurgical result of the child treated with NAM

Table 24.3: Timing for staged reconstruction of cleft deformities

Sr. No.	Procedure	Timing mentioned in the literature
1.	Cleft lip repair	After 10 weeks
2.	Cleft palate repair	9–18 months
3.	Pharyngeal flap/pharyngoplasty	3–5 years or later based on speech development
4.	Alveolar reconstruction with bone graft	6–9 years based on dental development
5.	Cleft orthognathic surgery	14–16 years in girls, 16–18 years in boys
6.	Cleft rhinoplasty	After age 5 years, but preferably at skeletal maturity; after orthognathic surgery when possible. Nowadays the concept is primary rhinoplasty at the time of lip correction, preschool rhinoplasty and final procedure at 15–18 years is practiced.
7.	Cleft lip revision	Anytime once initial remodeling and scar maturation is complete. Best done after 5 years.

- The surgical procedure itself may be easier when the child is slightly older, and the anatomic landmarks more prominent and well defined.
- The anesthetic risk-related data, historically suggested that the safest time period for surgery in this population of infants could be outlined simply by using the 'rule of 10.'

Rule of 10:

- 10 weeks old
- 10 pounds in weight
- With a minimum hemoglobin value of 10 dL/mg.[32]

Note: When anesthetic facilities were not adequate the rule of ten was followed, but now barring hemoglobin other criteria can be relaxed to certain extent and the surgeries can be performed safely.

Presurgical evaluation: Before the patient undergoes surgical intervention a presurgical evaluation of the patient is mandatory regarding fitness for surgery by pediatrician/physician (as applicable) and the anesthetist. Routine hematological investigations are required including (complete blood count, serum profiles, sickling, blood grouping, hepatitis B). According to 'rule of ten', patient must have at least 10 gm percent of hemoglobin, blood grouping is must if any transfusion is planned during surgery or immediately after surgery for which compatible blood should be ready before surgery. All patients should be evaluated by the anesthesiologist the day before surgery. Patients requiring general anesthesia should receive maintenance fluids at least 12 hours before surgery, with strict attention paid to urinary output and weight. Preoperative assessment of the patient should include checking for signs of vaso-occlusion, fever, respiratory tract infection and dehydration. The laboratory and physical examination results should be reviewed to identify abnormalities in the heart, liver, kidneys, brain and lungs. Through the clinical examination and relevant investigations must be done in all cases as the patients may have associated congenital anomalies like VSD, ASD, PDA, Dextrocardia. It is preferable to ascertain the ASA grading. Normally patients beyond ASA grade II require high degree of care and monitoring and relative operative risk is high. The parents must be taken in confidence and explained about the same. In high risk group, if the underlying anomaly is treatable, it should be treated first and then the definitive cleft repair can be undertaken to minimize the risk of surgery, e.g. repair of ASD/VSD/PDA should be undertaken prior to the cleft repair if it is significant.

After ascertaining the fitness for surgery, the patient preparation is undertaken. The counseling of the parents or the patient himself in cases of adults is done. Patient is kept nil by mouth (NBM) for at least 4 hours before surgery in case of children and at least 6 hours in case of adults.

Intra- and Postoperative Monitoring

Surgical procedures that have an increased probability of ischemia or hypoxia, hypotension and hypothermia deserve special attention.

All patients should be monitored with at least an ECG and have a determination of inspired oxygen concentration by pulse oximetry or blood gas testing. A warm temperature should be maintained in the operating room. General anesthesia should aim for a mild respiratory alkalosis (pH about 7.45) and a normothermic, well-hydrated patient. The patient should receive a minimum of 50 percent oxygen in combination with the anesthetic agent. Blood replacement for significant intraoperative blood loss is recommended. The children are very susceptible for fluid and electrolyte imbalance as the regulatory functions are not well established. Hence, calculation of fluid requirement should be done meticulously. The pediatric influsion pumps are very useful during the administration of IV fluids at appropriate rate and in desired quantity. The selection of appropriate fluid like Ringer's lactate and isolyte-P should be done, unless other fluids are specifically indicated.

Postoperatively, oxygen should be administered until the effects of anesthesia have worn off. In cleft patients, surgical wounds interfere with the respiration and hence requires an extended administrator of oxygen. Continued monitoring is recommended in the intensive care unit. Postoperative parenteral hydration should keep the patient at 1 to 1½ times maintenance. Aggressive respiratory care is necessary in sickle cell disease to minimize pulmonary complications. After the repair of the palate the wide open airway gets narrowed and the child takes time to get accustomed to the new situation. The air way patency should be ensured. Placing a tongue stitch to prevent tongue fall is recommended. Similarly, vigorous suction directly over the repaired palate should be avoided as the fragile mucosa can get avulsed and bleeding can occur. Blunt tipped catheters should be used and direct suction over the suture line should be avoided. The children are also prone to develop the broncospasm as the airway is hyper reactive and minor aspiration can lead to broncospasm, hence this should be prevented. Use of safer anesthetic drugs like sevofluorane, intravenous inducing agents like propofol/ketamine and muscle relaxants like veccuronium/atracurium should be used in place of conventional drugs, in spite of their higher cost to ensure smooth induction, uneventful recovery and preventing complications like malignant hyperthermia.

SURGICAL PROCEDURES FOR CLEFT LIP AND PALATE

- Primary
  - Closure of the lip/anterior palate repair.
  - Closure of the palate.
- Secondary
  - Rhinoplasty and scar revision of the lip.
  - Closure of the palatal fistulae.
  - Pharyngoplasty.
  - Alveolar bone grafting.
  - Orthodontic treatment.
  - Orthognathic procedures.

SURGICAL PROCEDURES FOR CLEFT LIP REPAIR

Various procedures have evolved over the period of time. The first procedure to be based on sound surgical principles was the straight line repair of Rose and Thompson.[33,34] Other commonly used techniques are:

- Straight line repair (when it was noticed that scar on lip contracts and notching is produced, the other techniques came in existence)
- Quadrangular flap technique.[35]
- Triangular flap technique (Tennison[36] and Randall[37] triangular flap repair) (*see* Figs 24.27 and 24.28)
- Rotation flap technique (Millard[38] rotation and advancement repair) (*see* Figs 24.29 and 24.30)
- Delaire technique.[39]

Straight Line Repair

Straight line repair is not a commonly practiced technique for the unilateral cleft lip deformities as the scar contractures invariably results in the notching of the lip. As in case of the bilateral cleft lip deformity in prolabium segment has inadequate tissue and the mobilization or advancement/rotation is not possible, generally it is resorted to straight line repair and the bilateral scars produced thereof are considered as philtral columns (Figs 24.31A and B).

Tennison and Randall Triangular Flap Repair

The repair of cleft lip deformity by tennison and Randall Triangular flap technique is shown in Figures 24.32A and B.

- Preoperative picture with marking
- Intraoperative with both side flap raised
- Final closure.

Advantages

- Lengthens both the lip segments of cleft as well as non-cleft sides
- It results in final symmetric, balanced lip with a well defined Cupid bow
- Only a small amount of tissue is discarded

- It also contributes to correction of nasal deformity
- This technique is comparatively easier for inexperienced surgeons.

Disadvantages

- It results in a final horizontal scar on the lip
- Precise matching of the incisions on both the sides are essential for both muscle and mucosa
- All layers to be sutured on the basis of triangular flap. If any mistake done in marking or incision it cannot be recorrected
- Procedure is difficult for revision during secondary surgical procedures.

Millard Rotation Advancement Repair

The markings and technique of cleft lip closure by Millard rotational advancement repair is shown in Figs 24.33A and B.

Advantages

- This procedure allows adjustments at the time of surgery (cut as you go)
- Minimal amount of tissue is discarded
- Places scar in anatomically correct position, i.e. scar line forms philtral ridge on cleft side
- Nostril sill is reinforced and built up with this procedure
- Revision is easy at time of secondary surgeries.

Disadvantages

- This technique is difficult to master, especially in wide clefts
- Major bulk of lip segments is in center and not on lower free border giving pouting appearance in wide clefts
- Difficulty in obtaining adequate lip length
- It has got a tendency toward vertical scar contracture
- It forms constricted nostril toward the cleft side.

Delaire's Philosophy to Repair Cleft Lip and Palate

This philosophy given by Professor Jean Delaire, who has developed philosophy concerning the significance, relationships and interactions of various structures from which he derived a rationale for treatment of cleft lip and palate deformities (Fig. 24.34). According to him:

- Careful muscular reconstruction and alignment is key to good esthetics

A

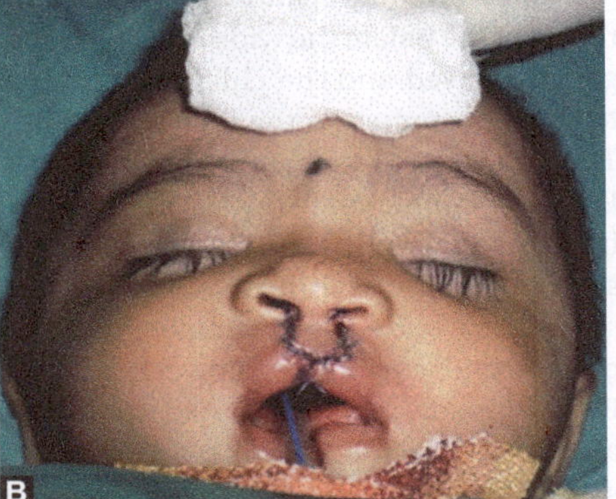

Figs 24.31A and B: (A) Preoperative photograph for straight line repair of bilateral partial cleft lip; (B) Final closure photograph

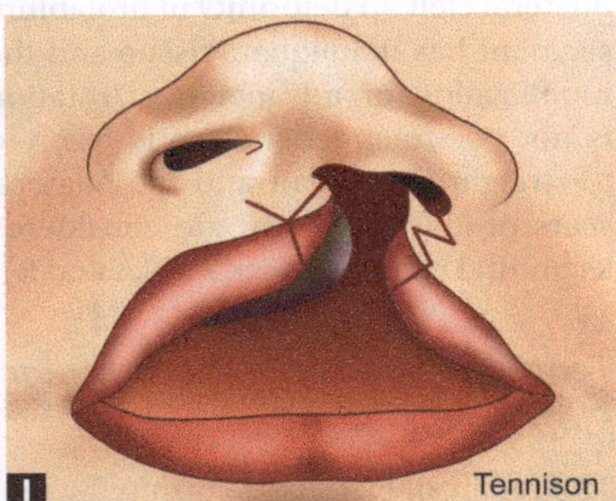

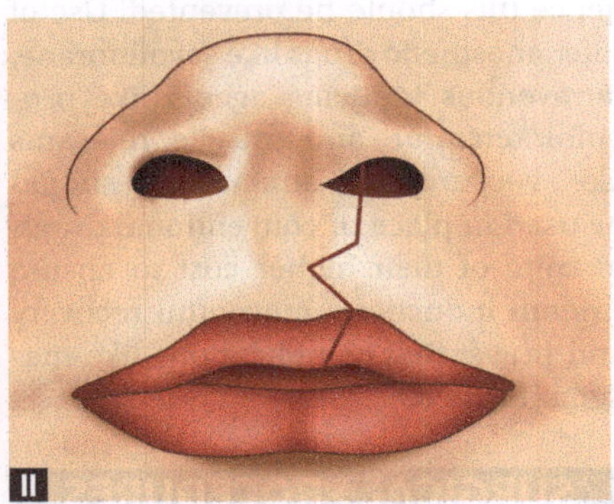

Fig 24.32A: Marking for incisions and final suture line of a triangular flap

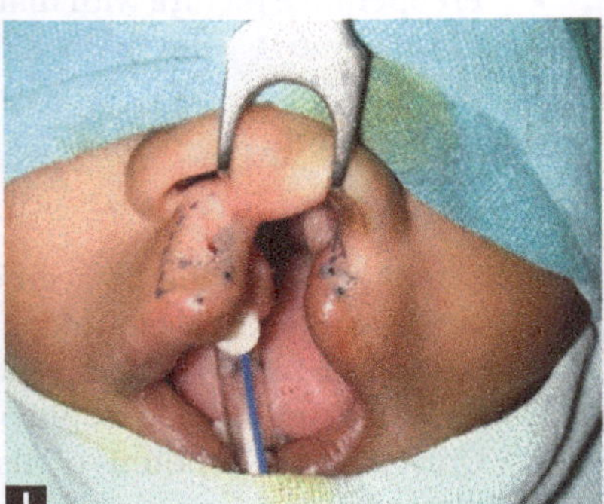

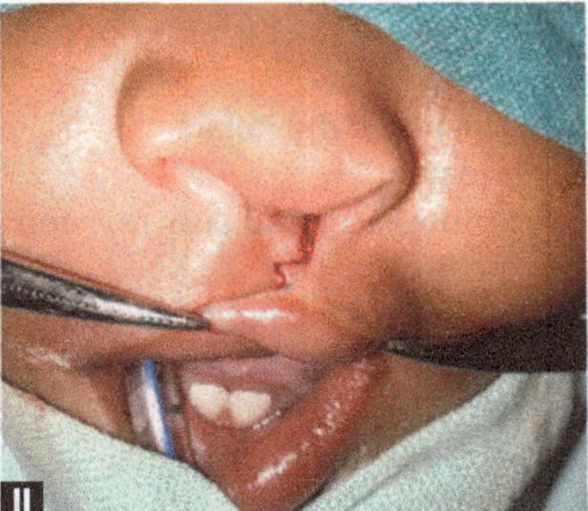

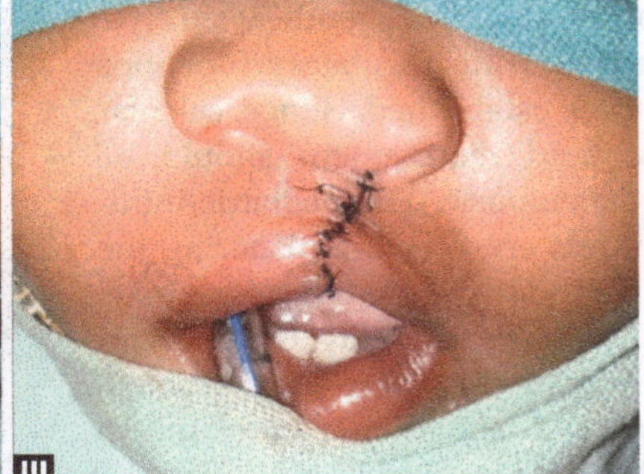

Fig. 24.32B: Triangular flap technique

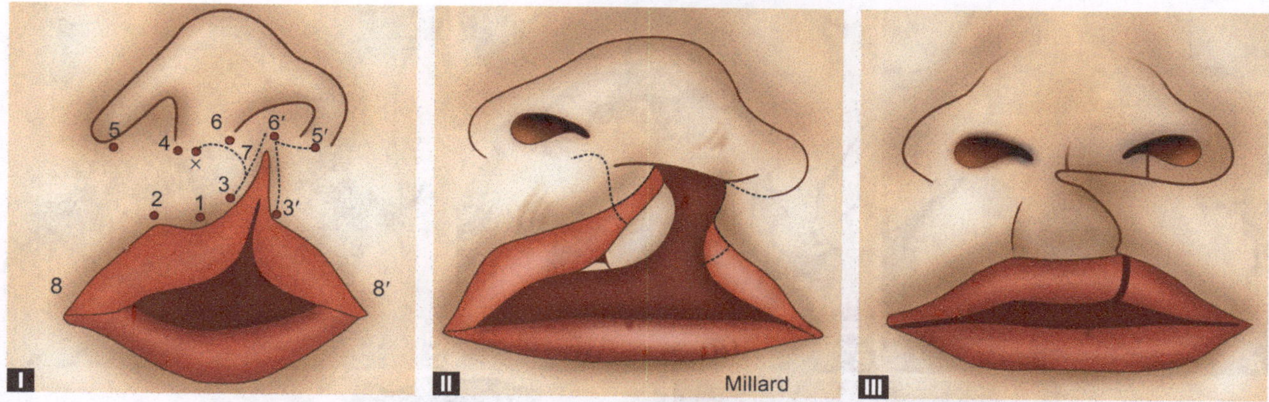

Fig. 24.33A: Marking for incisions and final suture line of a Millard rotational flap technique (1. Deepest point of Cupid's bow; 2. Highest point of Cupid's bow on noncleft side; 3 and 3′ High points of Cupid's bow of cleft; 4 and 6′ Located at base of columella; x-Midpoint of columella; 5 and 5′ Represents the alar base, 8 and 8′ Represents the corner of lip)

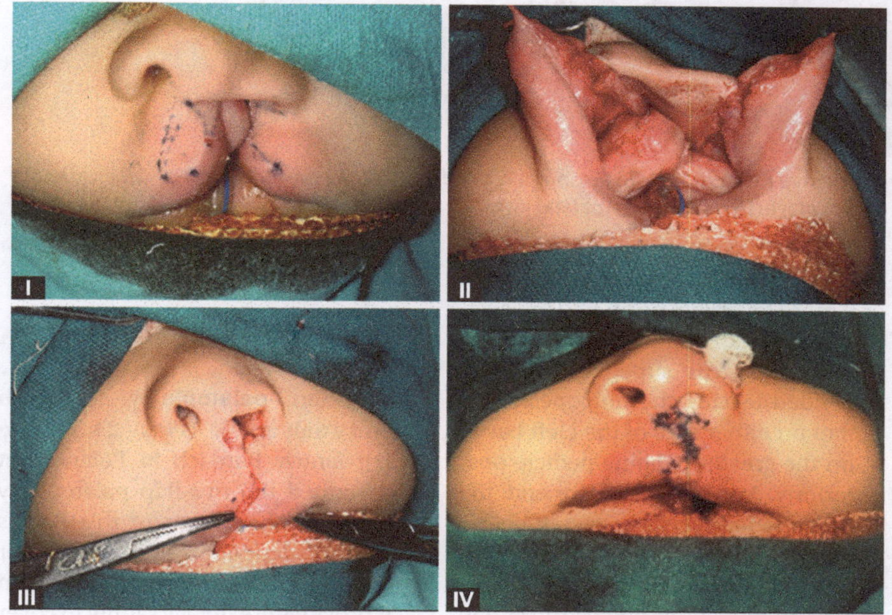

Fig. 24.33B: Millard rotational flap technique

and function of the soft palate, lip and nose.

- The concept of primary functional cheilorhinoplasty is launched.
- Subperiosteal undermining of the cleft-sided cheek is considered a prerequisite for tension free suturing of the nasolabial musculature with the extended subperiosteal undermining of anterior maxilla, the nasal pyramid and the lower orbital border.
- Hard palate closure is performed with bipedicled flaps of only fibromucosa of the palatal shelves, leaving the maxillary fibromucosa untouched. When the cleft is narrow, undermining of the palatal fibromucosa and paring of the edges is sufficient.
- The two stage closure of all wide palatal flaps (soft palate first) and the one stage closure of narrow

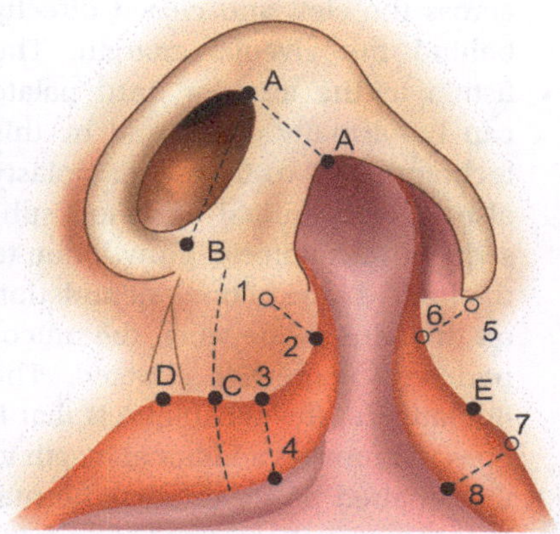

Fig. 24.34: Marking of Delaire technique for cleft lip (A. Upper corner of the noncleft nostril; A′ Upper corner of the cleft nostril; B. Base of columella at the noncleft side; C. Center line of the philtrum and of the future Cupid's bow; D. Peak of Cupid's bow at the noncleft side; E. End of the mucocutaneous rim (white roll) on the lateral lip segment; 1. Landmark on the base of the columella on the cleft side, at a distance from the midline that is equal to the distance from the midline to B (the line B-1 will be parallel to the line A-A′); 2. Landmark at which the continuation of the line; B-1 intersects the mucocutaneous rim; 3. Landmark on the mucocutaneous rim the distance of which from the midline of the philtrum is just a little than that of the distance C-D (in fact, account must be taken of the transverse retraction of the skin); 4. Landmark on border between vermillion and the wet mucosa, the distance of which to the median frenum is equal to the distance C-3; 5. Base of the nasal ala on the cleft side; 6. Intersection of the mucocutaneous rim by a perpendicular to it originating from landmark 5; 7. Landmark of greatest vermillion height on the cleft side, where the mucocutaneous rim begins to diminish (future lateral peak of Cupid's bow); 8. Landmark on the wet line, marked by the perpendicular to the mucocutaneous rim originating in landmark 7)

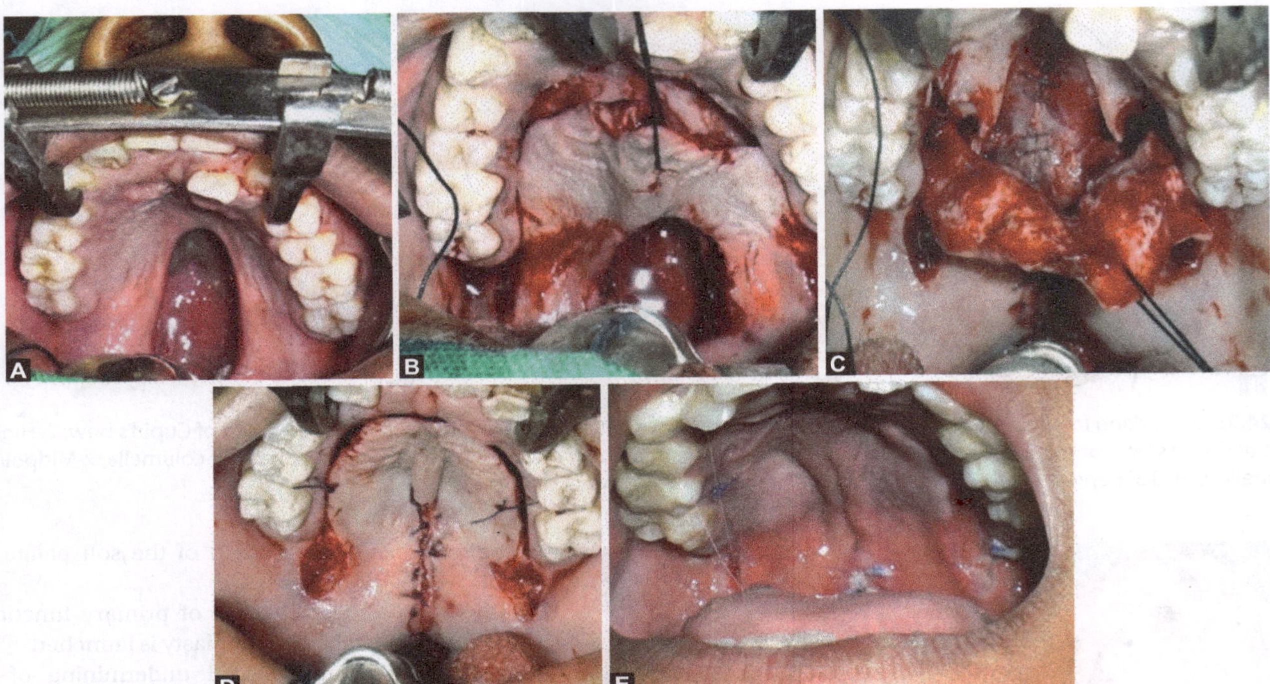

Figs 24.35A to E: Push-back technique: (A) Preoperative photograph; (B) Freshening of edges and palatal incision; (C) Mobilization of flap and closure of nasal layer; (D) Closure of palatal layer; (E) Healed palate

palatal clefts using the fibromucosa of the palate shelves.

Closure of the soft palate at 7 months and the hard palate at 16 to 18 months. Hard palate repair can be postponed till the age of 3 years, if closure necessitates the transposition of maxillary fibromucosa.

Surgical Procedures of Cleft Palate Repair

Hard Palate and Soft Palate

- **Veau-Wardill-Kilner or VY pushback palatoplasty (Figs 24.35A to E):** Veau-Wardill-Kilner or V-Y pushback palatoplasty is derived from a modification of the von Langenbeck technique. It can be used to increase the palatal length. The Veau-Wardill-Kilner pushback palatoplasty can be suitably used for incomplete clefts of the hard palate. The flap design is similar to the von Langenbeck palatoplasty. The essence of this technique is the V to Y incision and closure on the hard palate. The pushback technique has the advantage of lengthening the palate and repositioning the levator muscle in a more favorable position. However, this modification involves extensive dissection. The superior pedicle is divided leaving the mucoperiosteal flap on either side of the cleft based on the greater palatine pedicle posteriorly. At the free anterior end, the mucoperiosteal flaps can then be approximated directly or in a V-Y closure to lengthen the soft palate. This modification allows more flap advancement than the von Langenbeck technique and enables posterior lengthening of the palate, thus improving velopharyngeal competence. The Wardill-Kilner pushback palatoplasty offers significant longterm improvement in speech in terms of nasality and nasalance score. The pushback palatoplasty has several disadvantages. The denuded palatal bone from which the mucoperiosteal flaps are raised adversely affects midfacial growth in cleft palate patients. This technique also has a higher rate of fistula in complete cleft palate than other techniques because it provides only a single nasal mucosa layer anteriorly.
- **von Langenbeck[40] (Figs 24.36A and B)**
- **Two-flap palatoplasty (Bardach and Salyers[41]) (Figs 24.37A to D):** Janusz Bardach in Poland first described the two-flap palatoplasty in 1967. The design of this flap is entirely dependent on the greater palatine neurovascular pedicle and it provides greater versatility to cover the cleft. In a complete unilateral cleft, the mucoperiosteal flap from the medial segment can be shifted across the cleft and closed directly behind the alveolar margin. The fistula in the anterior hard palate can be virtually eliminated by this technique. Two-flap palatoplasty also has a minimal effect on subsequent maxillofacial growth due to the limited area of bone denudation on the hard palate when the mucoperiosteal flaps are elevated. The limitation of this technique is that it does not provide additional length to the repaired palate to allow normal speech production. A variation from

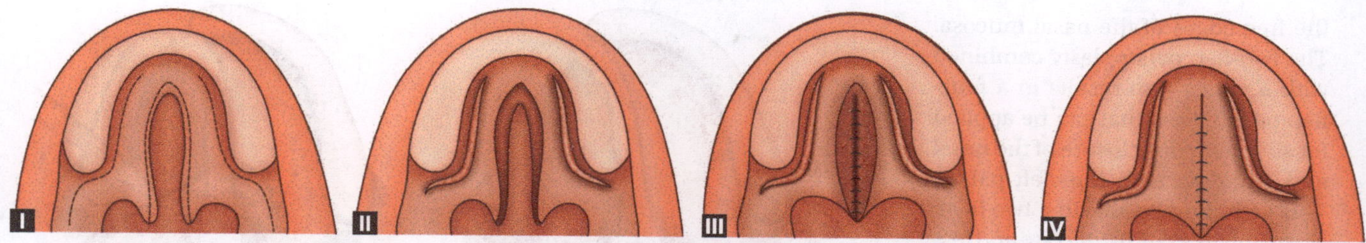

Figs 24.36(A) I to IV: Technique of von Langenbeck procedure: (I) Marking of incision; (II) Flap raised; (III) Nasal layer closure; (IV) Oral layer closure

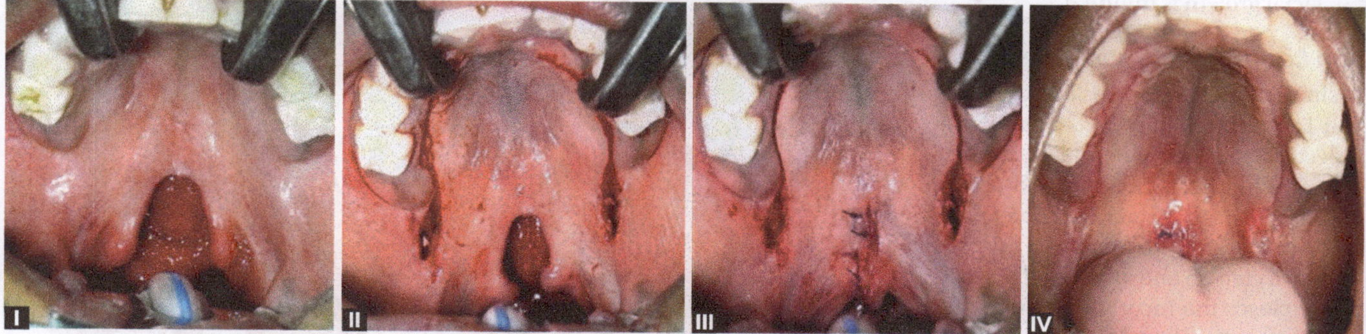

Figs 24.36(B) I and IV: von Langenbeck procedure: (I) Cleft soft palate; (II) Incision; (III) Closure; (IV) Postoperative view

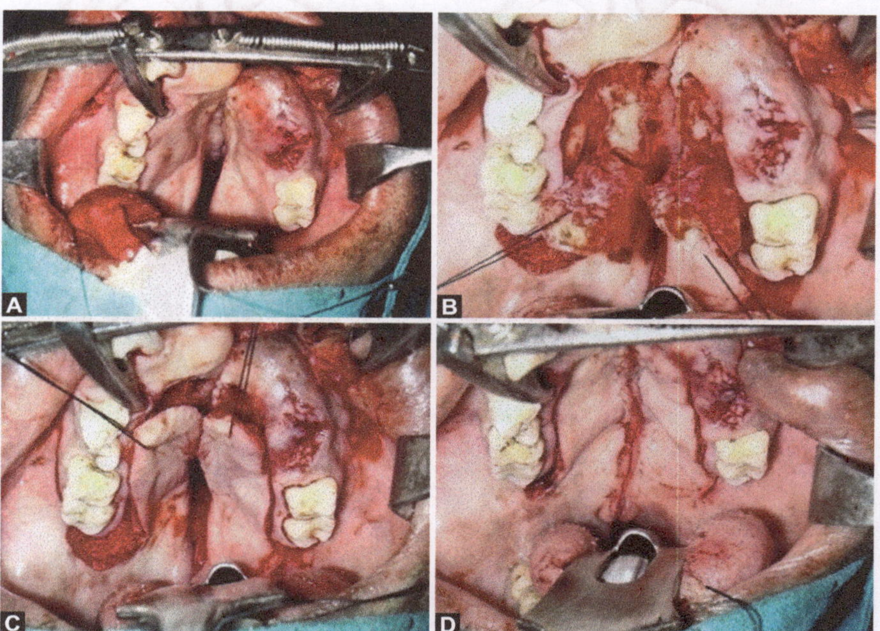

Figs 24.37A to D: Two-flap palatoplasty technique: (A) Preoperative; (B and C) Mobilization of flap; (D) Closure of nasal and oral layers

the standard technique of two flap palatoplasty has been reported using supraperiosteal flaps instead of the mucoperiosteal technique for palatal closure. Although this new approach improves speech outcome, it still requires further evaluation in a larger series to ascertain its applications. Nevertheless, the goal of palatal lengthening in palatoplasty is still considered essential to reduce the space in the posterior pharyngeal wall. Presently, widely accepted methods to reduce velopharyngeal insufficiency include retropositioning and reorientation of the velar muscles by performing either an intravelar velopasty or Furlow double opposing Z palatoplasty.

- **Vomer flaps:** In 1926, Pichler introduced the use of a vomer mucoperiosteal flap for palatal closure. The original vomer flap was inferiorly based. It was raised by an incision made high on the nasal septum and reflected downward to provide a single-layer closure on the oral side. This flap has a high incidence of maxillary retrusion, presumably from injury from vomer-premaxillary sutures, and a high fistula rate. However, similar problems have not been commonly found in a superiorly based vomer flap. This technique involves reflecting the mucosa from the septum close to the cleft margin with limited dissection to allow adequate closure of the nasal mucosa on the opposite site. In a bilateral complete cleft palate, a midline incision along the free margin of vomer is required to create two septal-mucosal flaps in opposite directions. These two flaps are used to bridge the gap between the free edges of the nasal mucosa. The two-flap palatoplasty combined with a vomer flap results in a four-flap palatoplasty that can be applied for simultaneous closure of the nasal and oral defects in the cleft palate. This technique results in a two layer closure with a low fistula rate and less maxillary growth retardation. The long-term effect of this technique on facial growth is minimal.

von Langenbeck Procedure

A simple palatal closure introduced by von Langenbeck in 1859 is possibly the oldest palatoplasty still widely used today. The von Langenbeck palatoplasty is commonly used for an incomplete cleft of the secondary palate without the presence of a cleft lip and alveolus. This technique closes the incomplete cleft of the hard and soft palates without lengthening the palate by mobilizing bipedicled mucoperiosteal flaps medially. The cleft margins can be approximated with a lateral relaxing incision that begins posterior to the maxillary tuberosity and follows the posterior portion of the alveolar ridge. Modifications of the von Langenbeck technique include repair of the levator palatini muscle and intravelar veloplasty to reproduce the normal muscle sling. von Langenbeck repair can also be used in combination with a Furlow double opposing Z-palatoplasty to increase palatal length with minimal mucoperiosteal undermining. Advantage with this technique is it does not leave any scarring in the anterior palate region, which Bardach's method leaves, but disadvantage with these techniques is they leave denuded areas of palatal bone at the lateral releasing incisions, midline longitudinal scar with risk of contracture, tendency towards anterior fistula formation and little palatal lenghthening.

Two Flap Palatoplasty

Two flap palatoplasty technique is shown in Figures 24.37A to D.

Soft Palate Repair

- Double opposing Z-plasty (Furlow[42]) (Figs 24.38 and 24.39)

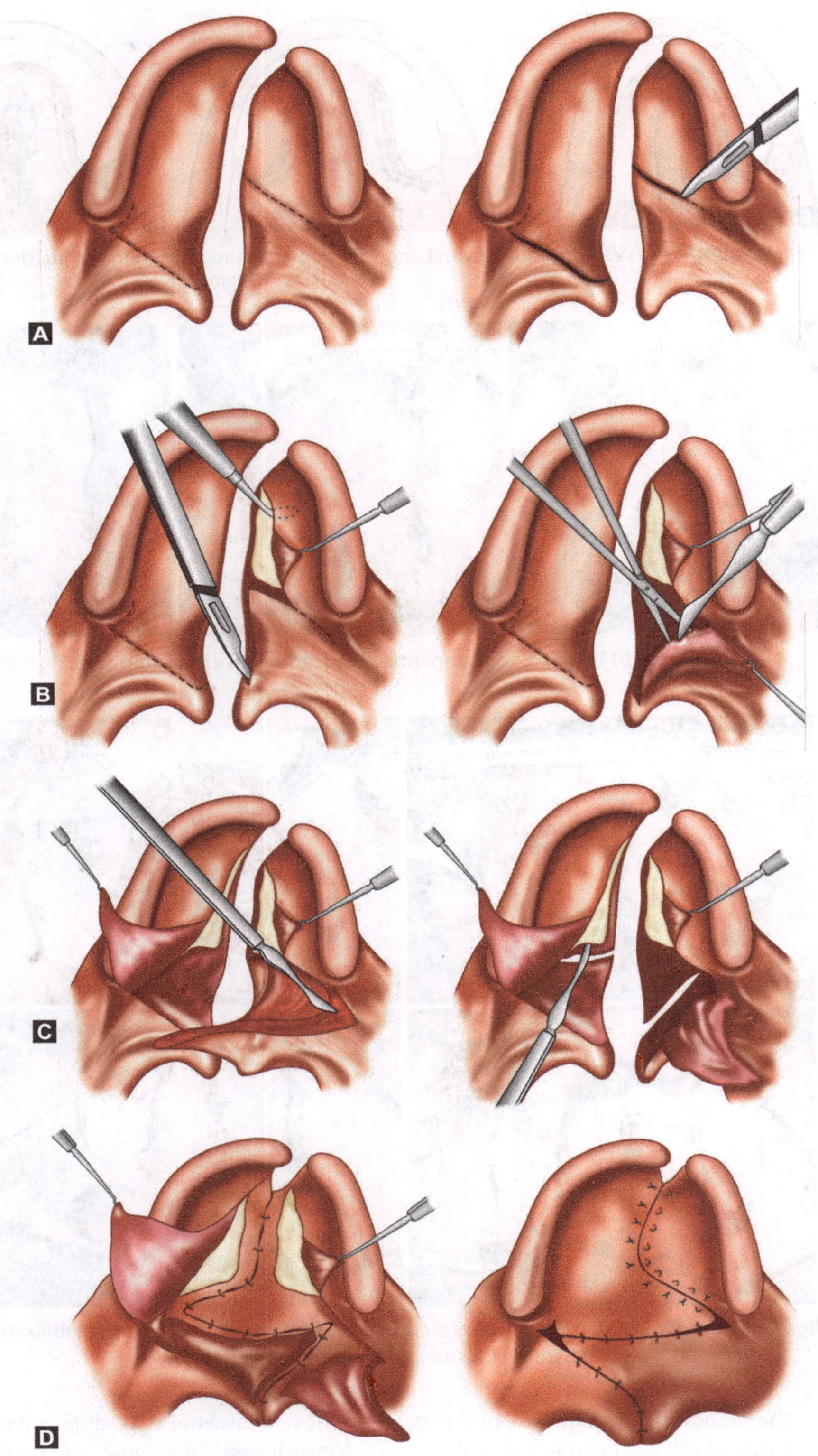

Figs 24.38A to D: Furlow's technique: (A) Marking and incision; (B) Flap raised on one side; (C) Both sides flap raised; (D) Nasal layer closure and then final closure; (*Source:* Salyer and Bardach's Atlas of Craniofacial and Cleft Surgery: Craniofacial Surgery, Vol. 1 by Kenneth E Salyer, Janusz Bardach)

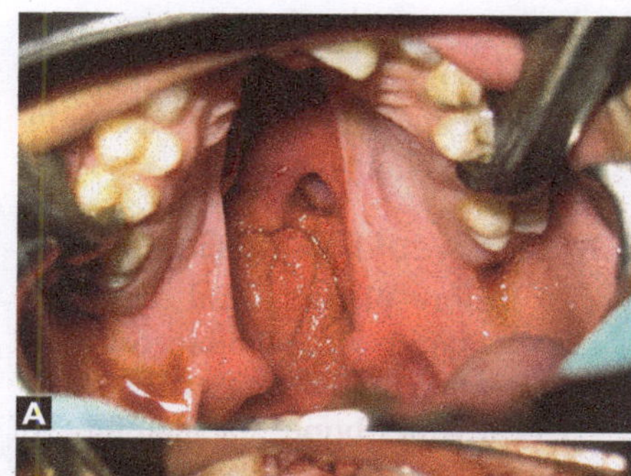

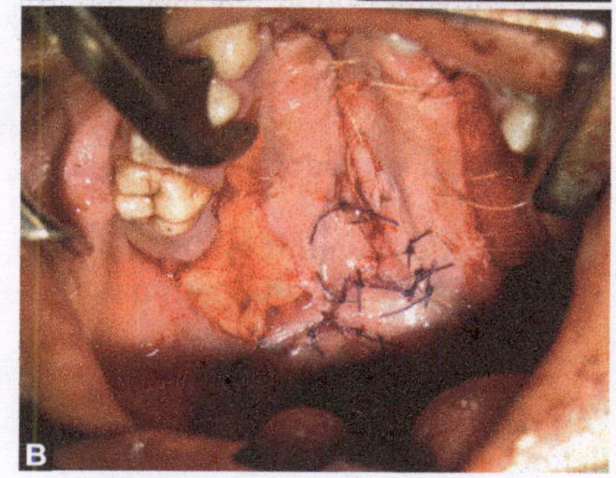

Figs 24.39A and B: (A) Unilateral cleft palate; (B) Repair by Furlow's technique

- Intravelar veloplasty (Sommerland[43])
- Microscopic repair of cleft palate (Sommerland[44])

Furlow Double Opposing Z-palatoplasty

Furlow technique is shown in Figures 24.38A to D. In 1978, Leonard T. Furlow Jr. unofficially introduced the double opposing Z-palatoplasty and much of his work was later published in 1986. This technique involves alternating the reversing Z-plasties of the nasal and oral flaps and repositioning the levator veli palatini muscle within the posteriorly mobilized flaps. With this technique, there is no need to raise large mucoperiosteal flaps from the hard palate. At the same time, the soft palate can be lengthened within the substance of the soft palate together with palatal muscle reorientation. This technique has shown early success in both speech outcomes and midfacial skeletal growth. Furlow Z-palatoplasty is effective for primary closure of a submucous cleft palate and secondary correction of marginal velopharyngeal insufficiency. Palatal closure in Furlow Z-palatoplasty is not anatomic and completely ignores the small longitudinal uvula muscle, but overall speech results are comparable to or better than those with other techniques. Problems may be encountered when this technique is used to close a very wide cleft palate, in which the distance traversed by the Z-plasty may be excessive. Modification of this technique to overcome excessive tension during closure involves extension of the relaxing incisions anteriorly to the cleft margin to create an island flap based on the palatine vessels. This maneuver provides greater mobility and shifts the closure to the side of the posteriorly based flap. Other ancillary procedures for tension free closure in a wide cleft palate include a combination of Furlow Z-palatoplasty with any of the following maneuvers: hard palate mucoperiosteal undermining, careful dissection into the space of Ernst, infracture of the hamulus or stretching of the greater palatine neurovascular bundles.

SECONDARY PROCEDURES

Speech Therapy

Adequate speech usually requires speech therapy and the speech pathologist sees the child frequently until age seven.

Factors Addressed by the Speech-Language Pathologist

- Feeding
- Hearing
- Cognitive ability
- Development
- Language
- Articulation
- Velopharyngeal function.

Factors Affecting Speech Impairment in Patients with Cleft Lip and Palate

- Articulation errors
- Velopharyngeal insufficiency (VPI) leading to:
  - Resonance
  - Nasal air emission
  - Low oral pressure
- Hearing loss
- Malocclusion
- Nasal obstruction.

Despite the extensive training provided, up to 20 percent of patients still require pharyngoplasty to reduce VPI.

Orthodontic Treatment

Presurgical orthodontics is done in cases, which has alveolar asymmetry especially in very wide cleft. Orthodontic treatment begins at the age of eruption of the permanent teeth. The final stage of orthodontic treatment includes the use of fixed appliances, which consist of bonded brackets and full banded molars.

Goals of Orthodontic Treatment Stage

- To obtain an adequate arch form and alignment
- To achieve the best occlusion and function
- To maintain or to improve the sagittal and transverse relationship between arches
- To avoid or to correct cross-bites
- To prepare for orthognathic surgery if needed or receive a prosthetic restoration.

Prosthetic Considerations

- Absence of lateral incisor in the cleft area is common, prosthetic restoration of the tooth in the treatment plan should be included.
- Transpalatal retainer with an acrylic tooth can be used to aid in maintaining the surgical result and provide a better dental appearance.
- If desired, fixed prosthetic appliance can be used 6 months after surgery (Figs 24.40A and B).
- A four-unit fixed bridge can be used, but an implant-borne prosthesis in a bone grafted alveolus gives the best result. Bone grafting of the alveolar cleft in cases in which the lateral incisor is missing should be performed with the aim of providing enough bone for a dental implant.

Alveolar Bone Grafting

Alveolar bone grafting is to reconstruct cleft alveolus with bone grafts. This

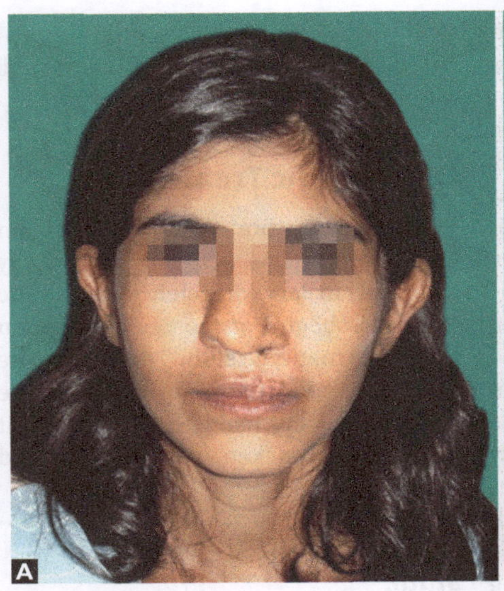

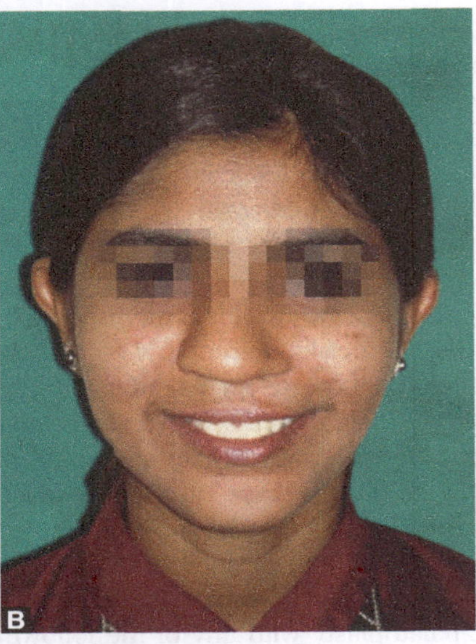

Figs 24.40A and B: Fixed prosthetic appliance for the missing lateral incisor: (A) Pre-treatment: (B) Post-treatment

method popularized by Abyholm[45] in 1981. In literature bone grafting was done in 1901 by Von Eiselberg[46] who used pedicled bone to fill the alveolus, in 1908 Lexer[47] tried using free bone grafts. By 1950's bone grafting was well accepted was performed routinely before patient's first birthday. Rib grafts were used to fill the defects. But by 1960's there was evidence that primary bone grafting is hampering facial growth due to dissection around vomeromaxillary suture, which is primarly midfacial growth center. Then it was cosidered that secondary bone-grafting during mixed dentition period is preferable and prefered sites for bone-grafting are iliac crest and tibia as rib grafts were too dense hence eruption of tooth was delayed. In wide clefts corticocancellous bone grafts are preferred. Overcorrection with cancellous bone graft is done since 25 percent of bone graft gets resorbed after surgery. Calvarial grafts has been recommended by some as an alternative to iliac crest grafting. However success rate of calvarial graft is not better than iliac crest graft, as bone grafts consisting of diploic bone have shown to be more successful, than those grafts harvested using a high speed rotary device to shave off primarily cortical bone from the surface of the calvaria.

Problems Faced by Patients Having Cleft Alveolus

Problems faced by patients having cleft alveolus are as follows:

- Patient may complain of food/fluid regurgitation from nose
- An inability to blow balloon or suck a straw
- A persistent smell and discharge from their nose
- Poor speech
- Missing or extra teeth in cleft area
- Lack of support for alar base, columella and lip.

Aims of Alveolar Bone Grafting

- To restore physiological continuity of dental arch to enable oral and dental health to be maintained
- To provide bone for stability of dental arch, to allow eruption of unerupted teeth or placement of implant
- To allow orthodontic alignment of teeth
- To provide support for lip and nose and to close persistent oronasal fistula.

Procedure (Figs 24.41A to F)

Before bone grafting, radiographs should be taken to evaluate the status of the canine and lateral incisor, if present. This is well visualized using a panoramic tomogram, periapical radiographs of the cleft side and a occlusal view of anterior maxilla. Bone grafting is mostly performed at approximately one-half to two-thirds root development of the tooth about to erupt into the cleft side.

Mostly iliac crest grfats are used as adequate cancellous bone can be

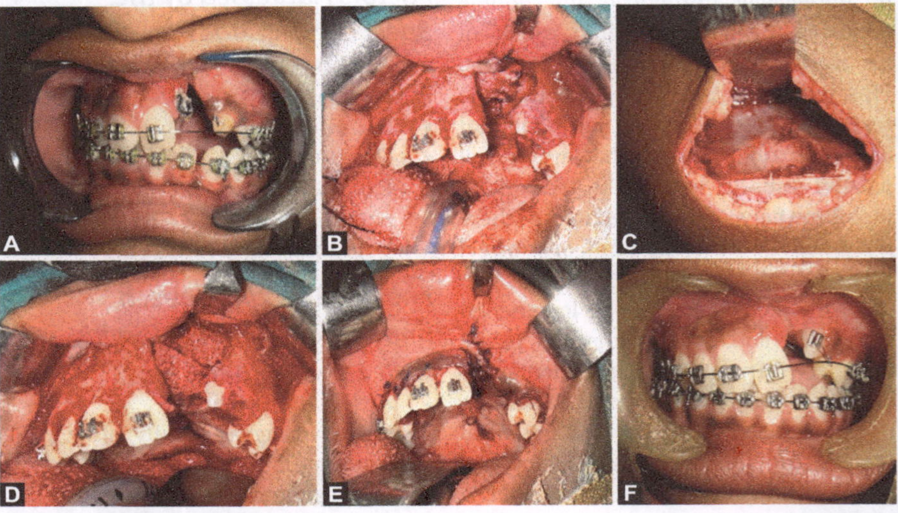

Figs 24.41A to F: Alveolar bone grafting: (A) Preoperative photograph; (B) Nasal layer closed and recipient site for graft prepared; (C) Exposure illiac crest; (D) Bone graft placement into the alveolar defect; (E) Closure of surgical site after graft placement; (F) Eruption of canine through the grafted bone

harvested from this site. In children under the age of 9 to 10, cancellous bone is not as much in quantity as in adults since apophysis of iliac crest is still largely cartilagenous. The first step requires development of full thickness mucoperiosteal buccal flaps. After the soft tissue flaps are developed by giving incisions on alveolus and palatal and nasal linings are mobilized. The nasal lining is sutured to provide base for the graft. Then bone graft is harvested from iliac crest site by giving either a medial or an incision just lateral to the anterior iliac crest spine, as it cannot be given on bony prominence of iliac crest spine, keeping in mind that lateral cutaneous nerve is present 1 cm lateral to the iliac crest spine. If any damage to the nerve, it can lead to complications in future. The graft is harvested from the iliac crest donor site by trap door technique in which both cortical plates are kept intact. If any perforation of inner cortical plate occurs it leads to hematoma formation. The cancellous bone is harvested using bone gouge. After achieving the hemostasis, the donor site is sutured in layers. During donor site closure scarpa's fascia (deep thick fascia at iliac crest) should be closed carefully as it provides airtight closure, better protection and aids in preventing pain and limping. The cancellous bone graft is packed in the cleft alveolus defect and the palatal layer is also closed.

Complications

Complications, which can occur after surgery at the cleft site are:

- There can be persistent bleeding and pain.
- Low-grade infections, which can leads to wound breakage or bone loss.
- Any injury to adjacent teeth.

The donor site complications after surgery are:

- There can be persistent pain at the site.
- Any neurological complications can occur such as loss of cutaneous sensations due to injury to lateral cutaneous nerve. It also can leads to neuroma formation at the site of nerve injury and painful scar.
- Limping, while walking due to injury to lateral cutaneous nerve of thigh and improper closure of scarpa's fascia can occur.
- Hematoma formation if inner cortical table perforates during harvesting. Patient may present later with complaints like inability to stand and walk, pain at donor site and on examination patient may have persistent tachycardia with features of anemia.
- There can be unsightly scar and contour abnormalities.

All these complications can be reduced by practicing meticulous surgical technique.

Pharyngoplasty

The success of palatoplasty is measured primarily by quality of speech. Nasality of voice requires further surgical intervention to improve the function of velopharyngeal sphincter, which is formed by muscles of soft palate and by superior constrictor muscle of pharynx. The inability of velopharyngeal sphincter to separate the oropharynx from nasopharynx results in hypernasality and nasal air emission. Speech assessment by speech pathologist, nasal endoscopy and air flow studies are used to determine the necessity of performing pharyngoplasty. The main aim of pharyngoplasty is speech improvement.

The most commonly practiced technique for pharyngoplasty is Hogan's[48] (1973). The soft palate is split in the midline. A suture is inserted for better visualization of posterior pharyngeal wall. The incision is carried on posterior wall of pharynx to create a superiorly based flap. The flap is raised over nasal surface of soft palate and it is dissected and turned upwards. Pharyngeal flap is sutured to the edges of soft palate on nasal side. Mucosal flap is raised on nasal surface of soft palate is used to close raw surface at its base. Superiorly based pharyngeal flap is closed at nasal surface of soft palate, mucosal flap raised on nasal side of soft palate is used to close the defect at its base. Defect on posterior pharyngeal wall is closed by simple approximation of tissues. The oral layer of soft palate is closed, resulting in large portion of coverage of soft palate. This will prevent shrinkage of pharyngeal flap and change in size of lateral ports (Figs 24.42 and 24.43).

Distraction Osteogenesis

Distraction osteogenesis (DO) (Figs 24.44A to D) was propagated by llizarov for orthopedic surgeries and popularized for correction of the craniofacial skeleton in the early 1990s. McCarthy et al. reported using distraction to lengthen the mandible in patients with hemifacial microsomia.[49] Figueroa and Polley[50] reported success with no significant complications when DO was used to advance the maxilla in children with cleft lip and palate. Recently, DO was used to advance the maxilla in patients with cleft palate. A well-known modality is surgically assisted maxillary expansion in adults that transversely distracts the hard palate through the midpalatal suture. This technique reduces the complications of rapid maxillary expansion, which relies on tooth abutments alone without surgical assistance and can result in gingival recession, ankylosis, and root resorption. The scarred tissue in repaired palate limits the advancement of the osteotomized maxilla and tends to pull them pack after the advancement leading to relapse. With the use of distraction osteogenesis in such, this problem is avoided. The distractors can be either extraoral or intraoral distractor (Figs 24.45 and 24.46).

Orthognathic Surgery

The correction of maxillary hypoplasia is achieved by the orthognathic surgery. Indications for the orthognathic surgery in the cleft patients are:

- Concave profile after repair of a cleft lip and palate.
- Disproportion between middle and lower thirds of the face.
- Underdevelopment of the maxilla and relatively greater growth of the mandible.
- It has been estimated that 25 to 60 percent of all patients born with

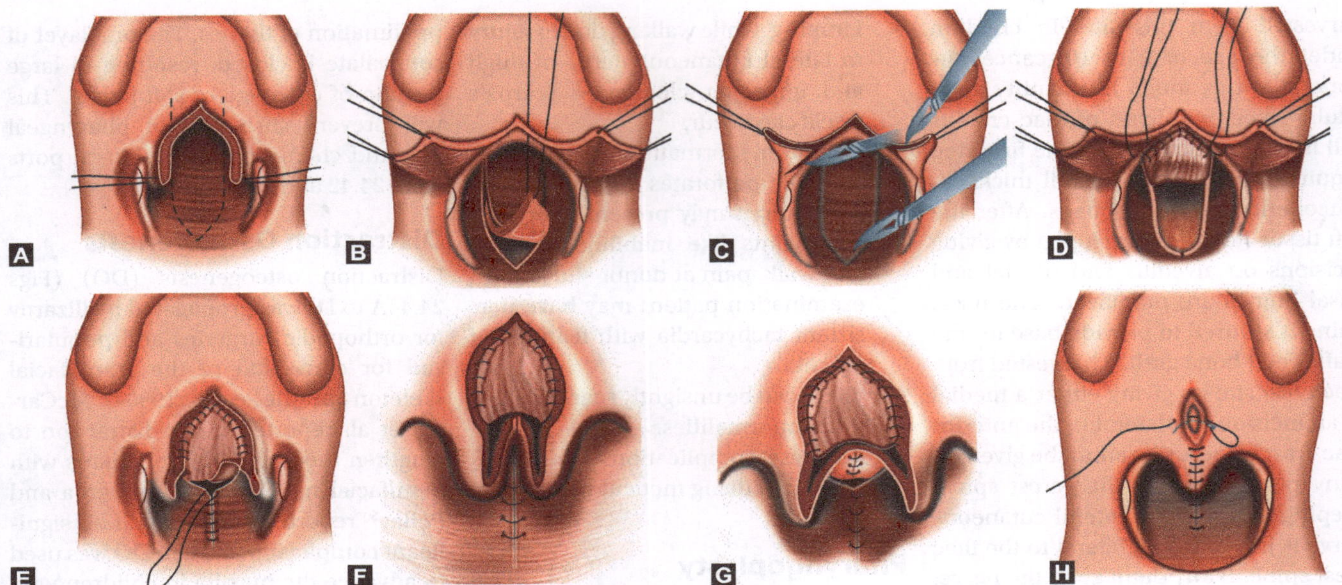

Figs 24.42A to H: Pharyngoplasty technique: (A) Incision on posterior wall of pharynx; (B and C) Soft palate flaps raised; (D) Pharyngeal flap sutured at nasal layer of soft palate; (E) Pharyngeal defect is closed; (F to H) Closure of soft palate (*Source:* Salyer and Bardach's Atlas of Craniofacial and Cleft Surgery: Craniofacial Surgery, Vol. 1 by Kenneth E Salyer, Janusz Bardach)

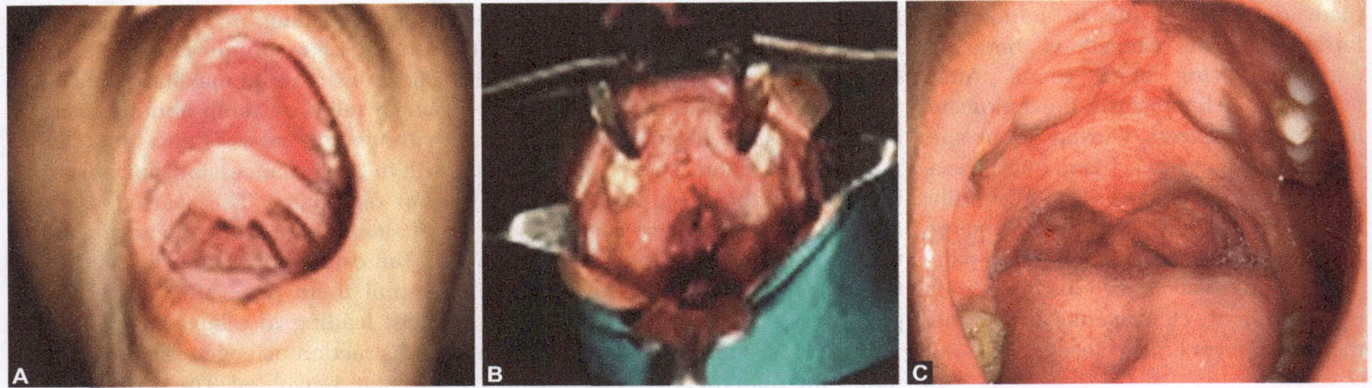

Figs 24.43A to C: Pharyngoplasty technique: (A) Preoperative; (B) Intraoperative; (C) Postoperative views

complete unilateral cleft lip and palate require maxillary advancement to correct the maxillary hypoplasia and improve esthetic facial proportions.

Timing of Surgery

It is prudent to delay surgery until complete maturation is achieved. Delaying surgery until the canine and second molars have erupted minimizes the risk of injury to the teeth during osteotomy.

Procedures

Maxillary osteotomy at Le-Fort I level is usually adequate and the Le-Fort II osteotomy is seldom needed, However, in cases of significant deformity, high Le-Fort I osteotomy could be required to correct concave facial deformity.

- Genial osteotomies

Osteotomies for cleft patients (Figs 24.47 and 24.48)

Because the skeleton is always asymmetrical in cleft patients, osteotomy design is important for maximum improvement of esthetics. The osteotomy cuts may require modifications and may not be symmetrical and are based on the need of individual case. It is advisable to do alveolar bone grafting before planning for orthognathic surgery. If for some reason, alveolar bone grafting was not done, then it can be done in the same surgery when orthognathic surgery is planned, but this should be avoided.

Use of Bone Grafts in Midface Advancement

- The bone graft can be wedged into the defects in the lateral maxillary walls after the maxillary advancement, which helps maintain the position of the maxilla during healing.

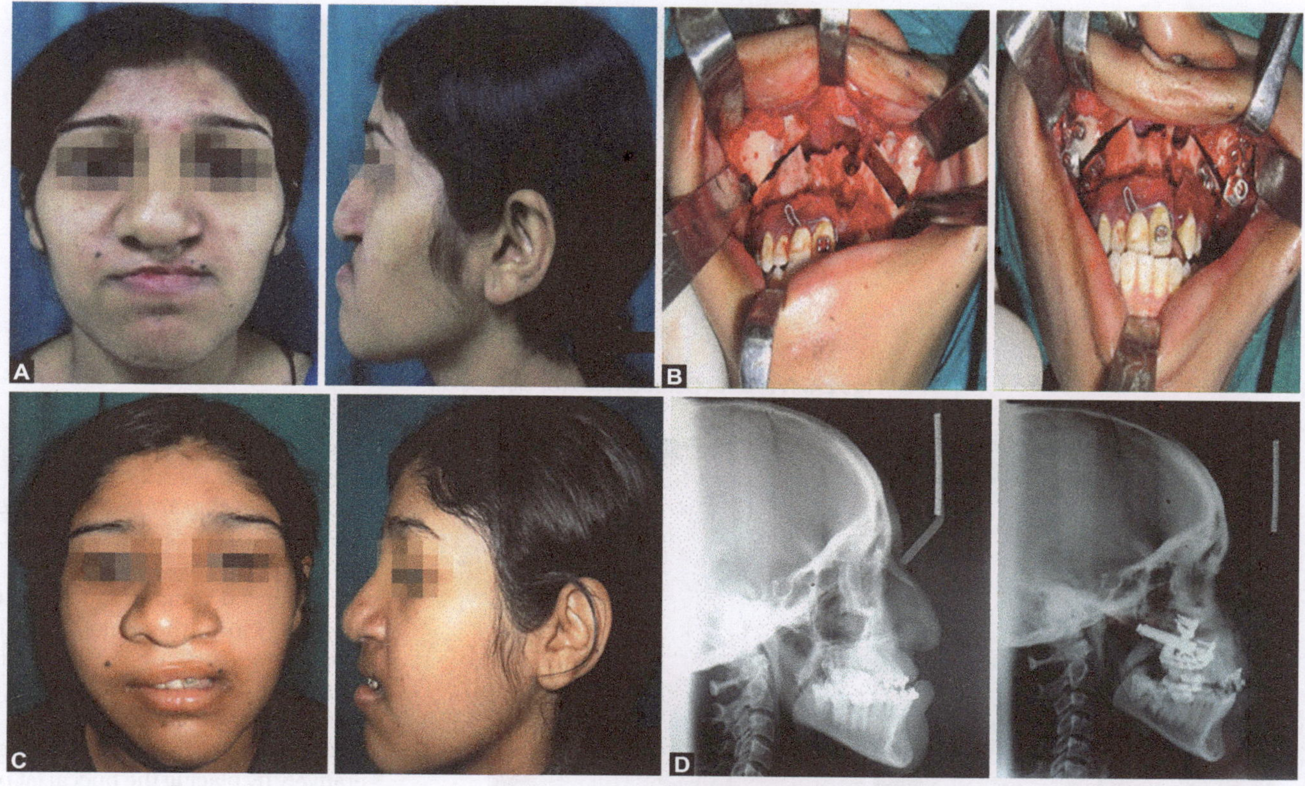

Figs 24.44A to D: (A) Preoperative frontal and profile views; (B) Osteotomy cut; (C) Postoperative frontal and profile views; (D) Prelateral and postlateral ceph X-rays

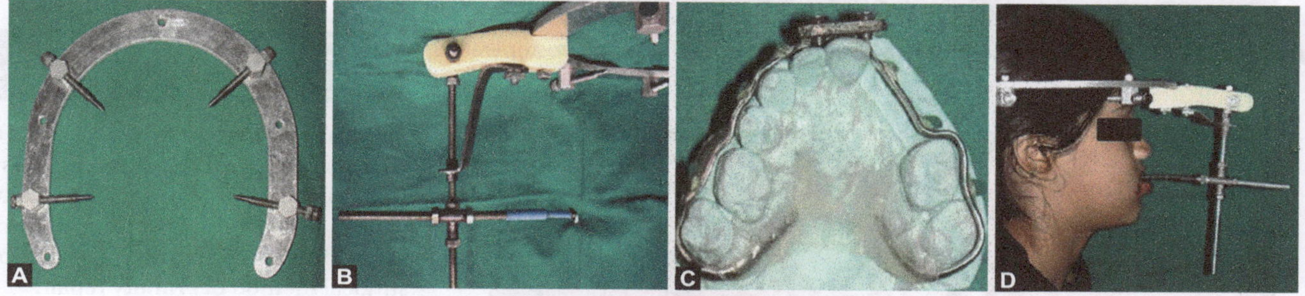

Figs 24.45A to D: Extraoral distractor components

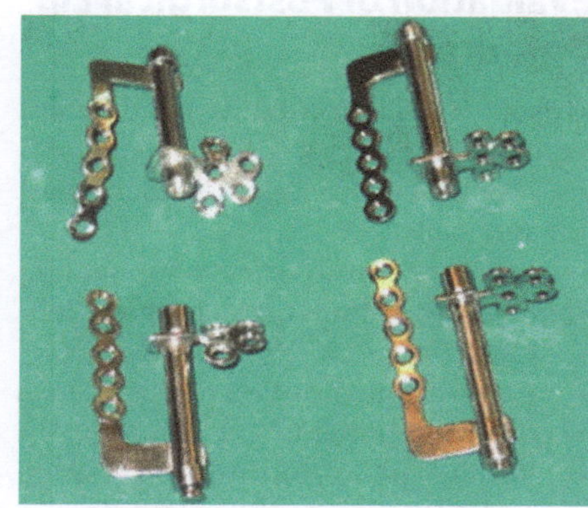

Fig. 24.46: Intraoral distractors

- The bone graft also encourages bone healing and reduces the risks of the fibrous union.
- The third use of bone grafts in midface advancement is to contour the middle face.

PALATAL FISTULA

The operated cases of palate should be examined after 1 year of surgery for presence of any palatal fistula due to break down of the palatal repair and the treatment if needed should be given. Palatal fistula if present should be repaired as per the demand and requirement of the patient. The patient should not be encouraged to undergo surgery for fistula unless the patient is having problem like nasal regurgitation, speech problems, etc.

Techniques of Fistula Repair

- Local tissue flaps (Figs 24.49A to D)
- Tongue flaps (Figs 24.50A and B)
- Extraoral flaps.

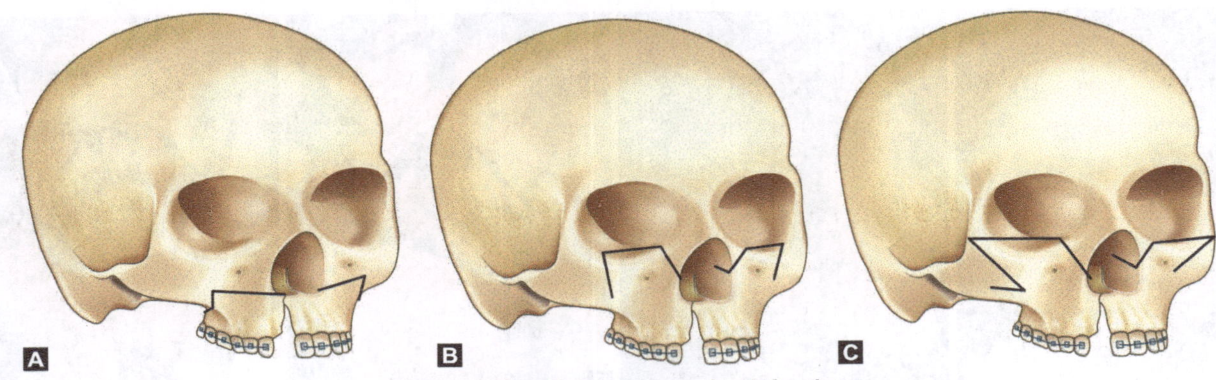

Figs 24.47A to C: Osteotomies for cleft palate

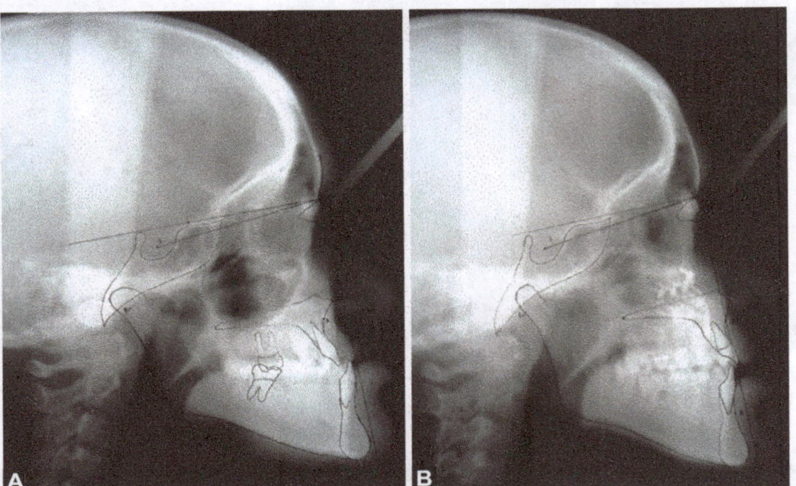

Figs 24.48A and B: Lateral cephalometric X-ray: (A) Preoperative; (B) 6 months postoperative

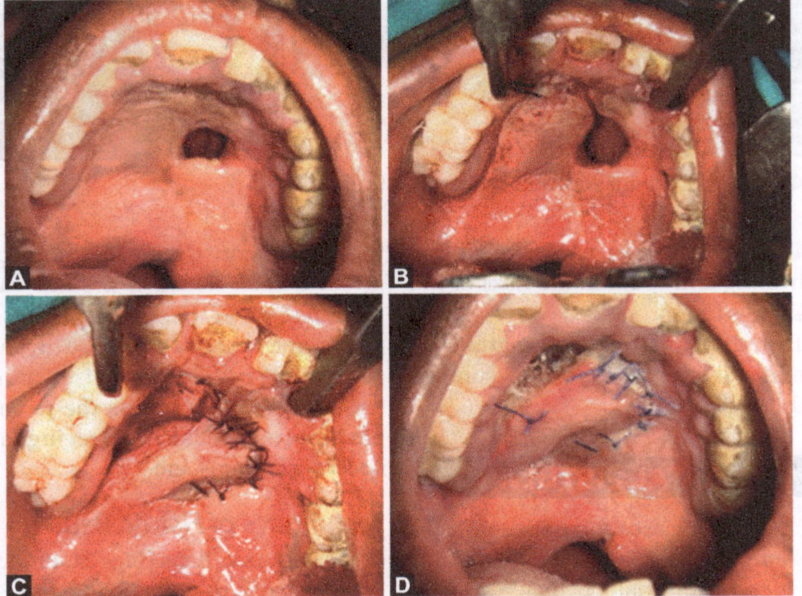

Figs 24.49A to D: (A) Preoperative photograph of fistula; (B) Palatal flap raised; (C) Palatal flap rotated and sutured to close the fistula; (D) Postoperative photograph

- Interpositional grafts.
- Buccal fat pad (Figs 24.51A to C)
- Local tissue flap from the adjacent site of the palate can be used to close the fistula.
- The pedicled tongue flap is widely used to close the palatal fistula. After the closure of the fistula the division of the tongue flap is done on postoperative 21st day.
- Buccal fat pad can also used intraoperatively by placing the buccal fat pad in between the deficient nasal layer and the oral layer in cases of wide cleft to avoid fistula formation in future.

SCAR REVISION OF THE CLEFT LIP

Surgical intervention to revise scar in CL must be based on complete analysis of the problem. Evaluating lip deformities should take into account ethnic variations, original deformity and previous surgical method of primary repair.

Evaluation of Postsurgical Lip Deformities

Wilson[51] (1985) looked at six different aspects of the lip:

- Amount of lip tissue present post surgically.
- Freedom of movement of upper lip.
- Equality of bulk over complete length of lip.
- Cupid's bow position and presence of all components.
- Width of philtrum, direction of scars, and relocation of philtral ridges.
- Alignment of circumoral muscles.

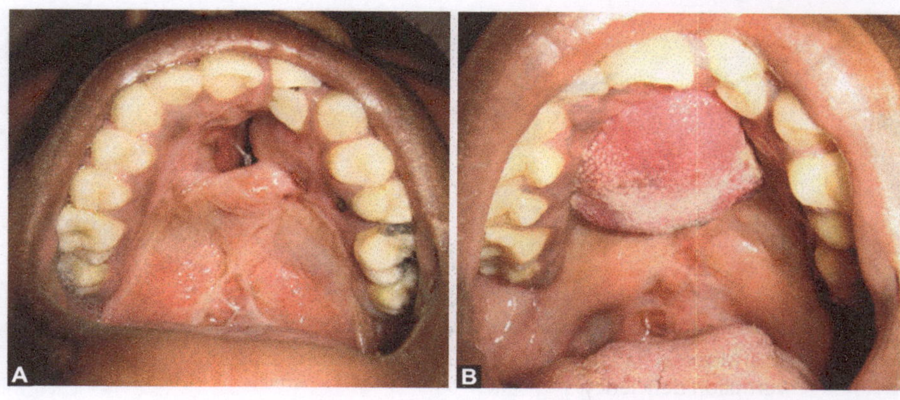

Figs 24.50A and B: (A) Anterior palatal fistula; (B) Tongue flap to close the fistula

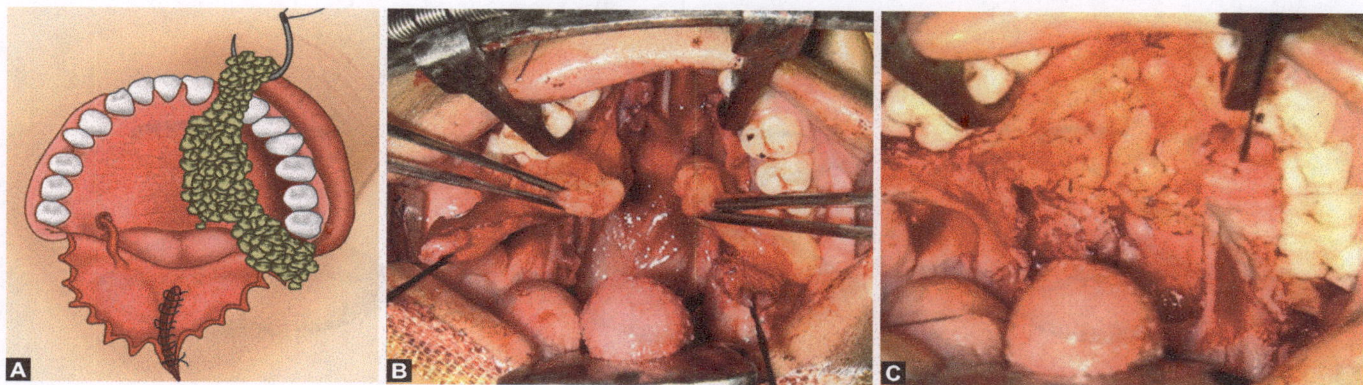

Figs 24.51A to C: (A) Buccal fat pad to close palatal fistula; (B) Harvesting of the BFP; (C) BFP used to close the fistula

Then in 2002, and Doonquah and Ogle[52] evaluated various deformities of lip present postsurgically under following categories:

- Lip volume defects
- Mobility defects
- Lip architectural deficiencies.

Procedures for Lip Scar Revision

Various procedures commonly practiced for scar revision are:

- **V-Y advancement flap:** This technique is routinely practiced for correcting vermillion deficiencies or deformities. The deformity can be a mismatch of the vermillion margins, vertical notching deformity or absent vermillion ridge. In cases of bilateral cleft lip, the classic 'whistle deformity' or central notching defect of vermilion is common (Figs 24.52 and 24.53). This technique can also be used for lengthening of the short bilateral lip (Figs 24.54A to C).

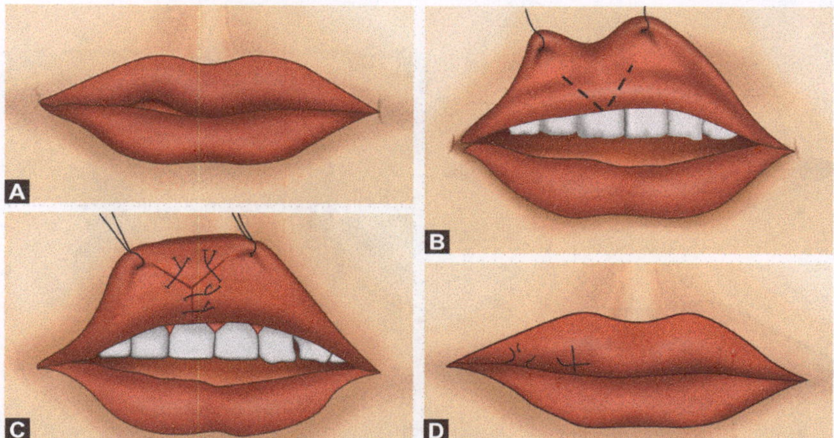

Figs 24.52A to D: V-Y advancement to recruit tissue into the areas of vermilion deficiency (*Source:* TB of Plastic Surgery Vol. 4 by Joseph G McCarthy)

- **Z-plasty:** The Z plasty technique is usually carried out for correction of minor misalignment of the vermilion border or step deformities of vermilion (Figs 24.55A to C).
- **Abbe flap:** Correction of marked horizontal deficiencies with gross lip disproportion may require an Abbe flap (Figs 24.56A and B). The cross flap was initially described by Sabbatini (1838) and was subsequently modified by Estlander (1872) and Abbe (1898). The flap is basically a composite transfer of skin, muscle and mucosa based on a pedicle containing the labial vessels. There is

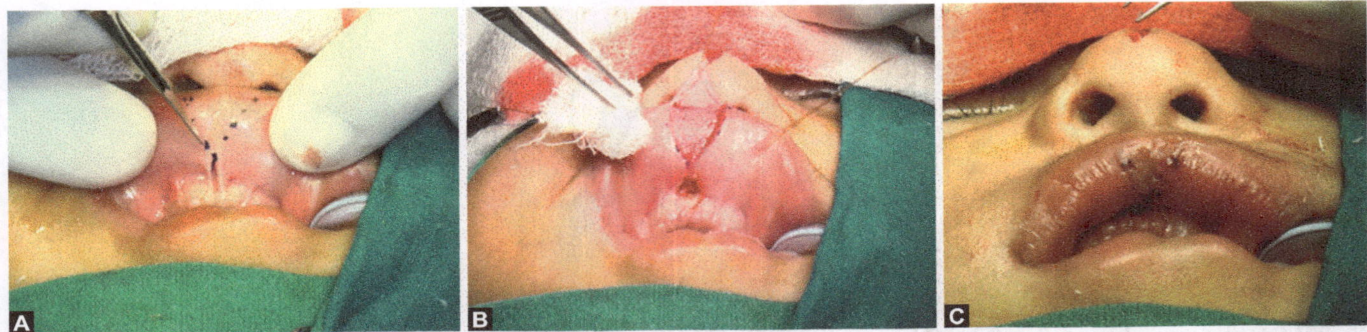

Figs 24.53A to C: (A) Marking for V-Y advancement; (B) Mucosal flap raised; (C) Closure done recruit tissue into the areas of vermilion deficiency

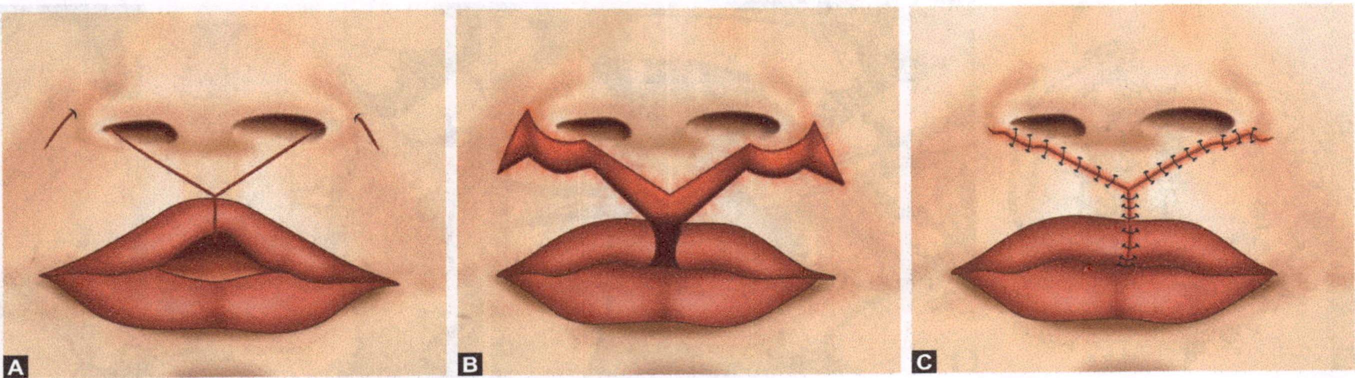

Figs 24.54A to C: Lengthening of the short bilateral lip with a V-Y procedure: (A) The design of the incisions enables lengthening of the midportion of the lip and narrowing of the alar bases; (B) Incisions are carried through all lip layers and a hook is inserted at the midline to pull the lip inferiorly, lengthening the midportion and approximating the lateral lip elements; (C) Completed procedure

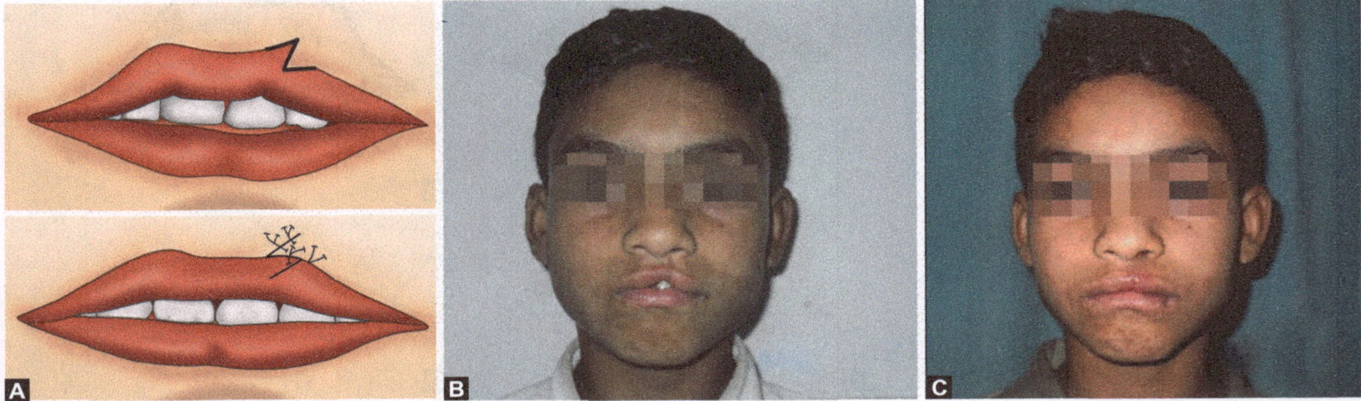

Figs 24.55A to C: (A) Z-plasty for correction of step deformity of vermilion border; (B) Preoperative; (C) Postoperative views (*Source:* L Doonquah, OE Ogle/Oral Maxillofacial Surg Clin N Am 2002;14:425-37)

180° rotation of flap and always better to make a triangular flap, as it has a advantage of closer apposition to the upper lip orbicularis oris muscle superiorly. It is more commonly practiced in the management of bilateral cleft lip deformities, where there is gross deficiency of the tissue for undertaking repair.

- **Kapetansky-Juri advancement flaps:** This technique is used to create a central lip tubercle by over-rotation of the pendulum flaps on both sides in the midline (Figs 24.57A and B).

RHINOPLASTY

For many cosmetic surgeons rhinoplasty is one of the most challenging surgical procedures. A clear understanding of nasal anatomy is critical in order to

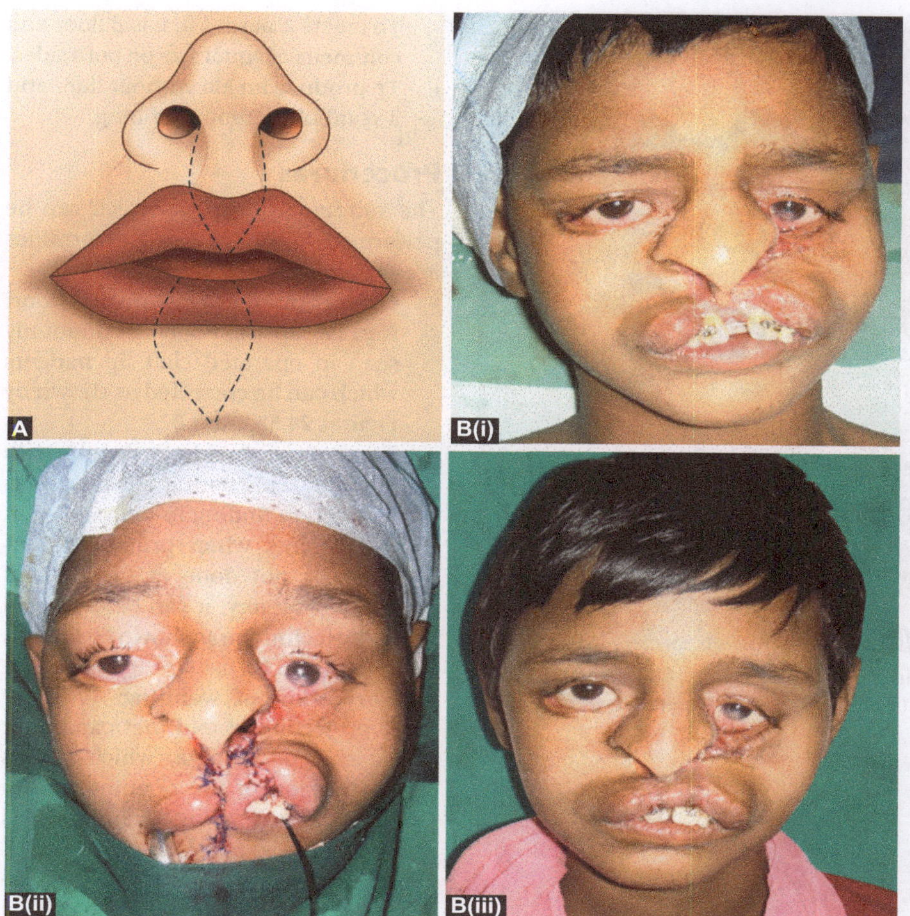

Figs 24.56A and B: (A) Abbe flap is used for lip volume defects in which cross-lip transfer is done. Flap is divided after 3 weeks postoperative approximately; (B) Abbe flap is used for replacement of the midline vermilion defect. Flap is divided after approximately 3 weeks postoperative

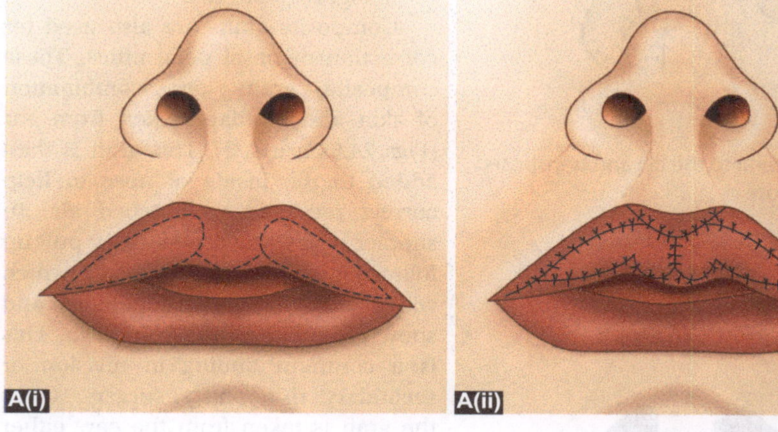

Fig. 24.57A: Kapetansky-Juri advancement flap (design and suturing) for cupid's bow correction

provide an esthetic result that does not compromise nasal function. Numerous rhinoplasty techniques have been described. Rhinoplasty can be:

- **Primary rhinoplasty:** It is done at the time of lip repair in this lower lateral cartilage is repaired.
- **Secondary rhinoplasty:** It is done after age of 15 years till that time growth of septal and nasal cartilage is over. In this procedure septal cartilage is repaired.

The various nasal deformities, which can be seen in cleft patients are:

- Slumping of lower lateral cartilage
- Lateral vestibular webbing
- Laterally displayed alar base.

OBJECTIVES OF CORRECTIVE SURGERY

- To restore the symmetry of alar cartilages.
- To produce a cosmetically acceptable nose and a harmonious relationship between the repaired lip and the nose.

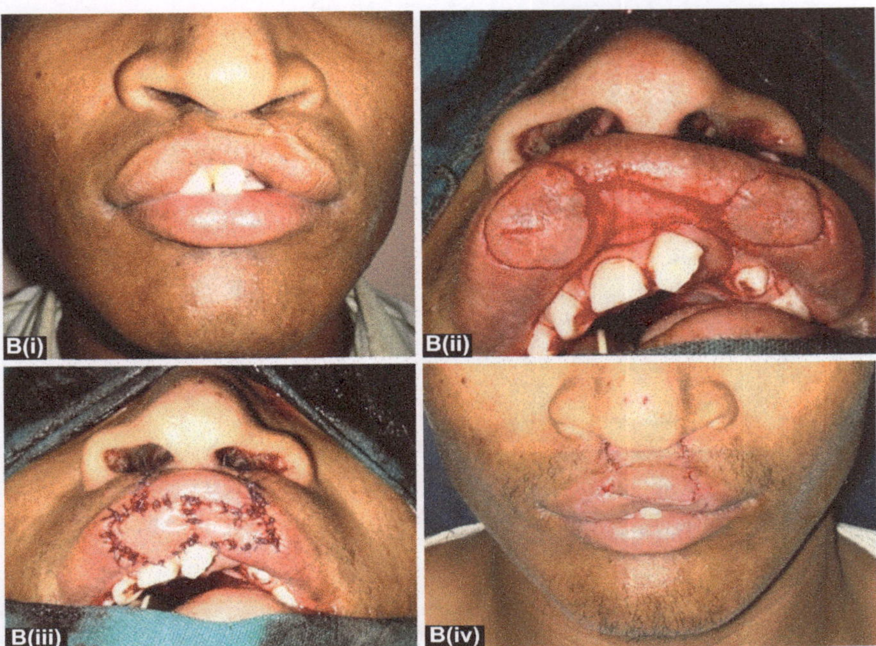

Fig. 24.57B: (i) Preoperative view with midline vermilion defect; (ii) Design for the Kapetansky-Juri advancement flap; (iii) Closure; (iv) Postoperative view

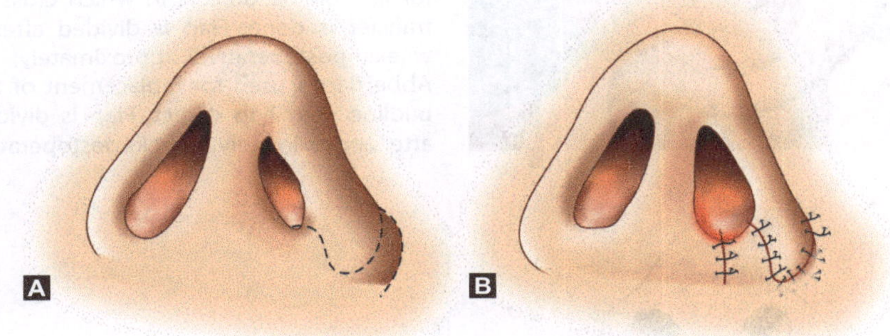

Figs 24.58A and B: Design of flap taken from the area lateral to the ala and transposed into floor of the vestibule of nose

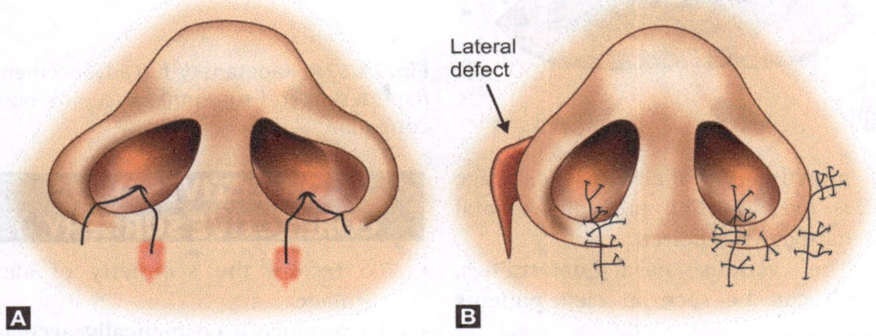

Figs 24.59A and B: Correction of the wide flaring nostrils: (A) Flap is raised from the floor of the nasal vestibule. An incision frees the alar base; (B) The alar base flap is rotated and sutured at floor of the nasal vestibule

- To create a nasal sill, nasal floor and columella of equal size on both sides.
- To produce an ala without flare and a vestibule without webbing.

Procedures

The various procedures, which can be performed for above listed deformities are as follows:

- **Correction of narrow nostril floor:** Narrow nostril floor is commonly seen in operated cleft lip patients which can be corrected as shown by Figures 24.58A and B.
- **Correction of wide flaring nostril:** Similarly wide flaring nostrils also is a common finding in operated cleft lip patients when primary rhinoplasty is not done at the time of cleft lip surgery, it can be corrected using technique as shown by Figures 24.59A and B.
- **Correction of webbing:** Webbing is projection of fold that can either be skin or mucosa, which causes obstruction of the opening. It can be corrected using techniques as shown by Figures 24.60A to C.
- **Columella lengthening:** The columella may need lengthening using one of the many methods described in Figures 24.61 to 24.63.

Composite grafts are also used for correction of nasal deformities. These composite grafts are combination of skin and cartilage taken from ear (Figs 24.64A and B). This graft is then added to the inside of nose to help correct retracted or notched ala. In simpler terms, the nostrils may pull up following rhinoplasty surgery, which will reveal the nostril openings and show too much of the columella. This is a common finding in revision or secondary rhinoplasty surgery. Once the graft is taken from the ear, either the defect (area where the skin/cartilage has been removed) is stitched together (Fig. 24.64C) or in some cases a piece of skin (full thickness skin graft) is taken from behind the ear and then placed in the defect (Fig. 24.64D) where composite graft was removed. This usually heals with minimal to no visible

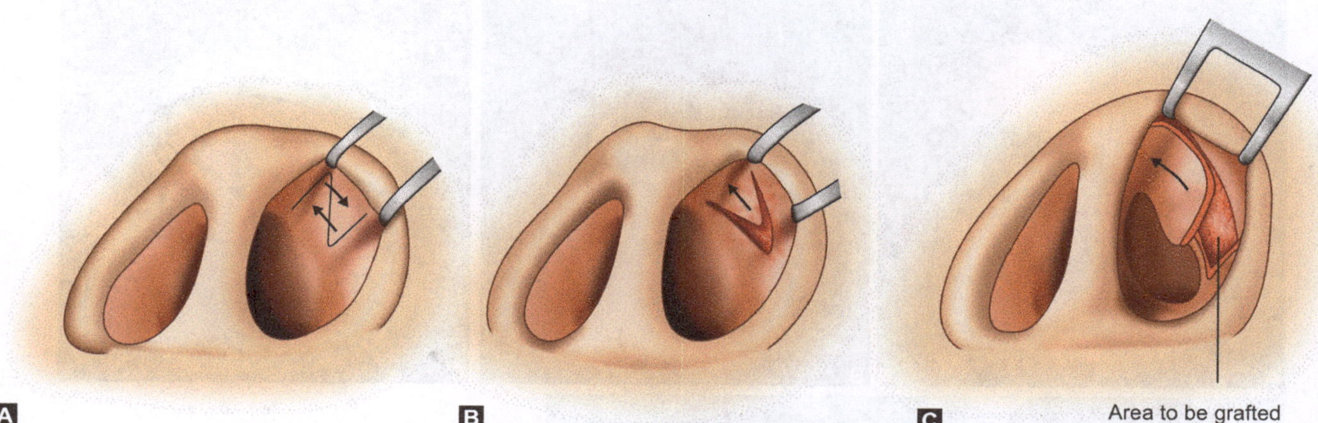

Figs 24.60A to C: (A) Z-plasty; (B) V-Y advancement; (C) Medial advancement. A full-thickness skin graft is placed in the resulting lateral defect

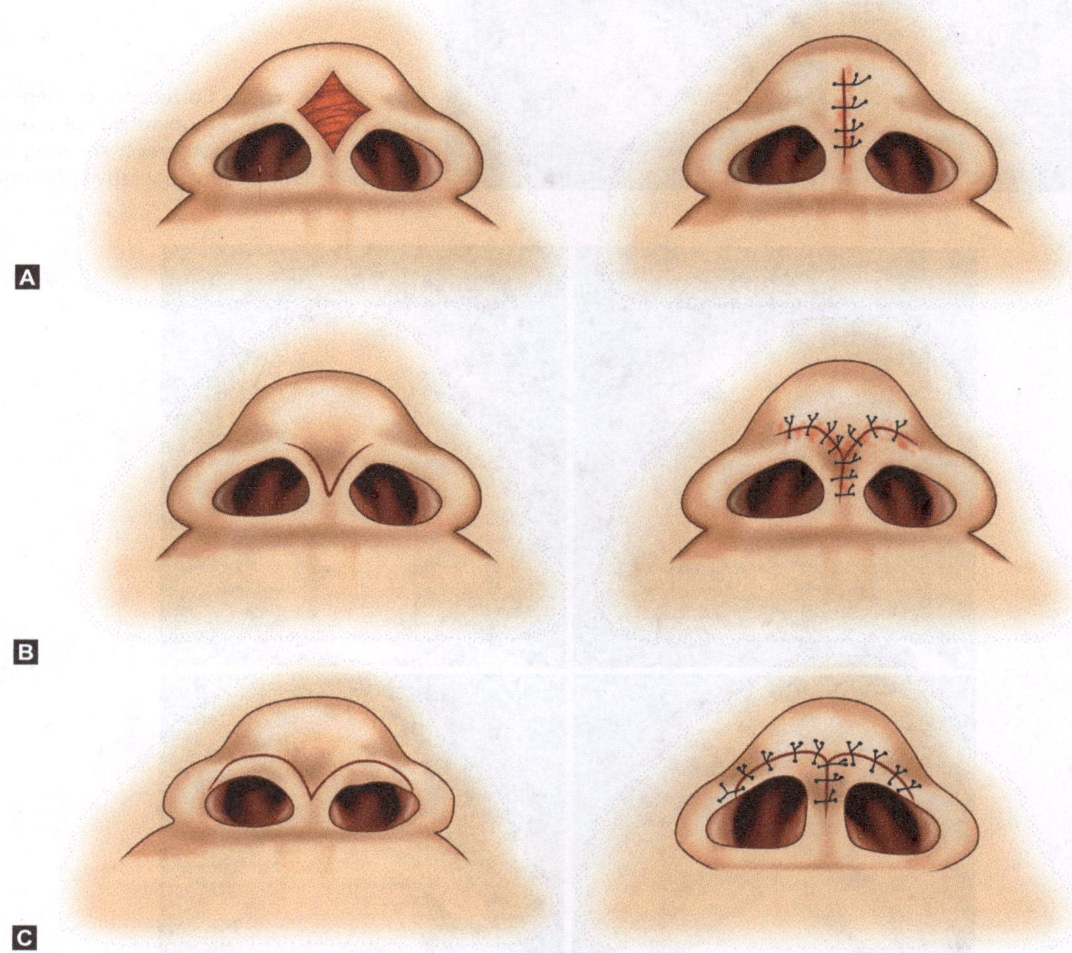

Figs 24.61A to C: Various methods for columella lengthening: (A) Diamond-shaped excision; (B) V-Y advancement of the tip; (C) Bilateral alar wing flap

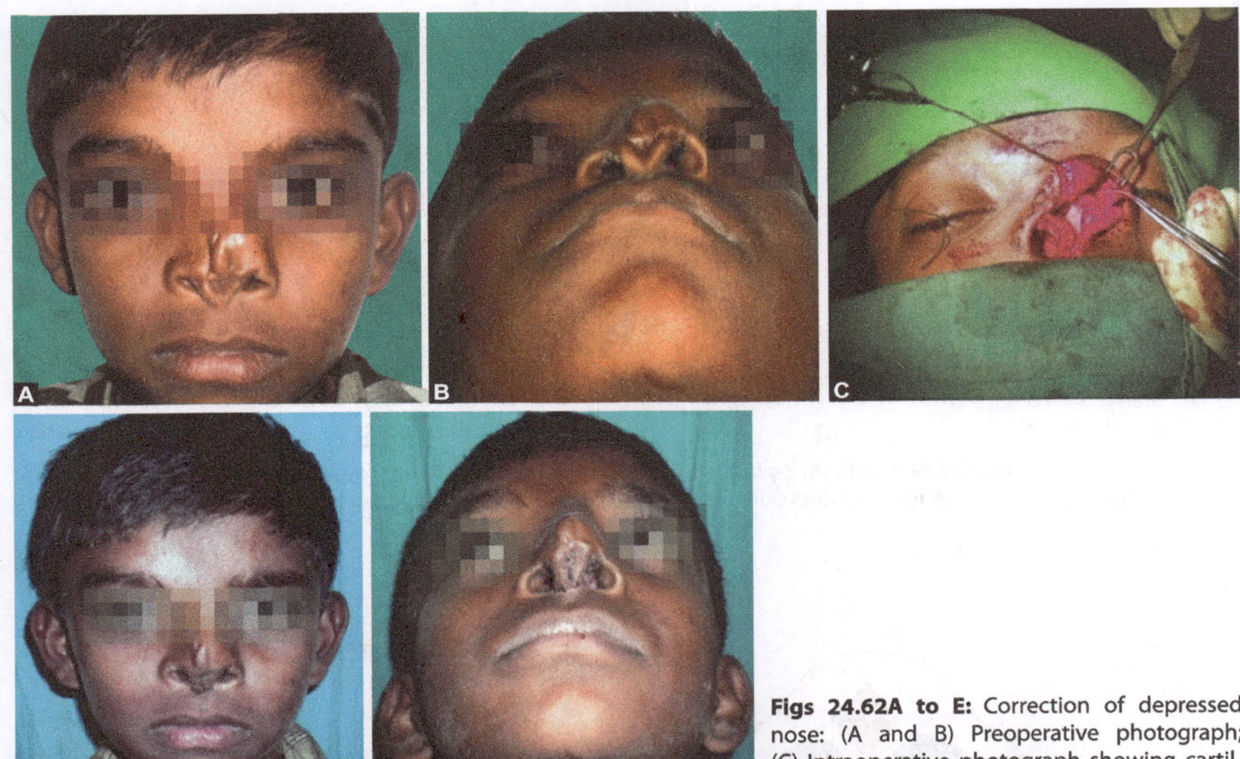

Figs 24.62A to E: Correction of depressed nose: (A and B) Preoperative photograph; (C) Intraoperative photograph showing cartilage repair; (D and E) Postoperative photograph

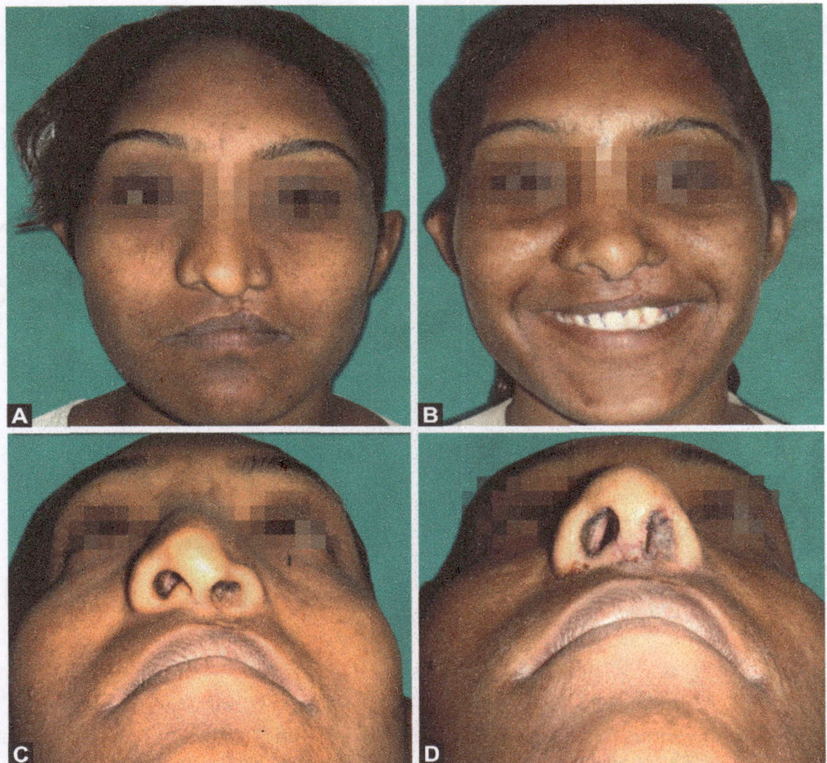

Figs 24.63A to D: (A) Preoperative frontal photograph; (B) Postoperative frontal photograph; (C) Preoperative worms view; (D) Postoperative worms view

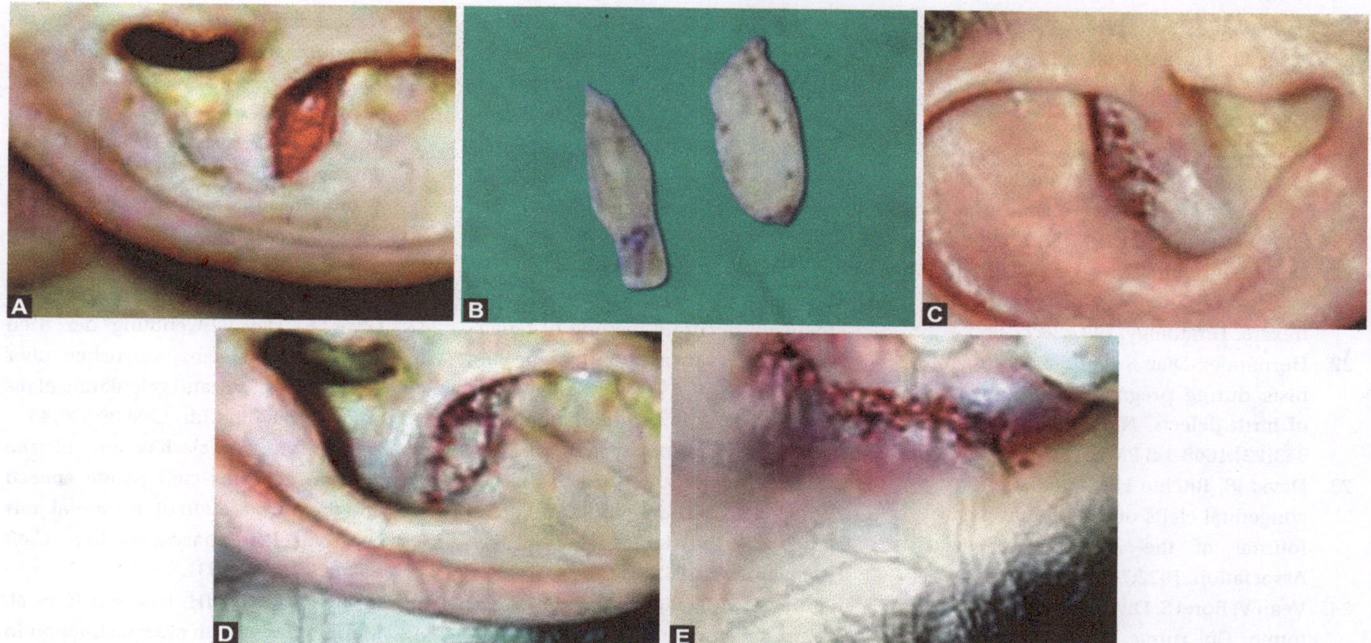

Figs 24.64A to E: (A) Composite graft taken from left ear; (B) Composite grafts; (C) Graft site stitched together; (D) Full thickness skin graft inserted into defect; (E) Behind ear where full thickness skin graft is harvested (*Source: www.rhinoplasty specialist.com*)

scar (Fig. 24.64E). The graft is inserted into the nostril and with time, will heal and becomes part of ala/nostril. Occasionally, the graft can become swollen up to approximately 3 months and there is a small risk that the graft will not survive.

CONCLUSION

Cleft lip and palate is not a cosmetic surgery and it is moreover a functional repair. Religious counseling of parents for regular follow-up, good relation between surgeon and parent, timing of surgery and support from other faculty is very important for a team approach for better life of the child. Basically now it is an era when we can have isolated clinics for cleft lip and palate because it is one deformity, which can be corrected to a level so that there is no postsurgical morbidity and deficiency.

REFERENCES

1. Boo-Chai K. An ancient Chinese text on a cleft lip. Plast Reconstr Surg. 1966;38(2):89-91.
2. Carolus JMF. La chirurgie de Maitre Jean Yperman. F and E. Gyselynck, Gand; 1954.
3. Blair VP, Brown JB. Mirault operation for single harelip. Surg Gynec Obstet. 1930;51:81-98.
4. Hagedorn, M. Uber eine Modification der Hasen schartenoperation. Zhl Chir. 1884;11.756.
5. Tennison CW. The repair of unilateral cleft lip by stencil method. Plast Reconstr Surg. 1952;9:115-120.
6. Millard DR Jr. A radical rotation in single harelip. Am J Surg. 1958;95:318.
7. Franco P. Traite des Hernies. Lyon, Thibauld Payan; 1561.
8. von Graefe CF, Bericht über die erste Staphyloplastik, Hufeland's Journal 44 (1817), p. 116.
9. Stephenson J. Repair of cleft palate by Philibert Roux in 1819. Plast Reconstr Surg. 1971 Mar;47(3):277-83.
10. Dieffenbach, J. F. Uber das Gaumensegel des Menschen und der Saeugethiere. Litt Ann d ges Heilk. 1826.
11. von Langenbeck B. Beitraege zur Osteoplastic. Deutsch Klin. 1859;2:471.
12. Von Langenbeck B. Die Uranoplastik Mittels Ablösung des Mukös-periostalen Gaumenüberzuges. Arch Klin Chir. 1861;2:205.
13. Stanier P, Moore GE. Genetics of cleft lip and palate: syndromic genes contribute to the incidence of non-syndromic clefts. Hum Mol Genet 13. (Review Issue Number 1): R73-R81.2004
14. Ferguson MW. The mechanism of palatal shelf elevation and the pathogenesis of cleft palate. Virchows Arch A Pathol Anat Histol. 1977; 375(2):97-113.
15. Zingade ND. The prevalence of otological manifestations in children with cleft palate. Indian Journal of Otolaryngology and Head and Neck Surgery. 2009;61(3):218-22.
16. Bonaiti-Pellié C, Smith C. Risk tables for genetic counselling in some common congenital malformations. J Med Genet. 1974;11:374-7. PMID:4613831.
17. Lammer EJ, Shaw GM, Iovannisci DM, et al. Maternal smoking and the risk of orofacial clefts: Susceptibility with NAT1 and NAT2 polymorphisms. Epidemiology. 2004; 15(2):150-156. Ref ID: 263.
18. Shaw GM, Lammer EJ. Maternal periconceptional alcohol consumption and risk for orofacial clefts. Journal of Pediatrics. 1999;134(3):298-303.

19. Park-Wyllie L, Mazzotta P, Pastuszak A, et al. Birth defects after maternal exposure to corticosteroids. Teratology. 2000;62:385-92.
20. Puhó EH. Drug treatment during pregnancy and isolated orofacial clefts in hungary. Cleft Palate Craniofac J. 2007;44(2):194-202. PMID: 17328645.
21. Darab DJ. Pathogenesis of median facial clefts in mice treated with methotrexate. Teratology. 1987:36:77-86.
22. Hernández-Díaz S. Folic acid antagonists during pregnancy and the risk of birth defects. N Engl J Med. 2000; 343(22):1608-14. PMID: 11096168.
23. Davis JS, Ritchie HP. Classification of congenital clefts of the lip and palate. Journal of the American Medical Association. 1922;79:1324.
24. Veau V, Borei S. Division Palatine, Anatomie, Chi rurgie, Phonétique. Paris: Masson; 1931.
25. Fogh-Andersen P. Inheritance of Harelip and Cleft Palate. Copenhagen: Arnold Busck; 1942.
26. Kernahan DA, Stark RB. A New Classification for Cleft Lip and Palate. Plast reconstr Surg. 1958;22:435.
27. Kernahan DA. The striped Y: A symbolic classification of cleft lips and palates. Plast Reconstr Surg. 1971;47:469.
28. Balakrishnan C. Indian classification of cleft lip and palate. Ind J Plast Surg. 1975;8:23-4.
29. Tessier P. Anatomical classification of facial, cranio-facial and latero-facial clefts. J Maxillo-Facial Surg. 1976;4:69.
30. Benacerraf BRMD. Fetal cleft lip and palate: sonographic diagnosis and postnatal outcome. Plast Reconstr Surg. 1993;92:1045-51.
31. Grayson BH, Santiago PE, Brecht LE. Presurgical nasoalveolar molding in infants with cleft lip and palate. Cleft Palate Craniofac J. 1999;36(6):486-98.
32. Gillies H, Millard DR. The Principles and Art of Plastic Surgery. Vol. 1. Boston:Little, Brown and Co.; 1957.
33. Rose W. On Harelip and Cleft Palate. London: HK Lewis, 1891.
34. Thompson JE. An artistic and mathematically accurate method of repairing the defect incases of harelip. Surg Gynecol. Obstet. 1912;14:498.
35. Le Mesurier AB. A Quadrilateral Mirault flap operation for harelip. Plast and Reconstruct Surg. 1955;16:422.
36. Tennison CW, The repair of unilateral cleft lip by the stencil method. Plast Reconstr Surg. 1952;9:115.
37. Randall P. A triangular flap operation for primary repair of unilateral clefts of the lip. Plast Reconstr Surg. 1959; 24:331-47.
38. Millard DR. A radical rotation in single harelip. Am J Surg. 1958;95:318.
39. Markus AF, Delaire J. Functional primary closure of cleft lip. Br J Oral Maxillofac Surg. 1993;31:281.
40. Von Langenbeck B. Die uranoplastik mittels ablosung des mukos-periostalen Gaumenuberzuges. Arch Klin Chir. 1861;2:205.
41. Bardach J, Salyer KE (Eds). Surgical techniques in cleft lip and palate. 2nd edn. St Louis, Mosby Year Book, 1991.
42. Furlow LT. Cleft palate repair by double opposing Z-plasty. Plast Reconstr Surg. 1986;78:724–36.
43. Sommerlad BC. A technique for cleft palate repair. Plast Reconstr Surg. 2003;112(6):1542-8.
44. Sommerlad BC. The use of the operating microscope for cleft palate repair and pharyngoplasty. Plast Reconstr Surg. 2003;112(6):1540-1.
45. Åbyholm F, Bergland O, Semb G. Secondary bone grafting of alveolar clefts. Scandinavian Journal of Plastic and Reconstructive Surgery. 1981;15:127–40.
46. von Eiselberg F. Zur Technic der Uranoplastik. Archiv Klin Chir. 1901;64: 509-29.
47. Lexer E. Die Verwendung der frien knochenplastic nebst versuchen uber gelenkversteifung and gelenktransplantation. Arch Klin Chir. 1908;86:939-43.
48. Hogan VM. A clarification of the surgical goals in cleft palate speech and the introduction of the lateral port control (LPC) pharyngeal flap. Cleft Palate J. 1973;10:331.
49. Hollier LH, Kim JH, Grayson B, et al. Mandibular growth after distraction in patients under 48 months of age. Plast Reconstr Surg. 1999;103:1361-70.
50. Figueroa AA, Polley JW, Ko EW. Maxillary distraction for the management of cleft maxillary hypoplasia with a rigid external distraction system. Seminars in Orthodontics. Distraction Osteogenesis. 1999;5(1):46-51.
51. Wilson LF. Correction of residual deformities of the lip and nose in repaired clefts of the primary palate (lip and alveolus). Clin Plast Surg. 1985;12(4): 719-33.
52. Doonquah L, Ogle OE. Scar revision of the cleft lip. Oral Maxillofac Surg Clin North Am. 2002;14(4):425-37.

25 Orthognathic Surgery

Borle Rajiv M, Bhola Nitin, Vibhute Pawan J

INTRODUCTION

The facial deformity caused by asymmetry has long been of great mutual interest to the orthodontist and the oral and maxillofacial surgeon. The deformities of maxillofacial region are readily expressed as a profile disfigurement, since the soft tissues of the face depend on the jaws for their contour. The selection of the proper type and site of osteotomies in orthognathic surgery is based on the extent of the dentofacial deformity, the degree of the desirable jaw movement and the anticipated soft tissue changes following surgical intervention. Clinically, deformities of the middle and lower third of face range from simple dentoalveolar discrepancy (malocclusion) to severe facial asymmetry and disfigurement. Facial disfigurement causes social embarrassment and often results in compromised masticatory and speech function. Furthermore, it often has a severe impact on the patient's self-esteem and jeopardizes his or her quality of life.

DEFINITION

Orthognathic surgery is the art and science of diagnosis, treatment planning and execution of treatment by combining orthodontics and oral and maxillofacial surgery to correct musculoskeletal, dento-osseous and soft tissue deformities of the jaws and associated structures.

The word orthognathic comes from the Greek word *'Ortho'* meaning to straighten and *'Gnathia'*, meaning jaw. Orthognathic surgery thus, means to straighten a jaw.

HISTORICAL ASPECTS

Hullihen[1] in 1849 performed the first anterior mandibular osteotomy in USA for the patient of distortion of face due to severe burns. The first description of Orthognathic surgery (Box 25.1) of the maxilla documented in the literature in 1859 is credited to Von Langenbeck.[2] He did it for the removal of nasopharyngeal polyps. Cheever[3] in 1867 did first maxillary osteotomy for correction of complete nasal obstruction secondary to recurrent epistaxis for which right hemimaxillary down fracture was used, this was the first maxillary osteotomy reported in America. In 1897, Blair performed osteotomy of the mandibular body (St. Louis operation). In 1907, he described several operative techniques for the correction of maxillofacial deformities.[4] Wassmund[5] in 1927 first described LeFort I osteotomy for the correction of midface deformities. However, total mobilization of the maxilla with immediate repositioning was performed in 1934 by Axhausen.[6]

Box 25.1: History of orthognathic surgery

1921	:	Cohn Stock[7] : Anterior maxillary osteotomies (Two stage)
1935	:	Wassmund : One stage anterior maxillary osteotomy.
1952	:	Converse[8] : Step osteotomy of the mandibular body for the correction of mandibular prognathism.
1954	:	Caldwell- Letterman[9] : Vertical subsigmoid osteotomy of ramus.
1955	:	Schuchhardt[10] : Developed posterior maxillary osteotomy.
1955	:	Obwegeser[11] : Intraoral sagittal split of the mandible.
1958	:	Dalpont[12] : Modified intraoral sagittal split technique.
1959	:	Kole[13] : First to describe bimaxillary surgery for the correction of bimaxillary protrusion. Proposed surgeries for open bite closure and for genioplasty procedures.
1968	:	Hunsuck[14] : Further modified sagittal split osteotomy.
1969	:	Obwegeser : Presented a large series of Le Fort I osteotomy.
1970	:	Obwegeser : Two jaw surgery.
1974	:	Spiessl : First to apply rigid fixation in orthognathic surgery.
1979	:	Luhr : Introduced the miniplate fixation in orthognathic surgery.

CLASSIFICATION OF FACIAL DEFORMITIES

Maxillary Deformities

- **Maxillary anteroposterior (AP) excess:** Protrusive maxilla where there is an overgrowth in an anterior horizontal direction. There is often a class II molar relationship, sometimes combined with mandibular protrusion (bimaxillary protrusion).
- **Maxillary AP deficiency:** Inadequate growth of the maxilla in an anterior direction with a class III malocclusion.
- **Vertical maxillary excess:** Overgrowth of the maxillary alveolus in the inferior direction, creating excess teeth and gingival display and often associated with an incompetent lip seal, without mentalis muscle strain.
- **Vertical maxillary deficiency:** Edentulous appearance showing no teeth, often combined with a deep bite in the mandible and prominent 'chin button' and a short lower face.
- **Alveolar clefts:** The alveolar defects usually present with maxillary constriction in AP and transverse dimensions. The defects are more pronounced in the patient with cleft palate deformity and in the cases of ankylosis.

Mandibular Deformities

- **Mandibular AP excess (hyperplasia):** It is characterized by mandibular Prognathism with class III malocclusion.
- **Mandibular AP deficiency (hypoplasia):** This is characterized by deficient anterior growth of mandible (retrognathia) with class II malocclusion.
- **Mandibular asymmetry:** It is as a result of lack of growth on one side of the mandible, often the condylar process, but sometimes ramus and body may be involved. It is seen in Temporomandibular joint ankylosis, condylar hypolasia/hyperplasia, hemifacial microsomia or tumors of the condyle. Malocclusion may or may not be present depending on any compensatory growth in the maxilla which may or may not have occurred.
- **Chin deformities:** The deformities of the chin are often associated with other mandibular deformities.
- **Macrogenia:** Overgrowth of chin in vertical or anterior direction.
- **Microgenia***:* Chin deficiency in vertical and/or anterior direction.

Short Face Syndrome

- **Brachy facial:** It is a deficient lower facial growth in the vertical dimension. It is often associated with low mandibular and occlusal plane angles. Usually there is Class II malocclusion with mandibular AP deficiency, but it is sometimes combined with vertical maxillary deficiency.
- **Long face syndrome:** Dolicofacial—there is excess of lower facial height usually associated with increased occlusal and mandibular plane angles. There is often a combination of vertical maxillary excess and mandibular hypoplasia.
- **Apertognathia:** It is characterized by anterior open bite. It is associated with long face syndrome or simply increased posterior facial height.
- **Lower facial asymmetry:** It is usually caused by unbalanced aberrant growth in the mandible, e.g. condylar hyperplasia/hypoplasia.

Uncommon Dentofacial Deformities

These are often associated with rare craniofacial syndromes. Some of the conditions wherein the facial deformities are commonly seen are as follows:

Cleft Lip and Palate

- Pierre Robin sequence
- Treacher-Collins syndrome
- Apert's syndrome.

Facial Asymmetry

- Hemifacial atrophy (Parry-Romberg syndrome)
- Hemifacial microsomia (Goldenhar syndrome)
- Hemifacial hypertrophy
- Neurofibromatosis (von Recklinghausen's disease).

Midface deficiencies

- Craniosynostoses
- Apert's syndrome
- Crouzon's syndrome
- Pfeifer syndrome
- Binder's syndrome
- Achondroplasia dwarf
- Cleidocranial dysplasia.

Mandibular deficiencies

- Pierre Robin sequence
- Treacher-Collins syndrome (oto-mandibulofacial dysostosis)
- Hemifacial microsomia (Goldenhar syndrome).

Mandibular prognathism

- Gorlin-Goltz syndrome
- Osteogenesis imperfacta
- Marfan syndrome
- Klinefelter syndrome.

PATIENT EVALUATION AND PLANNING

General Patient Evaluation

The following evaluation criteria should be thoroughly implemented while planning an orthognathic surgery:

- **Medical history:** Some of the deformities are associated with syndromic conditions and often have other associated congenital anomalies which need to be corrected or may compromise the treatment plan. Such conditions must be identified prior to the planning of the ortognathic surgery. Facial deformities are also associated with the endocrinal disturbances (e.g. Acromegaly) and unless the underlying disorders are not brought under control the relapse can occur and thus they must be treated prior to the orthognathic surgery.
- **Dental evaluation and dental health:** The facial esthetics is incompletely addressed unless the osseous and the dental components

are considered intandem. Mobilization of the jaw bones often alter the dental relationship and may result in unsatisfactory occlusion, malfunction and secondary TMJ complications. Teeth also serves as an excellent guide in planning the orthognathic surgery and for retention and fixation of various appliances for stabilizing of the osteotomized jaw segments and thus, thorough dental evaluation and necessary orthodontic interventions are mandatory while planning an orthognathic surgery.

- **Radiological evaluation:** Panoramic or full-mouth periapical radiographic evaluation for studying the jaw bones and dentoalveolar segment.
- Social and psychological evaluation.
- Esthetic facial evaluation.
- Frontal facial analysis.
- Profile analysis.
- Cephalometric analysis.
- Soft tissue profile analysis.
- Skeletal relations.
- Dental relations.

OCCLUSAL EVALUATION AND MODEL ANALYSIS

A satisfactory and functional occlusal relationship is necessary for the successful completion of the orthognathic surgery apart from the facial esthetic corrections. Hence, it is necessary to study the occlusion, existing descripancies, and compensatory changes as a result of the deformity. The need for the pre- and postsurgical orthodontic interventions required to achieve an acceptable, functional occlusion and esthetic alignment of the dental arches and teeth must be planned.

- Dental occlusion
- Dental arch form/length
- Dental alignment/symmetry
- Tooth mass relation.

The muscle imbalance is often associated with the dentofacial deformities as a compensatory mechanism. The repositioning of the jaw bones in the desired position alters the muscle equilibrium which might lead to relapse or malfunction. Similarly the TMJ is also subjected to stress and malfunction owing to abnormal maxillomandibular relationship. Surgical repositioning will further alter the muscle balance, position, alter the condylar position which may lead to malfunction of the masticatory apparatus or would lead to relapse following surgical correction and hence, it is necessary to evaluate the muscular activity, TMJ functioning prior to surgery and also the likely alterations in them following the surgery so as to make proper planning.

PROFILE ASSESSMENT

Apart from the routine profile photographs additional photographs like Symmetry view, Submental view; superior view and three-quarter view are useful in ascertaining the facial profile, its descripancies and the need for the correction. Computer assisted analysis and video manipulation are useful in comprehensive evaluation and predicting the surgical out come. The photographs can be used as a record to facilitate comparison of results.

Additional evaluation comprising of the following may be done as indicated in each case:

- Three dimentional CT scan reconstruction
- Diagnostic occlusal splint
- Velopharyngeal evaluation
- Speech evaluation
- Nasoendoscopy
- Clinical evaluation of tongue and its posture and also the radiographic evaluation of tongue posture.
- Final treatment plan
- Presurgical orthodontics
- Surgical plan
- Postsurgical orthodontics and maintenance.

General Evaluation

Medical and Dental Evaluation

Orthognathic surgery is mostly an elective procedure hence, a thorough evaluation of the medical condition of the patient should be done as the patient should be fit to undergo the procedure under suitable anesthesia.

After medical history, consideration is given to dental history, dental health, and periodontal status of the patient. Before the surgery, restorative orthodontic, periodontal and facial pain control therapy should be done. Before the surgical procedure is undertaken, healthy dentition should be established by dental prophylaxis and proper home care.

Inadequate attached gingival and acute periodontal disease must be managed before surgery.

Psychological Evaluation

In the psychological evaluation, patient's expectation about the surgery should be evaluated and it is the duty of the surgeon to give the brief idea of the outcome of the surgery to the patients. Patients who come for orthognathic surgery are mainly of two types. The first group includes patients who want to improve their facial appearance for esthetic reasons. These patients are self-motivated and are more reliable. The other group includes patients who attribute their social and personal problems to their facial appearance, so esthetic correction alone does not correct their personality problem. These patients remain unhappy even after the good surgical results. The patients at times have a very high expectations about the results of the orthognathic surgery. The surgeon must counsel the patients and explain him/her the realistic outcome of the surgery.

Esthetic Facial Evaluation

The patient is asked to sit or stand in upright position at the eye level of clinician during complete evaluation. At the time of examination the Frankfort horizontal plane and interpupillary lines should be parallel to the floor. Teeth should be in centric position and the lips reposed.

All the photographs are taken with Frankfort horizontal plane and interpupillary lines parallel to the floor for records and photographic analysis. The frontal analysis and profile analysis are the most useful facial analysis.

Frontal Face Analysis

The face is divided into three equal parts for vertical facial analysis. Upper third extends from the hairline to the glabella, middle third extends from glabella to subnasale and the lower third extends from subnasale to soft tissue menton (Figs 25.1A and B).

The frontal view evaluation should include 14 anatomic relationships which are as follows:

- The forehead, eyes, orbits and nose are evaluated for symmetry, size and deformity.
- Normal intercanthal distance is 32 ± 3 mm.
- Normal interpupillary distance is 65 ± 3 mm.
- The intercanthal distance, alar base width and palpebral fissure width should be equal.
- The width of the nasal dorsum should be one-half the intercanthal distance and width of the nasal lobule should be two-thirds the intercanthal distance.
- A vertical line through the medial canthus and perpendicular to the papillary plane should fall on the alar bases ± 2 mm.
- The upper lip length is measured from subnasale to upper lip stomion. The normal upper lip length is 22 ± 2 mm for males and 20 ± 2 mm for females.
- The facial midline, nasal midline, lip midlines, dental midlines, and chin midline all should be congruent, and the face should be reasonably symmetric, vertically and transversely.
- A normal upper tooth-to-lip relationship exposes 2.5 ± 1.5 mm of incisal edge with the lips in repose
- If the lips of the patient are overclosed, the jaws should be opened until the lips just begin to separate. The condyles should remain seated in the centric relation. The true lip length and tooth-to-lip relationship then may be evaluated.
- **Smile line:** During smiling, the vermilion of the upper lip should fall at the cervicogingival margin with no more than 1 to 2 mm of exposed gingival. Patient should be asked to give full smile to detect 'gummy smile'.
- The lower eyelid should be level with or slightly above the most inferior aspect of the iris. Sclera between the inferior aspect of the iris and lower lid (scleral show) may indicate infraorbital hypoplasia or exophthalmos.
- The distance from glabella to subnasale and subnasale to menton should be approximately in a 1:1 ratio, providing that the upper lip length is normal.
- The length of the upper lip should be one-third the length of the lower facial third, i.e. lower lip stomion to soft tissue menton should be twice the vertical dimension of the upper lip, provided that the upper lip is normal in length.

Lateral or Profile View

Vertical and anteroposterior plane problems of the jaws can be determined by evaluating the lateral plane.

The facial profile can be classified into convex, concave or straight (Fig. 25.1C). The various parameter that are taken into account are:

- The distance from the glabella to sub-nasale and from subnasale to soft tissue menton should be in a 1:1 ratio if the upper lip length is normal.
- With the maxilla in normal AP position and the upper lip of normal thickness, ideal chin projection is 3 ± 3 mm posterior to a line through subnasale that is perpendicular to clinical Frankfort horizontal plane.
- The morphologic characteristics and relationships of the nose, lips, cheeks and chin are evaluated.
- The cervicomandibular angle is evaluated in reference to chin position
- The length of the upper lip should be one third the length of the lower facial third, i.e. lower lip stomion to soft tissue menton should be twice the vertical dimension of the upper lip if the upper lip is normal in length

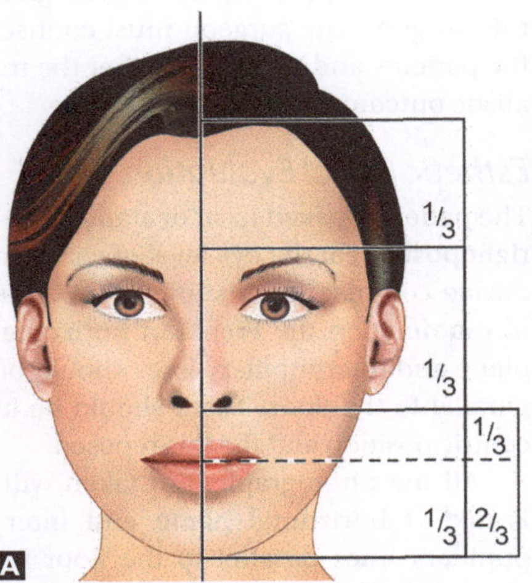

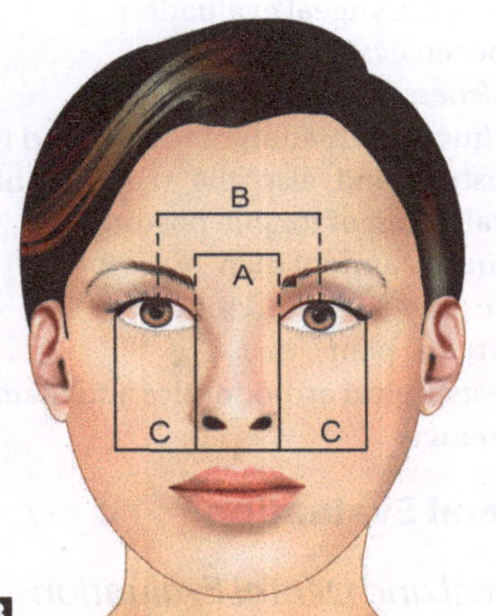

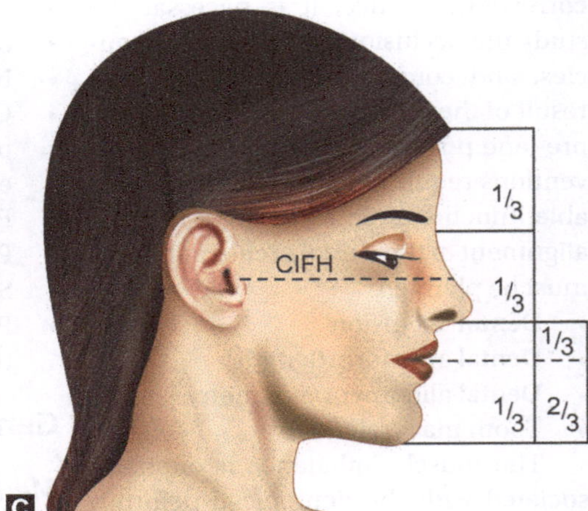

Figs 25.1A to C: Normal facial proportions in: (A) Frontal view; (B) Frontal view analysis: The transverse facial balance; A—The normal intercanthal distance—32 mm ± 3 mm; B—Normal interpupillary distance—65 mm ± 3 mm; C—The width of the palpebral fissures should be equal to the intercanthal distance; (C) Profile view

- Upper lip supralabrale should be 1 to 3 mm anterior to subnasale.
- A line perpendicular to Frankfort horizontal and tangent to the globe should fall on the infraorbital soft tissue ±2 mm.

CLINICAL FEATURES

Mandibular Excess—Prognathic Mandible

Facial Features

- Prominent chin is a dominant feature (prominent lower third of face)
- A concave profile
- Severe cases show lip incompetence
- Steep mandibular plane which may be parallel to high mandibular plane (angle over 35° normal is 25°)
- Obtuse gonial angle
- Middle third of the face appears relatively deficient
- Labiomental fold may be diminished or absent
- Nasolabial angle may be acute
- Anterior facial height may be increased.

Dental Features

- Angle's Class III malocclusion is present
- Reverse horizontal overjet in the incisor region
- Anterior cross bite
- Mandibular anterior teeth may be inclined lingually or may be upright
- Maxillary anterior teeth may be protrusive
- An anterior open bite may be present.

Mandibular Deficiency/Mandibular Retrognathism/Micrognathism

Facial Features

- A convex profile
- Retruded chin
- *"Bird Face Deformity"* in very severe cases
- Short upper lip, curled or protrusive at rest
- An everted lower lip, curled under the protrusive upper incisors with deep mentolabial fold
- Acute gonial angle
- The lip strain will be evident on closure with hyperactive mentalis muscle.

Dental Features

- Angle's Class II molar relationship
- Increased overjet
- Accentuated curve of spee of lower anteriors
- Lower anterior teeth may be tipped anteriorly (fanning) or crowded
- Skeletal deep bite may be present.

Maxillary Excess (Long Face Syndrome): Vertical Maxillary Excess

Facial Features

- Increased height of lower third of the face
- Recessive paranasal areas
- Narrow alar base
- Prominence of infraorbital rim, cheek bones, prominent nose
- Large interlabial gaps (more then 4 mm) incompetent lips
- Excessive incisor display—typical 'Gummy Smile'
- Retroposition or recessive chin
- Steep mandibular plane.

Dental Features

- An Angle's class II molar occlusion
- A high arched palate
- 'V' shaped maxillary dental arch
- Accentuated curve of spee.
- Further, there are two variants:

1. *With anterior open bite*—excessive posterior maxillary growth. A short or normal ramus. Two-third of the patients have anterior open bite.
2. *Without anterior open bite*—dental compensation with over eruption of incisor (an increased ramus height).

Maxillary Deficiency/Vertical Maxillary Deficiency (VMD)

Facial Features

- A short square shaped face with edentulous appearance
- Decreased lower facial height
- The mandible appears square and prominent due to overclosure
- Deep mentolabial fold 'Knobby' appearance of the chin (prominent chin button)
- Overclosure of lips.

Dental Features

- Angle's Class I or Class II molar relation
- Deep over bite
- Mandibular incisor frequently occlude with the palatal gingival
- Severe attrition of the teeth may be seen.

Skeletal Bimaxillary Protrusion with or without Anterior Open Bite

Facial Features

- Convex profile
- Extreme protrusion of maxillary and mandibular teeth
- Anterior teeth prominent and visible in the frontal and profile views
- Lip strain is evident, if the mouth is closed
- Lip incompetence
- Thick looking lips, with an everted vermilion border and rolled appearance
- Apparent chin deficiency.

Dental Features

- Anterior open bite or edge to edge bite may be present.
- Mild to severe crowding or spacing may be seen.
- May be associated with severe tongue thrust habit.
- When severe protusion of maxillary incisors is seen, accentuated curve of spee with mandibular incisors crowding and deep bite may follow.

Nasomaxillary Hypoplasia Associated with a Prognathic Mandible

Facial Features

- Flatening of face
- Sunken appearance of face
- Prognathic mandible
- Upper lip is flat and relatively short
- No display of upper incisors
- Deepened nasolabial fold

Dental Features

- Anterior and posterior cross bite
- Maxillary incisors tend to be protrusive in relation to hypoplastic maxilla
- Mandibular incisors upright to the mandibular basal bone
- Mandibular posterior teeth have an exaggerated lingual inclination
- Maxillary posterior teeth tend to lean outward.

Nasomaxillary Hypoplasia Associated with Cleft Lip-palate Deformities

Facial Features

- Severe mid face hypoplasia
- Short, distorted upper lip
- Asymmetry of nose (typical speech 'nasal twang')
- Mandible appears relatively prognathic (pseudoprognathism).

Dental Features

- Angle's Class III molar relation
- Constricted maxillary arch
- Anterior cross bite
- Crowding of maxillary teeth.

Conditions with Facial Asymmetry

Features

- Asymmetrical mandibular prognathism
- With or without anterior open bite
- Unilateral condylar hypoplasia
- Hemimandibular elongation
- Hemimandibular hyperplasia
- Hemifacial hypertrophy (rare).

Oral Examination

The following parameters must be ascertained during the comprehensive evaluation of the oral structures. The evaluation comprises of:

- Occlusal relationship (Class I, Class II, Class III)
- Anterior openbite or posterior Open bite
- Anterior overjet and any crossbites
- Health of the dentition
- Tooth size discrepancies
- Curve of Wilson
- Curve of Spee
- Dental crowding or spacing
- Missing, decayed, retained primary, nonsalvageable teeth
- Discrepancies between centric occlusion and centric relation
- Periodontal evaluation
- Transverse, anteroposterior or vertical asymmetries
- Anatomic or functional tongue abnormalities
- Recording of any masticatory difficulties
- Any other pathologic processes.

Temporomandibular Joint

Any signs of TMJ dysfunction or pathosis, in the form of hypermobility, hypomobility, subluxation, propping, clicking, pain, etc. should be detected *prior* to surgery.

Nasal and Pharyngeal Evaluation

Any nasal trauma, nasal airway obstruction, allergies, sinus pathologies, predominant mouth breathing, etc. are evaluated. Similarly in the cases of mandibular or maxillary hypoplasia the pharyngeal airway is compromised. It may be associated with snoring and sleep pathologies such as sleep apnoea syndrome. In severe cases the sleep studies and through evaluation of air way should be done. McNamara analysis is useful in assessing the pharyngeal airway.

Similarly, after a major setback surgery the pharyngeal space may get compromised, leading to sleep apnea. Thus preoperative assessment should be done and the problems must be anticipated and addressed.

Radiographic Evaluation

The radiographs used in the diagnosis of dentofacial deformities are:

- The lateral and PA cephalometric radiographs
- The panoramic radiograph
- The periapical radiograph.

Lateral and PA cephalometric radiographs are used to analyze skeletal, dentoalveolar and soft tissue relationships in the anteroposterior (AP), transverse, and vertical dimensions. Panoramic and periapical radiographs can be helpful to determine tooth alignment, root angulation and existing pathology.

CEPHALOMETRIC ANALYSIS

Hard Tissue Analysis

The hard tissue analysis helps in:

- Establishing two-dimensional relationships of craniofacial components.
- Classifying skeletal and dental abnormalities with respect to cranial base, skeletal pattern, inter- and intra-arch dental relationships and soft tissue profile.
- Analyzing growth and development responsible for dentofacial pattern, whether for cranial base configuration, congenital abnormalities, pathologic conditions, or facial asymmetry.
- Planning treatment for orthodontic and/or surgical procedures.
- Analyzing changes after treatment effectiveness of different treatment modalities and effectiveness of retention.
- Determining dentofacial growth changes after treatment.
- Predicting hard and soft tissue contours before initiation of treatment.

Hard Tissue Landmarks (Fig. 25.2)

- **Sella (S):** The center of pituitary fossa.
- **Nasion (N):** The most anterior point of the nasofrontal suture in the midsagittal plane.
- **Articulare (Ar):** It is a point at the junction of the posterior border of ramus and inferior border of basilar part of the occipital bone.
- **Anterior nasal spine (ANS):** The anterior most midsagittal point on the tip of sharp bony process of maxilla.
- **Prosthion (Pr):** The lowest and most anterior point on the alveolar bone in the middle between the

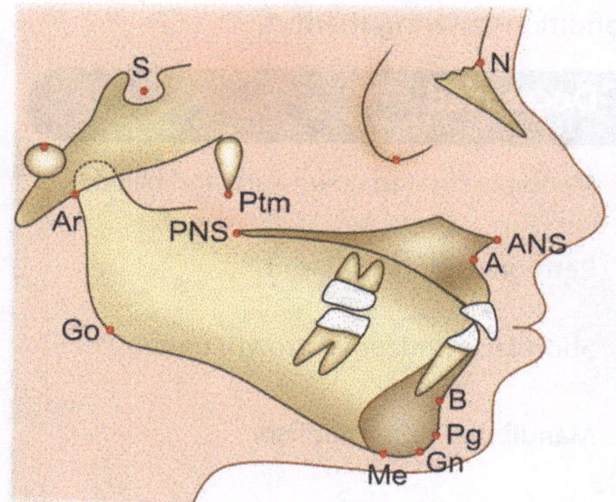

Fig. 25.2: Hard tissue landmarks

upper central incisors. It is also called supradentale.

- **Subspinale (A):** The deepest midsagittal point on the concavity between Anterior Nasal Spine and Prosthion.
- **Supramentale (B):** The deepest point in mid sagittal plane on the concavity between infradentale and pogonion.
- **Pogonion (Pg):** Most anterior mid sagittal point on the contour of the chin.
- **Gnathion (Gn):** Constructed by bisecting the Facial plane and tangent to lower border of mandible.
- **Menton (Me):** Most inferior point on the inferior contour of the chin.
- **Pterygomaxillary fissure (Ptm):** The most posterior point on the anterior contour of the maxillary tuberosity.
- **Posterior nasal spine (PNS):** The most posterior point on the contour of the palate.
- **Gonion (Go):** The most inferior, posterior, and lateral point on the external angle of the mandible.

DENTAL RELATIONS

There are four measurements for dental analysis relationships (Table 25.1).

Position of Upper Molar

A vertical line perpendicular to the Frankfort plane and passing through the posterior aspect of the pterygoid plate is drawn and the horizontal distance from the pterygoid vertical to the most distal aspect of the first molar crown is measured. This measurement helps to determine the maxillary molar position and to relate this position to the malocclusion. The value is misleading when maxillary teeth have been extracted (Fig. 25.3A).

Normal value:

- Age of the patient in years ± 3 mm
- Adult women: 18 ± 3 mm
- Adult man: 21 ± 3 mm.

Lower Incisor Protrusion

The normal distance from the tip of the lower incisor to the A-Po line in perpendicular is 1 ± 2 mm. This value helps to determine the protrusion of the lower arch (Fig. 25.3B).

Lower Incisor Inclination

Normally, the angle between the long axis of the lower incisor and N-Po line is 22 ± 4 degrees. The angulation gives the amount of tipping of the lower incisors (Fig. 25.3C).

Interincisal Angle

This is the angle formed by the long axis of the upper and lower central incisors. Normal value: 130 ± 6 degrees. Low angle indicates protrusion of the incisors and high angle is associated with retroclination with deep bite (Fig. 25.3D).

Skeletal Analysis

Following skeletal measurements for the skeletal analysis are commonly used (Table 25.1 and Fig. 25.4).

Facial Axis Angle

A line is drawn from the basion to the nasion. Another line is drawn from the gnathion to the posterosuperior point of the pterygomaxillary fissure (facial axis). The inferior angle formed when these two lines intersect is called the facial axis angle. The normal value is 90 ± 3 degrees.

Decreased value:

- Recessive chin, or
- Vertically excessive face.

Increased value:

- Prominent chin
- Vertically deficient face.

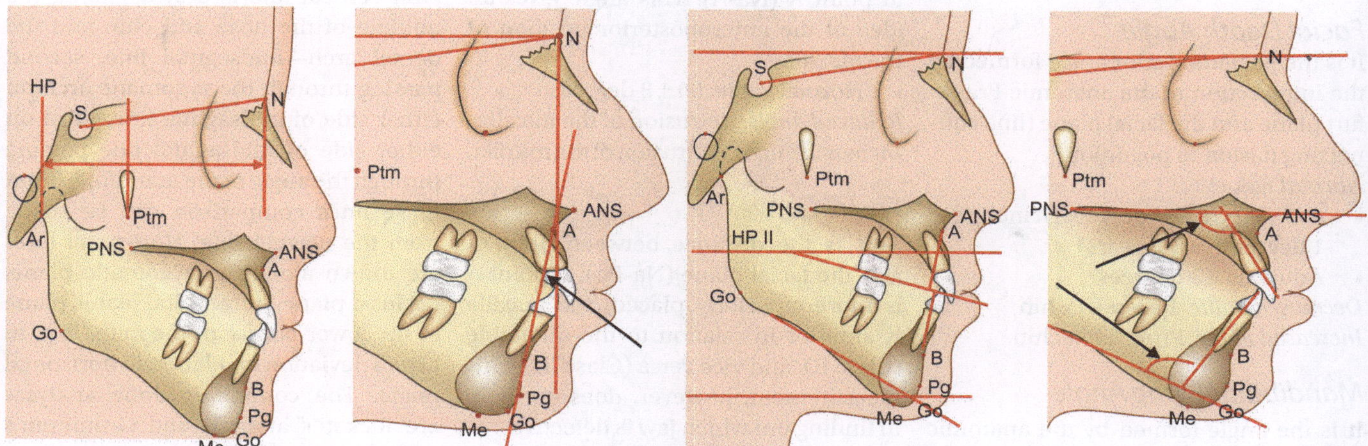

Figs 25.3A to D: Dental relations: (A) Relation of molar to the malocclusion; (B) Lower incisor protrusion; (C) Lower incisor inclination; (D) Interincisal angle

Table 25.1: Skeletal parameters along with their normal values and conditions altering them

Sr. No.	Parameter	Normal value	Increased	Decreased
1.	Facial-axis angle Ba.Na-Ptm.Gn	90° ± 3.5°	Mandible rotated forward and upward	Mandible rotated downward and backward
2.	Facial depth N.Pog-Fh	87° ± 3°	Prognathic mandible	Retrognathic mandible
3.	Mandibular plane angle	25°	Long face/vertical growth pattern	Short face/horizontal growth pattern
4.	Maxillary depth angle	90°		
5.	Facial convexity Na.A- A.Pog	0 ± 8.5	Mandibular prognathism	Mandibular retrognathism
6.	Maxillary length Co-Point A	100 mm	Prognathic maxilla	Retrognathic maxilla
7.	Mandibular length Co-Gn	131 mm	Mandibular prognathism	Mandibular retrognathism
8.	N perp to A point	0 ± 8.7	Prognathic maxilla	Retrognathic maxilla
9.	Jarabaks ratio S.GO/N.Me	(62%–65%)	Short face/horizontal growth pattern	Long face/vertical growth pattern

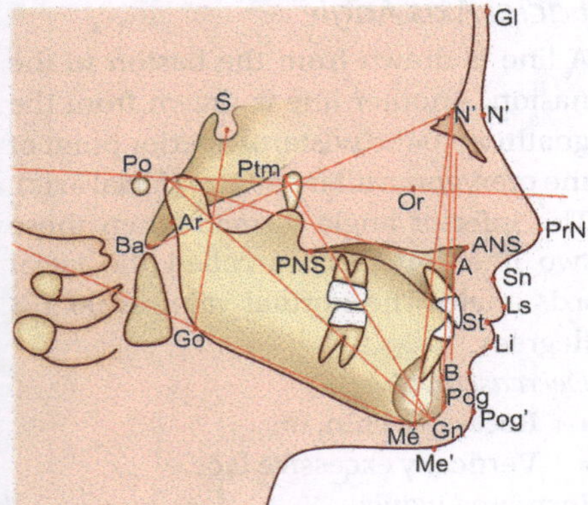

Fig. 25.4: Hard tissue cephalometric analysis for orthognathic surgery

Facial Depth Angle

It is the posteroinferior angle formed by the intersection of the anatomic Frankfurt plane and the facial plane (line connecting nasion to pogonion).

Normal value:

- At 9 years : 87 ± 3 degrees (It increases 1 degree every 3 years)
- Adult: 89 ± 3 degrees

Decreased value: Recessive chin

Increased value: Prominent chin.

Mandibular Plane Angle

It is the angle formed by the anatomic Frankfurt plane and the mandibular plane (A line tangent to the symphysis and the gonial portion of the mandible). This angle relates the posterior facial height to the anterior facial height.

- **Normal value:** At 9 years: 26 ± 4 degrees (It decreases by 1 degree every 3 years)
- **Adult:** 24 ± 4 degrees

High angle: Weak musculature and open bite

Low angle: Strong musculature and deep bite.

Maxillary Depth Angle

It is the angle formed by the anatomic Frankfurt plane and the line from nasion to point A (Na-A). This angle gives an idea of the anteroposterior position of the maxilla.

- Normal value: 90 ± 3 degrees

Reduced angle: Retrusion of the maxilla

Increased angle: Protrusion of the maxilla.

Facial Convexity

This is the distance between point A and the facial plane (Na-Po). If point A is more anteriorly placed, the maxilla is anterior in relation to the mandible (Class II), and vice versa (Class III). This measurement, however, does not help in finding out which jaw is defective.

- Normal value: 1 ± 2 mm.

Maxillary Length: Mandibular Length

The ratio, measured from the condylion to point A (maxillary length) and from the condylion to gnathion (mandibular length) is 1:1.3.

This helps in finding out the relative length of each jaw, independent of any vertical discrepancy.

POSTEROANTERIOR CEPHALOMETRIC ANALYSIS

The main indication of Posteroanterior (PA) analysis is asymmetry and deviation. First vertical line is drawn joining the midline of the nose and chin and the dental arch—midsagittal line, second passing through the zygomatic arch on either side of midsagittal line, third on either side of midsagittal line passing through the angle of the mandible. From these lines comparison can be made from the normal side. Horizontal lines are drawn along the zygomatic plane, occlusal plane, infraorbital plane, plane of the lower border of the mandible, to assess deviation in relation to horizontal plane. The commonly done analyses are Rickett's analysis and Grummon's analysis.

Important Planes in Cephalometric Analysis

Cranial Base

The base line for comparison of most of the data in this cephalometric analysis is a constructed plane called horizontal plane (HP). It is constructed by drawing a line 7° from the line SN (Burstone's cephalometric analysis for orthognathic surgery). It is a substitute to Frankfurt plane. Most of the measurements are made from projections either parallel or perpendicular to horizontal plane. The length of the cranial base is measured from Ar to N and parallel to HP. This measurement is not an absolute value, but a skeletal baseline to be correlated to other measurements such as maxillary or mandibular length. For example, a patient with cephalometrically large maxilla and mandible should have a normal appearance because of large cranial base.

Horizontal Skeletal Profile Analysis

Horizontal skeletal profile analyses are made parallel to HP. These are very important because most surgical corrections are primarily made in the anteroposterior direction. The McNamara analysis, Tweed analysis, Bustone analysis, Down's analysis and Steiner analysis are commonly done which include both the horizontal and vertical skeletal profile analysis, based on skeletal proportions and linear measurements.

Degree of Skeletal Convexity

The angle of facial convexity is measured by the angle formed by the line NA and the line from A to PoG. The N-A-PoG angle gives an indication of the overall facial convexity, but does not specify the diagnosis that whether the maxilla or the mandible is at fault.

A positive angle of convexity denotes convex face and a negative angle denotes concave face. A clockwise angle is positive (+ve), a counterclockwise angle is negative (–ve).

A line perpendicular from HP is dropped through N. Horizontal position of A is measured from this perpendicular line. This measurement describes the apical base of the maxilla in relation to N, and enables to determine if the anterior part of the maxilla is protrusive or retrusive. Similarly position of point B from this perpendicular line describes the horizontal position of the apical base of the mandible in relation to N. When inferior anatomical landmark is measured in relation to the superior structure, positive sign (+) denotes anterior and negative sign (–) posterior.

Thus, these measurements are useful in the planning of treatment of maxillary or mandibular advancement or reduction.

N-Pog is measured in the same manner as NA and NB and indicates the prominence of the chin. These measurements determine if there is horizontal genial hyperplasia or hypoplasia and useful in the planning of treatment of augmentation and reduction genioplasty, of anterior mandibular horizontal advancement or reduction, and total mandibular horizontal advancement or reduction.

Vertical Skeletal Profile Analysis

Vertical skeletal discrepancy may reflect anterior, posterior or complex dysplasia of the face. Therefore, vertical skeletal cephalometric measurements are divided into anterior and posterior components.

- **Anterior component:** The anterior component is subdivided into measurements of: (i) the middle third facial height (distance from N to ANS) that is measured perpendicular to HP, and (ii) the lower third facial height which is the measurement from ANS to Gn and is measured perpendicular to HP.
- **Posterior component:** Posterior maxillary height is the length of a perpendicular line dropped from HP intersecting the PNS. The divergence of the mandible posteriorly is shown by the mandibular plane angle (MP-HP), which is the angle formed between Go and Gn and HP. This angle helps in relating the posterior facial divergence with respect to the anterior facial height.

Vertical skeletal measurements help in the diagnosis of inferior posterior and total maxillary hyperplasia or hypoplasia and also clockwise or counterclockwise rotation of the maxilla and mandible.

Surgical correction of these problems includes total maxillary vertical advancement or reduction, anterior maxillary vertical augmentation or reduction, posterior maxillary vertical augmentation or reduction, combination of anterior and posterior maxillary vertical augmentation or reduction, and mandibular ramus rotation and ramus height reduction.

SOFT TISSUE CEPHALOMETRIC ANALYSIS

Soft Tissue Landmarks (Fig. 25.5 and Table 25.2)

- **Glabella (G):** The most prominent point in the midsagittal plane of the forehead.
- **Soft tissue nasion (N'):** The point of greatest concavity in the midline between the forehead and nose.
- **Columella point (Cm):** The most anterior point on the columella of the nose.
- **Subnasale (Sn):** The point at which the columella merges with the upper lip in the midsagittal plane.
- **Labiale superius (Ls):** A point indicating the mucocutaneous border of the upper lip.
- **Labiale inferius (Li):** A point indicating the mucocutaneous border of the lower lip.
- **Soft tissue pogonion (Pg'):** The foremost point on the soft tissue chin in the midsagittal plane.
- **Soft tissue menton (Me'):** The lowermost point on the soft tissue chin in the sagittal plane.
- **Angle of throat (C):** The intersection of the horizontal and vertical tangents to the profile of the soft tissue throat.

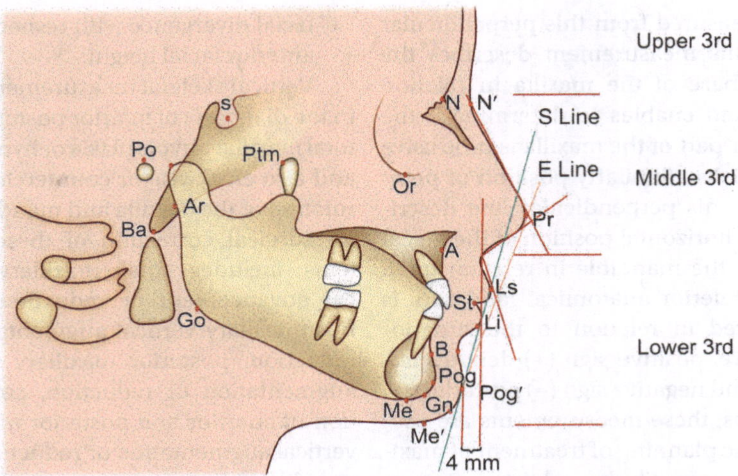

Fig. 25.5: Soft tissue landmarks

Presurgical Orthodontics

Goals of Presurgical Orthodontics

- The basic goal is to position the teeth upright over basal bone while satisfying the spatial requirements. In simple words it is decompensation of nature's compensation, e.g. when a patient has a retrognathic mandible the anterior teeth tend to procline which is a nature's compensatory mechanism to maintain a normal dental relationship on an abnormal basal bone framework. In such situation without presurgical orthodontics if the surgery is attempted to advance the mandible, these flared anterior teeth would cause a interference. Hence, by doing presurgical orthodontics we would like to upright the teeth so as to achieve a normal tooth to basal bone relationship and then go for a surgical correction
- To position of the teeth over their respective basal bones
- To position the long axis of the maxillary central incisors so that the final position would be approximately 22° to the NA line, with the labial face of the incisors 4 mm anterior to that line
- Position the mandibular central incisors so that final position will be approximately 20° to the NB line, with the labial face of the incisors 4 mm anterior to that line
- To align and level the teeth
- To adjust for tooth discrepancies
- To relieve arch crowding
- Closure of diastemas
- To correct rotated teeth
- To correct divergence of roots adjacent to surgical sites
- To achieve root paralleling to create space for segmental osteotomies
- To eliminate gross dental interferences
- Co-ordination of upper and lower arch width and to correct the transverse discrepancies without compromising stability and dental health.

Advantages of Presurgical Orthodontics

- Relapse tendencies are controlled. Most oftenly sugical relapse and orthodontic relapse are compensatory to each other, since dentition is decompensated before surgery
- Total treatment time is reduced
- Results in proper intraoperative interdigitation (occlusion)
- Allows quick and easy postsurgical orthodontic correction
- Allows effective surgical correction
- Improves results in terms of stability and occlusion.

Table 25.2: Soft tissue cephalometric parameters, standard values and conditions altering them

Sr. No.	Parameter	Normal value	Increased	Decreased
1.	Nasolabial angle	102° ± 4°	Lips retrusive	Protruded lips
2.	Nasomental angle	120° to 132°	Protrusive chin and retrusive nose	Retrusive chin and prominent nose
3.	Chin prominance	–1 to –4 mm	Prominent chin	Retrusive chin
4.	E Line: Upper lip	–4 mm	Prominent lips	Retrusive lips
	Lower lip	–2 mm	Retrusive lips	Prominent lips
5.	S Line: Upper lip	0 mm	Prominent lips	Retrusive lips
	Lower lip	0 mm	Retrusive lips	Prominent lips
6.	Facial symmetry: Upper 1/3	Equal three parts in vertical proportion		
	Middle 1/3		Maxillary excess	Maxillary deficiency
	Lower 1/3:		Maxillary excess	Maxillary deficiency

Presurgical Aids in Orthodontics

While performing orthognathic surgery, if any surgical procedure is considered to help the treatment, it is known as surgical aid to orthodontics. Following are some of the common surgical aids to orthodontic treatment:

- Serial extractions
- Therapeutic extractions
- Surgical removal or surgical exposure of unerupted teeth
- Extraction of submerged deciduous molars, removal of odontomes
- Correction of diastema
- Corticotomy.

Postsurgical Orthodontics

Four-to-six weeks after the surgery, when the surgeon confirms the satisfactory bony healing, the stabilizing arch wires are replaced by light arch wires and occlusion is allowed to settle.

Goals of Postsurgical Orthodontics

- Closure of residual spaces
- Root paralleling at the extraction sites
- Maximum interdigitation
- Finer tooth alignment
- Retention of the reoriented oral musculature to prevent relapse
- To establish ideal overbite and overjet
- To stabilize the results obtained through the surgery.

Dental Model Surgery—(Mock Surgery)

Mock surgery gives three dimensional understanding of the postoperative relationship of the jaws (Figs 25.6A and B). Cephalometric analysis cannot reproduce three-dimensional view of the patient's dental arch.

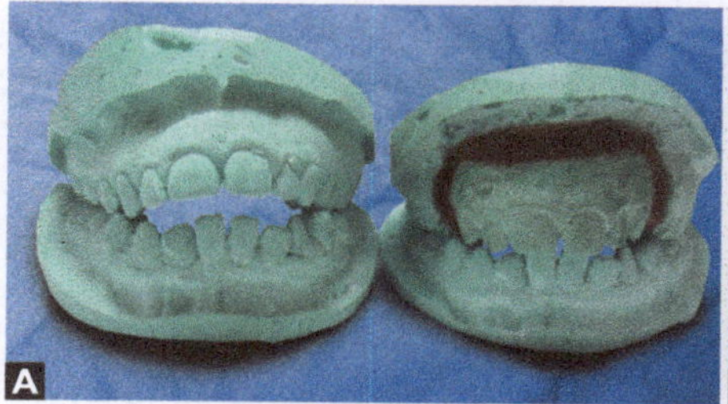

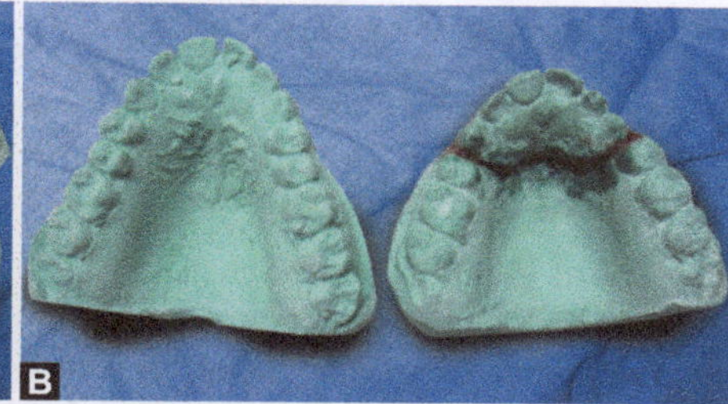

Figs 25.6A and B: Cut for correcting anterior open bite on cast for mock surgery

Aims of Model Surgery

- To determine the feasible surgical plane, extent of bone/arch advancement or reduction required in the surgery
- To determine vertical change that will be achieved at the time of surgery in such a way that it can be accurately duplicated intraoperatively
- To determine the direction in which dento-osseous segment moves
- To obtain measurements of osteotomies
- To get postoperative relationship of the jaws, dentition and occlusion
- To decide about postsurgical orthodontic treatment
- Fabrication of splints for stabilization after surgery.

Indications

Model surgery is used in double jaw surgery, as well as in single jaw surgery where unoperated jaw will act as a template.

Advantages

- The simulation of the patient's facial structure functionally and spatially in three dimensions
- The surgeon can correlate the relevant information and arrive at the surgical prediction in three dimensions
- Model surgery gives an accurate 1:1 replica of the patient's dentition allowing an increased accuracy of prediction when compared to the 10 percent discrepancy seen in cephalometric distortion
- Model platform and block is capable of accurately measuring articulator mounted models in three planes of space allowing the surgeon to carry out accurate model surgery movements on a full sized anatomic articulator.

Disadvantages

Condyles are never perfectly symmetrical therefore:

- Model surgery performed on the mounted casts gives slightly inaccurate reading
- There can be errors related to the actual model orientation itself
- There can be measurement errors related to instruments and perspective.

Technique

First the models are positioned in the required jaw relationship using semi-adjustible articulators. The models are cut exactly similar to the planned surgery, avoiding root apices. Detect the problem areas like proximity of roots, bony interference, etc. Observe rotation and expansion of the dento-osseous segment. Achieve maximum interdigitation and measure anteroposterior (AP), transverse and interdental changes and re-evaluate and compare with prediction tracing measurements.

Surgical Splints

Surgical splints are also known as occlusal wafer splints. They are utilized in the operating room to position the teeth and add to stabilization. They are used during the surgery as well as postsurgically.

Advantages

- Provide a clearly visualized goal for the surgeon at the operating table
- Aids in positioning bone fragments correctly to aid healing
- Possible to put teeth in a planned position at surgery, even if they do not interdigitate perfectly without a splint.

Surgical splints are utilized in the following procedures:

- Maxillary surgery
- Mandibular ramus surgery

- Segmental jaw surgery
- Dual jaw surgery.

Construction of Splints

The splint is made on the casts as they have been related by mock surgery on models. After they have been checked by the surgeon and orthodontist, the following steps are undertaken:

- Stabilize cast with plaster or stone, so that no shift occurs as splint is fabricated
- Articulator is opened to allow for enough thickness of splint material
- Self-curing acrylic is formed into the desired U-shaped configuration. Care is taken to avoid rolling the acrylic excessively, as this causes cracks and bubbles
- Lay the U-shaped roll of uncured acrylic on the lower occlusal surface. The casts are then closed onto it, when the acrylic is still soft. At this point, the casts must be firmly secured to the articulator. If the casts shift, splint dictates wrong position at surgery
- While the acrylic is still soft, scissors/ scalpel is used to trim the excess on the labial aspect. Ensure that it does not tear away while carrying out this procedure
- After the acrylic has cured, a semi-trimmed splint with occlusal indentations is obtained
- Trim away excessive bulk of acrylic, labially and lingually with burs. Buccal aspect of splint must be contoured to avoid interference with orthodontic appliances and to allow visual determination of proper seating during surgery. The acrylic should be relieved on lingual aspect of anterior teeth and distal aspect of buccal segment cusp tip to allow a smooth arc of closure
- Trim occlusal surfaces so that only shallow occlusal indentations remain
- Finally, place bur holes along labial and buccal surface for attaching splint to the arch wires
- Routine finishing and polishing must be carried out for patient's comfort and maintenance of oral hygiene.

Various surgical procedures done for the correction of the jaw deformities are shown in Box 25.2.

Principles of Surgical Treatment

- Psychological preparation of the patient.
- Maintenance of blood supply through the appropriate pedicle.
- Care of nerves, vessels, teeth and bone.
- Minimum periosteal stripping.
- Rotary instruments or saws should be used under copious saline irrigation to prevent thermal damage of the bone.
- Osteotomy cuts should be 3 to 5 mm away from the apices of the teeth.
- Osteotomized fragments should be approximated in class I canine and molar relation (ideal).
- Bone grafts should be used if bone defect is created.
- Short term immobilization to prevent movement of osteotomy site.
- Postsurgical care includes balance of fluid intake and output, control of infection, edema and pain.
- Maintenance of oral hygiene.
- Regular follow-up.

Box 25.2: Surgical procedures

Maxillary procedures
Subapical osteotomies
- Anterior
- Posterior

Le Fort I osteotomy with modifications
Le Fort II osteotomy
Le Fort III osteotomy
Mandibular procedures
- Body procedures
  - Body osteotomy
  - Genioplasty
  - Inferior border osteotomy
- Ramus procedures
  - Sagittal split osteotomy
  - Intra oral vertical ramal osteotomy (IVRO)
  - C osteotomy
  - Subsigmoid osteotomy
  - Condylectomy
- New techniques
  Mid facial and mandibular distraction osteosynthesis using Ilizarov's technique.

OPERATIVE PROCEDURES

Maxillary Osteotomies

The Le Fort I osteotomy, anterior subapical osteotomies, and posterior subapical osteotomies are commonly performed in maxilla and Le Fort II and Le Fort III osteotomies are done in cases with severe mid facial hypoplasia. According to the clinical situation modifications can be done in these procedures and these can be combined with other procedures also.

Le Fort I Osteotomy

This is the most versatile procedure used to correct the deformities of maxilla in all planes and with low complication rate. The maxilla may be mobilized and repositioned and its survival continues as long as the mobilized maxilla remains attached to a broad soft tissue pedicle. Even if the maxilla is segmented in several pieces, healing will occur as long as the vascular pedicle is maintained. The necrosis occurs when the vascular pedicles are damaged or compromised (Figs 25.7 and 25.8).

Indications

- It is used most commonly in such deformities coexist in multiple planes.
- Shortening of maxilla, especially at premolar extraction sites, is possible and was commonly performed until awareness of the tendency to flatten the upper lip was recognized.
- Superior repositioning of the maxilla was noted to increase the stability of anterior open bite and offered significant cosmetic benefits, especially in long faced patients.
- Inferior repositioning and widening of maxilla are also possible.
- Three dimensional repositioning of the maxilla is possible, but this requires that the maxilla be segmented.
- In all cases of apertognathia, Le Fort I osteotomy should be given consideration because of stability issues.

Surgical Procedure

Before the surgical procedure the head of the patient is elevated approximately 10 degrees. Hypotensive anesthesia

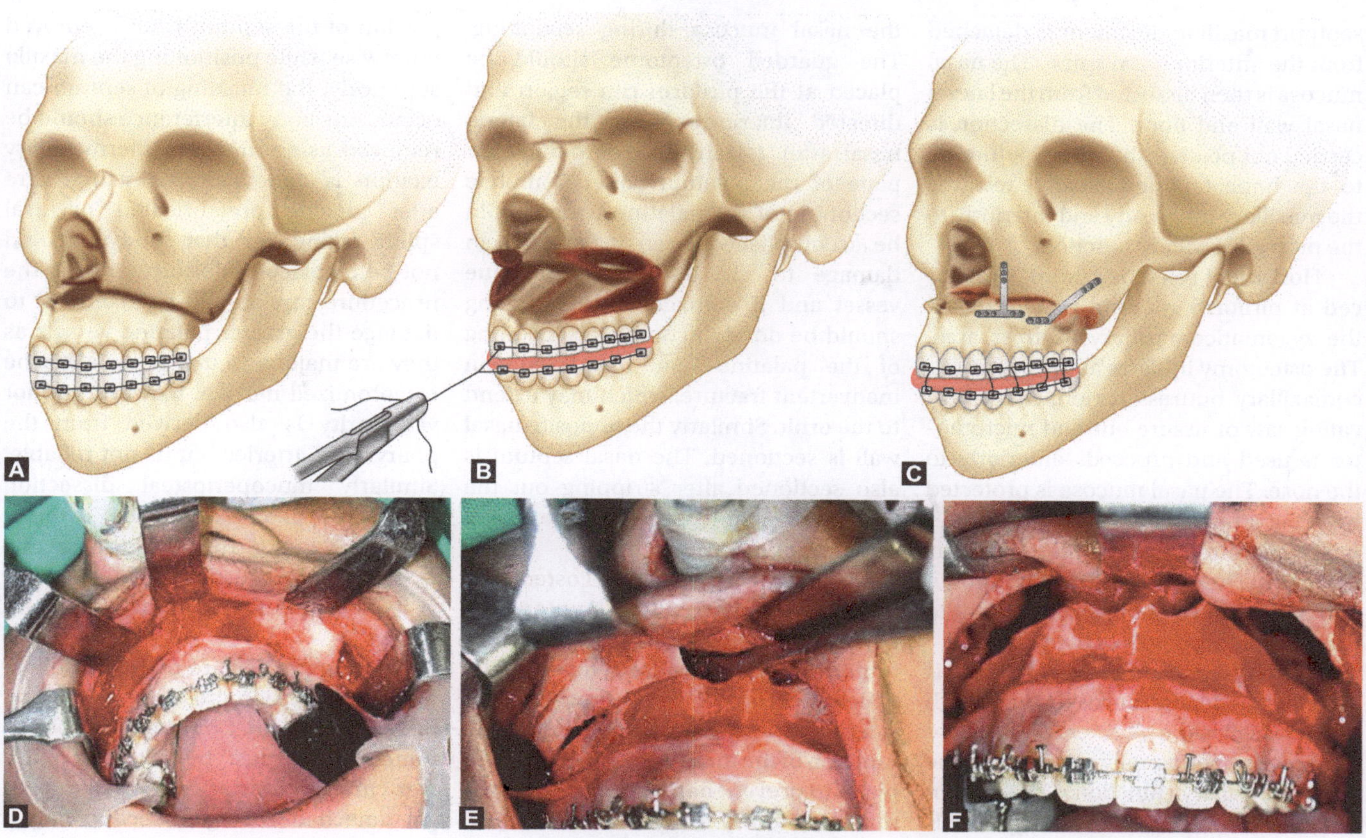

Figs 25.7A to F: Le Fort I osteotomy

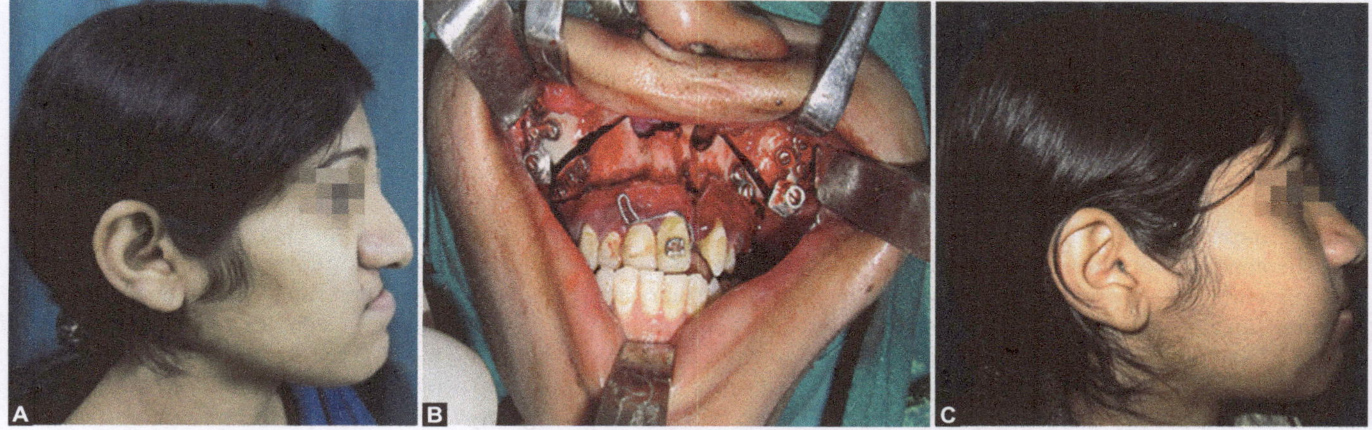

Figs 25.8A to C: Preoperative, intraoperative and postoperative photographs of a case treated with Le Fort I osteotomy

technique is preferred (systolic blood pressure of 90 mm of Hg), to reduce the blood loss during the surgery. A diluted solution of 2 percent lignocanine hydrochloride with 1:100,000 epinephrine is infiltrated into the buccal vestibule of the maxilla on either sides. Palatal infiltration is not adviced since it can compromise the palatel perfusion of blood to the maxilla.

Incision is placed high in the mucobuccal fold of the upper lip, extends from the zygomatic buttress region above the first molar to the midline. The incision is carried through the mucosa, muscle, and periosteum of the bone. Some surgeons do not take a continuous incision but, leave a band of tissue in the region of nasal aperture in the midline to maintain additional vascular pedicle to maxilla. The maxilla is exposed by reflecting the tissue subperiosteally from the buttress region to the anterior nasal spine. The subperiosteal dissection carried upto the infraorbital rim taking care not to damage the infraorbital nerve. The anterior nasal spine and piriform rim are identified and septopremaxillary ligament is detached from the anterior nasal spine. The nasal mucosa is then dissected from the lateral nasal wall and floor. The dissection is carried out posteriorly, strictly adhering to the bone (subperiosteally) towards the maxillary tuberosity and inferiorly to the pterygomaxillary junction.

Horizontal reference points are placed at piriform aperture region and at the zygomaticomaxillary buttress area. The osteotomy initiates at the zygomaticomaxillary buttress region. A reciprocating saw or fissure bur and micromotor is used and proceeds anteriorly to the nose. The nasal mucosa is protected by using a periosteal elevator or copper malleable retractor while cutting the piriform rim. The cut should be made about 3 to 5 mm above the apex of the root to preserve blood supply of the teeth.

The posterolateral wall of the maxilla is sectioned under the mucosal tunnels with direct visualization. A reverse L retractor is placed subperiosteally extending to the pterygomaxillary junction. The osteotomy cut decends inferiorly as it proceeds posteriorly from the buttress region to the junction of the maxilla and the pterygoid plate. This minimizes the risk of damaging the internal maxillary artery or any of its terminal branches as they descend from the pterygopalatine fossa, after the posterior wall is cut, saw is reversed so that the blade is placed into the maxillary sinus and osteotomy is completed from the sinus to the outside.

If the impacted third molar is present, the osteotomy is not altered and third molar is removed after maxilla is down fractured. Ideally the third molars are extracted 2 to 3 months prior to the surgery so that the cuts can be taken more precisely. When the bone cuts are complete the region is packed with moistened gauze, soaked in the solution of saline and adrenaline in a dilution of 1:200000. The same steps are repeated on the opposite side from the incision onwards.

The lateral wall of the nasal cavity is to be sectioned next. A periosteal elevator or copper malleable retractor is placed subperiosteally on the medial aspect of the lateral wall of the nose. This protects the nasal mucosa during sectioning. The guarded osteotome should be placed at the piriform rim region and directed inferiorly along the lateral nasal wall toward the perpendicular plate of the palatine bone. Complete sectioning of the palatine bone should be accomplished, even if it results in damage to the descending palatine vessel and if damage occurs packing should be done. Incomplete sectioning of the palatine bone can result in inadvertent fracture, which may extend to the orbit. Similarly the opposite nasal wall is sectioned. The nasal septum is also sectioned after stripping out the mucoperiosteum on either side, using double guarded osteotomes.

The final step in Le Fort I osteotomy is separation of maxilla from pterygoid plates. Pterygoid chisel or curved osteotome is used to separate the maxilla, which is directed anteromedially and inferiorly at the lowest part of the junction of the maxilla and the pterygoid plate, to prevent damage to the internal maxillary artery or its branches. Index finger is placed at the hamular notch on the palate which helps to direct and orient the cut. The osteotome is malleted to achieve bony separation which can be felt by placing the index finger in the palatal region. On the opposite side same step is repeated. Nowadays, the classical disjunction of maxilla and pterygoid plates is not done. The cut is place vertically in the region of the maxillary tuberosity and the disjuction is done at the tuberosity, i.e. anterior to the pterygomaxillary junction. It is considered safe and as effective as the classical pterygoid disjuction. Maxilla is down fractured after all the bony cuts are over. The maxilla is gently depressed at the anterior aspect with hand pressure. As the maxilla moved downwards and if any attachment of nasal soft tissues are present, they should be dissected free. Excess bone from the nasal crest, vomer, medial wall of maxillary sinus, etc. is removed by using rongeur forceps and burs. If superior repositioning is planned anterior nasal spine is removed. The portion of the septum is also removed otherwise while positioning the maxilla superiorly, the buckling of septum can occur. Any bony interference should be removed using rongeur. Intermaxillary fixation is done using 26-gauge wire after placing prefabricated occlusal splint, taking care that condyle should not be displaced inferiorly. During the procedure care should be taken not to damage the greater palatine vessels as they are major vascular pedicle for the osteotomized maxilla. However, minor vascularity is also derived from the pharyngeal arteries but its not reliable. Similarly mucoperiosteal dissection over the palate should be avoided (Figs 25.9 and 25.10). After the maxilla is brought in the desired position, it is fixed with suitable mini plates and screws.

During the closure of any maxillary degloving incision crossing the midline taken for Le Fort I or subapical osteotomies, care must be taken to place alar cinch sutures as the alar cartilages get detached during dissection and if the alar cinching is not done flaring of the nose can result. Secondly, lip lengthening can also be done while closing these incisions by doing simple V-Y closure in the midline.

High Le Fort I Osteotomy

The high Le Fort I osteotomy is indicated for correction of the maxillary deficiency along with paranasal hypoplasia. The osteotomy cut starts at the upper level at the lateral rim of pyriform aperture and then in a step like manner descends to the zygomaticomaxillary buttress area over the anterior surface of the maxilla. Rest of the procedure remains same as the classical Le Fort I osteotomy.

Le Fort II Osteotomy

Severe paranasal hypoplasia extending to the infraorbital rims necessitates a Le Fort II osteotomy as described: Henderson and Jackson (1973), but it should be understood that this is not a common occurrence.

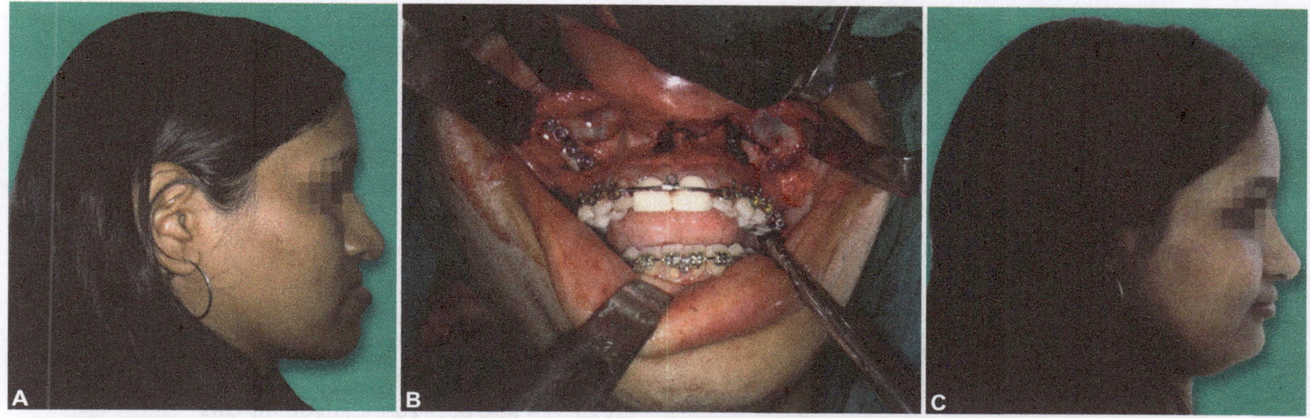

Figs 25.9A to C: Case of maxillary retrusion treated with Le Fort I advancement: (A) Preoperative photograph; (B) Intraoperative photograph; (C) Postoperative photograph

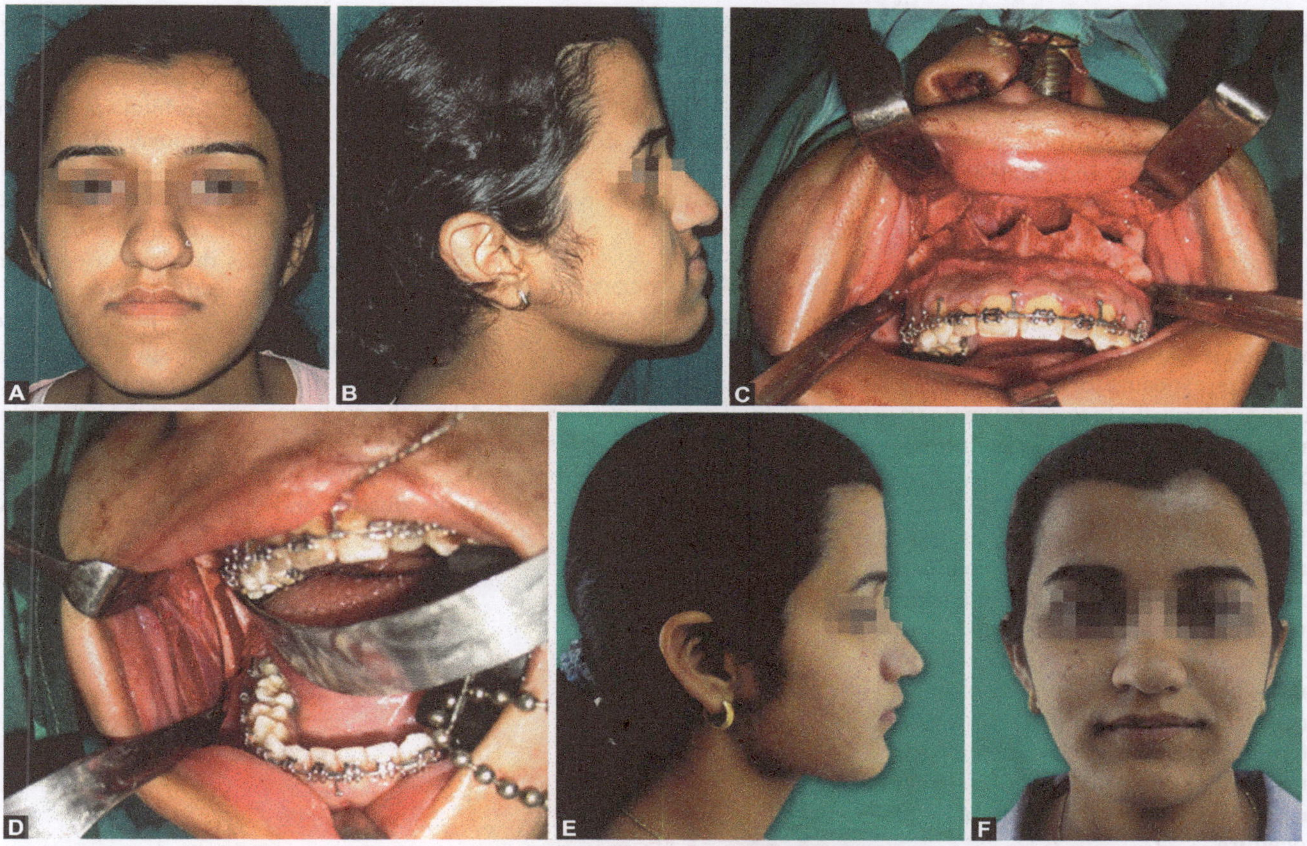

Figs 25.10A to F: Case of maxillary hypoplasia with mandibular prognathism treated with mandibular set back by BSSO and maxillary advancement by Le Fort I osteotomy. (Bijaw surgery) (A and B) Preoperative photographs; (C and D) Osteotomy cuts; (E and F) Postoperative photographs

Exposure is gained through a bicoronal incision or bilateral paranasal incisions (Figs 25.11A and B). The former is a more extensive procedure, possibly entailing medial canthal disruption; the latter results in potentially visible external scar. Intraoral access was also described for Le Fort II osteotomy (Figs 25.12A and B).

The medial orbital floor, infraorbital rim, medial orbital wall, and lacrimal sac are exposed in a subperiosteal plane. Medial canthal tendons are left undisturbed. An osteotomy is made with a side-cutting bur down the medial orbital wall behind the lacrimal groove. It is extended medially to the infraorbital nerve area through the orbital floor, over

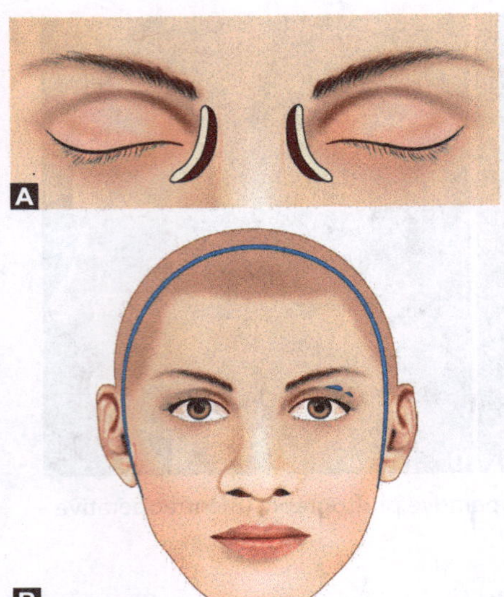

Figs 25.11A and B: (A) Paranasal access incision; (B) Bicoronal incision

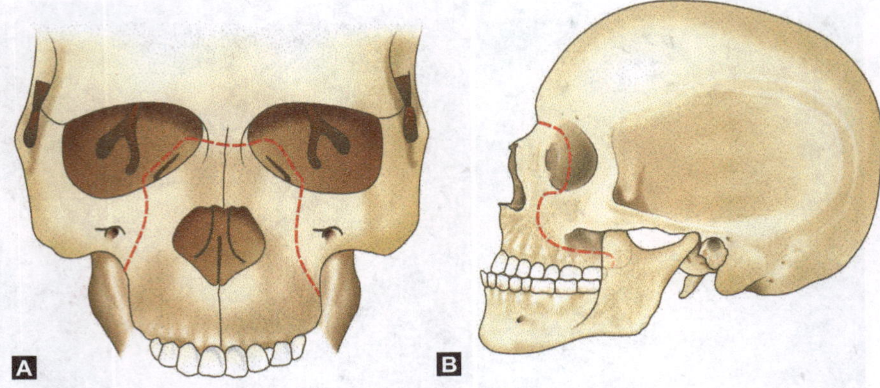

Figs 25.12A and B: Le Fort II osteotomy cuts

the anterior maxilla, and caudally as far as possible. Aufricht retractor is inserted from one paranasal incision to the other to retract the dorsal nasal skin, and the osteotomies are connected to the nasal dorsum using a reciprocating saw. Any unconnected areas are cut with a fine osteotome; exposure for the osteotomies is improved with the bicoronal approach. Through a posterior buccal sulcus incision, osteotomy cuts are located and are extended across the maxillary tuberosities till the pterygomaxillary fissures. Maxillary tuberosities are separated from the pterygoid plates with a curved osteotome. To complete the osteotomy, a curved osteotome is placed in transverse cut across the nasofrontal junction and is driven posteriorly and inferiorly to separate the vomer from the anterior skull base. Mobilization of the maxilla is achieved as in the Le Fort I procedure.

The infraorbital rim defects are accurately bone grafted through the paranasal incisions. Anterior osteotomy sites are filled with inlay and onlay bone grafts using the buccal sulcus approach. Split cranial bone grafts are readily available when a coronal approach is used (Jackson, Pellett and Smith, 1983). Wire or multiple screws and miniplates placed from the frontal bone to the nasal skeleton provide secure fixation of the central maxilla to the skull. If nasal height is lacking, a split cranial bone graft can be placed beneath the dorsal nasal skin and secured with two screws or wire to provide a cantilever type of dorsal graft.

Le Fort III Advancement Osteotomy (Figs 25.13A and B)

Gillies and Harrison (1950–51) reported the first high maxillary (a modified Le Fort III) osteotomy in a patient with craniofacial dysostosis. Through external incisions they performed transverse osteotomies that separated the nasal bones from the frontal bones. Osteotomy of the orbital floor was placed immediately within the infraorbital margin and extended across the floor of the orbit to the lateral orbital wall anterior to the lacrimal groove. Osteotomies were also performed through frontal processes of the maxilla to diminish the width of the nose. Temporal process of the zygoma was divided on each side. An osteotome was then introduced into the pterygomaxillary junction. Anterior to the greater palatine foramen, an incision was made transversely across the mucoperiosteum of the hard palate, extending laterally and posterior to the alveolar ridge. The hard palate was divided and the line of osteotomy was

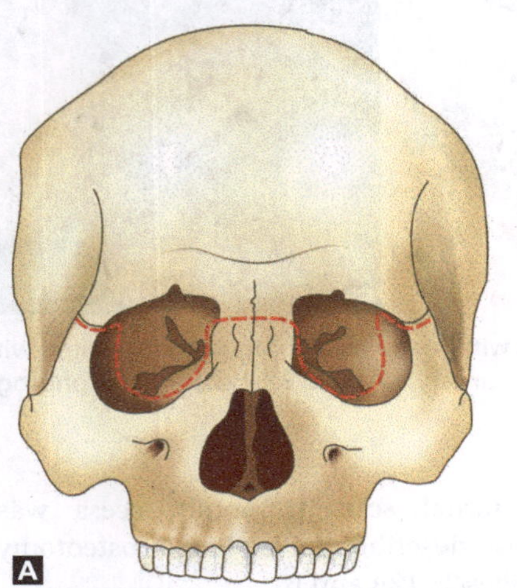

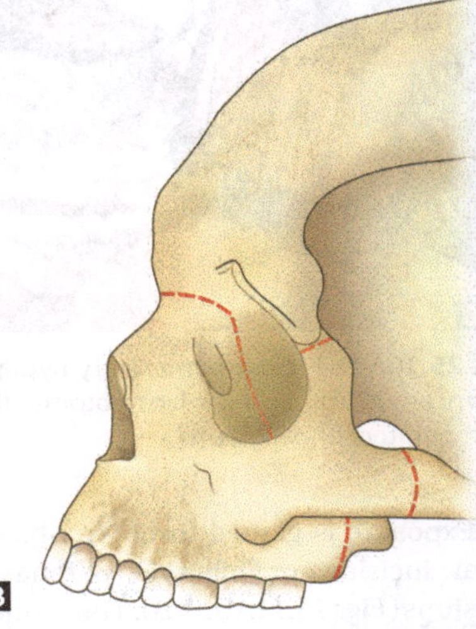

Figs 25.13A and B: Le Fort III osteotomy cuts for total advancement of zygomatic complex

rejoined at the pterygomaxillary junction. In this way, spatial relationships of the soft palate were undisturbed. The operation was completed by severing the septum with a pair of large scissors introduced through the osteotomy line at the root of the nose. Intermaxillary fixation was established.

Segmental Maxillary Osteotomy

Indications

- Transverse discrepancies between the dental arches
- Vertical steps in the maxillary occlusal plane
- Space remaining in the maxillary arch.

Single Tooth Osteotomy

Indications

- Tooth malposition
- Dental ankylosis
- For closure of diastema.

Advantages

- Treatment time is reduced
- Dental relapse is less.

Disadvantages

- Chances of injury to adjacent teeth
- Periodontal compromise of treated tooth
- Chances of devitalization of the teeth.

Surgical Procedure

A horizontal incision is given in the vestibule and a mucoperiosteal flap is reflected upto the attached gingival to preserve the blood supply. The anterior nasal spine and pyriform rim/aperture of the nose are to be exposed.

If the diastema is present at more than one place then multiple vertical interdental incision can be taken.

Osteotomy cut is then made with the bur in the vertical direction in the labial cortex from the nasal floor to the level of the attached gingival. 5 mm above the apices of the teeth, so that the vitality of the pulp is maintained. Then cut extended up to the palatal cortex. Then with the help of the fine osteotome alveolar crest bone is sectioned. Separate horizontal cut can be made if sufficient bone is present in between the nasal floor and the root apex. The segment is then mobilized into the correct position and then splint is placed and closure done.

Anterior Maxillary Osteotomy

Indications

Excess in vertical and/or anteroposterior dimension of maxillary alveolar process in patients with acceptable posterior occlusion (Figs 25.14 and 25.15).

The most common indication is correction of bimaxillary protrusion when it is combined with mandibular subapical osteotomy.

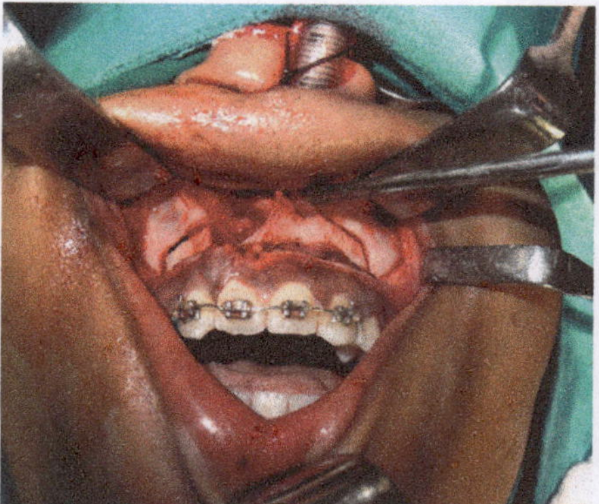

Fig. 25.14: Segmental osteotomy cut

Other indications include:

- For correction of marked protrusion of maxillary teeth
- Correction of anterior open bite
- To correct anterior teeth proclination
- When tooth movement with orthodontic therapy is not indicated.

In 1921 Cohn-Stock first reported segmental maxillary osteotomy procedure. Wassmund in 1935 and Wunderer in 1962 modified the procedure which were widely accepted and used till today.

Wassmund Technique

After infiltration with lignocaine 1:100,000 epinephrine, a vertical incision is given between canine and first premolar extending to the nasal floor and the mucoperiosteum is reflected. The first premolar is extracted if required and the palatal mucosa is reflected by

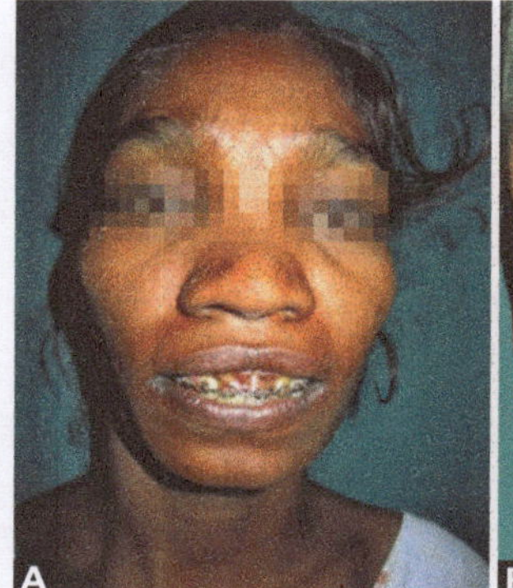

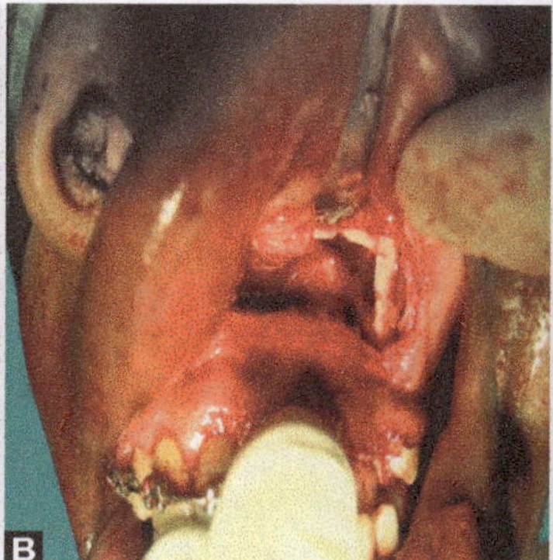

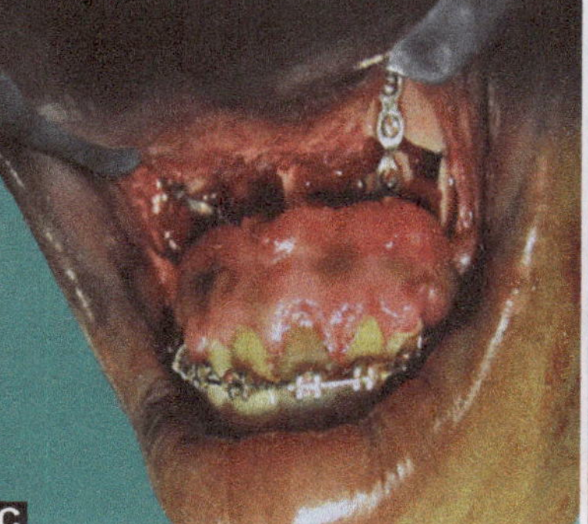

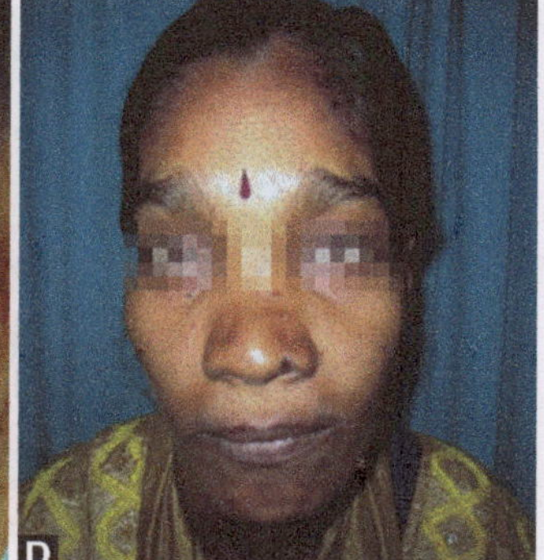

Figs 25.15A to D: A case of anterior maxillary osteotomy showing anterior osteotomy cuts with postoperative results: (A) preoperative photograph; (B) Intraoperative photograph showing down fracture of the osteotomized segment; (C) Osteotomy segment fixed in superior and posterior position; (D) Postoperative photograph

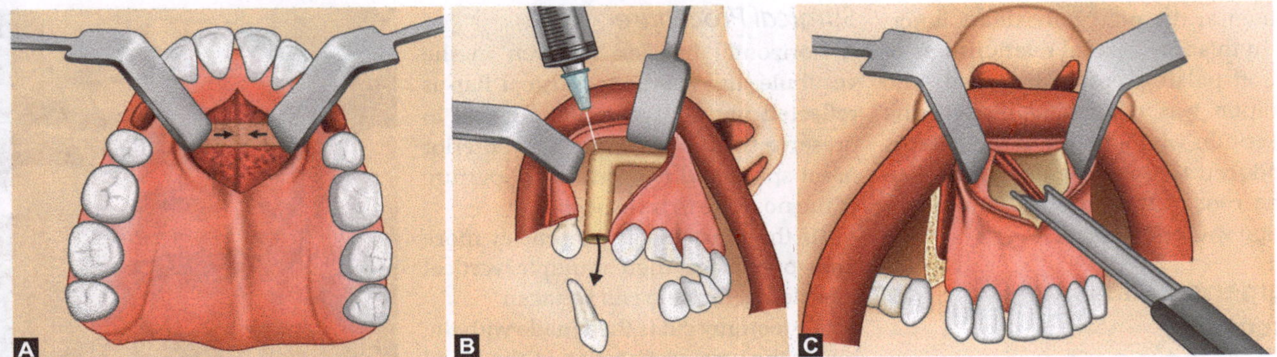

Figs 25.16A to C: (A) Midpalatine split; (B) Buccal cut through canine and premolar; (C) Vertical incision given at anterior nasal spine

tunneling past midline. Now with the help of the bur or reciprocating saw and under copious saline irrigation buccal cut is made in the vertical direction 5 mm above the apex of the canine and turned medially at the level of pyriform rim region. Then through the mid palatine incision in the anteroposterior direction (Figs 25.16A to C), the palatal bone is removed from the alveolus to the midline taking care not to damage the palatine soft tissues. Similar procedure is repeated on the opposite side. A vertical incision is then given over the anterior nasal spine and the mucoperiosteum is reflected, then with the help of nasal osteotome septum is separated from the anterior maxillary segment.

This procedure can be completed without taking the vertical labial incision and palatal incision, as described in the original technique. A degloving incision is taken in the labial vestibule and the gingiva over the premolar can be tunnelled inferiorly both, labially and palatally. The premolar is extracted and then the vertical osteotomy cuts can be placed below the tunnelled gingiva. The operator keeps a finger palatally while taking vertical and horizontal cuts and feels the bur or osteotome movement. This avoids injury to the palatal pedicle. This technique provides additional blood supply to the osteotomized maxillary segment through the labial pedicle (*see* Fig. 25.14).

After completion of all the osteotomies, the anterior maxillary dento-osseous segment can be repositioned and the prefabricated occlusal splint is fitted to the dental component. Closure done with 3-0 vicryl.

Wunderer Technique

The labial osteotomy procedure is similar to the Wassmund technique. The advantage of this technique is that it provides good access to the palate region. This osteotomy technique relies on the intact buccal pedicle for its blood supply (Figs 25.17A to C).

After the buccal surgical procedure the palatal surgical procedure is started by giving the transverse incision at the planned osteotomy site. The soft tissue reflection is done posteriorly behind the planned osteotomy site. The osteotomy procedure is then performed with the help of the saw or bur under copious saline irrigation. After the completion of the osteotomy cuts, osteotomy segment is mobilized and separated from the nasal septum. The segment is then positioned after placing the prefabricated occlusal splint and closure done with 3-0 vicryl.

Posterior Maxillary Osteotomy

Schuchardt in 1959 described this procedure for the correction of open-bite

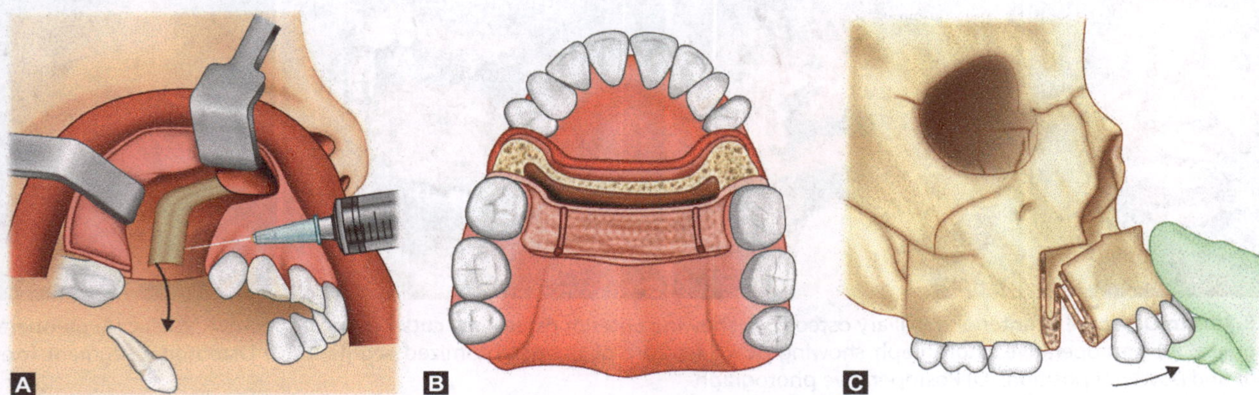

Figs 25.17A to C: (A) Buccal osteotomy cut; (B) Transverse palatal cut; (C) Down fracture with separation at nasal septum

deformities. Bilateral osteotomies can be performed at a time to correct the deformities.

Indications

- Posterior maxillary alveolar hyperplasia
- Total maxillary hyperplasia (when combined with AMO)
- Posterior open bite
- Transverse excess or deficiency
- Distal repositioning of the posterior maxillary alveolar fragment
- Spacing in the dentition.

Surgical Technique

The buccal vestibular incision is given from canine to the second molar region below the zygomatic buttress. The mucoperiosteal flap tunneling is done superiorly and inferiorly. The lateral maxillary wall and region posterior to the pterygoid plates is exposed (Fig. 25.18).

The horizontal osteotomy cut is started 5 mm above apices of the posterior teeth using bur or saw from the location of the anterior vertical osteotomy to the maxillary tuberosity. The vertical cut is done either between the adjoining teeth (interdentally) or if preplanned then in the extraction socket region. About 1 mm of bone support is kept along the root surfaces of the adjacent teeth in order to prevent the formation of a periodontal defect. Vertical and horizontal cuts are completed through the palatal cortex by keeping the index finger on the palate to prevent the soft tissue damage. A small curved osteotome is used to separate the entire posterior segment from the pterygomaxillary junction and downfractured it, which is pedicled on the palatal mucosa. Now under the direct vision palatal bone can be removed (Fig. 25.19).

After completion of all the osteotomy the segment is well mobilized, the prefabricated splint is fitted and wired to the teeth. If large gap is to be created at the osteotomy site, then bone grafts are used.

Complications

- Loss of vitality of teeth
- Periodontal defect of teeth adjacent to vertical osteotomy site
- Infection
- Wound dehiscence
- Necrosis of segment
- Relapse.

Variations of Posterior Segmental Maxillary Osteotomy

In 1970, Kufner made only a horizontal incision above the apices of the involved teeth, gaining access to the palatal aspect (Figs 25.20A and B).

Perko in 1972 and later Bell in 1975 made a hockey stick incision along the midline of the palate as far forward as the incisive papilla and then carried it out laterally anterior to the proposed osteotomy site (Figs 25.21A to C).

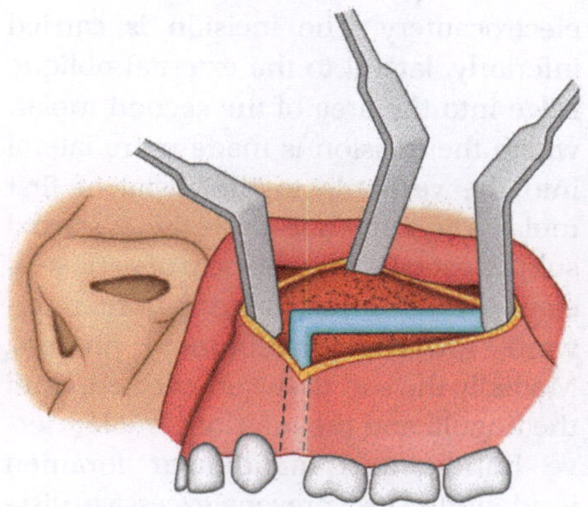

Fig. 25.18: Limited buccal incision with combined horizontal and anterior vertical osteotomies

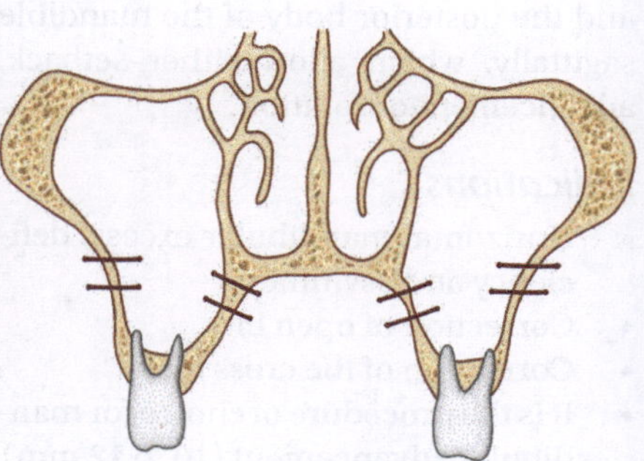

Fig. 25.19: Coronal view indicating bone and cuts

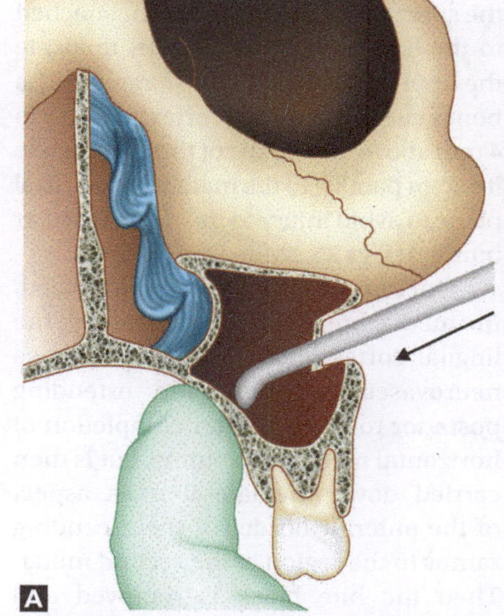

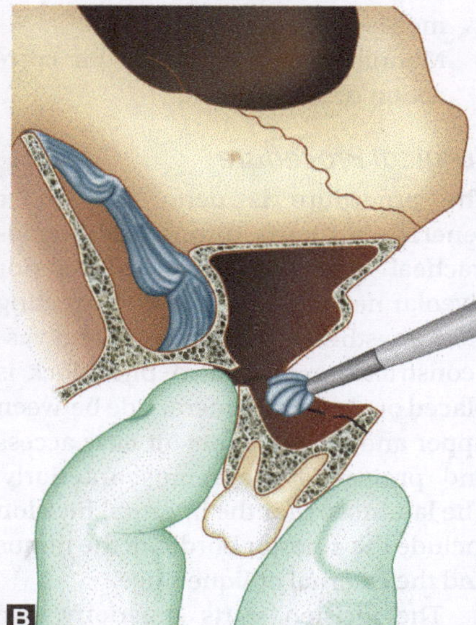

Figs 25.20A and B: (A) Coronal view—Transantral palatal osteotomy via chisel following lateral sinus wall osteotomy; (B) Transantral palatal osteotomy trimming of bone segment

Sagittal Split Osteotomy

The sagittal split osteotomy (SSO) of the ramus of the mandible was described by Obwegessor. Later the technique was modified by his student Dal Pont to make it more versatile. The SSO is one of the most commonly practiced surgical procedures to correct the mandibular deformities due to its versatility.

Bilateral Sagittal Split Osteotomy (BSSO)

It is the surgical procedure for the correction of lower jaw deformities. This is

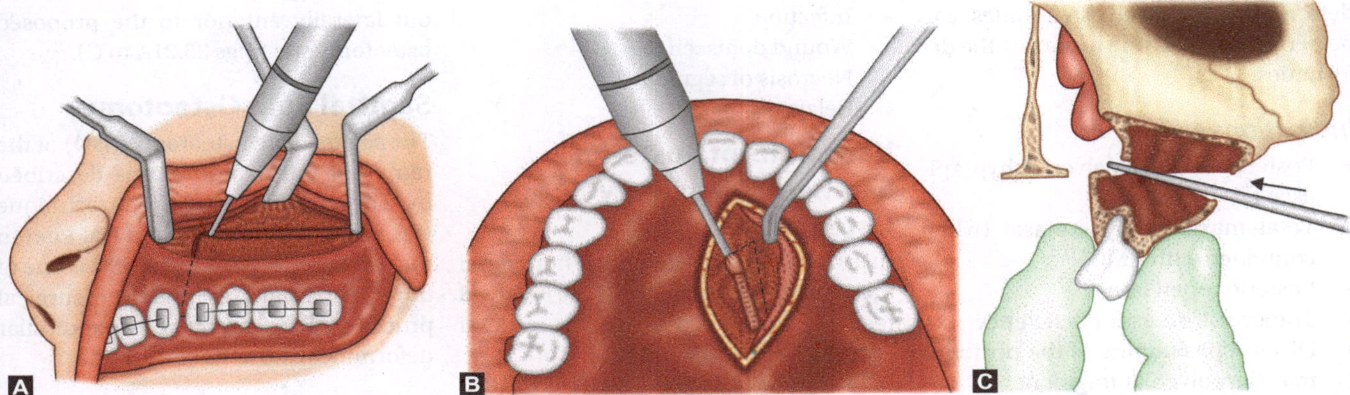

Figs 25.21A to C: (A) Limited buccal incision with combined horizontal and vertical osteotomies; (B) Palatal incision located medial to planned lateral palatal osteotomy; (C) Coronal view: bone cuts with transantral medial nasal wall osteotomy

accomplished through transoral incision. The osteotomy splits the ramus and the posterior body of the mandible sagittally, which allow either setback, advancement or rotation.

Indications

- Horizontal mandibular excess, deficiency and asymmetry
- Correction of open bite
- Correction of the cross bite
- It is the procedure of choice for mandibular advancement (10 to 12 mm)
- Excellent operation for a mandibular setback of small to moderate magnitude (7 to 8 mm)
- Procedure of choice for minor asymmetries.
- Mandibular advancement for correction of sleep apnea.

Surgical Procedure

The procedure is performed under general anesthesia through nasoendotracheal intubation. Bilateral inferior alveolar nerve blocks with a long acting local anesthetic (Bupivacaine) and vasoconstrictor are given. A bite block is placed on the contralateral side between upper and lower molars for easy access and projecting the ramus anteriorly. The landmarks for the intraoral incision include the anterior border of the ramus and the external oblique ridge.

The incision starts superiorly, two thirds up the anterior border of the ramus over the bone, an incision is made through mucosa with a sharp scalpel or electrocautery. The incision is carried inferiorly, lateral to the external oblique ridge into the area of the second molar, where the incision is made more lateral into the vestibule to the distal of first molar. The soft tissue dissection is started subperiosteally with the help of periosteal elevator, along the anterior border upward, towards the coronoid process. Medially the soft tissue is reflected, until the lingula and the inferior alveolar nerve bundle and mandibular foramen is identified (to prevent excessive dissection and easy identification of the foramen, a blunt nerver hook can be passed along the bone and hooked around the neurovascular bundle and the sphenomandibular ligament attached to the lingula of the mandible, to locate the level of the mandibular foramen. The boney cut on the medial cortex is taken 3 to 4 mm above the handle of the probe while it is kept parallel to the madibular occlusal plane to avoid injury to the neurovascular bundle) (Figs 25.22A to D).

Once the lingula has been visualized, the medial bone cut is made through the lingual cortex about 3 to 4 mm above neurovascular bundle and extending posterior to lingula. After completion of horizontal medial osteotomy, cut is then carried down the lateral most aspect of the anterior border of the ascending ramus to the region of the second molar. Then the bite block is removed and dissection is carried along the ascending ramus, inferiorly and laterally. For advancement vertical cut is placed in the first molar or premolar region to ensure good overlap during advancement and for setback procedures, the vertical osteotomy cut is placed lateral to second molar. The vertical cut is completed through the lateral cortex only. The cut extends through both the cortical plates at the inferior border of the mandible. (Taken circumferentially around the inferior border keeping the channel retractor at the inferior border to retract the soft tissue and facial artery away from the bone). The bony cuts are checked for completeness with osteotome, the segments are separated with Smith's bone spreader. The two beaks of the spreader are on the buccal side and single third beak is on the lingual side to prevent the fracture of the thinner buccal cortex due to pressure. While using the spreader controlled force should be used to gradually spread the bone. In case of excessive resistance the cortical cuts should be rechecked for completeness. A spatula osteotome can be used which is gently tapped in the cancellous bone and intermittently rotated to separate the buccal and lingual cortices. The osteotome can be used in tandem with the spreader. Some surgeons do not prefer to use the osteotome as it may traumatize the inferior alveolar nerve. The bone is spread gentally and the neurovascular bundle is visualized as the bone is spreading. This is the best method of avoiding trauma it. Usually after the proper cut the neurovascular bundle lies in the distal segment but

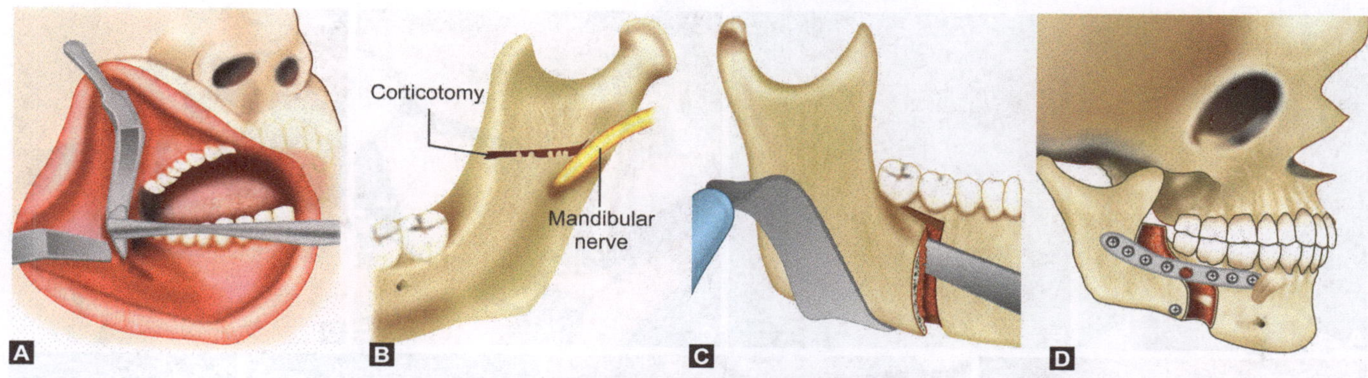

Figs 25.22A to D: Sagittal split osteotomy

occasionally it may be seen clinging to the proximal segment, in such cases it should be carefully separated from the bone. The same procedure is repeated on other side (Figs 25.23 and 25.24).

After the bone is spread, the impacted third molars, if present, should be removed. It is preferable that the impacted third molars should be electively removed 3 to 4 months before the surgery to ensure proper bony healing so that the osteotomy cuts are placed properly and there is no hindrance due to the impacted third molars.

For the setback procedure, the distal fragment is pushed back, there will be overlap of the buccal cortex of proximal fragment in the molar region. The excess bone on the proximal fragment is cut off by taking another vertical cut on the buccal cortex, distal to previous cut. The fragments should be checked for proper approximation and fixation of fragments done by intraosseous wiring or lag screws or by bone plates. Care should be taken not to cause too much rotation of mandibular condyles as it may cause joint pain later. In case of advancement distal fragment is advanced and fixed into desired position and fixation is carried out using mini plate and screws. When the mandibular setback is done the mandibular tray gets reduced and the tongue is not accommodated. In such cases there is a possibility of the tongue getting pushed backwards causing enchroachment on the pharyngeal space and obstructing the air way or there can be tongue bite and due to the pressure there can be more relaspse. It is therefore recommended that if the tongue is large and is not properly accommodated in the reduced mandibular tray, a reduction glossectomy should be done (Figs 25.25A to C).

Advantages

- Transoral procedure well accepted by the patients.
- Mandibular augmentation in excess of 10 mm possible.
- Correction of obtuse gonial angle is possible during correction of skeletal class III deformities.

Complications

- Malpositioning of condyle leading to TMJ pain syndrome.
- Malocclusion, open bite
- Lateral shift
- Unfavorable splits (Bad split)
- Proximal segment fracture
- Distal fragment fracture
- Excessive inflammatory edema which may extend to the larynx and cause respiratory embarrassment
- Relapse following surgery. The chances are more if the amount of augmentation or set back is excessive or the surgery is attempted in the growing age before growth maturity.
- Injury to the inferior alveolar nerve (most common), rarely injury to the lingual nerve.
- TMJ dysfunction and hypomobility
- Hemorrhage/hematoma

Modification of Sagittal Split Osteotomy

Trauner and Obwegeser (1957) made horizontal cut just above the mandibular foramen on the mesial side of ramus. The vertical cut was taken down the anterior border of ramus of the mandible. An oblique cut was made through the lateral cortex towards angle of the jaw. It is a good technique for mandibular setback but had poor bone contact with mandibular advancement. Avascular necrosis of angle due to extensive

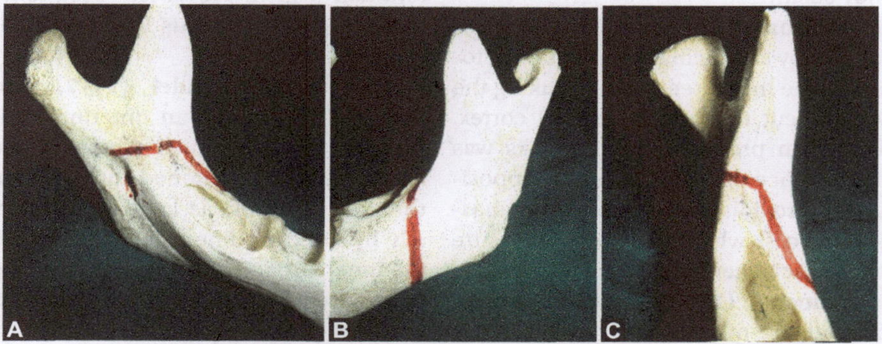

Figs 25.23A to C: Osteotomy cuts for SSO on mandible

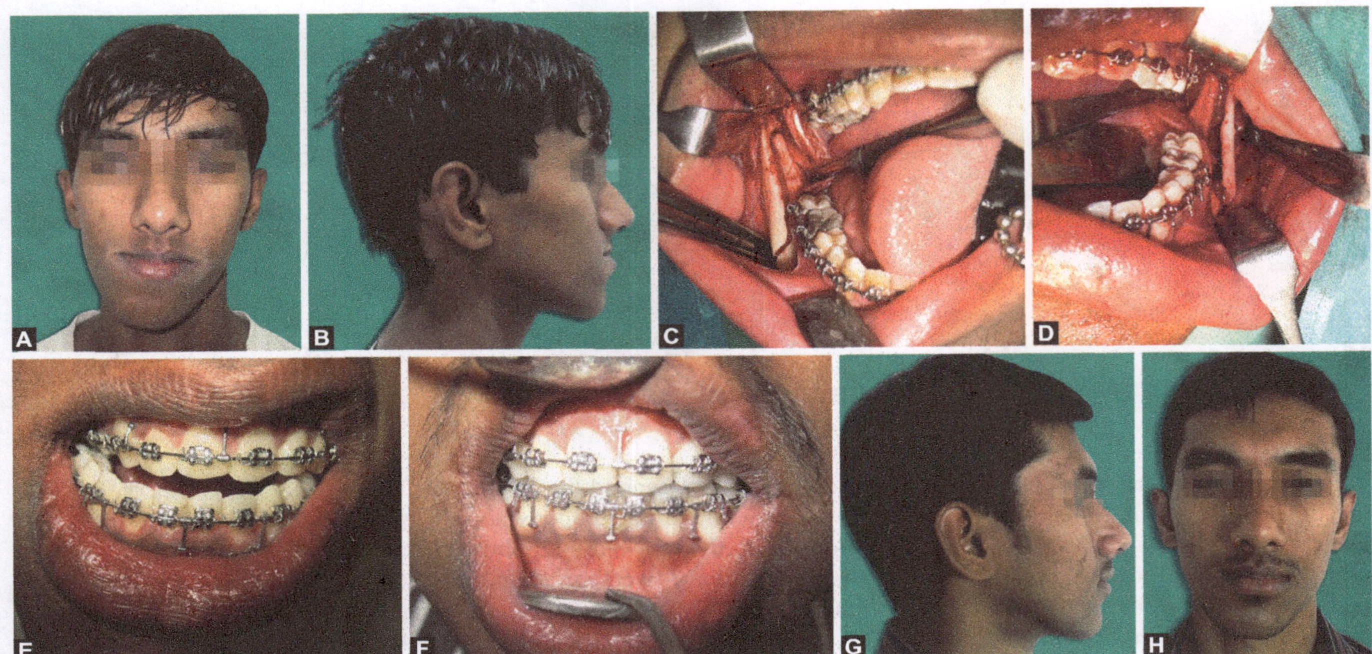

Figs 25.24A to H: Clinical case of BSSO for mandibular set back and midline correction: (A and B) Preoperative photographs; (C and D) Intraoperative photographs showing split; (E and F) Pre- and postoperative occlusion; (G and H) Postoperative photographs

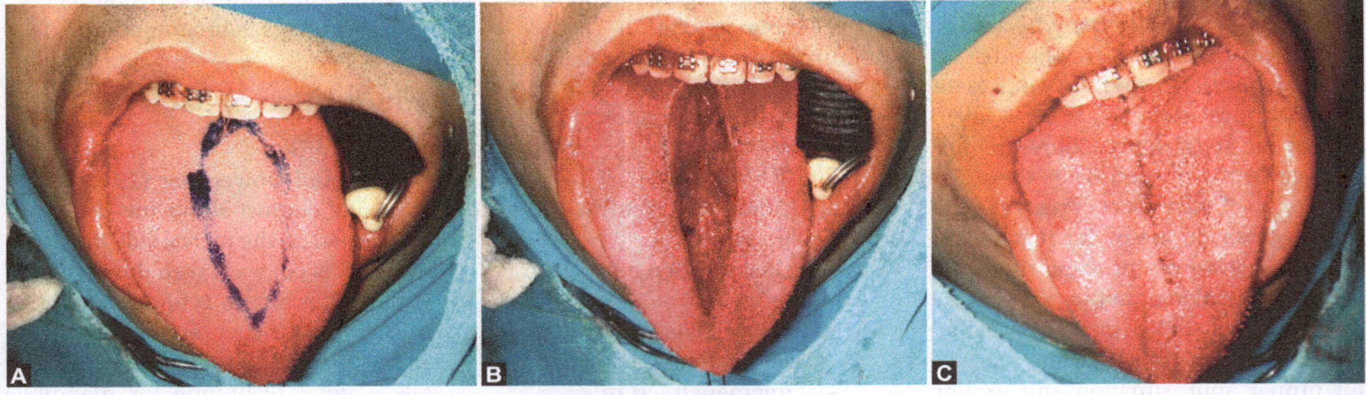

Figs 25.25A to C: Reduction glossectomy: (A) Marking of the incision; (B) Excision of the myomucosal tissue in an elliptical manner; (C) Closure of the defect with absorbable suture by placing inverted sutures

stripping of the pterygomasseteric sling may occur.

Dalpont (1961) modified the sagittal split by advancing the oblique cut towards the molar region and making the vertical cut through the lateral cortex. The main problem with setbacks was interference between main retropositioned proximal fragment and the mastoid process where occasional pressure on the facial nerve may occur as well.

Hunsuck (1968) shortened the cut through the medial cortex of the ramus by taking it only as far as the mandibular foramen which prevented occasional shattering of the ramus in mandibular setbacks.

Bell and Schendel (1977) and Epker (1978) made an anterior vertical cut, through which whole of the lower border is sectioned through and through. The split is kept more laterally by directing fine osteotomes down the inner surface of the lateral cortex to produce easier splitting. *Epker* included minimal stripping of the masseter muscle and limited medial dissection. These modifications decreased postoperative swelling, hemorrhage, and manipulation of the neurovascular bundle. Blood supply to the ramus is preserved as the need to strip the pterygomasseteric sling is eliminated and intraosseous ischemia and necrosis of the proximal segment were significantly reduced.

Spiessel (1976) advocated rigid internal fixation of the BSSO to promote healing, restore early function and attenuate relapse.

Inverted 'L' Osteotomy

It is described by Trauner and Obwegeser in 1957 as an intraoral procedure, but it can also be accomplished through submandibular incision. It is a versatile procedure to treat severe mandibular deformities. The inverted- L osteotomy is particularly well suited to secondary correction of proximal segment malrotation following sagittal split ramus osteotomy (SSRO), as well as simultaneous advancement and lengthening of the ramus in cases of severe ramus under development (e.g. Treacher Collins syndrome, Goldenhar's syndrome). It is best suited method for mandibular advancement.

Surgical Procedure

The ramus is approached by submandibular incision. The approximate length of the incision is 6 cm. The inferior border of the mandible is reached, care is taken to avoid damage to the marginal mandibular nerve. The dissection is further continued to expose the sigmoid notch by reflecting the masseter muscle. The vertical cut is made at least 7 mm anterior to posterior border of ramus upto the inferior border of angle of mandible to ensure that the cut is posterior to the mandibular foramen and to avoid cutting through it. Horizontal cut is made above the anticipated position of the inferior alveolar foramen. Once cuts are completed medial periosteum may have to be elevated from some of the distal fragment to allow its advancement. Similar procedure is repeated on other side and IMF is done. Next step depends on the type of mandibular movement. If the distal segment is set back, then proximal segment has to be overlapped laterally. If the mandibular advancement is done cancellous bone graft is packed in the gap between the proximal segment and the advanced distal segment (Fig. 25.26B). Fragments are secured with mini plates or lag screws and closure done in layers. Extraoral pressure dressing is maintained for 24 to 48 hours (Figs 25.26A and B).

C–Ramus Osteotomy

This technique was first described by Caldwell and colleagues in 1968.

Indications

The C osteotomy is preffered for treatment of horizontal mandibular deficiencies and to correct anterior open bite.

Surgical Procedure

Except the inferior horizontal cut in the C osteotomy as shown in Figures 25.27A and B, the surgical procedure for inverted L and C osteotomy is almost the same. Both the procedures are primarily indicated for mandibular advancement.

Intraoral Vertical Ramus Osteotomy

Indications

- In patients with horizontal mandibular excess in whom a good profile, arch and dental relationship can be obtained by retruding the intact mandibular arch.
- Mandibular asymmetry which requires largely rotational movement of one or both mandibular rami to achieve correction of deformity.
- To achieve vertical correction in the mandibular arch.
- To correct minor occlusal discrepanies resulting after isolated Le Fort I osteotomy.
- In patients with significant temporomandibular joint (TMJ) complaints.

Contraindications

- Advancement of the distal, tooth-bearing mandibular segment.
- Recent condylar fractures.

Surgical Procedure

This is the technique indicated for correction of the mandibular prognathism (Class III) the procedure can be done intraorally by taking an incision along the anterior border of the coronoid process extending from the tip to the molar area. The lateral side of the ramus is degloved completely by the sub periosteal dissection, detaching the masseter completely. The posterior border of the ramus and the sigmoid notch are identified. The soft tissue is retracted using channel retractors placed over the posterior border and the sigmoid notch. For performing this osteotomy procedure intraorally oscillating saw is mandatory. The ramus is osteotomised roughly 7 to 8 mm anterior

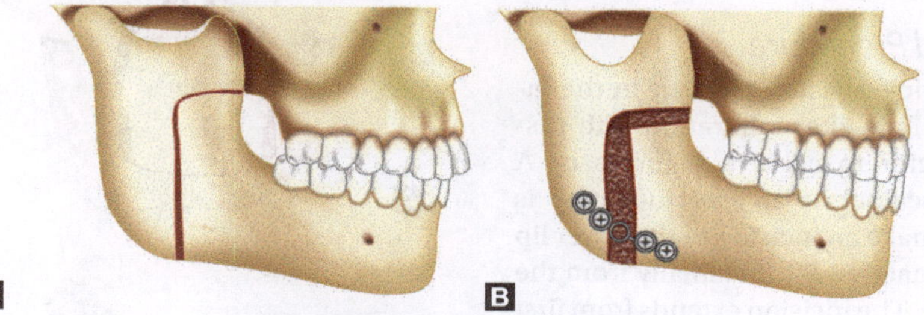

Figs 25.26A and B: Inverted L osteotomy

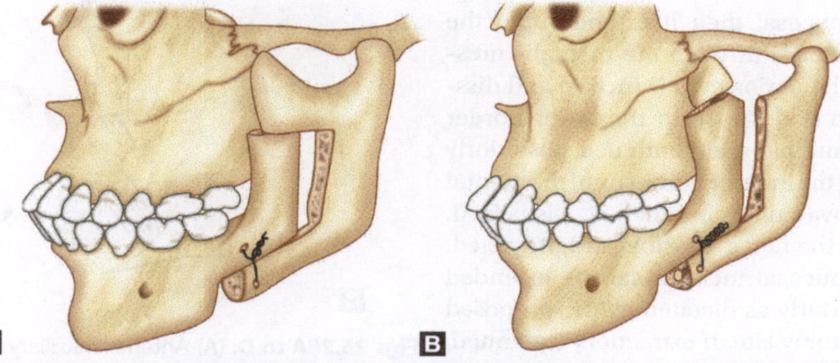

Figs 25.27A and B: Caldwell, Hayward and Lister (1968) presented 'vertical L osteotomy' which was later modified to conform to a 'C osteotomy'

to the posterior border of the ramus, to ensure that it is posterior to the mandibular foramen to avoid injury to the neurovascular bundle and extends vertically from the sigmoid notch to the inferior border. After the osteotomy, the distal mandibular segment is placed backward and medially while the proximal segment lies laterally. The distal and proximal segments need not be fixed rigidly but only IMF in desired position as guided by guiding splints for four weeks is enough. If the oscillating saw is not available, this procedure can be done extraorally through small extraoral Risdon's incision.

Complications

- Bleeding
- Inferior alveolar nerve injury
- Unfavorable osteotomy.

Anterior Mandibular Subapical Osteotomy

Indications

- Correction of mild anterior open bite.
- Correction of mandibular dentoalveolar proclination and dental arch asymmetry.
- Leveling an accentuated curve of spee.

Surgical Procedure

A degloving incision is given in the labial vestibule after infiltration with vasoconstrictor to achieve hemostasis. A No. 15 scalpel or an electrucautery is used to make an incision in the lower lip approximately 1.5 mm labially from the vestibule. The incision extends from first premolar to the first premolar of other side and is initially carried only through the mucosa, then it extends upto the periosteum through the mentalis muscle. The periosteum is incised and dissection is done up to the lower border of mandible and continued posteriorly along the inferior border until the mental neurovascular bundle is visualized. Once the nerve is visible and protected, the mucosal incision can be extended posteriorly as dictated by the proposed osteotomy site. If extraction is planned, it can be performed at this time.

If the vertical osteotomy cut is proximal to the mental foramen, it will be necessary to reposition and retract the mental nerve (Figs 25.28A to D). The osteotomy is accomplished with rotary instrument or with microsaws. After completing the vertical osteotomy cut, a horizontal cut is made, connecting the vertical cuts at their inferior extent. Horizontal osteotomy cut should be made atleast 5 mm below the apices of teeth to prevent devitalization.

The segment is mobilized by using an osteotome. A preformed surgical splint should be used to guide the segment into its predetermined position. All bony interferences should be removed. The segment is secured by transosseous wires or with miniplates. The incision is closed in two layers, i.e. the muscle and a mucosal layer and a pressure dressing is given externally.

Complications

- Loss of bone and/or teeth in the osteotomized segment
- Root damage and devitalization of the teeth if bone cuts are too close to roots
- Mental nerve damage
- Nonunion or malunion if segments are not properly fixed.

Total Mandibular Subapical Osteotomy

Hullihen in 1849, described a procedure similar to subapical osteotomy who

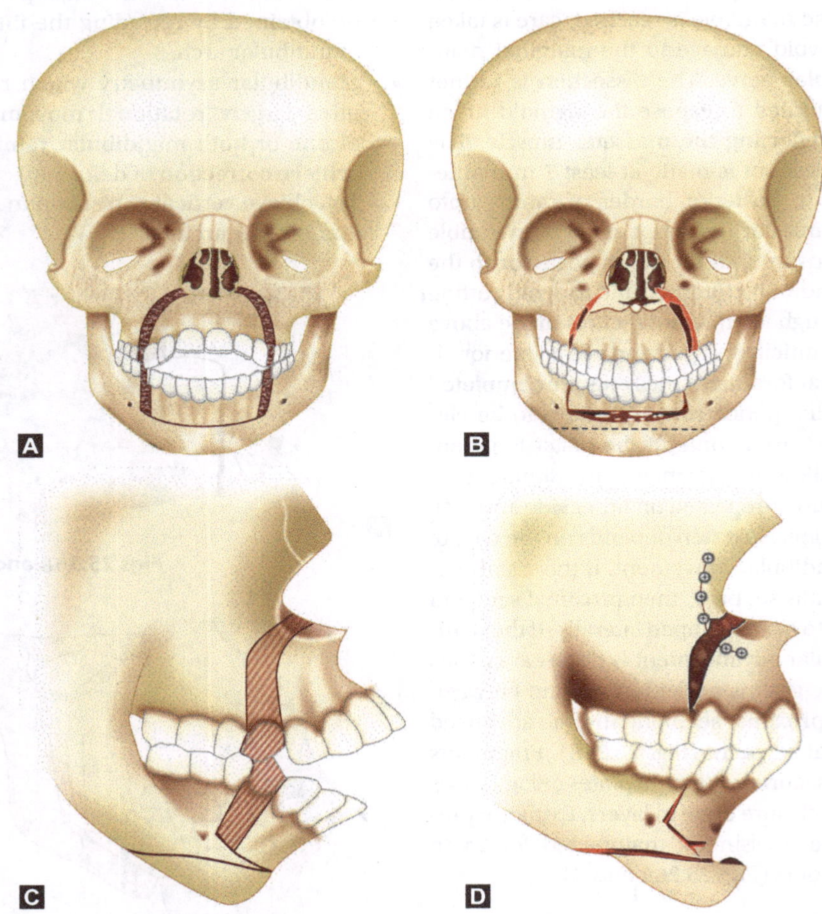

Figs 25.28A to D: (A) Anterior maxillary subapical ostetomy; (B and C) Anterior mandibular subapical osteotomy with genioplasty and (D) Final positioning of the osteotomized segments

used it to treat "elongation of the underjaw". Hofer and Kole described the modifications of the procedure. This is not performed routinely.

Indications

- Malocclusion caused by a mandibular dentoalveolar deformity with appropriately positioned maxillary and mandibular skeletal bases.
- It is used to reposition entire mandibular dentoalveolar segment anteriorly, posteriorly or superiorly.

Surgical Procedure

A circumvestibular incision is made from retromolar area of one side of mandible to other side; care is taken to incise mucosa and submucosa only. The mental neurovascular bundle is identified and skeletonized with blunt dissection to avoid damage. Anterior to neurovascular bundle, the incision is carried out into the anterior vestibule (as for a genioplasty). Dissection is then completed in the subperiosteal plane while protecting the mental neurovascular bundle (Figs 25.29A and B).

The buccal cortical bone above and below the neurovascular canal is cut with fissure bur, then removed with an osteotome. This cortical bone can be morselized and replaced in strategic locations later. Before beginning horizontal osteotomy, vertical reference marks are made anteriorly and posteriorly. The actual osteotomy site is marked by taking direct measurement from the occlusal plane. The horizontal osteotomy started from symphysis region and continued posterior to the last molar. Care must be taken when completing the horizontal osteotomy to prevent damage to the lingual vascular pedicle; this is accomplished by placing the guiding finger on the lingual side. The horizontal osteotomy is completed 0.5 cm or more from the apices of the teeth in order to preserve pulpal circulation.

A vertical osteotomy is performed through an extraction socket or between the adjacent teeth using bur, saw or osteotome. Care must be taken to prevent damage to lingual nerve. The buccal cut is then completed through only outer cortex and remainder of the lingual cortex adjacent to and below the bundle, is fractured with the osteotome.

Vertical Subsigmoid Osteotomy (VSO)

Caldwell–Letterman in 1954 first proposed this procedure through extraoral approach.

Indications

- It is limited to deformities requiring mandible to be setback for mandibular horizontal excess or to be rotated for mandibular asymmetry.
- Large mandibular setbacks of greater than 10 mm.

Surgical Procedure

Extraoral approach is used for VSO; however the procedure can also be accomplished intraorally. Submandibular or postramal incision is given; sharp and blunt dissection is used to reach the lower border of the mandible. Care is taken to avoid damage the marginal mandibular branch of the facial nerve. With the help of periosteal elevator periosteum is reflected and the ascending ramus, sigmoid notch and coronoid process are exposed. Mandible is pulled downwards with the help of the bone forceps applied at the angle of the mandible (Figs 25.30A and B).

The osteotomy cut is started from the sigmoid notch above the level of mandibular foramen through both the cortices. Then the cut is started from inferior border going up to the level of mandibular foramen, both the cuts then joined together. Care is taken to protect the medial tissues. Similar procedure is carried out on the opposite side. After that proximal fragments placed over distal fragments and tempory IMF is done. Decortication of the distal segment is carried out on the lateral aspect of the overlap area and the proximal segment on the medial aspect. The proximal segment is fixed laterally to the distal segment overlapping it with intraosseous wiring, lag screws or bone plates.

Mandibular Body Osteotomy

Blair in 1907 first described body osteotomy as an extraoral procedure. Later Dingman used a combination of intraoral and extraoral access with preservation of the inferior alveolar neurovascular and bone grafting to assist bony union. This was one of the earliest procedures used for mandibular prognathism. Since the advent of the ramus procedures the body osteotomy has lost popularity (Figs 25.31A to D).

Indications

- Mandibular setback
- Progenia correction

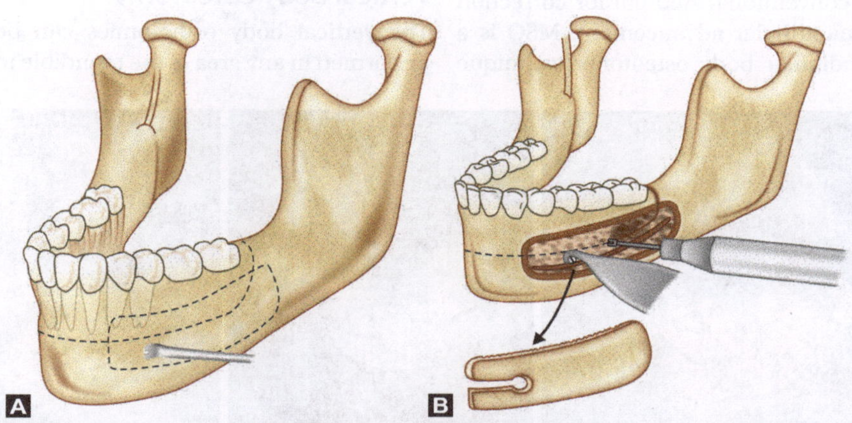

Figs 25.29A and B: Osteotomy cut for total mandibular subapical ostetomy. Prior to this ostetomy cut buccal cortical plate graft is harvested and then osteotomy cut is completed above neurovascular bundle but below apices of tooth and then buccal graft is placed back in position

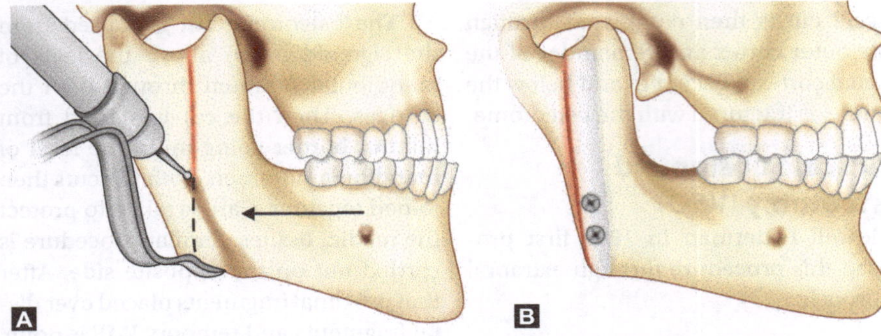

Figs 25.30A and B: Vertical subsigmoid osteotomy

- Mandibular advancement
- Anterior open bite closure and curve of spee reduction.

Surgical Technique

Mandibular Step Osteotomy

Von Eiselburg first described the mandibular step osteotomy (MSO) technique for correction of mandibular retrognathia in 1906. Shortly after, Pichler (in 1918) described the use of MSO for correction of mandibular prognathism. They both performed the technique through an extraoral route with no intention of preserving the mental nerve. In 1948, Dingman combined the intraoral and extraoral approaches for correction of mandibular retrusion. Converse and Shapiro were the first to perform MSO using a pure intraoral approach. They recommended different step designs for the correction of a variety of mandibular deformities; this included the conventional step-cut for correction of mandibular advancement. MSO is a mandibular body osteotomy technique that involves a step-cut made anterior to the mental foramen. It is indicated for correction of mandibular prognathism by either using the space from extraction of a posterior tooth or by closing an existing edentulous space (Figs 25.32A and B). MSO is different from ramus osteotomy in that it allows further modification of the dental arch form vertically for closure of anterior open bite or correction of reverse curve of spee and transversely for arch constriction. The stability of the osteotomy is enhanced mechanically by the step-cut design, which provides a favorable fracture pattern as well as maximal bony approximation. Fixation can be easily achieved by single miniplate on each side. The basic disadvantage with this technique is chances of damage to the neurovascular bundle and necessity for extraction of the functioning premolars.

Vertical Body Osteotomy

The vertical body osteotomies can be performed in any area of the mandible to move the anterior segment of the mandible posteriorly, or alter the vertical and transverse position (Figs 25.33A and B). The main disadvantage of this technique is less bone contacts and in the past owing to lack of the rigid fixation the results were unstable. The chances of damage to the neurovascular bundle are high.

Genioplasty

It is the surgical procedure done for corrrecting the deformities of the chin. The deformities of the chin like chin excess, chin retrusion and chin deviation can be corrected with this procedure and the genioplasty is typed accordingly. It is also indicated for the correction of chin asymmetry following the TMJ ankylosis and case of condylar hyperplasia or hypoplasia.

- **Augmentation genioplasty**—the augmentation could be either vertical or horizontal. This technique is used for the correction of the hypoplastic or retruded chin. (bilateral TMJ ankylosis, micrognathia) as shown in Figures 25.34A and B.
- **Reduction genioplasty**—for the correction of excess in the vertical or horizontal directions. (Skeletal class III or prognathism) as shown in Figures 25.35 and 25.36B.
- **Sliding genioplasty**—it is indicated for the correction of the asymmetry of lower jaw due to deviation of the chin on one side (unilateral TMJ ankylosis, unilateral condylar hyperplasia, etc.) (Figs 25.37, 25.38 and 25.36C)
- **Flip genioplasty**—it is the process which is generally done for the

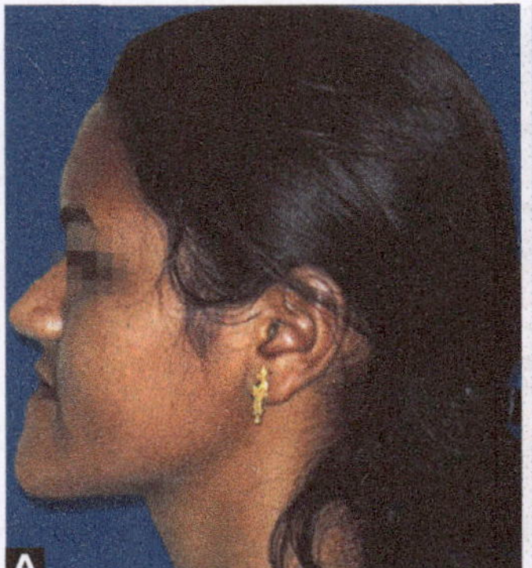

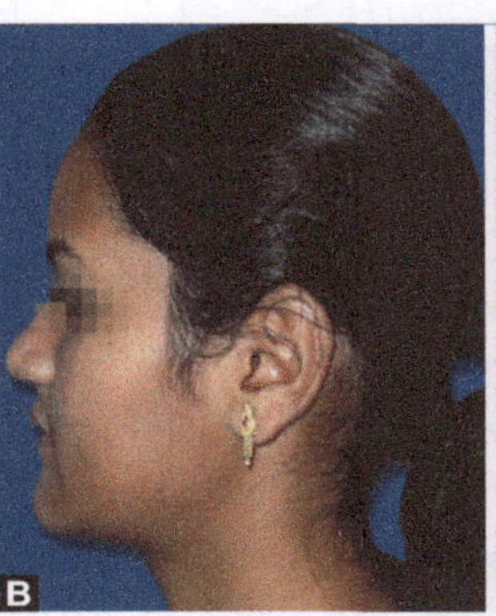

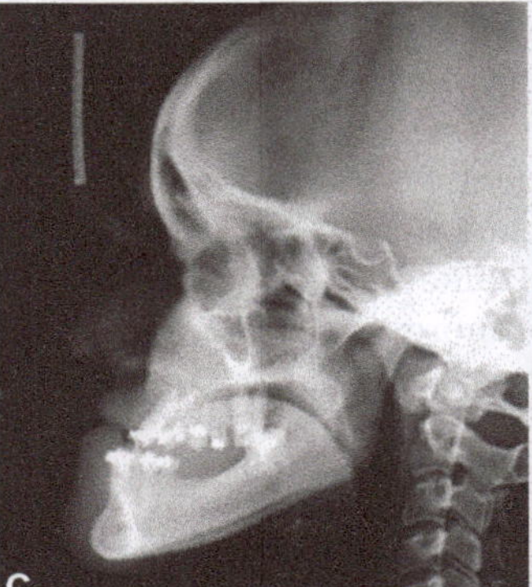

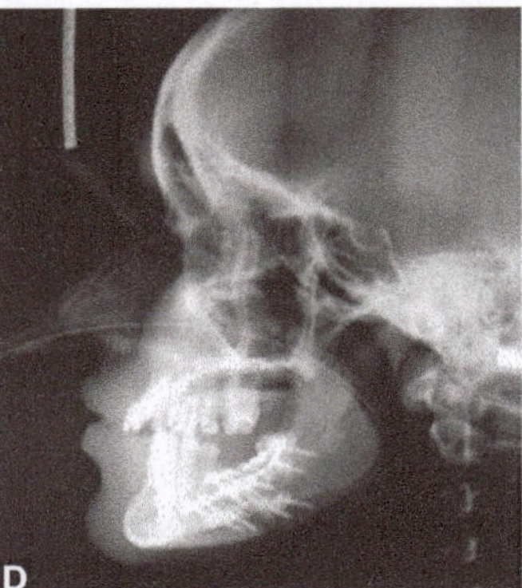

Figs 25.31A to D: Body osteotomy: (A) Preoperative photograph; (B) Postoperative photograph; (C) Preoperative radiograph showing Class III malocclusion; (D) Postoperative radiograph showing surgical correction and bone plates in place

correction of the deformity of the chin following the TMJ ankylosis. The genioplasty cut is taken and based on the geniohyoid pedicle the osteotomized segment is twisted 360° and flipped to other side. It produces good cosmetic results but the acute twisting of the pedicle may lead to avulsion of the segment or avasular necrosis if the vascularity is compromised (Fig. 25.36D).

- **Double sliding genioplasty**—it is used to treat severe deficiency of the chin, when occlusion is stable. The chin is moved in multiple segments in a stepwise manner rather than moving it forward in one block. The advantage is that there is gradual incremental augmentation of the chin which gives good profile. But, the disadvantage being that there can be loss of vascularity of smaller fragments (Fig. 25.37).
- **Sandwitch genioplasty**—when the gap between the fragments is more and bone contact is less, to facilitate the bone healing cancellous bone graft is placed between the two fragments (Fig. 25.38).
- **Alloplastic augmentation genioplasty**—it is a simple procedure which is dien transorally. A vestibular incision is placed in the anterior region, protecting the mental nerves. An implant biopore, silicone, silastic is placed over the bone as an overlay, after carving it to the desired shape and secured in place with screws. The basic disadvantage is rejection of the implant. This technique is not very popular as most of the chin deformities can be corrected with augmentation, reduction or sliding genioplasty, without any need for the alloplastic implants (Fig. 25.39A and B).

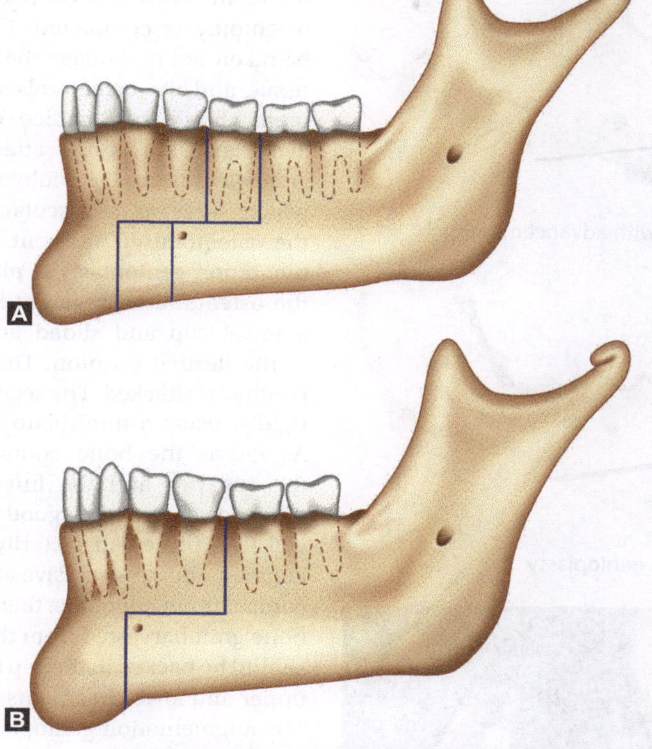

Figs 25.32A and B: Mandibular step osteotomy

Procedure

The procedure is essentially done intraorally through a degloving incision in

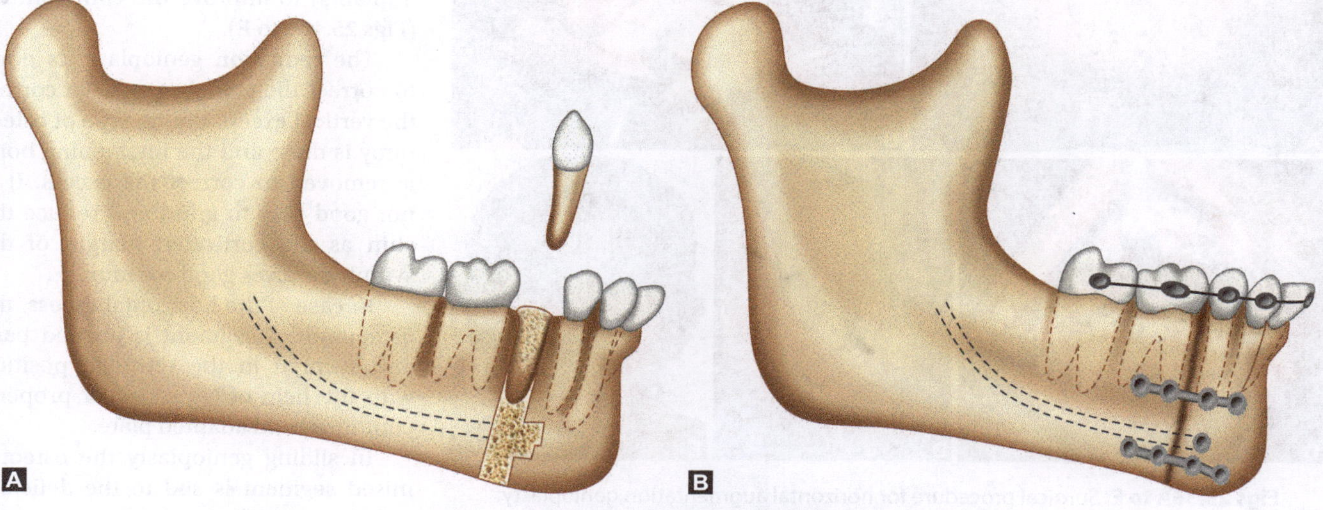

Figs 25.33A and B: Vertical body osteotomy

the labial vestibule of the lower jaw, extending from the premolar to premolar (Figs 25.36A to N). Care should be taken to avoid damage to the branches of the mental nerve. The sharp and blunt dissection is carried out to expose the symphyseal area from mental foramen to mental foramen on either side. The mental nerve is carefully retracted. The labial soft tisse is retracted using the chin retractor. The dissection is carried out up to the inferior border to expose it. A chin retractor is used to retract the soft tissue and the lower lip. The genioplasty cut is marked using the recroprocting saw or a fine bur. The cut extends from mental foramen to mental foramen without damaging the mental nerve and goes below the apices of the teeth. The cut is deepened and the osteotomy is completed. Care should be taken not to damage the lingual soft tissue and the osteotomised chin segment should be handled carefully to avoid avulsion of the attachments of genioglossus and geniohyoid muscles which serve as a vascular pedicle to the osteotomised segment. If the augmentation genioplasty is planned then the osteotomised segment is held with a towel clip and slided anteriorly up to the desired position. The soft tissue contour is checked. The segment is fixed rigidly, using a mini plate and screws. As far as the bone contact between the superior and the inferior (osteotomized) segments is good the healing will take place satisfactorily, but if the augmentation is excessive and the bone contact is not adequate, then cancellous bone graft harvested from the iliac crest should be packed in the gap between the upper and lower fragments (Fig. 25.38). The augmentation genioplasty can also be done by giving overlay graft (Figs 25.39A and B) or implants (medpore implants) to improve the chin contour (Figs 25.40A to E).

Figs 25.34A and B: Horizontal genioplasty with advancement

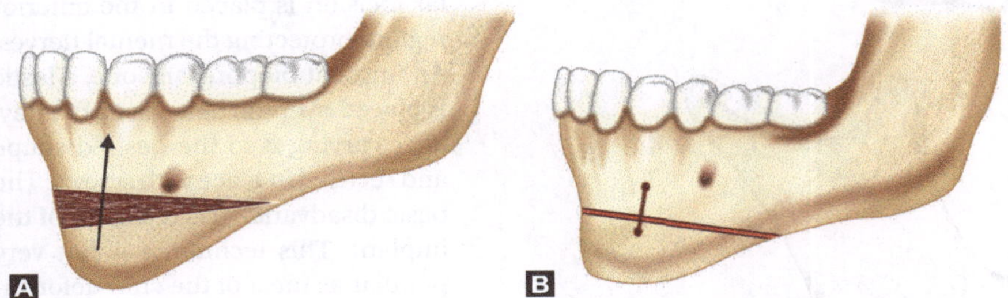

Figs 25.35A and B: Vertical reduction genioplasty

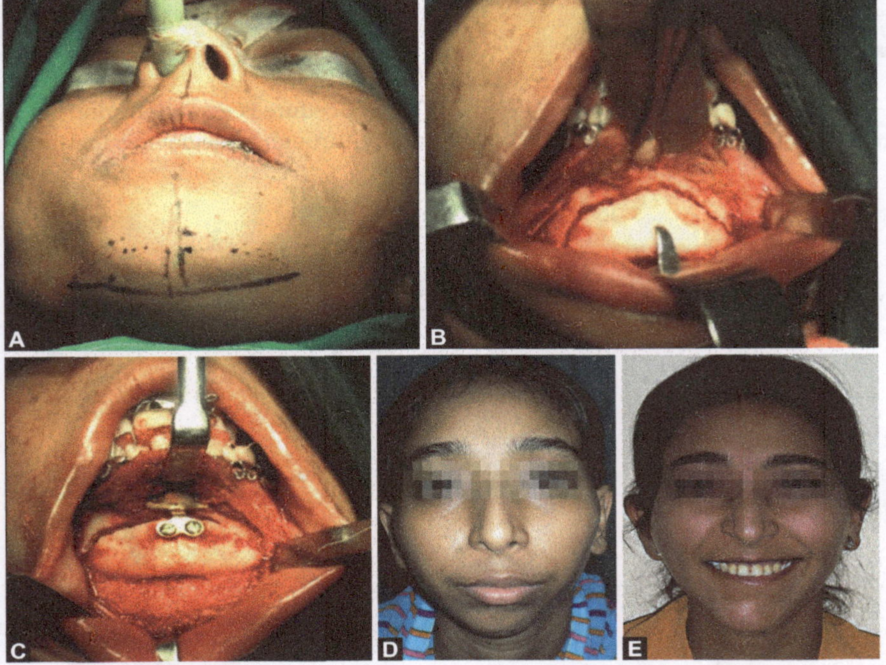

Figs 25.36A to E: Surgical procedure for horizontal augmentation genioplasty: (A to C) Intraoperative photographs; (D) Preoperative photagraph; (E) Postoperative result

The reduction genioplasty is done to correct the genial excess. To correct the vertical excess similar type of osteotomy is done and the intervening bone is removed to correct the excess. It is not good idea to grind and reduce the chin as the corticated margin of the symphysis gives good contour.

In case of the horizontal excess, the osteotomised segment is pushed back and secured in the retruded position with the help of lag screw or properly contoured and adapted plate.

In sliding genioplasty the osteotomised segment is slid to the deficient side to correct the asymmetry.

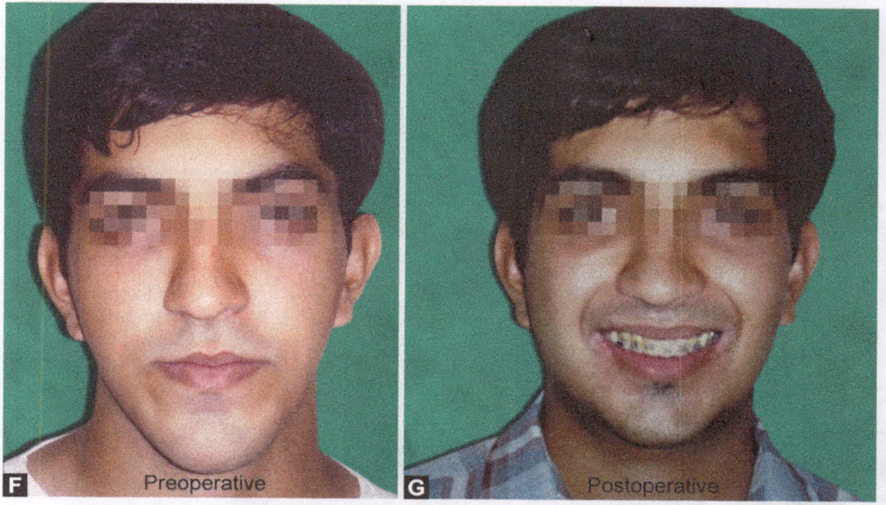

Figs 25.36F and G: Surgical procedure for vertical reduction genioplasty: (F) Preoperative; (G) Postoperative photographs

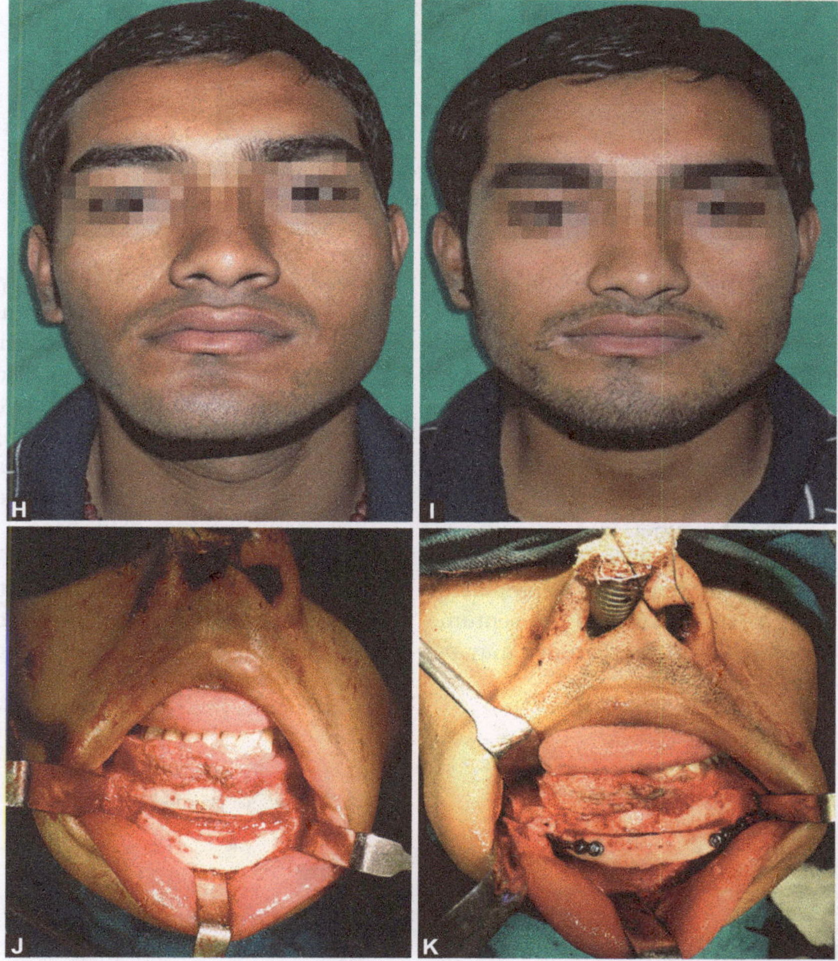

Figs 25.36H to K: Sliding genioplasty: (H) Preoperative photograph; (I) Postoperative photograph; (J) Osteotomy cut; (K) Sliding genioplasty, segment fixed with screw and plates

COMPLICATIONS OF ORTHOGNATHIC SURGERY

The immediate complications are:

- **Vascular complications:** Hemorrhage occurs due to damage to regional vesssels like inferior alveolar artery, posterior superior alveolar artery, pterigoid plexus of veins, greater palatine artery or branches of internal maxillary artery. Care should be taken to do the dissection in a subperiosteal plane and the soft tissue should be properly guarded and retracted during the surgery.
- **Edema, hematoma, airway edema:** The edema is the common complication following the sagittal split osteotomy and Le Fort osteotomies. It is due to the fact that the surgeries are performed transorally and the wounds are closed primarily. The osteotomy site lies in the closed compartment and there is no natural decompression/drainage. Thus, the edema accumulates and distends the tissue. Minor oozing of the blood at the surgical site leads to hematoma formation. The edema can spread to the adjacent areas like pharynx and larynx causing respiratory obstruction. To avoid excess of edema perisurgical steroid therapy with hydrocortisone or dexamethasone is helpful. The incision is closed with loose sutures so that it works as natural drainage site. The judicious use of the vacuum drains also helps in reducing the edema and hematoma. The hemostasis should be meticulous. Periodic evaluation of the airway for patency and airway edema should be done especially in the initial 24 to 48 hours. In case the excessive edema is anticipated the nasal endotracheal tube may be left indwelling for 24 hours to ensure respiratory passage patency.
- **Dental and periodontal injuries** are more common in cases of subapical osteotomies and body osteotomies.
- **Sensory and motor nerve injuries:** Injury to inferior alveolar during the sagittal split osteotomy or

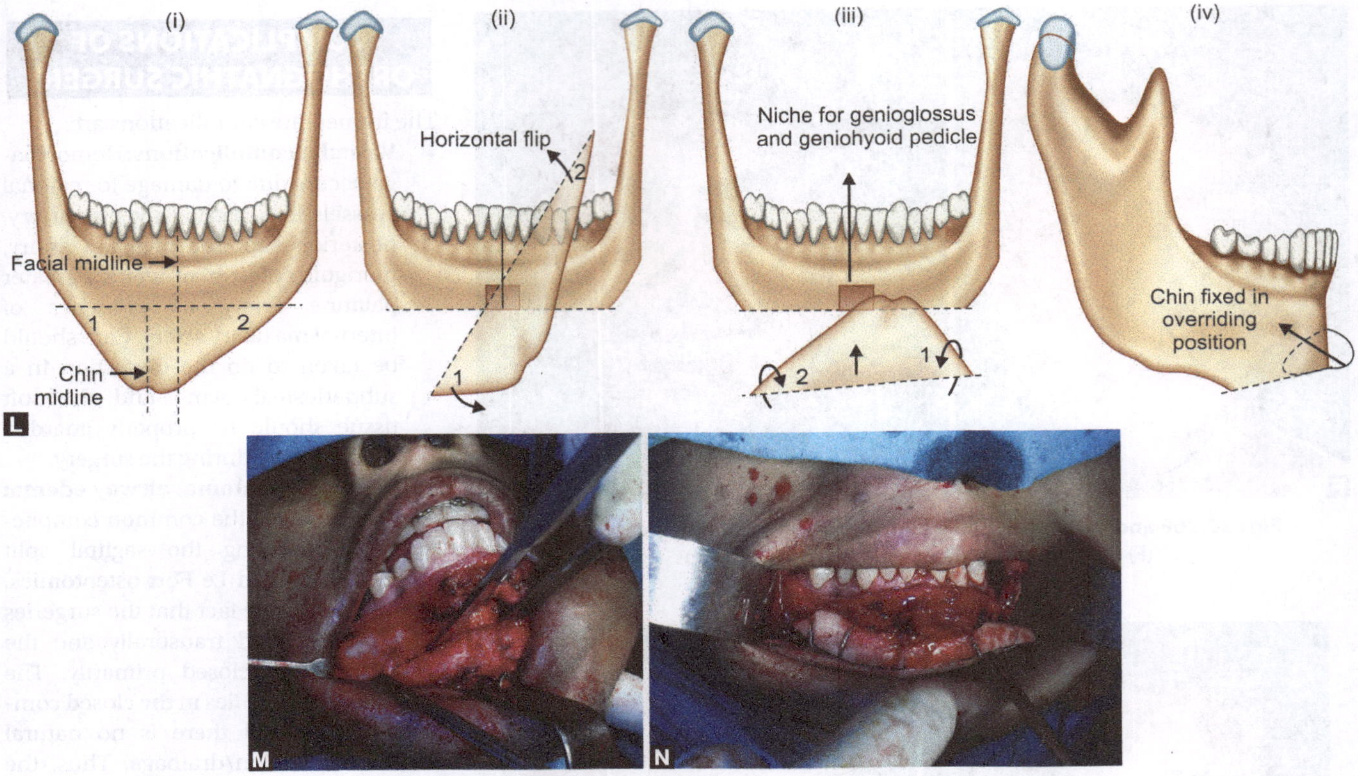

Figs 25.36L to N: Case of flip genioplasty: (L) Diagrammatic representation of the flip genioplasty; (M) Osteotomy cut; (N) Flipped segment secured in place

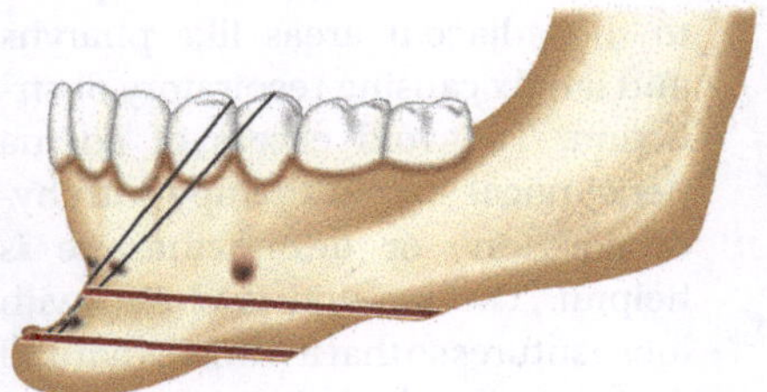

Fig. 25.37: Double sliding horizontal genioplasty

distraction, ramal osteotomies and mental nerve during genioplasty or anterior segmental osteotomy of mandible are possible. Even after adequate precautions minor neurological disturbances may occur which usually recover within few weeks. The chances of inferior alveolar nerve injuries are more during the mandibular body osteotomies, but, these procedures are seldom performed.

- **Alteration in nasal septum, nasal valve, alar base:** Following the Le Fort osteotomies of maxilla the septal osteotomy is done and after placing the maxilla in the desired position the septum is repositioned. If care is not taken the septal deviation and obstruction/narrowing the nasal passage may result creating subsequent nasal obstruction. During the superior positioning of the maxilla a wedge of septal bone/cartilage is removed (septoplasty) to prevent buckling of the septum. Alternatively a deep groove may be created in the maxilla (floor of pyriform fossa) to reposition the septum.

  The alar cartilages are detached during the degloving incision taken for the Le Fort osteotomy. During the closure alar cinch is done by placing a non absorbable suture engaging bases of both the alar cartilages to prevent flaring and distortion of the nose.
- **Proximal segment fracture:** The proximal fragment during the sagittal split osteotomy are often thinner and weak as the vertical cut

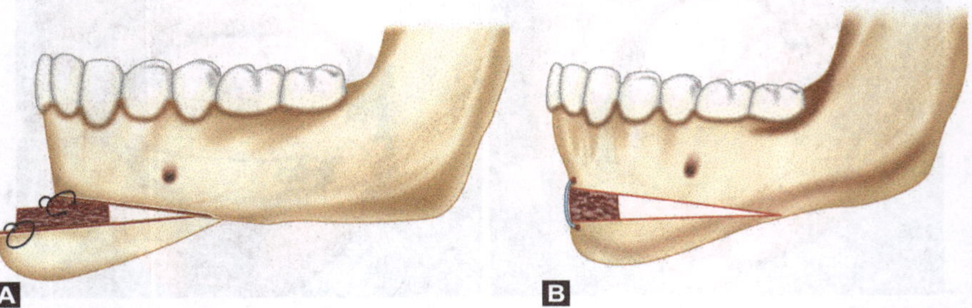

Figs 25.38A and B: Sandwitch genioplasty. (A) Vertical as well horizontal augmentation; (B) Verticle augmentation, by sandwiching the cancellous bone graft

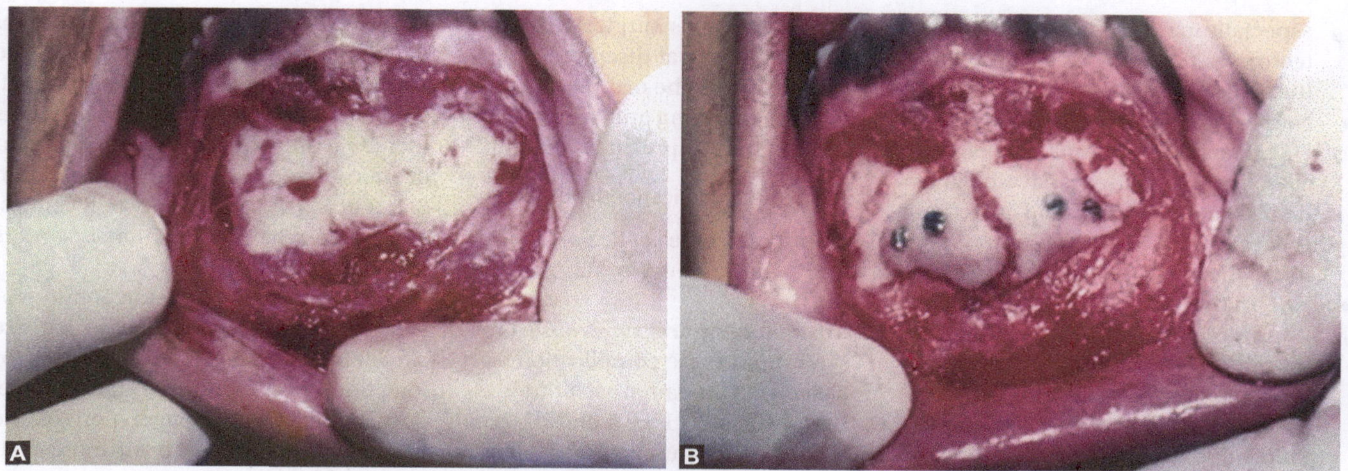

Figs 25.39A and B: Overlay grafting for augmentation genioplasty: (A) Exposure of surgical site; (B) Overlay iliac crest graft, fixed with screws

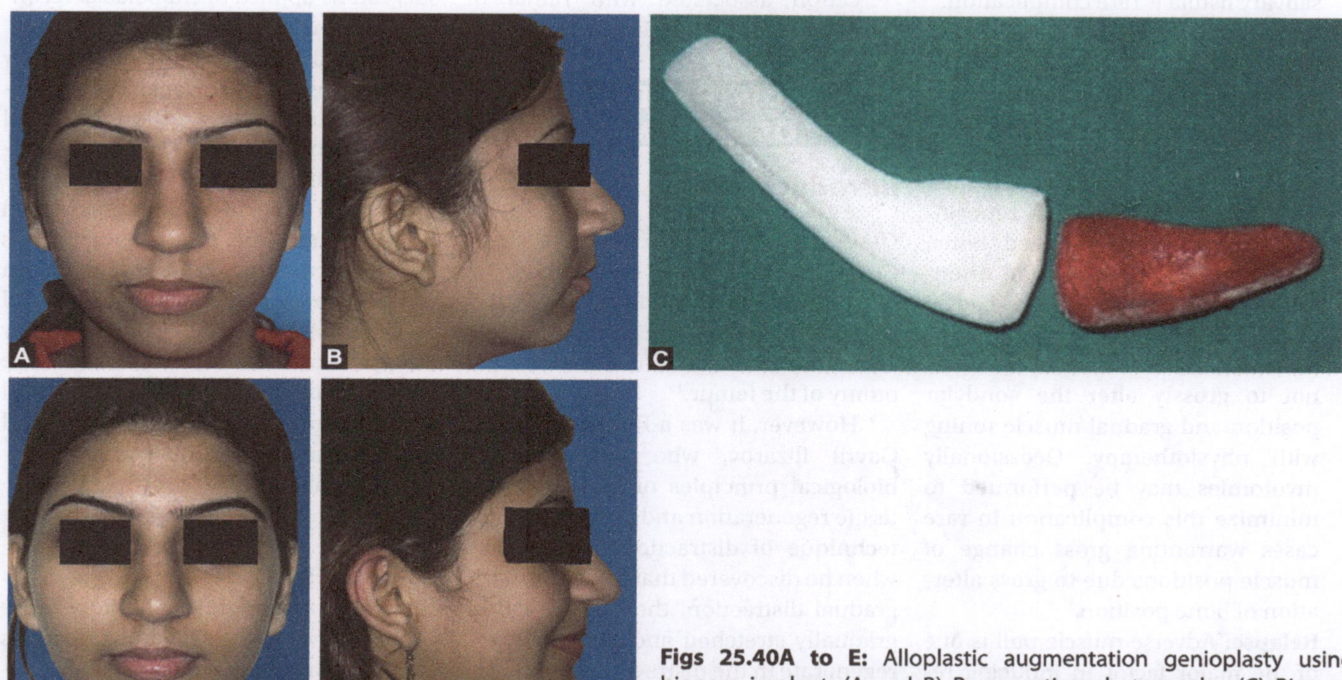

Figs 25.40A to E: Alloplastic augmentation genioplasty using biopore implant: (A and B) Preoperative photographs; (C) Biopore implant carved as per the need of the patient; (D and E) Postoperative photographs. (*Source:* Dr Sanjay Deshpande, MS, MCh, Mumbai)

is taken more buccally to prevent injury to the inferior alveolar nerve. Injudicious application of the force with bone spreader may lead to fracture of proximal segment.

- **Lingual segment fracture:** A bad split due to the inadequate cortical cuts, excessive force or anatomical variations such as thin ramus may occur. Meticulous evaluation, planning and patient approach during the split without using undue force can avoid such complications.
- Excessive lateral displacement or rotation of the proximal segment may occur during the sagittal split osteotomy or VRO and mandibular set back. It leads to abnormal condylar position and subsequent TMJ complications. To avoid the same excess of the overlapping bone on the buccal cortex of the proximal segment should be trimmed to ensure that the displacement is not in excess of 10 degrees.

Delayed Complications are:

- **Loss of vascularity:** Loss of vascular pedicle due to injudicious handling leads to such complications especially in maxillary segmental osteotomies, Le Fort osteotomies and the genioplasty.

- **Necrosis of hard and soft tissues:** Due to excessive trauma, loss of vascular pedicle and excessive edema, hematoma formation and infection of surgical site, the soft tissue or bony fragments may undergo necrosis.
- **Nonunion or delayed union:** Improper immobilization/fixation, infection and avascular necrosis of the osteotomised bone ends can lead to healing complications like delayed union, fibrous union, or non union.
- **Fistulas:** Oronasal and oroantral fistulas could be the commonest fistulas following maxillary osteotomies. The salivary fistula is rare complication.
- **Infection:** Surgical site complication is a common complication following any surgical procedure. It can be prevented by meticulous planning, aspetic precautions, judicious tissue handling and prophylactic antibiotics.
- **TMJ dysfunction:** Due to repositioning of the osteotomized bone, altered muscle position and orientation and change of the codyle position, the TMJ dysfunction can be precipitated. Care should be taken not to grossly alter the condylar position and gradual muscle toning with physiotherapy. Occasionally myotomies may be performed to minimize this complication in rare cases warranting gross change of muscle positions due to gross alteration of bone position.
- **Relapse:** Adverse muscle pull is one of the major factor in inducing relapse. Certain degree of relapse is unavoidable. The relapse is more significant when the advancement or setbacks are significantly high. Selective myotomy (muscle stripping) may avoid the relapse. However, if the augmentation is more, distraction should be preferred over osteotomy to get more lasting and stable results.
- **Occlusal discrepancies:** Even after meticulous planning and presurgical orthodontics minor occlusal disharmony may remain which can be corrected by postsurgical orthodontics. The occlusal discrepancies are more severe if the orthodontic evaluations, planning and interventions are not done in presurgical period.

Miscellaneous complications could be:

- Epiphora in cases of Le Fort II osteotomy due to injury to nasolacrymal duct.
- **Auriculotemporal syndrome:** Frey's syndrome is rare complication associated with the ramal osteotomies.
- **Facial scars:** Le Fort II and III osteotomy necessitates incisions on skin and can leave behind scars. Most of other procedures are done transorally.
- **Salivary injuries:** It is rare complication associated with ramal or maxillary osteotomies.

DISTRACTION OSTEOGENESIS

Introduction

Historical Background

Codivilla from Italy is credited for having performed the first lengthening procedure by applying skeletal traction through a calcaneal pin, following osteotomy of the femur.[15]

However, it was a Russian surgeon, Gavril Ilizarov, who pioneered the biological principles of bone and soft tissue regeneration and popularized the technique of distraction osteogenesis, when he discovered that under slow and gradual distraction, the callous will be gradually stretched and new bone will regenerate in the distracted gap.[15]

Starting in the early 1950s, he worked in a village in Siberia, Kurgan, unknown to the rest of the world. Subsequently, in 1982, he successfully treated a famous Italian explorer "Carlo Mauri" for a resistant nonunion of his tibia and it was only then when his principles were made known to the Western World.

Mandibular distraction was first performed in 1973 in a canine model (Snyder et al., 1973). However, it was only in 1992 when it was first reported in humans (Mccarthy et al., 1992). Currently, both extraoral and intraoral devices may be used depending on the condition to be treated (Goldwaser et al., 2011).[15] Commonly treated conditions include craniofacial deficiencies, syndromic craniosynostosis, Pierre Robin Sequence, post-traumatic deformities, and sleep-related breathing disorders (Vander Kolk et al. 2001).[15]

The concepts of distraction osteogenesis in the maxillofacial region are similar in many respects to those used for long bones, yet differences in the shape, development and configuration of the bones of the face make its use more challenging than traditional osteotomies. Distraction osteogenesis (DO), a useful technique to generate bone and soft tissue, can be applied to craniofacial reconstruction, including orthognathic surgery, cleft lip and palate reconstruction, a new mandibular condyle regeneration, a dentoalveolar unit reconstruction for dental implants and transport DO for discontinuity defects.

The principles of distraction as refined by Ilizarov and other orthopedic surgeons and they continue to be refined when used by orthopedic and maxillofacial surgeons. An almost bewildering array of appliances is available to distract the bones of the face, including intraoral and extraoral appliances, univectors and multivectors, and tooth-borne and bone-borne appliances.

Concept of Distraction Osteogenesis

Regardless of the surgical site, adherence to the following basic Ilizarov principles is the key to surgical success:

- Osteotomy of the bone site with minimal periosteal stripping
- Latency period: 3, 5, or 7 days, depending on the surgical site
- Distraction rate: 1.0 mm per day (0.5–2.0 mm)
- **Distraction rhythm:** Continuous force application is best, yet device activation twice a day is more practical and allows for better patient compliance
- **Consolidation:** Until a cortical outline can be seen radiographically

across the distraction gap, usually 6 weeks.

Using distraction rates of 0.5, 1, or 2 mm/day and different distraction frequencies with both osteotomies and closed techniques, Ilizarov found that a distraction rate of 1 mm/day led to the best results for bone, fascia, skeletal muscles, smooth muscle, blood vessels, nerves and skin regeneration (lengthening). He observed that the greater the distraction frequency, the better is the outcome. He concluded that the best results were obtained with preservation of periosseous tissues, bone marrow and blood supply at the time of osteotomy, stability of the distractor (external) and a rate of 1 mm/day with a rhythm of four turns per day.[16]

Histology

From a histologic evaluation, when distraction is completed, new bone forms in parallel columns that extend in both directions from the osteotomy. The distraction process can be divided into three phases. During the latency period (first phase), histologic and molecular events are similar to those seen during fracture healing, with the osteotomy site surrounded by a hyaline cartilage external callus. In the distraction phase (second phase), chondrocytes are stretched along the tension vector and become fibroblast-like in shape.

As distraction is advanced (third phase), the cartilaginous callus is progressively replaced by a bone callus first by endochrondral ossification; later new bone is directly formed by intramembranous ossification.

During distraction, several molecules of the bone morphogenic protein super family have been noted. Several studies have noted increased blood flow and vessel formation within the zone of distraction. Pacicca and colleagues showed two different angiogenic factors localized at the leading edge of the distraction gap where new bone was forming.[17] They also found these factors to be maximal during active distraction.

Variables in Distraction

Rate and Rhythm

In practice, most surgeons use a 3 to 5 days latency period followed by a rate of 1 mm/day with a twice-a-day rhythm in the mandible. A shorter latency is used in the maxilla.[16,17]

Age of the Patient

In a pediatric population, Hollier and colleagues were able to eliminate the latency period and successfully distracted the mandibles of 22 patients at a rate of 2 mm/day. Most surgeons use a shorter latency in pediatric patients and a more rapid rate of expansion.[16] One of the complications of a long latency or a slow distraction rate in a pediatric population is premature consolidation.

Systemic Factors

The ideal management of patients with history of smoking and alcohol use involves eliminating or markedly reducing their use before surgery.

Indications

- Severe deficiency of maxilla and mandible (bilateral or unilateral)
- Jaw bone deficiency related to syndromes
- Cases in which large amount of advancement is required which cannot be corrected by orthognathic surgery.[17]

Contraindications

As a method of new bone formation in patients with osseous dysplasia.[17]

Type of Distractors

Fundamentally, external distractors are less stable than internal ones. Under biomechanical testing that external distractors failed with permanent deformation of the pins rather than fracture of the model, as seen in the ones with internal distractors. The situation becomes more complex when soft tissue considerations are made. The position in which the distractor is placed to simulate soft tissues affects the distraction vector.

Vector

Vector is the direction that the segment is moved. Extrinsic and intrinsic vectors must be considered when planning a case. In the case of a single vector ramus distractor, the primary vector is the direction that the tram is pointed. Intrinsic vectors (the masseter and medial pterygoid muscles) are more resistant to vertical movement of the segment than the suprahyoid musculature is to anterior movement of the mandible.[18]

In contrast to vertical distraction of the ramus with mandibular advancement the suprahyoid musculature exerts a vertical pull on the distal segment as the mandible is advanced. To counteract these intrinsic vectors, the distracters should be directed in a slightly upward direction toward the maxillary dentition.

Treatment Planning

As with orthognathic surgery, treatment planning for distraction osteogenesis includes predicting the amount and trajectory of the planned bone movement.

Although the DO device may be activated 1.0 mm per day, this does not translate to 1.0 mm of bone advancement per day. The amount of actual bone movement is always less than the distance that is indicated on the distraction device, therefore the clinician monitors the patient's progress closely, including radiographs. The surgical approach and technique are similar to orthognathic surgery. When locating and positioning the bone cut, also consider the placement and orientation of the distraction device. Mark the planned osteotomy. Then create a corticotomy, verifying the ability to place the distractor in the proper orientation. Make the screw fixation holes for the distraction device, and remove the device. The corticotomy is then converted atraumatically to an osteotomy and the distraction device is refixed in place. The device is activated to ensure impedance-free advancement of the distraction segments. Remove any bony interferences and return the device to its closed neutral position. Prior to initial device orientation and placement, activate the distractor 1.0 to 2.0 mm. Thus, after the osteotomy and the device are secured into place, the DO device can be "closed" 1.0 to 2.0 mm, reducing and minimizing the initially created distraction gap.[16]

DISTRACTION DEVICES AND OPTIONS

Midface and Maxilla

Submerged Versus Nonsubmerged

The basic distractor is a tram that allows expansion in one or more directions that has some sort of attachment to the bone, teeth, or both.

- **Submerged device**: The submerged device is designed to be internal, self-retaining and remains fully buried in the tissue after the distraction is complete and thus, can be used as retentive device as well during the consolidation phase (Figs 25.41 and 25.42). The important design features that improve the performance and ease of use include:
  - Internal, submergible design to allow prolonged fixation period.
  - Self-retention to eliminate problems with fixation screw loosening.
  - Bilateral, parallel distraction vector to decrease unfavorable forces at anchorage sites.
  - It is torque calibrated to allow control of distraction forces.
  - Permanently implantable or readily removable.
- **Nonsubmerged device:** The device utilizes a skeletally (cranial) fixed distraction device that is fully adjustable and offers the ability to change the vertical and horizontal vectors of distraction at any time without patient discomfort during the distraction process. The important design features that improve the performance and ease of use include:
  - It controls the vector of distraction relative to the maxillary center of resistance.
  - The vector can be made to pass through or above the center of resistance of maxilla.
  - It is not necessary to wait until skeletal maturity to treat severe midface hypoplasia.
  - Patient tolerance to the device is less.

Technique

A complete Le Fort I osteotomy is performed with pterygomaxillary and septal disjunction followed by mobilization. Once the maxillary osteotomy is complete the halo portion of the device is adjusted to the width of the neurocranium and is rigidly fixed around the head with two or three scalp screws per side. The screws must be over solid bone about 2 to 4 cm above helix of the ear. Vertical bar of the device should be centered with mid sagittal plane, parallel to the facial plane and sufficiently anterior to allow desired amount of distraction. After the halo is secured, the vertical facial bar is removed since distraction is not begun 3 to 5 days after surgery. Once the latent phase is over, the vertical rod is replaced and the tooth borne appliance is attached to it and is activated periodically to distract the maxilla at the rate of 1 mm per day.

Bone-borne Versus Tooth-borne

Appliances that are applied to the teeth usually create a moment arm resulting in uneven distraction because they are not at the center point of segment to be distracted. Tooth-borne appliances in the maxilla usually are custom made and cemented to teeth before surgery. The most common use is to widen the maxilla by surgically assisted rapid palatal expansion. Anteroposterior intra-arch distraction, however, can be done for arch length discrepancies in the maxilla with and without crowding.

Mandible

Submerged Versus Nonsubmerged

Like the maxilla, the desired movement of the mandible seldom is in one direction. Deficiencies may be in vertical ramus length and sagittal anteroposterior deficiency with some patients presenting with a component of both deficiencies.

Submerged distractors can be accessed by a transcutaneous or intraoral approach. The ramus may be vertically lengthened, the body can be horizontally lengthened, or both.

Transcutaneous distractor for vertical lengthening of the ramus can be manipulated extraorally to achieve an ideal position. They usually come in a right and left side. Distractors for the body come in different designs and can be adapted to the body or ramus depending on the desired access and surgeons preference.[19]

- **Submerged device:** It is a device that can be attached to the mandible with 1.9 or 2.3 mm self-tapping monocortical or bicortical screws. The bone plate component of the device can be contoured or shortened intraoperatively to accommodate the local anatomy. The important design features that improve the performance and ease of use include:
  - Antiback activation screw provides excellent stability and offers adjustment of mediolateral vector of distraction during unilateral or bilateral mandibular lengthening.
  - Device is suitable for children, adolescents and the adults with hemifacial microsomia.
  - After consolidation approximately 3 months later a second surgery is required for device removal (Figs 25.43A to E).
- **Nonsubmerged device:** The device essentially consists of an angulation joint and two geared rods of variable lengths. It can be a hinge joint or a double ball joint (Figs 25.44A to E). The important design features that improve the performance and ease of use include:
  - The pin holders facilitate movement of the riders in different direction.
  - The device can be adapted according to individual anatomic situation.
  - Bony segments can be moved in almost any direction.

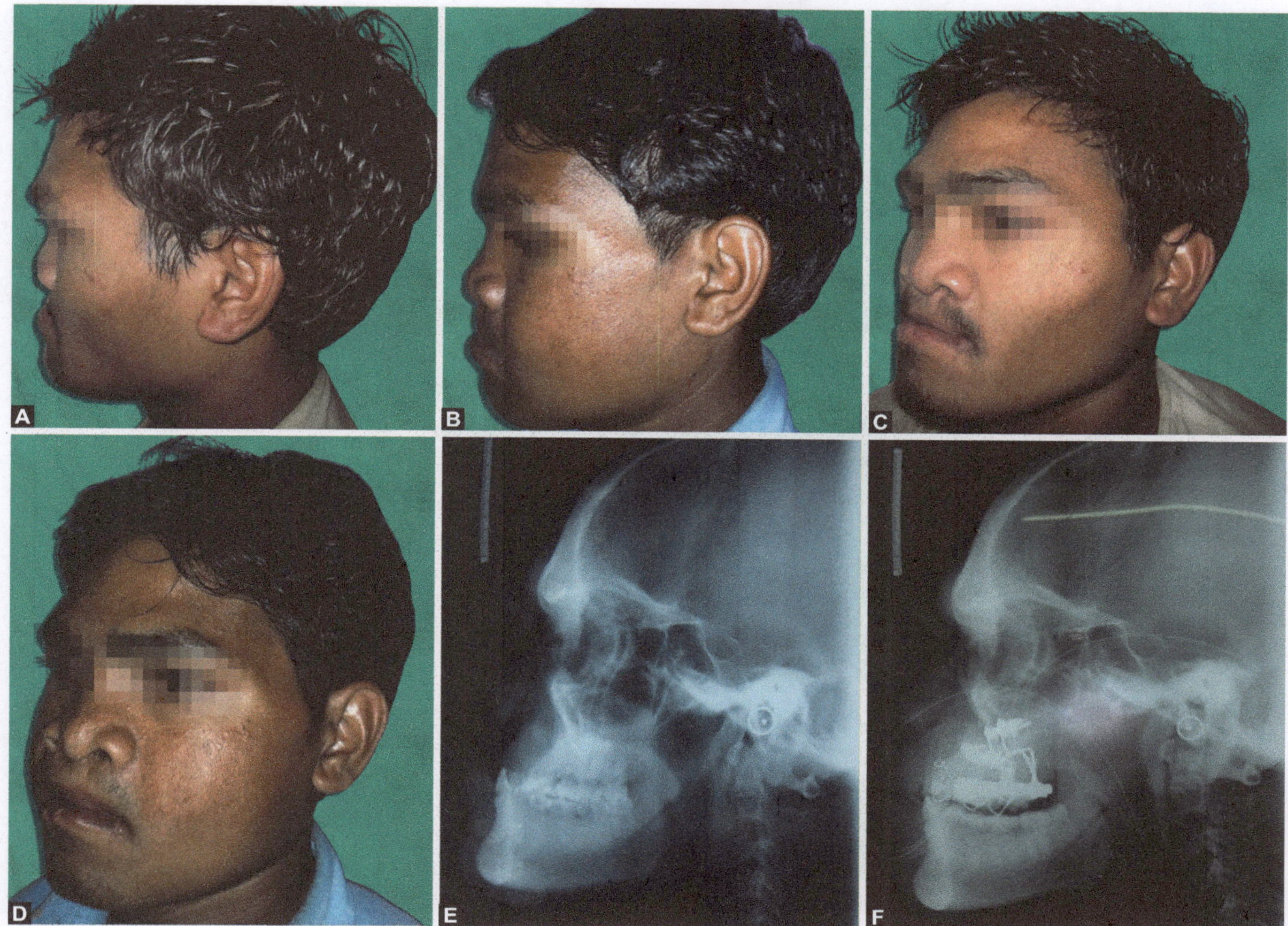

Figs 25.41A to F: A case of maxillary hypoplasia secondary to cleft lip and palate treated with maxillary distraction: (A) Preoperative photograph showing midface deficiency (frontal view); (B) Postdistraction advancement of maxilla (frontal view); (C) Preoperative photograph (three quarter view); (D) Postdistraction advancement of maxilla (three quarter view); (E) Preoperative lateral cephalogram; (F) Postoperative lateral cephalogram with maxillary advancement

Bone-borne Versus Tooth-borne

Several of the tooth-borne distracters are for intra-arch distraction of the mandible. The most popular type of intra-arch distraction is at the symphysis to increase arch length while simultaneously resolving crowding. They produce symmetric distraction of both the alveolar crest and the inferior border. They can be used when the teeth are healthy and the crown to root ratio is adequate. Bone borne distraction devices should be considered when there is poor bony support to the teeth on which the distraction device would be placed. Other indications include patients with mixed dentition stage.

Dancing Distraction

Perform "dancing" of the distraction segment if a discrepancy occurs in planned distraction, such as bilateral mandibular advancement for asymmetries.

Initially, both segments are advanced at the planned distraction rate. When the larger, less asymmetric side reaches its final position, this segment becomes the dancing side, i.e. advancing the larger segment in the morning and then turning it back the same amount in the evening. In the meantime, the lesser more asymmetric segment continues to be advanced at the planned rate until it catches up with the contralateral side. Carry out any final adjustments to the mandibular positioning when the asymmetry has been corrected by advancing or dancing of the two sides as needed.[16]

Mandibular Distraction

For patients with craniofacial microsomia, mandibular distraction of the affected side is a useful technique for generating both bone and soft tissue. The surgical approach is similar to a sagittal osteotomy. Intraoral distracters (Figs 25.43 and 25.45) are preferred to

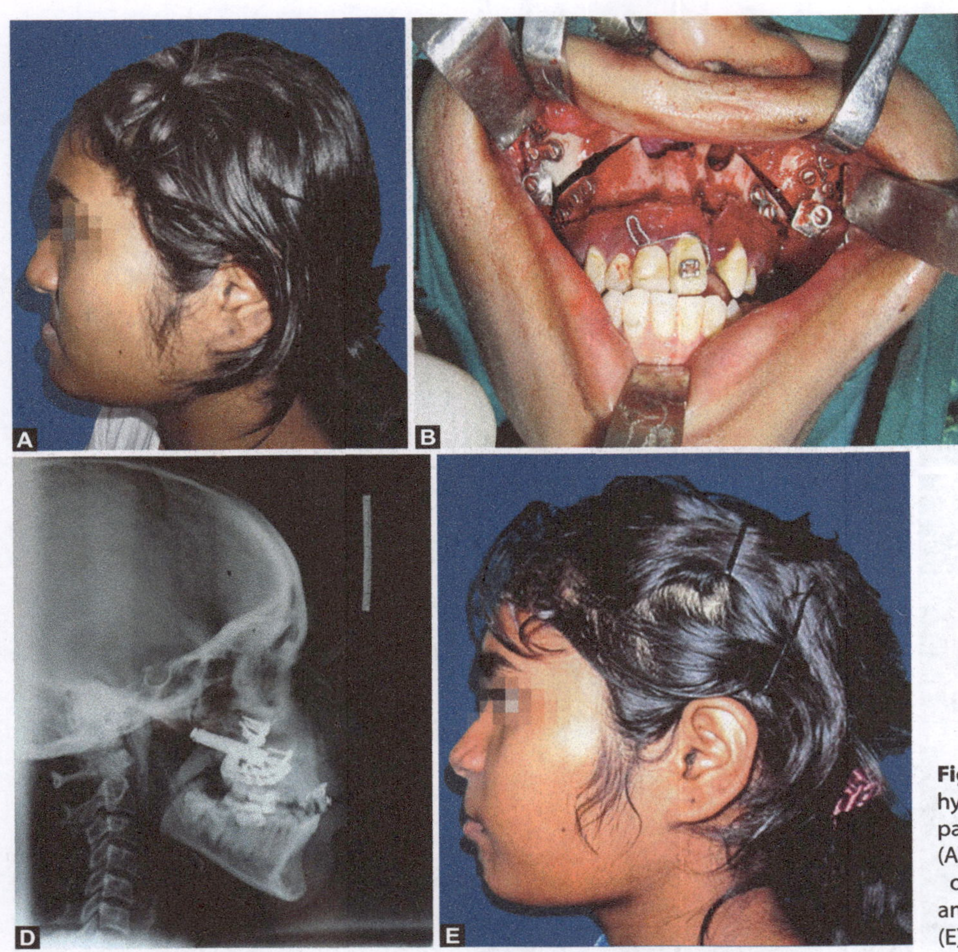

Figs 25.42A to E: Case of maxillary hypoplasia secondary to cleft lip and palate treated with maxillary distractor. (A) Preoperative e photograph; (B) Le Fort I osteotomy cut; (C and D); Preoperative and postoperative lateral cephalograms; (E) Postoperative photograph.

external devices (*see* Figs 25.44A to E) to decrease scarring. Compared with a completely submerged device, DO devices in which the distraction mechanism is intraoral yet extramucosal, allow the clinician to monitor the distractor directly without the need for radiographs. The vector of distraction is calculated based on the trajectory of the bone segment and on the local anatomy, including bone stock, tooth buds and/or roots, and position of the inferior alveolar nerve. The chin point correction is achieved by vertical distraction of the ramus. The distraction process continues 1.0 mm per day until the mandibular asymmetry is corrected.[16]

EXTRAORAL DISTRACTOR

Mandibular Widening

Distraction osteogenesis is a useful tool to create space for severe mandibular crowding, it is often combined with maxillary transverse widening and surgically assisted palatal expansion.

Distraction is a treatment alternative when transverse mandibular deficiency is too large for conventional orthodontic or surgical procedure. The goal of symphyseal osteodistraction is to create new bone and soft tissue. Distraction may avoid inherent limitations of bone graft and permit a better adaptation of surrounding soft tissue in the area, thus avoiding the soft tissue flap. Since distraction is a slower procedure, less trauma is caused to the TMJ when compared to the conventional orthognathic surgery.

Indications

- When it is necessary to significantly after the mandibular arch form and treatment requirements exceeds the limits of conventional surgery (> 4 mm).
- Most applicable when chin appears narrow clinically.
- Arch length inadequacy.
- Crowded anterior teeth.
- Absolute bone deficiency.

A horizontal vestibular incision is made like for the genioplasty from canine to canine. The dissection is directed obliquely through the mentalis muscle to reach the bone. A subperiosteal dissection is then performed until the inferior border of the mandible is exposed, taking care not to damage the mental nerves. Tooth root prominences are either visualized or palpated in order to mark the location of the vertical interdental osteotomy. This is often between the central incisor or sometimes between roots of the canine and lateral incisors, depending upon the amount and location of crowding and the site with the maximum interdental bone. Midline osteotomy is preferred.

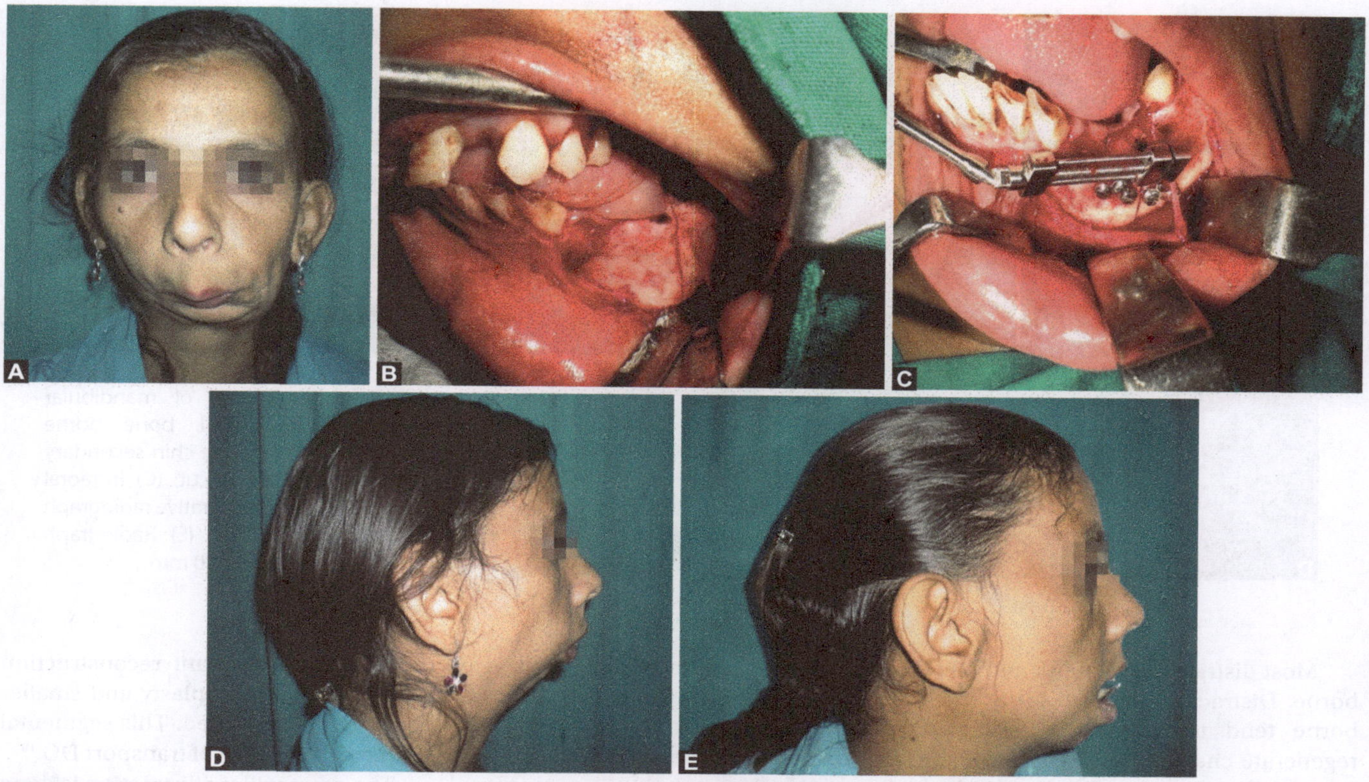

Figs 25.43A to E: Case of TMJ ankylosis, residual deformity treated by mandibular distraction: (A) Preoperative photograph; (B) Osteotomy cut; (C) Distractor placement; (D) Preoperative (E) Postoperative profile photograph

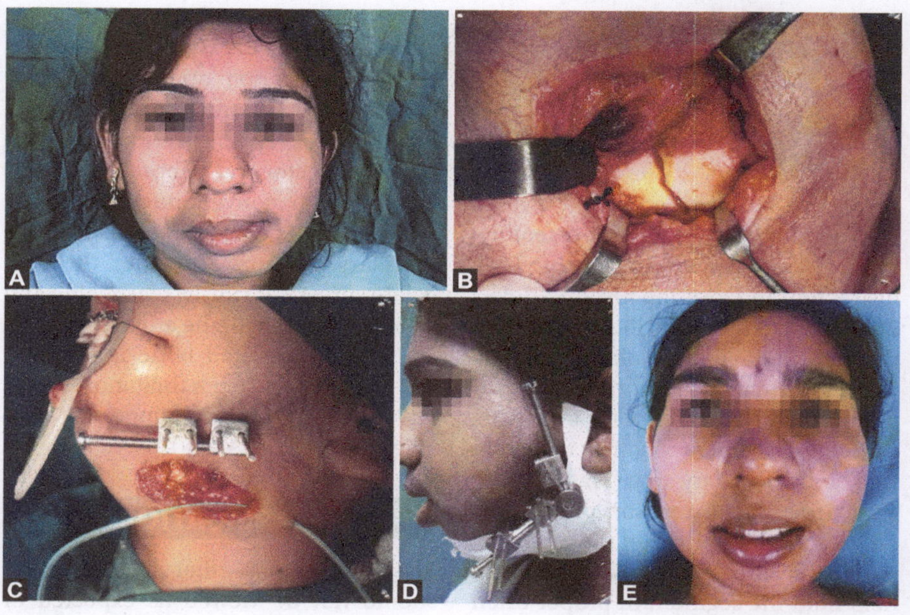

Figs 25.44A to E: A case of unilateral TMJ ankylosis with deviation of chin treated with extraoral mandibular distraction device: (A) Preoperative profile photograph; (B) Osteotomy cut; (C) Distractor placement; (D) Extraoral distraction device in place; (E) Postoperative profile photograph

A complete osteotomy is performed below the level of the roots of the incisors with a reciprocating saw blade. The labial alveolar bone cortex is then sectioned with a Lindemann bur, while the superior flap is reflected with a hook. An osteotomy is used to complete the lingual osteotomy of the alveolus, taking care not to injure the tooth roots and the gingival tissue.

When the roots are too close to the superior aspect of the osteotomy, the remainder of the upper osteotomy is completed by using an expansion forceps (spreader) inserted at the inferior aspect of the symphysis, immediate expansion without tearing the gingival tissue is performed to ensure that the vertical interdental osteotomy is complete. The mini plates incorporated in the device are then adapted to the symphysis. Screws near the midline transmit the most amount of force. The mucosa is closed by interrupted 3-0 vicryl sutures, leaving the upper part of the device uncovered.

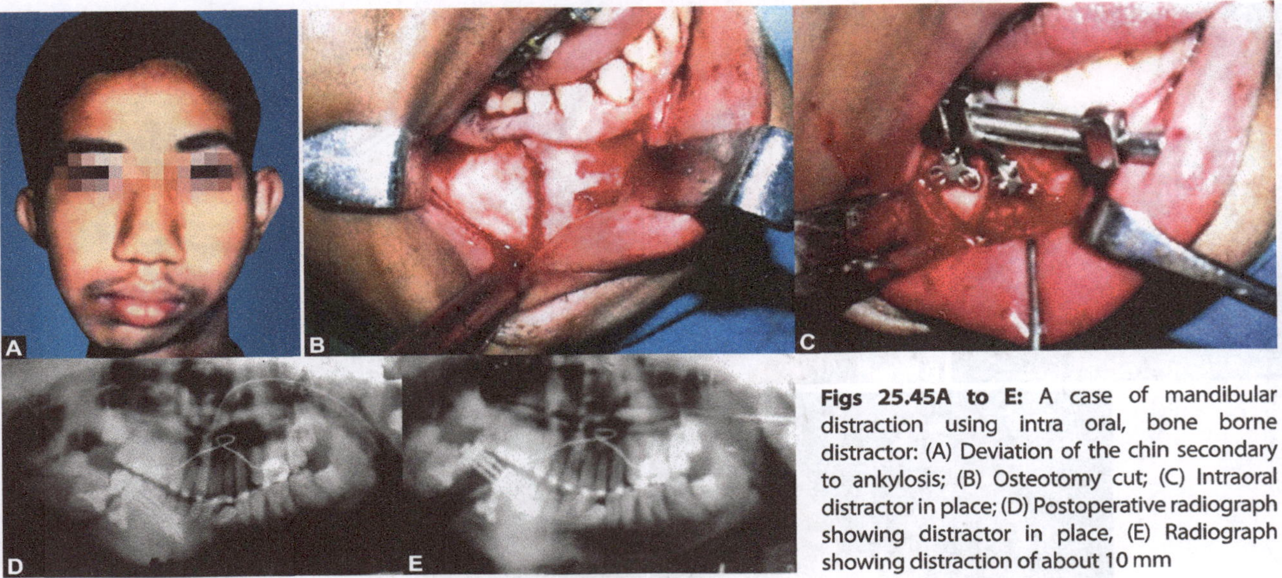

Figs 25.45A to E: A case of mandibular distraction using intra oral, bone borne distractor: (A) Deviation of the chin secondary to ankylosis; (B) Osteotomy cut; (C) Intraoral distractor in place; (D) Postoperative radiograph showing distractor in place, (E) Radiograph showing distraction of about 10 mm

Most distractors are tooth and bone borne. Distractors that are solely bone borne tend to produce a V-shaped regenerate chamber, with more widening at the level of the alveolus and less widening at the level of the inferior border. After DO, the surgeon may place a plastic pontic tooth in the gap between the central incisors to stabilize the teeth and to prevent their central migration. To prevent migration of the teeth into the DO gap, include these teeth in the orthodontic arch wire, with the possible placement of a light spring. Remove the distractor once a cortical outline can be seen on the radiograph. Place a lingual arch to help stabilize the new transverse dimension.[16]

Maxillary Distraction

This technique is especially useful for patients with large advancements or in patients postpalatoplasty for cleft lip and palate whose scarring causes inadequate tissue or difficulty in moving the maxilla. The surgical approach is similar to conventional orthognathic surgery, with the osteotomy at the Le Fort I level. The maxilla is freed but not completely down-fractured. The distractors are precontoured to facilitate device placement. The zygomatic buttress region is a good point for device fixation. Ideal trajectory would locate the two distractors that are parallel to each other and the midsagittal plane. Ensure that the resultant movement arm of the two distractors will not counter each other as the distractors reach their maximal length. Use anterior traction elastics to guide the maxilla to its proper position (Figs 25.45A to F).

Maxillary Segmental Distraction

In patients who have a wide alveolar cleft, perform a segmental osteotomy in the lesser segment, advancing it via distraction to close the alveolar defect. The bone cut is usually located between the bicuspid and the molar teeth of the lesser segment. Use of orthodontic appliances and the arch wire allows the distraction segment to follow the curvature of the maxillary arch (Figs 25.46A to F). During postdistraction phase place an orthodontic spring on the arch wire, paralleling the regenerate chamber to help hold the segment in proper orientation. Within 1 to 2 weeks after distraction ossification, move the bicuspid and cuspid teeth orthodontically back to their correct position into the ossified DO bone, leaving the anterior dentoalveolar unit for implant reconstruction or for final periosteoplasty and smaller bone graft, if indicated. This segmental distraction is a form of transport DO.[16]

The premaxillary distraction is done in case of severe maxillary hypoplasia secondary to the cleft palate. The anterior segmental osteotomy is performed and a custom made distractor devise is fabricated using the Hyrax screw placed in anteroposterior orientation rather than the lateral orientation as it is placed for the arch expansion. It is a type of tooth borne distractor and is more effective as compared to conventional osteotomy as the scarred palatal tissue restricts the maxillary advancement after the cleft palate surgery. It causes reasonable and stable distraction of the anterior maxilla and the regenerated bone is used for the prosthodontic rehabilitation of the patient with implant supported prosthesis (Figs 25.46A to F).

COMPLICATIONS

The complications that arise from DO should not be viewed as expected or acceptable side effects of the technique. Ilizarov has pointed out that 'there are no complications with the technique, there are only inexperienced surgeons causing problems for their patients.'[19]

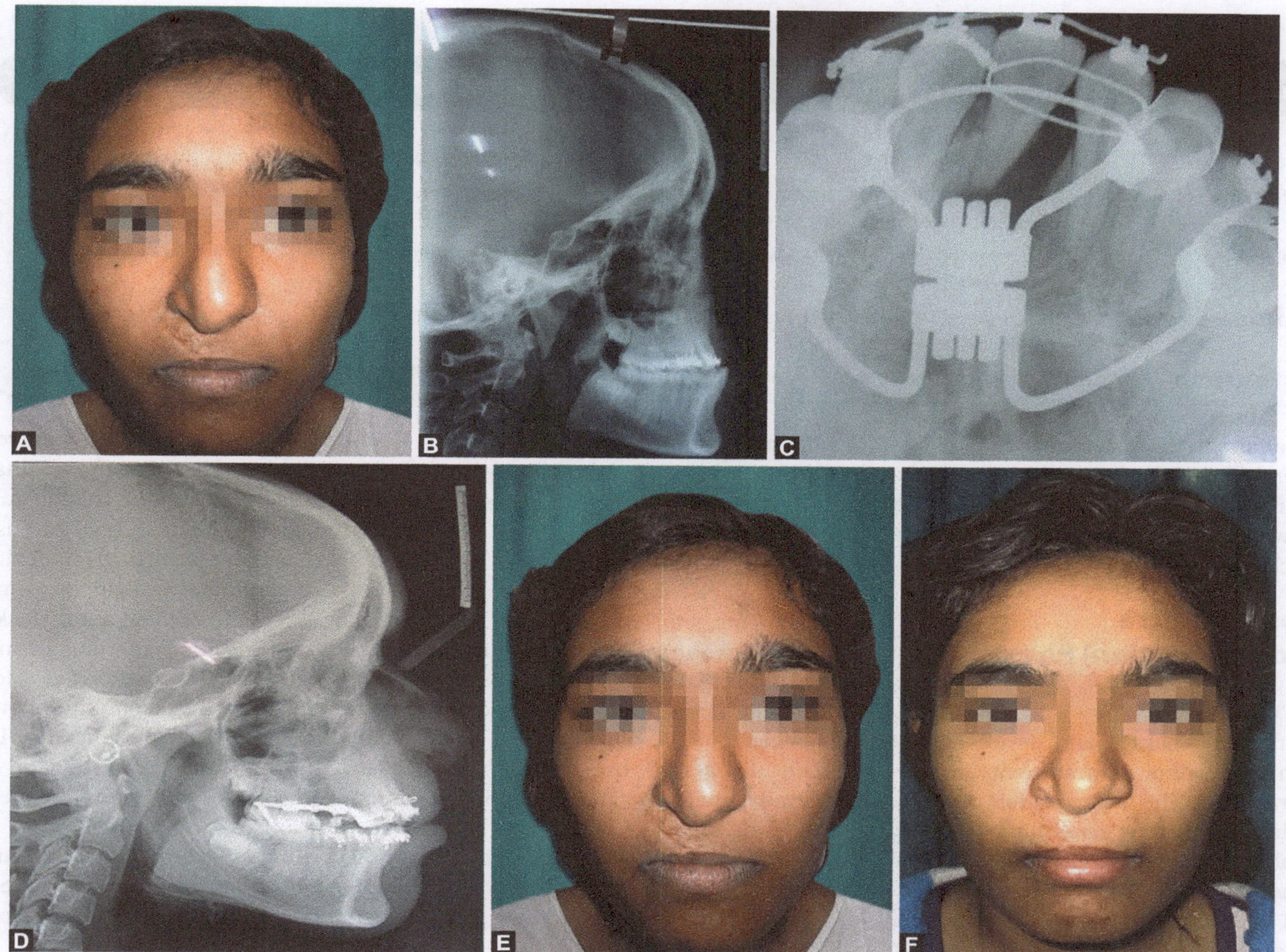

Figs 25.46A to F: A case of maxillary hypoplasia secondary to cleft lip and palate treated with tooth-borne intraoral distraction device: (A) Preoperative photograph; (B) Preoperative lateral cephalogram; (C) Occlusal radiograph of tooth-borne distractor; (D) Lateral cephalogram showing advancement of maxilla; (E and F) Preoperative and postoperative profile photographs

Cherkashin and Samchukov have defined a complication of DO as 'an unexpected deviation from the treatment plan that, without appropriate correction, will lead to worsening of the existing, development of a new, or recurrence of the initial pathologic process.'[19]

Preoperative (Planning) Phase

Patient Selection

The surgeon must select patients who are willing and psychologically and physically capable of activating the distraction device on a daily basis. The surgeon must be prepared to counsel and encourage the patient (and family) on a regular basis during the distraction phase.

Distraction Vector

Malocclusion that results from an incorrect vector of distraction is a common complication. As with other techniques in orthognathic surgery, success or failure of DO is often determined by the accuracy of the preoperative planning. Clinical examination and analysis of photographs, radiographs (lateral and anteroposterior cephalograms, orthopantomogram, and three-dimensional CT images) and dental casts are currently used to determine the desired vector of distraction and approximate the magnitude of bone lengthening required.

Operative (Distractor Placement) Phase

Anatomic Complications

Intraoperative surgical complications are similar to those seen with traditional mandibular procedures, including bleeding, injury to inferior alveolar or lingual nerves, damage to teeth or tooth buds, improper position of corticotomy or osteotomy, or incomplete corticotomy or osteotomy.

If the device placement, execution of proper vector, the orientation and

Table 25.3: Distraction osteogenesis versus orthognathic surgery[20]

Feature	Distraction osteogenesis	Orthognathic surgery
Stability	More stable outcome	Relatively less stable
Effect on tissue	Bone and soft tissue advancement possible • Better adaptability of soft tissues	Only hard tissue advancement • Acute changes lead to stretching of tissues
Relapse	Less common (up to 15 mm advancement can be done)	More common (Maximum 10 mm advancement can be done)
Operative procedure	Technique sensitive and tedious (parallelism of vectors)	Less cumbersome
Patient compliance	Of utmost importance for success of therapy	Better compliance as correction is done in single step

location of the osteotomy and placement of the device are incorrect, the resultant distraction vector produces a new malocclusion or makes the existing occlusion worse.

Postoperative (Postdistraction) Phase

Device Failure

Hardware breakage and device failures can occur, although these events are rarely reported. This complication often requires a secondary surgical procedure to replace the nonfunctional device. External pins may fracture or become mobile. Buried or semiburied screw-fixated devices rarely become loose if applied incorrectly. Once the regenerate has consolidated, it is common to have loosening of the device with no adverse consequences.[19]

Inadequate Distraction

Anatomic Factors

The movement of the proximal and distal fragments during mandibular DO, especially in patients with abnormal morphology of the ramus/condyle unit (e.g. hemifacial microsomia), can be complex. Accurate visualization of the proximal and distal fragments or prediction of their movements is not always appreciated on plain radiographs. Pain may result when the coronoid process collides with the skull base, for example.

Infection

Although reported rates of infection range between 5 and 30 percent in the orthopedic literature, the infection rate in the craniomaxillofacial region seems to be much lower.

Inadequate Regenerate

Inadequate bone formation is a risk in older patients, smokers, irradiated jaws and persons with poor oral hygiene. Even under these circumstances, if the device is left in place for a prolonged period the bone regeneration is often poor.[20]

The distraction osteogenesis has certain advantages over the conventional orthognathic surgeries at the same time it also has few disadvantages which are summerized in Table 25.3.

Distraction osteogenesis is an exciting and promising technique for skeletal expansion. It is technically demanding, however and requires precise planning and a significant commitment on the part of the surgeon, patient and family. Most complications arise from poor patient preparation and compliance, inadequate preoperative planning and inaccurate surgical execution. In the future, technical complications will be minimized by more accurate three-dimensional planning systems and surgical navigation during the distraction phase.

Transport Bone Distraction Osteogenesis

This technique was first introduced by Ilizarov for treating long bone defects resulting from trauma, oncological resection, and other severe congenital or acquired deformities. The distraction osteogenesis occurs under the influence of tensional stress and a typical bony regenerate is formed between the residual host bone segment and the trailing end of the transport segment. After the transport bone segment reaches the opposite or residual target bone segment, compression forces are applied at the docking site until the bony margins of the transport and target segments are fused. Several bone transport techniques have been developed and are included in Ilizarov's classification of distraction—compression osteosynthesis and related osteogenesis method.

According to Ilizarov, the technique are divided into three groups based on the number of distraction/compression sites:

- Monofocal
- Bifocal
- Trifocal.

Monofocal osteosynthesis is used primarily in cases with small osseous defects of up to several millimeters, where healing of the two bone ends is abnormal, resulting in nonunion. In cases not requiring an increase in limb length, compression forces are applied and the pathologic tissue undergoes reparative remodelling, which results in reparative callus formation and fusion of both the bone ends. This is termed monofocal compression osteosynthesis. Conversely an increase in limb length, distraction forces are applied to separate the bone ends. As distraction continues, the pathologic tissues are gradually transformed into regenerate bone. This is termed 'monofocal distraction osteosynthesis.

Bifocal bone transport is used for larger bone defects having one distraction and one compression site. During bifocal osteosynthesis, a free bone segment (TS) (transport segment) is created by performing an osteotomy, from one of the residual segments, i.e the host bone segment (RHBS). This transport disk is then moved from the residual host segment (from which the transport disk is created) to the residual target bone segment (RTBS) (the end towards the transport segment is distracted). This technique involves the gradual movement of a free segment also known as the transport segment of bone across the osseous defect. The transport segment has two ends the leading end and the trailing end. The leading end of the transport segment faces the residual target segment and forms part of the docking site. During movement of the transport segment, new bone is formed between the residual host bone segment and the transport segment (Fig. 25.47). Once the transport segment reaches the residual target bone segment, compressive forces are applied at the docking site (final destination point). At the docking site, the compressive forces stimulate gradual fusion of the contacting bony margins into solid bone regenerate. This technique is commonly used in maxillofacial surgery to reconstruct moderate sized defects of the mandible secondary to tumor resection.

Trifocal distraction is used in very large bony defects, the two transport segments are created from both residual bone segments and simultaneously moved centripetally toward each other so that they meet in the center of the defect. It is characterized by two simultaneously formed distraction regenerates at the docking site in the center of the defect (Fig. 25.48).

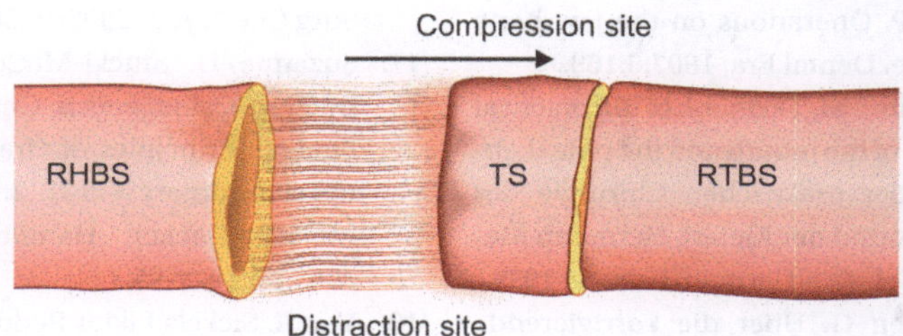

Fig. 25.47: Bifocal transport distraction

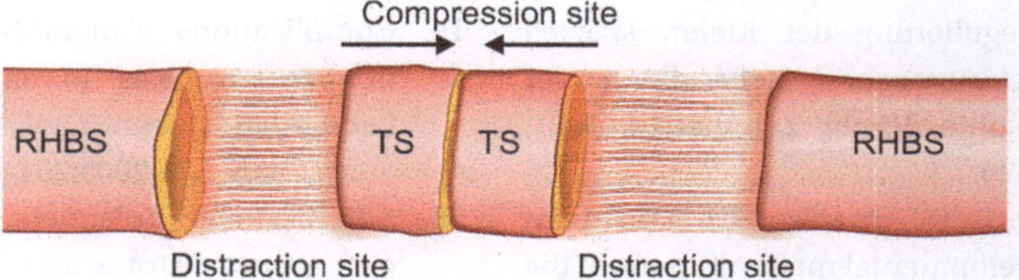

Fig. 25.48: Trifocal transport distraction

Surgical Technique

The surgical procedure is minimally invasive and can be performed in an outpatient setting. A small standard submandibular incision is placed to create an access to the bone. Using tunnelling technique, the lateral border of the mandible is exposed with minimal periosteal stripping on the buccal cortex and no periosteal stripping is done on the lingual cortex as it serves as the vascular pedicle. Using a fissure bur or a reciprocating saw, a corticotomy is created through the lateral cortex and inferior border of the mandible, approximately 15 mm from the distal end of the proximal bone stump. Care is taken to avoid violating the inferior alveolar neurovascular bundle.

The transport device is then applied using bicortical screw fixation. To avoid a significant scar on the facial skin, the pins are placed through individual stab incisions rather than through the submandibular incision. In an effort to minimize the visibility and magnitude of the screw-tract scars, the external screw should be introduced through the skin low in the neck while pinching the skin between the screw site and lifting the skin superiorly. The device is then attached to the screw, verifying the vector and trajectory of the planned transport segment. The device is adjusted to fit passively onto the fixation screws and locked so that further adjustment is not possible and then removed. The corticotomy is then gently converted to an osteotomy using a chisel placed at the inferior mandibular border. The distraction device is reattached to the screws in the same orientation and activated to verify that the transport disk is mobile. The device is then closed until the bone edges touch, following by closure of the surgical site in layers.

Normally, a 5-day latency period is observed for bone transport. Since the purpose of the latency period is to allow the formation of the reparative callus and to allow the wound to enter into the next phase of healing. After latency, the transport disk is distracted at a rate of 0.5 mm twice per day. In cases of vascularity compromised tissues, a rate of 0.25 twice per day is indicated. If blanching is noticed during distraction then rate should be changed to 0.25 mm four times per day. The consolidation period may range from 4 months to 6 months depending on the size of the defect.

The reconstruction of the mandible is often challenging. The transport distraction is good modality of bone regeneration for reconstructing small to moderate mandibular defects along with regeneration of the soft tissues. The reconstruction of the mandibular defects spanning across the midline is far more challenging with the conventional modalities like reconstruction plate and

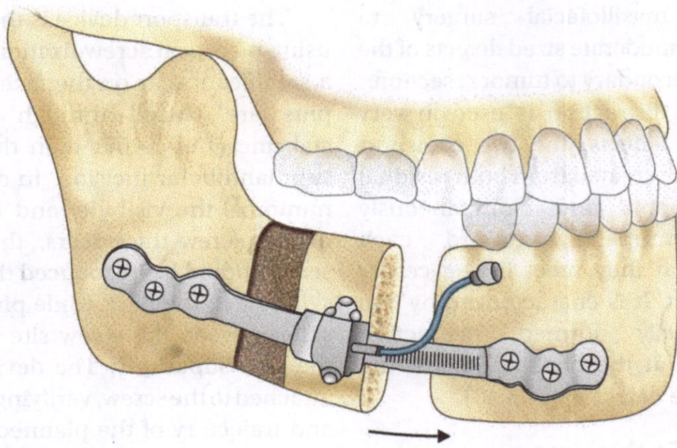

Fig. 25.49: Plate guided, intraoral mandibular transport distractor

bone grafts due to typical stress pattern in this region. The transport distraction is a good modality to reconstruct such bony defects along with the regeneration of the soft tissues.

Intraoral Transport Distraction Device

The first intraoral distraction device for mandibular bone transport was developed in 1987 by Wolfson. The device consisted of a slotted reconstruction plate attached to the residual bone segments by screws. The treaded distraction rod rotated inside the plates slot thereby translating the sliding clamp attached to the transport bone segment (Fig. 25.49).

More recently, different intraoral devices were developed for correction of large mandibular continuity defects, reconstruction of neocondyles and cleft palates.

The advantange of intraoral transport bone distracters includes minimal patient discomfort although the regeneration of large defects takes a long time. The placement of the device is barely noticeable. The surgery is less complicated and leaves no facial scars and can be performed in an ambulatory setting.

The transport devices can be custom made using the stereolithographic models.

REFERENCES

1 Hullihen SP. Case of elongation of the underjaw and distortion of the face and neck by burn, successfully treated. Am J Dent Sac. 1849;9:157..

2. Von Langenbeck, B. Die Uranoplastik. Arch Klin Chir. 1861;2:252..

3. Cheever DW. Nasopharyngeal polypus attached to the basilar process of occipital and body of sphenoid bone successfully removed by a section, displacement and subsequent replacement and reunion of superior maxillary bone. Bost Med and Surg J. 1867;8:162..

4. Blair VP. Operations on the jaw-bone and face. Dental Era. 1907;6:169..

5. Wassmund M. Textbook of the practical surgery of the mouth and the pine [Lehrbuch der praktischen Chirurgie des Mundes und der Kiefer], Hermann Meusser, Vol. 1, in German, Leipzig, 1935..

6. Axhausen G. Uber die korrigierende Osteotomie am Oberkiefer. Dtsch Z Chir. 1936;248:515.

7. Cohn Stock H. Die chirurgische Immediatregulierung der Kiefer, speziell der chirurgischen Behandlung der Prognathie, Vjschr Zahnheilkd. 1921; 37.p.320.

8. Converse JM, Shapiro HH. Treatment of developmental malformations of the jaws. Plast Reconstr Surg. 1952;10:473.

9. Caldwell JB, Letterman GS, Vertical Osteotomy in the Mandibular Rami for Correction of Prognathism. J Oral Surg. 1954;12:p.185.

10. Schuchardt K. Experiences with the surgical treatment of deformities of the jaws: prognathia, micrognathia, and open bite. In: Wallace AG, ed. Second. Congress of International Society of Plastic Surgeons. London: E and S Livingstone, 1959.

11. Obwegeser H. In: Zur Operationstechnik bei der Progenie und anderen Unterkieferanomalien. (In Germany) Dtsch. Z. Mund Kiefer. Gesichtschir. 1955;23:1.

12. Dal Pont G. Retromolar osteotomy for the correction of prognathism. J Oral Surg Anesth Hosp Dent Serv. 1961;19: 42-7.

13. Kole H. Surgical operations on the alveolar ridge to correct occlusal abnormalities. Oral Surgery, Oral Med and Oral Pathology 1959;12:515-29.

14. Hunsuck EE. A modified intra-oral sagittal splitting technique for correction of mandibular prognathism. J Oral Surg. 1968,26;pp.250-3.

15. Reggie C. Hamdy, Juan S Rendon, Maryam Tabrizian. Distraction Osteogenesis and Its Challenges in Bone Regeneration "Bone Regeneration" edited by Haim Tal, ISBN 978-953-51-0487-2, InTech, 2012.

16. Distraction Osteogenesis: Advancements in the Last 10 Years Joseph E. Van Sickels, DDS Oral Maxillofacial Surg Clin N Am. 2007;19:565-574.

17. Suzanne U. Stucki-McCormick, Distraction Osteogenesis Chapter 62 Peterson's Principles of Oral and Maxillofacial Surgery Vol II. 2nd edn. Publ by BC Decker, Hamilton Ontario. 2004;pp.1277-95.

18. Van E. Sickels Likith Reddy V. Distractor Design and OptionsJoseph, Atlas Oral Maxillofacial Surg Clin N Am. 2008;6:159-67.

19. Complications of mandibular distraction osteogenesis Maria J. Troulis, Leonard B. Kaban, Oral Maxillofacial Surg Clin N Am. 2003;251-64.

20. Adi Rachmeil. Treatment of maxillary cleft palate: Distraction osteogenesis vs Orthognathic surgery. Annals of Oral and Maxillofacial Surgery. 2012;2(2): 127-30.

Section 9

Temporomandibular Joint

26 Temporomandibular Joint Disorders

Borle Rajiv M, Arora Aakash, Singh Divya

The temporomandibular joint (TMJ) is complex articulation between condylar head of the mandible and glenoid fossa of the temporal bone. Over the course of evolution it has evolved to a more complex structure. This joint is not only involved in the inflammatory pathologies, but also involved secondary to the stress and the psychological disorders due to the mandibular parafunctions. In the present chapter the common pathologies involving the TMJ are discussed.

TEMPOROMANDIBULAR JOINT ANKYLOSIS

Ankylosis is defined as '*a pathological fusion between two articulating surfaces of a joint*'. The TMJ ankylosis is '*the pathological fusion between the glenoid fossa of the temporal bone and the condylar process of the mandible*' (Fig. 26.1). It is more commonly seen in developing countries like India, but its incidence is less in Western countries.

Applied Surgical Anatomy

The temporomandibular joint (TMJ) is a synovial joint and is described as ginglymodiarthroidial type of joint, due to two different types of movements that occur in it, i.e. translatory and rotatory. The injuries of the chin due to fall are common during the childhood, which cause indirect injuries to the mandibular condyle. The condylar head in the children is covered by fibrocartilaginous

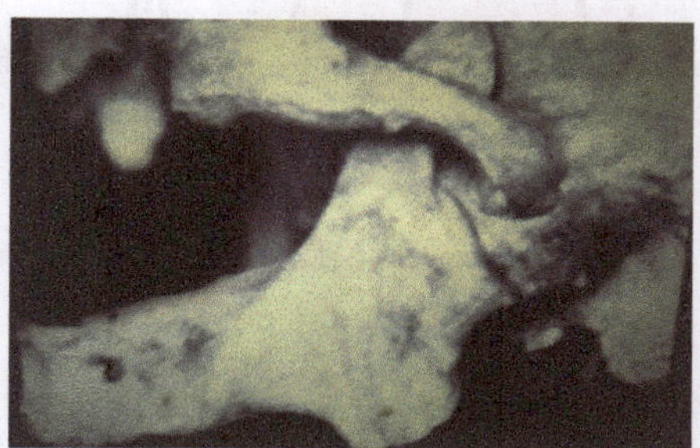

Fig. 26.1: Cadaveric specimen of TMJ ankylosis, notice the hypertrophy of the coronoid process (*Courtesy:* Kurt H Thoma, TB of Oral surgery)

tissue, which is traversed by numerous, tiny capillaries. In the event of trauma these capillaries rupture and effusion of blood takes place in the joint (*hemarthrosis*) and if not treated properly, it results in fibrous adhesions, leading to fibrous ankylosis, which in due course of time gets ossified and changes into bony ankylosis.

The superficial temporal artery and vein is present deep to the superficial temporal fascia. The artery bifurcates into temporal and transverse facial branches. The incisions for exposing this joint are placed in such way that they lie in the bifurcation and do not damage these vessels. The facial nerve emerges from the anterior border of the superficial lobe of parotid gland and lies below the lobule of ear inferior to its attachment to the facial skin. If the incision is extended beyond this point, the nerve is likely to be damaged. The zygomaticotemporal branch of the facial nerve crosses the zygomatic arch and runs in between the two layers of the deep temporal fascia in the fat lobules, near their attachment to the zygomatic arch. Fat lobules are present between these two layers of the fascia, which give valuable indication of proper plane of dissection during the TMJ surgery (Figs 26.2A and B). The cartilaginous external auditory canal lies posterior to the joint and if proper care is not taken during the dissection it may get damaged and result into its stenosis or painful perichondritis. The auriculotemporal nerve fibers are present anterosuperiorly to the joint in the preauricular area and may get damaged if the incision is taken anterior to the preauricular fold, producing numbness of skin of the preauricular area. The internal maxillary artery, one of the terminal branches of the external carotid artery, originates in the substance of parotid gland and passes deep to the neck of the condyle (Figs 26.2A and B). It also gives the inferior alveolar branch which descends inferiorly to the mandibular foramen and enters the inferior alveolar canal. This artery also lies medial to the condylar neck and is likely to be damaged if a guard is not kept medially, during the release of ankylosis. In the chronic, severe cases of ankylosis the ramus is so short that while releasing the ankylosis the inferior cut in the bone may damage the inferior alveolar artery and cause profuse bleeding. The coronoid process becomes elongated in ankylosis and the temporalis muscle becomes

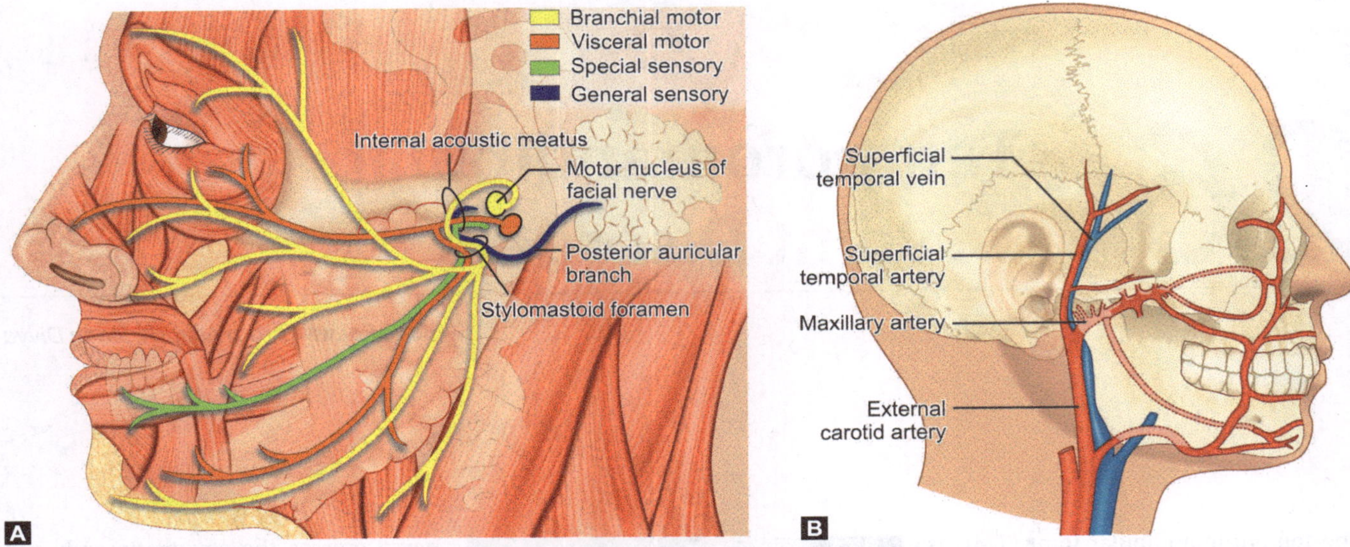

Figs 26.2A and B: Branches of: (A) Facial nerve; (B) External carotid artery (superficial temporal and internal maxillary) in relation to TMJ

atrophic. It restricts the mandibular excursions even after adequate release of ankylosis and the coronoid process is required to be excised for achieving free and passive movements of the mandible and get good postoperative mouth opening.

Etiopathogenesis (Box 26.1)

The trauma or infection in the joint tends to heal by fibrosis if not treated properly. The childhood falls on chin lead to indirect TMJ injuries and joint effusions, which lead to fibrous

Box 26.1: Etiology of ankylosis

1. Trauma
   a. Fall on the chin leading to indirect injuries to TMJ like hemarthrosis, contusion.
   b. Intracapsular and extracapsular fractures of condyle.
   c. Birth trauma—application of forceps during labor.
2. Infections
   a. Middle ear infections—CSOM
   b. Septic fractures of condyle, zygomatic arch
   c. Osteomyelitis of condyle
   d. Mastoiditis
   e. Hematogenous infections
   f. Specific infections—tuberculosis, syphilis, actinomycosis, etc.
3. Inflammatory joint pathologies—Osteoarthritis, rheumatoid arthritis, rheumatic arthritis.

adhesions and subsequently the ankylosis. The condylar fractures/injuries are often treated inadequately and lead to subsequent ankylosis. The hemarthrosis makes the environments in the joint space hypoxic, which facilitates calcification and may result in ankylosis.

The second most common cause of the TMJ ankylosis is chronic suppurative otitis media (CSOM). The middle ear infections are rampant in India. Apart from poor personal hygiene in rural population, the social customs like putting medicated oil in the external auditory meatus of newborn and children is a common practice not only in rural area, but also in the urban areas of India. This practice predisposes the middle ear infections. The middle ear infections are not always attended by specialists and are often inadequately treated leading to chronic course of the infection and its spread to adjacent TMJ leading to infective damage to the growing condylar head and healing by fibrosis, which results in ankylosis.

During the labor, when the fetus has vertex presentation and the labor is obstructed, the vaginal delivery is facilitated by application of delivery forceps. The beaks of the forceps are often applied over the preauricular region and not on the head as the skull bones are not fully ossified and can get damaged leading to gravious injury. The application of the forceps beaks can lead to damage to the tender, fibrocartilagenous condylar heads, leading to ankylosis. Although this problem was more common in the past, but in recent times as the procedure of labor has refined and as majority of pregnancies are precious and the facilities of caesarian sections are available even at smaller towns, majority of deliveries are carried out by caesarian section, to ensure the safety in difficult cases, the incidence of forceps assisted deliveries has drastically reduced and so has the incidence of TMJ ankylosis secondary to this cause.

Classification (Box 26.2 and 26.3)

- **True ankylosis or intra-articular ankylosis.**
  - Fibrous
  - Bony.
- **False or extra-articular ankylosis**
  - Fusion of coronoid process with the zygomatic arch.

Box 26.2: Topazian's classification

Stage-1: Ankylotic bone limited to condylar process.

Stage-2 : Ankylotic bone extending to sigmoid notch.

Stage-3 : Ankylotic bone extending to coronoid process.

Box 26.3: Approaches to the TMJ

- Preauricular
  - Hockey stick
  - Angulated vertical
  - Al-Kayat Bramley's.
- Postauricular.
- Endaural.
- Submandibular.
- Retromandibular (Hind's).
- Uni and bicoronal.

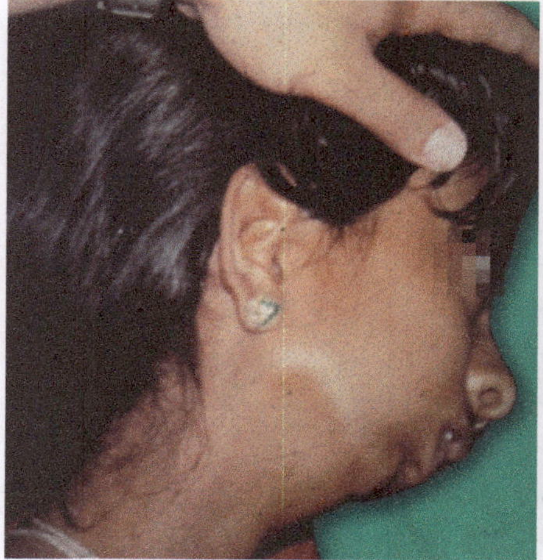

Fig. 26.4: Prominent gonial angle and accentuated antegonial notch

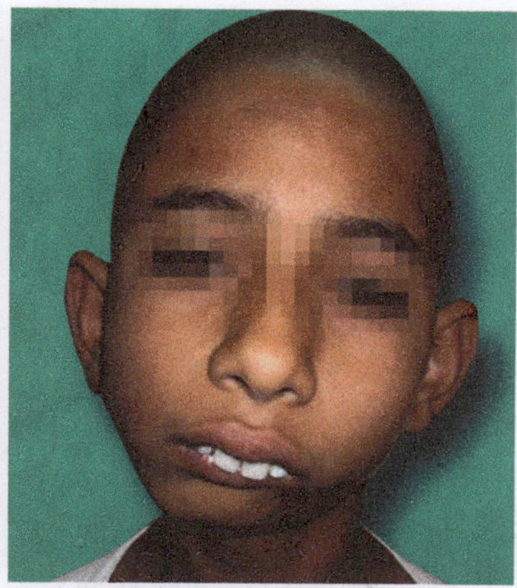

Fig. 26.5: Deviation of the chin to the affected side (right)

- Muscle fibrosis
- Myositis ossificans
- Oral submucous fibrosis
- Trismus hystericus
- Neurogenic—tetanus, tetany, meningitis, bulbar paralysis, etc.
- Congenital—Pierrie-Robins syndrome
- Miscellaneous—pericoronitis, depressed zygomatic fractures, oral
- Malignancy with retromolar extension or infratemporal extension, etc.

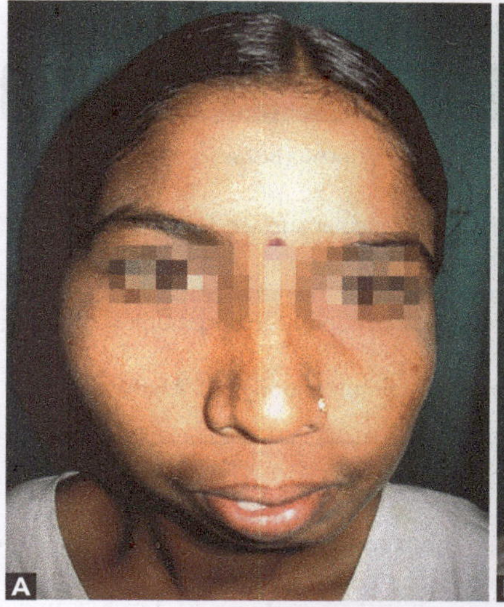

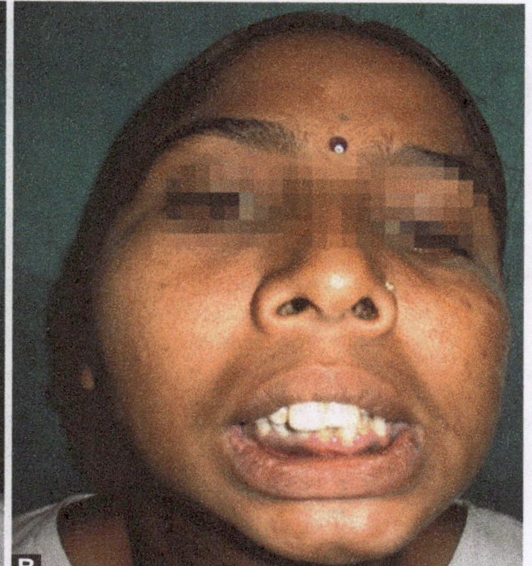

Figs 26.6A and B: Unilateral TMJ ankylosis of left side

Clinical Features

- Trismus—the mouth opening is gradually decreased. It is severely restricted in bony ankylosis as compared to fibrous ankylosis (Fig. 26.3).
- The TMJ movements are severely restricted in all excursions, i.e. protrusion, lateral excursion, including the opening. The joint movements are poorly palpable. In case of fibrous ankylosis, the joint movements are better felt as compared to bony ankylosis. In children the false joint movements are palpable due to stretching in the cranial sutures during forced opening.
- Restricted vertical growth of ramus.
- Prominent gonial angle with accentuated antigonial angle, due to pull from supra hyoid group of muscles (Fig. 26.4).
- Deviation of chin to the affected side, in case of unilateral ankylosis due to restricted vertical and horizontal growth of the mandible on the affected side, while as the other side keeps on growing normally (Figs 26.5 and 26.6).
- 'Bird face deformity' in case of bilateral ankylosis (Figs 26.7A and B).
- Fullness of face on the affected side, while the normal side is flattened.
- Convex facial profile.
- Poor oral hygiene.
- Rampant caries and periodontal problems.
- The coronoid process gets elongated due to atrophy of the temporalis muscle and the chronic pull exerted on it. The anatomy of the ramus, condyle and the coronoid process is distorted and the distortion becomes more conspicuous with the

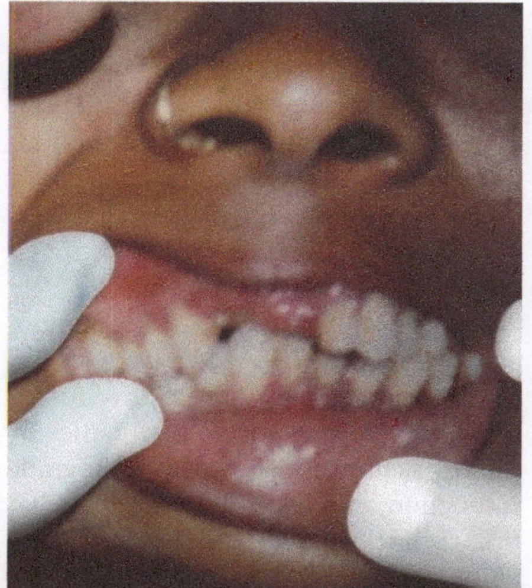

Fig. 26.3: Severe trismus, deep bite and loss of anterior teeth due to caries

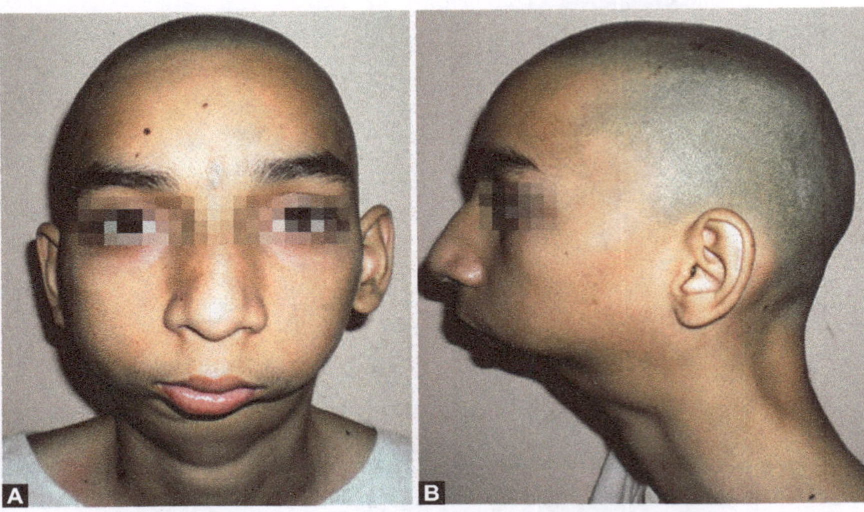

Figs 26.7A and B: Severe bird face deformity due to bilateral TMJ ankylosis

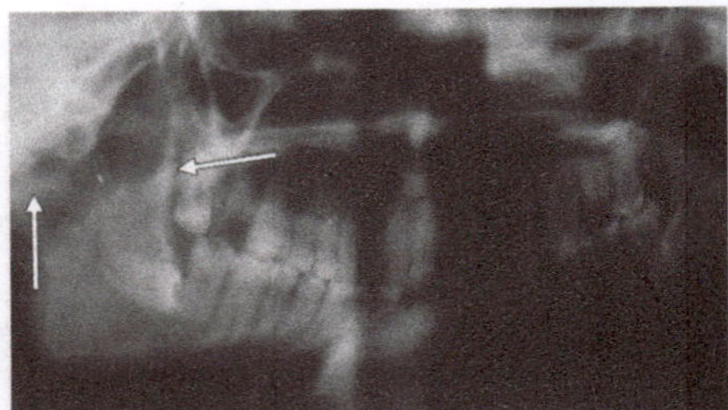

Fig. 26.8: Panoramic radiograph showing severe bony ankylosis with coronoid elongation

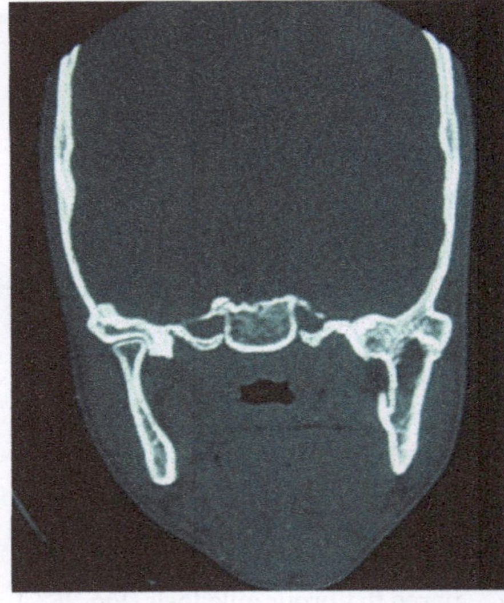

Fig. 26.9: CT scan showing deformed condyle and ankylosis

Table 26.1: Sawhney's grading

Sawhneys (1986) grading of TMJ ankylosis	
Type-1:	Condylar head is present without much distortion, fibrous adhesions make movement impossible.
Type-2:	Bony fusion of misshaped head of condyle and articular surface. No involvement of sigmoid notch and coronoid process.
Type-3:	A bony block bridging across the zygomatic arch and the ramus. Medially an atrophic, dislocated fragment of former head of condyle. Elongation of coronoid process seen.
Type-4:	Normal anatomy of TMJ is totally destroyed by complete bony block between ramus and skull base.

chronicity of the ankylosis. In long standing ankylosis the boney morphology is totally lost and replaced by a block of bone at the base of the skull. Depending on the radiological picture of the lesion, Sawhney (1986) has proposed the grading of the TMJ ankylosis as shown in Table 26.1.

- Crowding of teeth, the lower incisors often exhibit supraeruption and fanning and often tend to touch the palatal mucosa, especially in long standing cases. It is the compensatory phenomenon as the mandible is too far posteriorly placed as compared to the maxilla.
- The over all physical growth of the child is restricted due to malnourishment.
- Snoring in case of bilateral ankylosis cases due to decrease in posterior pharyngeal space
- The patient suffers from psychological problems due to the facial disfigurement.

Investigations

- X-rays—PA view of mandible, panoramic view of the mandible (Fig. 26.8), lateral oblique view of the mandible, transcranial and transpharyngeal views of the TMJ.
- CT scan, 2D or 3D reconstruction are very useful as they show the medial extent of the ankylosis properly, which is not otherwise visualized on conventional radiographs (Figs 26.9 and 26.10).
- X-ray chest to rule out pulmonary pathology and study the ribs in case costochondral graft or sternoclavicular joint graft is planned.
- Proper preoperative assessment of respiratory passage is required preoperatively as the intubation is often difficult due to trismus.
- Routine preoperative investigations are done to rule out any medical compromise, which may adversely affect the outcome of the surgery.

Anesthesia

As these patients have trismus laryngoscopy is not possible, hence the endotracheal intubation is extremely difficult. Thus, the patient is intubated either by blind nasal intubation or by retrograde intubation or by using fiberoptic intubating bronchoscope/laryngoscope (Fig. 26.11). When such skill or facilities are not available, elective tracheostomy may be done to intubate the patient for safe

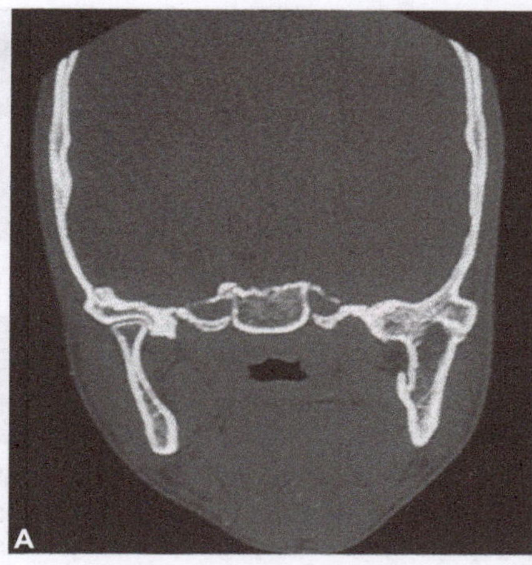

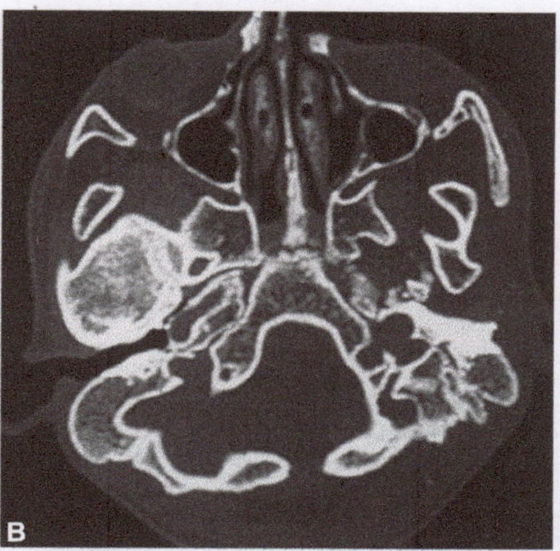

Figs 26.10A and B: (A) Coronal section showing severe bony ankylosis on left side; (B) Axial section showing large bony mass replacing condyle in a severe case of ankylosis the ankylosis is almost extending to the sphenoid bone

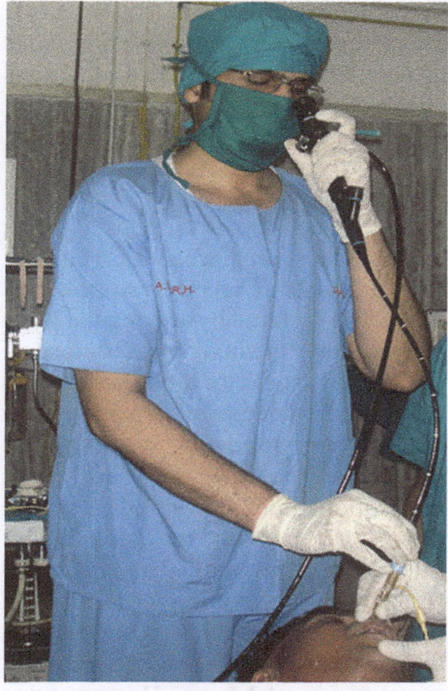

Fig. 26.11: Endotracheal intubation using a fiberoptic bronchoscope

administration of general anesthesia. If the tracheostomy is done the cuffed PVC tracheostomy tube is used to administer the anesthesia through it, as it seals the trachea. The cuff makes the tube self-retaining and prevents aspiration.

Surgical Access to the TMJ

The surgical access is created by giving various incisions. The ideal requirements of the incision are:

- It should give good, passive access to the surgical site.
- The scar should be hidden in the skin folds or hair line to get good cosmetic results.
- It should avoid damage to the important structures like superficial temporal vessels and facial nerve.

The following incisions are recommended for the TMJ surgery.

- *Preauricular incisions*
  - Angulated vertical incision[1]—the vertical limb lies in the preauricular fold and is angulated 45° to the vertical incision in the hairline, which goes in the bifurcation of superficial temporal vessels. The exposure is often inadequate with this incision.
  - Hockey stick incision[2,3]—the vertical limb lies in the preauricular fold and bends on the zygomatic arch. The incision is too inadequate, leaves an unsightly scar in the zygomatic arch and the chances of damage to zygomaticotemporal branch of the facial nerve are very high.
  - Al-Kayat Bramley's incision[4] (reverse question mark incision)—it is one of the most commonly practiced incisions as it gives an excellent access without damaging the important anatomical structures and is cosmetically acceptable (details of this incision are given in Chapter 3).
- *Unicoronal or bicoronal incisions*—give good exposure and facilitate coronoidectomy and temporal muscle interposition.
- *Endaural incision*—the incision is curled in the external ear to hide the scar.
- *Postauricular incision—not commonly practiced.*
- Submandibular incision (Risdon's)—this incision is *(discussed in Chapter 3—Incisions in Maxillofacial Surgery)*.
- Retro-mandibular extension (Hind's) This incision is *(discussed in Chapter 3—Incisions in Maxillofacial Surgery)*.

The last two incisions are seldom used for the management of ankylosis, but are commonly used for fixation of subcondylar fractures of other ramal surgeries (Figs 26.12A to D).

Management of TMJ Ankylosis

Various treatment modalities have been proposed for the management of the TMJ ankylosis as shown in the Box 26.4. The treatment should be comprehensive ensuring long-term, recurrence free management with adequate, sustainable mouth opening and correction of the facial deformities for improving esthetics and social acceptance. The aims of the TMJ ankylosis are summarized in Box 26.5.

Kaban's Protocol

Kaban[5] proposed (Box 26.6) a comprehensive protocol for the effective management of TMJ ankylosis, which is popularly known as Kaban's protocol.

Brisement Force

Brisement force is the forceful mouth opening, under general anesthesia, using heavy mouth gags. It is a treatment modality for treating the fibrous ankylosis. The assessment of the condylar head and the joint space is very critical before opting for this treatment modality. When the condylar head is not deformed and joint space is not severely narrowed, this method may be used. But, when the condyle is deformed and the joint space is severely narrowed it should be considered as transition from fibrous to bony ankylosis and condylectomy should be performed as the chances of recurrence are very high. However,

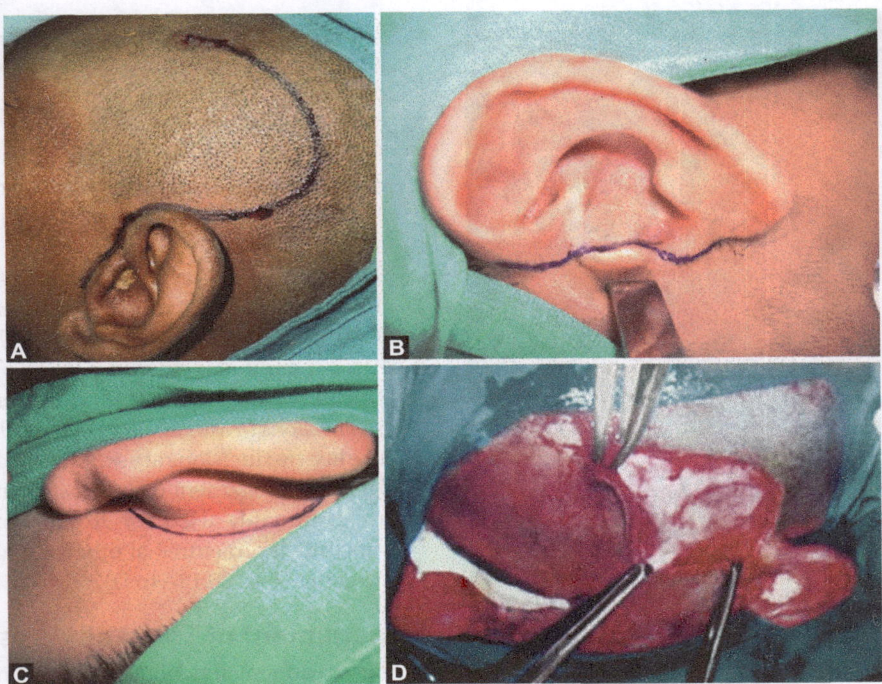

Figs 26.12A to D: Various approaches for TMJ: (A) Al-Kayat Bramley incision; (B) Preauricular incision; (C) Postauricular incision; (D) Unicoronal incision

Box 26.4: Treatment modalities

- Brisement force
- Condylectomy
- Gap arthroplasty
- Interpositional arthroplasty with reconstruction of the joint.

Box 26.5: Aims of treatment

- Release of ankylosis
- Prevention of re-ankylosis
- To restore vertical height of mandible
- To facilitate growth
- Correction of residual facial deformities.

Box 26.6: Kaban's protocol

- Aggressive surgical resection creating gap of minimum 1.5 cm
- Ipsilateral coronoidectomy
- Contralateral coronoidectomy (minimum mouth opening of 35 mm)
- Interpositioning
- Aggressive postoperative physiotherapy
- Regular follow-up
- Rehabilitation.

such assessment is not often possible on routine radiographs and CT scans are more suitable investigation (Fig. 26.13).

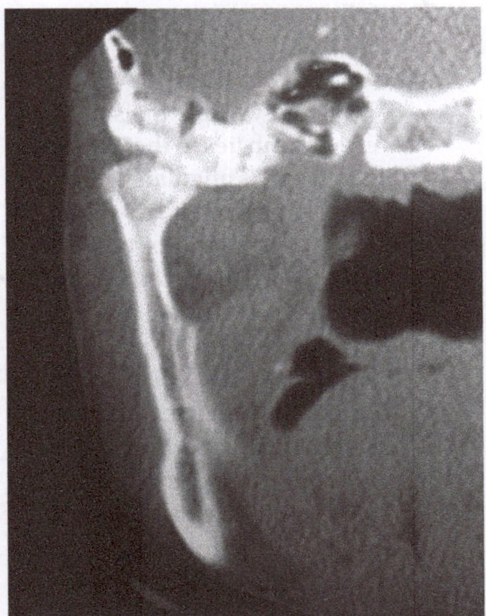

Fig. 26.13: Fibrous ankylosis with distortion of the condylar head, an indication for condylectomy

Condylectomy

When the outline of the glenoid fossa and condyle is identifiable, the superior osteotomy cut is placed at this level of glenoid fossa and the condyle is resected by completing the osteotomy by taking the inferior cut at the neck. This procedure is done in early cases of bony ankylosis and cases of fibrous ankylosis where the condyle is deformed (Fig. 26.14).

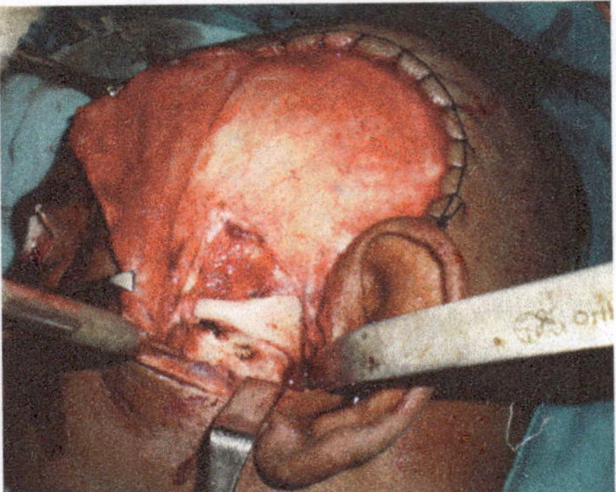

Fig. 26.14: Exposure of ankylosed joint and insertion of the condylar retractor as a guard to prevent injury to blood vessels present medially

Gap Arthroplasty

The joint is exposed surgically using any of the above approaches. The joint morphology is invariably disturbed and the joint is replaced by an irregular bony mass. Usually the bony mass is more on the medial aspect than the lateral. The root of the zygomatic arch is identified; the superior osteotomy cut is placed just below it to ensure that accidental perforation into the middle cranial fossa. After marking the superior cut the inferior cut is marked about 1 to 1.5 cm inferiorly to get a good clearance. The intervening bone is removed, and the gap is created. It is desirable to create a gap of 1.5 cm. However, due to long standing, severe ankylosis as seen in India, the height of the ramus is so short that the inferior cut lies near the inferior border of the mandible or one is likely cut through the impacted third molar present in the ramus, thus, a gap of 1 cm should be regarded as adequate (Figs 26.15A to C). While doing the osteotomy with a bur or saw care should be taken to prevent damage to the internal maxillary artery and its descending branch, the inferior alveolar artery, which lies medial to the condylar

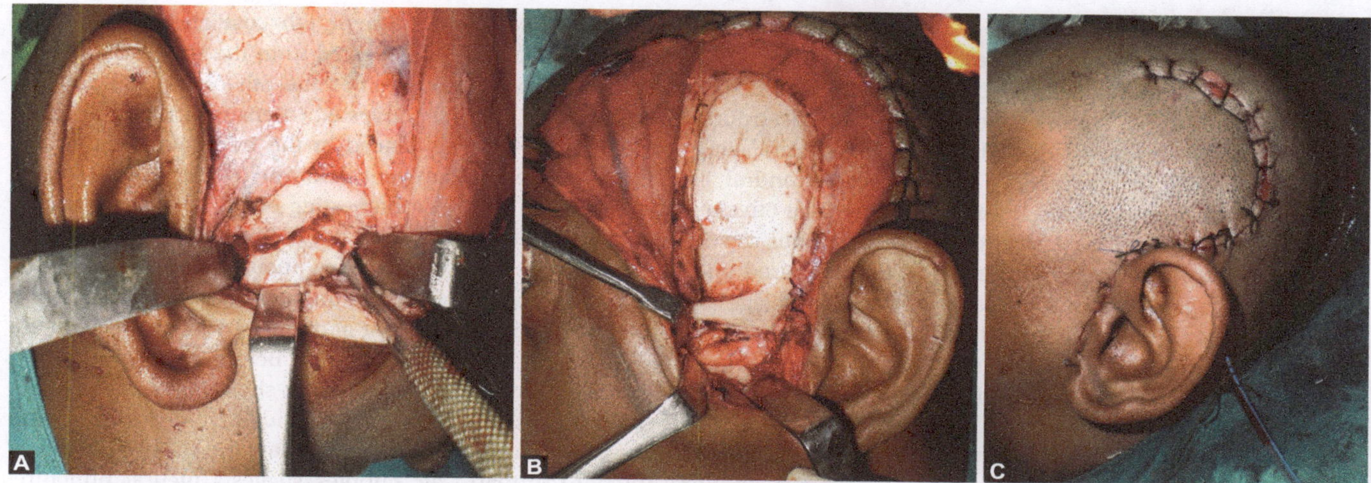

Figs 26.15A to C: Marking superior and inferior cuts for gap arthroplasty and final gap arthroplasty with interposition

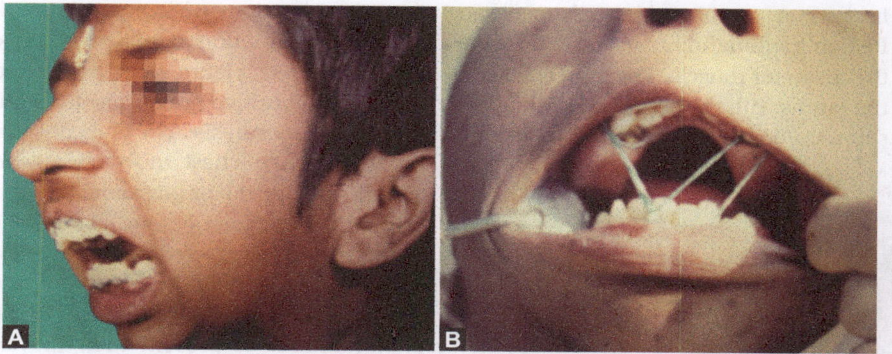

Figs 26.16A and B: Open bite deformity due to shortening of ramus after bilateral gap arthroplasty

neck, by keeping a guard (condylar retractor). After the complete release of the ankylosis, the mouth opening is verified on the table by forceful opening with the help of a mouth gag. The mouth opening of minimum 35 mm is considered to be adequate, which gradually improves with postoperative physiotherapy. The raw edges of the bone are smoothened and the posterosuperior edge of the ostetomized ramus should be rounded off to prevent obstruction during the mandibular opening. Free, unobstructed movements of the mandible should be elicited by manually moving the mandible. If the mouth opening is not adequate and the mandibular movements appear to be obstructed when the mandible is moved in different excursions by the operator, the coronoidectomy is indicated. The wound is closed in layers, keeping a drain in place. The main disadvantage with gap arthroplasty is recurrence. The gap tends to get narrowed due to upward pulling of the mandible due to muscle pull and fibrosis during the healing phase. It is more conspicuous in cases of bilateral ankylosis where shortening of ramus following creation of the gaps and upward pull of mandible leads to anterior open bite deformity (apertognathia). The mechanics of the mandible get altered and changes from a class I lever to the class III lever. This can be prevented to certain extent by giving the patient a hypomochlion and anterior inter maxillary guiding elastics (Figs 26.16A and B). All the cases of TMJ ankylosis are essentially followed up postoperatively by long-term, aggressive physiotherapy, to prevent re-ankylosis.

Interpositional Arthroplasty

After the drawbacks of gap arthroplasty became evident, efforts were made to prevent the reankylosis by interposing a barrier between the two osteotomized bony ends to prevent the bony growth and reunion. According to Verneuil, the first arthroplasty was made by Percy and Barton in 1826. In 1860 Verneuil was the first to suggest the interpositional arthroplasty.[6] Many materials were tried for the interposition with varied degree of success and the choice of the interpositional material varies from surgeon to surgeon. The interpositional materials can be classified as:

Alloplastic Material

Titanium, teflon, silastic, stainless steel, acrylic, silicon, etc.[7-9]

The use of silastic[10] was very popular in the mid seventies, but due to its high failure rate it lost its popularity. The acrylic, teflon and titanium have been used with varied degree of success. The use of metallic condyle for reconstruction of joint was recommended. However, the metallic condyle tends to erode the roof of the glenoid fossa and cause perforation into the middle cranial fossa.[11] The total joint replacement with metallic glenoid fossa and the condyle is also recommended.

Autogenous Material

Full thickness skin,[12] cartilage,[13], fascia lata,[14] temporal muscle-fascia,[15] costochondral joint (CCG), sternoclavicular joint,[16] metacarpal joint, etc. have been used as interpositional material.

The surgical procedure remains similar to that of gap arthroplasty, except that the interpositional material is interposed in the gap. When the ankylosis is released by performing an osteotomy both the superior and inferior ends of the bone are raw and are likely to reunite due to bone formation as it is seen during the healing of the fracture. The interpositional material prevents the proliferation of bone and subsequent reankylosis by serving as a subsequent materials like CCG, sternoclavicular joint, metacarpal joint, help in restoration of vertical height of ramus and prevent the open bite deformity. The CCG is a popular interpositional material, either alone or with temporal muscle and fascia. The cranial surface of the osteomized bone is lined by a pedicled temporal muscle-fascia–pericranium flap, keeping the pericranium facing cranially and then a costochondral junction is harvested from 5th or 6th rib on the right side. The cartilaginous cap over the rib is trimmed and contoured and not more than 3 to 4 mm of cartilage is kept, (2 mm according to new protocol by Kaban) because the costochondral junction is fragile and tends to fracture under stress if kept longer. Some surgeons prefer to preserve a strip of periosteum and perichondrium over the costochondral junction to impart it strength. The CCG is interposed either through the same incision or is tunneled in proper position through separate Risdon's submandibular incision, below the masseter muscle. The graft is fixed to the ramus with the help of SS or titanium screws. For harvesting the CCG usually the 5th or 6th costochondral junction is harvested from the right side. In case of females the 6th or 7th CC junction is harvested to ensure that the incision is placed in the inframammary fold to prevent deformity of the breast. During the harvesting of the CCG, care should be taken not to injure the parietal pleura as it leads to pneumothorax (Figs 26.17A to D). An intercostal drain should always be kept as a standby in case the pleura is perforated. Before closing the chest incision, saline should be sprayed at the surgical site and the anesthetist should be asked to inflate the chest, presence of air bubbles suggests pleural puncture. All the cases where the CCG is harvested should be evaluated postoperatively for detecting the signs of pneumothorax if the small perforation is missed on table or the eroded pleura gets perforated later due to positive pressure ventilation during the anesthesia. The clinical signs like diminished chest movements and air entry, surgical emphysema, hyper-resonant percussion note should be noted and in suspected cases PA view of the chest should be done to rule out pneumothorax (Fig. 26.18). If the pneumothorax is present then the air in the pleural space should be drained by inserting an intercostal drain (under water seal) and advising blowing exercises to the patient.

Advantages of CCG

- Restores the vertical height of mandible.

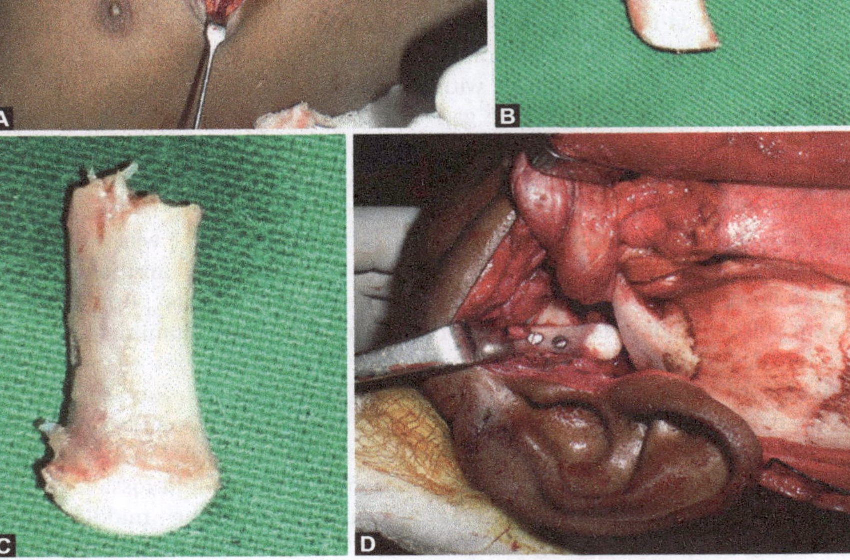

Figs 26.17A to D: (A) Incision and exposure of the 6th rib and CC junction; (B) Harvested CC graft; (C) Reduction of the cartilage cap to 3 to 4 mm to prevent fracture; (D) Fixation of CCG with screws to the lateral aspect of the ramus

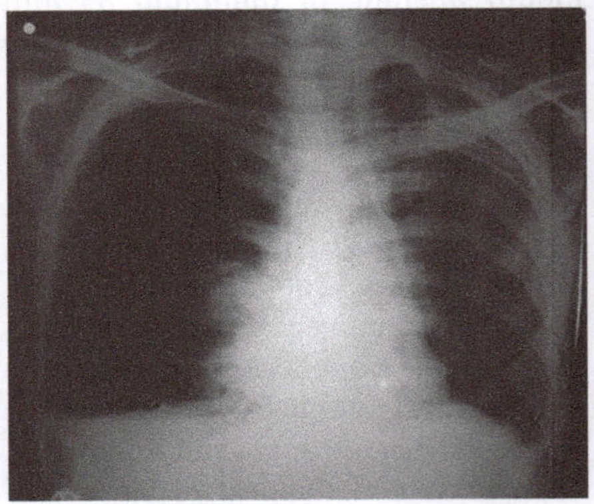

Fig. 26.18: X-ray chest showing pneumothorax (absence of lung shadow on the right side)

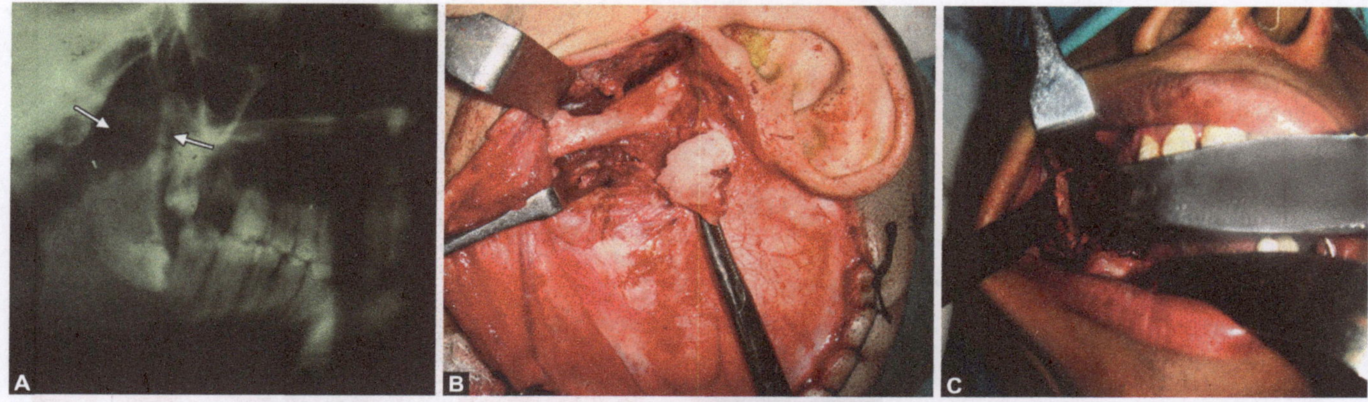

Figs 26.19A to C: Ipsilateral coronoidectomy through the same incision and contralateral coronoidectomy by transoral approach

- Facilitates the growth of mandible by growing like a natural condyle.

Disadvantages of CCG

- Infection
- Fracture of CC junction
- Rejection
- Over growth especially in growth spurs and during pregnancy in females.
- Pleural puncture while harvesting the graft may lead to pneumothorax.

Role of Coronoidectomy

The coronoid process often gets elongated and deformed in cases of long standing TMJ ankylosis. The temporalis muscle inserted onto the coronoid process is also severely atrophic and restricts the mandibular opening even after the ankylosis is adequately released. During the surgery the wasting of the temporalis is evident in the form of thinning out of the muscle. In order to achieve the satisfactory mouth opening of minimum 35 mm following the release of ankylosis, it becomes imperative to excise the ipsilateral coronoid process and evaluate the mouth opening. If the mouth opening and the jaw excursions are still inadequate then the contralateral coronoid process should also be excised. The ipsilateral coronoid process can be excised through the same incision taken for the release of ankylosis and the contralateral coronoid process can be easily excised through a transoral incision taken over the anterior border of the coronoid process (Figs 26.19A to C). After excision of the coronoid processes not only the interincisal opening is assessed, but the passive mandibular excursions should also be demonstrable. It is not always necessary to remove the resected coronoid process and only release of the coronoid process (coronoidotomy) is adequate to overcome the restraining effect of the atrophic temporalis muscle. The moment the coronoid process is resected the strong pull of the atrophic temporalis muscle retracts it superiorly in the infratemporal fossa. Although there is no fixed criterion to decide when the coronoidectomy should be done, but it becomes necessary if the duration of ankylosis is more than 2 years as this time is adequate to induce atrophic changes in the temporalis muscle. The most appropriate decision is taken on table by assessing the interincisal opening and passive mandibular excursions, following release of ankylosis.

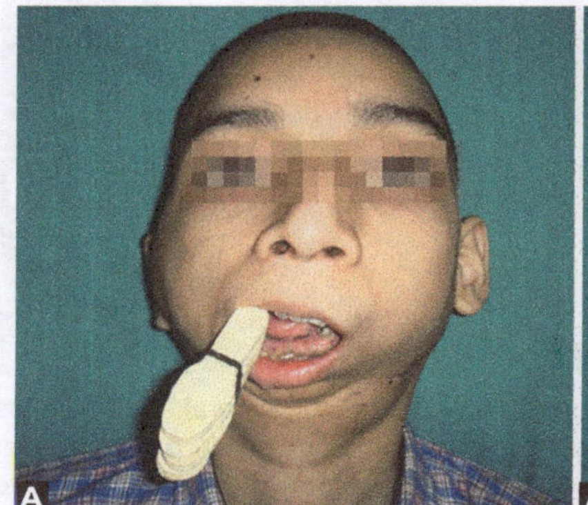

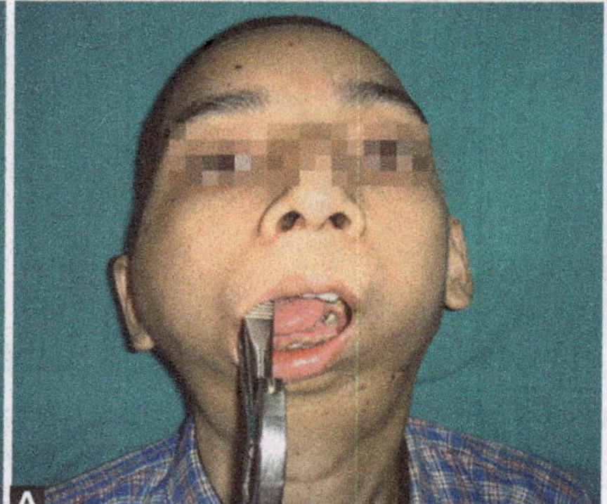

Figs 26.20A and B: (A) Passive jaw exercises using ice cream sticks; (B) Heister's jaw exercises

Role of Physiotherapy

The postoperative physiotherapy is of vital importance to improve and maintain the results achieved by the surgery. Most of the failures following the surgery are due to inadequate efforts taken by the surgeon to highlight the importance of physiotherapy to the patient or due to noncompliance of the patient. The physiotherapy should be started after 7 to 10 days of latency period postoperatively and should be continued for a period of 2 years following the surgery. During the initial phase the physiotherapy is started with ice cream sticks and later the Heister's jaw exerciser is a good instrument to impart physiotherapy. Periodic follow up and supervision of the physiotherapy is mandatory (Figs 26.20A and B).

Apart from the forceful jaw opening exercises, physiotherapy in form of TENS is indicated to treat the accidental damage to the facial nerve (neuropraxia) during the TMJ surgery.

Surgical Photos of Cases

Case 1: Figures 26.21A to H
Case 2: Figures 26.22A to I
Case 3: Figures 26.23A to J
Case 4: Figures 26.24A to E

Complications

The complications associated with TMJ surgery are:

- Infection.
- Hemorrhage—due to damage to superficial temporal vessels, internal maxillary artery, inferior alveolar artery, internal jugular vein.
- Reankylosis.
- Open bite deformity.
- Damage to the facial nerve and auriculotemporal nerve (Figs 26.25A and B).
- Stenosis of external auditory canal.
- Perforation in middle cranial fossa.

Management of Mandibular Deformities

The mandibular growth is severely restricted in ankylosis, which results in severe deformities like retrusion of chin, deviation of chin, reduced vertical height, crowding, malocclusion, etc. These deformities can be corrected by orthognathic surgical procedures like genioplasty, sagittal split osteotomy, distraction osteogenesis, orthodontic therapy, etc. depending the merit of each case. The details of these procedures are discussed in the Chapter 25 (Orthognathic Surgery).

The distraction osteogenesis is more commonly practiced modality for correcting the mandibular deformity following the TMJ ankylosis. The distraction can be done preoperatively or postoperatively. The advantage of preoperative distraction is that the distraction vector is more controlled. In case of postoperative distraction the proxymal fragments tends to move cranially, reducing the gap created during the release of ankylosis, thus enhancing the

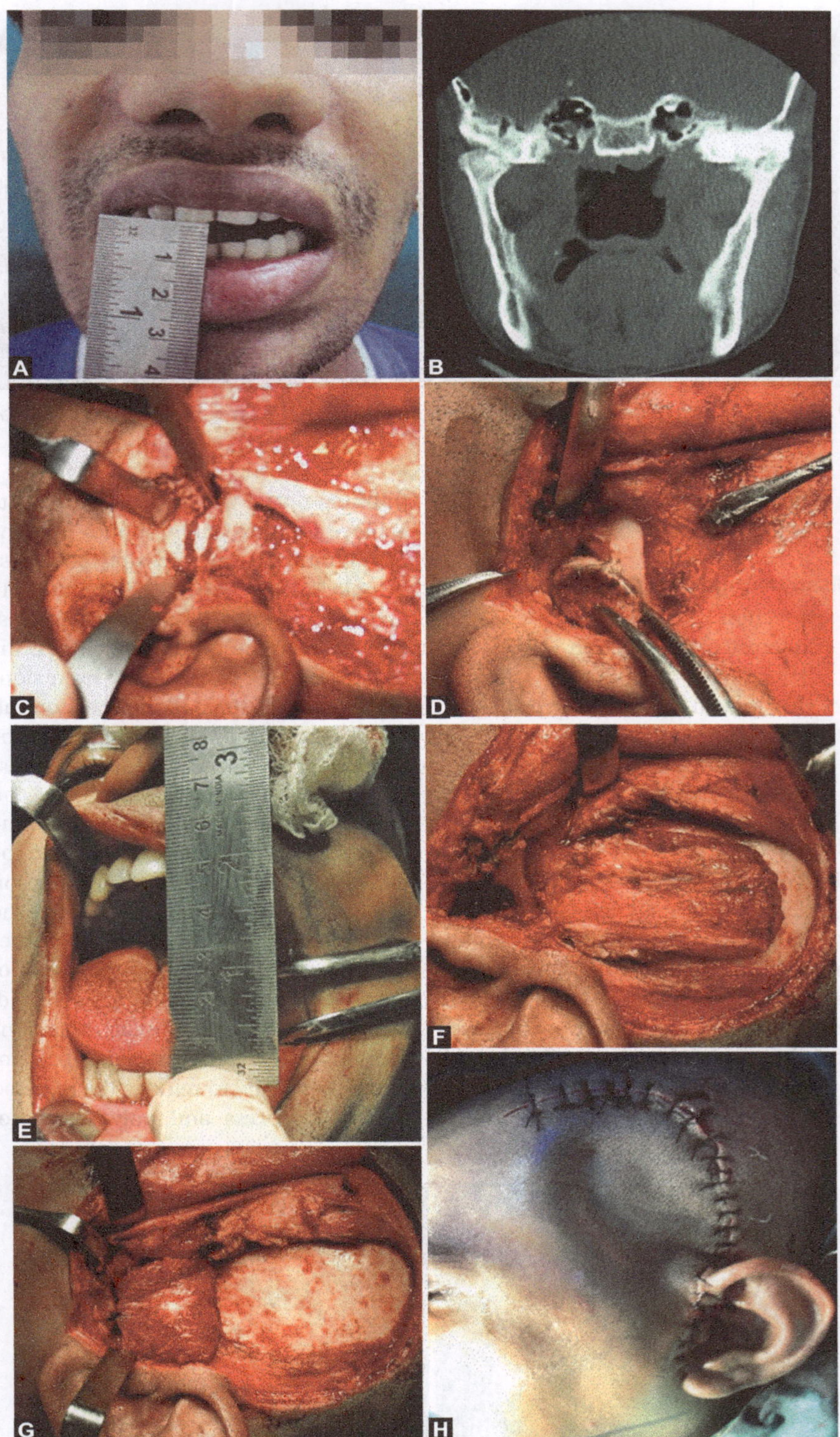

Figs 26.21A to H: (A) Mouth opening restricted in a case of bilateral TMJ ankylosis; (B) CT scan showing bony ankylosis on left side and early fibrous union on right side in coronal cuts; (C) Osteotomy cuts for gap arthroplasty; (D) Ankylotic bony mass removed; (E) Mouth opening achieved after gap arthroplasty; (F) Temporalis muscle harvested for interpositional arthroplasty; (G) Temporalis muscle sutured over the zygomatic arch; (H) Final closure with activated drain

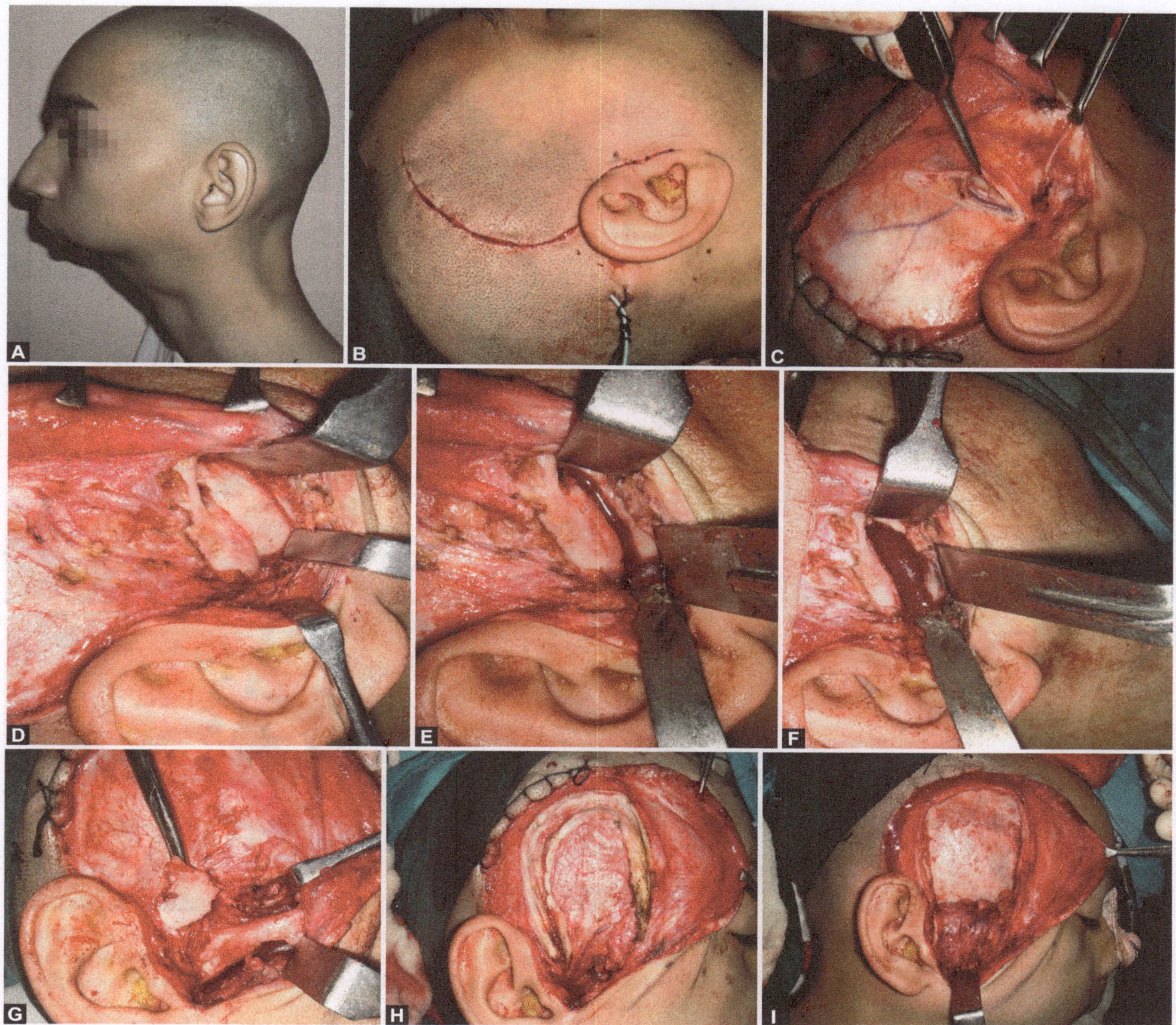

Figs 26.22A to I: A case of bilateral TMJ ankylosis with surgical photos: (A) Bilateral ankylosis; (B) Al-Kayat Bramley's incision; (C) and (D) Splitting the layers of deep temporal fascia to prevent damage to the facial nerve and exposure of ankylotic area; (E and F) Osteotomy cut below the root of the zygomatic arch and creation of gap and release of ankylosis; (G and H) Coronoidectomy through the same incision and harvested temporal muscle-fascia-pericranium flap; (I) Interpositioning of temporal muscle fascia pericranium flap in the gap

chances of reankylosis. The other problem with the postoperative distraction is that once the mouth opening is achieved by release of ankylosis, the patients do not report for the correction of deformity in the Indian circumstances. The distraction can be two dimentional, i.e. the verical ramal height can be increased along with the horizontal elongation of the atrophic mandible.

OTHER TEMPOROMANDIBULAR JOINT DISORDERS

Arthritis

Traumatic Arthritis, Hemarthrosis

The TMJ is often subjected to indirect trauma. The fall on the chin thrusts the mandible backward and upward and the intervening soft tissues like the capsule, meniscus and synovial membrane get contused and undergo inflammation. The inflammatory reaction makes the joint painful and hypomobile. The effusion of the joint space by the inflammatory exudates and or blood takes place, because of which the condyle gets pushed downwards

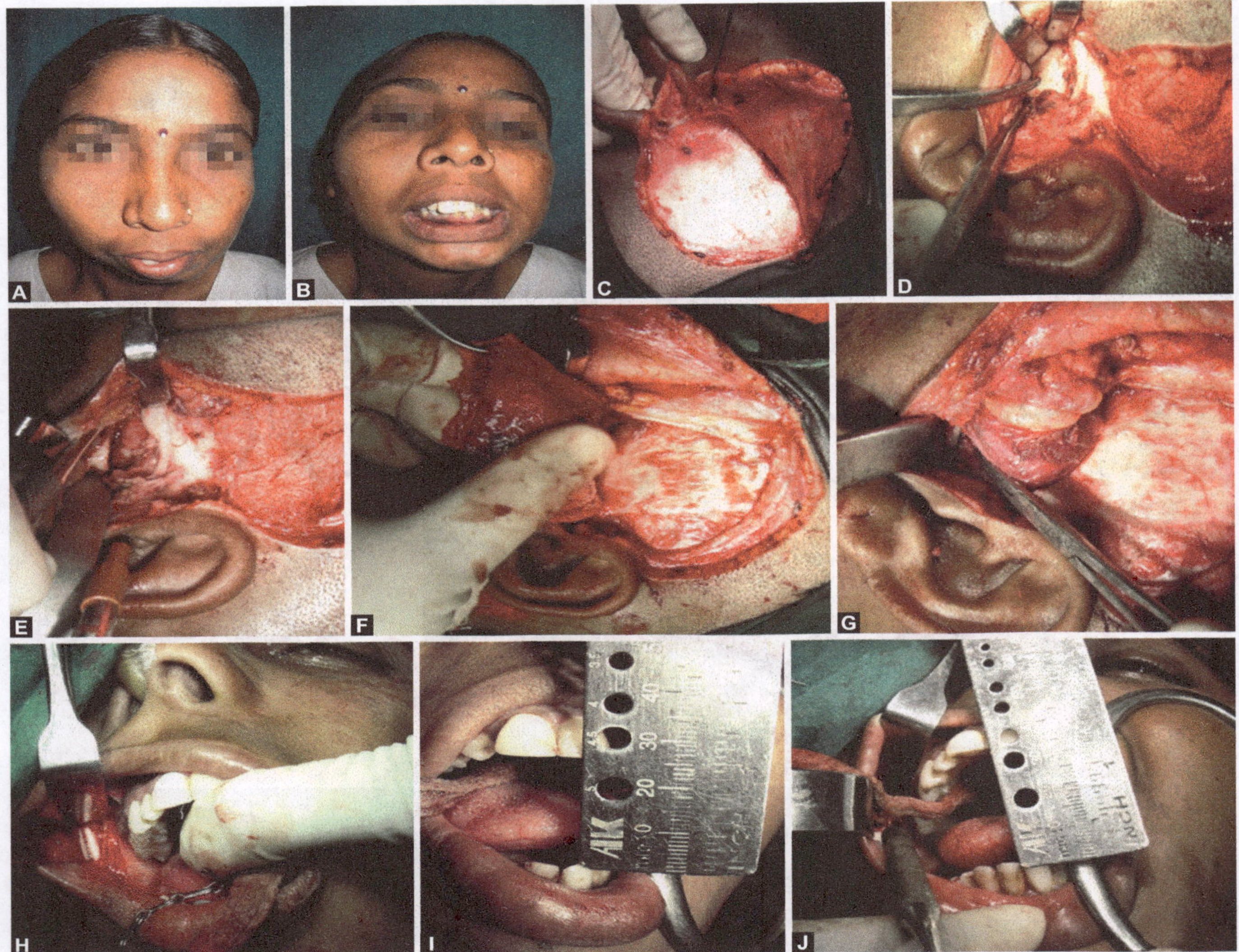

Figs 26.23A to J: Surgical management of ankylosis with interpositional arthroplasty: (A and B) Preoperative photographs; (C) Exposure of deep temporal fascia; (D) Exposure of ankylotic mass; (E) Release of ankylosis; (F) Harvesting temporal muscle fascia flap; (G) Interpositioning temporal muscle fascia flap; (H) Ipsilateral coronoidectomy; (I) Interincisal opening; (J) Improved interincisal opening after contralateral coronoidectomy

and produces open bite on the involved side.

The clinical features of the traumatic arthritis are:

- Positive history of trauma.
- Pain tenderness and swelling over the TMJ.
- Trismus and restricted excursions.
- There is open bite on the involved side due to effusion of exudates or blood (hemarthrosis) in the joint space.
- X-ray shows widening of the joint space.

Management

In the acute phase of inflammation the inflamed joint needs rest and thus, the jaw movements should be restricted by placing inter maxillary elastics or by placing temporary IMF for a period of a week. Supportive treatment in the form of prescription of anti-inflammatory drugs is started. If there is hemarthrosis, then drugs like trypsin, chymotrypsin, serratiopeptidase may be helpful. Prophylactic antibiotics to prevent secondary infection can be considered. The patient is prescribed liquid and soft diet. Exercises are contraindicated in acute phase and physiotherapy in the form of diathermy may be prescribed. The heat induces vasodilatation and helps in clearing the inflammatory reaction. Once the acute phase subsides, the patient is advised active physiotherapy to prevent adhesions and ankylosis.

Osteoarthritis (Degenerative Joint Disorder)

Osteoarthritis is a noninflammatory disorder characterized by joint deteriorat-ion and proliferation. It is also thought

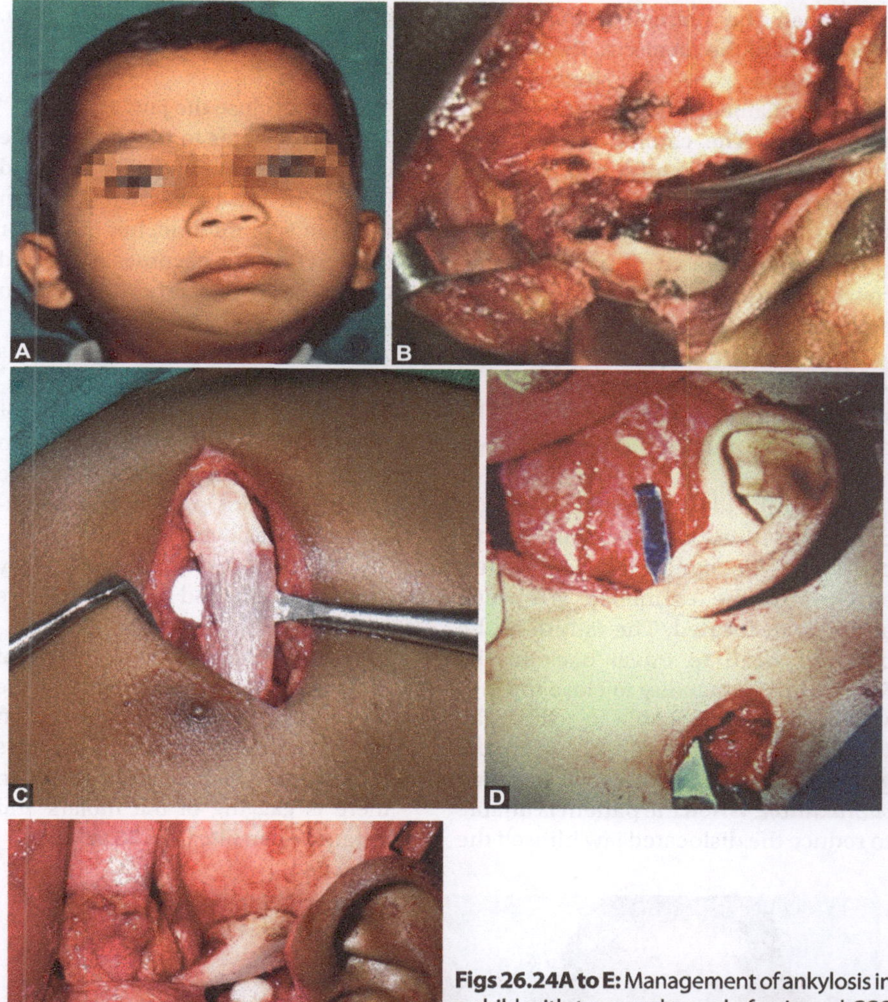

Figs 26.24A to E: Management of ankylosis in a child with temporal muscle fascia and CCG interposition: (A) Preoperative photograph; (B) Release of ankylosis; (C) Harvesting CCG; (D) Preparation of the tunnel through the separate submandibular incision; (E) Fixing the CCG to the ramus with screws

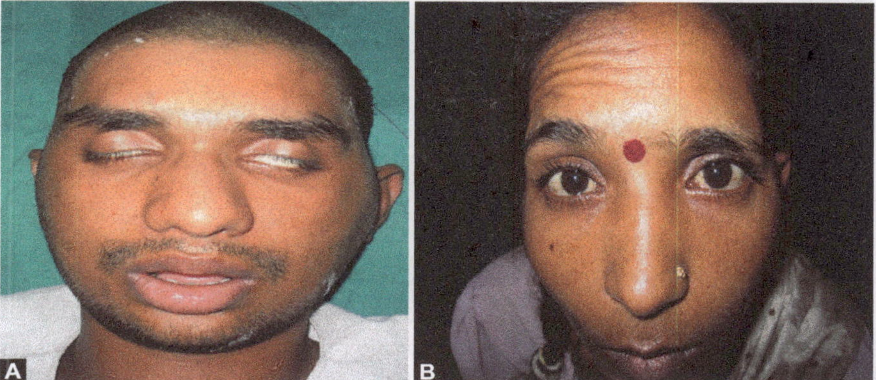

Figs 26.25A and B: Damage to the zygomaticotemporal branch of facial nerve leading to loss of wrinkling over forehead and incomplete closure of upper eyelid

to be the most common type of arthritis. Although the etiology is unknown it is a disease associated with aging process.

Clinical signs and symptoms are remarkably absent even in the phase of histological changes in the joint. Since the TMJ is not a weight-bearing joint, changes here are insignificant even though arthropathy may be present in other joints. Patient may complain of pain on palpation and movements, which is associated with muscle spasm. The onset of these symptoms may be sudden or gradual and symptoms may disappear spontaneously, only to return in recurring cycles.

Radiographic features

When the patient is in maximum intercuspation, the joint space may be narrow or absent. Flattening of condylar head may be evident. Loss of cortex or erosion of the articulating surfaces of the condyle or temporal component are characteristic of this disease. 'Ely cysts', small round radiolucent areas with irregular margins surrounded by increased density, are visible. In the advanced stage of the disease bony proliferation occurs at the periphery of the articulating surface area. This new bone, which is formed is known as osteophyte. The broken osteophytes lie within the joint space, known as 'joint mice'.

Treatment

Treatment is directed towards relieving joint stress-splint therapy, relieving secondary inflammation with anti-inflammatory drugs and physiotherapy. Arthrocentesis has been effective in washing out noxious metabolites and 'bone sand' that are present in the joint and can produce symptomatic relief from pain. Intra-articular injections of corticosteroids also produce symptomatic relief. In severe cases high conylotomy (condylar shave) or excision of the affected condyle and join replacement can be done.

Rheumatoid Arthritis

Rheumatoid arthritis is an autoimmune inflammatory condition in which the inflamed and hypertrophic synovial membrane grows onto the articulating surfaces.

The TM joint is frequently involved in rheumatoid arthritis. Ganik and Williams reported 65 percent patients with juvenile arthritis have TM disorder. Haandes et al reported that more than half of the cases involved TM joints.

It is more common in females and may occur at any age, but there is increase in the incidence with increasing age. Usually small joints of the hands, wrist, knees and feet are affected in a bilateral, symmetric fashion, similarly TM joint involvement usually occurs bilaterally and symmetrically. Patients with TM joint involvement complain of swelling, pain, tenderness, stiffness on opening, limited range of motion and crepitus. Bilateral destruction of joint may lead to anterosuperior positioning of condyles, which may further lead to anterior open bite.

Radiographic features

Diminished width of a joint space due to destruction of disk may be visible. bony erosion of the condylar anterior or posterior surfaces may occur giving a 'sharpened pencil' appearance of the condyle. Erosive changes sometimes are so severe that entire condyle is destroyed.

Treatment

Treatment is directed towards pain relief-analgesics, reduction or suppression of inflammation-NSAID or corticosteroids and physiotherapy. High condylotomy or joint replacement in the patients with severe joint destruction may be required.

Hypermobility, Subluxation and Dislocation

The inherent weakness in the joint capsule, the laxity anteromedially, makes it susceptible to hypermobility and related disorders. Normally during the opening of the jaw, the condyle translates up to the posterior slope of articular eminence. When the capsule is lax, the restraining action on the condyle is lost and the condyle moves ahead of the articular eminence. This condition is clinically manifested as hypermobility. The jaw opens more than the normal. The posterior attachment of the meniscus, the fibers of the bilamellar zone, gets stretched and become inflamed, which produces pain in the joint. The chronic stretching in the fibers makes them lax and meniscus condylar disharmony may be precipitated, leading to clicking, painful joint.

The management of hypermobility consists of restraining the excessive jaw movements by advising the patient not to open the mouth wide or support the lower jaw at the chin, while yawning. In severe cases the jaw movements can be restrained by placing the intermaxillary elastics.

A step ahead of the hypermobility is the subluxation or dislocation. In this condition the condylar head travels anterior to the eminence articularis and gets dislocated. The failure of the condylar head to travel back in the fossa, leads to inability to close the jaw. When the patient is able to reduce the condyle in its normal position in the glenoid fossa of his own, it is called *subluxation*. When the patient is unable to reduce the dislocated jaw himself the condition is described as *dislocation*. The clinical features of the dislocation are as follows:

- Inability to close the jaw.
- The jaw deviates to the normal side in case of unilateral dislocation and in case of the bilateral dislocation the chin is in midline, but the lower third of the face becomes elongated due to open bite. The lips remain parted (Fig. 26.26A).
- The saliva dribbles as the patient is unable to swallow.
- The patient complains of pain over the joint. The pain produces spasm of the periarticular muscles and the spastic muscles prevent the reduction of the dislocated jaw.
- The glenoid fossae appear empty on inspection and palpation (Figs 26.26B and C).
- Occlusal derangement—in case of unilateral dislocation the teeth on the involved side are in open bite and on the contralateral side there is cross bite. In case of bilateral dislocation there is gagging of the molars and anterior open bite (Fig. 26.26D).

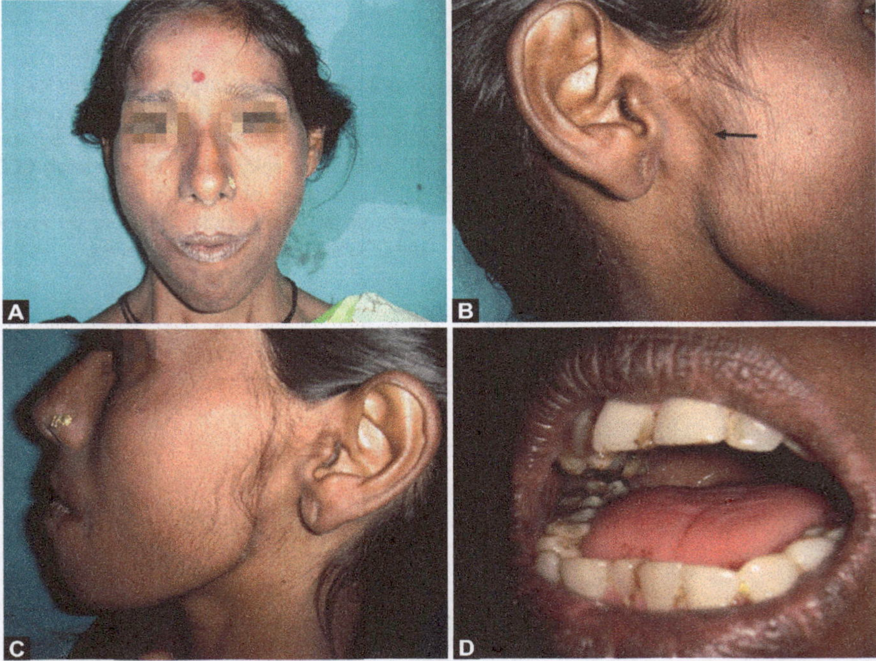

Figs 26.26A to D: A case of bilateral TMJ dislocation showing inability to close the jaw, elongation of the face, open bite with gagging of the posterior teeth, hollowing in the TMJ region

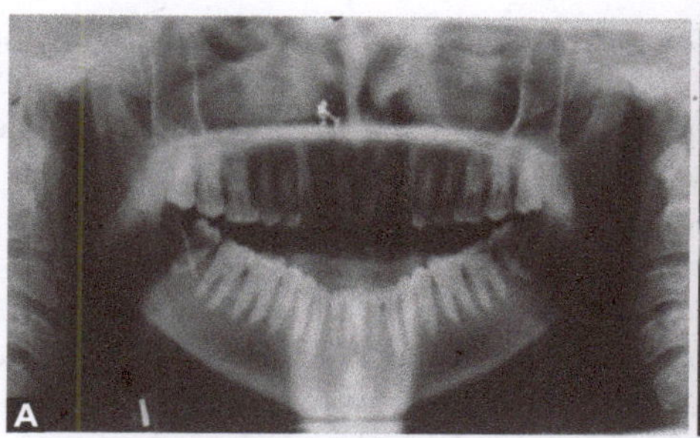
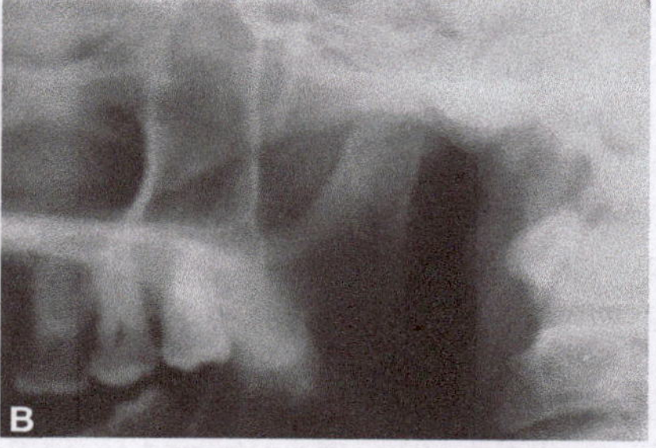

Figs 26.27A and B: The X-rays show the condyle anterior to the articular eminence

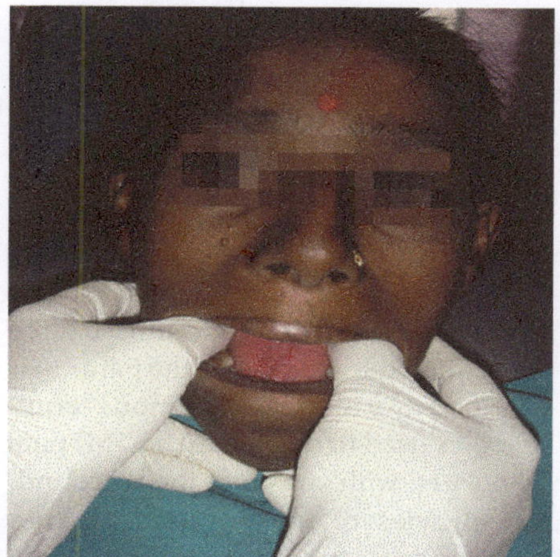

Fig. 26.28: Reduction of the dislocation

- X-ray shows empty glenoid fossae and condyle lies ahead of articular eminence (Figs 26.27A and B).

Management

In acute condition the dislocation can be reduced by manipulation of the lower jaw. The patient is made to sit in the dental chair with the occiputes supported by head rest. The operator stands in front at 7 o'clock position and holds the mandible by keeping the thumbs on the molars and the index and middle fingers on the inferior border. The mandible is then drawn slightly anterior, down wards and then pushed backwards and upwards to reduce the dislocated condyles back in the fossae (Fig. 26.28). This maneuver helps in negotiating the articular eminence. This procedure is usually done without anesthesia. When the muscle spasm or pain is present administration of the sedatives, analgesics and muscle relaxants may be required. In the cases where the acute pain and severe muscle spasm is present, which prevents the reduction or where the dislocation is relatively old or if the patient is apprehensive the reduction may be attempted under GA with full muscle relaxation. Once the reduction is achieved, to prevent the recurrence, the lower jaw is supported by giving extraoral barrel or four tailed bandage or intermaxillary elastics are given in patients with recurrent dislocation. The patient is educated and instructed to support the jaw, while yawning and prevent wide opening.

In cases with chronic dislocation fibrous adhesions develop, which prevent the reduction of the dislocated jaw in spite of attempts under GA. In such cases surgical treatment like eminectomy or condylectomy may be required.

The preventive treatment in cases of recurrent subluxation or dislocation comprises of:

- **Capsule plication procedures:** The plication (tightening) is achieved by injecting corticosteroids in the joint space. The steroids not only reduce the inflammation, but also induce fibrosis in the capsule and make it stiff. The intra-articular injections with sclerosing agents like sodium morrhuate are also indicated. Surgical exploration of the joint and placement of plicating stitch with nonabsorbable material is also advocated.[17,18]
- **Removal of barrier:** The articular eminence serves as a barrier and prevents the reduction of the condylar head in the glenoid fossa. If this barrier is removed then the condyle will not get locked and will travel freely to and fro and the subluxation or dislocation will not take place. This is achieved by reducing the height of the articular eminence by exposing it surgically through a preauricular incision and reducing it with a bur. This procedure is called as 'eminectomy' (Figs 26.29A and B).

  The alternative to eminectomy is reducing the height of the condyle. This is done by entering the joint space and shaving off the superior condylar surface. This is called condyloplasty or high condylectomy or condylar shave procedure.[19]
- **Creating a barrier:** The dislocation or subluxation results due to too far anterior translation of the condyle during opening. If this anterior translation is prevented mechanically by creating a barrier, the dislocation can be prevented. This barrier is created by:

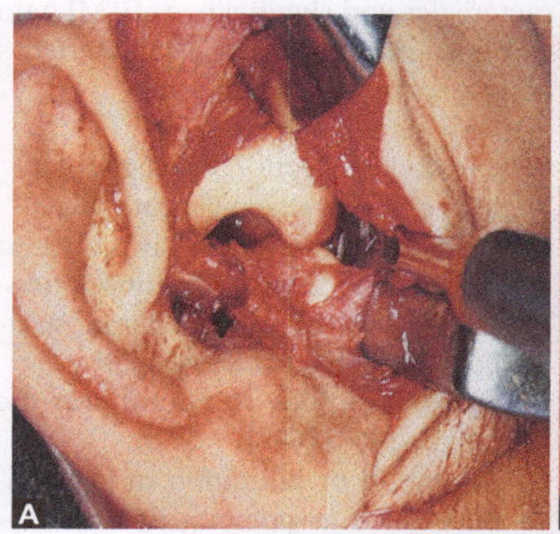
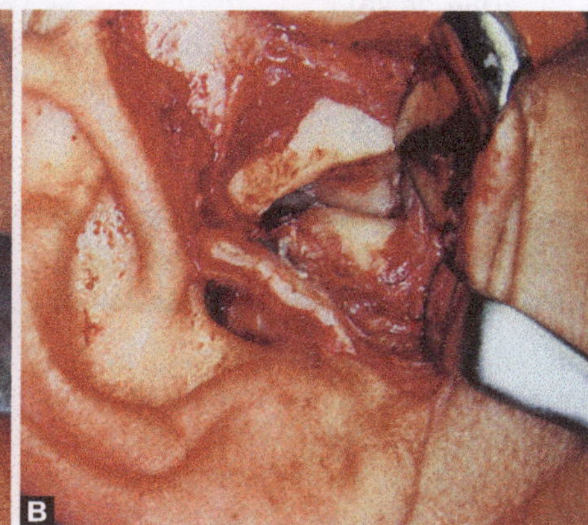

Figs 26.29A and B: Eminectomy to remove the barrier

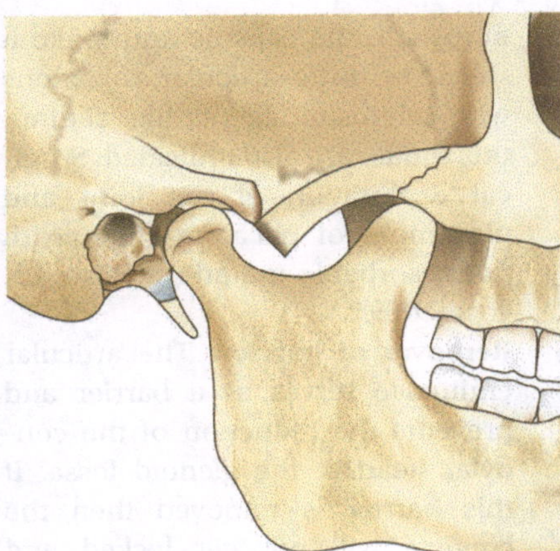

Fig. 26.30: Dautry's procedure to create a barrier

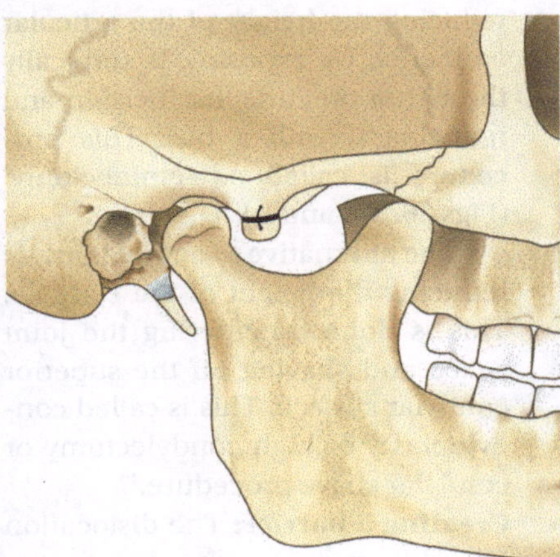

Fig. 26.31: Overlay graft to create a barrier

- Implanting titanium pins in the articular eminence
- Down fracturing of the zygomatic arch as its root and fixing it at lower level (*Dautry's procedure*) (Fig. 26.30).
- Overlay bone grafts to augment the height of the articular eminence (Fig. 26.31).

MYOFACIAL PAIN DYSFUNCTION SYNDROME

This entity has been identified in the clinical practice since a long. It was described by Coston[20] in 1934 as the pain in TMJ associated with ankylosing spondilitis, occlusal disharmony and was called Coston's syndrome. He correlated bite over closure (due to loss of posterior teeth), as well as ear and sinus problems including diminished hearing, tinnitus, dizziness, burning and occipito vertex headache to it. Although, proved inaccurate it acknowledged the fact that the TMJ symptoms and occlusion often seem intimately related. The relationship was referred to as the 'TMJ syndrome'. Later Schawrtz 1952, drew attention to the fact that the sufferers of the TMJ syndrome were symptomatic because of the masticatory and perimasticatory muscle spasm. He expanded the syndrome to the 'TMJ pain-dysfunction syndrome' and perceptively noted that many sufferers had an altered or unusual psychological make up as well. This represents a transition from the age of strict occlusal etiology to the age in which occlusion plus the entire suspensory jaw apparatus and the patient's psychological make up are seen as causative. Travell[21], 1960 showed how pain could be referred from one area of head and neck to another, through the use of injections of isotonic saline solutions, intramuscularly. He described sore points in the periarticular muscles as 'Trigger points'. He also noted that whenever the pain is associated with skeletal muscle spasm, it almost always gets referred a distance from the muscle, i.e. its source, trigger areas are often easily located by palpation. Since there is lowered pain threshold deep pressure on the trigger zone leads to referred pain.

Laskin[22] (1969) summarized the characteristics and significance of TMJ pain dysfunction theory. The characteristics of pain according to him are:

- Unilateral pain
- Located in preauricular region
- May be referred in all directions
- Often described as dull and constant
- Mostly associated with muscle tenderness, which could be demonstrated clinically by careful palpation.
- Clicking or popping sound over the affected TMJ (66%)
- Alteration or limitation of jaw function seen as opening deviation or restricted movement, unilaterally or bilaterally.

In summary the clinical signs can be listed as:

- Pain
- Muscle tenderness
- Alteration of limitation of motion.

Besides having one or more of the four cardinal symptoms the patient considered to have the syndrome must also have these negative characteristics.

- Absence of clinical, radiological or biochemical evidence of organic changes in TMJ.
- Lack of tenderness in the TMJ when palpated via the external auditory meatus.

The significance of these negative characteristics in establishing the diagnosis lies in their indication that the primary site of problem is in the musculature rather than the structure of the joint.

There are many synonymous terminologies used to designate the TMJ pain associated with spasm of the surrounding muscles of mastication and they are Coston's syndrome, myofacial pain dysfunction syndrome, myelogelosen interstitial myofibrosities, non-articular rheumatism, TMJ dysfunction, myalgia, etc. However, myofacial pain dysfunction is the most accepted terminology. The condition is characterized by unilateral facial pain secondary to the TMJ disorder, which is often associated with periarticular muscle spasm and pain with dysfunction of the spastic muscles.

Etiological Factors

The etiological factors for the MPDs are:

- **Intracapsular causes**—internal derangements like:
  - Anterior disc dislocation with reduction and without reduction
  - Disc perforation
  - Disc adhesions.
- **Extracapsular causes**
  - Occlusal disharmony
  - Psychosis
  - Muscular imbalance
  - Hypermobility, subluxation
  - Whiplash injury
  - Muscle over extension due to restorations or prosthesis, which

Flow chart 26.1: Etiopathogenesis of MPDS

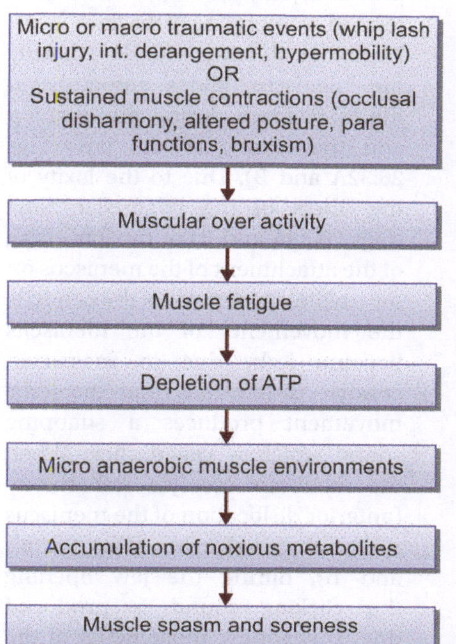

encroach on the intermaxillary space (high points)

- Muscle overcontraction–loss of posterior teeth.
- Parafunctions–bruxism, clenching, grinding, etc.

The etiopathogenesis is shown in (Flow chart 26.1).

The occlusal disharmony due to malocclusion, malunited fractures, post-orthognathic surgery, alters the mandibular posture, which leads to abnormal resting position of the jaw and the TMJ, muscle over activity. The para functions like tongue thrusting, lip biting, excursive movements, bruxism, etc. lead to muscle over activity. The fatigued muscle is depleted of ATP. The muscle metabolism becomes anerobic due to relative hypoxic environment as the O_2 consumption is increased and it is not readily available. Thus, the noxious metabolic end products like lactic acid accumulate in the muscle and the muscle become spastic, sore and stiff. It leads to further altered posture, further stretching, fatigue and the vicious cycle of pain-spasm is created.

The internal derangements in the joint like meniscus dislocation, meniscus perforations, meniscus adhesions and degenerative changes in the joint, produce pain in the joint. Secondary to the pain, a protective myospasm sets in, which leads to altered posture, fatigue, soreness and all the events are repeated in a cyclic manner.

The development of muscle spasm, pain, limitation of motion results in minor shift in the rest position of the jaw so that the teeth do not occlude properly. The teeth may gradually shift to accommodate this malocclusion. But, when the spasm is relieved the patients develop another occlusal imbalance. The initial muscle spasm indicates homeostatic protection against injury. This protective splinting of myospasm, however, tends to get more momentum so that increasing number of related muscle groups develop spasm and the pathways of pain-spasm-pain chain reaction becomes extensively facilitated. Apart from these two organic changes, degenerative arthritis and fibrosis of preauricular tissue are seen.

Clinical Features

- Pain, which is usually unilateral and is aggravated on chewing, yawning and opening. The pain and the restricted jaw movements are some times more pronounced in the morning and wanes off as the day progresses. This is often designated as morning stiffness.
- Pain in temples, vertex, occipital areas, headaches, neck and shoulder aches are common.
- Restricted joint excursions—there is not only trismus, but the other joint excursions like protrusion and lateral excursions are painful and restricted. The jaw movements are not steady and there may be deviation due to muscle spasm and imbalance during

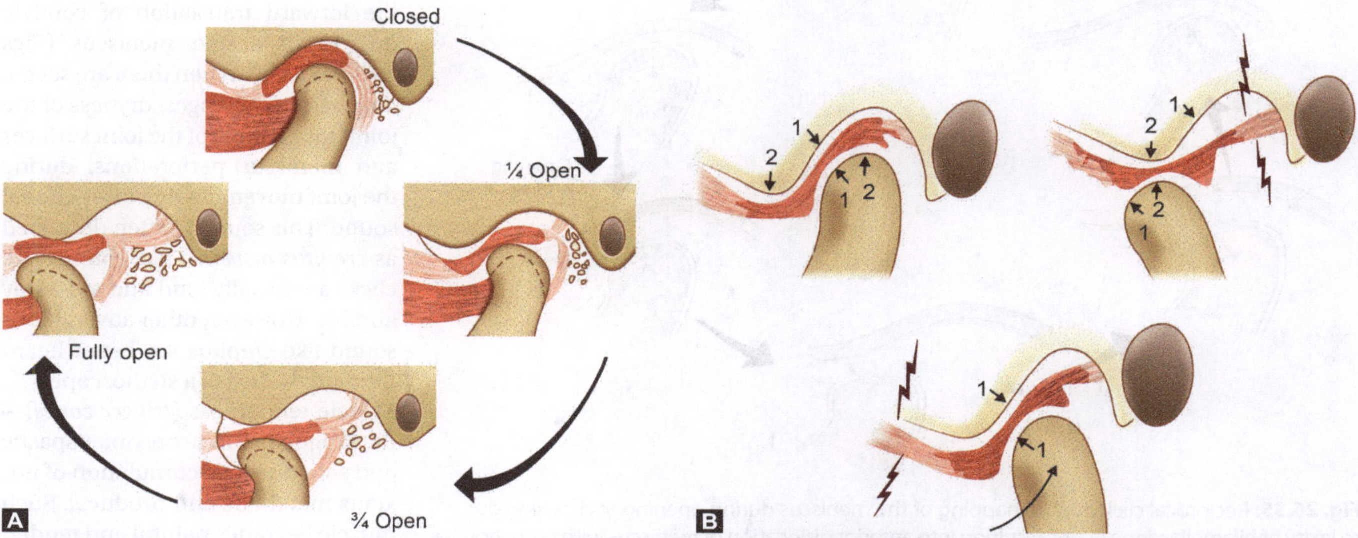

Figs 26.32A and B: (A) Normal condyle meniscus complex movements during opening; (B) Tension is generated in the bilamellar zone while opening due to stretching and it also balances the pull of lateral pterygoid contraction while closing

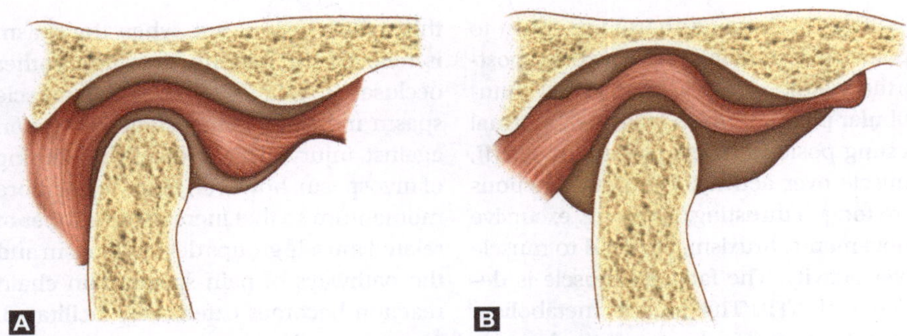

Figs 26.33A and B: Laxity of bilamellar zone

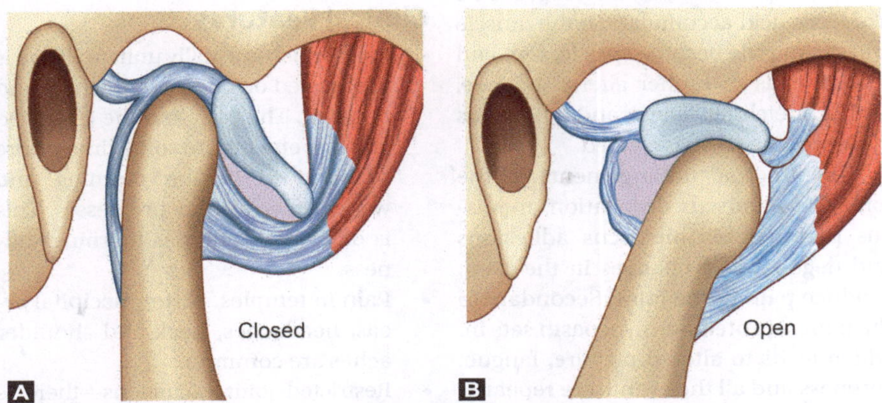

Figs 26.34A and B: Anterior lock with reduction: (A) Anteriorly dislocated meniscus; (B) Reduction of the dislocated meniscus during opening

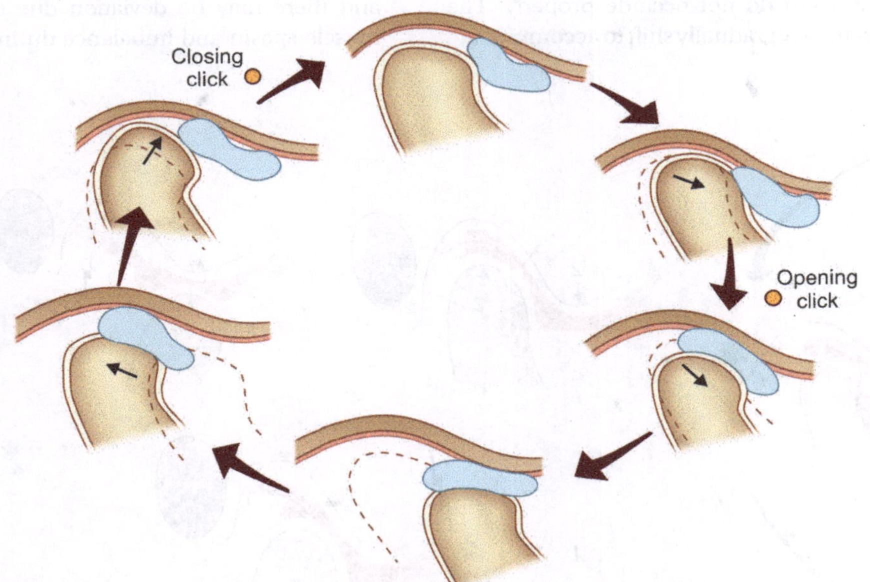

Fig. 26.35: Reciprocal click due to snapping of the meniscus during opening and closing due to laxity of bilamellar zone fibers, resulting into anterior dislocation of meniscus with reduction

the opening. The meniscus dislocation produces jerky jaw movements often termed as 'propping of the jaw'.

- Pathological joint sounds—Usually the meniscus glides smoothly in the joint space during the opening and the closing of the jaw (Figs 26.32A and B). Due to the laxity of the fibers of the bilamellar zone (Figs 26.33A and B) or the loosening of the attachment of the meniscus on the mediolateral poles of the condyle, the movements of the meniscus become jerky due to meniscus-condyle disharmony and the jerky movement produces a snapping sound which is called click. When the meniscus condyle disharmony (anterior dislocation of the meniscus with reduction) exists (Figs 26.34A and B), during the jaw opening the clicking sound is produced due to snapping movements of the meniscus. This clicking sound is also heard on closing and when it is present on both the opening and closing it is called reciprocal clicking (Fig. 26.35). Then the bilamellar zone is severely damaged and the meniscus gets dislocated anteriorly, without reduction, it creates an anterior lock. In such cases the previously noisy joints become silent but the restricted mouth opening is present due to the obstruction to the forward translation of condyle due to dislocated meniscus (Figs 26.36A and B). When there are severe degenerative changes, dryness of the joint, roughening of the joint surfaces and meniscus perforations, during the joint movement there is frictional sound. This sound is often described as *crepitus or velcro* like sound. The clicks are usually loud and are easily audible. However, other adventitious sound like crepitus are better heard through the bell of a stethoscope.
- Muscle tenderness (*trigger zones*)—the fatigued muscle becomes spastic and sore due to accumulation of noxious metabolic end products. Such muscle becomes painful and tender.

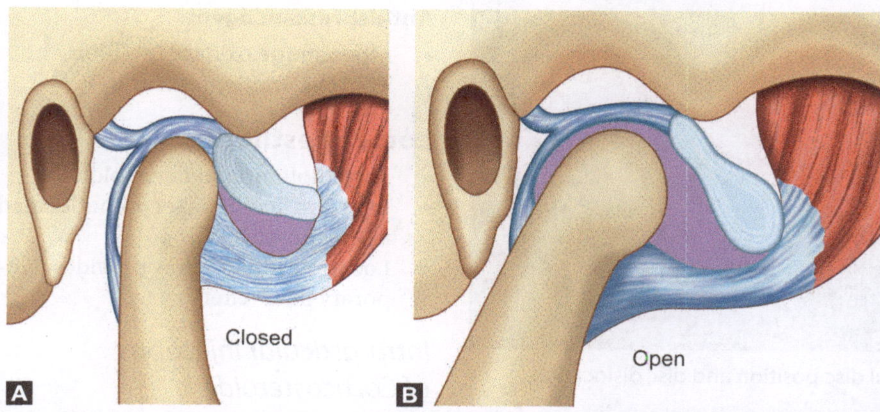

Fig. 26.36A and B: Anterior dislocation of meniscus without reduction: (A) Anteriorly dislocated meniscus; (B) During opening it does not get reduced but forms a mass of dislocated meniscus, obstructing the forward translation of the condyle, resulting in restricted mouth opening

On palpation definite tender points are elicited over these periarticular muscles like masseter (70%), temporalis (49%), medial (35%) and lateral pterygoid (84%) cervical, scalp and facial muscles (43%). Tenderness is also elicited on the condylar neck above maxillary tuberosity, at angle of the mandible and at the temporal crest.

- Otologic symptoms like ringing in ear, heaviness in the ear.
- Referred dental pain.
- Subluxation or dislocation (17%).
- Vertigo (7%).
- Altered psychosis—the patients with psychosis commonly have the habit of parafunctions like lip biting, bruxism and mandibular parafunctions. It leads to strain in the muscle, spasm and soreness. Other findings of stress like acid peptic disorders, migraine, headache, dermatitis, significant elevation of urinary steroid levels and catecholamines may be present. Hence, psychological evaluation and management of the patient with MPDS is also very important aspect of the management.
- Occlusal discrepancies—the occlusal discrepancies in the form of crowding, premature contacts, attrition, deep bite, loss of teeth leading to over closure and straining of the joint may be present. These discrepancies may be developmental or acquired as a result of malunited fracture, postorthognathic surgery.

Clinical Examination

- Palpation of TMJ.
- Palpation of muscle of mastication and neck muscles for detecting the sore points (Trigger areas) in the spastic muscles (Figs 26.37A to F).
- Assessment of range of movement, deviation of mandible and smoothness or jerky movements (popping).
- Assessment of clicking/grating/synchrony of joint movements.
- Intraoral examination of deflective occlusal contacts, occlusal discrepancies, prematurities, interferences, attrition, wear facets, missing/mobile teeth, anterior open bite, cross bite, reduced vertical dimension.

Investigations

The radiographic evaluation is needed to rule out associated pathologies of TMJ:

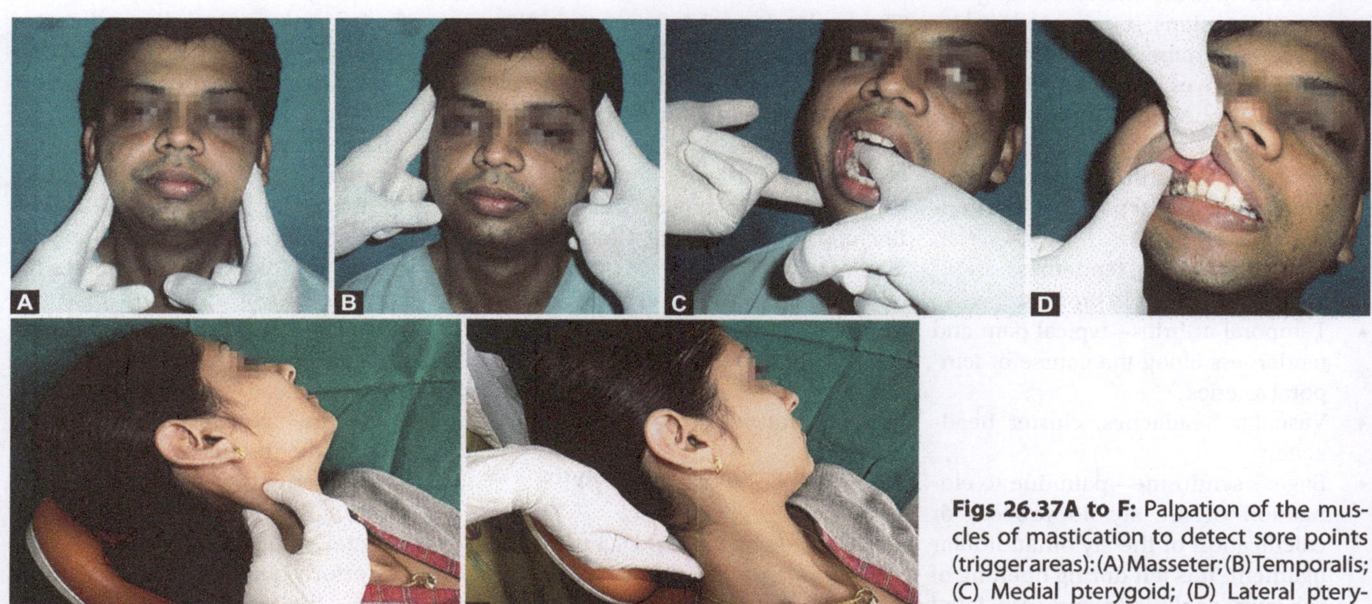

Figs 26.37A to F: Palpation of the muscles of mastication to detect sore points (trigger areas): (A) Masseter; (B) Temporalis; (C) Medial pterygoid; (D) Lateral pterygoid; (E) Sternomastoid; (F) Trapezius

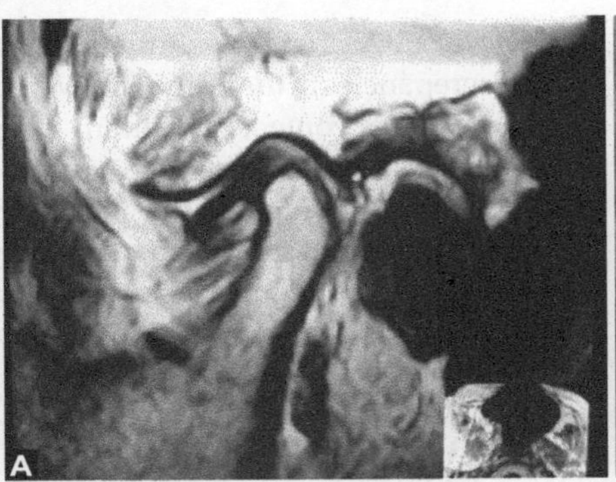

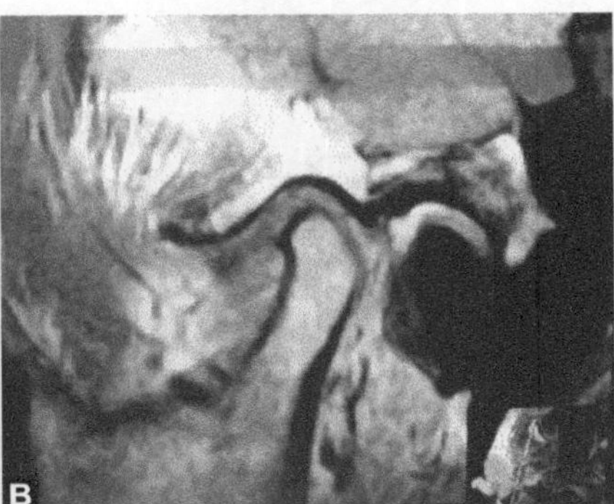

Figs 26.38A and B: MRI showing normal disc position and disc dislocation

- OPG
- Transpharyngeal view
- Transcranial view
- MRI is the most appropriate investigation to asses the internal soft tissue pathologies of the joint (Figs 26.38A and B).

Differential Diagnosis of the Myofacial Pain Dysfunction Syndrome

Various conditions associated with the head and neck region may mimic the pain secondary to myofacial pain dysfunction syndrome (MPDS) and thus, they warrant consideration for ruling them out.

- Migraine—more commonly seen in females, pain is severe in the morning, associated with nausea, vomiting and visual abrasions. It is precipitated by stress, gastrointestinal upsets, oral contraceptives, menses, consumption of alcohol, candies, chocolates.
- Otitis media—chronic condition, associated with purulent ear discharge, predominantly ear pain, hearing impairment.
- Mastoiditis—pain, tenderness, swelling over the mastoid process.
- Temporal arthritis—typical pain and tenderness along the course of temporal arteries.
- Vascular headaches, cluster headache.
- Eagle's syndrome—pain due to elongation of the styloid process or calcification of the stylomandibular ligament. It is felt during opening of the jaws, deglutition and associated with caratodynia. The elongated styloid process can be felt on transoral palpation in the retromolar area medial to the ramus and can also be visualized on X-rays.

Management

- Pharmacological modalities.
- Intra-articular injections.
- Occlusal splints.
- Physiotherapeutic modalities.
- Stress management.
- Biofeedback and relaxation therapy.
- Psychologic modalities.
- Surgical management.

Pharmacological Modalities

Anti-inflammatory drugs

The analgesic anti-inflammatory drugs like ibuprofen, diclofenac sodium and salicylates provide relief from the pain and reduce the inflammation.

Muscle relaxants

Centrally acting muscle relaxants like Baclofen 10 to 25 mg, Chlorzoxazone 500 mg, Metaxalone, Methocarbamol 500 mg, etc. can be prescribed to relive the muscle spasm. These drugs reduce skeletal muscle tone by selective action on the cerebrospinal axis without altering consciousness.

Stress reduction with anxiolytic agents

- Alprazolam: 0.25 and 0.5 mg HS
- Diazepam: 2 to 5 mg HS. It also works as a skeletal muscle relaxant.

Antidepressant agents

- Monoamine oxidase inhibitor
- Tricyclic antidepressant.

Local anesthetics

- Auriculotemporal nerve block
- Injection at the trigger points located in the muscles
- Local anesthetic spray provides temporary pain relief.

Intra-articular Injections of Corticosteroids

The injection of corticosteroids (hydrocort) in upper joint space with local anesthetics should be given under strict aseptic precautions. The intra-articular steroids help in reducing the inflammation within the joint and bring down the pain. The codylar irregularities are also remodelled to certain extent and thus, it is also called 'chemical condylotomy'. Steroids should not be injected very frequently and there should be a gap of about 5 to 6 months between the two injections.

Occlusal Splints

The occlusal splints are given to serve the following purpose:

- To create balanced joint-tooth relationship.
- To reduce spasm, contracture, hyperactivity of musculature.
- To improve vertical dimension and prevent the over rotation of the condyle during the closure so as to prevent stretching of the fibers of bilamellar zone.
- As the mandible is pushed down by the splint, the condyle also gets pushed inferiorly increasing the space within the joint, which facilitates the free movement of the inflamed and edematous meniscus without getting traumatized and helps in reducing its inflammation (Figs 26.39A and B).
- **Anterior repositioning splint:** When the meniscus is anteriorly dislocated, the anterior repositioning splints are indicated. The lingual ramp glides the mandible anteriorly and the condyle glides over the dislocated meniscus

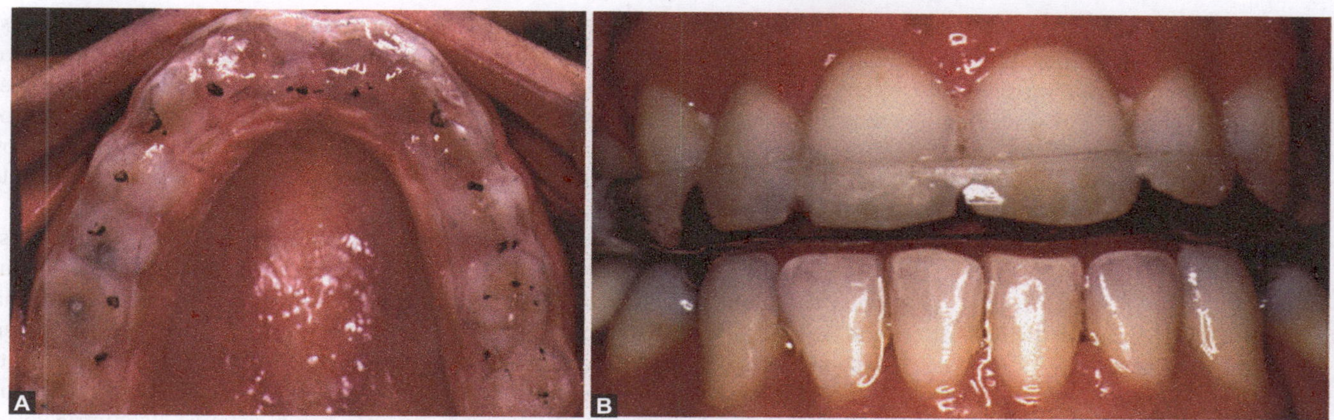

Figs 26.39A and B: Occlusal splint

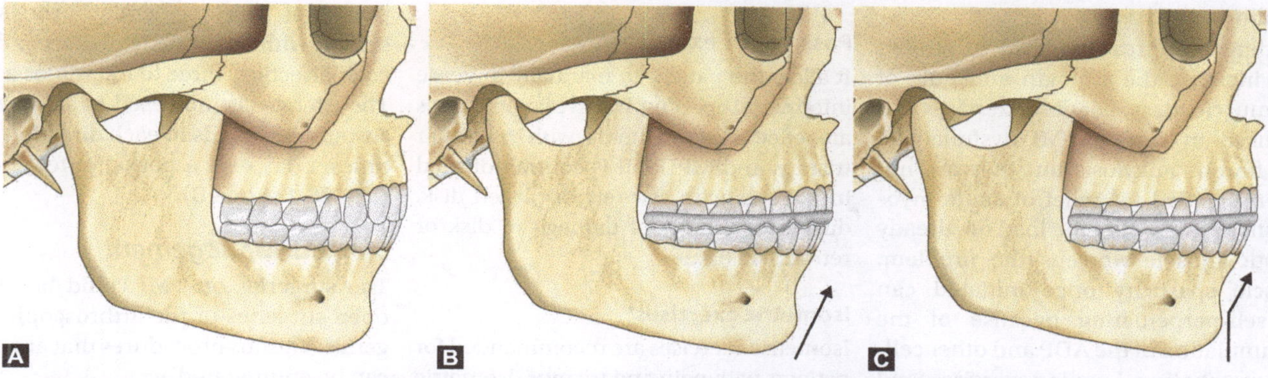

Figs 26.40A to C: Anterior repositioning splint: (A) Anteriorly displaced disc; (B) Splint in place and teeth are occluded; (C) The mandible is pushed anteriorly and the condyle glides anteroinferiorly

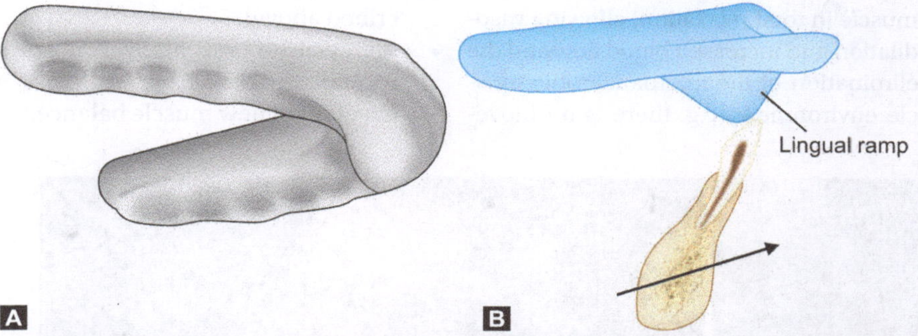

Figs 26.41A and B: Anterior repositioning splint with lingual ramp for positioning the mandible anteriorly

anteroinferiorly. This prevents abnormal posturing of the mandible, muscle imbalance and pain due to muscle fatigue. It also helps in reduction of the meniscus in its normal position (Figs 26.40 and 26.41).

Physiotherapeutic Modalities

- Acute stage—no active physiotherapy is advisable in an acute stage, but the joint should be provided rest.
- Chronic stage.
  - *Infrared diathermy*: The electromagnetic waves that generate heat and provide deeper penetration of the heat.
  - *Short wave diathermy*: It is a high frequency alternating current and the heat energy is obtained from the wave. The frequency is 27,120,000 cycles per second and the wavelength is 11 meter and provides deeper penetration of heat in the periarticular muscles.
  - *Ultrasonic therapy*: These electromagnetic waves are different from sound waves. The frequencies of waves are between 500,000 and 3,000,000 cycles/sec.
  - *Microwave diathermy*: They are the electromagnetic waves with a wavelength between infrared rays and short wave diathermy waves, and the wavelength is 12.25 cm with frequency of 2,450 cycles/sec.

During the conventional hot fomentations, the heat does not penetrate the deeper structures like muscles and the joint. The shorter the wavelength, deeper is the heat penetration. Hence, microwave diathermy produces deeper heat penetration than the short wave diathermy.

Exercises

Exercises of the TMJ can be divided into:

- Loading exercises.
  - Active jaw exercises.
  - Passive jaw exercises.
- Isometric exercises.

Loading exercises

Loading exercises are used to stretch and increase the strength and bulk of the muscle mass. Loading exercises can be used in certain TMJ dysfunctions like fibrous ankylosis but they are not recommended for relief of acute myospasm as increasing the load on already spastic muscle worsens the problem. Muscle spasticity once initiated can be self-perpetuating because of the accumulation of the ADP and other cellular metabolites. Loading exercises tend to increase ADP and other anaerobic metabolites, thus increasing myospasm.

Active jaw exercise/kinetic exercises

Using patient's musculature allow the patient to activate for example, their suprahyoid muscle (geniohyoid, mylohyoid, digastric and stylohyoid), thereby inactivating the elevators of the jaw (medial pterygoid, masseter, temporalis). This may allow relaxation of the hyperactive muscles of mastication and assist in achieving maximal interincisal opening. In the active stretch phase patient is asked to open the mouth for several seconds and relax. They are advised to open the mouth till they perceive pain and keep the mouth open for several second and to repeat this exercise several times in a day. In the active protrusion, patient stands in front of the mirror and protrudes the mandible forward stretching lateral pterygoid bilaterally.

Passive jaw exercises

It allow the patient to manually increase interincisal opening. Passive jaw exercises are effective in patients with muscular trismus and MPDS. It is contraindicated in patients with severely displaced disk, due to possibility of damage to disk or retrodiskal tissue.

Isometric exercises

Isometric exercises are recommended for patients with pain and trismus. Isometric exercises work on the principle of reflex-relaxation, as one group of the muscle is in total contracture, the other group of the muscle in total relaxation, allowing vasodilation and increased blood flow and the elimination of the microanaerobic muscle environment, e.g. there is no movement in these exercises while the depressor muscles are activated, allowing for relaxation of the opposite elevator muscles (medial pterygoid, masseter, temporalis). These exercises are performed by holding the mandible stationary, while the muscles are activated isometrically.

For isometric exercises, patient is asked to visualize the jaw as working in four separate directions—open-closed and right-left. Isometric exercises are then accomplished as the patient attempts to move the jaw in all these directions against the resistance. Isometric exercise, to be effective, should be done with great effort and be sustained for short period of time. Generally, exercise is started with three sustained seconds in each direction, three to four times a day. The exercise is increased to six to eight sustained seconds in each direction four times a day over a period of few weeks (Figs 26.42A and B).

Surgical Management

The surgeries on TMJ could be either open surgeries or the arthroscopic surgeries. Various procedures that are done can be enumerated as:

- Arthrocentesis.
- Capsule tightening procedures.
- Creating mechanical obstacle (described above).
- Removal of mechanical obstacle (described above).
- Creation of new muscle balance.

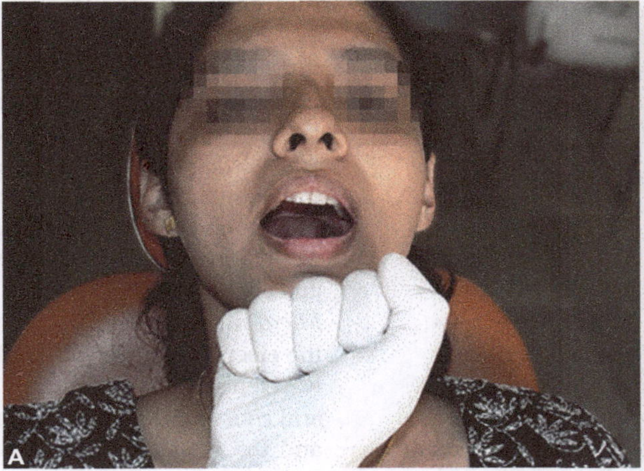

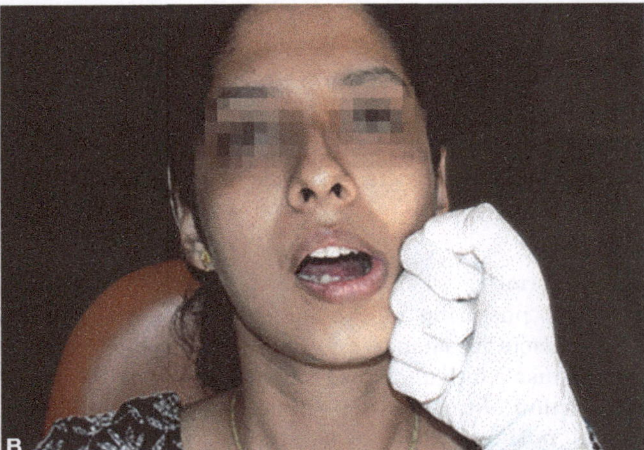

Figs 26.42A and B: Isometric jaw exercises: (A) Opening the jaw against resistance, (B) Lateral excursion against resistance applied by clenched fist

TMJ arthrocentesis

Arthrocentesis is traditionally defined as a procedure in which the fluid in a joint cavity is aspirated with a needle and a therapeutic substance is injected. The procedure is generally performed under local anesthesia and strictly sterile conditions. Because of its simplicity, it may be performed repeatedly if necessary. Alarcón-Segovia[23] reported how Mexican prehispanic physicians used therapeutic arthrocentesis in swollen unwounded knees. Swollen knees were punctured with a thorn to relieve pain and restore function.[24] Fray Bernardino de Sahagún gathered this information through direct interviews with the surviving Aztec nobility in México city in the 16th century and realized that an inflamed joint was potentially harmful and were the first to perform therapeutic arthrocentesis using an unspecified thorn. They also described the nature of the aspirated fluid, which they compared with the viscid fluid from the leaves of the nopal cactus. Numerous studies have shown the exceptional diagnostic and therapeutic value of arthrocentesis, while emphasizing the low incidence of associated complications, including joint contamination and local irritation caused by introduction of foreign materials. Most studies on TMJ arthrocentesis refer to temporomandibular disorder (TMD), which comprises a wide variety of disorders of the TMJ, the masticatory muscles, or both. Pain and dysfunction of the TMJ itself accounts for a small proportion of TMD conditions, and are often insufficiently diagnosed. The prime suspects in symptomatic synovial joint are intra- and extra-articular overloading and immobilization. Microscopic analysis of the synovial fluid is also a valuable diagnostic tool. Identification of crystals allows innocuous effusion caused by osteoarthritis to be differentiated from that which is caused by crystal-induced inflammation and the vastly more dangerous septic arthritis. Determining total white blood cell count and the percentage of polymorphonuclear cells in synovial fluid may distinguish between inflammatory and noninflammatory disease and is essential for judging therapeutic success. The presence of succinic acid and to a lesser extent lactic acid or depressed glucose concentrations in synovial fluid is a useful marker in diagnosing septic arthritis. Measuring total protein, albumin and individual immunoglobulins permits mechanical, acute inflammatory and chronic inflammatory processes to be distinguished, especially when compared with serum values. However, the value of biochemical studies of synovial fluid has often been challenged.

Indications for TMJ arthrocentesis

- Diagnostic: Biochemical and microbial analysis of synovial fliuid.
- Toileting of the joint space to flush away the accumulated chemical mediators of inflammation, thus reducing pain and inflammation.
- Instillation or administration of drugs (hyaluronic acid, Steroids)

Murakami and colleagues[25] offered the first systematic description of TMJ arthrocentesis, which they termed manipulation technique after pumping and hydraulic pressure. Arthrocentesis of the TMJ is a modification of the traditional method, whereby two needles instead of one are introduced into the upper joint space. This adaptation permits massive lavage of the joint, in addition to aspiration and injection.

The patient is seated at a 45 degree angle, with the head turned to the unaffected side to provide an easy approach to the affected joint. After proper preparation of the target site, the external auditory meatus is blocked with cotton soaked in mineral oil. A line is drawn from the middle of the tragus to the outer canthus. The posterior entrance point is located along the canthotragal line, 10 mm from the middle of the tragus and 2 mm below the line. The anterior point of entry is placed 10 mm farther along the line and 10 mm below it. These markings over the skin indicate the location of the articular fossa and the eminence of the TMJ. A local anaesthetic is injected at the planned entrance points, avoiding penetration into the joint and injection into the synovial fluid. A 19-gauge needle connected to a syringe filled with lactated Ringer's solution is then inserted into the superior compartment at the articular fossa (posterior point) aided by palpation. The solution is injected and immediately aspirated. The fluid in the syringe is often sucked into the joint space, which normally has negative pressure. Then 2 to 3 mL lactated Ringer's solution or bupivacaine, 0.5 percent, are injected to distend the upper joint space and anesthetize the adjacent tissues. A second 19-gauge needle is then inserted into the distended compartment in the area of the articular eminence to enable free flow of Ringer's solution through the superior compartment. Due to lavage, the pain mediators prostaglandin E2 and leukotriene get washed out, reducing the inflammation and pain. The inability of disc to slide can readily be reversed by lavage. The injected fluid distends hydraulically, the joint space and enables the disc to slide. During the lavage, the mandible is moved through opening, excursive and protrusive movements to facilitate lysis of adhesions. At the end of the procedure and after one needle is removed, medication can be injected into the joint space. Temporary facial paresis or paralysis caused by the use of a local anesthetic or swelling of the neighboring tissues caused by perfusion of Ringer's solution may occur during arthrocentesis. However, these effects are transient and disappear within a few hours (Figs 26.43A and B).

Advantages of Arthrocentesis

- Simple and less invasive technique.
- Minimum armamentarium and less expensive.
- Therapeutic advantage.

Capsule tightening procedures

Placation stitch, intracapsular injection of steroids, sodium morrhuate.

Disc plication

- Full thickness excision of wedge shaped tissue of posterior portion.
- Partial thickness excision of superior retrodiskal lamina—in this

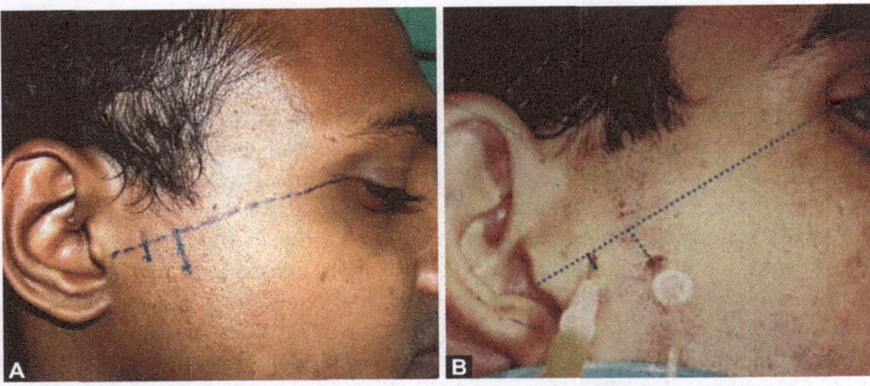

Figs 26.43A and B: (A) Markings for insertion of the needles during arthrocentesis; (B) Arthrocentesis in process

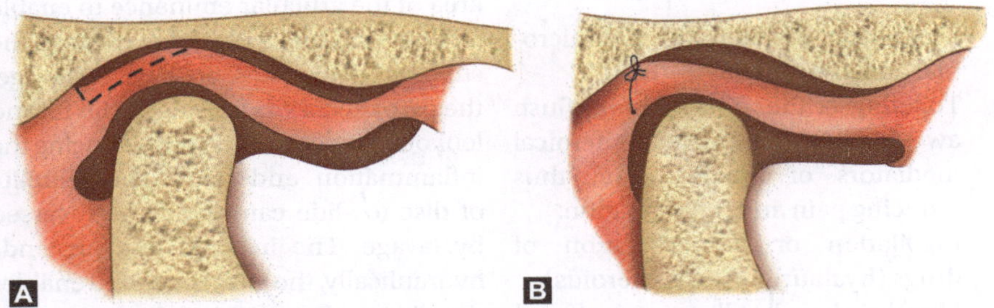

Figs 26.44A and B: Full thickness excision of superior retrodiskal lamina

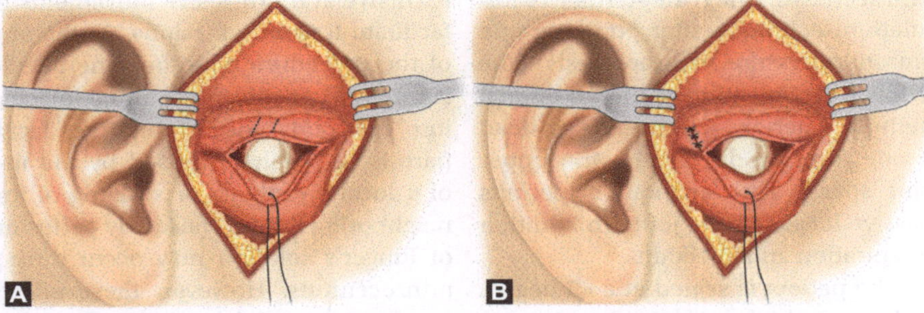

Figs 26.45A and B: A full thickness wedge shaped portion of posterior attachment is removed and lateroposterior tissues are approximated

procedure, a partial thickness excision of superior lamina of retrodiskal tissue is done and its posterior attachments are removed. The lateroposterior tissues are approximated (Figs 26.44 and 26.45).

- The disk repositioning is achieved by plication of posterior attachment or disk is sutured to lateral capsular ligament.

REFERENCES

1. Kurt H Thoma. Hyperostosis of the mandibular condyle: with report of two cases. American Journal of Orthodontics and Oral Surgery. 1945;31(10):597-607.
2. Blair VP. Operative Treatment of Ankylosis of the Mandible With a History of the Operation and Ankylosis of 212 Cases. Surg Gynecol Obstet. 1914;19: 436-51.
3. Blair, Ivy, Brown. Essential of Oral Surgery. CV Mosbv Co., 2nd edn. 1936.
4. Al-Kayat A, Bramley P. A modified preauricular approach to the temporomandibular joint and malar arch. Br J Oral Surg. 1979;17:91-103.
5. Kaban LB, Perott DH, Fisher K. A Protocol for Management of Temporomandibular Joint Ankylosis. J Oral Maxfac Surg. 1990;48:1145-51.
6. Orhan Güven. A clinical study on temporomandibular joint ankylosis. Auris Nasus Larynx. 2000;27(1):27-33.
7. Güven, Orhan. A Clinical Study on Temporomandibular Joint Ankylosis in Children. Journal of Craniofacial Surgery. 2008;19(5):1263-9.
8. Ahmad QG. Interposition arthroplasty in temporomandibular joint ankylosis. Indian Journal of Otolaryngology and Head and Neck Surgery. 2004;54(1):5-8.
9. Spiessl B, Schmoker R, Mathys R. Treatment of ankylosis by a condylar prosthesis of the mandible. New Concepts in Maxillofacial Bone Surgery (1976) Springer, Berlin.
10. Richard W DeChamplain. Autopolymerizing silastic for interpositional arthroplasty. JOMS. 1988;46(6):522-5.
11. Westermark A. Condylar replacement alone is not sufficient for prosthetic reconstruction of the temporomandibular joint. International Journal of Oral and Maxillofacial Surgery. 2006; 35(6):488-92.
12. Chossegros C, Guyot L, Cheynet F, et al. Full-thickness skin graft interposition after temporomandibular joint ankylosis surgery. A study of 31 cases. Int. J Oral Maxillofac Surg. 1999;28:330-4.
13. Lei Z. Auricular cartilage graft interposition after temporomandibular joint ankylosis surgery in children. J Oral Maxillofac Surg. 2002;60:985-7.
14. Paterson AW, Shepherd JP. Fascia lata interpositional arthroplasty in the treatment of temporomandibular joint ankylosis caused by psoriatic arthritis. Int J Oral Maxillofac Surg. 1992; 21(3):137-9.
15. Kim Su-Gwan. Treatment of temporomandibular joint ankylosis with temporalis muscle and fascia flap. Int J Oral Maxillofac Surg. 2001;30(3):189-93.
16. Wolford LM, Cottrell DA, Henry C. Sternoclavicular grafts for temporomandibular joint reconstruction. J Oral Maxillofac Surg. 1994;52(2):119-28; discussion 128-9.
17. Bruce Sanders. Surgical treatment for recurrent dislocation or chronic subluxation of the temporomandibular joint. Int J Oral Surg. 1975;4(5):179-83.

18. Raja Kummoona. Surgical reconstruction of the temporomandibular joint for chronic subluxation and dislocation. Int J Oral Maxillofac Surg. 2001; 30(4):344-8.
19. Robert D Marciani. Healing following condylar shave in the monkey temporomandibular joint. JOMS. 1988; 46(12):1071-6.
20. Costen JB. A Syndrome of Ear and Sinus Symptoms Dependent upon Disturbed Function of the Temporomandibular Joint. Ann Otol Rhinol. 1934;43:1.
21. Travell JG, Simons DG. Myofascial pain and dysfunction: The trigger point manual. Baltimore: William Wilkins, 1983;4(544):103-64.
22. Laskin DM. Etiology of the pain-dysfunction syndrome. J Am Dent Assoc. 1969;79(1):147-53.
23. Alarcón-Segovia D. Descriptions of therapeutic arthrocentesis and of synovial fluid in a Nahuatl text from prehispanic Mexico. Ann Rheum Dis. 1980; 39:291-3.
24. Sahagún B. Historia General de las Cosas de Nueva España (3 volumes). Introduction, paleography, glossary and notes by López Austin A, García Quintana. J Mexico: Conaculta, 2000.
25. Murakami K, Hosaka H, Moriya Y, et al. Short-term treatment outcome study for the management of temporomandibular joint closed lock. A comparison of arthrocentesis to non-surgical therapy and arthroscopic lysis and lavage. Oral Surg Oral Med Oral Pathol Oral Radiol Endodontics. 1995; 80(3):253-7.

Section 10

Neoplastic Conditions of Head, Neck and Face

27 Odontogenic and Nonodontogenic Cysts of the Maxillofacial Region

Borle Rajiv M, Gadbail Amol, Singh Divya

> *'A surgeon should be a pathologist who does operations'.*
> —*Eric Carlson*

ODONTOGENIC CYSTS

Definitions

A cyst is defined as *'a pathological cavity, which may or may not be lined by epithelium, and contains liquid, semi-solid or gaseous contents'*.

All odontogenic cysts arise from remnants related to embryonic development and therefore termed as developmental cysts. The etiology of the cyst ranges from the embryonic remnants to the parasitic infections. For example, the thyroglossal cyst or the branchial cleft cyst originates from the embryonic remnants, while the hydatid cyst is formed secondary to the parasitic infection. The traumatic bone cyst is an empty cavity, while the dermoid cyst may contain the hard tissues like teeth. The sebaceous cyst and the mucocele are types of retention cyst. The sebaceous cyst has semisolid contents while the mucocele contains mucoid contents. The aneurismal bone cyst contains frank blood while most of the odontogenic cysts contain straw or amber colored fluid.

A majority of cysts which are seen commonly in the oral cavity are odontogenic in origin and are centrally located within the bone. The non-odontogenic cysts of the oral cavity are seen both centrally (fissural cysts like globulomaxillary cysts, median palatine cyst) or peripherally in the oral tissues (mucocele, ranula, thyroglossal, sublingual dermoid, etc).

DEVELOPMENT OF A CYST

The common behavioral feature of all cysts is the stimulation of residual developmental epithelial cells leading to proliferation, but not invasion of the adjacent tissues (Table 27.1).

CLASSIFICATION OF THE CYST OF ORAL CAVITY

Although in the past many researchers tried to classify the cysts of the orofacial region (Robinson[1] 1945, Gorlin[2] 1964, (Box 27.1) Pindborg and Karmer[3] 1992) in an attempt to categorize the cystic lesions, the recent being the WHO

Table 27.1: Development of cyst in relation to stage of development of tooth

Stage of tooth	Defect	Pathology
Initiation	Failure of initiation Basal cell offshoots	Primordial Midpalatal cyst Gingival cyst of newborn
Bud stage	Failure of layer formation	Primordial cyst, OKC
Cap stage	Degeneration of stellate reticulum	Primordial cyst, OKC
Bell stage	Degeneration of stellate reticulum	Primordial cyst, OKC
Apposition	Failure of apposition Cell rests of HERS	Primordial cyst Lat periodontal cyst
Maturation	Hypoplasia of enamel	Dentigerous cyst Lat periodontal cyst
Eruption	After eruption from epithelial rests	Eruption cyst Gingival cyst of adult ? OKC, Dentigerous cyst

Box 27.1: Classifications of cyst—Gorlin (1964)

A. Odontogenic cysts
- Dentigerous cyst
- Eruption cyst
- Gingival cyst of newborn infants
- Lateral periodontal and gingival cyst
- Keratinizing and calcifying cyst
- Radicular cyst
- Primordial cyst
- Multiple cysts of jaws and multiple cutaneous nevoid basal cell carcinoma and skeletal anomalies

B. Nonodontogenic and fissural cysts
- Globulomaxillary cyst (premaxilla maxillary cyst)
- Nasoalveolar (Nasolabial Klestadt's cyst)
- Nasopalatine (median anterior maxillary) cyst
- Median mandibular cyst
- Anterior lingual cyst
- Dermoid and epidermoid cyst
- Palatal cyst of newborn infants

C. Cysts of neck and oral floor and salivary gland
- Thyroglossal duct cyst
- Lymphoepithelial (bronchial cleft) cyst
- Oral cysts with gastric or intestinal epithelium
- Salivary gland cyst
- Mucocele and ranula

D. Pseudocyst
- Aneurysmal bone cyst
- Static (developmental latent) bone cyst
- Traumatic (hemorrhagic solitary) bone cyst

classification[4] 2005, (Box 27.2) which is widely accepted.

Box 27.2: Classifications of cysts (WHO 2005)

Developmental odontogenic cysts

a. Primordial
b. Gingival cyst of infants
c. Eruption cyst
d. Dentigerous cyst (folicular)
e. Gingival cyst of adults
f. Lateral periodontal cyst
g. Glandular odontogenic cyst, sialo-odontogenic cyst

ETIOPATHOGENESIS

The odontogenic cysts originate from the odontogenic epithelium. The etiopathogenesis of the odontogenic cysts is related closely to the development of the tooth (Tables 27.1 and 27.2). The stage at which the pathological changes are initiated leads to formation of a particular type of cyst, i.e. if the cystic changes occur at the bud or cap stage the further development of the tooth does not take place and in its place a cyst is formed which is called primordial cyst. If the cystic changes occur after the completion of the crown then a dentigerous cyst will occur. The other odontogenic cysts originate from the remnants of the odontogenic epithelium in the jaws.

GENERAL CLINICAL FEATURES OF ODONTOGENIC CYSTS

Before the individual cysts are discussed, their general features like behavior, presentation in oral cavity and management, are discussed.

- The cysts are slow growing, painless and asymptomatic, unless secondarily infected or are very large in size and cause pressure signs.
- They usually cause expansion of the bone. As they grow slowly, the pressure due to growth will cause resorption of the adjacent bone from inside and as reparative phenomena, bone apposition will occur simultaneously at the periphery, causing expansion of the bone. The expansion is more commonly seen at the buccal cortex; however in very large cysts both the buccal and lingual cortices may get expanded. This could be a differentiating feature between the ameloblastoma and a cyst, as in the former expansion of all the four cortices is seen, i.e. buccal, lingual inferior border and alveolar bone. The odontogenic keratocyst also causes bony expansion, but the expansion is not as conspicuous as the other varieties of the odontogenic cysts. It is common to see an odontogenic cyst infiltrating a large area of the bone without any significant facial asymmetry or bone expansion. This is due to the infiltrative nature of the OKC (Fig. 27.1).
- The overlying bone is thinned out and becomes paper thin and on palpation crackles under pressure producing classical "*egg shell crackling*". When the cortex is completely perforated then the fluctuations can be elicited.
- The teeth in the involved area are usually displaced and may become mobile at a later stage due to resorption of the roots.
- The X-ray shows a classical radiolucent lesion, surrounded by well sclerotic/corticated borders, due to bone apposition at the edges (Fig. 27.1). The radiolucency could be uniloculated or multiloculated. In the latter case fine bony septa can be seen in the lesion, which divide the cystic cavity in different compartments (locula). The inferior

Table 27.2: Stages of cyst formation and type of cyst formed

Stage of development of tooth	Tissue	Type of cyst formed
Bud stage, cap stage, bell stage	Odontogenic epithelium	Primordial cyst, OKC
Formation of crown	Reduced enamel epithelium	Dentigerous cyst, eruption cyst
After root formation	Cell rests of Malasez	Periapical cyst, residual cyst
Odontogenic remnants of dental lamina	Cell rests of Malasez, the remnants of dental lamina	OKC, CEOC

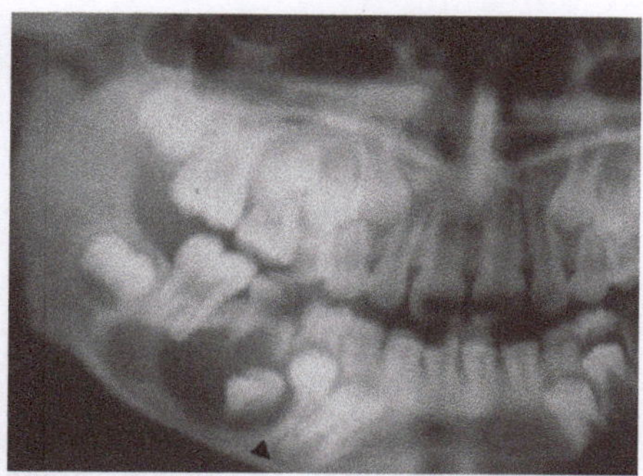

Fig. 27.1: Cystic lesions in mandible showing a radiolucent lesion with well-corticated borders, displacement of the teeth and resorption of the roots

alveolar canal is displaced due to the pressure created by cysts within the mandible.

- The aspiration of the cystic lesion is important aid in the diagnosis of the cyst. The color of the aspirate can give idea regarding the nature of the cyst, e.g. the dentigerous cyst contains the straw-colored fluid, while the OKC contains cheesy material and the ABC contains frank blood. Further the aspirated material can be subjected for cytological examination or biochemical examination (protein contents) for reaching a diagnosis. The OKC has more protein content than the other odontogenic cysts.[1] However, histopathology is the most appropriate and confirmatory diagnostic aid.

THEORIES OF CYST ENLARGEMENT

Harris[5] in 1974 classified cyst theories:

- Mural Growth
  - Peripheral cell division.
  - Accumulation of cellular content.
- Hydrostatic enlargement
  - Secretion.
  - Transudation and exudation.
- Bone resorbing factor.

Mural Growth Theory

Mural growth in the form of epithelial proliferation is one of the essential processes by which the surface area of the sac increases. This is achieved by either peripheral cell division or accumulation of cellular contents.

Peripheral Cell Division

Proliferation of local groups of epithelial cells brings about multicentric growth pattern, e.g. keratocyst. High mitotic rates of certain epithelial linings resulting in *unremitting growth* and cystic enlargement, e.g. Keratocyst. Accumulation of cellular content occurs by collegenase activity (*increased collagenolysis*) could also result in cyst expansion, e.g. primordial cyst and radicular cyst. *Low-grade infection* stimulates cells such as cell rests of Malassez to proliferate and form arcades, e.g. radicular cyst.

Hydrostatic Cyst Enlargement

Certain cysts have lining which secrete mucin. Accumulation of mucus increases the cyst volume and hence the enlargement, e.g. mucus secreting cyst.

Transudation and Exudation

Inflammatory cells (which are present in cases of infection) release cofactors, lymphocytes release lymphokines, osteoclast activating factor (OAF), and monocytes release IL-1. All these factors stimulate fibroblast to release prostaglandin (Pg). This produces a hyperosmolar cyst fluid. Increased hyperosmolarity draws fluid from surrounding. This increases hydrostatic pressure leading to cyst enlargement, e.g. inflammatory cysts like radicular cyst, residual cyst, paradental cyst.

Bone Resorption

Enlarging cysts often release bone resorbing factors from cyst capsule which stimulate osteoclastic, e.g. prostanoids PGE2 and PGI2, leucotrienes. Differences in size of various cystic lesions could possibly be dependent on the quantity of these osteoclastic factors.

To summarize the growth of cyst, there is proliferation of residual developmental epithelial cells leading to formation of solid mass of epithelial cells. As the mass enlarges, the epithelial cells in the center become positioned further from blood supply at periphery of the mass (Fig. 27.2).

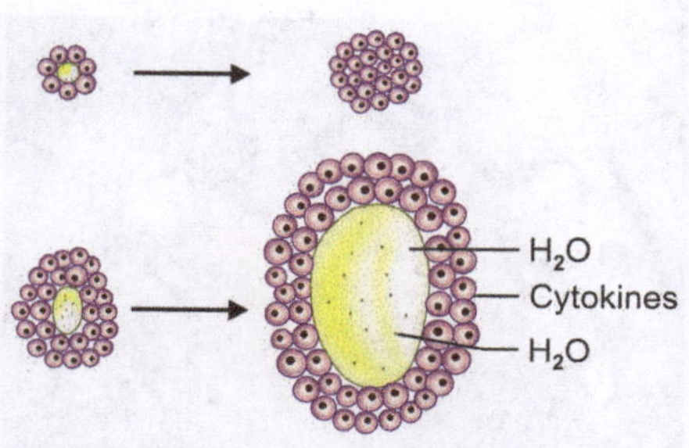

Fig. 27.2: Growth of the cyst

As the distance increases (usually 0.18 to 0.2 mm), the cells at center get too far shifted from nearest blood vessel to survive by nutritional diffusion. They degenerate, thus creating a lumen in the center. Their intracellular products make lumen hypertonic, which transudates fluid into the lumen (Fig. 27.2). This creates hydrostatic pressure, producing bone resorption, clinical expansion and sometimes mild paresthesia or pain. As additional cells die, their slough perpetuates the hypertonic state and the hydrostatic pressure. The cell membranes and nuclear membranes are high in cholesterol, hence presence of *cholesterol clefts* in cyst lumen or wall.[2]

DIAGNOSIS OF THE CYST

The cystic lesion in the jaw may simulate the tumors like ameloblastoma and other cystic neoplasms. Sometimes, the presentation is so similar that on clinical findings alone the diagnosis may be difficult. Other nonodontogenic conditions, aneurysmal bone cyst (ABC), osteoclastoma and cherubism may produce expansion of the bone and a radiological picture similar to that of a cyst and need to be differentiated from the cyst. Accidental opening into an ABC may lead to a catastrophic hemorrhage. Thus, a definitive methodology needs to be followed while diagnosing a cyst.

- **Clinical examination:** A cyst will be slowly growing, painless, expansile lesion. The expansion of buccal cortex is commonly seen in small to moderate sized cystic lesions, unlike the ameloblastoma where all the

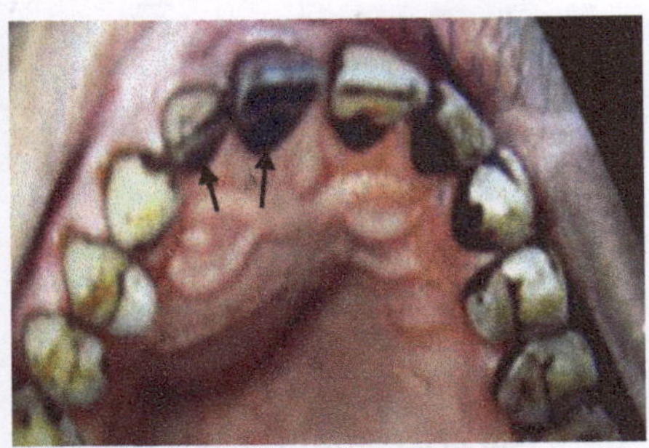

Fig. 27.3: Radicular cyst associated with nonvital tooth

cortices are expanded. The teeth are displaced due to the pressure and sometimes fail to erupt in the oral cavity due to the pressure. The neurovascular bundle is also displaced and in spite of the large size the neurological deficit is seldom present. The overlying bone is paper thin and produces egg shell crackling on palpation. When the bone is perforated, fluctuations may be present. The radicular/periapical cyst is usually associated with the nonvital tooth (Fig. 27.3).

- Radiologically the cyst presents as a well corticated, uniloculated or multiloculated, redioluscent lesion. The bone is expanded. The teeth in the region are displaced and resorption of the roots may be seen (Fig. 27.4).
- The aspiration of the cyst yields yellowish fluid, which shows presence of cholesterol crystals. The OKC has protein content (<4 mg/dL). Cytology is usually non-conclusive.
- When it is difficult to make a definitive diagnosis on clinical, radiological and aspiration to establish a correct diagnosis can be achieved by incisional biopsy. Such a difficulty is often encountered while dealing with large multiloculated lesions where it is difficult to differentiate between OKC and an ameloblastoma. The ameloblastic changes in the lining of the cyst cannot be diagnosed on clinical grounds alone and the biopsy is of critical value as the treatment modalities for the cyst and the ameloblastoma are different.[1]

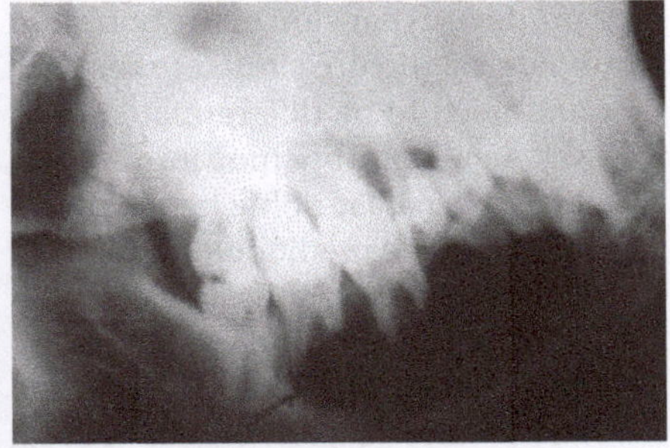

Fig 27.4: Multiloculated cystic lesion with displacement and resorption of the roots

The incisional biopsy is not required for smaller lesions as the treatment is otherwise also going to be same, i.e. enucleation, irrespective of the type of the cyst.

TREATMENT MODALITIES OF THE CYST[6]

The cyst can be treated by following modalities:

- Enucleation
- Marsupialization (*Partsch operation*)
- Combination of marsupialization and enucleation (*Waldron operation*)
- Enucleation with chemical cauterization of the base
- Enblock excision
- Segmental resection.

The later two are rarely practiced in the large lesions where the bone is severely undermined, if there is pathological fracture or suspicion of ameloblastic transformation.

Enucleation

Separation of a lesion from bone, with preservation of bone continuity, by virtue of the lesion's containment within an encapsulating or circumscribing connective tissue envelope derived from the lesion or surrounding bone (Figs 27.5A to F).

It is the most commonly practiced modality where the whole cystic lining is removed from the bony cavity, either *in toto* or in piecemeal. Most of the cystic lesions are slowly growing and the bony cavity has smooth cortication all around. A complete enucleation will show a cavity in bone devoid of any soft tissue lining. In OKC the nature of the cyst is infiltrative and thus the cavity may not appear smooth after the enucleation of the lining and thus may need further curettage or carbolization of the base.

The advantage of the enucleation is that the whole pathological lining is removed completely, thus the chances of recurrence and neoplastic transformation are minimal. The disadvantage is that in large cystic lesions when it is in close proximity with the vital structures, these structures may get traumatized. The enucleation produces big defect which heals slowly by secondary intention and needs to be packed open and maintenance of good local hygiene.

Surgical Procedure

The procedure of enucleation comprises of reflection of mucoperiosteal flap, removal of overlying bone to create an access (corticotomy) the lining is then carefully separated from the bone and removed with the help of the sharp curette. The cavity is carefully inspected and any remnants are enucleated easily and the lining is removed *in toto*. But, the cysts which have thin, friable lining (e.g. OKC) or where the lining becomes friable due to secondary infection, is removed in piecemeal. The residual bony defect is packed with gauze soaked in iodoform or whitehead varnish. This procedure is called *"packing the cavity open"*. The pack initially helps in hemostasis and also protects the wound from contamination. Primary closure of the wound is often unsuccessful as the mucoperiosteal flap often lies on the bony defect and is unsupported and invariably leads to dehiscence (gaping) of the suture line. Rather than keeping the whole cavity open, the defect should be packed with roll gauze and the flap is then sutured keeping an area open, through which the end of the pack is drawn out. The pack is changed daily after gently irrigating the wound and also reduced progressively in size to facilitate healing. The packing may be discontinued after 8 to 10 days as during this period the

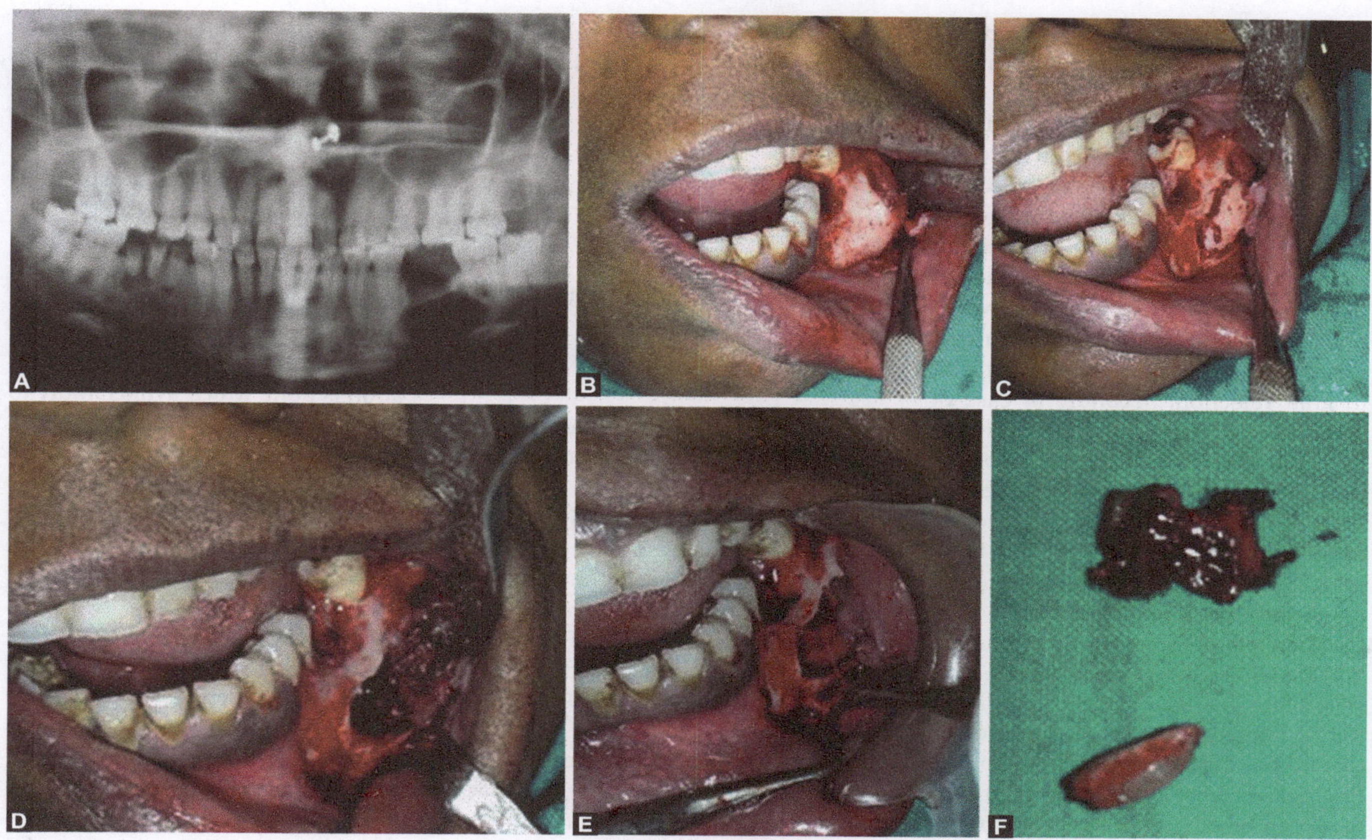

Figs 27.5A to F: (A) Radiograph showing cystic lesions; (B) Cortical expansion; (C) Buccal decortications; (D) Enucleation cystic lining; (E) Cystic cavity after enucleation; (F) Specimen of enucleated lining

base of the cavity gets granulated and subsequently, epithelized and does not require further protection. Only the local hygiene needs to be maintained. To prevent the food particles from entering in the cavity an acrylic obturator may be fabricated and placed.

In case of OKC, the cystic lining is fragile and thus the chances of incomplete removal of lining are high. Secondly, the cyst has a high recurrence rate and being infiltrative in nature infiltrates in the medullary bone. To avoid the recurrence and to eliminate the residual lining, after the enucleation the adjoining bone is thoroughly curetted and the base of the cavity is cauterized using 1 percent carbolic acid solution or using a Carnoy's solution.[7]

Time dependent depth penetration in different tissues on application of Carnoy's solution for 5 minutes as shown in Table 27.3.

Table 27.3: Time dependent depth penetration in different tissues on application of Carnoy's solution for 5 minutes

Tissue	Depth of penetration (mm)
Nerve	0.15
Mucosa	0.51
Bone	1.54

Uses

Some of the uses of Carnoy's solution are:

- Applied directly following enucleation for the treatment of keratocystic odontogenic tumors.
- Enhancing lymph node detection during dissection of cadavers.
- Immunohistochemical fixation and detection of NMDA receptors within the murine hippocampus.
- In some cases direct application following enucleation for certain kinds of unicystic ameloblastomas. This appears to decrease the likelihood of recurrence over enucleation alone. Protein coagulation is thought to limit uptake of these toxic materials by surrounding tissues, however it is this fact that limits its usefulness as a treatment agent in general.
- As a fixative for pap smear samples.
- As a fixative agent for both nuclear and mitochondrial DNA in various tissues.

Carnoy's solution penetrates to a predictable, time-dependent depth without injuring the neurovascular structures. Five minute application penetrates bone to a depth of 1.54 mm, nerve to a depth of 0.15 mm and mucosa to a depth of 0.51 mm.[8]

Primary bone grafting in the defect following the surgical removal is debatable topic. Some surgeons may recommend it, but the risk involved is that the chances of graft infection and rejection are optimum as the watertight closure of the defect is not always possible which may lead to oral contamination and infection which may subsequently result in graft rejection. Secondly in case of cysts like OKC there is a high recurrence potential and unless the recurrence is not ruled out by reasonable length of follow-up, primary grafting may not be a good idea. Instead secondary bone grafting is considered to be safe. The enucleated cystic lining must be sent for the histopathological examination and the entire lining must be screened thoroughly by histological examination to rule out any ameloblastic changes, so that in case of positive histopathological findings an appropriate follow-up protocol can be advised to the patient and remedial steps can be taken earlier in case of any recurrence.

Advantages of Enucleation

- Primary closure of the wound is possible
- Healing is rapid
- Postoperative care is reduced
- Thorough examination of whole cystic lining is possible.

Disadvantages of Enucleation

- Unerupted teeth in dentigerous cyst will be removed with the lesion
- Large cyst removal will make the jaws prone to fracture
- Damage to adjacent vital structures
- Pulp necrosis and nonvitality of the adjacent teeth.

Marsupialization

The word *marsupial* is derived from the Greek for *"pouch"*. It is the surgical exteriorization of a lesion by removal of overlying tissue to expose its internal surface to the oral cavity or another body cavity, by excision of a portion of the lesion (deroofing) bordering that surface or cavity. It is the procedure in which the cystic lining is not removed fully, but instead a small portion of the cystic lining along with the overlying oral epithelium is excised, the contents are evacuated and the cystic lining is sutured to the oral mucosa (Fig. 27.6). The cavity is packed gently with a guaze soaked in the antiseptic solution and the pack is changed daily with reducing size. Alternatively, an impression of the defect is made after the base has granulated and an acrylic obturator with a bulb is fabricated. The bulb projects in the lumen and the size of the bulb is gradually reduced by trimming as the cyst heals. As the cyst is deroofed, the pressure in the cystic cavity drops and the further growth of the cyst is arrested and the cyst begins to shrink with simultaneous healing at the periphery. After few months the cyst heals completely and the cystic lining merges with the oral mucosa. This procedure is also called as a Partsch's operation.

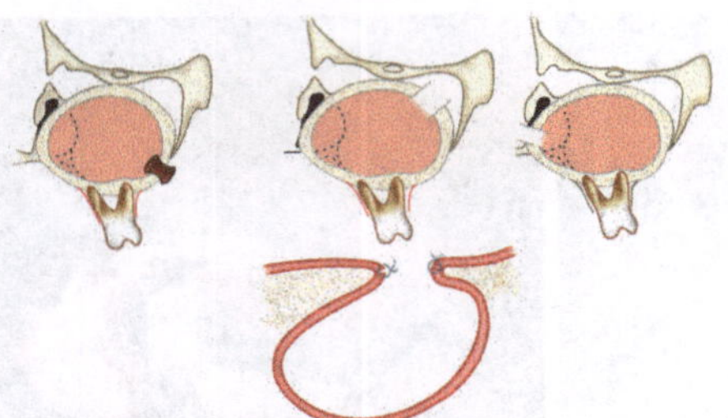

Fig. 27.6: Diagrammatic representation of marsupialization

The indications of marsupialization are:

- Large cystic lesions where enucleation may cause weakening or pathological fracture of the bone.
- Cystic lesions in close proximity with the vital structures, where enucleation may damage the vital structures.
- Dentigerous cysts associated with tooth which is required to be preserved or the tooth is in such a position that their eruption in the oral cavity can be facilitated, e.g. maxillary canine.
- Cysts with very thin and friable lining which is difficult to be removed completely, e.g. sublingual ranula.
- Medically compromised patients where the major surgical procedure or exposure to general anesthesia is contraindicated.
- As a combination with the enucleation in cases of large lesions. Initially, the marsupialization is done and the cystic size is allowed to shrink and subsequently the enucleation is done which avoids injury to the vital structures in the vicinity and the ensuing surgical defect is also smaller and manageable. This also prevents the weakening and fracture of the bone. This procedure also called *Waldron operation.*

Advantages of Marsupialization

- It is technically simple
- Spares vital structures
- Allows eruption of teeth
- Prevents oronasal, oroantral fistula
- Prevents pathologic fracture
- Reduces operating time
- Helps shrinkage of cystic cavity and allows for endosteal bone formation.

Disadvantages of Marsupialization

- The demerit of this procedure is that the pathological tissue, i.e. the cystic lining is left behind, which can lead to the recurrence and neoplastic transformations.
- Histologic examination of entire cystic lining not possible.
- Postoperative care is required for long time.
- Prolonged follow-up is required to maintain larger opening than underlying cavity (formation of slit like pocket that may harbor foodstuffs).
- Secondary surgery may be required with risk of invagination and new cyst formation.[2]

Waldron's Method[9] (1941)

In this technique the cyst is first marsupialized and then enucleated subsequently.

Due to deroofing of the cyst there is decrease in the osmotic pressure which in return decreases the osteoclastic activity around the cyst resulting in the gradual decrease in the size of the cyst due to healing at the periphery.

- Large cysts contain multiple septae so during marsupialization the cavity is converted into single one. This causes ease in the complete enucleation process.
- Vital structures in approximation with the cysts are protected.

Advantages

- Development of thickened cystic lining which makes enucleation easy
- Spares adjacent vital structures
- Combined approach reduces morbidity
- Accelerated healing process
- Allows histopathological examination of residual tissue.

Disadvantages

It requires secondary surgery for removal of residual pathological lining.

Other Modalities

Segmental Resection

Segmental resection is done when the bone is severely thinned out and multiple perforations are present, in cases of pathological fractures and ameloblastic transformation within the cyst. In such advanced cases, the cyst extends to adjoining soft tissue and attempts for its enucleation are usually inadequate leading to the recurrence in the soft tissue. This is more relevant and applicable to the OKCs as compared to the other odontogenic cysts as the former behave more aggressively. In cases where the lesions are extensive, the bone is so severely thinned out that it becomes virtually impossible to preserve it and during the surgery itself multiple pathological fractures occur warranting the segmental resection of the thinned out bone (Fig. 27.7).

Chemical Cauterization

Enucleation followed by chemical cauterization—the presence of epithelial islands within mucosa overlying the cyst and the bony cavity have prompted the use of various surgical strategies to treat the surrounding tissue adjunctively in effort to eradicate residual disease and minimize recurrence. Chemical cauterization followed by enucleation serves the purpose. Carnoy's solution is a popular chemical tissue fixative.

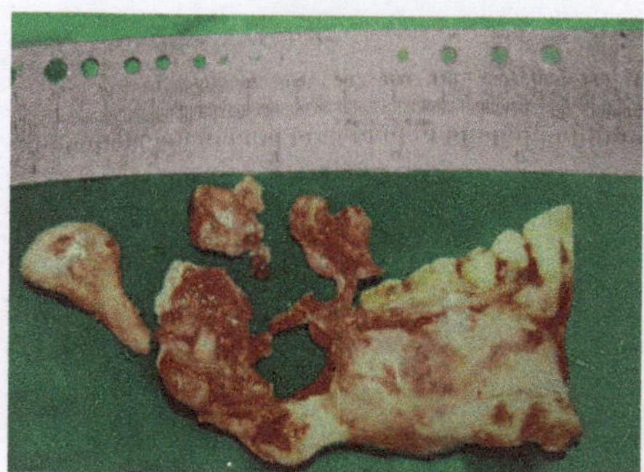

Fig. 27.7: Specimen of resected mandible, severely undermined by OKC showing multiple pathological fractures

Cryosurgery[10]

Cryosurgery is an adjunct to the surgical treatment of benign cyst and tumors of jaw. Similar to cryotherapy it allows for removal of cyst by enucleation and curettage followed by treatment of the surrounding structures. Cryosurgery for osseous lesions produce cellular necrosis in bone, while maintaining the inorganic osseous frame work. Predictable cell lysis occur at the temperature below 20°C and is caused by:

- Direct damage to the intracellular and extracellular ice crystal formation
- Osmotic disturbance
- Electrolyte imbalance.

DEVELOPMENTAL CYSTS OF ODONTOGENIC ORIGIN

Primordial Cyst

The primordial cyst is formed as a result of the cystic degeneration in the tooth bud of a developing tooth as early as the bud, cap or early bell stage. Thus, the involved tooth fails to develop and is missing. It can originate from the tooth of the normal series or from the bud of the supernumerary tooth. As it originates quite early state of odontogenesis, the age of occurrence is also quite early in the life, i.e. the late first or second decade of life. Clinically it may vary widely in size. This cyst is relatively docile in nature and seldom recurs after adequate surgical removal. The cyst produces a well circumscribed, radiolucent lesion and often does not grown to a large size. The management comprises of enucleation.

Histopathologically, most of the cases of primordial cysts, diagnosed on the basis of clinical features, turned out to be odontogenic keratocysts (Para or Orthokeratinized). In view of the same the terminology "primordial cyst" is not used for histopathogical diagnosis if the evidence of keratinization is present. In such cases it will be reported as odontogenic cyst and on clinical correlation it will be primordial cyst formed at the initiation stage of tooth development.

Dentigerous Cyst

A dentigerous cyst is the cyst which encircles the crown of an unerupted tooth. At least two types of dentigerous cyst. Dentigerous cyst arising due to degeneration of stellate reticulum in early stages of tooth development, enamel hypoplasia is a ensuing feature. Dentigerous cyst also can arise after tooth formation by accumulation of fluid within the reduced enamel epithelium or just below it; enamel hypoplasia may not be a feature. Other theories of dentigerous cyst include enamel hypoplasia which diminishes the adherence of reduced enamel epithelium to crown and provides starting point for development of cyst. Crown of a permanent tooth sometimes erupts into a radicular cyst of its deciduous predecessor. This is rare as cystic condition in primary dentition is seldom seen.

Shibata et al.[11] (2004) conducted a retrospective study on 70 patients, who had histologically confirmed dentigerous cyst in anterior region. They concluded that inflammatory changes at the apex of a deciduous tooth may be responsible for initiating a dentigerous cyst of the permanent successor. It is the cyst that surrounds the crown of an unerupted tooth. It is formed as a result of accumulation of the fluid between the reduced enamel epithelium and the crown of the tooth.

Clinical Features

Dentigerous cysts is commonly seen in early part of life, i.e. second decade. It is most commonly seen in maxillary canine and mandibular third molar area, but can occur with any tooth including the supernumerary tooth may be displaced as low as the inferior border. Dentigerous cysts associated with supernumerary teeth are rare and estimated to constitute 5 to 6 percent of all dentigerous cysts. They resemble the usual dentigerous cysts in terms of sex predilection and age distribution. The vast majority, about 90 percent, are associated with a maxillary mesiodens.[6] The incidence of association dentigerous cyst with an impacted tooth increases with age. It is characterized by missing tooth with hard swelling. It is usually painless unless and until secondarily infected or very large. It may lead to failure of eruption of adjacent tooth due to pressure. There is no neurologic deficit even though the neurovascular bundle is grossly displaced. Expansion of cortices especially buccal cortex (Fig. 27.8B). Sometimes in case of lower molars lingual cortex and if the cyst is very large both the cortices get expanded. If cyst is rapid growing cortices become paper thin and on palpation there is egg shell crackling. Fluctuation can be elicited on palpation when the bone is perforated. The maxillary canines can also be severely displaced up to the infraorbital margin due to the pressure from the cyst. The cyst causes expansion of the bone and the involved tooth is often missing as it is displaced away from the alveolar bone due to pressure exerted by the cyst. The adjacent teeth may also be displaced due to the pressure. The overlying cortical bone is thinned and cortex is expanded more often.

Three varieties of the dentigerous cyst have been described namely central, lateral and circumferential. The ameloblastic transformations are more common in a dentigerous cyst. The rapid growth, expansion of other cortices, multilocular appearance may suggest ameloblastic transformation. Malignant transformation is comparatively less common than the ameloblastic transformation. The malignancy associated with the dentigerous cyst is squamous cell carcinoma and possibly the mucoepidermoid carcinoma than the ameloblastic carcinoma.

Radiograghic Features

Dertigerous cysts presents as smooth well-corticated radiolucency, commonly unilocular or multilocular if infected. It is associated with unerupted tooth attached at cemento enamel junction (Fig. 27.8C). It mostly causes displacement of roots, but if lesion is fast growing or is of long, standing duration it may lead to resorbtion of roots and may also cause displacement of the neurovascular bundle. The involved tooth gets severely displaced due to pressure from the growing cyst and may be present at the inferior border of the mandible or very high in the orbital floor in maxillary cysts (Figs 27.8A and C).

Dental follicle may expand to produce radiographic appearance of following:

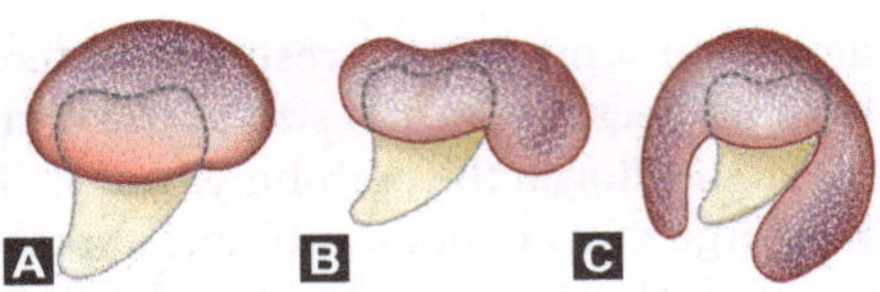

Figs 27.9A to C: Varieties of dentigerous cyst. (A) Central; (B) Lateral; (C) Circumferential type

- Central
- Lateral
- Circumferential types of dentigerous Cysts (Figs 27.9A to C).

Aspiration

Aspiration is done using a wide bore (18 gauge) needle. The dentigerous cyst usually contains a straw colored fluid. The cystic fluid contains cholesterol crystals and is rich in protein on biochemical investigation.

Incisional biopsy is indicated only in large cysts to rule out ameloblastic changes in the cystic lining. However, the preoperative incisional biopsy in small and moderate cases is usually unnecessary.

Differential Diagnosis

- Ameloblastoma and ameloblastic fibroma
- Adenomatoid odontogenic tumor occurs in maxilla.

Management

The treatment of choice is enucleation along with removal of the involved tooth. The lining is thick and has nice capsule which facilitates the removal of the cyst in Toto. When the tooth is not severely displaced and can erupt in its normal position and needs conservation, in such

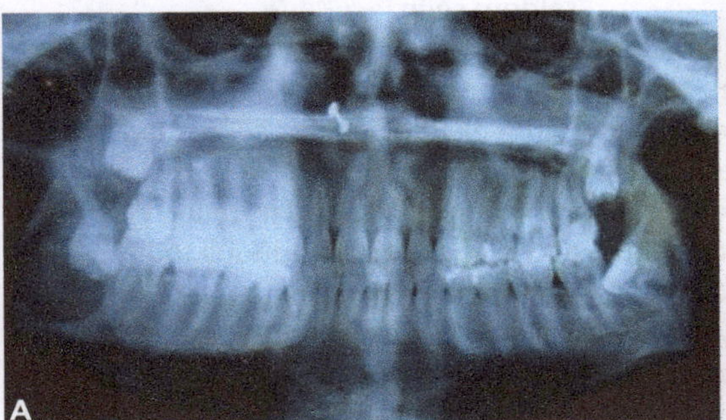

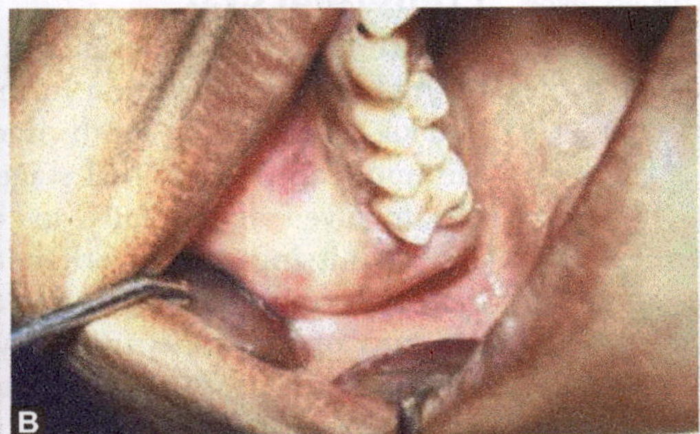

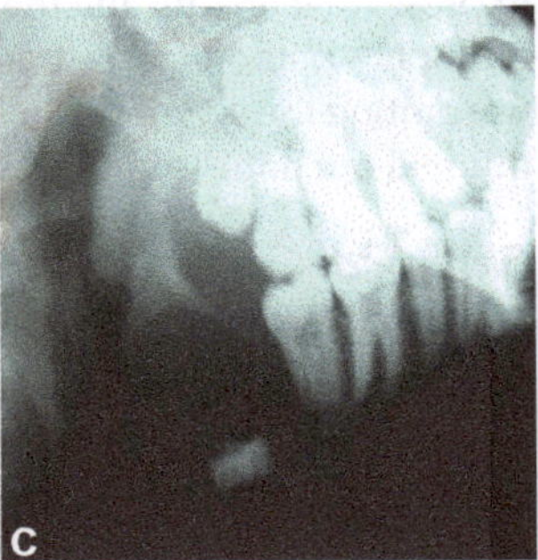

Figs 27.8A to C: Dentigerous cyst with severely displaced unerupted molars

cases marsupialization can be done. The eruption of the tooth can be assisted orthodontically. The lining must be sent for histopathological examination to rule out ameloblastic changes, especially in large cysts (Figs 27.10, 27.11 and 27.12). The cyst does not recur after adequate surgical procedure. According to most authors, the common treatment for the dentigerous cysts has been total elimination of the cyst including the tooth involved; however if the lesion is present in young patients during the eruption period and the radiographic and clinical features are suggestive of dentigerous cysts an alternative treatment is the maintenance of the permanent tooth and enucleation of the lesion alone, stating

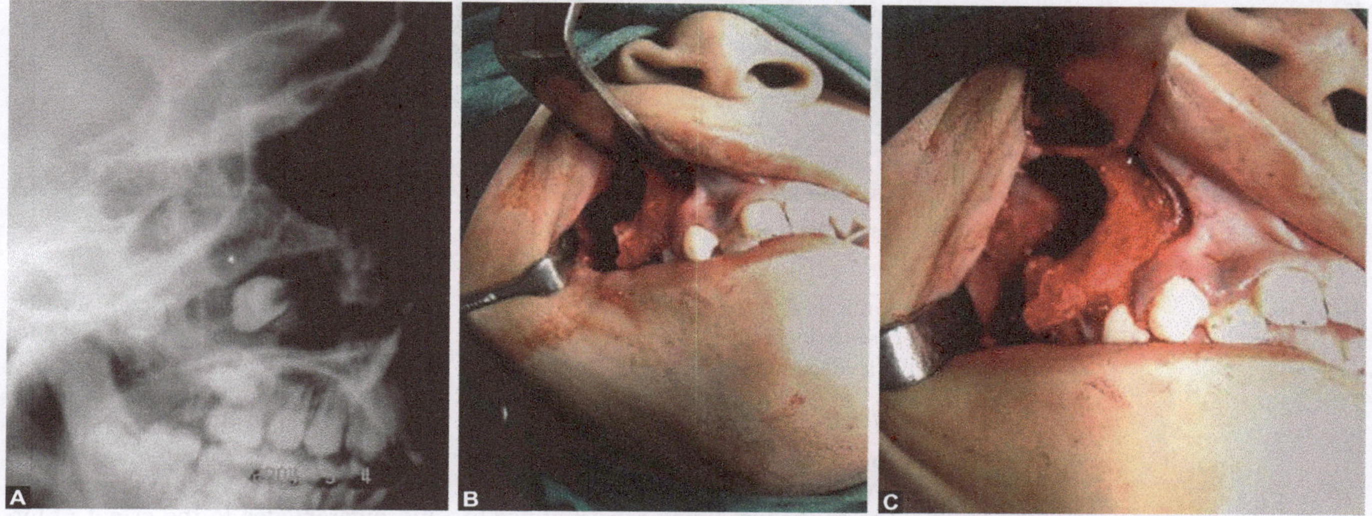

Figs 27.10A to C: Dentigerous cyst with maxillary premolar managed by enucleation

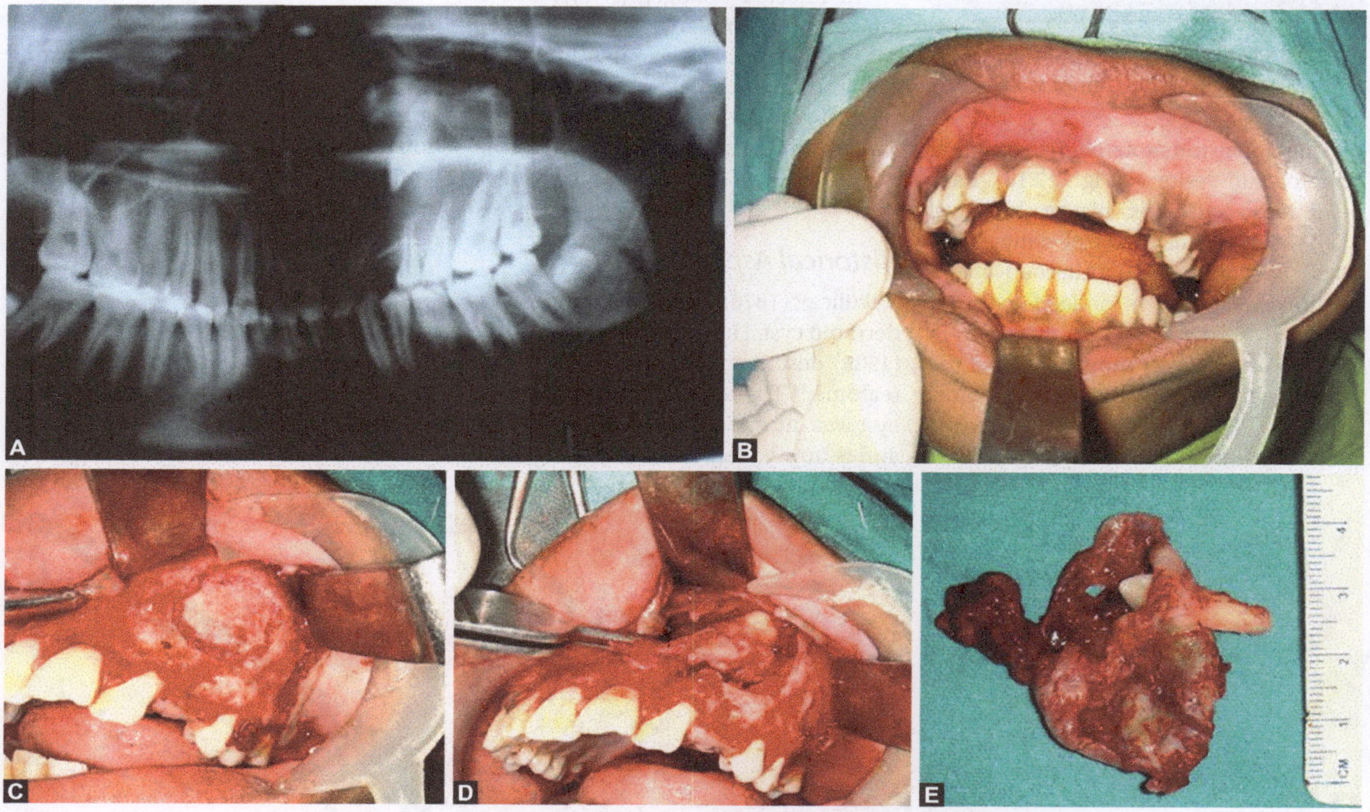

Figs 27.11A to E: Dentigerous cyst with maxillary canine treated with enucleation

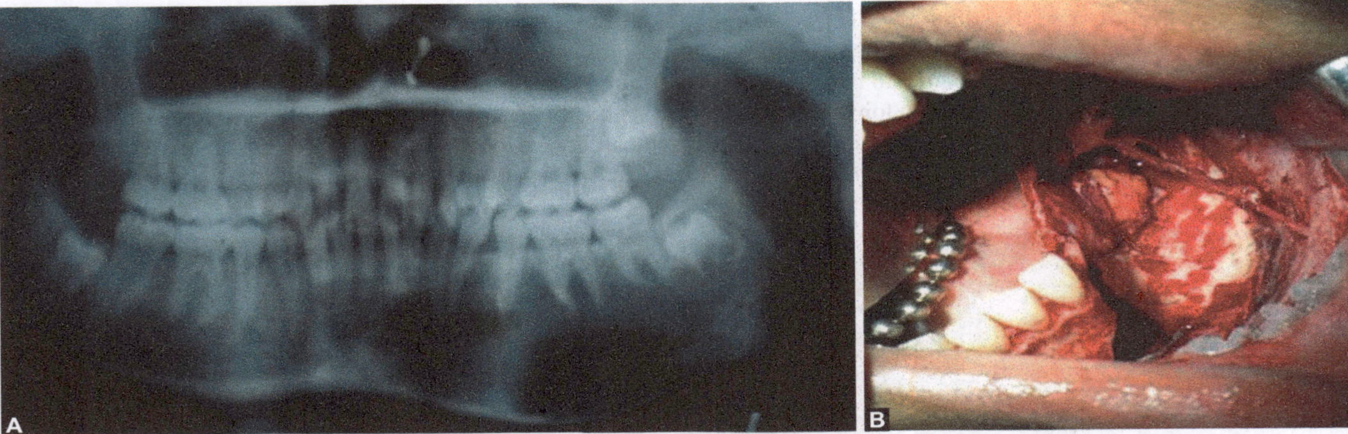

Fig. 27.12: Enucleation of dentigerous cyst in the mandibular body and ramus with preservation of neurovascular bundle

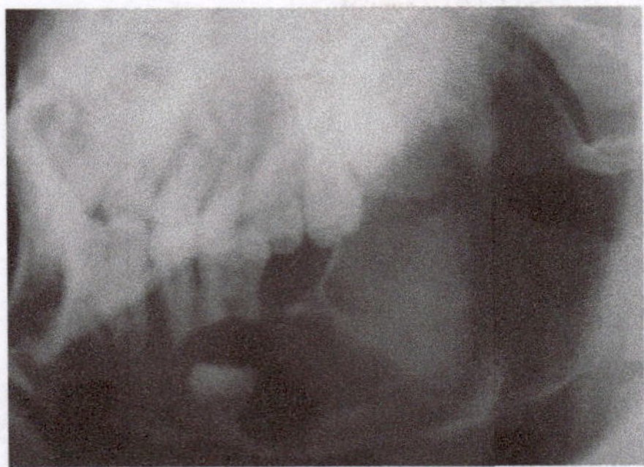

Fig. 27.13: Dentigerous cyst undergoing ameloblastic changes

that ameloblastomatous changes or other odontogenic lesions (Fig. 27.13) have been ruled out after histopathological analysis and a diagnosis of dentigerous cysts is confirmed.[12] Alternatively if the involved tooth is noticed to be in favorable position for its eruption in the oral cavity in a young individual the marsupialization of the cyst may be done. As the pressure from the growing cyst drops the tooth starts erupting. Orthodontic assistance may be required in such cases to facilitate the eruption of the tooth in its desired position.

Histopathological Findings

The lesions consist of a fibrous connective tissue wall which is loosely arranged. The epithelium lining consist of two to three layers of cuboidal epithelial cell.

In infected dentigerous cyst due to infection the fibrous wall become more collagenized, with a variable infiltration of chronic inflammatory cell along with some areas of hyperplastic squamous epithelial lining was seen (Figs 27.14A to C).

Odontogenic Keratocyst (OKC)

Historical Aspect

Mikulicz[13] (1876), described the OKC as a dermoid cyst. Hauer (1926) and Kostecka (1929) described keratocyst as a cholesteatoma.[14] The term odontogenic keratocyst was introduced by Philipsen[15] (1956) and is now widely used. The designation keratocyst was used to describe any jaw cyst in which keratin was formed to a large extent.

The odontogenic keratocyst (OKC) is the term coined by Phillipsen (1956) to describe a class of odontogenic cyst where the lining epithelium proliferates and differentiates to the extent of formation of keratin.

Etiology and Pathogenesis

Paul Stoelinga[16] stated in the past that OKC was considered to originate from primordium of tooth before mineralization has taken place, remnants of dental lamina or basal cell hamartias. It may arise from the cell rests of Malassez, remnants of dental lamina or in the lining of other odontogenic cysts.

Enlargement of Keratocyst

Scharfetter et al.[17] (1989) found that invasive growth of keratocyst was likely to be a result of active growth of the connective tissue wall. Toller[18] (1970) suggested

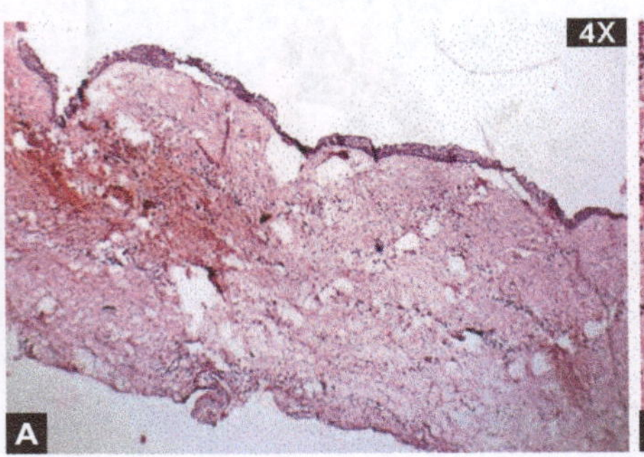

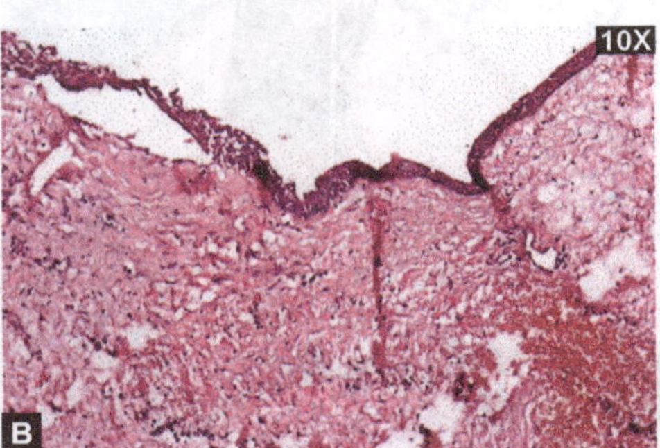

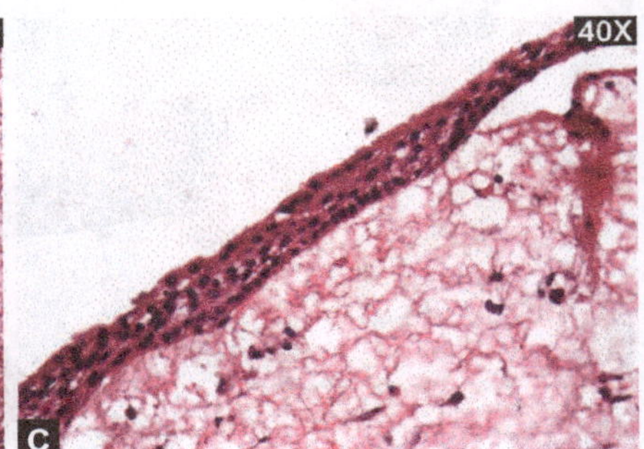

Figs 27.14A to C: Photomicrograph showing the lining of a dentigerous cyst

that osmolality plays an important role in expansive growth of OKC. Main[19] (1970) suggested that mural growth in the form of epithelial proliferation causes expansion of OKC. The rate of growth of keratocyst varies from 2 to 14 mm a year, with average of about 7 mm^2. Browne[20] (1970) and Kramer[21] (1974) proposed that multilocular outlines is due to proliferation of local groups of epithelial cells against the semisolid cyst content. Fenestrated capillaries in OKC cause expansion.

Clinical Features

- It occurs as early as 1st decade and as late as 9th decade, with pronounced peak frequency in 2nd and 3rd decade of life. There Bimodal age distribution with 2nd peak in 5th decade or later.
- There is a male predilection.
- Whites races are more affected than blacks.
- Mandible is commonly involved than maxilla. Approximately half of all keratocysts occur in angle and extends to varying distances into the ascending ramus and forward into body. Pain, swelling and discharge may present with paraesthesia of lower lip. The cyst can attain large size involving maxillary sinus, entire ascending ramus including condylar and coronoid process (Fig. 27.15).
- There may be displacement and/or resorption of teeth.
- When maxillary sinus is involved there can be displacement and destruction of floor of orbit and proptosis of eyeball.

Fig. 27.15: Site predilection for occurrence of OKC

- When cyst occurs entirely on gingiva it is known as peripheral odontogenic keratocyst.
- In 60 percent of cases there is bony expansion, more on buccal than lingual side. In 39 percent perforation of bone is also noted. However it is observed that the OKC usually attains a large size without causing a conspicuous bony expansion.
- The cyst may even extend from maxilla to base of skull behaving like a low-grade squamous cell carcinoma. Neurological symptoms occasionally noted.
- The cyst has high rate of recurrence after incomplete inucleation and the patients are required to be kept under long term postoperative follow-up.
- Multiple OKC are seen in case of "Jaw cyst—Basal cell nervus – Bifid rib syndrome" and the Gorlin – Goltz syndrome.

The recurrence rate is very high in OKC due to:

- Thin and fragile lining.
- Infiltrative nature.
- Incomplete removal of cyst lining.
- Retention of daughter cysts/microcyst or epithelial islands in the wall of original cyst.
- There is development of new keratocysts from epithelial offshoots of the basal layer of oral epithelium and infiltrative nature of the cyst.

Types of Keratocyst (Fig. 27.16)

- Replacement
- Envelopmental
- Extraneous
- Collateral.

Odontogenic Keratocysts Reclassified as Keratocystic Odontogenic Tumor

The odontogenic keratocyst is regarded as a developmental abnormality and is generally known for its aggressive nature and high recurrence rate, especially in comparison with other developmental odontogenic cysts. In addition to a distinctive clinical aggressive biological

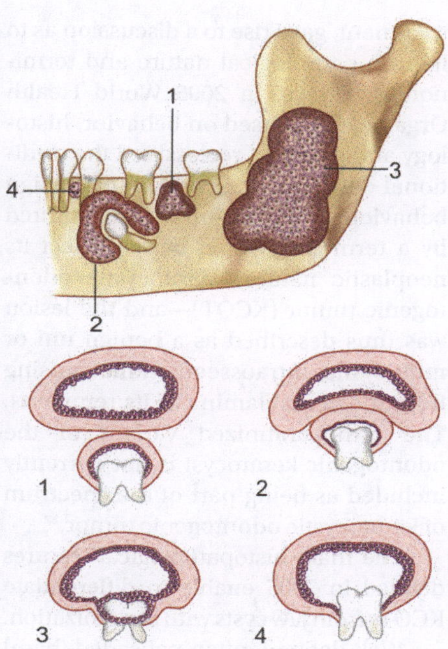

Fig. 27.16: Types of keratocyst

behavior, the expression of various proliferation markers in the epithelial lining and over expression of p53 protein and mutations in p53 and PTCH genes (tumor suppressor genes) have led several investigators to consider odontogenic keratocyst as a benign cystic neoplasm. The components of the connective tissue in KCOT revealed some resemblance with the stromal components of aggressive tumors such as ameloblastoma: high frequency of stromal myofibroblasts, differences in the collagen fibers of the extracellular matrix, high enzymatic activity with increased matrix metalloproteinases (MMPs) and mast cell tryptase, and increased expression of receptor activator of nuclear factor-κB (RANK), RANK ligand (RANKL), osteoprotegerin (OPG) and tumor angiogenesis. Focusing on the importance of the epithelial-mesenchymal interactions in odontogenic tumors, previous studies supported that the stroma of keratocysts should not be regarded just a structural support of the cyst wall, but rather as portraying the features of a "tumoral stroma". However, its growing potential to a large size before manifesting clinically and the tendency to recur following surgical treatment, gave rise to a discussion as to its true pathological nature and terminology. Hence, in 2005 World Health Organization, based on behavior, histology and genetics, reclassified the traditional designation, stressing the benign behaviour of this lesion was substituted by a term that would better reflect its neoplastic nature—keratocystic odontogenic tumor (KCOT)—and the lesion was thus described as a benign uni or multicystic, intraosseous tumor arising from the dental lamina or its remnants. The orthokeratinized variant of the odontogenic keratocyst is not currently included as being part of the spectrum of keratocystic odontogenic tumor.[22]

The main histopathological features defined in 2005 enable to differentiate KCOTs from jaw cysts with keratinization.

- Well defined, often palisaded, basal layer of columnar or cuboidal cells
- Intense basophilic nuclei of the columnar basal cells oriented away from the basement membrane
- Parakeratotic layers with an often corrugated surface
- Mitotic figures frequently present in the suprabasal layers.

Histopathological Findings

The epithelial lining and connective tissue wall of the odontogenic keratocyst (OKC) is characteristically thin and friable, thus causing the specimen to fragment when treated. Grossly, the lesion often has a bosselated, gray, cystic appearance mimicking the appearance of a glove.

In 1962, Pindborg and Phillipsen and Henriksen established strict histologic criteria for the diagnosis of an odontogenic keratocyst (OKC). These criteria include an epithelial lining that is usually thin and uniform in thickness, with little or no evidence of rete ridges; a well-defined basal cell layer, the component cells of which are cuboidal or columnar in shape and often fashioned in a palisaded arrangement; a thin, spinous cell layer which often shows a direct transition from the basal cell layer; spinous-cell layer intracellular edema; surface keratinization that is corrugated and predominantly parakeratotic; and a fibrous connective tissue cyst wall that is thin and usually uninflamed. Additionally, satellite cysts, solid epithelial proliferations, odontogenic rests, and basal layer budding have been described in association with the odontogenic keratocyst (OKC).

The histologic variants of the odontogenic keratocyst (OKC) are: (1) parakeratinized (2) orthokeratinized, and (3) combined. The recurrence rate is much higher in the parakeratinized variant than that the orthokeratinized variant (Figs 27.17A and B).

Contents of Cyst

Heparin sulfate, Chondroitin 4 sulphate, Hyaluronic acid, GAG. On aspiration there it is whitish, cheesy material with Keratin flecks. There is low protein content (< 4 mg/dL), with specific gravity 1.018. Histologic differential diagnosis from cystic ameloblastoma, dentigerous cyst, glandular odontogenic cyst, lateral periodontal cyst. The OKC is also known to undergo ameloblastic transformations. Multiple OKC are seen in case of 'Jaw cyst-basal cell nervus-bifid rib syndrome' and the 'Gorlin-Goltz syndrome'.

Radiologically the cyst has a classical multiloculated appearance with sclerotic borders. The classical scalloping of the borders is seen in this cyst and the loculi are separated by fine bony septae. The loculi are variable in size and the cyst extends between the roots of the teeth (Figs 27.18A to D). The CT scans provide more accurate information regarding the perforation of cortex and extraosseous spread of the lesion. This information is more vital as the extraosseous spread warrants more comprehensive surgical management to prevent soft tissue recurrence (Figs 27.19 and 27.20). The cyst initially contains a straw-colored

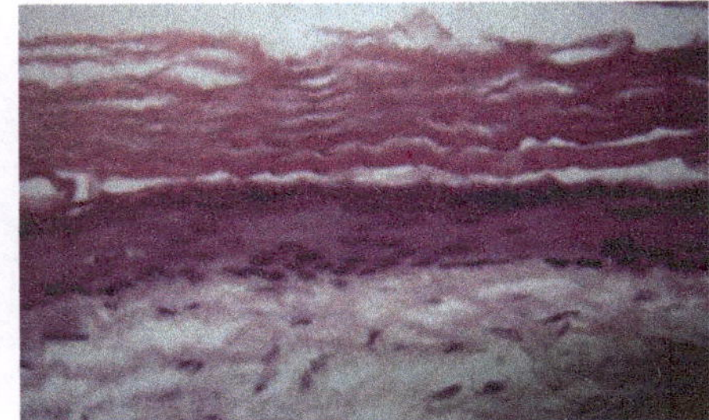

Fig. 27.17A: Orthokeratinized OKC

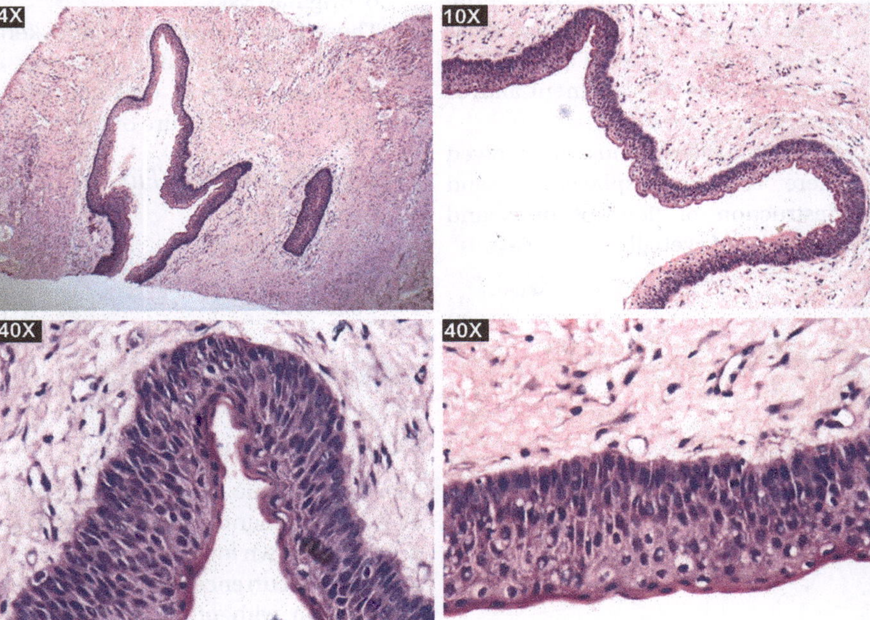

Fig. 27.17B: Photomicrograph of Parakeratinized OKC (Keratocystic odontogenic tumor)

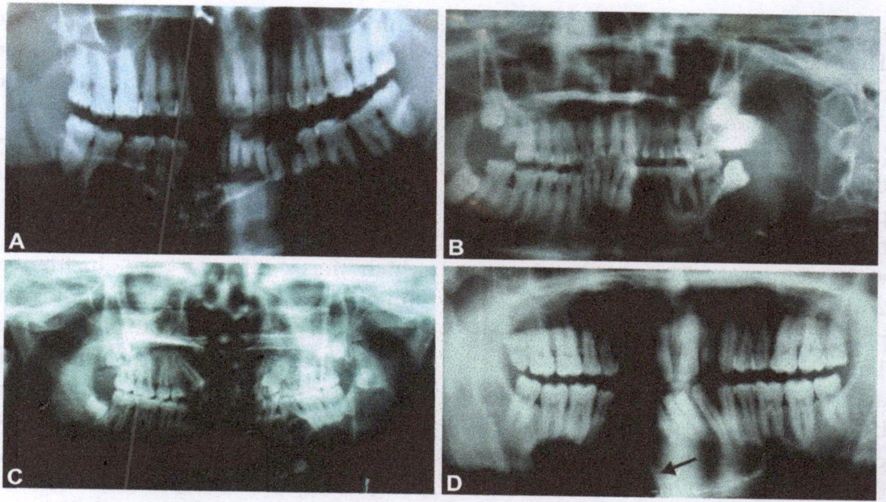

Figs 27.18A to D: Keratocyst showing multiloculated radiluscent appearance

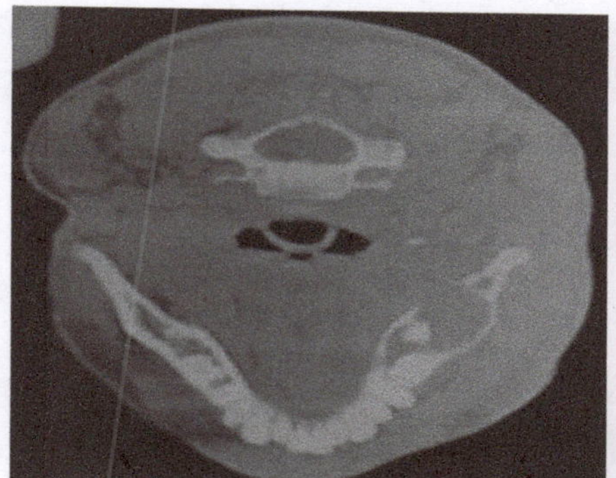

Fig. 27.19: Multiloculated lesion, with bony septae CT scan showing perforation of lingual and scalooping of the border cortex

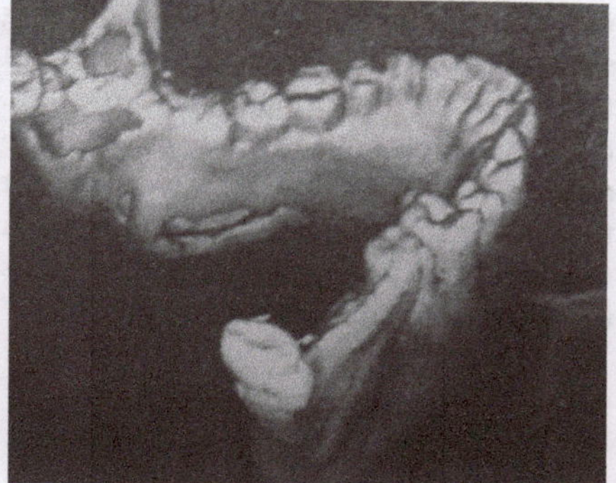

Fig. 27.20: 3-D CT scan showing multiple cortical perforations

fluid, which changes into cheesy material due to accumulation of the exfoliated keratin in its lumen. This may be differentiating feature of the OKC from the ameloblastoma, as both may appear similar radiographically.

Management

The different modalities that are proposed for the management are:

- Enucleation and curettage
- Enucleation and peripheral ostectomy
- Marsupialization
- Osseous resection
- Cryotherapy
- Excision of overlying mucosa in conjunction with cyst enucleation and treatment of bony defect with Carnoy's solution.

The selection of the appropriate treatment modality is based on various factors like age of the patient, location of the lesion, extent of the lesion and presence of cortical perforation and extension of the cyst in the adjacent soft tissue.

The OKC is treated with more aggressive way due to its high rate of recurrence. The treatment modalities are:

- Enucleation with vigorous curettage of the adjacent bone.
- Enucleation with chemical cauterization of the base of the bony cavity. Many authors recommend the use of Carnoy's solution, a tissue fixative that is applied to the bone cavity following the enucleation and curettage of the cyst lining and bone cavity.
- Segmental resection in case of multiple perforations of the cortex, pathological fracture, where the bone so severely thinned out that it is difficult to conserve it. The spillage of the cyst in the soft tissue also requires attention as the cyst is known to recur in the soft tissue as well. If the perforation in the soft tissue is encountered, excision of soft tissue upto the next anatomical boundary is recommended and the excised tissue be subjected for frozen sections to determine adequacy of surgical margins.
- Marsupialization is mentioned in the literature as the treatment modality, but it is a poor choice of therapy as the cyst is aggressive and it is dangerous to leave behind the pathological difficulty is that during the marsupialization all the loculi, especially the smaller ones may not be opened and the cyst will start growing again. The daughter cysts may proliferate and cause recurrence. The risk of ameloblastic changes is always there. Marsupialization followed by enucleation is also recommended in the literature in the management of the large lesions however it is not a popular treatment modality for the obvious reasons. Decompression of cyst involves any technique that relieves the pressure within the cyst that causes it to grow. Growth of cysts is believed to occur by a combination of osmotic pressure and pressure resorption, coupled with release of prostaglandins and growth factors. Decompression, by any means, appears to change to environment and decreases the amount of interleukin-α which is released. Decompression can be performed by making a small opening in the cyst and keeping it open with a drain. Marsupialization, on the other hand, involves converting the cyst into a pouch. By converting the cyst to a pouch, the lesion is decompressed, but this is a more definitive treatment for the cavity and exposes the cyst lining to the oral environment. Mandibular cysts are normally marsupialized into the oral cavity, although maxillary

cysts can also be marsupialized into the maxillary sinus or nasal cavity, as well as the oral cavity.[8] The basic limitation of the marsupialization is that the cyst is multiloculated and has many loculi and even daughter cysts in the lining. The marsupialization may lead to decompression of the major locule, but other loculi may remain unaddressed and thus the treatment with this modality may not be adequate to treat the large lesions.

- Long-term follow-up is mandatory after any treatment to detect the recurrence early.

The enucleated lining should be submitted for the histopathlogcial examination to confirm the diagnosis and to rule out other changes.

Calcifying Epithelial Odontogenic Cyst (Gorlin's Cyst)

Calcifying epithelial odontogenic cyst (CEOC) was first described by Gorlin and associates[23] in 1962 and thus eponymously named as Gorlin's cyst. The cyst is commonly seen in the mandible (Fig. 27.21A). The central CEOCs are more common than peripheral lesions (3:1) and they are usually diagnosed in the second decade of life, whereas the peripheral ones are usually noted after the age of 50. The CEOC may associated with odontoms.[9] The age incidence is 2nd and 3rd decades of life with equal predelection to males and females. There are two variants of CEOC, a cystic and neoplastic variant. It is considered to be the oral counterpart of the cutaneous calcifying epitelioma of Malherbe. Both the lesions are characterized by the presence of *"ghost cells"* histologically. The main histopathologic criteria for the diagnosis of the calcifying odontogenic cyst are well-established. The cyst lining should show proliferation to the point that it resembles ameloblastoma, (i.e. columnar cells over which are stellate and spindled cells in an arrangement that suggest stellate reticulum). Within this proliferation of epithelium, cells undergo the characteristic *'ghost cell'* keratinization (Figs 27.22A to C). The other lesion which also shows presence of the ghost cells is craniopharyngeoma. The ghost cells are degenerating epithelial cells. The presence of patchy foci of calcification within the lesion is another peculiarity of this cyst. It warrants differentiation from the CEOT, which has different age incidence, clinical behavior and histopathological features. The radiological picture is a well-corticated radiolucent lesion with patchy foci of dystrophic calcification in it (Fig. 27.21B). The diagnostic incisional biopsy may be conclusive in establishing the preoperative diagnosis in case of large lesions. The treatment of choice for the CEOC comprises of enucleation (Fig. 27.21C). The recurrence rate after adequate enucleation is low.

Gingival Cyst and Midpalatal Raphae Cyst of Infants

It was first described by Moscow and Bloom[24] 1983. During the morphodifferentiation (*late bell stage*), disintegration of the *dental lamina* begins to

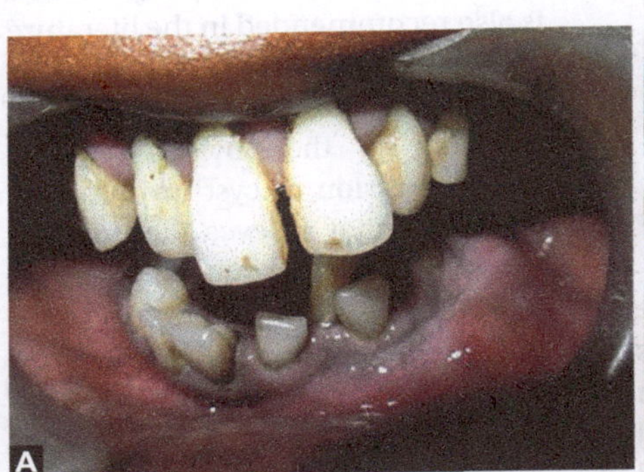

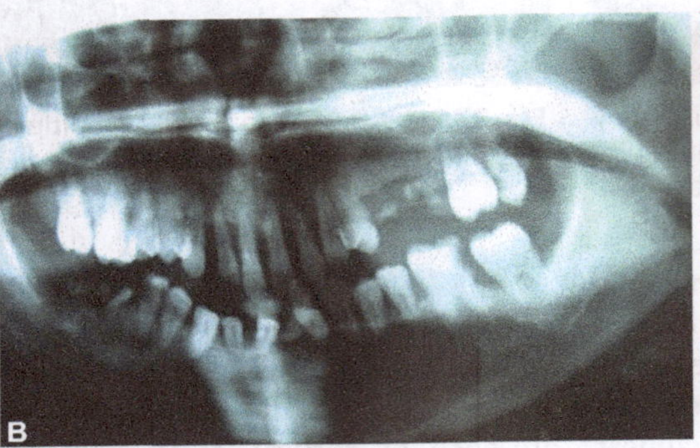

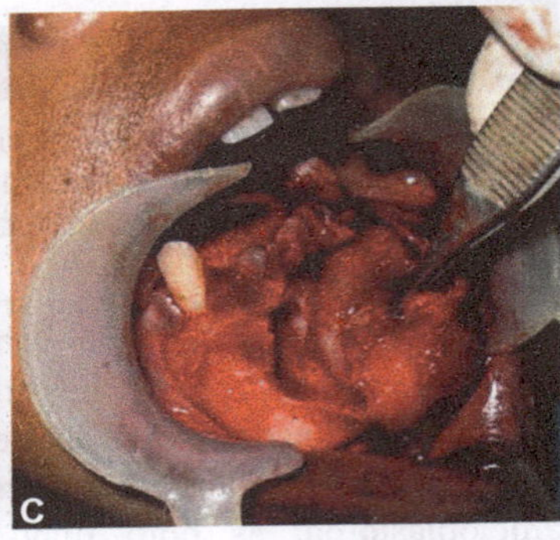

Figs 27.21A to C: CEOC: (A) Clinical appearance; (B) Radiographic appearance; (C) Treatment with enucleation

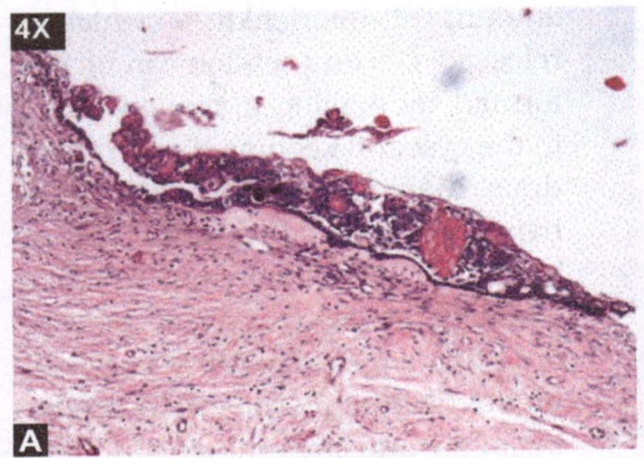

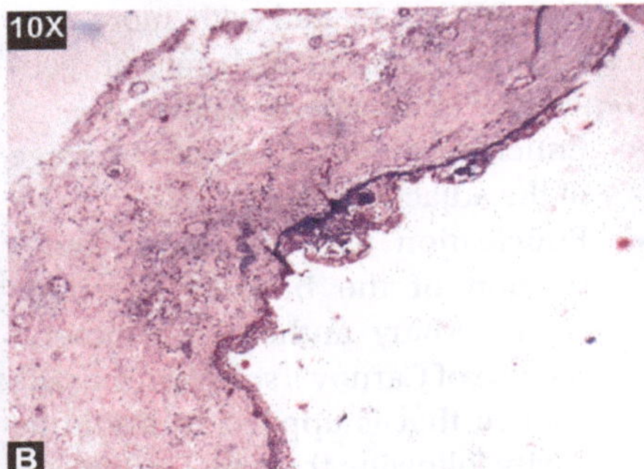

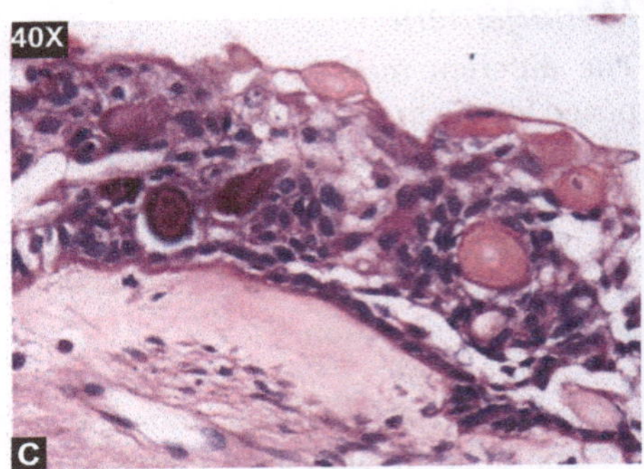

Figs 27.22A to C: Photomicrograph showing the proliferation of the lining epithelium with palisaded, hyperchromatic columnar nuclei, stellate reticulum—like area and sheets of ghost cells (H and E stain)

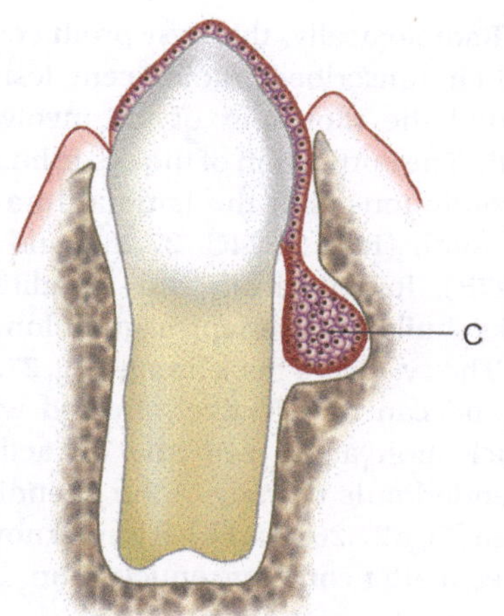

Fig. 27.23: Lateral periodontal cyst

occur and numerous islands and strands of odontogenic epithelium are seen in the corium between the tooth germ and the oral epithelium, remote from the alveolar process. Those dental lamina remnants which had already evolved into small cysts, expanded rapidly at this stage (15–20 weeks) and there was thinning of overlying oral epithelium.

Lateral Periodontal Cyst

Lateral periodontal cyst is uncommon, but well-recognized type of developmental odontogenic cyst. It arises from odontogenic epithelial cell rests, traumatic implantation of surface epithelium or cystic degeneration of deep projections of surface epithelium (Fig. 27.23).

Histopathological Features

The lateral periodontal cyst is composed of a cystic cavity with a connective tissue wall. The cyst lining of the lateral periodontal cyst is generally composed of 1 to 5 cell layers of cuboidal to stratified, nonkeratinized, squamous epithelium, with focal plaque like thickenings that appear as whorls and mural protrusions. Shear and Pindborg suggested that these thickenings represented an example of the odontogenic epithelium establishing original morphology under pathologic conditions, akin to the thickening of stomatodeal ectoderm in the formation of dental lamina during early odontogenesis.

The Botryoid odontogenic cyst has a similar histology to that of the lateral periodontal cyst, except for more pronounced plaquelike thickenings, mural protrusions, and a multilocular pattern histologically. The thickened areas are usually separated by thin, fibrous septa. Microscopic assessment is necessary to distinguish lateral periodontal cyst from other odontogenic cysts and pathologic processes.

Eruption Cyst

Eruption cyst is essentially a dentigerous cyst occurring in the soft tissues. Crown of the tooth associated with an eruption cyst usually projects into cyst lumen, derived from reduced enamel epithelium.

ODONTOGENIC CYST OF INFLAMMATORY ORIGIN

Radicular Cyst

The origin of cyst epithelium lies in cell rests of malassez. The products of pulpal infection and necrosis spill out into the periapical tissues, initiating an inflammatory response. The inflammatory cells secrete lymphokines to neutralize, immobilize and degrade bacteria.

These cells are thought to elaborate many other factors that either directly or indirectly act as epithelial growth factors, stimulating the proliferation of rests of Malassez.

A radicular cyst is an inflammatory cyst which is usually associated with a non-vital tooth. The tooth is either carious, fractured or attrided, causing exposure of the pulp. The pulp becomes inflamed, necrotic and the tooth becomes non-vital. The repeated infection leads to chronic periapical infection. The remnants of the root sheath of Hertwig get irritated and they proliferate to give rise to a radicular cyst. The cyst seldom more than 1 cm in diameter. But larger lesions are also seen in some patients. The cyst causes expansion of the bone and the overlying cortex becomes thin and eroded to produce egg shell crackling in cases of larger cysts (Figs 27.24 and 27.25). As the cyst is inflammatory in origin, dull pain is associated with this cyst. Long standing periapical cysts may present as a

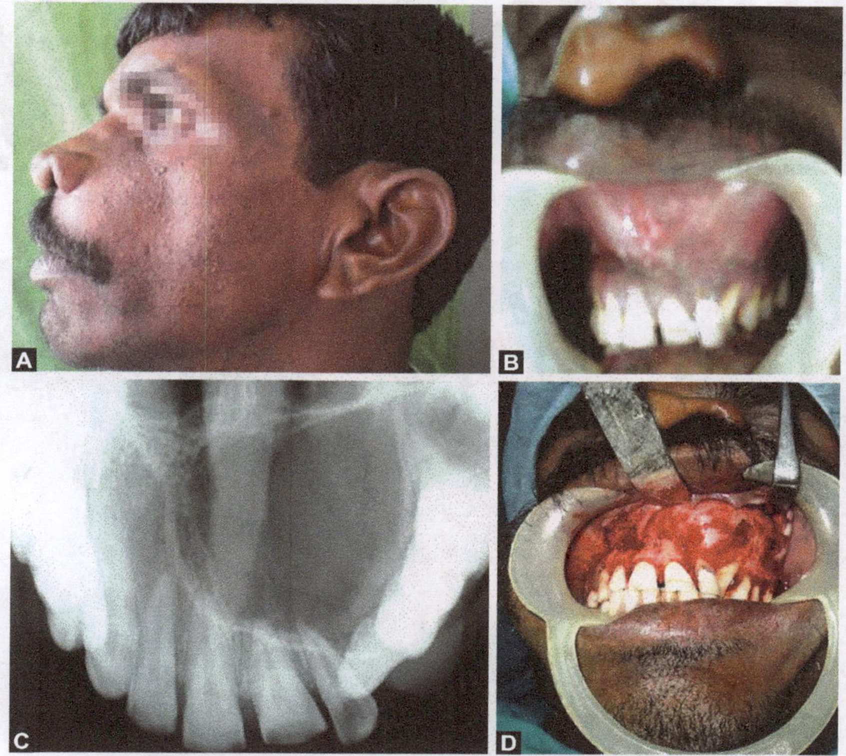

Figs 27.24A to D: Radicular cyst: (A and B) Clinical presentation; (C) Radiographic appearance; (D) Surgically exposed lesion

gingival sinus, draining pus intermittently (Fig. 27.27A). Acute exacerbation of the infection may produce throbbing pain and the clinical picture could be similar to a periapical abscess.

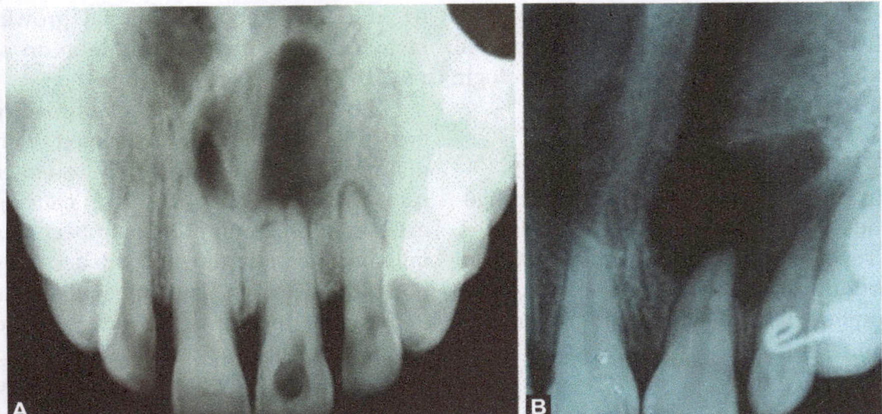

Figs 27.25A and B: Radicular cyst with nonvital maxillary incisors, a common clinical entity

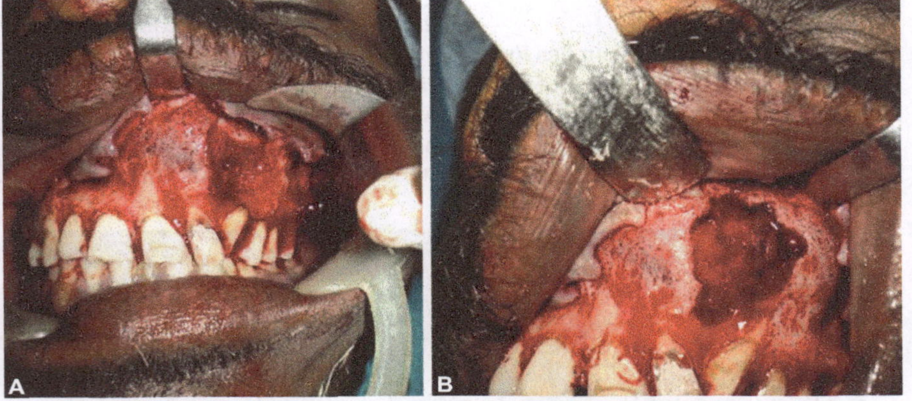

Figs 27.26A and B: Management of a large radicular cyst with enucleation

Radiologically, this cyst produces a well-circumscribed, radiolucent lesion around the root apex of the involved tooth. The cortication of the cystic lining is continuous with the lamina dura of the tooth (Figs 27.24C, 27.26A and B, 27.27B). Radiologically, this condition looks similar to a periapical granuloma.

The cyst has a thick lining (Fig. 27.24 D) and can be effectively treated with enucleation along with the extraction or endodontic therapy of the offending tooth (Figs 27.26A and B). It is not known to recur after complete enucleation.

Macroscopic Findings

The gross specimen may be spherical or ovoid intact cystic masses, but often they are irregular and collapsed. The walls vary from extremely thin to a thickness of about 5 mm. The inner surface may be smooth or corrugated.

Histopatholgical Findings

The histopathological studies shows following features:

Epithelial lining: Almost all radicular cysts are lined by stratified Squamous Epithelium and range in thickness from 1 to 50 cell layers. The only exception to this is in those rare cases of periapical lesions of Maxillary Sinus. In such cases, cyst is then lined with a pseudo stratified cilliated columnar epithelium or respiratory type of epithelium. Rushton's

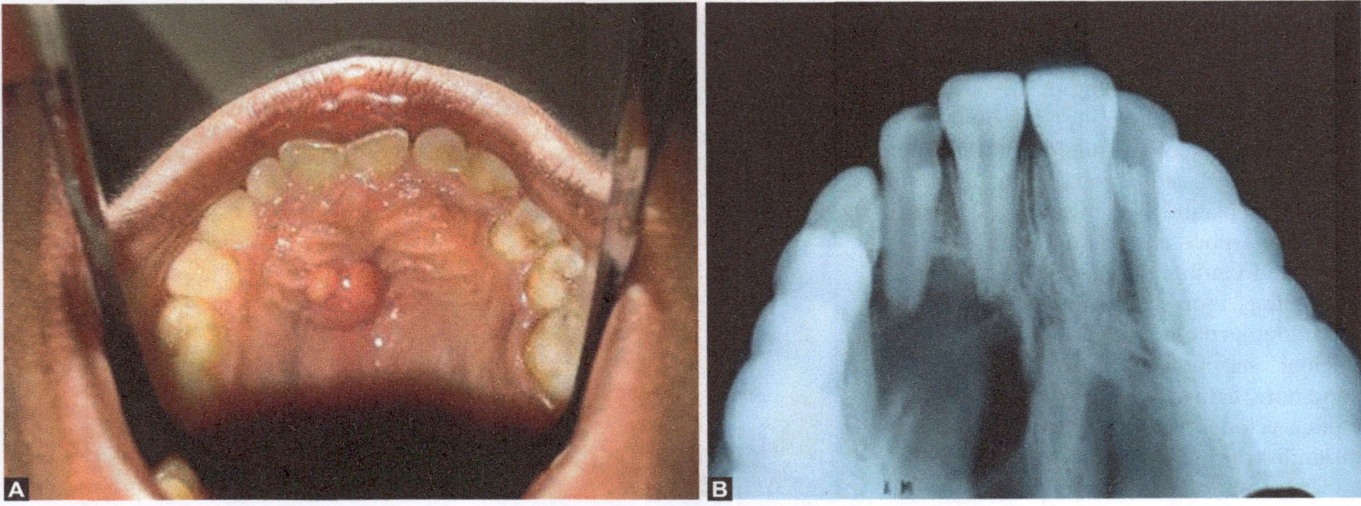

Figs 27.27A and B: Radicular cyst with incisors presenting as a palatal sinus

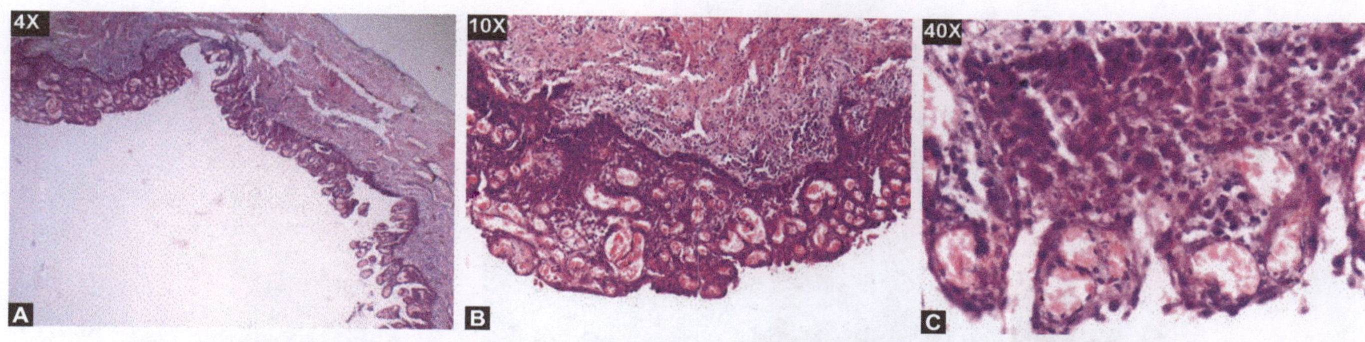

Figs 27.28A to C: Photomicrograph of radicular cyst, note chronic inflammatory cell infilteration in the lining

Hyaline bodies are found in epithelial linings. Very rarely they are found in Fibrous capsule.

Fibrous capsule: Fibrous capsule of radicular cyst is composed of mainly condensed parallel bundles of collagen fibres peripherally and a loose connective tissue adjacent to epithelial lining. Deposition of cholesterol crystals are found in many radicular cysts, slow but considerable amount of cholesterol accumulation could occur through degeneration and disintegation of lymphocytes, plasma cells and macrophages taking part in inflammatory process, with consequent release of cholesterol from their walls. Acute inflammatory cells are present when epithelium is proliferating. Chronic inflammatory cells are present in connective tissue immediately adjacent to epithelium (Figs 27.28A to C).

Residual Cyst

Residual cyst refers to an inflammatory cyst of the jaws that fails to involute after root canal therapy or tooth removal (Fig. 27.29). Although, it is conceptualized as resulting from tooth extraction that did not include removal of an associated radicular cyst. But more commonly it occurs due to failure of endodontic treatment or misdiagnosed accessory canal.

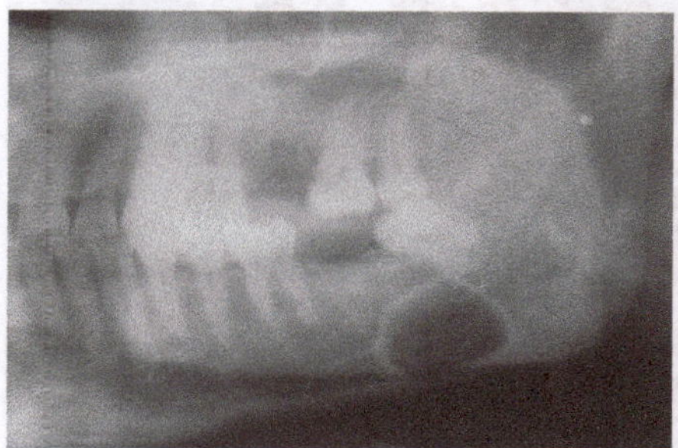

Fig. 27.29: X-ray showing residual cyst in lower left second molar region

NON-ODONTOGENIC CYSTS

Inclusion Cysts

Midpalatal Cysts

They arise from epithelial inclusions at the line of fusion of palatal folds and nasal processes. After birth these epithelial inclusions usually atrophy and are absorbed. Some however produce keratin containing keratocyst which extend onto the surface. Burke et al.[25] 1966 suggested possibility of abortive glandular differentiation leading to cyst formation. The exact cause of the epithelial proliferation and the cyst formation is not known.

The median palatal cyst is located in the midline of the hard palate between the lateral palatal processes. The cyst may become large to be visible clinically as a midline palatal swelling. It produces a well-circumscribed radiolucent lesion on the palatal radiograph (Figs 27.30A and B).

Globulomaxillary Cyst

The globullomaxillary cyst has been described as an intrabony fissural cyst between the maxillary lateral incisor and the canine teeth. Radiologically, it is a well corticated, heart shaped radiolucent lesion causing the divergence of the adjacent teeth.

The globulomaxillary cyst forms at the junction of the globular process of the medial nasal process and the maxillary process. The globulomaxillary fissure is present between the lateral incisor and the canine teeth (Fig. 27.31). It is often asymptomatic clinically and is detected on routine radiographs or during the orthodontic treatment. The treatment comprises of surgical removal, sparing the adjacent teeth.

Traumatic Bone Cyst

(*Synonyms—Traumatic, simple, hemorhagic, solitary, simple, idiopathic bone cyst, extravasation cyst, unicaramel cyst*).

The traumatic cyst is an unusual lesion which occurs with considerable frequency in jaws as well as in other bones.

Traumatic Theory

After trauma to an area of spongy bone containing hemopoietic marrow enclosed by a layer of dense cortical bone there is a failure of organization of the blood clot and for some unexplained reason, subsequent degeneration of the clot occurs that eventually produces an empty cavity within the bone. In the development of the lesion, the trabeculae of bone in the involed area becomes necrotic after degeneration of the clot and the bone marrow, although some viable tissue must persist to initiate the resorbtion of the involved trabeculae. The expansion tends to cease when the cyst reaches the cortical bone, thus there is no cortical expansion.

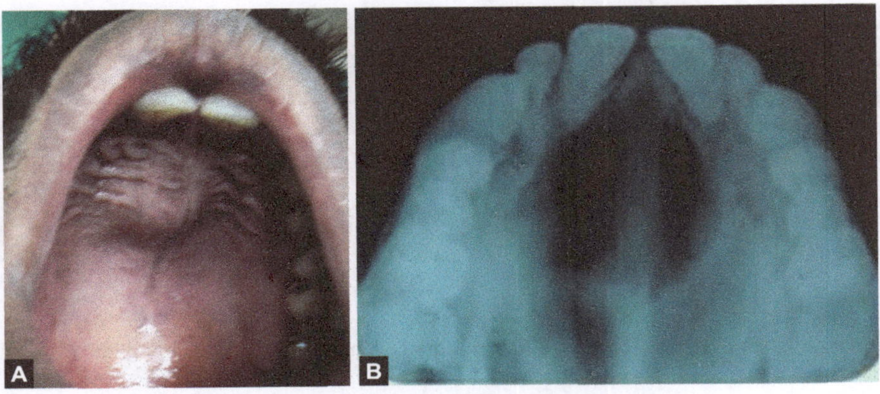

Figs 27.30A and B: Median palatal cyst

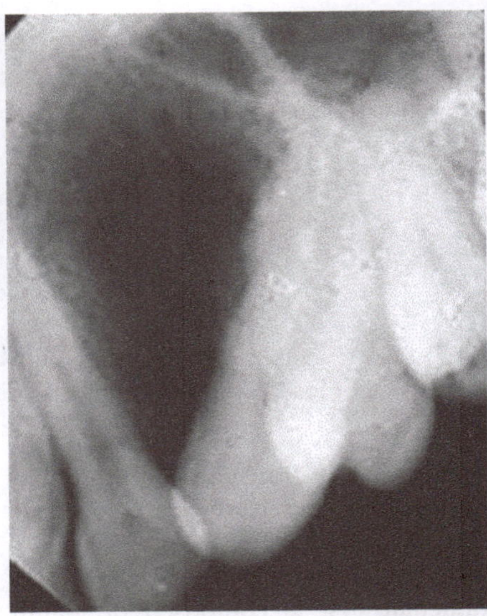

Fig. 27.31: Globulomaxillary cyst between the lateral incisor and canine producing pear shaped shadow

Other Theories of Origin

- Origin from bone tumors that have undergone cystic degeneration
- A result of calcium metabolism such as that induced by parathyroid disease
- Necrosis of fatty marrow due to ischemia
- Low grade chronic infection
- Trauma creating unequal balance of osteoclasis and repair of bone.

Clinical Features

The traumatic bone cyst usually occurs in young patients. Males are more frequently affected than females probably because they are more exposed to trauma. Mandibular molars are more common site although cases with anterior mandible have also been reported which may be probably due to presence of hematopoietic marrow (Figs 27.32A to C). The traumatic bone cyst occurs in mandible and very seldom in maxilla.

The teeth in the involved region are generally vital. When the cavity is surgically opened, it is found to be an empty which may contain either small amount of straw-colored fluid, shreds of necrotic blood clots, fragments of connective tissue or nothing.

The hydrostatic pressure in cystic lumen is exceptionally low as compared to other cysts.

Radiographic Features

It reveals a rather smoothly outlined radiolucent area of variable size which may be lined by sclerotic bone depending on the duration of the lesion. The size may be small in centimeter or may be large enough to involves the whole of body or ramus. The cavity may be lobulated or scalloped if it involves root apices. The cyst in the molar region should be differentiated from lingual salivary gland depression which is located below mandibular canal where as solitary cyst is present above it.

The histopathologic features are a thin connective tissue membrane lining the cavity.

Treatment

Since the definitive diagnosis of the solitary bone cyst cannot be established

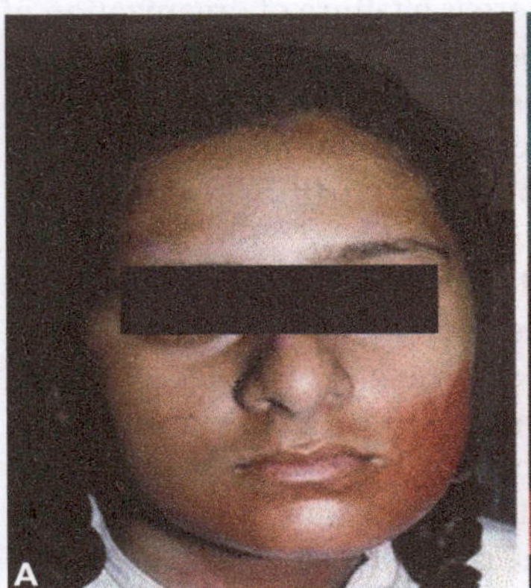

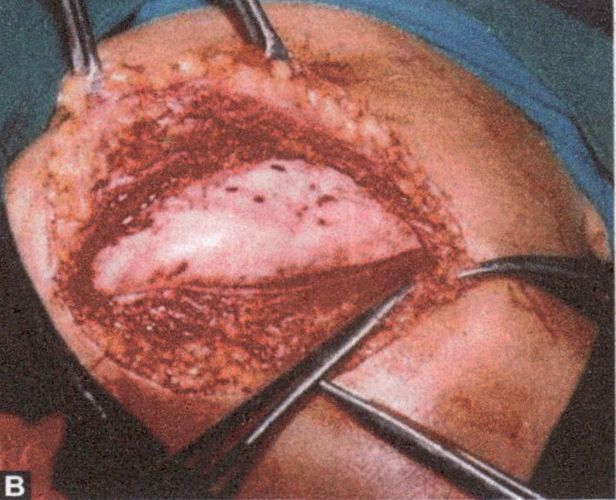

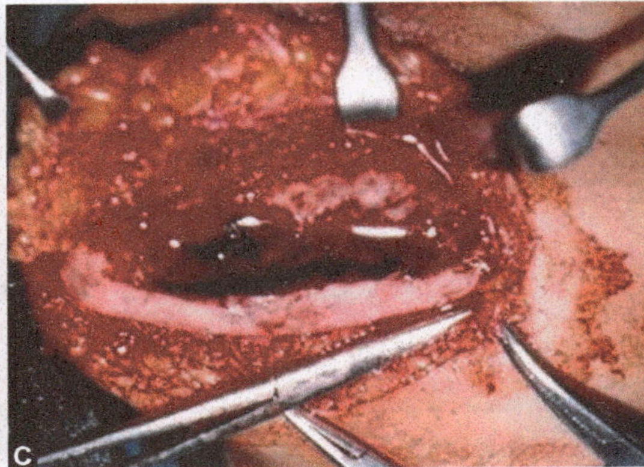

Figs 27.32A to C: (A and B) A case of traumatic bone cyst in a young girl of 15 years age watch the bony expansion; (C) Empty cavity without lining

without surgical exploration. So attempts to enucleate the lining and in course of manipulation reestablish bleeding into the lesion should be attempted. If the cavity is then closed, it has been found that healing and filling of the space by bone occur in 6 to 12 months. If the space is large, cancellous bone chips and hydroxyl appetite crystals can be used to fill the defect. The platelet rich plasma when added with the cancellous bone chips facilitiates the faster healing of the bony defect.

Aneurysmal Bone Cyst

The aneurysmal bone cyst is an interesting entity described by Jaffe and Lichtenstein[26] (1942), they coined the term anuerysmal bone cyst to describe the characteristic blow out of the bone seen in the radiograph.

Clinical Features

The cyst is rarely found in jaws. It is generally fond in 1st and 2nd decade with female predilection. The common sites of involvement are mandibular and maxillary molar region and also involve angle and ascending ramus region. Aneurysmal cysts of jaws produce firm swelling which may be associated with tenderness. Swelling may be associated with malocclusion and displacement of teeth. It may enlarge to perforate the cortex being covered by periosteum or thin shell of bone and may be associated with egg shell crackling. The intraoperative findings are characteristic in a way that typical welling of the blood from the tissue is encountered on entering the lesion. The involved tissue is often described as '*blood soaked sponge*' with large pores representing the cavernous spaces of the lesion.

Four phases of the pathogenesis have been identified as follows:

- Initial osteolytic phase.
- Active growth phase, characterized by rapid destruction of the bone and a subperiosteal blow out pattern.
- Mature stage, also known as stage of stabilization, which is manifested by the formation of a distinct peripheral bony shell and internal bony septae and trabaculae that produce the classic soap bubble appearance.
- Healing phase, with progressive calcification (*formation of the phleboliths*) and ossification of the cyst and its eventual transformation into a dense bony mass with a irregular structure.

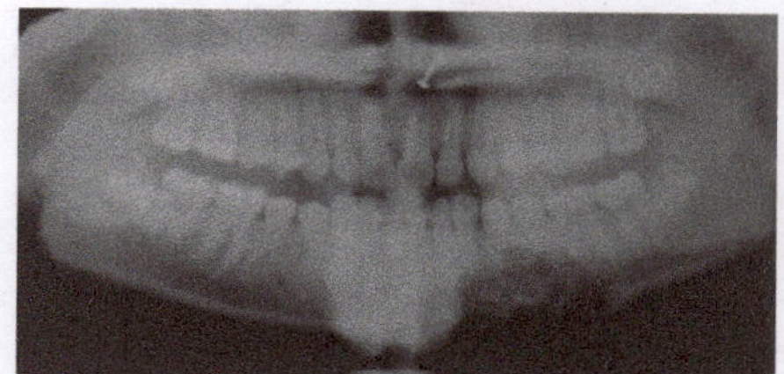

Fig. 27.33: A case of aneurismal bone cyst (ABC) showing Honey comb appearance on radiograph

Thus, the lesion is known to regress spontaneously after incomplete removal.

Radiographic Features

The radiological picture is a radiolucent area which produces ovoid or cruciform expansion of the bone. It is generally unilocular or may be multilocular or have honey comb appearance (Fig. 27.33).

Histopathological Features

Aneurysmal bone cysts' histopathological features show mixture of benign stromal tissue consisting of large *vascular lacunae* separated by septa in which numerous giant cells are found and filled with clotted blood (blood-filled spaces with bland fibrous connective tissue septa) that resembles cranberry sauce; cavernous spaces vessel lack walls and normal features of blood vessels; stroma has histiocytes, fibroblasts, scattered giant cells, hemosiderin and occasional inflammatory cells; giant cells; ABC may be difficult to distinguish from that of giant cell tumor of bone; large amounts of hemosiderin.

Secondary aneurysmal bone cysts occur in conjunction with other lesions (e.g., chondroblastoma, osteoblastoma, osteosarcoma, nonossifying fibroma).

Pathogenesis

Various reasons have been postulated. In may be due to persistent local change in the hemodynamics, leading to increase venous pressure leading to development of dilated engorged veins. It has also been explained as exuberant attempt to repair hematoma of bone similar to central giant cell granuloma. But in cases of aneurysmal bone cyst it is postulated that the hematoma maintains circulatory connection with damaged blood vessels. The slow flow of blood thought the lesion leading *welling* of the lesion when entered. It has been associated with solitary cyst, giant cell tumors or osteosarcomas.

Treatment

Surgical curettage of the lesion is advised. The flow pattern is evaluated and if possible the feeding vessels are ligated. High flow lesions may require interventional radiological support by way of embolization of the feeding vessels using enbutyl cinoacrylate or polyvinyl alcohol particles or micro coils to reduce vascularity and then the lesion is treated by surgical curettage within 24 hours. Low-dose radiation has also been used. But, the possibility of radiation sarcoma is always a hazard.

CYST OF SOFT TISSUE OF HEAD, NECK AND FACE

Sebaceous Cyst

A sebaceous cyst is a closed sac or cyst below the surface of the skin that has a lining that resembles the uppermost part (infundibulum) of a hair follicle and fills with a fatty white, semisolid material called sebum.

If the duct or mouth of the sebaceous gland becomes blocked, the gland becomes distended with its own secretions and forms sebaceous cyst. It is retention cyst and is also called epidermoid cyst as it is lined by superficial squamous cells. It contains sebum which is yellowish pultaceous material with unpleasant smell. Such material contains sebum, fat and desquamated epithelial cells. It may be seen anywhere in the body, but is commonly seen in parts of body with plenty of sebaceous glands like the face and the scalp.

It presents as typical cystic swelling which is spherical in shape and varies in shape from few millimeters to 5 cm in size. It has smooth surface and there is bluish spot or punctum which indicated the blocked opening of the duct (Figs 27.34A to C). Sebaceous cyst is always fixed to the skin and is cystic in consistency. It indents to finger due to the presence of sebum. In large cyst, fluctuation is positive. This cyst is freely mobile over the underlying structures. It is non-tender till it gets secondarily infected.

Total excision is the treatment of choice. If infected, antibiotic should be given and excision should be performed only when the infection subsides.

Two types of surgical methods for excision are recommended:

1. **Dissection method:** Elliptical incision is made on the skin including the punctum. The cyst is gradually dissected from the surrounding skin till the entire cyst can be removed intact as it may recur if removed incompletely. This method is suitable when the cyst is infected previously as this makes the cyst wall thick and well defined (Figs 27.35A to D).
2. **Incision avulsion technique:** Under local anesthesia, incision is made through the skin into the cyst and some contents of the cyst are squeezed out. The cyst wall is then held with pair of disseting forceps and cyst is avulsed out.

Branchial Cyst

Development

Branchial cleft cysts are congenital epithelial cysts, which arise on the lateral part of the neck from a failure of obliteration of the second branchial cleft in embryonic development. At the 4th week of embryonic life, the development of four branchial (or pharyngeal) clefts results in five ridges known as the branchial (or pharyngeal) arches, which contribute to the formation of various structures of the head, the neck and the thorax. The second arch or the hyoid arch grows caudally as well as ventrally and at greater pace than the third and fourth arch at the end of the 5th week. The ridge produced by this arch grows downward and meets caudally a small bridge termed as the epipericardial ridge just above the pericardium. According to some, it meets the fifth arch and the two fuse. A small depression is formed which lies superficial to the 3rd and 4th arch and deep to the second arch. This depression is called precervical sinus. Ultimately this sinus disappears, but if it persists, it forms a cystic swelling in the upper part of the

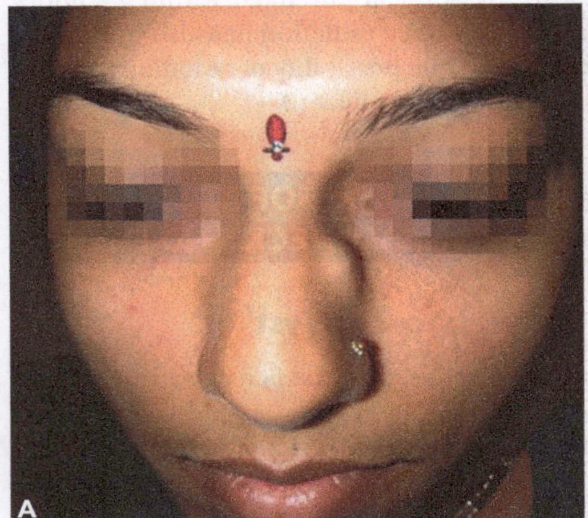
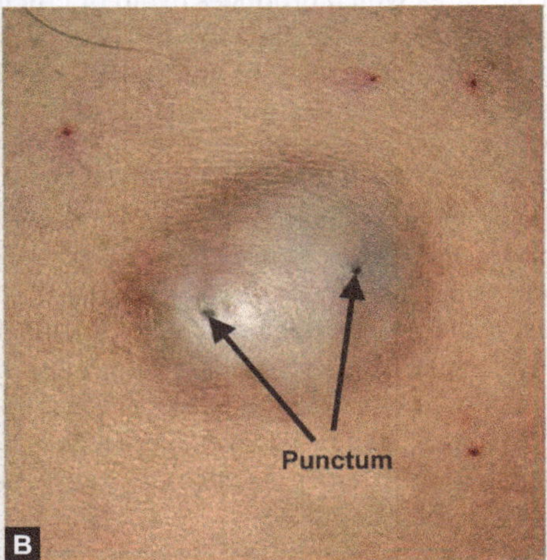

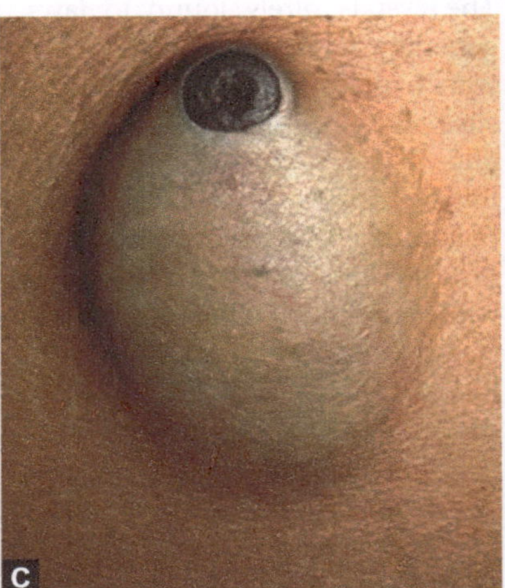

Figs 27.34A to C: Sebaceous cyst, note the classical black punctum

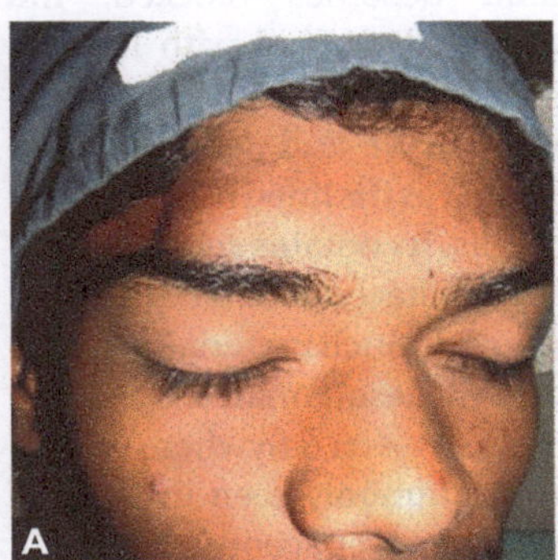
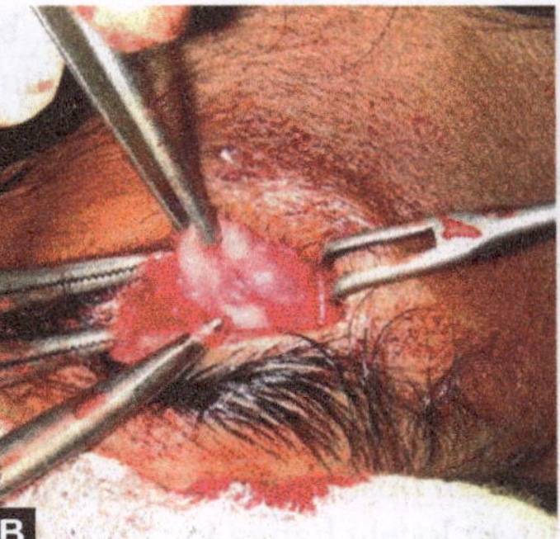
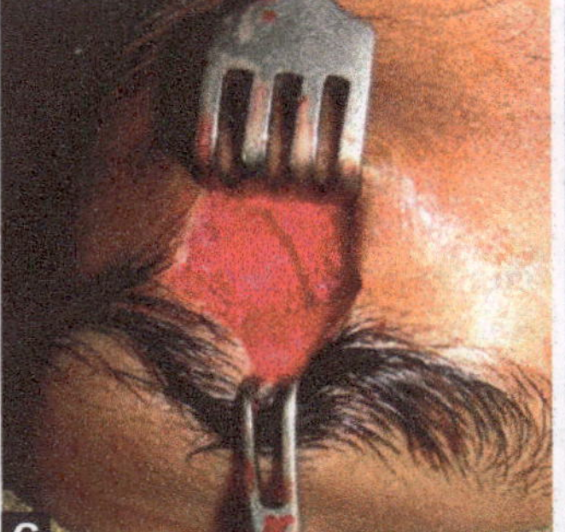
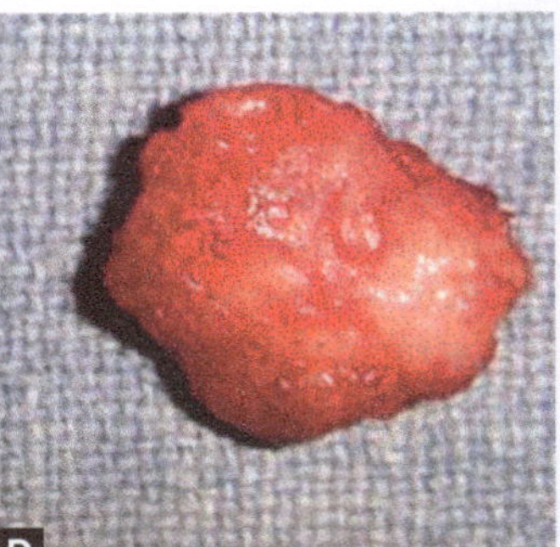

Figs 27.35A to D: Excision of the sebaceous cyst

neck, which is called brachial cyst. If the second arch fails to fuse with the 5th arch or epipericardial ridge, a fistula develops and it connects the precervical sinus and is called the brachial sinus or fistula.

According to Illingworth theory it develops from inclusion of the parotid epithelium in the upper deep cervical lymph node.

Pathology

The cyst is usually lined by stratified squamous epithelium. If it arises from the internal branchial furrow the epithelium may be columnar and ciliated. The striking feature of this cyst is that its wall contains large amount of lymphoid tissue. For this, the cyst is prone to infection and this has laid to Illingworth's theory of inclusion of ectopic epithelium in upper deep cervical lymph nodes. The contents are viscid, mucoid, cheesy material and cholesterol crystals in large numbers.

Clinical Features

Age incidence

Though congenital, yet it does not manifest itself before puberty. Majority of the patients are between 20 to 25 years or even later. This is because the fluid which it contains takes this time to accumulate. There is equal distribution of sex is noticed.

Symptoms

Painless swelling in the upper and the lateral part of the neck is the main symptom. If manifested the swelling may be painful and it becomes difficult to differentiate from acute lymphadenitis, chronic lymphadenitis or tuberculosis lymphadenitis and cold abscess.

Physical Examination

- **Site:** Branchial cyst occupies upper and lateral part of the neck deep to the upper third of the sternomastoid muscle. It protrudes from beneath the anterior border of the sternomastoid. The sternomastoid muscle develops from the migrated myotome in the ridge of the second branchial arch which covers the precervical sinus. The branchial cyst develops from the precervical sinus. So it will always be deep to the sternomastoid muscle. It may be round, but is usually oval in shape with its long axis running forwards and downwards. It is of variable sizes and may attain size of an orange, majority are of sizes between 5 to 10 cm in diameter (Fig. 27.36A).
- **Surface:** It is smooth and edge is distinct, but yields under the palpating fingers. The overlying skin looks normal, though its infected, may be red and angry looking.
- **Consistency:** It is soft, when the content is under tension, feel may be firm or even hard, fluctuation test will be positive. Transillumination test is usually negative, but may be positive if the content is clear fluid. The lump is not freely movable as it is particularly deep to sternomastoid. Regional lymph nodes are usually not palpable, unless the cyst is not infected. The cyst cannot be reduced or compressed. On aspiration cholesterol crystals can be demonstrated in the aspirated fluid. Cysts containing cholesterol crystals are branchial cyst, dental cyst, dentigerous cyst, cystic hygroma, old hydrocele, thyroglossal cyst.

Treatment

Excision is the treatment of choice, incision is made parallel to the skin crease, one must be particular not to leave behind a portion of the cyst wall, to ensure this, dissection must be made carefully (Figs 27.36B and C). Some amount of the content may be aspirated before the dissection so that the wall of cyst may be grasped with forceps without injuring it. Sometimes, it extends between the origins of the internal and external carotid arteries upto the pharyngeal wall. Hypoglossal and glossopharengeal nerves lie deep into the cyst and they should be protected. The cyst usually lies deep to the posterior belly of daigastric. The spinal accessory nerve also lies deep to the cyst and should be protected.

Sclerotherapy with OK-432 (picibanil) has been reported to be an effective alternative to surgical excision of branchial cleft cysts by some groups.[27]

Thyroglossal Tract Cyst

Thyroglossal tract cyst is a swelling in the remnants of thyroglossal tract (Fig. 27.37A). The development is from the ventral portion of the entoderm

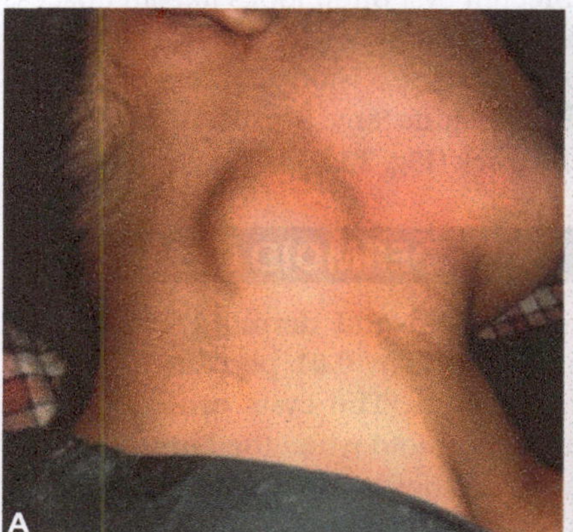
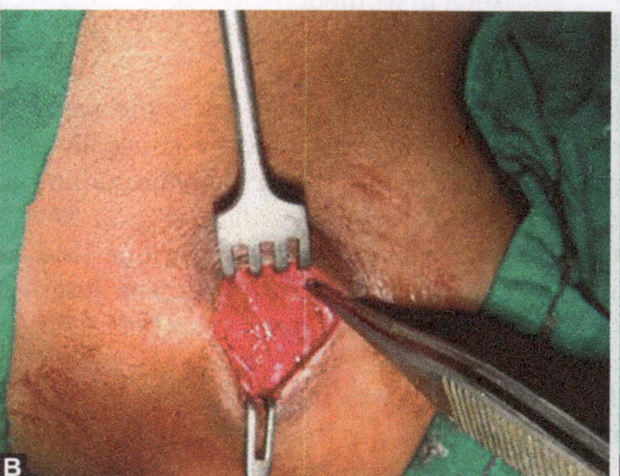
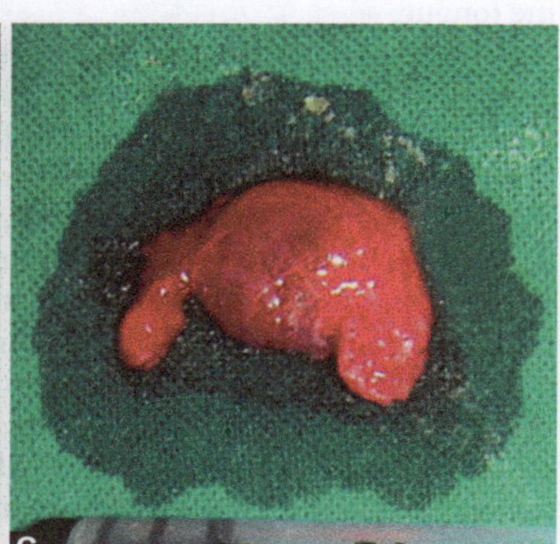

Figs 27.36A to C: Excision of branchical cleft cyst

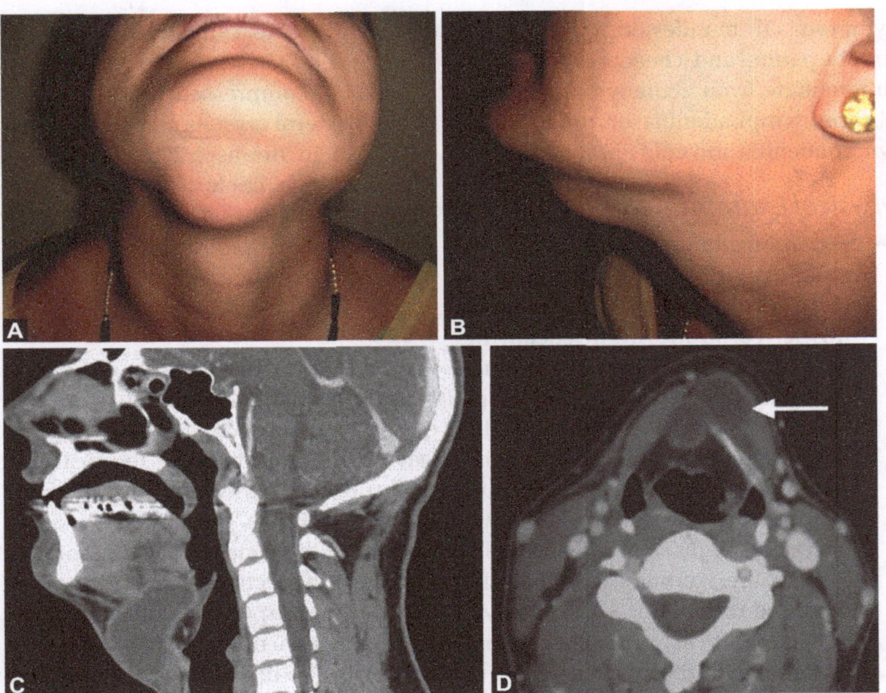

Figs 27.37A to D: (A and B) Thyroglossal cyst; (C and D) CT scan showing thyroglossal cyst

between the first and second branchial arch, a divercation is made which extends downwards and forms the median thyroid diverticulum. The diverticulum moves downward and comes infront of the thyroid cartilage to form the isthmus and the pyramidal lobe of thyroid gland. This tract is known as thyroglossal tract. The hyoid bone which is developed from the second and the third branchial arches comes in very close relation with this tract. The entoderm from where the tract or the thyroglossal duct has started ultimately forms the foramen ceacum of the tongue.

The course of the thyroglossal tract or duct—the thyroglossal duct passes down from the foramen caecum of the tongue between the genoglossus muscles, then it passes along the midline downwards, it descends either infront of the hyoid bone or it hooks below and behind the hyoid bone and then descends downwards along the midline to the upper border of the thyroid cartilage. It then moves slightly to the left and ultimately ends in the pyramidal lobe of the thyroid gland.

Pathology

The thyroglossal cyst is lined by pseudostratified ciliated columnar epithelium, there may be squamous lining and mucous glands. There may be some lymphoid tissue outside the epithelial lining, for which the cyst is prone to get infected. It may contain thyroid tissue.

Clinical Features

- **Age:** Thyroglossal cyst may appear at any age, but majority of the patients are between 15 to 30 years of age.
- **Sex:** The cyst is more commonly seen in women.

Symptoms

The commonest symptom is the painless swelling in the neck; it is usually a midline swelling except when the midline is below the thyroid cartilage (Figs 27.37A and B). where it may shift to one side, more commonly to the left. The lump may be present for many years before the patient comes to the doctor, it is actually the swelling which gets the patient to the clinician. Pain in the cyst is almost always associated with infection of the cyst. Systemic symptoms are never seen in this condition.

Examination

Position: A thyroglossal cyst may develop anywhere along the thyroglossal tract, starting from the Foramen Caecum to the isthmus of the thyroid gland, but according to frequency its position may be as follows subhyoid position, in the region of thyroid cartilage, suprahyoid position, at the level of carotid cartilage, in the floor of the mouth; beneath the foramen caceum. Thyroglossal cyst is spherical or oval with the long axis along the thyroglossal tract. The cyst may become tender if it is infected. Though it is a cystic swelling, yet it's consistency is often firm or hard depending upon the tension of fluid within the cyst. Paget's test should be done. It may occasionally be positive, when a cyst is a small one, but due to the thick content with epithelial debris it is usually negative (Paget's test—A solid tumor is hardest in the center, whereas the cyst is least hard in the center). The cyst can be moved sideways, but not vertically, the cyst moves with deglutition, it moves with protrusion of the tongue. Regional lymph nodes are usually not enlarged unless they are infected. The cyst can be best visualized on MRI scan as it is a soft tissue pathology. The MRI also gives information regarding the relation of the cyst to the adjacent vital structures (Figs 27.37C and D).

It should be excised routinely, as due to the presence of the lymphatic tissue in the wall infection is inevitable, an infected cyst often looks like an abscess and a incision will lead to the formation of a sinus, excision of the cyst should also include any persistent portion of the track (Fig. 27.37B).

DERMOID CYST

Epidermoid and dermoid cysts represent less than 0.01 percent of all oral cavity cysts. The cysts can be defined as epidermoid when the lining presents only epithelium, dermoid cysts when skin adnexa are found and teratoid cysts when other tissue such as muscle, cartilage and bone are present.

A dermoid cyst can be described as a sac-like growth that is present at birth.

A dermoid cyst is a cystic teratoma that contains developmentally mature skin complete with hair follicles and sweat glands, sometimes luxuriant clumps of long hair and often pockets of sebum, blood, fat, bone, nails, teeth, eyes, cartilage and thyroid tissue. Because it contains mature tissue, a dermoid cyst is almost always benign.

There are four types of dermoid cyst:

1. Sequestration dermoid.
2. Implantation dermoid—acquired variety.
3. Tubulodermoid.
4. Teratomatous dermoid.

Sequestration Dermoid

Sequestration dermoid is congenital variety of dermoid cyst, which is formed by inclusion of the epithelium buried in the line of the embryonic fusion. It contains white pultaceous desquamated material with or without hairs. It is mixture of sebum, sweat and desquamated epithelial cells. It is commonly seen in midline of the body particularly in the neck, above the angle of the eye at the line of fusion of frontonasal and maxillary processes, postauricular and at the midline of the face particularly at the root of the nose.

At the line of the embryonic fusion, a few ectodermal cells are sequestrated into the deeper layer which proliferate and form sequestration dermoid cyst. It lies near the mesoderm from where the bones develop.

It may be noticed at birth, but is usually seen sometimes afterwards as it takes sometime to form the cyst. It presents as painless swelling which is slow growing and is present at the areas of the embryonic fusion. They remain small in size, i.e. around 2 cm in diameter and are usually ovoid or spherical in shape with smooth surface and soft in consistency. It may indent with pressure as the content is thick pultaceous material. It is non-compressible, non-reducible and is not attached to the skin as well as underlying structures. There may be bony indentations, if the bone lies exactly deep to the cyst which may be palpated. Transillumination test is always negative. Surgical excision is the treatment of choice.

Implantation Dermoid

Implantation dermoid is a acquired dermoid and arises from the indriven epithelium beneath the skin due to the puncture injury, e.g. needle prick or thorn prick. It is lined by stratified squamous epithelium and contains white cheesy material formed by desquamated epithelial cells and sebum. Hair is usually absent. It usually painful.

Tubulodermoid

Tubulodermoid is epidermal cyst, but develop from the unobliterated portion of congenital ectodermal duct or tube. It is usually formed by the accumulation of secretion of the lining ectodermal cells of the unobliterated portion of the embryonic duct, e.g. thyroglossal cyst which develops from thyroglossal duct.

Teratomatous Dermoid Cyst

Teratomatous dermoid is a cystic swelling which develop from the totipotent cells with ectodermal predominance. It usually contains mesodermal elements like bone, cartilage, etc. hairs are always present in such cyst.

Dermoid cysts grow slowly and are not tender unless ruptured. They usually occur on the face, inside the skull, on the lower back, and in the ovaries. It present as a solitary or occasionally multiple, hamartomatous tumor. The tumor is covered by a thick dermis like wall that contains multiple sebaceous glands and almost all skin adnexa. Hair and large amounts of fatty masses cover poorly to fully differentiated structures derived from the ectoderm.

Depending on the location of the lesion, dermoid cysts may contain substances such as nails and teeth, cartilage and bone like structures. If limited to the skin or subcutaneous tissue, dermoid cysts are thin-walled tumors that contain different amounts of fatty masses; occasionally, they contain horny masses and hairs.

Pathophysiology

The pathogenesis of midline cysts of the floor of the mouth is not well established and dysontogenetic, traumatic and thyroglossal anomaly theories have been suggested. Histologically, Meyer divided the cysts of the floor of the mouth into three groups: Epidermoid, dermoid and teratoid. Although dermoid cysts represent a separate entity, the term "dermoid" is typically used to indicate all three categories. In fact, dermoid cysts occur primarily in the testes and ovaries and the most common location in the head and neck is the external third of the eyebrows.

Race

No racial predilection is apparent; however, most cases of dermoid cysts in the literature are described in white persons.

Sex

Dermoid cysts of the ovary or omentum are sex restricted, i.e. they occur only in the female population. In other dermoid cysts, no sex predilection has been found.

Age

Dermoid cysts generally present with slow and progressive growth and even if they are congenital, the diagnosis is usually possible in the 2nd or 3rd decade of life. Dermoid cysts are described in persons of all ages.

Dermoid cysts on the face, neck or scalp are subcutaneous cysts that are usually present at birth. Intracranial or perispinal dermoid cysts are most often found in infants, children or young adolescents. Intra-abdominal dermoid cysts are described in females aged 15 to 40 years. Most dermoid cysts on the floor of the mouth occur in individuals aged 10 to 30 years. Only a few cases describe oral dermoid cysts in newborns or children.

History

Dermoid cysts that are congenital and localized on the neck, head or trunk are usually visible at birth. The intracranial, intraspinal, or intra-abdominal dermoid cysts may be suspected after specific or non-specific neurologic or gynecologic symptoms occur. In these instances, imaging studies may help in distinguishing dermoid cysts from other tumors or organ malformations. A congenital intracranial frontotemporal dermoid cyst may be first evident as a cutaneous fistula, although intracranial extension and cutaneous sinus tract formation are rarely seen with these dermoid cysts.

Unilateral upper eyelid swelling may be the first sign, with imaging studies demonstrating a soft tissue orbital dermoid cyst arising from the lacrimal gland.

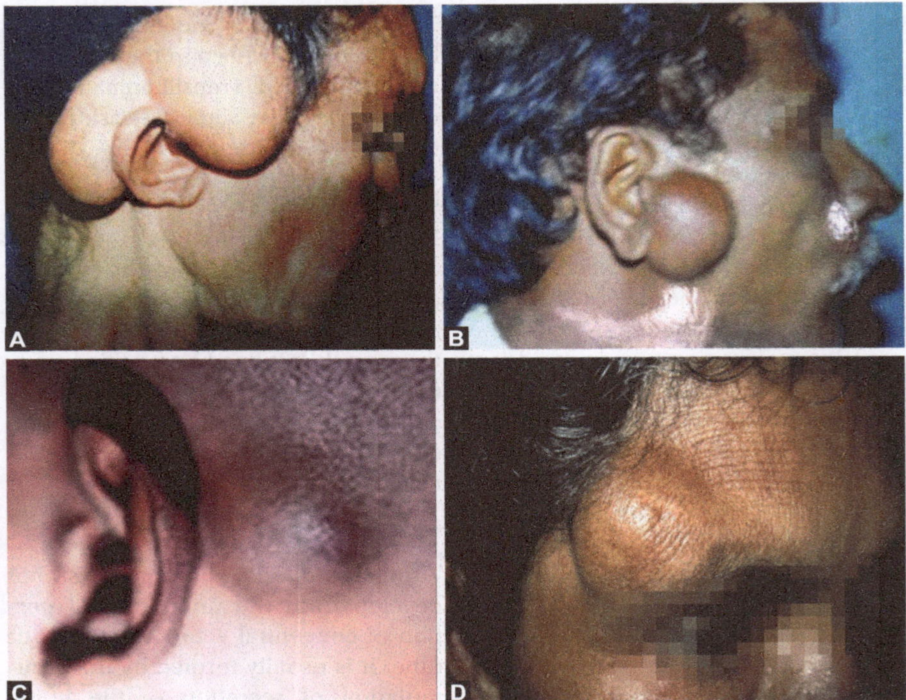

Figs 27.38A to D: Dermoid cysts of the head neck area

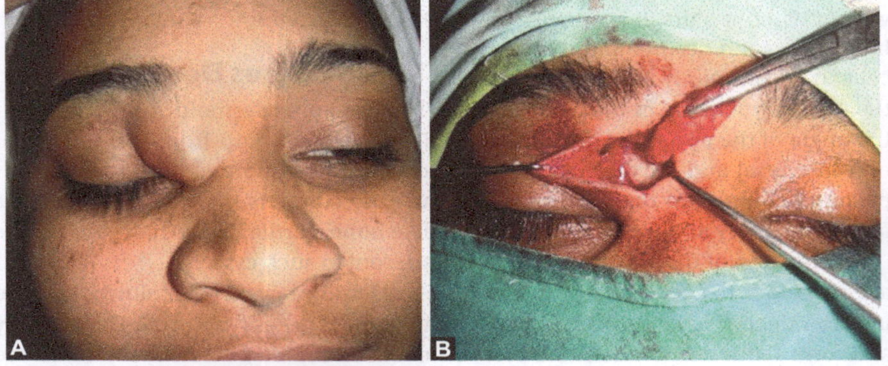

Figs 27.39A and B: (A) Dermoid cyst near the medial canthus of eye; (B) Excision of a dermoid cyst

Physical Examination

Dermoid cysts can appear as cutaneous cysts on the head, as cysts on the floor of the mouth or elsewhere in the head (Figs 27.38A to D and 27.39A).[15]

Cutaneous cysts most commonly occur on the head, mainly around the eyes. Occasionally, they occur on the neck or in a midline region. When on the head, dermoid cysts are often adherent to the periosteum. The usual diameter of the lesions is 1 to 4 cm.

Dermoid cysts on the forehead and brow are known to cause pressure-related erosion of the underlying bony tissue, and surgical intervention may be helpful. Occasionally, skin-related dermoid cysts are multiple and develop over periods as long as 20 years. In many patients, dermoid cysts occur on the floor of the mouth or elsewhere in the mouth.

The differential diagnosis of sublingual lesions includes: Infectious process, ranula, lymphatic malformation, dermoid cyst, epidermoid cyst, heterotopic gastrointestinal cyst and duplication foregut cyst. For this reason, bimanual palpation and conventional radiography are not always sufficient in making differential diagnoses. In these cases, it is necessary to use ultrasonography, computed tomography or magnetic resonance imaging together with cytologic examination by fine-needle aspiration biopsy.

Causes

Dermoid cysts are true hamartomas. Dermoid cysts occur when skin and skin structures get entrapped during fetal development. Histogenetically, dermoid cysts are a result of the sequestration of skin along the lines of embryonic closure.

Epidermoid cysts may be classified as congenital or acquired, even if there is no difference between the two on presentation or histologically. Many etiopathogenetical theories have been proposed. Congenital cysts are dysembryogenetic lesions that arise from ectodermic elements entrapped during the midline fusion of the first and second branchial arches between the 3rd and 4th weeks of intrauterine life. Alternatively, they may arise from the 'tuberculum impar of His' which, with each mandibular arch, forms the floor of the mouth and the body of the tongue. Acquired cysts derive from traumatic or iatrogenic inclusion of epithelial cells or from the occlusion of a sebaceous gland duct. Moreover, other authors proposed that midline cysts may represent a variant form of thyroglossal duct cyst.

Congenital cysts of ectodermal origin are uncommon in the oral cavity (1.6%), with epidermoid cysts occurring rarely.

Radiography, CT scanning and MRI are helpful in making the correct differential diagnosis of dermoid cysts. Ultrasonography represents the first choice of imaging technique because it is reliable, economical and without X-ray exposure, thus, it is easily suitable for young patients also. Computed tomography and magnetic resonance imaging allow more precise localization of the lesion in relationship to geniohyoid and mylohyoid muscles and they also enable the surgeon to choose the most appropriate surgical approach, especially for very large lesions.

Histologic Findings

Dermoid cysts are a result of the sequestration of the skin along the lines of embryonic closure. In contrast to epidermal cysts, dermoid cysts in the skin are lined by an epidermis that possesses various epidermal appendages. As a rule, these appendages are fully mature. Hair follicles containing hairs that project into the lumen of the cyst are often present. The dermis of dermoid cysts usually contains sebaceous glands; eccrine glands and, in many patients, apocrine glands. Occasionally, the lining epithelium may proliferate as papillary boundaries extend externally or inward toward the lumen of the cyst. This proliferation may have some superficial resemblance to epidermal carcinomatous proliferation and the growth may be misclassified as a cancer. A congenital dermoid together with a bronchogenic cyst of the tongue is extremely rare, but has been described in a few patients.

Treatment

The treatment of dermoid cysts of maxillofacial region is surgical and can be by an intraoral or extraoral approach (Fig. 27.39B), according to the localization and the size of the mass. There are no rules regarding the timing for operation; because dermoid cysts are mainly congenital, they can appear in every age of life, so the time when they appear (generally with dysphagia, dysphonia and dyspnea) is generally the right time to operate on them. Also, in very young patients, a problem can arise from the anesthesiologic risk, which is generally quite low in patients weighing more than 20 kg.

The extraoral approach is generally preferred in the case of median geniohyoid or very large sublingual cysts, whereas the intraoral approach is typically used for smaller sublingual cysts.

In some patients, surgery should be performed even more carefully than usual because the fatty content of the cyst may spread to the surrounding tissues or anatomic structures, especially if the cyst is infected with bacteria. The spread of these contents can cause foreign body reactions and severe complications.

Recently, minimally invasive surgical techniques have been successful in removing dermoid cysts from difficult locations, such as those on the tongue or the floor of the mouth. Intralingual dermoid cysts lead to lingual motility defects and speech problems. These cysts should be surgically removed to restore normal lingual function and to correct speech problems.

Intracranial, intramedullary and ovarian dermoid cysts are difficult to treat and sophisticated neurosurgical or gynecologic surgical techniques are often needed to remove the lesion and prevent possible complications.

In some patients with dermoid cysts on the forehead and brow, successful excision with endoscopy-assisted surgery has been described.

In the reported cases, no complications (e.g. paresthesia or numbness on the scalp) occurred. The absence of visible scarring is an additional advantage of endoscopy-assisted surgery.[13,14]

HYDATID CYST

Hydatid disease of the head and neck is rare. It accounts for only two out of every thousand cases of hydatid disease. Most hydatid cysts are "silent," but become clinically apparent because of their mass effects, when they rupture or if they become super infected. Hydatid disease is a worldwide parasitic disease, particularly in areas where livestock and subsistence farming are practiced. *Echinococcus* infection may cause serious morbidity and even death in the intermediate host. It is an endemic disease in many parts of the world including the Mediterranean, the Middle East, South America, Australasia and is highly endemic in sub-Saharan Africa. Of the three forms of hydatid disease, *Echinococcus granulosis* is most common and gives rise to cystic hydatid disease. *Echinococcus granulosis* is a small tapeworm, 3 to 5 mm in length, comprising three to four segments. It lives in the small intestine of the definitive host, the dog. The oldest segments at the end of the worms produce eggs, which are excreted in feces. Intermediate hosts ingest contaminated feces. Humans are accidental intermediate hosts. The eggs hatch in the intestine of the intermediate hosts, cattle, sheep and pigs. Humans are also a susceptible intermediate hosts and as dogs are common house hold pets, may accidently ingest the ova and the embryo migrates through the intestinal wall into the portal system. Most embryos (65%) lodge in the liver. Some (25%) escape this first filter and lodge in the lung. A small percentage escape to the systemic circulation where they may lodge in any organ, most commonly the spleen, kidneys, heart, bone, muscle or central nervous system.

Clinical Features

Hydatid cyst is more common in liver, but also reported in lung, bones and brain. Liver involvement causes hepatomegaly and jaundice. Pulmonary involvement may cause shortness of breath and hemoptysis. Hydatid cysts have been reported in a variety of sites in the head and neck region including salivary glands (most commonly submandibular gland and parotid), orbit, thyroid gland, superficial temporal muscles, paraspinal muscles, cervical soft tissues, sternocleidomastoid muscle, retropharyngeal tissues, tongue, mastoid, infratemporal fossa, pterygopalatine fossa, and posterior cranial fossa. They do not appear to have a predilection for any particular site. Only 2 percent of the hydatid cysts are located in the skeleton and of these only 3 to 4 percent are in the skull. Oral hydatid cysts presents as painless, progressively increasing, soft elastic and well-circumscribed fluctuant swelling. They may pose speech and mastication problems.

Histological Features

The hydatid cysts are initially of microscopic dimensions, but enlarge progressively. The natural cyst consists of three layers; an outer layer of host origin and two inner layers of parasitic origin. The host layer consists of fibrous tissue in which there is an infiltrate of chronic inflammatory cells, eosinophils and giant cells. The intermediate layer is white, non-nucleated and consists of numerous delicate laminations. It usually shrinks away from the outer fibrous layer when the tension within the cyst is relieved. Finally, there is the inner nucleated germinal layer. The cyst fluid is relatively clear, albumin free and contains the so called *"hydatid sand"* consisting of brood capsules and scolices. These brood capsules or daughter cysts develop originally as minute projections of the germinative layer which develop central vesicles and become minute cysts. Scolices of the head of the worm develop in the inner aspects of the brood capsules. It is when they separate from the germinative layer that they form of the "Hydatid sand". The hydatid cyst of the maxillofacial area are the rare entity occasional cases have been reported in the literature.

Diagnosis

Radiographically calcification of cysts wall may be visualised in 50 percent of cases. USG may reveal daughter cysts and hydatid sand. CT scan furnishes useful information, investigations include blood examination, which will reveal eosinophilia in 20 to 25 percent cases.

Of the serological tests, the indirect hemagglutination test, Casoni's test and complement fixation would be positive. Casoni's test includes intradermal injection of 0.2 mL of fresh sterile aspirated cystic fluid which produces a wheel of 5 cm in diameter within 30 minutes. Problems with Casoni's test are that it may cause false positive result and produce anaphylaxis. This stands to reason as to aspiration is usually avoided in these cases as it may result in spillage of the cystic content and result in fatal anaphylaxis.

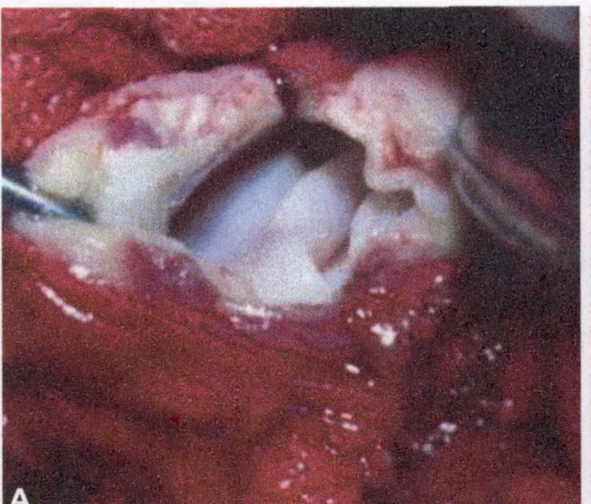

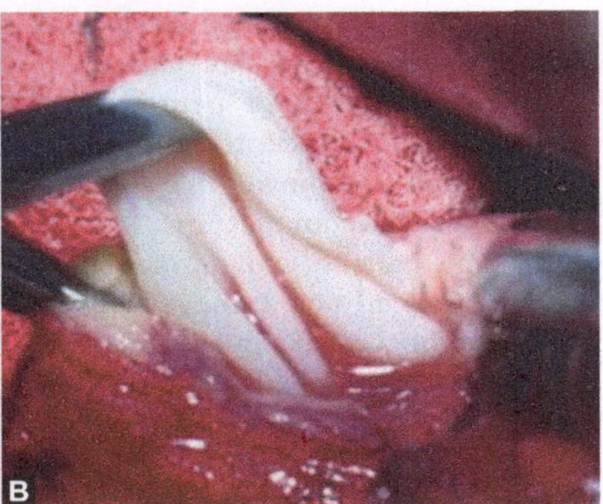

Figs 27.40A and B: Whitish lining of the hydatid cyst

Treatment

Treatment is primarily surgical (excision). Excision of the hydatid cyst using the natural cleavage plane which exists between germinative layer and the surrounding tissue. Care should be taken to avoid accidental rupture and spillage of the contents of the cystic cavity. Fatal anaphylaxis on spilling the contents of the cyst has been reported. The surgical strategy varies widely between radical clearance followed by lavage and simple instillation of scolicide. Chlorhexidine, 80 percent alcohol and 0.5 percent cetrimide solution may be instilled into the cystic cavity which destroys 80 to 90 percent of scolices. Supplementary chemotherapy, such as mebendazole or albendazole, can also be used.

If the cyst gets infected secondarily, all the parasites die and the treatment becomes much easier and needs to be treated like an abscess by incision and drainage. The whitish lining sloughs out and should be curetted (Figs 27.40A and B).

REFERENCES

1. Robinson HBG. Classification of Cysts of the Jaws. Am J Orthodontics and Oral Surg. (Oral Surg Sect). 1945;31:370.
2. Gorlin RJ, Pindborg JJ, Redman RS, et al. The calcifying odontogenic cyst: A new entity and possible analogue of the cutaneous calcifying epithelioma of Malherbe. Cancer. 1964;17:723-9.
3. Karmer IRH, Pindborg JJ, Shear M. Histological typing of odontogenic tumours: WHO International Histological Classification of Tumours (ed 2). Springer. 1992.
4. The new WHO classification of tumors of the head and neck. What has changed? J Oral Pathol Med. 2005;34(9): 558-64.
5. Harris M, Toller P. The pathogenesis of dental cysts. Br Med Bull. 1975;31: 159-63.
6. Gold L, Upton G, Marx R. Standardized surgical terminology for the excision of lesions in bone: An argument for accuracy in reporting. J Oral Maxillofac Surg. 1991;49(11):1214-7.

7. Morgan TA, Burton CC, Qian F. A retrospective review of treatment of the odontogenic keratocyst. J Oral Maxillofac Surg. 2005;63(5):635-9.
8. Bell R, Dierks E. Treatment options for the recurrent odontogenic keratocyst. Oral and Maxillofacial Surgery Clinics of North America. 2003;15(3):429-46.
9. Waldron CW. Tumors of the Upper Jaw. Surg Gynec and Obst. 1971;72:503.
10. Dr Makoto Toida. A simple cryosurgical method for treatment of oral mucous cysts. Int J Oral Maxillofac Surg. 1993;22 (6):353-5.
11. Shibata Y, Asaumi J, Yanagi Y, et al. Radiographic examination of dentigerous cysts in the transitional dentition Dentomaxillofaial Radiology. 2004; 33:17.
12. Anthony Pogrel M. Treatment of Keratocysts: The Case for Decompression and Marsupialization. J Oral Maxillo Surg. 2005;63(11):1667-73.
13. Mikulicz J, Beitrag zur Genese der Dermoide am Kopfe, Wien Med Wochenschr. 1876;26:pp. 953-6.
14. Kostecka F. Ein Cholesteatom im Unterkiefer Ztschr f Stomatol. 1929;27:1102.
15. Philipsen HP. Om keratocyster (kolesteatomer) I kaeberne. Tandlaegebladet. 1956; 60.pp.693-7.
16. Stoelinga PJW. Long-term follow-up on keratocysts treated according to a defined protocol. Int J Oral Maxillofac Surg. 2001;30:p.14.
17. Scharfetter, Balz-Hermann C, Lagrange W, et al. Proliferation kinetics—study of the growth of keratocysts. J Cran-Max-Fac Surg. 1989;17:226-33.
18. Toller PA. Protein substances in odontogenic cyst fluids. Br Dent J. 1970; 128(7):317-22.
19. Main, DMG. The enlargement of epithelial jaw cysts. Odontologisk Revy. 1970; 21:29-49.
20. Browne RM. The odontogenic keratocyst: Clinical aspects. Br Dent J. 1970;128:225.
21. Kramer IR, Toller PA. The use of exfoliative cytology and protein estimations in preoperative diagnosis of odontogenic keratocysts. Int J Oral Surg. 1973;2(4):143-51.
22. Barnes L, Eveson JW, Reichart P, et al. World Health Organization Classification of Tumors. WHO Histological classification of odontogenic tumors. Lyon: IARC Press; 2005.pp.306-7.
23. Gorlin RJ, Pindborg JJ, Clausen FP, et al. The calcifying odontogenic cyst—a possible analogue of the cutaneous calcifying epithelioma of Malherbe. 1963; pp.249-51.
24 Moscow BS, Siegel K, Zegarelli EV, et al. Gingival and lateral periodontal cysts. Periodontol. 1970;41:249-60.
25. Burke GW, Feagans Jr. WM, Elzay RP, et al. Some aspects of the origin and fate of midpalatal cysts in human fetuses. J Dent Res. 1966;45:159-64.
26. Lichtenstein L. Aneurysmal Bone Cyst. J. Bone and Joint Surg. 1956;38-B:310-1.
27. Kim MG, Kim SG, Lee JH, et al. The therapeutic effect of OK-432 (picibanil) sclerotherapy for benign neck cysts. Laryngoscope. 2008;118(12): 2177-81.

28 Odontogenic Tumors

Borle Rajiv M, Singh Divya

INTRODUCTION

Odontogenic tumors comprise a group of lesions of the jaw derived from the primordial tooth forming tissues (*odontogenic epithelium*) and presenting a large number of histologic patterns. Some of these lesions, particularly the odontomas are now interpreted as developmental malformations or hamartomatous lesions rather than true neoplasms. Other lesions such as ameloblastoma are accepted as true neoplasms and must be diagnosed and treated as such. Odontogenic tumors share two major characteristics, namely they arise from the tissues with the potential for differentiation into tooth or periodontal structures and are therefore found exclusively in the mandible and maxilla and, on rare occasions, the gingiva. Another variable, but distinctive feature includes formation of tooth related extracellular substances some of which may calcify and be visible on radiographs; they are products of epithelial-mesenchymal interaction.

The most common sites for these tumors are mandibular molar region and the maxillary cuspid region. They are usually slow growing and asymptomatic. Certain odontogenic tumors have a predilection for particular age, gender, geographic location and race. (Sawyer et al.[1] 1985; Assael.[2] 1992).

ACCORDING TO WHO

"Odontogenic tumors and tumor-like lesions constitute a group of heterogeneous diseases that range from hamartomatous or non-neoplastic tissue proliferations to benign malignant tumors with metastatic potential. They are derived from epithelial, ectomesenchymal and/or mesenchymal elements of the tooth forming apparatus. Odontogenic tumors are rare, some even extremely rare, but can pose a significant diagnostic and therapeutic challenge."

Broca,[3] a French physician, first described an odontogenic neoplasm in 1868 and since then various authors have proposed classifications for such neoplasms based on different criterias.

Malassez[4] (1885) and Sutton[5] (1888) included numerous odontogenic neoplasms within their all encompassing term odontome. In 1946, Thoma and Goldman[6] introduced a classification based on the germ cell layer of origin and they classified tumor in three categories, i.e. epithelial, mesenchymal and mixed. Spouge[7] (1968) tried to correlate tumor histogenesis with odontogenesis and suggested that odontogenic tumors arise from various components of the odontogenic apparatus at one phase or stage of odontogenesis. Since then, many authors have tried to correlate sequential changes in odontogenesis with tumor formation.

It was in 1971, when a five-year collaborated effort organized by World Health Organization resulted in the first consensus on taxonomy of odontogenic tumors. The appearance of this first authoritative guide to the classification of odontogenic tumor marked the start of an era of quite intensive interest for studying this particular field of tumors. In 1971, WHO gave histological typing of odontogenic tumors,[8] jaw cysts and allied lesions which was based on the concept suggested by Pindbord and Clausen that the characteristic interaction between epithelium and mesenchymal tissue elements occurring during normal tooth development to a certain extent also operates in pathogenesis and histodifferentiation of odontogenic tumors.

A wealth of new information which provided new variants and entities, led to the proposal of second edition of histological typing of odontogenic tumors by WHO in 1992,[9] which provided an updated classification. The WHO classification was further updated in 2004 and the latest edition being in 2005.[10]

WHO CLASSIFICATION OF ODONTOGENIC TUMORS[10]

Tumors (neoplasms) and tumor-like lesions in the jaws.

(Including non-neoplastic, non-inflammatory jaw lesions)

Odontogenic tumors (modified 2005 WHO classification).

Benign

- Odontogenic epithelium with mature, fibrous stroma without odontogenic ectomesenchyme
  - Ameloblastoma (solid/multicystic, extraosseous/peripheral, desmoplastic, unicystic)
  - Squamous odontogenic tumor
  - Calcifying epithelial odontogenic tumor (Pindborg's tumor)
  - Adenomatoid odontogenic tumor
  - Keratocystic odontogenic tumor*.
- Odontogenic epithelium with odontogenic ectomesenchyme with or without hard tissue formation
  - Ameloblastic fibroma
  - Ameloblastic fibrodentinoma
  - Ameloblastic fibro-odontoma
  - Odontoma
    a. Complex type
    b. Compound type
  - Odontoameloblastoma
  - Calcifying cystic odontogenic tumor
  - Dentinogenic ghost cell tumor
- Mesenchyme and/or odontogenic ectomesenchyme with or without odontogenic epithelium
  - Odontogenic fibroma
  - Odontogenic myxoma (myxofibroma)
  - Cementoblastoma

Malignant (Examples)

- Odontogenic carcinomas
  - Malignant ameloblastoma
  - Ameloblastic carcinoma
  - Primary intraosseous carcinoma
  - Clear cell odontogenic carcinoma
  - Ghost cell odontogenic carcinoma
- Odontogenic sarcomas
  - Ameloblastic fibrosarcoma
  - Ameloblastic fibrodentinosarcoma
  - Ameloblastic fibro-odontosarcoma

*This is the odontogenic keratocyst. You will find it in the classification of odontogenic cysts.

Other Jaw Tumors (Neoplasias)

- Benign
  - Ossifying fibroma (cemento-ossifying fibroma)
  - Osteoma
  - Osteoblastoma/osteoid osteoma
  - Chondroma
  - Chondromyxoid fibroma
  - Desmoplastic fibroma (intraosseous non-odontogenic fibroma)
  - Melanotic neuroectodermal tumor of infancy
  - Others (neurofibroma, neurilemmoma, hemangioma (angio), leiomyoma, etc.)
- Malignant
  - Osteosarcoma
  - Chondrosarcoma
  - Metastatic tumors to the jaws
  - Others (Ewing's sarcoma, myeloid and lymphoid neoplasias, etc.)

Non-neoplastic Jaw Lesions

- Fibro-osseous dysplasias
  - Fibrous dysplasia
  - Focal osseous dysplasia (focal cemento-osseous dysplasia)
  - Florid osseous dysplasia (including familial gigantiform cementoma)
  - Periapical cemental dysplasia (periapical fibrous dysplasia)
- Others
  - Cherubism
  - Central giant cell lesion (granuloma) (incl. hyperparathyroidism)
  - Aneurismal bone cyst
  - Simple bone cyst (traumatic bone cyst, hemorrhagic bone cyst, solitary bone cyst)
  - Tori and exostoses
  - Langerhans cell histiocytosis.

AMELOBLASTOMA

Introduction

The ameloblastoma is the most common neoplasm arising from odontogenic epithelium. According to WHO, *"it is a true neoplasm of enamel organ type tissue, which does not undergo differentiation to the point of enamel formation"*. In 1992, WHO classified ameloblastoma as a benign, but locally invasive epithelial odontogenic neoplasm, which has a strong tendency to recur. According to Robinson,[11] "it is usually unicentric, non-functional, intermittent in growth, anatomically benign and clinically persistent" type of tumor. Churchill[12] suggested the term ameloblastoma in 1934 to replace the term adamantinoma coined by Malassez[4] in 1885, since the latter term implies the formation of hard tissue and such material is not necessarily present in this lesion.

Pathogenesis

The resemblance between the odontogenic apparatus and the ameloblastoma is well documented. The ameloblastoma has a varied origin; however the stimulus for ameloblastic transformation in the odontogenic epithelium is not understood. Thus, the tumor is thought to develop from:

- Residual epithelium of the tooth forming apparatus such as the cell rests of enamel, remnants of the Hertwig's root sheath and the remnants of dental lamina.
- Epithelium of odontogenic cysts, particularly the dentigerous cyst and the odontomas. In different studies, it has been reported that the incidence of ameloblastoma developing from a follicular (dentigerous) cyst associated with the impacted tooth is approximately 17 percent.
- Basal cells of the surface epithelium.
- Disturbances of the enamel organ.
- Heterotropic epithelium from extra-oral sites such as the pituitary gland.

Incidence

It accounts for 1 percent of all oral tumors and for 9 to 11 percent of all odontogenic tumors. It occurs over a broad range of age; cases have been reported in children younger than 10 years to adults and older persons than 90 years of age.[13] The occurrence in the mandible is 4 times higher than in maxilla. Within the mandible, the molar angle ramus[14] area is involved 3 times more commonly than are the premolar and anterior regions combined.

In the literature, the average age of occurrence is in the third or fourth decade (Joseph and Savage,[15] 1992), both men and women being afflicted equally (Robinson,[11] 1937; Burkhard, 1991: Richert and Philipson 1999). However, some Nigerian and one Indian study showed a male preponderance with a male:female ratio of 1.7:1.

Small and Waldron[16] (1955) showed that 47 percent of maxillary ameloblastomas occur in the molar region, 33 percent in the antrum and floor of the nose, 9 percent both in premolar region and in the canine region and 2 percent in the palate. Ameloblastomas also have been reported to arise primarily in the sinonasal region without overt evidence of origin from the tooth bearing alveolar bone.[17] When comparing large studies, it appears that maxillary tumors tend to occur in slightly older patients than do mandibular lesions. Asians seem to have fewer tumors involving the ramus than do whites or blacks, whereas blacks have an increased frequency of tumors in the anterior mandible compared with other 2 groups.[18]

The ameloblastoma is notorious for its slow growth, the histological benign appearance, local invasiveness and a high incidence (50–72%) of local recurrence (Infante-Cossio et al.[19] 1998). Malignant features and metastasis are rare, exhibiting various kinds of histology and clinical behavior.

- Slowly growing painless swelling (Figs 28.1A to G).
- All the cortices expand, viz. buccal, lingual, inferior cortex (Fig. 28.2A).
- Thinning of the bone with egg shell crackling (Fig. 28.2C). If the tumor perforates the cortex the cystic variants show fluctuations while the solid variant is firm in consistency (Fig. 28.2B).
- Displacement and resorption of the roots of the teeth involved in the region of the tumor.
- Aspiration yields straw colored fluid in cases of cystic variants and is negative in solid tumors.

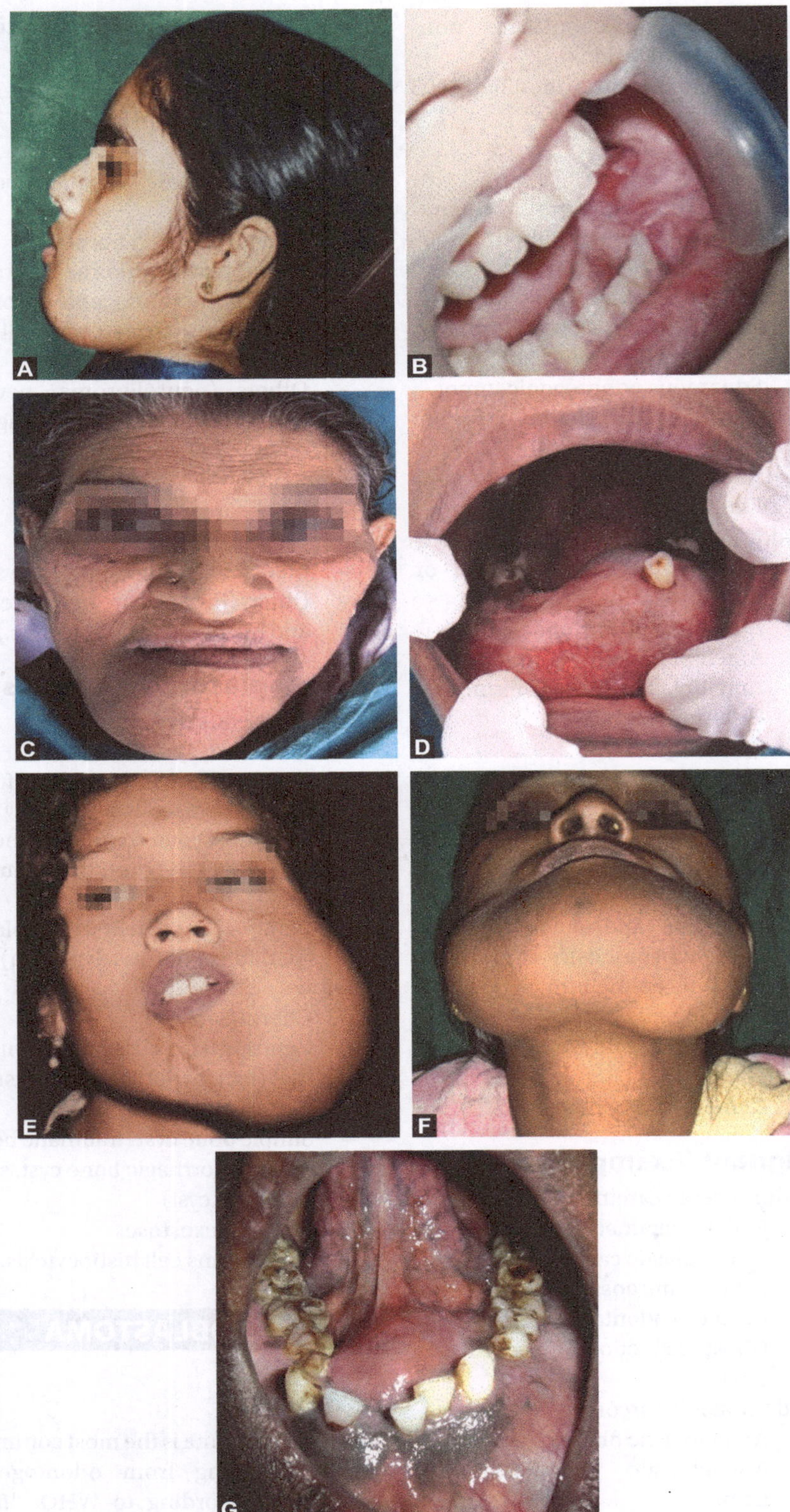

Figs 28.1A to G: Different clinical presentations of the ameloblastoma

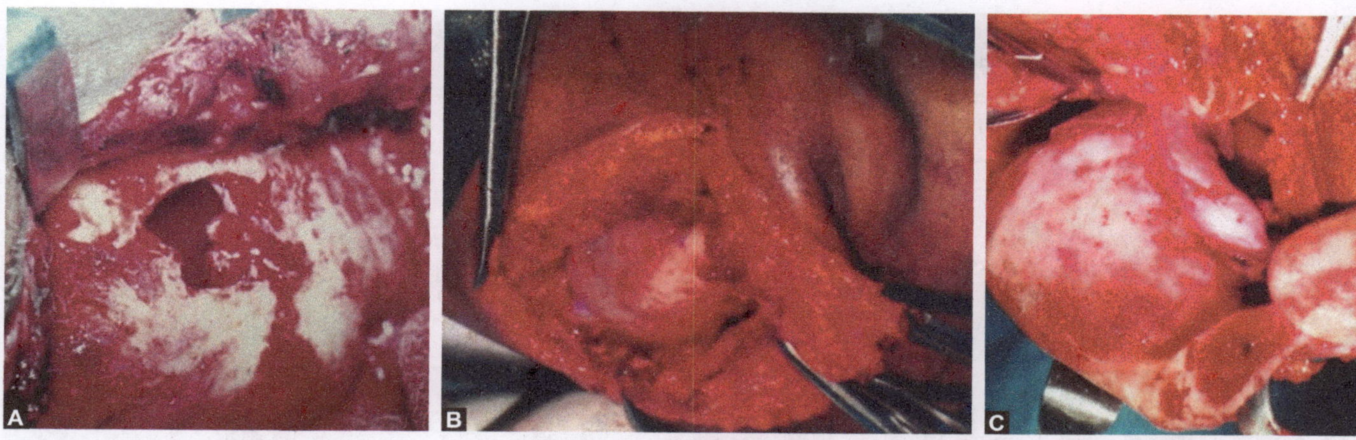

Figs 28.2A to C: (A) Ameloblastoma showing severe thinning of the cortex; (B and C) Cortical expansion due to ameloblastoma and paper thin cortices

Radiological Features

Radiologically, ameloblastoma exhibits a multiloculated radiolucent lesion with expansion of the bone. The loculi are of variable size (*Soap bubble appearance*).[20] In case of unicystic lesions, a large uniloculated radiolucent lesion is seen with bony expansion and well corticated borders (Figs 28.3A to I). If the ameloblastoma has developed secondary to a dentigerous cyst, a displaced tooth is often seen associated with the lesion. A mixed lucent-opaque radiographic appearance in a lesion histopathologically diagnosed as ameloblastoma signals the presence of desmoplastic type of ameloblastoma. This variant was first described in 1984 by Eversole et al.[21] The unicystic ameloblastoma mimics the cystic lesion.

According to WHO, ameloblastoma can be divided clinically as:

- Solid or multicystic
- Unicystic
- Peripheral (extraosseous)
- Desmoplastic.

The distinction between these variants of ameloblastoma is important clinically.

Diagnosis

The diagnosis is based on the clinical and radiological presentation. However, the diagnosis is confirmed on histopathological examination of the biopsied specimen. An incisional biopsy is required to make an accurate diagnosis as sometimes the clinical picture may mimic the odontogenic keratocyst, giant cell granuloma, dentigerous cyst and other slow growing, multiloculated, expansile lesions. The treatment for ameloblastoma is more radical as compared to the lesions mentioned in the differential diagnosis and the radical treatment needs to be justified.

The definitive diagnosis is established only after incision, excision or intraoperative frozen section biopsy and histopathologic analysis. The specific biopsy technique is selected after careful assessment of the patient (age, physical health, emotional status) and of the use of local sedation or general anesthesia to ensure patient cooperation, gain access to the lesion, and obtain sufficient tissue for study. Intraoperative frozen section should be used to study questionable soft tissue encountered in areas not sampled by incisional biopsy and to examine the adequacy of the boundary between lesion and host bone and/or soft tissue in instances in which extensive resection is not planned. The frozen sections are useful in ascertaining adequate peripheral clearance especially when the tumor has perforated the cortical bone and spilled in the adjacent soft tissues. The preparation of a good frozen section is technique sensitive and requires proper specimen orientation and avoidance of incorporated dense bone (*which nicks the microtome blade and disrupts the tissue section*).

The biopsy is an important procedure and must be planned and conducted carefully. Because of its key role in the diagnotic process and later in the surgical procedure, some aspects of the biopsy are discussed here:

- The lesion is approached, with radiographic guidance, by incision through intact crestal mucosa over bone, in order to preserve 'non-contaminated' mucosal soft tissue that may be used for wound closure after a postbiopsy surgical procedure.
- The lesion is aspirated through the intact bone to rule out a vascular lesion masquerading as an odontogenic tumor (other potential radiographic imitators of odontogenic tumor includes aneurysmal bone cyst, giant cell lesion and fibro-osseous disease).
- Aspiration of the cystic fluid neither confirms nor disproves the presence of a cystic odontogenic tumor; the fluid may or may not be retained for a cell block preparation.
- Entrance through the bone to the lesion should be selected and obtained without injury to nerve or teeth, if possible.
- If the radiographs indicate variations in the lesion (solid, cystic or calcified areas), a sufficient number of tissue samples should be removed for thorough histologic study, including

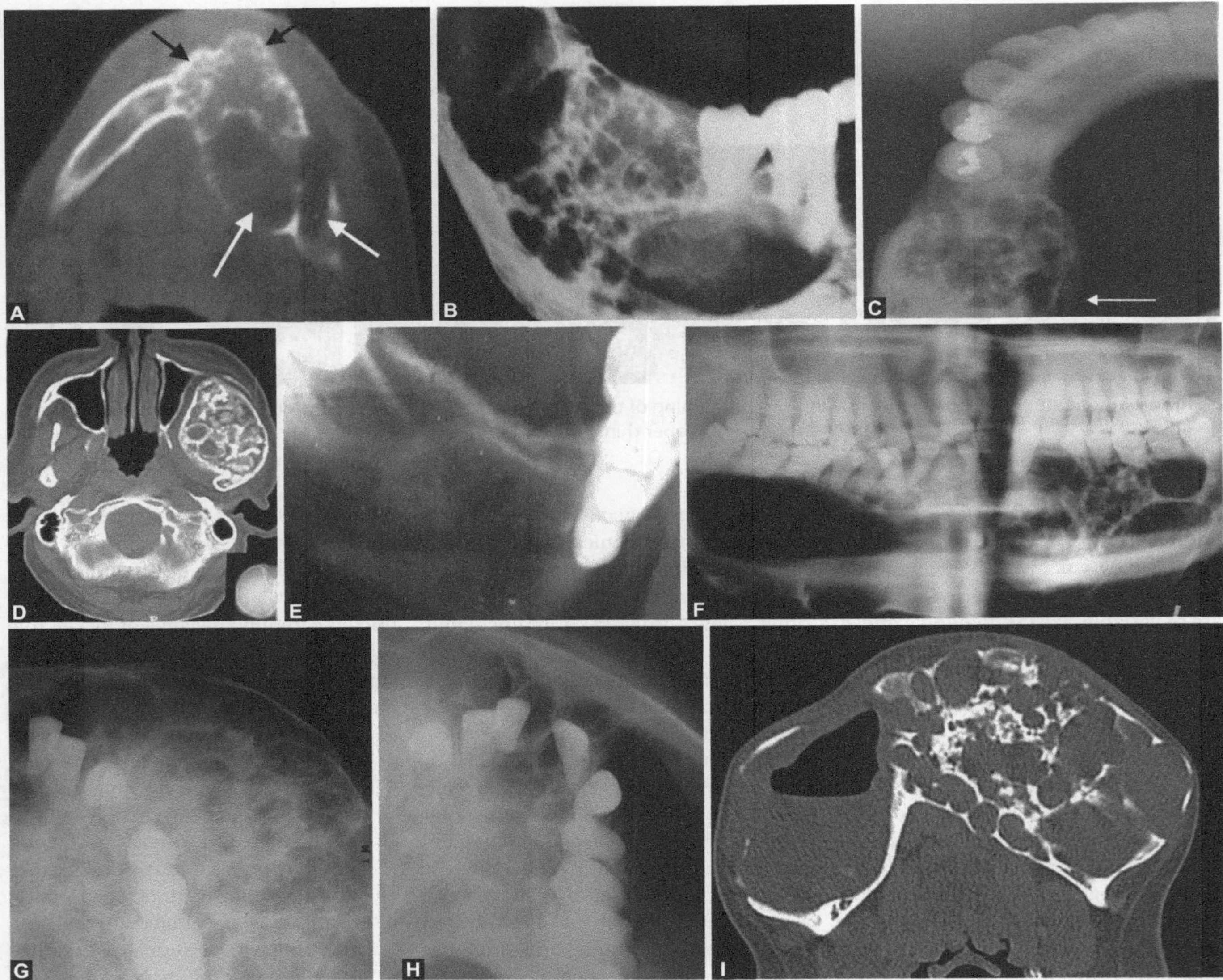

Figs 28.3A to I: Radiological pictures of ameloblastoma: (A) CT scan showing multiloculated lesion; (B and C) Radiograph showing the multiloculated lesion; (D) CT scan showing the multiloculated ameloblastoma in the ramus; (E) Expansion of the bone with bony septae in the lesion; (F) Multiloculated radiolucency; (G and H) Soap bubble appearance; (I) CT scan of ameloblastoma involving entire mandible

tissue bordering the lesion-host bone interface. The specimens are incised for removal and not crushed with forceps or hemostats.

- Before suture closure of the biopsy incision, if desired, a non-resorbable tissue barrier can be placed over the bone entrance to the lesion, to prevent fluid or lesional cell escape into non-involved periosteum or mucosa.

Ameloblastoma: A Benign or Malignant Tumor?

Ameloblastoma is justly considered the most unexplainable of odontogenic tumors, because of its clinical and histological features, intriguingly contradictory, paradoxical and incongruent, if its benign histological aspect and its invasive and destructive clinical behavior are considered, besides the reported capacity of establishing pulmonary metastases, a possible, though infrequent, occurrence.

These characteristics of the ameloblastoma simulate the basal-cell carcinoma, a known malignant neoplasm. The similarities between the ameloblastoma and the basal cell carcinoma are that both are locally invasive, seldom metastasize, radioresistant and exhibit similar histopathological characteristics in some cases. Ameloblastoma is known to be benign by its histological aspect, nevertheless, presents a highly aggressive behavior and, despite its slow growth, it is extremely invasive, as are malignant tumors and produces occasional metastases. The final result, in both cases, is exactly the same.

Basal cell carcinoma is a neoplasm, which develops exclusively in the skin, from the epidermal basal layer or root sheaths of hair follicles, never occurring in the mucosa (Shafer et al. 1983). As the basal layer of the epidermis is composed of cells potentially capable of differentiating into tiny of the skin appendages, aborted attempts to produce these types of structures are at times seen in basal cell carcinomas.

Ameloblastoma is equally a tumor derived indirectly from the epithelial basal layer, however from the covering of the gingival mucosa, perhaps from embryonic remnants of that which could be considered grossly as gingivo-maxillary appendages; the teeth.

The histology of a typical basal cell carcinoma is very similar to that of primordial or basaloid type of ameloblastoma. The follicular aspect observed in many of the cellular islets of the tumor represents only an aborted attempt of the neoplastic tissue to form teeth, in the same manner in which the basal-cell carcinoma also attempts to form hair follicles. Both the tumors are locally invasive and capable of inflicting damage to the local hard and soft tissues, do not metastasize and are radioresistant.

This analogy of clinical behavior as well as the histological picture between the two tumors was what led Willis[22] (1948) to categorically affirm that "attempts to distinguish benign and malignant adamantinomas are futile; they are all malignant in that they are locally invasive and prone to recur".

In a small number of cases, a tumor of ameloblastoma type forms outside the bone presumably from some of the numerous epithelial residues lying between the periosteum and the oral epithelium. Such tumors may show no fusion with the epithelium of the oral mucosa.

The reason for the neoplastic change in the epithelium from which the ameloblastoma develops is not known. It has been suggested that, trauma, infection or the tissue changes associated with the tooth eruption may be involved. However, these factors are so often present, whether or not a turn over develops, it is difficult to show that there is anything more than the random association. The similar tumors arising in the parapituitary epithelium (Craniopharyngioma of Rathke's pouch) residues are not associated with these factors.

Tumor Spread

Ameloblastoma spreads slowly by infiltration through the medullary spaces and may erode the cortical bone. Eventually, it will resorb the cortical plate and may extend into the adjacent soft tissues. Tumors of the posterior maxilla tend to obliterate the maxillary sinus, extend to ethmoidal air cells, infratemporal fossa and subsequently extend intracranially.

Histopathological Types

The ameloblastoma has 6 histopathological subtypes namely:[13,18,23]

1. Follicular
2. Acanthomatous
3. Granular cell
4. Plexiform
5. Basal cell
6. Desmoplastic.

Reichart et al. have shown that these histological subtypes have different clinical behavior and have bearing on the treatment and prognosis. The follicular ameloblastoma shows highest recurrence rate (29.5%) while the acanthomatus has 4.5 percent recurrence rate. The plexiform variety shows 16.7 percent recurrence rate and the desmoplastic ameloblastoma has recurrence rate in the range of the other histological subtypes of ameloblastoma.[13]

Management

The basic modality of the management of the ameloblastoma is surgery. Wide local excisions with at least 1 to 1.5 cm margins of normal bone are recommended for the central tumors. The tumor is known to recur after incomplete excision. Fonseca[24] has emphasized the role of radical treatment for the ameloblastoma and went on to state that "anything short of radical resection for the management of ameloblastoma amounts to the planned recurrence". However, in spite of the fact that ameloblastoma needs to be treated radically, in the clinical practice occasionally conservative treatment is opted in the interest of the patient with a calculated risk of recurrence (e.g. very young patients, unicystic nature and medically compromised patients). The various surgical modalities for the management of the ameloblastoma are:

Enucleation and Curettage

It is usually an inadequate treatment and has high incidence of recurrence, primarily due to the infilterative nature of the tumor. The tumor invades the adjoining cancellous bone and thus enucleation and curettage is inadequate. In exceptional cases where the lesion is very large and encroaching upon the vital structures, medically compromised patients, extreme ages, i.e. very old or very young patient who are not willing to undergo segmental resection of the bone, the enucleation may be done along with the cauterization of the base with Cornoy's solution. Such patients require long-term, periodic postoperative follow-up to detect any recurrence. While opting for such treatment, the clinician must remember that this is not what is ideally required and the tumor could recur and it has been done due to compelling circumstances and not by choice. The patient needs to be counseled for regular follow-up.

The unicystic ameloblastomas, which mimic the cyst in its clinical presentation are intentionally or unintentionally treated with enucleation (see Figs 28.12D and E). When the lesion is diagnosed as a cyst and no preoperative biopsy is done, the natural treatment choice becomes enucleation. Even if the preoperative biopsy is done and if the representing area is not included in biopsy, the lesion is diagnosed as a cyst and treated conservatively by enucleation. It must be remembered that in cases of mural ameloblastoma the ameloblastic changes may not be present throughout its lining and thus, the preoperative diagnosis of ameloblastoma is not always possible unless the biopsy includes the representative area. Moreover in younger patients where the segmental resection is more morbid, most of the surgeons prefer to treat the unicystic ameloblastomas conservatively and keep the patients under long-term follow-up to rule out recurrence. The enucleation and cauterization of the base is often an adequate treatment for the unicystic ameloblastomas.

Irradiation

There is a lack of well-documented evidence in the literature concerning the relative radioresponsiveness or radioresistance of ameloblastomas, although they are generally considered radioresistant. It has been recommended as one of the modalities of the treatment of ameloblastoma in the older literature.[25] Although radiotherapy can reduce the size of an ameloblastoma, primarily that part of the tumor which has expanded the jaw or broken into the soft tissues, it does not appear to be an appropriate treatment for an operable ameloblastoma. Its main use is in inoperable cases, primarily in the posterior maxilla. In the recent times, this treatment modality for ameloblastoma has become obsolete.

Resection of the Mandible

- **Resection with continuity:** Marginal mandibulectomy or wedge mandibulectomy is the method of maintaining the continuity of the bone at the same time excising the lesion. The ameloblastoma tends to infilterate the cancellous bone and the thick cortical plates are eroded but not invaded. The mandibular anterior has plenty of cortical bone and the ameloblastomas, which are relatively small and have not eroded the cortical bone significantly can be treated with marginal mandibulectomy. The large lesions which have severely undermined the cortex and are likely to sustain a pathological fracture require segmental resection.
- **Resection without continuity:** Segmental resection—when the tumor has grown sizably and the inferior border of the mandible is severely undermined the segmental resection is recommended (Figs 28.4A and B). The attempts to preserve the inferior border may compromise the surgical clearance and the chances of recurrence are very high. The thinned out inferior border does not serve any purpose as the chances of pathological fracture can occur. Moreover, it is better to treat the primary tumor radically than treating a nasty recurrence, especially in the ramal area.
- **Hemimandibulectomy:** A classical hemimandibulectomy comprises of resection of half of the mandible along with the disarticulation of the condyle. When an ameloblastoma involves the ramus extensively and surgical clearance is doubtful then the classical hemimandibulectomy with disarticlation of the conyle is undertaken (Figs 28.5A to D). Preserving the condyle by resecting the tumor at subsigmoid level helps in better reconstruction as the implant can be secured to the resected proximal fragment. However, it should not be the only consideration while treating the patient and attempt must be made to get an adequate clearance as the recurrence at this site is often very difficult to treat.
- Although the treatment is often discussed in terms of the bony clearance, it is equally important to address the soft tissue clearance. When the tumor is central in location and the bony cortex is not perforated, one can easily dissect in the subperiosteal plane around the involved bone and remove the tumor adequately. But, When the tumor perforates through the cortex and extends in the soft tissue the plain of dissection needs to be changed and safe resection margins must be established by excising the adjoining soft tissue. The frozen section biopsies may be very useful in such cases to ascertain adequate surgical clearance.

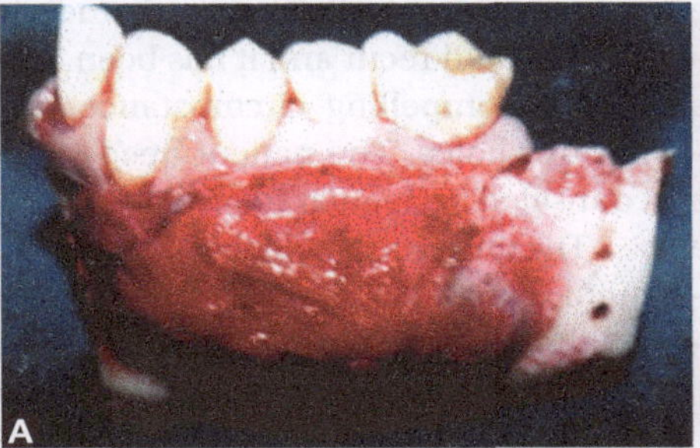

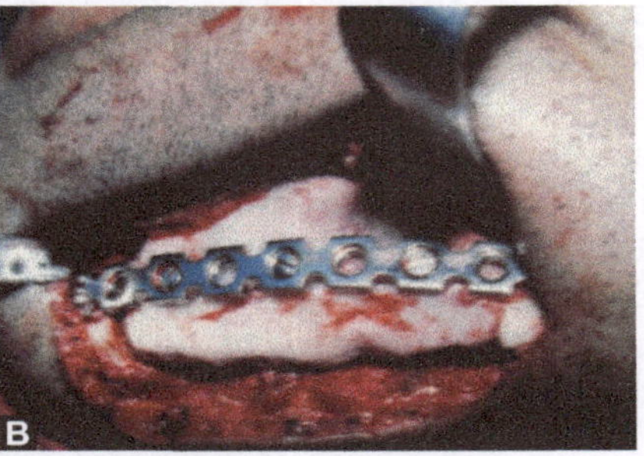

Figs 28.4A and B: Specimen of resected plexiform ameloblastoma the surgical defect reconstructed with reconstructed plate and iliac crest corticocancellous graft

Maxillary Tumors

- Subtotal/partial maxillectomy
- Total maxillectomy
- Extended maxillectomy.

The treatment in the maxillary tumors is more radical as the tumor invades the bone more commonly due to its spongy nature and the recurrence is more likely if the excision is inadequate. The proximity with air sinuses and subsequently through them to the cranial cavity makes the resection of the tumor more difficult if these structures are involved. Similarly, the perforation of the thin posterior wall of the maxilla facilitates the spread of the tumor in the infratemporal fossa where the proximity with the vital structures makes the tumor resection difficult. The recurrence in the maxilla could be very difficult to treat due to the proximity to the vital structures, especially to the skull base.

Specimen Radiography

It is generally accepted that the central ameloblastomas should be excised along with 1 to 1.5 cm margins of healthy bone to achieve adequate surgical clearance, as the tumor invades in the cancellous bone. Studies have shown that the tumor extends microscopically 5 to 6 mm beyond the radiological and 3 to 4 mm beyond the CT margins of the tumor. Thus, minimum 1 cm clearance in the normal bone is recommended. When the radiographs are taken in a patient there is certain amount of distortion and the tumor margins may not be accurate. Thus, after excision the specimen is radiographed to confirm minimum 1 cm margin beyond the radiological extent of the tumor (Figs 28.6A and B). If the margins are found to be inadequate then still the surgeon has the chance to resect additional small segment of the bone.

Reconstruction of the surgical defect is mandatory to prevent postoperative morbidity. As the majority of the patients are young, the reconstruction should fulfill following goals:

- Restoration of movements and equilibrium of mandible
- Maintenance of normal occlusal plane, floor of the mouth and tongue's anatomical position
- Restoration of near normal feeding
- Acceptable esthetics and function
- More favorable social acceptance

The reconstruction should ideally be done primarily to prevent deformity and collapse of the resected segments due to fibrosis. However, in certain cases where the primary reconstruction is not advisable due to uncertainty of the resection margins and higher chances of recurrence, the reconstruction can be done as a secondary procedure.

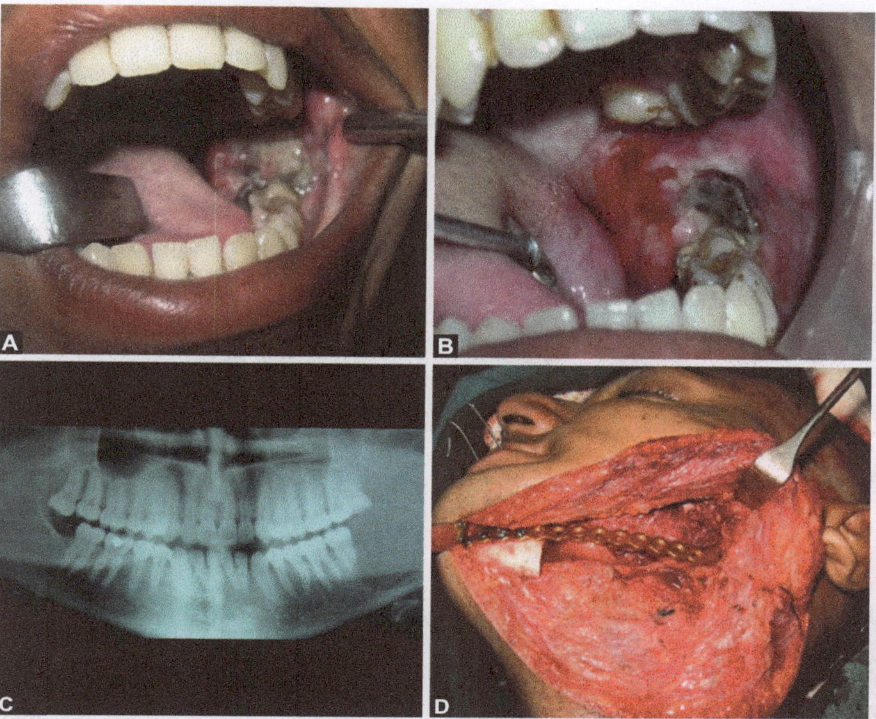

Figs 28.5A to D: Solid variant of ameloblastoma in ramus perforating the cortex and fungating through the mucosa. Treated with hemimandibulectomy and reconstruction with titanium plate

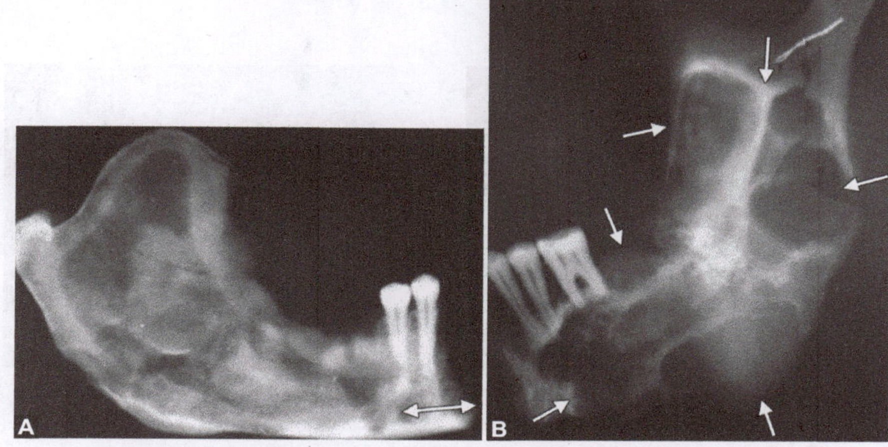

Figs 28.6A and B: Specimen radiographs showing adequate surgical margins of 1 cm

The various modalities for reconstructing the surgical defect in the mandible are:

- **Reconstruction plates:** The metallic reconstruction plates made up of titanium or stainless steel are commonly used. The plates effectively bridge the bony defect. The plates are contoured to match the facial profile and secured to the distal and proximal bony fragments with the help of the screws (Figs 28.7 and 28.8). A variety of reconstruction plates are available which are suitable in different situations. The reconstruction plates with condyle are also available for reconstructing the defect following hemimandibulectomy with disarticulation

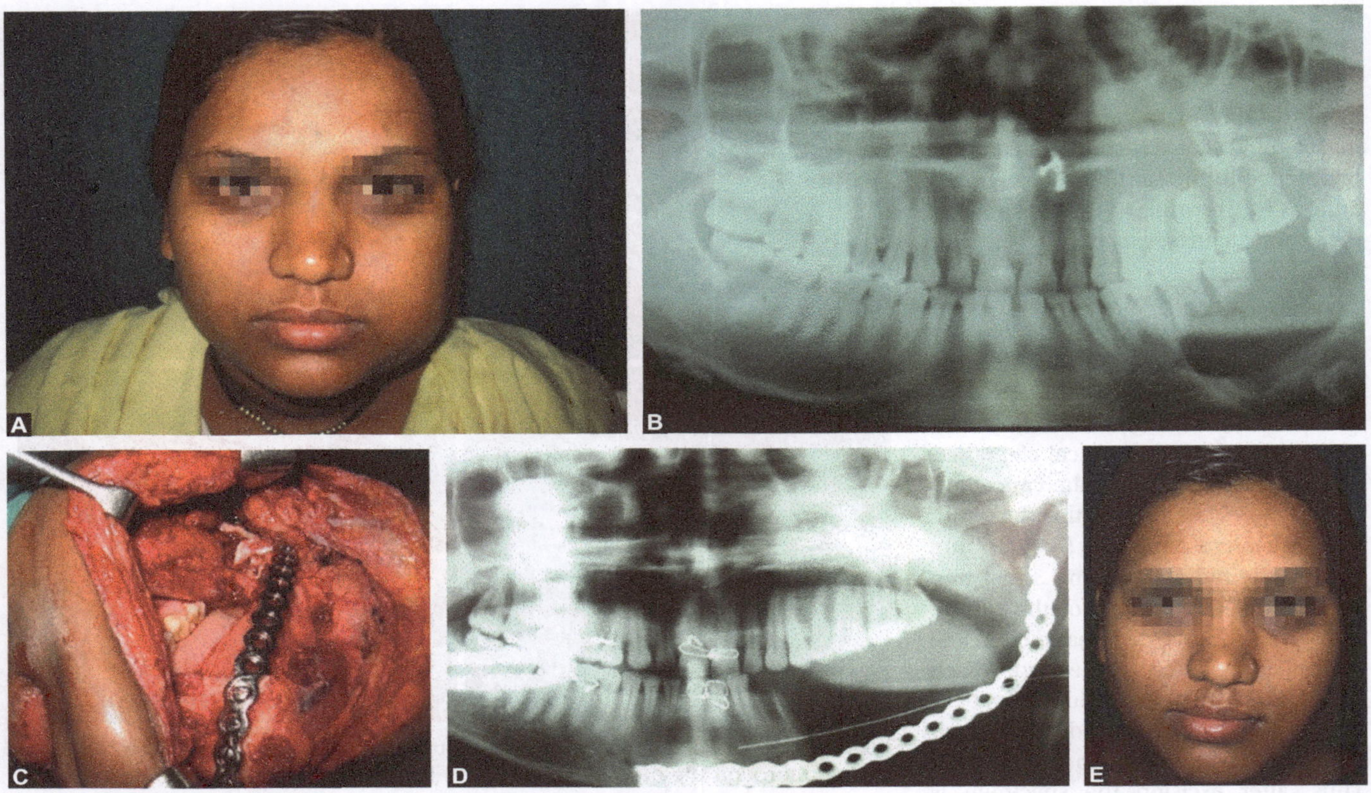

Figs 28.7A to E: Ameloblastoma of mandible treated with segmental resection and reconstruction with reconstruction plate: (A) Preoperative picture; (B) Preoperative OPG; (C) Fixation of recostruction plate; (D) Postoperative OPG; (E) Postoperative result

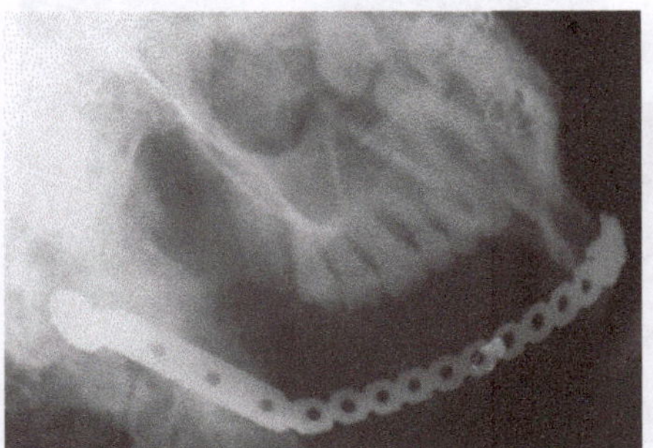

Fig. 28.8: Reconstruction plate with condylar prosthesis

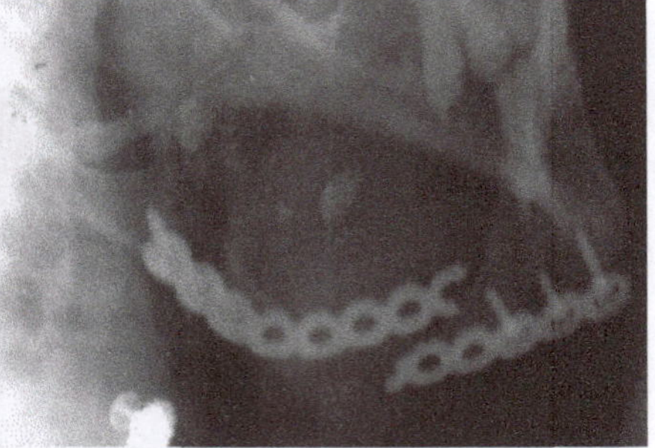

Fig. 28.9: Fractured reconstruction plate

of the condyle. The disadvantages of the reconstruction plate are:

- They help only in establishing the contour, but the masticatory function cannot be restored as the fabrication of the denture is not possible.
- The plates are liable to get loosened, infected and can evoke tissue reaction and need to be removed.
- The midline reconstruction with the plates is often problematic and dehiscence of plate is a common complication.
- The plates can fracture due to trauma or extreme stress (Fig. 28.9).

- **Bone grafts:** Corticocancellous bone grafts harvested from the anterior iliac crest (*See* Fig. 28.4B) or the rib grafts can also be used to reconstruct the mandible. The bone grafts can get rejected due to the infection and can undergo variable degree of resorption and thus are unpredictable. The free grafts can get infected and rejected.
- **Free microvascular fibular grafts:** Anastamosed to regional artery and vein, they are the best option to reconstruct the mandible and in selected cases maxillary defects (Figs 28.10 and 28.11). The graft provides adequate bone to restore the contour and in cases of deficient cover due to excision of the mucosa, the skin pedal can be harvested and used to bridge the soft tissue defect to provide adequate cover for the bone graft. Subsequently, dental rehabilitation can also be done by insertion of implants. However, the facilities for the (microvascular anastomosis) free tissue transfer are not universally available.

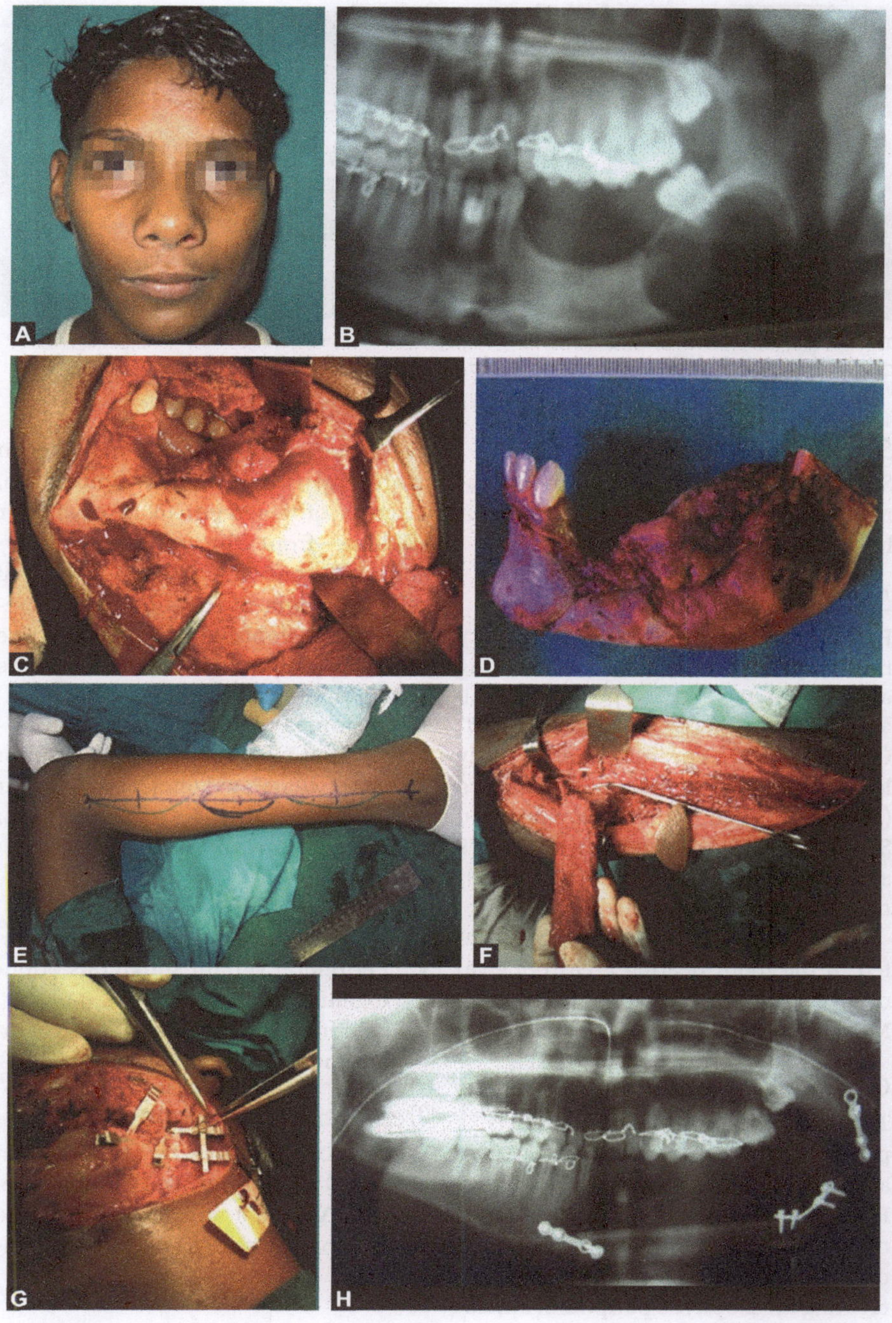

Figs 28.10A to H: Case of ameloblastoma of mandible treated with segmental resection and reconstruction of the defect with free fibular graft: (A) Preoperative photograph; (B) Preoperative radiograph; (C) Exposed tumor; (D) Resected specimen; (E) Marking of fibular graft and skin pedal; (F) Harvesting fibular graft on peroneal vessels pedicle; (G) Microvascular anastomosis of graft; (H) Postoperative radiograph showing graft in place

- **Custom made implants:** Using the stereolithography and rapid prototyping the custom made implants can be fabricated and used to reconstruct the surgical bony defects. It provides better results as compared to the reconstruction plate. However the other short comings are similar to the reconstruction plates.
- **Bone transport:** The transport technique using the Elizarow technique by means of distraction devices can be used to bridge smaller bony defects.

Reconstruction of the Maxillary Defects

The reconstruction of the maxillary defects is always challenging. The defects are large and complex. The common modalities for maxillary reconstruction after the maxillectomy are:

- Use of temporalis muscle fascia flaps
- Use of nasal septum to reconstruct the orbital floor.

Free vascularized flaps like fibula are not ideal as the vascular pedicle is short. However, with the insertion of implants in the fibular graft the dental rehabilitation is possible. For maxillary reconstruction, free scapular flaps are preferred because of the long vascular pedicle and good bone quality.

Obturators

The ensuing surgical defect following the maxillectomy performed for excising the ameloblastoma can be plugged using prosthesis in the form of an obturator.

Extraosseous/Peripheral Ameloblastoma

History

The peripheral ameloblastoma was first reported by Stanley and Krogh[26] in 1959 and has a histopathological appearance similar to the solid ameloblastoma. It is an uncommon lesion usually presenting as a painless, nonulcerated sessile or pedunculated gingival or alveolar lesion. The lesion shows an innocuous clinical behavior and is treated with local excision.

The tumor was first described by Kuru[27] (1911). In a review by Mintz et al.[28] (1999) covering the period between 1959 and 1989, only 33 cases were documented, while Redman et al.[29] (1994) found 55 cases in the Anglo-Saxon literature. Reichart et al.[13] (1995), in a review of 3677 cases of ameloblastoma, found only 2 percent to possess peripheral ameloblastomas. Likewise, Gurol and Burkes (Gardner 1996) reviewed

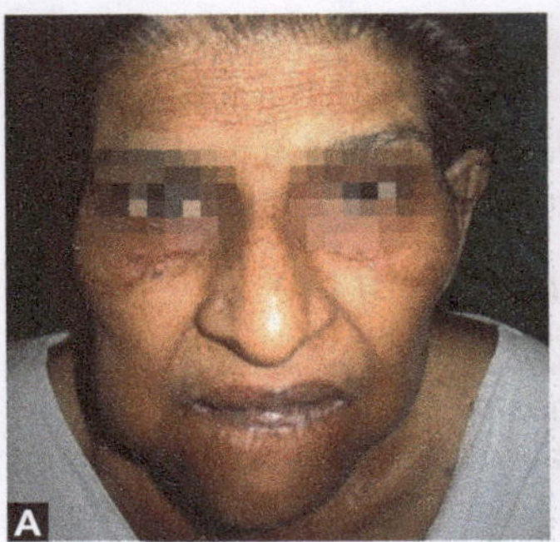

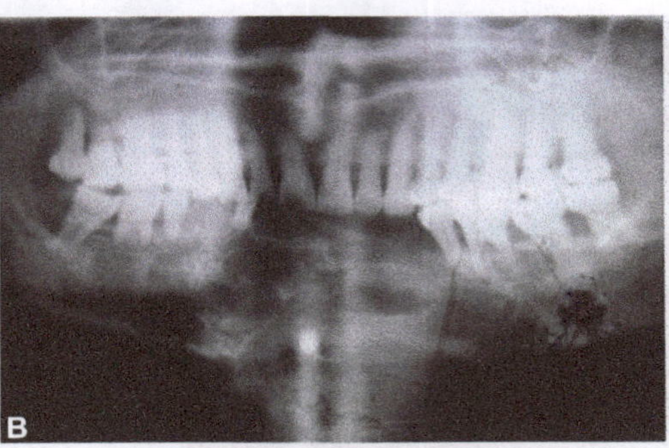

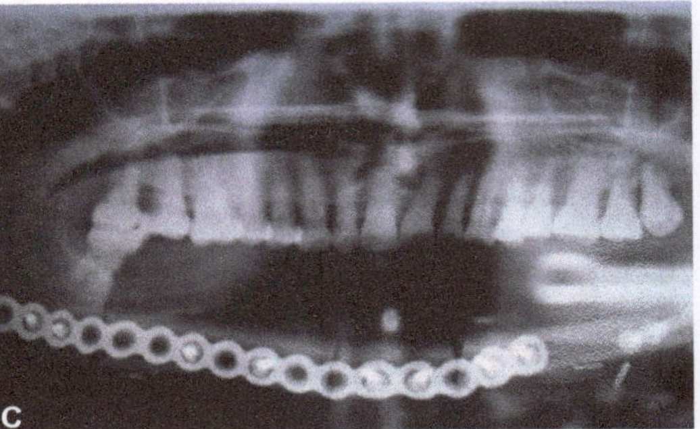

Figs 28.11A to C: Case of ameloblastoma of mandible in the anterior area treated with segmental resection and reconstruction of the defect with free fibular graft and reconstructed plate

205 ameloblastomas in the period from 1956 to 1994 and found only eight cases to correspond to peripheral ameloblastoma. In a 2002 review conducted by Philipsen et al. peripheral ameloblastoma was seen to account for 2 to 10 percent of all ameloblastomas. All these studies document the rarity of this variant of the ameloblastoma.

One of the main uncertainties regarding the origin of this tumor, is that it is believed to be derived directly from the lining epithelium or from remains of the dental lamina located in non-bony soft tissues (Moskow and Baden[30] 1982, Kaneko and Ueno[31] 1986, Horowitz et al.[32] 1987, Gurol and Burkes[33] 1995, Ide et al. 2002).

Histologically, peripheral ameloblastoma is similar to central ameloblastoma, although the former is less aggressive (Buchner and Sciuba[34] 1987).

The maximum incidence is observed between the fifth and sixth decades of life, with an average patient age at initial appearance of the lesion to be 50 years. A slight male predominance has been reported (Gardner 1996[35]). In most cases (65%), the lesion is located in the mandible, particularly on the lingual aspect of the premolar zone (representing 32.6% of all locations) (Philipsen et al. 2001[36]). In the upper maxilla the most frequent location corresponds to the anterior zone for Japanese patients, while in Caucasians it corresponds to the region of the tuberosity (Shiba et al. 1983, Orsini et al. 2000).

Synonyms

Soft tissue ameloblastoma, ameloblastoma of the mucosal origin, ameloblastoma of the gingiva.

Epidemiology

Peripheral ameloblastoma is a very rare odontogenic tumor, representing approximately 1 to 5 percent of all ameloblastomas (El-Mofty et al. 1991, Gardner 1996[35]). The lesion is exclusively located in the gingiva or oral mucosa (Guralnick et al.[37] 1983, Buchner and Sciuba[34] 1987). Age range varies from 9 and 92 years with 64 percent of all cases occurring in the 5th to 7th decade.

Peripheral ameloblastomas are located in the tooth bearing areas (gingiva) or alveolar mucosa in edentulous areas. Mandible: Maxilla ratio of 2.4:1 is noted.

Clinical Features/Imaging

The peripheral ameloblastoma is a painless, firm and exophytic growth with a smooth, pebbly or papillary surface. Rarely, intraosseous ameloblastomas may extend to the gingival tissues and merge with the gingival epithelium, creating an exophytic peripheral ameloblastoma like lesions.[38]

Histopathology

The peripheral ameloblastoma consists of odontogenic epithelium with the same histomorphic cell types and patterns as seen in central solid variant of ameloblastoma. Some lesions are located entirely within the connective tissue of the gingiva, showing no continuity with the surface epithelium, whereas others seem to fuse with or originate from the mucosal epithelium. It is generally believed that basal cell carcinoma of the gingiva and peripheral ameloblastoma represents the same neoplasm. Squamous cells in the acanthomatous areas of peripheral ameloblastomas may show ghost cell formation and in some parts of the tumor islands,[39] vacuolated or clear cells occur in discrete clusters. The stroma is that of a mature fibrous connective tissue.

Differential Diagnosis

- Peripheral odontogenic fibroma
- Peripheral variant squamous odontogenic tumor
- Odontogenic gingival epithelial hamartoma.

Treatment and Prognosis

It does not show invasive behavior and conservative excision is a treatment of choice. Although the recurrence rate is low, long-term follow-up is recommended.

Pituitary Ameloblastoma (Craniopharyngioma, Rathke's Pouch Tumor)

This is the tumor involving the central nervous system, which grows as a pseudoencapsulated mass. It is usually seen as suprasellar mass, but occasionally present as an intrasellar mass destroying the pituitary gland. The peak incidence is reported between 13 and 23 years of age. It is generally thought to originate from the unobliterated portion of the fetal craniopharyngeal duct, which itself originates from the Rathke's pouch. The epithelial remnants of craniopharyngeal duct are common in adults. These cells are pleuripotent and can give rise to histologically similar tumor-like ameloblastoma of the jaws.

The microscopic features of craniopharyngioma differ from ameloblastoma due to the almost universal presence of calcified foci and neoplastic bone or cartilage. It has histological similarity with the calcifying epithelial odontogenic cyst (CEOC) due to the presence of ghost cells. Tooth formation in a craniopharyngioma has also been reported.

The rate of growth of this tumor is different from the ameloblastoma and often presents with endocrine dysfunctions, drowsiness and toxic symptoms.

Unicystic Type (Synonym - Cytogenic Ameloblastoma)

History

The unicystic ameloblastoma represents an ameloblastoma variant, presenting as a cyst (WHO). The unicystic ameloblastoma was first described in 1977 by Robinson and Martinez.[40] This variant has a large cystic cavity with either luminal or mural proliferation of ameloblastic cells. It has been shown that this type of ameloblastoma has a low recurrence rate. Ackermann[41] advocated simple enucleation for cystic ameloblastoma, with more aggressive surgery if the connective tissue of the wall was shown to have invasive islands of ameloblastomatous epithelium.

The unicystic ameloblastoma tends to occur at an earlier age than the solid or multicystic forms (Gardner and Corio[42] 1984). It frequently presents as a unilocular well-defined radiolucency surrounding the crown of an unerupted mandibular third molar and may also mimic a dentigerous cyst. Ackermann et al.[41] (1988) described three distinct histological types as:

- Cyst lined by variable epithelium with no infiltration into the fibrous cyst wall.
- Cyst showing intraluminal plexiform epithelial proliferation with no infiltration.
- Cyst with invasion of epithelium into the cyst wall in either a follicular or a plexiform pattern.

Microscopically, it was demonstrated that in all types there is a basal layer of columnar preameloblasts with hyperchromatic nuclei polarized away from the basement membrane, with a clear basal cytoplasm and a more superficial loose stellate reticulum-like epithelium (Leider et al.[43] 1985, Li et al.[44] 2000, Philipsen and Reichart.[45] 1998, Neville et al.[14] 2002). Due to its clinical behavior, this lesion is commonly seen as an incidental finding on radiographs taken for other purposes. In these circumstances, some lesions could remain undiagnosed in the early stages of their development (Eversole et al.[46] 1984).

Epidemiology

The cases associated with unerupted tooth show a mean age of 16 years as opposed to 35 years in the absence of an unerupted tooth.[45] The mean age is significantly lower than that of solid ameloblastoma. There is no gender predilection. About 5 to 15 percent of all ameloblastomas are unicystic type. More than 90 percent cases involve mandible, usually the posterior region.

Clinical Features/Imaging

Some cases are asymptomatic and some present as a swelling of the posterior mandible (Fig. 28.12A). About 80 percent cases are associated with unerupted mandibular third molars. The lesion presents radiographically as a well corticated, unilocular, often pericoronal radiolucency (Fig. 28.12B).[46] Root resorption may occur.[47] The clinical radiographic diagnosis is frequently a dentigerous cyst (Fig. 28.12C). The differences between conventional and unicystic ameloblastoma are shown in Box 28.1.

The lesions vary in size and when removed intact, are typically cystic and generally attached to an unerupted tooth at the cementoenamel junction (Figs 28.13A and B). The cyst wall may contain one or more tumor proliferations extending into the lumen. These proliferations and other thickened areas must be selected for microscopic examination.

Histopathology

The unicystic ameloblastoma has two histopathological variants (Fig. 28.14).[41]

1. The luminal variant is a cystic lesion lined by ameloblastomatous epithelium. In addition, intraluminal extensions may occur. These extensions usually exhibit plexiform epithelial pattern. There is no tumor infiltration into the fibrous wall.
2. The mural variant, the cyst wall is infiltrated by ameloblastomatous epithelium that exhibits either a follicular or plexiform pattern. Sometimes, both variants may occur in the same lesion. The mural variant of unicystic ameloblastoma may be confused with either dentigerous cyst or dental follicles containing a lot of odontogenic epithelial remnants. These epithelial nests, however, do not show the typical histologic features of ameloblastoma, peripheral palisading and nuclear polarization.

   The ameloblastic changes in the lining may be focal and not generalized throughout the lining. In such cases even if the biopsy is done, it may not be from the representing site and the histopathological report may be a cyst. In such cases it is essentially treated by conservative approach, i.e. enucleation, rather than resection (Figs 28.15A to D).

Prognosis

Most unicystic ameloblastomas are enucleated with the preoperative clinical

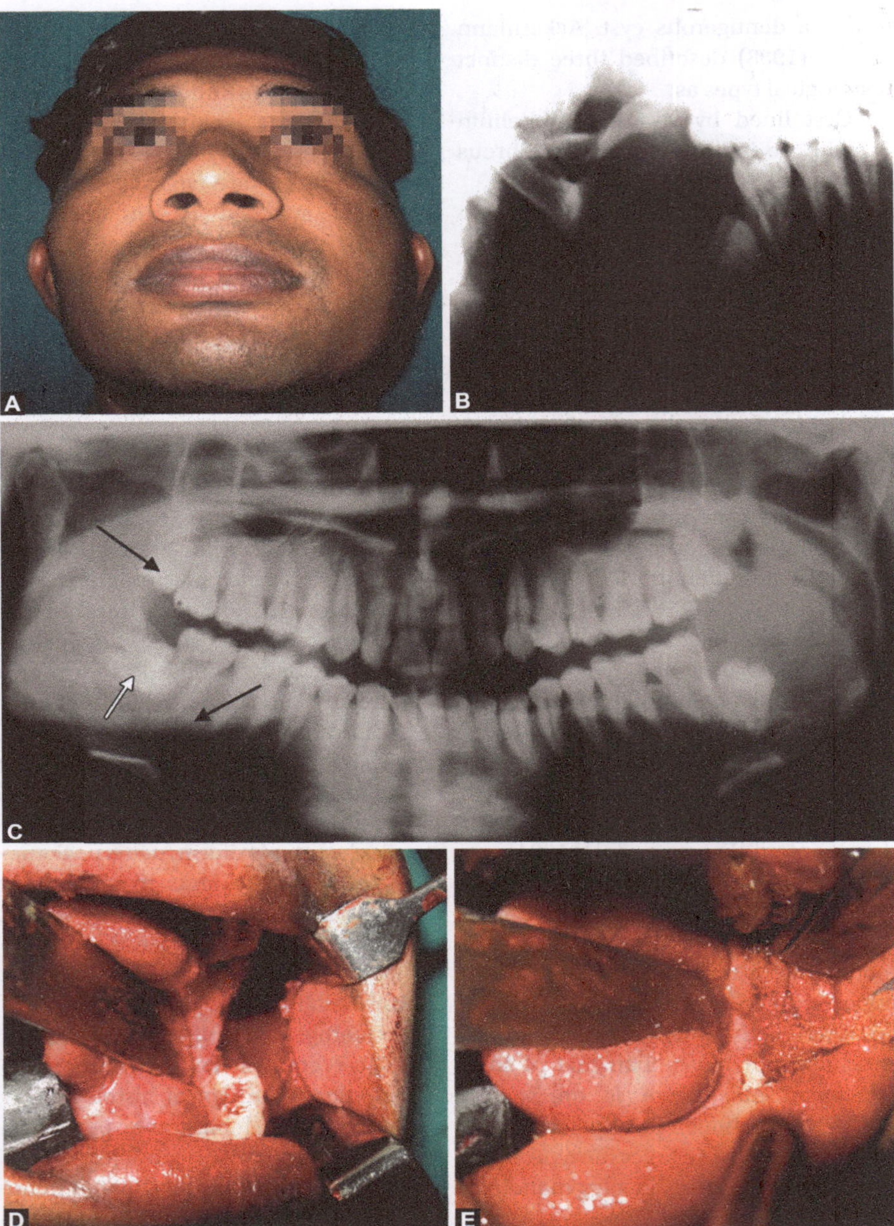

Figs 28.12A to E: A clinical case of unicystic ameloblastoma in the ramus managed by enucleation the cavity packed open for healing by secondary intention

Box 28.1: Differences between conventional and unicystic ameloblastomas

Conventional	Unicystic
Grows in its typical island, strand and cord-like patterns, but presents surgically as a largely solid tumor mass within the bone	Cystic areas nearly always noted, grows predominantly as a cystic lesion
More than 90% of all ameloblastomas	6–10% of all ameloblastomas
100% recurrence rate for that treated only by curettage, however most studies report lower rates, ranging from 50% to greater than 90%	Better prognosis, lesser recurrence (10.7–25%) (Philipsen and Reichart)

diagnosis of dentigerous cyst and it is only on pathologic examination of the enucleated lining that their true nature is determined. The luminal variant does not infiltrate the surrounding bone and as a result no further treatment is required for those lesions. Long-term follow-up is recommended to detect recurrence, if any (Figs 28.12 and 28.14).

Desmoplastic Ameloblastoma

Desmoplastic ameloblastoma is a variant of ameloblastoma with specific clinical, imaging and histological features (WHO). Desmoplasia is the term which refers to the presence of excessive connective tissue stroma.

Eversole was the first to describe it in English literature. Desmoplastic ameloblastoma has also been reviewed by Waldron CA et al.[48] in 1987 in his histopathological study of 116 ameloblastomas with special reference to the desmoplastic variant.

Desmoplastic ameloblastoma has also been reviewed by Ashman et al.[49] (1993) and in more detail by Philipsen et al. (1992) who analyzed the findings in 29 reported cases.

Desmoplastic ameloblastoma variant accounted for 1.4 percent of 1593 ameloblastomas reviewed by Reichart et al.[13] (1995).

Epidemiology

Desmoplastic ameloblastoma exhibits no gender predilection and occurs over a wide range. Most of the cases are diagnosed between 30 and 60 years of age. The maxilla: mandible ratio is 1:1 (Fig. 28.16A). The desmoplastic ameloblastomas are found predominantly in the anterior mandibular region.

Clinical Features

A painless swelling of the jaw bone represents the chief initial complaint. The size of the tumor varies between 1.0 and 8.5 cm in diameter. An extraosseous variant of desmoplastic ameloblastoma has not been reported. The lesional tissue has a gritty consistency and the cut surface is solid in most of the cases.

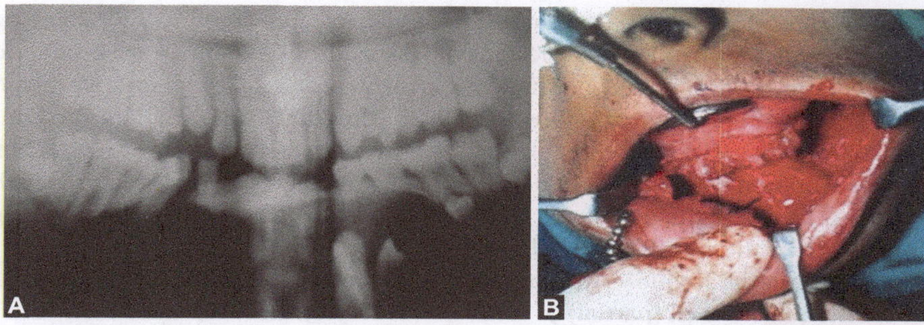

Figs 28.13A and B: Unicystic ameloblastoma involving the anterior mandible in a 16-year-old boy treated by enucleation

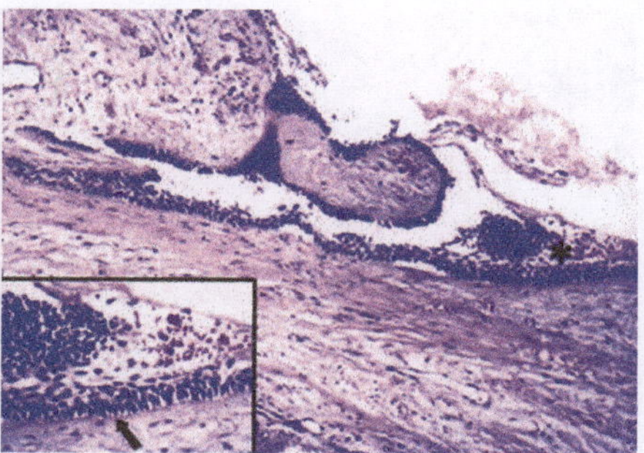

Fig. 28.14: Histological aspects of the unicystic ameloblastoma. Note that epithelial lining presents the overlying epithelial cells loosely disposed resembling stellate reticulum. In the insert a basal layer can be seen showing a hyperchromatic and polarized basal cells

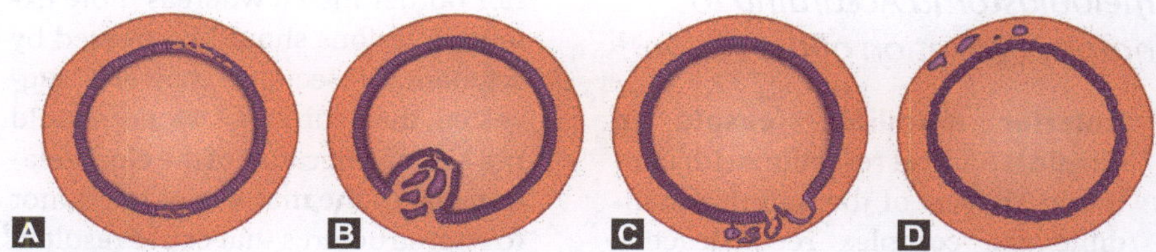

Figs 28.15A to D: Diagrammatic representation of various situations that may be found in unicystic ameloblastoma on histologic examination: (A) The lining epithelium is ameloblastomatous; (B) A nodule of ameloblastoma projects in the lumen; (C) The ameloblastoma has proliferated from the cystic lining into the connective tissue wall of the cyst; (D) Islands of ameloblastoma are present in connective tissue wall of an apparently non-neoplastic cyst

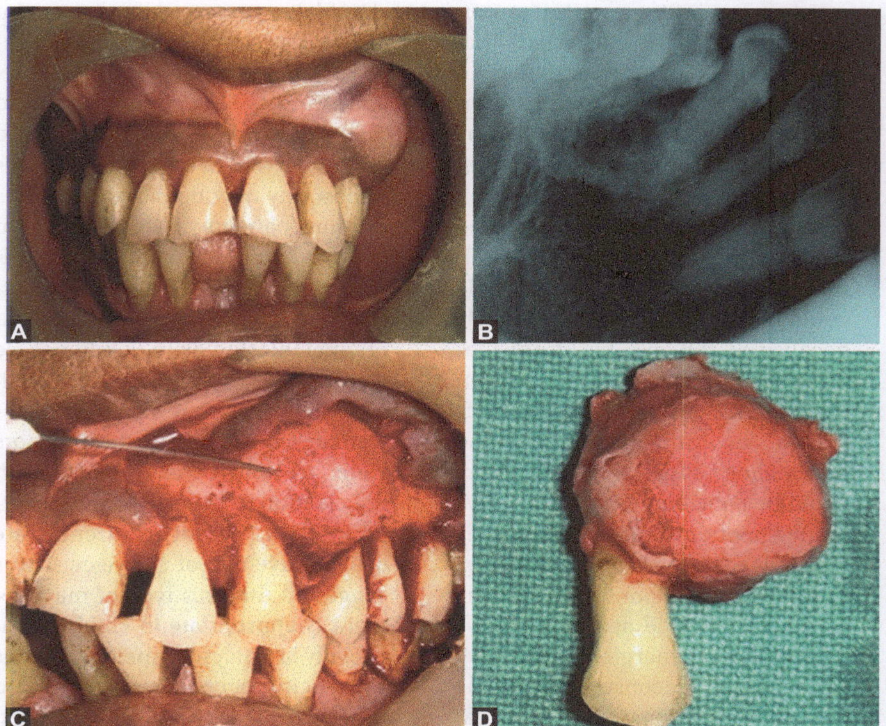

Figs 28.16A to D: Desmoplastic ameloblastoma involving the maxilla

Radiographically, about 50 percent of the desmoplastic ameloblastomas show a mottled mixed radiolucency/radiopacity with diffuse margins, suggesting a fibro-osseous lesion. Resorption of tooth roots may occur (Fig. 28.16B). The ill-defined borders of desmoplastic ameloblastomas make high resolution CT and MRI helpful in treatment planning.[50]

Histopathology (Fig. 28.17)

In desmoplastic ameloblastoma, the stromal component dominates compressing the odontogenic epithelial components. The epithelial tumor islands are very irregular or bizarre in shape with a pointed stellate appearance. The epithelial cells at the periphery of the islands are cuboidal with occasional hyperchromatic nuclei. Columnar cells with nuclear polarity are rarely conspicuous. The islands have a swirled, hypercellular center with spindle shaped or squamous epithelial cells. Microcytes may occur centrally. Myxoid changes in the juxtaepithelial stroma are often found. Formation of metastatic osteoid trabeculae (osteoplasia) may be present. A fibrous capsule is not present corresponding to the radiographically poorly defined tumor margin. A combination desmoplastic ameloblastoma with A-S/M is

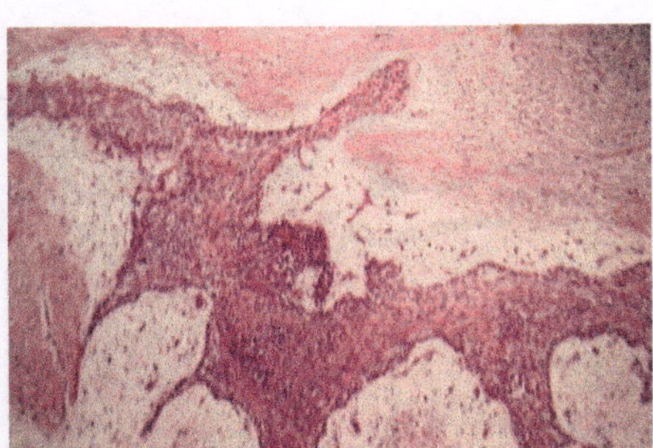

Fig. 28.17: Desmoplastic ameloblastoma. Irregularly shaped epithelial island surrounded by narrow zone of loose structures embedded in desmoblastic stroma

known and has been termed as hybrid lesion.[51]

Management

Present knowledge leads to recommendation to apply same treatment modality as for multicystic ameloblastoma (Figs 28.16C and D). Treatment decisions for ameloblastoma are based on the individual patient situation and the best judgment of the surgeons. The surgical plan should be influenced by whether the lesion involves maxilla or mandible. Maxillary lesions behave distinctly different from mandibular lesions. The higher cancellous bone percentage in the maxilla facilitates the spread of ameloblastoma, whereas the density of the cortical plates in the mandible tends to limit the spread of neoplasm. The location of the maxilla in the center of the maxillofacial complex allows greater ease of extension of the ameloblastoma into vital structures, sinus, orbit and skull base, resulting in increased morbidity and mortality rates.

Successful treatment is the treatment that renders an acceptable prognosis, complete eradication of the lesion, reconstruction of the resultant defect, causes minimal disfigurement and is based on the behavior and potential of the tumor, the growth patterns of the various physical forms, duration, the anatomic site of the occurrence, the clinical extent and size of the tumor and histological assessment. The treatment modality is also determined considering the general health and age of the patient.

The radical approach includes, resection and the excision of a lesion that includes a measurable perimeter of investing bone. In the mandible this could be done with (segmental) or without (marginal) continuity defect or extend to disarticulation if the TMJ is involved. In the maxilla, it would be defined by the anatomic extension of the excision in subtotal (partial) or total maxillectomy.

Surgical Management of Ameloblastoma According to Anatomic Location of the Lesion[52]

- **Anterior mandible (cuspid to cuspid):** Radical resection with continuity defects of the anterior mandible are complex reconstructive cases. If at all possible, attempts should be made to maintain the inferior border of the symphyseal region. The use of a marginal resection is made possible because the thickness of cortical bone in the symphyseal region is more resistant to infiltration by tumor. Mehlisch et al.[53] suggested that small lesions (less than 3 cm in diameter) located in the anterior part of the jaws could be treated by excision with cautery whereas larger lesions required 'segmental or en bloc resection'. Gardner reported that treatment of ameloblastoma in the anterior body of the mandible could be approached conservatively because of the distance from major anatomic structures. However, if curettage is used, recurrence should be anticipated. Holland and Mellor[54] suggested that cautery could be considered in conservative management even though scientific evidence to support its use is lacking. In summary, ameloblastoma of the anterior mandible at times can be treated by a marginal resection. Moreover, the reconstruction of the anterior mandibular defect, spreading across the midline is often unsatisfactory if the conventional reconstruction plates are used. The plates often erode the overlying skin in due course of time and dehiscence takes place. However, in the large lesions where the conservative excision is not possible, segmental resection is required with reconstruction of the defect using the free fibular graft.
- **Posterior mandible (bicuspid or condyle):** Gardner and Pecak[55] indicated that 'small lesions of the posterior mandible' should be treated by marginal resection leaving the posterior border intact, whereas more extensive lesions should be treated by segmental resection. They also suggested that curettage alone should not be done because of the close relationship of the margins of the tumor to vital structures that could result in a recurrence rate of 55 to 90 percent. Cryotherapy increased the chance of success by causing devitalization of the bone to a depth of 1 to 3 cm. Even though the follow-up period was short (10 years is the 'gold standard') they suggested that radical treatment should be preserved for treatment failure. Ueno et al.[56] reviewed 91 cases of ameloblastomas with follow-ups from 1 to 15 years and suggested that extensive resectioning of the mandible was over treatment. This philosophy may be particularly true in young patients where interruption in growth and development may interfere with future function and esthetics. Kahn found that 68.6 percent of ameloblastomas in young people were associated with impacted teeth and 72.2 percent of these were unilocular. The majority of these tumors were treated conservatively with enucleation or curettage and resulted in a 6.9 percent recurrence rate over an average of 5.2 years it was suggested that this type of management is appropriate in children, especially in unicystic ameloblastomas without tumor cell extension beyond the margins of the cyst wall. Stephen E Feinberg[57] believes on the basis of their clinical experience and the literature review, that treatment of solid

or multilocular ameloblastomas of the body and posterior mandible requires radical therapy. Marginal resection without continuity defect with 1 to 2 cm margins (maintenance of the inferior or posterior border when possible) should be the treatment of choice for solid multilocular lesions. Patients who undergo marginal resection with continuity defects might require maxillomandibular fixation if pathologic fracture is a possibility. Reconstruction plates should be adapted before segmental resection without continuity defect in order to maintain a normal anatomic relationship between the remaining distal and proximal segments. In contrast, unicystic ameloblastoma of the posterior mandible can be treated conservatively with curettage or peripheral ostectomy if adequate follow-up is possible. Most of the unicystic ameloblastomas are seen at an early age and are often associated with impacted teeth. They clinically adjoining cancellous bone and often diagnosed as the same and treated with enucleation and curettage. Only upon postsurgical histopathology of the specimen, diagnosis of unicystic ameloblastoma is arrived at adjoining cancellous bone is done preoperatively, considering the fact that the ameloblastic changes in the lining of the cyst may not be generalized, the biopsy need not be from this representing site and the histopathological diagnosis may come as dentigerous cyst. Under these circumstances the lesion is treated conservatively. In either cases the long term follow-up to detect recurrence is the only solution. As the unicystic ameloblastomas occur at an early age and are extensive at the time of the first diagnosis, a radical treatment comprising the segmental resection is too morbid for the patient. It does not only cause functional and cosmetic morbidity but also leads to retarded growth and also psycological problems to the affected child. The unicystic ameloblastomas have thick lining and it can be easily separated from the bone and can be removed completely. The authors strongly recommend and practice the conservative treatment for the unicystic ameloblatomas with reasonable success which comprises of enucleation of the lining, vigorous curettage of the adjoining cancellous bone followed by application of Cornoy's solution to the base (*see* Figs 28.12A to E and Figs 28.13A and B). The patients should be kept under long term follow-up and failures of conservative treatment should be treated with radical treatment like segmental madibulectomy and appropriate reconstruction.

- **Anterior maxilla (cuspid to cuspid):** Ameloblastomas of anterior maxilla represents approximately 2 percent of all documented occurrences. Gardner suggested that ameloblastoma of the anterior maxilla could be treated less aggressively than those of the posterior maxilla as sufficient distances from vital structures allow for less radical treatment. Data suggests that conservative treatment has the risk of occurrence with potential extension to the orbits, nasal cavity, and ethmoid cells. On the other hand, radical treatment (partial or total maxillectomy) may result in a significant deformity requiring complex reconstruction.
- **Posterior maxilla (bicuspid to pterygoid plates):** Approximately 47 to 50 percent of maxillary ameloblastomas are found in the molar region and 15 to 30 percent in the maxillary sinus region and the floor of the nose, it is generally felt that maxillary ameloblastomas are more dangerous than mandibular ameloblastomas because of a lack of maxillary cortical bone to contain the tumor and their difficulty in early detection in conjugation with their intimate relationship with complex regional anatomy, posterior maxillary tumors are not well confined by the thin maxillary cortical bone and can easily spread outside maxillary boundaries, which makes definitive treatment difficult. Bredenkamp et al.[58] described maxillary ameloblastomas as being locally aggressive, incurable and lethal, they found a 5-year survival rate of 16 percent when initial treatment consisted of a limited resectioning as their recurrences were treated with a maxillectomy or debulking procedure if total removal is impossible, it is clear that there is little support for conservative management of solid or multicystic ameloblastomas of the posterior maxilla. Initial treatment should include surgical margins of 1 to 2 cm. The surgical approach to obtain these margins, depending on the location and size of the tumor, may require a transoral resection or a maxillectomy could be done via a Weber-Fergusson incision to gain adequate exposure for tumor resection. Tumors of the infratemporal fossa and pterygomaxillary region would need combined surgical approach necessitating intraoral and bicoronal or hemi coronal incision. The maxillary ameloblastomas by and large require more aggressive treatment as the tumor infilterates the spongy maxillary bone and the attempts towards conservative excision invariably fail and recurrence is more common. The recurrence may be at a site, which is more difficult to excise surgically making it unresectable. Thus, the first attempt for the complete removal should be well planned and radical.

Use of Carnoy's Solution after Enucleation of Unicystic Ameloblastoma

- Carnoy's solution[59] was described in 1933 as a sclerozing agent for the treatment of cysts and fistulae and remains in use today as a fixative.
- The use of Carnoy's solution for this specific purpose in relation to unicystic ameloblastoma was initially suggested by Stoelinga and Bronkhorst[60] in 1988 and recently proposed again as a possible means

to diminish the recurrence risk after conservative treatment.

- Carnoy's solution is probably able to fix residual ameloblastoma tissue after enucleation of unicystic ameloblastoma with mural invasion and diminish the risk of recurrence, but based on the two studies this is unlikely to be effective for conventional multicystic ameloblastoma and some of the unicystic lesions with mural invasion. It was surprising to find the patients treated by enucleation, but without the application of Carnoy's solution experienced recurrence (100% recurrence). Carnoy's solution is effective in diminishing expected recurrence.
- Carnoy's solution was applied to the bony cavity for 3 minutes using cotton applicators or ribbon gauze soaked with Carnoy's solution. When mandibular nerve was visible in the bony cavity, contact with Carnoy's solution was avoided as far possible. This was followed by copious irrigation with normal saline. Bismuth iodoform paraffin paste (BIPP) impregnated gauze was then inserted into the bony defect and the wound kept open over the gauze pack.

Radiosensitivity of Ameloblastomas

It is usually accepted that ameloblastomas are radioresistant but this is incorrect. As they are well-differentiated epithelial tumors, they are quite radiosensitive, this is illustrated by the way therapeutic irradiation can reduce the extraosseous components of large ameloblastomas. However, tumors that are radiosensitive may not beds controlled by therapeutic irradiation; this is true of ameloblastomas that are basically infrabony tumors. Their intraosseous location makes them resistant to radiotherapy in the same way those squamous cell carcinomas are resistant to this modality once they have invaded bone.

Tumors, apart from therapeutic irradiation not being reliably effective in controlling ameloblastomas there are two other reasons why this modality should not be used other than in exceptional cases: First, the danger of osteoradionecrosis and second the risk inducing a malignant transformation.

Radiation and chemotherapy have been used for primary and recurrent tumors. Atkinson et al. did a retrospective study of 10 cases of ameloblastoma in which 7 were primarily treated with radiation alone and 3 patients had combined radiation and surgery; 9 patients treated initially with mega voltage radiation alone or radiotherapy surgery had successful treatment with only one recurrence noted. Based on their data, they suggested that radiation therapy could be used in cases when surgical treatment would be technically complex because of tumor bulk, location or medical status of the patient. Gardner felt that radiation therapy was unsuccessful for intraosseous ameloblastomas, but may be more beneficial in assisting in inoperable cases.

CALCIFYING EPITHELIAL ODONTOGENIC TUMOR

Introduction[61]

The calcifying epithelial odontogenic tumor (CEOT) is a locally invasive epithelial odontogenic neoplasm, characterized by the presence of amyloid material that may become calcified (WHO).

The calcifying epithelial odontogenic tumor was first introduced into the scientific literature almost 50 years ago by JJ Pindborg,[61] the term Pindborg's tumor, is now a universally recognized synonym for this neoplasm. The CEOT is a benign, though occasionally locally invasive, slow-growing, odontogenic neoplasm that is exclusively epithelial in its tissue of origin.

The tumor had, however, been reported prior to 1955 under different names such as:[62]

- Ameloblastoma of unusual type with calcification
- Calcifying ameloblastoma
- Malignant odontoma
- Adenoid adamantoblastoma
- Cystic complex odontoma
- As a variant of the simple ameloblastoma.

The Pindborg's tumor is classified as an uncommon, benign, odontogenic neoplasm that is exclusively epithelial in its tissue of origin.

Epidemiology[63,64]

The calcifying epithelial odontogenic tumor is generally considered a rare odontogenic neoplasm. The age range of all patients with CEOT varies between 8 and 92 years at the time of diagnosis with a mean of 36.9 years. However, if the tumor is divided according to the two topographical variants, the age ranges and means are as follows:

- Intraosseous type (range 8–92, mean 38.9 years)
- Extraosseous type (range 12–64, mean 34.4 years).

Almost two-thirds (64%) of the intraosseous variants are found in the third, fourth and fifth decades of life. The male : female ratio is almost same and there is no gender predilection. There is predilection for the premolar/molar region, although any site may be involved. Peripheral lesions usually occur in the anterior gingiva. Most cases are intraosseous and approximately 6 percent arise in extraosseous locations. Intraosseous lesions affect the mandible more often than the maxilla with a ratio of 2 : 1.

Clinical Features[65,66]

Pindborg tumor begins asymptomatically and consequently may be discovered only through routine radiographic examinations by the dentist. It is a slow-growing, painless, expansile, hard, bony swelling causing cortical bone to become egg-shell thin before perforation and subsequent soft tissue infiltration takes place.

Pindborg tumor may potentially cause associated tooth tipping, rotation, migration and/or mobility secondary to root resorption. Just as there is an uncommon peripheral variant of ameloblastoma, so there is also a distinctly uncommon peripheral variant of Pindborg tumor, limited to soft tissue only that presents clinically as a nodular mass on gingival mucosa, frequently in the anterior region.

Radiographic Features[67]

The Pindborg tumor displays a range of radiographic features with regards to lesion size and bone pattern. On examination of routine dental radiographic images (periapical, occlusal, panoral and plain film skull), Pindborg tumor may be completely radiolucent in character or in the case of more mature lesions, exhibit a mixed radiolucent and radiopaque appearance (Figs 28.18A to C).

When present, the radiopacities from the calcifications in this tumor are said to resemble 'wind driven snow' (Figs 28.19A and B), according to Pindborg.

Pindborg's tumor may be unilocular and cystic in appearance (Fig. 28.18B), often associated with an unerupted tooth or more characteristically demonstrate a mixture of small and large multilocular spaces described respectively as 'honeycomb' or 'soap bubble' in appearance (Figs 28.18A and B). In almost all cases, the radiographic border between tumor and surrounding bone appears to be well defined and circumscribed.

On CT examination, calcifying epithelial odontogenic tumor has been reported in the mandible as demonstrating expansion and thinning of buccal and lingual cortical plates by a well-defined mass containing scattered radiopaque areas of varying size and signal intensity.

When Pindborg tumor is analyzed by MRI, it reveals predominantly a hypo- intense lesion on T1-weighted images and a mixed hyperintense lesion on T2-weighted images.

Pathogenesis[68]

The tumor develops from the reduced enamel organ. Some have suggested that the epithelial cells of the Pindborg tumor are reminiscent of the sequestered cells in the stratum intermedium layer of the enamel organ in tooth development or odontogenesis. Therefore, based on this cytological similarity, the calcifying epithelial odontogenic tumor is supposed to arise from stratum intermedium cells. Furthermore, some oral and maxillofacial pathologists have suggested that amyloid deposition within Pindborg tumors is an immunologic response to these stratum intermedium cells that have been previously sequestered from exposure, which as neoplastic cells are now exposed and unrecognized as host tissue.

With the appearance of reported cases of intraosseous CEOT without an associated unerupted tooth and cases of the peripheral variant, it became evident that sources other than reduced enamel epithelium should be considered while discussing the histogenesis of CEOT.

The peripheral location strongly suggests the possibility that the tumor arises from remnents of the dental lamina or from the basal cells of the oral epithelium.

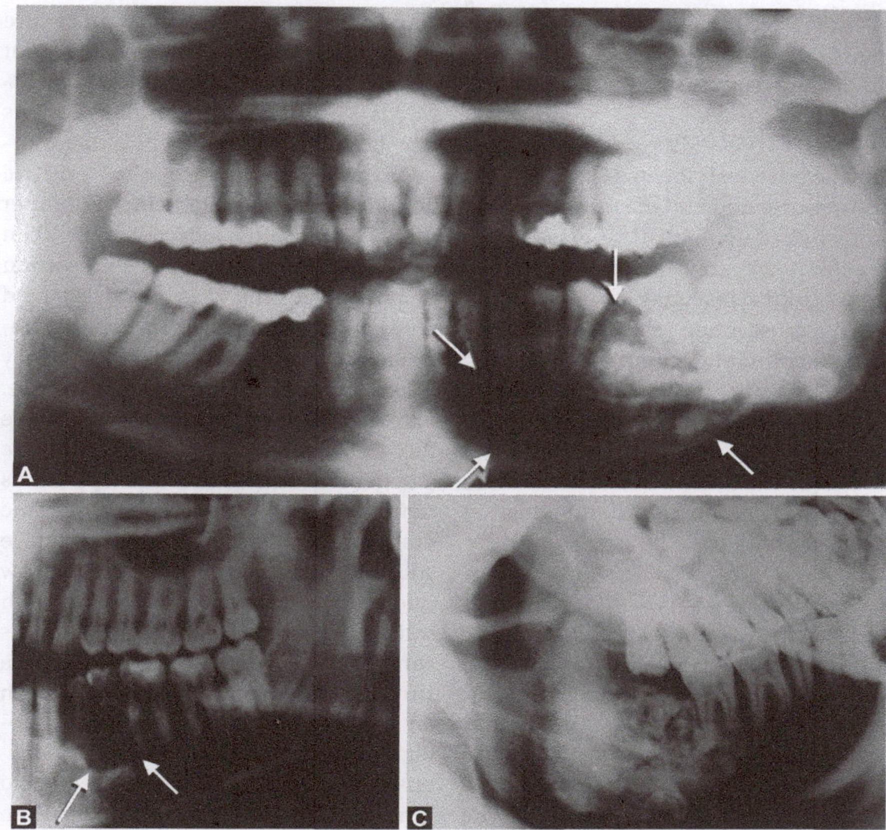

Figs 28.18A to C: Segment of panoramic radiograph showing mixed radiolucent and radiopaque lesion of the posterior body of the mandible

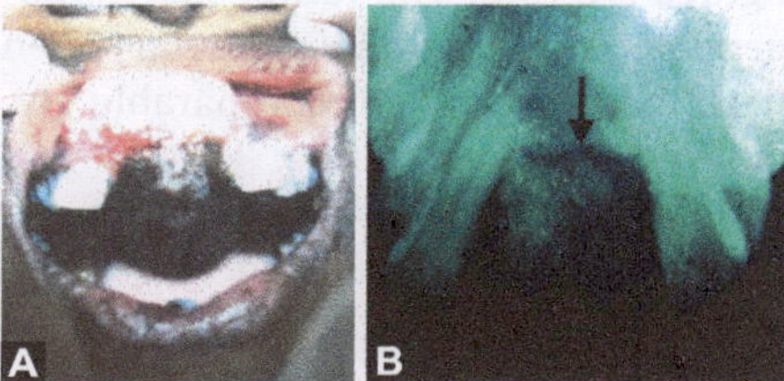

Figs 28.19A and B: Extraosseous CEOT involving anterior maxilla in 45-year-old female

In order to conceptualize a unified source of origin for the diverse locations of CEOT, one has to look for odontogenic epithelium with a widespread occurrence. Of all the possible candidates only one matches the requirements of widespread distribution, namely, the dental lamina complex or its remnants.

Disintegration of the complex system of dental lamina gives rise to a countless number of epithelial remnants persisting in the jawbones and gingiva after the completion of odontogenesis. The latter argument concerning the histogenesis seems relevant for several odontogenic tumors and hamartomatous lesions.

Gross Pathology

The intraosseously located CEOT is often easily enucleated and the tumor volume varies from 1 to 4 cm. The mass varies in color from grayish-white or yellow to tan pink. Bisecting the specimen reveals most often calcified particles giving a crunching sound while cutting. The tumor may be all solid or minute cystic spaces may be encountered. If associated with an unerupted tooth, the crown (or hard dental structures of an odontoma) can be found embedded in the tumor mass.

Microscopic Features

The calcifying epithelial odontogenic tumor consists of polyhedral epithelial cells, in either compact sheets or scattered small islands, in a fibrous connective tissue stroma. The cells have eosinophilic granular cytoplasm and prominent intercellular bridges. The nuclei are often hyperchromatic with pleomorphism. The giant nuclei and multinucleation is common but mitotic figures are rare. The tumor has homogeneous, eosinophilic material often described as amyloid, comparable glycoprotein, basal lamina, keratin and enamel matrix. The calcification in Liesegang fashion is present.

Treatment[69]

There are a variety of alternative surgical treatment methods to successfully manage Pindborg tumors. Treatment is dependent on the size and location of the neoplasm, the patient's overall medical condition or tolerance to withstand the surgical procedure and the skill or experience level of the operator.

Small, intrabony mandibular lesions with well-defined borders may possibly be cured by simple complete, but conservative tumor enucleation or curettage followed by judicious removal of a thin layer of bone adjacent to the tumor. This operation characteristically enjoys a significantly lower recurrence rate than could be expected for a similar procedure performed in treatment of a solid variant or multilocular ameloblastoma (10–15% versus 35–40%). Small maxillary lesions may be surgically excised by either thorough intrabony curettage or conservative en-bloc resection sacrificing a thinner margin of healthy adjacent bone than would normally be required for resection of ameloblastoma. Lesions designated recurrences following conservative approaches like intrabony curettage may in fact represent persistence of disease. Like ameloblastoma, small infiltrative foci of Pindborg tumor may insinuate along bony trabeculae and appear as uninvolved bone radiographically. Some oral and maxillofacial pathologists have suggested that even with an expected low rate of local recurrence compared with solid ameloblastoma, maxillary tumors can be treated more aggressively than a similar-sized lesion in the mandible, with an opportunity to confirm histopathologically tumor-free bone margins. Obviously, recurrent or persistent disease and tumors diagnosed late in the duration of their clinical course, which over an extended time have become larger and more extensive (greater than 4 cm), may not be curable by conservative surgical measures such as en-bloc resection only. Consequently, segmental resections such as partial or hemimandibulectomy or hemimaxillectomy—which leave a significant bone discontinuity requiring either distraction osteogenesis or, more likely, graft and reconstruction procedures may be required.

Treatment of histopathologically atypical or frankly malignant calcifying epithelial odontogenic tumors is limited by the paucity of cases reported. Robert K Goode[70] advocates early intervention before such a lesion could escape the confines of the involved mandible or maxilla (stage 1 and 2 disease). The size and extent of tumor determine the appropriate surgical operation needed to achieve complete assured removal of all neoplastic tissue with a generous histopathologically confirmed tumor-free margin in all directions. This generally requires radical resection of the affected jaw portion and any associated soft tissues with no less than 1 cm in every direction, as might be performed for any other variant of odontogenic carcinoma (carcinoma arising in a long standing odontogenic cyst, ameloblastic carcinoma or clear cell odontogenic carcinoma). Adjunctive external beam radiation therapy is advocated following determination of local spread to cervical lymph nodes and adjunctive chemotherapy may play some role in control of distant organ metastasis in some patients. Radiotherapy in lieu of surgical resection is contraindicated as a recommended treatment for Pindborg tumor, because osteoradionecrosis, xerostomia and radiation-induced malignancy present as serious complications of this therapy.

Treatment of peripheral Pindborg tumors as advocated by Houston and Fowler[71] is simple local excision based on their review of pertinent literature.

Prognosis

Most studies of Pindborg tumor report a local recurrence rate of between 10 and 20 percent following conservative, but complete removal of the lesion. Like ameloblastoma, the time interval between initial and recurrent tumor may be measured in years or decades, making routine annual follow-up examination with radiographic survey a prudent measure.

Bouckaert MMR, Raubenheimer EJ, Jacobs FJ[72] (2000) reported one case of advanced disease in the patient's maxilla resulted in local extension to the brain.

The incidence of malignant transformation to odontogenic carcinoma ex-Pindborg tumor is extremely low and should be considered distinctly rare. To date, only three such cases that either suggested this outcome or definitely rendered such a diagnosis have been reported in the literature. No follow-up information is available.

With regard to peripheral Pindborg tumors, no recurrence has been reported in the 11 cases known to have been treated with simple local excision.

SQUAMOUS ODONTOGENIC TUMORS

Introduction

The squamous odontogenic tumor is "*A benign, but locally infiltrative neoplasm consisting of islands of well-differentiated squamous epithelium in a fibrous stroma. The epithelial islands occasionally show foci of central cystic degeneration*" (WHO). It was first described by Pullon et al.[73] in 1975.

Before 1975, the squamous odontogenic tumor was reported under a variety of names such as:

- Benign epithelial odontogenic tumor
- Acanthomatous ameloblastoma
- Hyperplasia and squamous metaplasia of residual
- Odontogenic epithelium acanthomatous ameloblastic fibroma
- Benign odontogenic tumor, unclassified.

These names were given due to the presence of islands of squamous epithelium, which have a morphologic similarity to that seen in the follicular pattern of ameloblastoma. Its inclusion as a separate entity in a classification of odontogenic tumors is based on its characteristic histologic features and distinct biologic entity.

It is a rare, sometimes multifocal, benign epithelial odontogenic tumor, consisting of islands of stratified squamous epithelium that commonly contain microcysts and calcifications in a dense fibrous background.

History

Pullon et al.[73] (1975) called attention to the possible hamartomatous nature of the squamous odontogenic tumor because of multiple site involvement in one of their cases.

The multicentric lesions have typically exhibited a less aggressive biological behavior. Unal et al.[74] (1987) suggested using the term 'squamous odontogenic hamartomatoid lesion', for squamous odontogenic tumor-like islands in the walls of the odontogenic cyst. Most investigators believe that it is a hamartomatous epithelial proliferation, probably arising from cell rests of Malassez. Recurrences have been recorded by Pullon et al.[73] but they seem to be extremely rare and are most likely results of insufficient initial removal.

Histogenesis

The histogenesis of the squamous odontogenic tumor may be multifactorial.

Intraosseous

- The lesions associated with the alveolar process adjacent to the lateral root surface of the teeth: Rests of Malassez is the source of epithelial proliferation.
- The lesions developed in association with the crowns of unerupted or impacted teeth: dental lamina may be the source.

Extraosseous

Surface stratified squamous epithelium (dropping off effect) and from the Rests of Serres.[75]

Features

Clinical Features

The reported incidence peaks in third decade of life however; wide age range (8–74 years) is reported. It is more common in males than the females. It occurs throughout the alveolar processes of the maxilla and mandible with no site of predilection. A few patients have been reported to have multiple squamous odontogenic tumor that involved several quadrants of the mouth. It involves the maxilla and mandible with equal frequency. In maxilla incisor-cuspid area and in mandible bicuspid-molar area are more commonly involved. It presents as a painless or mildly painful gingival swelling associated with mobility of associated teeth as the most common complaint.

Radiographic Features

No radiographic features are sufficiently characteristic to suggest the diagnosis. The reported cases have exhibited a triangular or semicircular radiolucency located in the alveolar bone along the lateral surface of the roots with the narrow portion (apex) towards the alveolar crest. In some instances this suggests vertical bone loss. The radiolucent area is somewhat ill defined or may show well-defined sclerotic margins. They are mostly small lesions, up to 1.5 cm in diameter.

The tooth mobility may be a presenting symptom. If crestal bone has been destroyed, the lesion may mimic alveolar bone loss seen in chronic periodontitis. Other documented cases presented as pericoronal radiolucency associated with an impacted or unerupted tooth.

Peripheral lesions may cause saucerization of underlying bone, which is likely to be a pressure phenomenon rather than the result of true tumor infiltration.

No periodontal ligament can be visualized between the lesion and the root of the tooth, suggesting that lesion arises from cell rests of Malassez in the periodontal ligament or closely adjacent mucous membrane.

Some of the rare extensive lesions may have a multilocular appearance involving the body of the mandible or pushing aside the maxillary sinus.

Differential Diagnosis

Squamous odontogenic tumor may be overdiagnosed as:

- Ameloblastoma particularly acanthomatous and the desmoplastic variant
- Well-differentiated squamous cell carcinoma.

Acanthomatous and the Desmoplastic Variant

Both exhibit squamous differentiation within the tumor islands, but there is demonstrable ameloblastic change of the peripheral cells, including:

- Columnar shape
- Polarization of elongated nuclei away from the basement membrane
- Vacuolated or clear cytoplasm.

These changes are less evident in squamous odontogenic tumor. In which the peripheral cell layer is composed of flat to cuboidal cells.

The islands and strands of desmoplastic ameloblastoma often are thin and compressed rather than rounded and broad shaped as seen in squamous odontogenic tumor. The squamoid areas in desmoplastic ameloblastoma often exhibit swirls of squamous cells, which are not seen in squamous odontogenic tumor.

Well Differentiated Squamous Cell Carcinoma

- The islands in squamous odontogenic tumor are well defined and the cells lack variation in cell size, shape and nuclear staining characteristics that are seen in squamous cell carcinoma.
- Mitotic figures are rare to nonexistent in squamous odontogenic tumor and atypical, mitotic figures or chromatin abnormalities are not seen.
- Significant keratin formation also is not typical.
- Occasionally dentigerous, apical periodontal (radicular) cysts and periodontal granulomatous tissue exhibit foci of squamous odontogenic tumor-like proliferation. These characteristics have been interpreted as a neoplastic, reactive process that is secondary to cyst formation or inflammation.[74,76]
- Definitive criteria differentiating this reactive proliferation from the neoplastic process have not been established but Melrose[77] (1999) indicates that, the reactive islands seldom form microcysts or contain intraepithelial calcifications.
- Reactive foci of squamous odontogenic tumor within the connective tissue wall of odontogenic cysts do not appear to cause any alteration in the usual biologic behavior of the cyst and do not appear to develop into the tumor.

Treatment and Prognosis

Enucleation, curettage and local excision are treatment modalities that most often are described in case reports of squamous odontogenic tumor. Clinically, aggressive lesions have been treated by en bloc excision. Ide has reported a case in which a squamous cell carcinoma was associated with a squamous odontogenic tumor[78] and Norris[79] reported a case of bilateral maxillary squamous odontogenic tumor in a patient with a mandibular intraosseous carcinoma. It could not be confirmed that the mandibular squamous cell carcinoma developed within a squamous odontogenic tumor. In their review of literature, Baden et al.[80] noted two recurrences.

ADENOMATOID ODONTOGENIC TUMOR

Introduction

The adenomatoid odontogenic tumor (AOT) is included in classifications of odontogenic tumors because it occurs only in the tooth-bearing area of the jaws and because of its histomorphologic resemblance to components of the dental organ (tooth germ). The AOT is a locally invasive neoplasm characterized by ameloblastoma like islands of epithelial cells in a mature connective tissue stroma. Abberant keratinization may be found in the form of ghost cells in association with varying amounts of dysplastic dentin (WHO). AOT generally is considered to be an uncommon tumor. Its distinctive, although not pathognomonic, clinicopathologic profile is unique among odontogenic tumors because most lesions occur in association with an unerupted maxillary cuspid in teenage girls. The so-called 'duct-like structures' are a unique (although not always present) microscopic feature of AOT. No unequivocal recurrences have been reported despite known incomplete removal of some tumors.

Philipsen and Birn[81] in 1969 gave the name 'Adenomatoid Odontogenic Tumor' to this condition and previously it was described by variety of names such as adamantoma, 'adenoadamantoblastoma' or 'adamantoblastoma, adenoma type', 'adenoameloblastoma', 'adenomatoid ameloblastoma', 'adenomatoid odontoma', 'ameloblastic adenomatoid tumor', 'odontogenic adenomatoid tumor'.

Hamartoma Versus Neoplasm

Previously, the AOT was considered to be a hamartoma because of its limited size in most cases (attributed to its minimal growth potential) and lack of recurrence (even following definitely incomplete removal). AOT is considered to be a non-invasive benign neoplasm presumably because the limited size in most of the cases is due to the fact that they are detected early (often, on a routine dental radiograph) and removed before the slow-growing tumor reaches a clinically noticeable size. They also point to the considerable size of some reported cases that had gone undetected or untreated for many years. Additional support comes from the microscopic features of the lesional tissue that show greater departure from the arrangement of the normal odontogenic apparatus than should be expected in a developmental anomaly. AOT is "most appropriately considered a benign embryonal neoplasm."[82]

Epidemiology

The incidence and prevalence of odontogenic tumors is unknown, largely because most of them are benign and are not reported to local, regional or national tumor registries that compile and track malignant tumors. AOT accounts for approximately 3 to 7 percent[83,84] of odontogenic tumors that are accessioned by a variety of institutions around the world, which makes it the 4th or 5th among the odontogenic tumors, only surpassed by odontomas, myxomas, ameloblastomas and cemento-osseous tumors.

Demographic Features

Age[83,84]

Although AOT has been reported in patients from 3 to 82 years of age, its predilection for young patients is well-established.

It is unique among odontogenic tumors and unexplainable that:

- More than two-thirds (69%) are diagnosed between the ages of 10 and 19 years
- More than half (53%) are diagnosed in teenagers
- Twenty-one percent are diagnosed between ages 20 and 29
- Altogether, 88 percent are diagnosed in the second and third decades.

Pericoronal (dentigerous, follicular) AOTs are diagnosed at an earlier age than lesions that are not in a pericoronal relationship to a tooth, probably because affected patients seek consultation concerning failure of the associated tooth to erupt. The early detection of gingival (peripheral, extraosseous) AOTs is likely due to the discovery of a variably obvious anterior maxillary gingival mass. Although the average age at the time of excision of gingival lesions is 13 years (and ranges from 3 to 19 years), the fact that some lesions had already been present for 3 to 5 years suggests that gingival AOTs develop at an early age.

Gender[83,84]

The tumor is diagnosed approximately twice as frequently in women. Although in the third decade AOT is nearly four times more frequent in women, in patients who are older than age 30 it is diagnosed nearly twice as commonly in men. It also is interesting and unexplainable that the female : male ratio for gingival lesions is 1.4 : 1.

Location

The AOT appears in three clinicotopographic variations:

a. Intrabony or central (including both follicular and extrafollicular) constitute 96 percent of all AOTs, out of which, follicular are 71 percent.
b. Commonly found in maxilla than in the mandible with a total ratio of 2.1:1.

Peripheral

They are a rare type and constitute 4.4 percent of all reported AOT cases. They almost exclusively occur in the anterior upper jaw (88%). They are detected earlier than the AOTs of follicular or extrafollicular type as they are peripheral and more conspicuous.

The peripheral AOT are often found associated with unerupted permanent teeth. Unerupted permanent teeth found in association with the follicular AOT, are all four canines accounting for 59 percent and the maxillary canine alone for 40 percent.

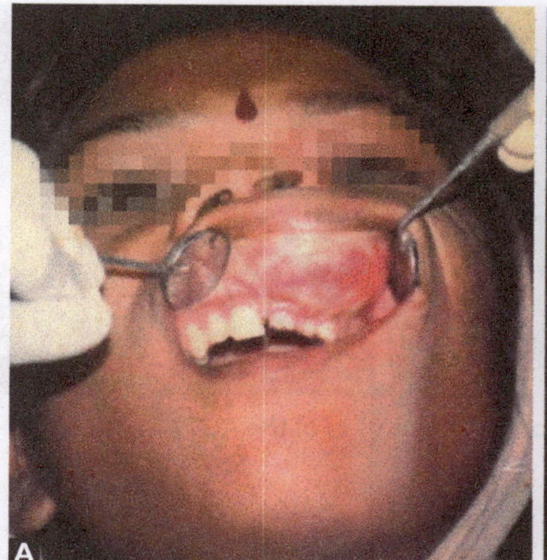

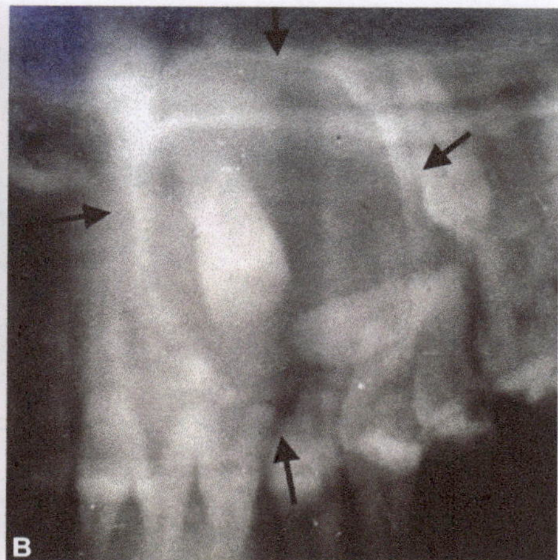

Figs 28.20A and B: AOT involving the maxillary anterior area in a 20-year-old female

Clinical Features

Usually, AOTs are asymptomatic; however, the tumor is commonly present in the anterior maxillary region, especially in younger patients. Patients may be aware of a gingival swelling or an area of jaw enlargement. The teeth in the involved area are missing as they are embedded in the lesion. Nasal obstruction is reported in conjunction with rarely encountered large maxillary lesions. Gingival lesions most often are painless and slow growing.

Clinical Signs

Most central lesions are discovered on routine dental radiographic examination; however, delayed eruption of (especially an anterior maxillary) permanent teeth or slow-growing bony expansion (with or without displacement of adjacent teeth) commonly leads to the discovery of the intragnathic AOTs. The mobility of teeth, swelling of the cheek[85] and asymmetrical facial swelling has been reported less frequently (Fig. 28.20A).

Peripheral lesions present as a gingival-colored mass that ranges from 1 to 1.5 mm in diameter (the size was listed in only 4 of 18 reported cases). They are 10 times more prevalent in the maxillary gingiva than in the mandibular gingiva; all but 3 of the 18 reported cases were located adjacent to an incisor—usually the maxillary central incisor.[84]

Clinical Differential Diagnosis

The diffuse swelling that can accompany central lesions is clinically indistinguishable from the maxillary or mandibular enlargement that may occur with:

- Central odontogenic cysts and tumors as well as
- Benign fibro-osseous lesions
- Benign mesenchymal neoplasms.

As a result, radiographic evaluation is indicated to narrow the differential diagnostic considerations.

Gingival lesions cannot be differentiated clinically from gingival fibromas, peripheral cemento-ossifying fibromas, peripheral giant cell lesions or from other peripheral odontogenic tumors such as odontogenic fibroma, ameloblastoma, calcifying odontogenic cyst and calcifying epithelial odontogenic tumor.

Diagnosis

Radiographic Features

A significant number of AOTs are discovered radiographically because more

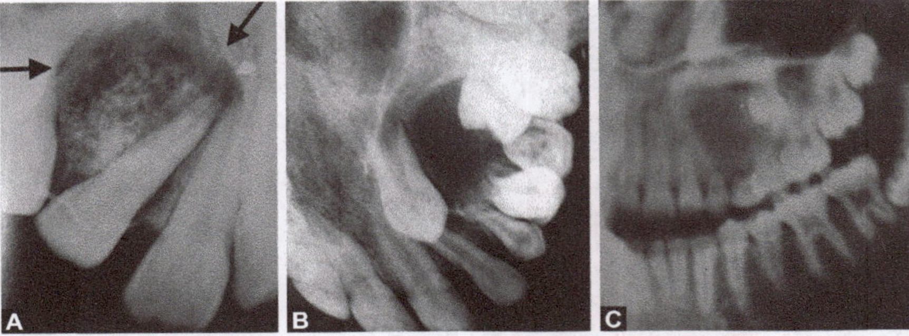

Figs 28.21A to C: Radiographic presentation of the AOT

than 95 percent occur intraosseously (centrally), usually as small asymptomatic lesions.

The central AOTs present as a well demarcated, almost always unilocular radiolucency that generally exhibit a smooth corticated border (Fig. 28.20B). Most lesions are pericoronal or juxta coronal, but the radiolucency may extend apically beyond the CE junction on at least one side of the root. Rare, multilocular cases have been reported and the scalloped borders are observed occasionally. Most cases are between 1 and 3 cm in the greatest diameter. About 65 percent of reported cases also demonstrate faintly detectable radiopaque foci within the radiolucent lesion. Occasionally, a more obvious intralesional radiopacity may be identified. Divergence of roots and displacement of teeth occurs more frequently than the root resorption.

About 71 percent of AOTs are associated with the crown of an unerupted permanent tooth, including about 6 percent that are associated with two or more unerupted teeth (Fig. 28.20B). Nearly 60 percent of AOTs are associated with cuspids—40 percent with the maxillary cuspids (Figs 28.21A to C).

Macroscopic Features

Unmagnified gross examination of most excisional surgical specimens of central AOTs reveal a soft, roughly spherical mass with a discernible fibrous capsule. Upon gross sectioning, the tumor may exhibit white to tan solid to crumbly tissue or one or more cystic spaces of varying size; minimal yellow brown fluid to semisolid material; fine, hard 'gritty' granular material; and one to several larger calcified masses.

Microscopic Features

The AOTs exhibit diverse histological features. The tumor is composed of multinodular proliferation of the spindle, cuboidal and columnar cells in a variety of patterns comprising of scattered duct-like structures, eosinophilic material and calcification in several forms, delimited by fibrous capsule of variable thickness. The typical feature of AOT is numerous duct-like structures with lumina of variable size, which are lined by single-layered cuboidal or columnar cells with the nuclei situated away from the lumen. The duct-like or microcyst lumina are frequently lined by a band of eosinophilic material of varying thickness called hyaline rings. Some AOTs contain varying amount of dysplastic dentin, dentinoid and osteodentin. Irregular round calcified bodies, which may exhibit areas with a concentric layered pattern (Liesegang rings) may be seen in the parenchymal or stromal zones.

Treatment

Surgical Findings

Although there may be expansion of the alveolar bone overlying central lesions, the cortex is almost invariably intact; however, on rare occasions, penetration of the cortical plate has been reported. Essentially all cases have a smooth, well-defined capsule of varying thickness.

Enucleation and Curettage

As the tumor is well encapsulated and usually present in the anterior maxilla, the surgical access is simple. The tumor is easily shelled out from the bone and in most of the cases can be enucleated in total.

Prognosis

Adenomatoid odontogenic tumor almost is always referred to as 'slow' or 'very-slowly growing' but no report of measurements of growth rate over a course of time could be located. The recurrence after adequate enucleation is not common.

AMELOBLASTIC FIBROMA

Ameloblastic fibroma is a relatively rare true mixed tumor in which epithelial and the ectomesenchymal elements are neoplastic. The lesion was first reported by 'Kruse'[86] in 1891. It is an uncommon tumor and represents only 2 percent of odontogenic tumors, but the data regarding its frequency are difficult to evaluate because (particularly in earlier reports) some lesions that are diagnosed as ameloblastic fibroma may actually have represented the early developing stage of an odontoma. It is characterized by the simultaneous neoplastic proliferation of the mesenchymal and epithelial components without formation of dental hard tissues namely dentin and enamel. Ameloblastic fibroma and related lesions were defined by the WHO as:

- Ameloblastic fibroma consists of odontogenic ecto-mesenchyme resembling the dental papilla and epithelial strands and nests resembling dental lamina and enamel organ.
- No dental hard tissue is present.
- If there is dentin formation, the lesion is referred to as ameloblastic fibrodentinoma.

In older literature, it is reported as '*soft mixed odontoma*' as it was believed that it could mature into an odontoma.

Pathogenesis

- It is believed to arise *de novo* during odontogenesis, possibly as a result of

overproduction of the basal lamina without odontogenic differentiation.
- Lesions composed of similar elements, but in which inductive change has resulted in the deposition of dentin alone or dentin plus enamel, are termed ameloblastic fibrodentinoma and ameloblastic fibro-odontoma respectively.

Controversy

Regarding the belief, that these lesions represent separate entities or are the same lesion in a continuum representing different stages of evolution. Cahn and Blum[87] (1952) postulated that ameloblastic fibroma represented the least histologically differentiated lesion that evolves from a moderately differentiated form, ameloblastic fibro-odontoma to odontoma. However, this concept is not widely accepted. Some investigators believe that ameloblastic fibroma and ameloblastic fibro-odontoma are variations of the same process. And some authors consider that ameloblastic fibro-odontoma is a variant of ameloblastic fibroma.

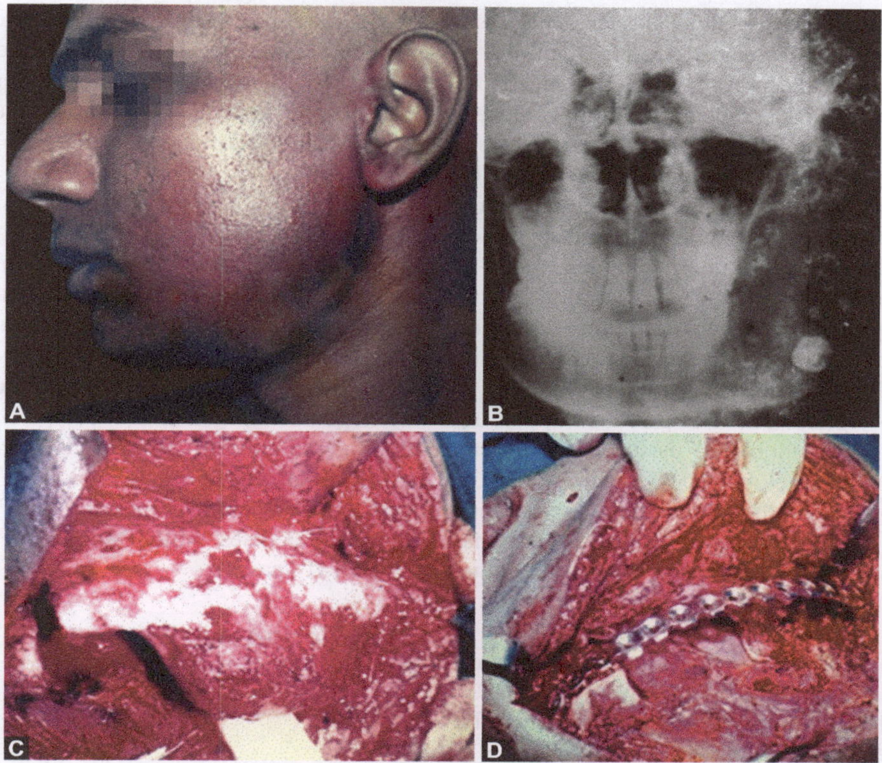

Figs 28.22A to D: Ameloblastic fibroma in a 35-year-old man

Clinical Features

It is predominantly found in children and young adults, usually within an age range of 6 months to 42 years (average age: 14.6–15.5 years), the mean age being 14.8 years.[88] It also has been reported in a 7-week-old infant (Mosby EL[89] 1998). Trodahl[90] (1972) reported that there is no gender predilection. Other authors reported a slight male bias. The posterior mandible is the most common site and about 70 percent of cases are located in the first permanent molar and second primary molar area while the remaining cases are in the posterior maxilla and rarely in the anterior region of the jaws (Figs 28.22A to D).[91]

Ameloblastic fibroma is a painless, slow growing and expansile neoplasm. About 20 percent of the lesions are discovered on routine radiography. Ameloblastic fibroma exhibits slower clinical growth than ameloblastomas and does not tend to infiltrate bone. It enlarges by gradual expansion so that the periphery of the lesion often remains smooth. Initial presentation may include pain, tenderness or mild swelling of the jaws. It is associated with an impacted tooth in about 75 percent of the cases.

Radiographic Features

It appears as a well-defined, unilocular or multilocular radiolucency with a smooth, well defined outline and often with a sclerotic opaque border. The large mandibular lesions are multilocular, whereas smaller lesions are typically unilocular (Fig. 28.22B). They may range in size from 1 to 8 mm.

Trodahl[90] reported no constant significant differences between the appearance of the simple ameloblastoma and that of ameloblastic fibroma. It may mimic a dentigerous cyst when associated with unerupted teeth. Radiographic evidence of cortical expansion of bone may not be seen in all cases.

Histogenesis

Ameloblastic fibroma arises from odontogenic epithelial and mesenchymal cells of the enamel organ and dental papilla, respectively. It appears to be a true mixed tumor and it is noticeable that, unlike the histologically somewhat similar, appearing ameloblastoma, malignant change in ameloblastic fibroma affects the mesenchymal component and not the epithelium.

Rare Variants of Ameloblastic Fibroma

Granular Cell Ameloblastic Fibroma

Couch et al.[92,93] 1962 reported 2 cases of central mandibular lesions composed of large round to polygonal stromal cells with finely granular, eosinophilic cytoplasm and small, often eccentrically located, ovoid to round nuclei. These granular cells were arranged in lobules separated by thin, fibrous connective tissue septa. Within the lobules of granular cells were small ovoid to sometimes elongated islands of cuboidal to columnar epithelial cells, with basal to centrally located nuclei. The center of large collections of epithelial cells had a loose stellate reticulum like appearance.

He concluded that, the lesions were ameloblastic fibromas characterized by differentiation of the mesenchymal component into granular cells and suggested the name 'granular cell ameloblastic fibroma'. White et al. (1978) thought that granular cell ameloblastic fibromas could not represent variants of the ameloblastic fibroma due to following reasons:

- The absence of primitive appearing mesenchymal tissue, characteristic of ameloblastic fibroma
- No proliferative activity of the strands of odontogenic epithelium or histodifferentiation towards enamel organ-like structures as observed in ameloblastic fibroma.

They called the lesion 'Central granular cell tumor of the jaws' (White DK[94] 1978). Others suggested: 'Central granular cell odontogenic fibroma' (Vincent SD[95] 1987) or 'Central odontogenic fibroma, granular cell variant' (Shiro BC[96] 1989).

Clinical features

The granular cell ameloblastic fibroma is most common in woman and occurs between 50 and 60 years of age. The mandible is more commonly involved than the maxilla. It is common in molar-premolar region and is mostly centrally located.

Radiological features

It presents as a radiolucent lesion, with well defined or sometimes irregular borders.

Histopathological features

The ultrastructural findings of granular cell ameloblastic fibroma, first reported by White et al. 1978, described that their findings indicated the granular cells were of connective tissue origin and identical to the cells in the granular cell myoblastoma. Takeda Y 199997 also reveals that, the granular cells were of mesenchymal origin. The presence of numerous intracytoplasmic lysosomal granules and absence of organelles in the granular cells may suggest the cells are degenerative rather than neoplastic in nature. Such hypothesis is supported by the fact that no recurrences after surgical treatment of the lesions have been documented in the literature.

Peripheral Ameloblastic Fibroma

The peripheral ameloblastoma is an extremely rare lesion. In making a histopathologic diagnosis of peripheral ameloblastic fibroma, a distinction between this lesion and the peripheral odontogenic fibroma of WHO type or odontogenic gingival epithelial hamartoma (hamartoma of the dental lamina) needs to be made. (Abughazaleh K[98] mentioned 3 cases, while Darling MR[99] mentioned 4 cases).

Interrelationship between Ameloblastic Fibroma and Other Mixed Odontogenic Tumors

Ameloblastic Fibrodentinoma

Ameloblastic fibrodentinoma is defined 'a neoplasm similar to ameloblastic fibroma, but also showing inductive changes that lead to the formation of dentin.' It is thought that ameloblastic fibrodentinoma is a histologic variant of ameloblastic fibroma in which dentin or dentinoid tissue has formed. In some cases diagnosed as ameloblastic fibrodentinoma, dentin matrix or dentinoid tissue is an area of hyalinization around epithelial component and some workers have suggested that such hyalinized zone may not represent a dentin formation.

In other cases a hyalinized area containing entrapped cells has been considered to be an abortive dentin or dentinoid tissue because of its proximity to odontogenic epithelium, the margins of such zone often shows radially arranged coarse fiber bundles with elongated cells and rarely found tubular structure. It is important to realize that there is no evidence that such ameloblastic fibromas with hyalinization or abortive dentin exhibit a different biologic behavior than ordinary ameloblastic fibroma.

In a revised WHO classification of odontogenic tumors, the term 'ameloblastic fibrodentinoma' and 'dentinoma' are used synonymously.

Ameloblastic Fibro-odontoma

Hooker[100] (1967) made an important contribution to the understanding of odontogenic tumors when he showed that two separate tumors with different clinical behavior were previously grouped, together under the term ameloblastic odontoma. He differentiated ameloblastic fibro-odontoma from the ameloblastic odontoma and used the term ameloblastic odontoma for the more aggressive tumors composed of an ameloblastoma and a compound or complex odontoma. The latter, which behaves in the typically invasive manner of the classic ameloblastoma, has been termed odontoameloblastoma.

The revised WHO classification of odontogenic tumor defines ameloblastic fibro-odontoma as *"a lesion similar to ameloblastic fibroma, but showing inductive changes that lead to formation of dentin and enamel."*

The lesion represents approximately 1 to 3 percent of odontogenic tumors, however, if patients younger than 16 years are considered, ameloblastic fibro-odontoma comprises about 7 percent of odontogenic tumors. About 80 cases have been reported in the literature, including a literature review of the 50 cases published by Slootweg[101] (1981).

Clinical features

Ameloblastic fibro-odontoma usually is diagnosed in the first two decades of life. Philipsen et al. 1997 reported that the average age in 86 cases was 9 years. It has a slight male predilection. Most tumors are found in the posterior mandible, the second most popular location being the posterior maxilla. It is an exclusively central or intraosseous lesion. It usually presents as a painless, slow-growing expansile lesion and often presents with swelling and failure of tooth eruption. Most ameloblastic fibro-odontomas are associated with an unerupted tooth.

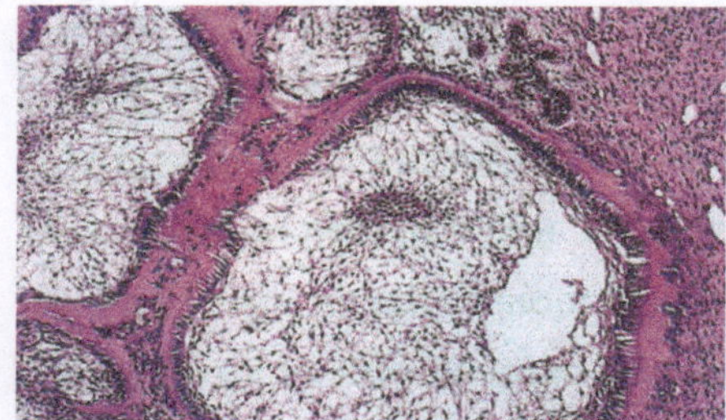

Fig. 28.23: Ameloblastic fibro-odontoma showing induction of a thin rim of atubular dentin in the stroma by the ameloblast-like cells

Radiographic features

Ameloblastic fibro-odontoma presents as a well-circumscribed expansile radiolucency that generally contains solitary or multiple small radiopaque foci, which represent the calcified product in the lesion.

- Most lesions are relatively small when first detected and are not more than 1 to 2 cm in size.
- Occasionally, large tumors involving the entire body and ramus of the mandible have been reported.
- Miller et al. (1976) described a case in which the calcified portion of the lesion alone measured 6 cm × 7 cm, causing significant facial deformity.

Histopathologic features

The tumor is composed of strands, cords and islands of odontogenic epithelium distributed in a cell-rich, dental papilla-like ectomesenchymal stroma. Varying amounts of osteodentin or dentin-like material and occasionally enamel matrix can be identified. The odontogenic epithelium adjacent to the enamel matrix seems to be preameloblast like. More calcified lesions exhibit mature dental hard tissues that resemble rudimentary teeth or a conglomerate of enamel and dentin (Fig. 28.23).

Treatment and prognosis

Conservative surgical enucleation is considered to be the treatment of choice with concurrent removal of the associated unerupted tooth. Extensive lesions causing severe undermining of the bone require segmental resection of the mandible (Figs 28.22A to D). When the hard tissue component in the tumor is minimal, the lesion should be removed conservatively without removal of the impacted tooth. A case of mandibular ameloblastic fibroma which was treated earlier by enucleation, and had recurrent tumor in the submadibular region, extending in the neck is shown in Figs 28.24A to E. The recurrent tumor was treated with excision. The tumor was perforating through the cortical perforation in the mandible and thus, has spillage in the soft tissue and recurrence. It is therefore recommended that when the ameloblastoma or its variants show cortical perforation, the dissection should be extended in the soft tissue to take care of the soft tissue extension of the tumor.

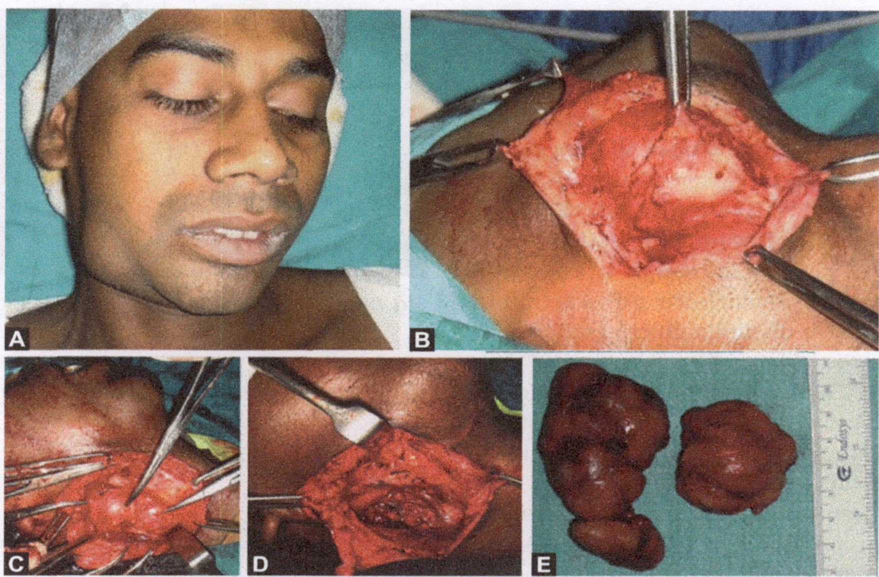

Figs 28.24A to E: Case of ameloblastic fibroma having recurrence locally and in the neck

ODONTOGENIC FIBROMA

Odontogenic fibroma has been included in the classification of odontogenic tumors dating back as early as 1941. In WHO classification of odontogenic neoplasm, the odontogenic fibroma appears under the subheading mesenchyme and/or odontogenic ectomesenchyme with or without odontogenic epithelium.

Definition

The odontogenic fibroma (OF) is a rare neoplasm characterized by varying amount of inactive looking odontogenic epithelium embedded in a mature, fibrous stroma (WHO).

Synonyms

Controversy[56] exists as to concept and definition. At present the term OF is applied to two histological types of lesions: The epithelium-poor type (formly termed simple type) and the epithelium-rich type (formerly termed complex or WHO type).

Epidemiology

- **Age:** When considering the epithelium—rich type, the age range was 11 to 66 years with a mean age of 40 years.
- **Gender:** Female predominance of 2.8:1.
- **Localization:** There were considerably more cases located in the mandible than in the maxilla, giving a maxilla to mandible ratio of 1:6.5. Of the mandibular lesions most involved were the molar and premolar areas and out of the maxillary lesions, only the anterior region was affected.

Pathogenesis

Some authors believe the central odontogenic fibroma to be derived from the ectomesenchymal tissue of the periodontal ligament, dental papilla or dental follicle. It is the epithelial component of the WHO type of central odontogenic fibroma and the fact that this tumor does not occur in an extragnathic location that provide the strongest argument for this tumor being of odontogenic origin. Gardner[102] stated that it is possible that the WHO type central odontogenic fibroma arises from the periodontal ligament, while the simple type is derived from the dental follicle, thus accounting for their dissimilar microscopic appearances.

The criteria for designating a central fibroma as odontogenic are still far from being defined. It may be difficult, if not impossible; to decide whether a central fibroma has arisen from the mesenchyme of the jaws rather than from the odontogenic apparatus. The presence of odontogenic epithelium embedded in the tumor tissue may be sufficient, because these structures are rarely found in the nonodontogenic jaw lesions. Some authors (WHO, Gardner) claim that the absence of odontogenic epithelial remnants does not preclude a central fibroma from being odontogenic.

Thus, the histoarchitecture of a particular central fibroma does not prove that the lesion is nonodontogenic unless the following characteristics are found: bundles of abundant collagen fibers separated by spindle-shaped fibroblasts with elongated or ovoid nuclei[103] combined with areas of delicate collagen fibers aggregating into focal tuft-like bundles and the absence of odontogenic epithelium and remanants of calcified material. If the morphologic pattern occurs in a central fibroma that has shown locally aggressive behavior, there is a considerable chance that the lesion is a non-odontogenic desmoplastic fibroma. It is, however possible that a central desmoplastic fibroma may infiltrate or expand into an unerupted tooth and in doing so be intimately associated with its crown. This situation should not be considered evidence of odontogenic origin, but must be regarded as coincidental.

Thus, the idea put forward by Gardner and supported by Slootweg and Muller that "every jaw fibroma is odontogenic if it does not clearly demonstrate the features (stated above) of a desmoplastic fibroma."

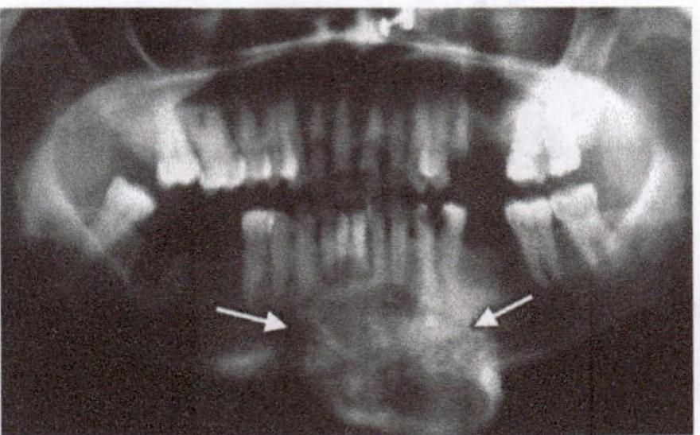

Fig. 28.25: Odontogenic fibroma involving anterior mandible

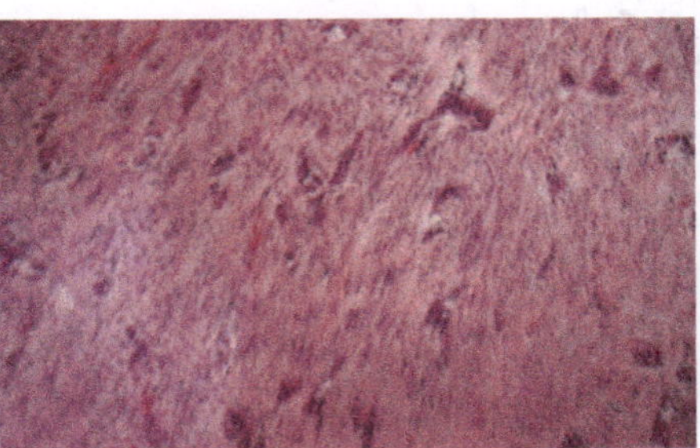

Fig. 28.26: Collagenous cell rich stroma with numerous strands of odontogenic epithelium without palisading of peripheral cells

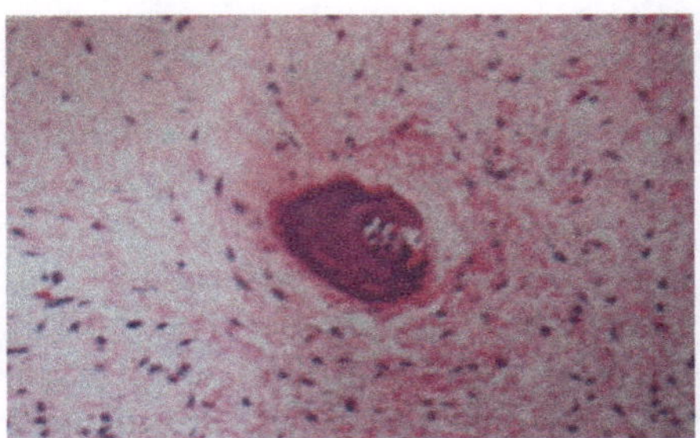

Fig. 28.27: Calcified material encircles and epithelial islands

Features

Clinical Features

The epithelium-rich type presents a slow growing, progressive but painless swelling, often with cortical expansion. The tumor is silent when small and painless swelling may announce its presence. A few patients may experience slight sensitivity. Janssen and Blijdorp[104] in their study reported an associated palatal depression. Flower et al. found that four of five lesions occurring in the anterior maxilla had a palatal cleft.

Radiographic Features

- The tumor appears as a unilocular radiolucent area with well-defined often-sclerotic borders (Fig. 28.25).
- Rarely, the occurrence of calcified material may produce a mixed radiolucent/radiopaque appearance.
- Larger lesions show scalloping of the margins.
- Many of the cases are locally aggressive and show external resorption of the roots, displacement of the tooth, tooth mobility, mucosal irritation and displacement of the inferior alveolar canal.
- Some tumors are associated with the crown of an unerupted tooth.

Histopathology

The epithelium-poor type of central odontogenic fibroma is a noninfiltrating connective tissue lesion resembling a dental follicle. It is minimally cellular with dispersed delicate collagen fibers. A considerable amount of ground substance produces a fibromyxoid quality to the background. Scattered remnants of inactive-looking odontogenic epithelium appear as small irregular islands and cords. Occasionally, variably formed calcifications occur (Figs 28.26 and 28.27).

The epithelium-rich type of central odontogenic fibroma is composed of cellular, fibroblastic connective tissue interwoven with less cellular and often vascular areas. Islands or strands of inactive—looking odontogenic epithelium are an integral component; they may be sparse but are often conspicuous. This shows foci of calcified material considered to be metaplastically produced dysplastic cementum/osteoid/dentin. A well-defined capsule is rare. Subvariants of both histological types of central odontogenic fibroma have been described.[105,106]

Histogenesis

It has been suggested that the epithelium poor type of central odontogenic fibroma is derived from the dental follicle whereas the epithelium rich type arises from the periodontal ligament. Existence of two types of central odontogenic fibroma has been challenged.

Treatment and Prognosis

Treatment for central odontogenic fibromas, irrespective of type, is enucleation by vigorous curettage. Long-term follow-up of a large series is not available, but the recurrence rate is considered low.

BENIGN CEMENTOBLASTOMA

Benign cementoblastoma (BC) or true cementoma was first described by Norberg in 1930.[107] It is a rare benign odontogenic tumor of the ectomesenchymal origin. It is considered to be the only true neoplasm of the cemental origin and is characterized by proliferation of the cellular cementum.

Definition

A cementoblastoma is characterized by the formation of cementum-like tissue in connection with the root of a tooth (WHO).

Epidemiology

A cementoblastoma occurs from the age of 8 to 44 years of age, the mean age being approximately 20 years.[108] There is no distinct gender preference. The male: female ratio was 1:1.2.[109]

Localization

The majority of cementoblastomas are located in the mandible, particularly related to the permanent first molar; association with a primary tooth is exceptional.

Features

Clinical Features

The most common finding is a painful swelling at the buccal and lingual/palatal aspect of the alveolar ridges. The vitality of the involved tooth remains intact. Lower-lip paresthesia or a pathologic fracture of the mandible is rarely reported. The benign cementoblastoma, intimately associated with a tooth root, generally presents as a slow-growing, unilateral swelling with the expansion of the affected bone. Ulmansky et al.[110] recorded swelling and expansion in 70 percent of their cases. In the survey published by Ulmansky et al. 61 percent of the patients had a history of pain. Of 15 cases of benign cementoblastomas reported by Jelic et al.[111] 9 were symptomatic and patients complained of pain. The type of pain is usually characterized as a tooth ache arising in the pulp.

Radiographic Features

Radiographically, benign cementoblastomas have a characteristic, almost pathognomonic appearance. The tumor is well-defined and is mainly of a radiopaque or mixed-density, surrounded by a thin radiolucent zone. Root resorption, loss of root outline and obliteration of the periodontal ligament space are common findings (Fig. 28.28).

Macroscopy Features

The tumor consists of a rounded or nodular mass attached to one or more tooth roots and is surrounded by a gray-to-tan layer of irregular soft tissue (Fig. 28.29).

Histopathology

A cementoblastoma consists of dense masses of acellular cementum-like material in a fibrous, sometimes rather vascular stroma containing multinucleated cells (Fig. 28.30). The tumor mass blends with the root of a tooth with simultaneous root resorption. In the more mature parts of the tumor, basophilic reversal lines may produce a Paget disease-like pattern. At the periphery, sheets of unmineralized tissue may be seen, often being arranged in a radiating column. The differential diagnosis includes osteoblastoma, the only distinctive criterion being the true connection with the surface of root of a tooth in case of a cementoblastoma.[112] An important differential diagnosis is osteosarcoma. Without radiographs it is difficult to properly diagnose a cementoblastoma. The diagnosis cannot be made on the biopsy alone.

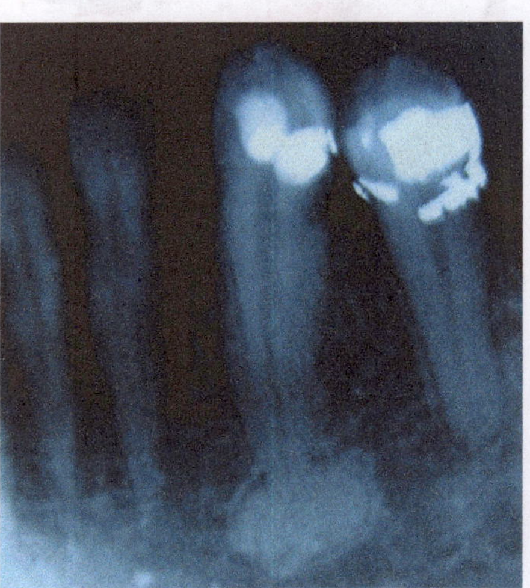

Fig. 28.28: Periapical dental radiograph showing benign cementoblastoma at the apex of the root of the mandibular canine

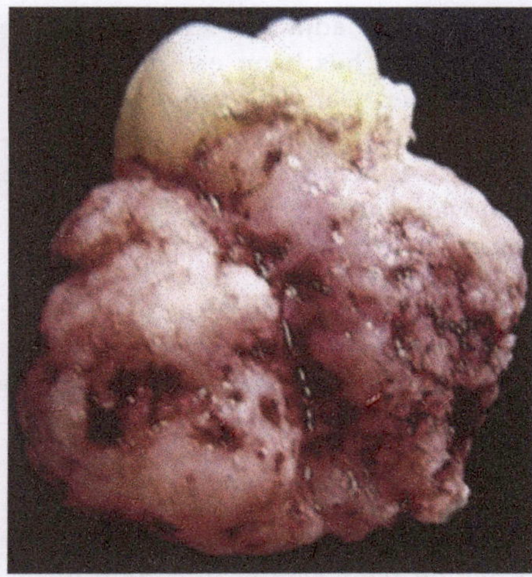

Fig. 28.29: Macroscopic view of the surgical specimen. The lesion is large and extends up to the cemento-enamel junction of the tooth

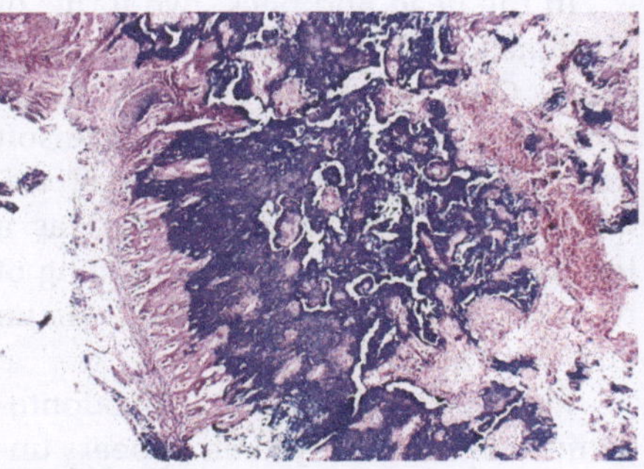

Fig. 28.30: Cementoblastoma. The root surface is largely destroyed by the cementum-like tissue, while the pulpal tissue of the tooth still remained vital

Treatment and Recurrence Rate

The recommended treatment of choice is early surgical removal due to the cementoblastomic capabilities for persistent growth, expansion and involvement of the adjacent structures. The growth rate has been estimated to be 0.5 cm per year. The tumor is readily enucleated and does not recur. 'Recurrence' is usually the result of incomplete removal. The affected tooth has been removed with the tumor in almost all the reported cases.

MYXOMA (ODONTOGENIC MYXOMA, FIBROMYXOMA)

Introduction

The myxoma (*fibromyxoma*), which is a benign neoplasm of uncertain histogenesis with characteristic histologic appearance, often behaves in a locally aggressive, infiltrating fashion.[113]

In the head and neck, two forms of myxomas or fibromyxomas are recognized: One is derived from the facial skeleton other is derived from the soft tissue. The WHO defines myxoma (*odontogenic myxoma, myxofibroma*) as a locally invasive neoplasm consisting of rounded and angular cells that lie in an abundant mucoid stroma.

In the WHO classification of odontogenic neoplasms, myxoma appears under the subheading 'odontogenic ectomesenchyme with or without included odontogenic epithelium'.[114]

Myxoma is of odontogenic origin that has been perpetuated by its:

- Almost exclusive occurrence in the tooth bearing areas of the jaws
- Frequent occurrence in young individuals
- Common association with an unerupted tooth or a developmentally absent tooth
- Histologic resemblance to dental mesenchyme, especially the dental papilla
- Occasional presence of sparse amounts of odontogenic epithelium.[115-118]

The neoplasms odontogenic derivation is believed to originate from the primitive mesenchymal portion of the developing tooth germ (*dental follicle, dental papilla* and *periodontal ligament*) as an inductive effect of nests of odontogenic epithelium on mesenchymal tissue or as a direct myxomatous change of fibrous tissue in an odontogenic fibroma.

Goldblatt's[119] ultrastructural study of a maxillary myxoma could not verify an odontogenic origin from primitive non-odontogenic mesenchymal rests.

Slootweg et al.[120] concluded from their biochemical study on a mandibular myxoma that the myxoma matrix differs from the matrix in dental pulp and periodontal ligament.

The uncertainty that the myxoma is strictly an odontogenic lesion is sustained by its origin in extragnathic locations and non-tooth bearing area of the jaws. This tumor occurs in sites separate from the odontogenic area, including the sinonasal tract, facial bones, extracranial skeleton, upper ramus and condyle of the mandible.[121-123]

Sinonasal myxomas probably arise from or within bone and the anterior maxillary sinus wall is a frequent location.[124]

Subclassifying myxomas that are derived from facial skeleton into:

- Odontogenic myxoma
- True osteogenic myxomas may better define their histogenesis.[125]

Features

Clinical Features

Kaffe et al.[126] reviewed 164 odontogenic myxomas of the jaws and found that 75 percent occurred between the second and fourth decades (patient age range, 1–73 years; mean 30 years). Seven percent of the patients were in the first decade of life. The female to male ratio was 1.5:1. There were 109 (66%) neoplasms in the mandible and 55 (34%) in the maxilla. Myxomas can occur anywhere in the jaws, but have a predilection for the molar and premolar regions of the mandible and maxilla. The odontogenic myxoma causes cortical expansion and perforation (Figs 28.31A and B). The maxillary myxomas often extend into the sinus. Small odontogenic myxomas are asymptomatic. Large odontogenic myxomas cause painless expansion. Unilateral sinonasal obliteration may mimic nasal polyposis.

The central myxomas are not seen in other bones except the jaw bones. The tumor is infilterative and has tendency to recur after surgical enucleation.

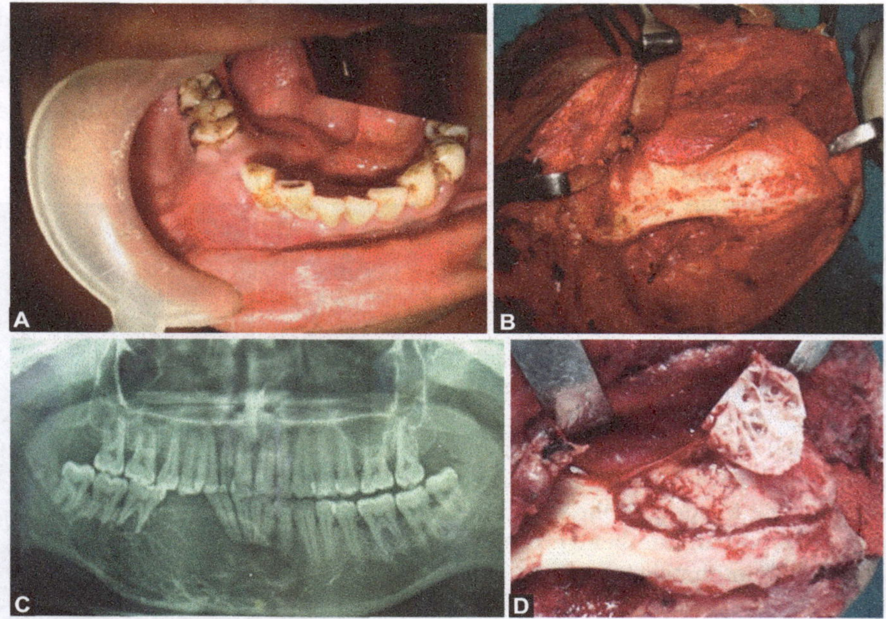

Figs 28.31A to D: Odontogenic myxoma of mandible: (A and B) Expansion of the bone due to the tumor; (C) Tennis racket appearance on the X-ray; (D) Tennis racket type bony trabaculae present on the inner side of the buccal cortical plate that produce typical 'tennis racket' appearance on X-ray

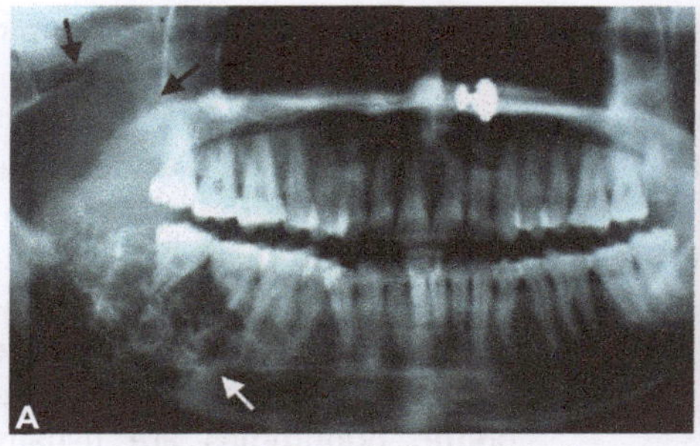

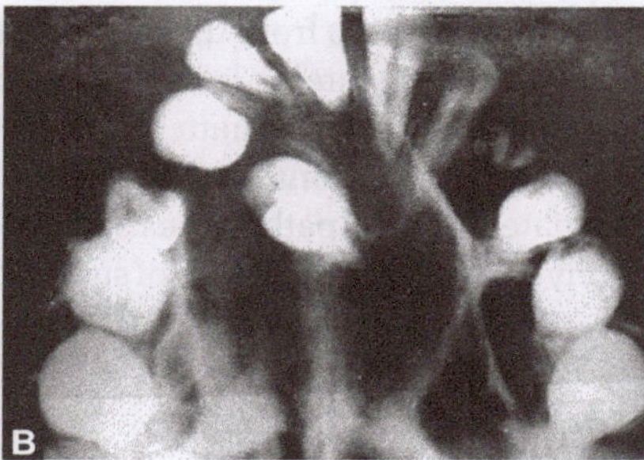

Figs 28.32A and B: Typical tennis racket appearance of odontogenic myxoma on X-ray: (A) Posterior mandible; (B) Anterior maxilla in 14 years old female

Radiographic Features

Periapical dental radiographs and panoramic radiographs are often the first indicators of myxomas of jaw. The radiographic features of the odontogenic myxoma are variable, ranging from small unilocular lesions to large multilocular neoplasms, which often displace teeth or less frequently, resorb roots.[117] The multilocular trabecular pattern has been described as 'honey comb', 'soap bubble', 'tennis racket', 'wispy' and 'spiderweb' in appearance (Figs 28.31C and D, Fig. 28.32A).

Odontogenic Myxoma of the Anterior Maxilla

Most multilocular myxomas are greater than 4 cm; unilocular myxomas tend to be smaller (Fig. 28.32B). Only 5 percent of myxomas are associated with unerupted teeth.[126] Kaffe et al. found that 12.5 percent of myxomas were mixed radiolucent and radiopaque and 7.5 percent were radiopaque.

Gross Pathology

The myxoma is usually a well-delineated, unencapsulated gray-white to tan-yellow mass that can be rubbery soft or gelatanious (slimy) in texture. The margins are usually ill defined in gelatinous specimens. On the cut surface, it is typically glistening, translucent and homogeneous.

Histopathology

Histologically, the myxoma is bland in appearance and is composed of loosely arranged, evenly dispersed spindle-shaped, rounded and stellate cells with a lightly eosinophilic cytoplasm in a mucoid rich, intercellular matrix, although some degree of mild nuclear pleomorphism or hyperchromatism may exist, including an occasional mitosis or binucleate cell, there which has no correlation with recurrence of the neoplasm (Fig. 28.33).[127]

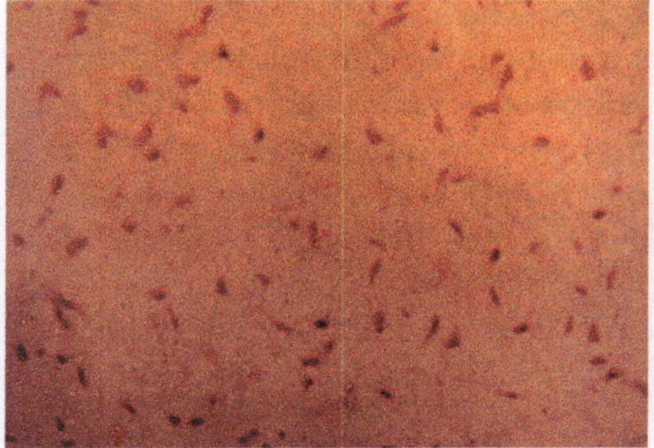

Fig. 28.33: Odontogenic myxoma, high power view of randomly arranged spindle-shaped, stellate and rounded cells in a loose myxoid stroma

Treatment and Prognosis

In Barkers review of literature, the overall recurrence for myxomas ranged from 10 to 33 percent. These high recurrence rates can be attributed to the subtal local invasion of the neoplasm between the cancellous bone, beyond radiographical visible margins and lack of incapsulation.[128] The production of mucoid ground substance is believed to be the cause for its growth, because enhanced mitotic activity and high proliferation rates are absent. This recurrence rate differences were related to the method of treatment. The standard treatment for myxomas is surgical exision. Radiation therapy and chemotherapy are inactive treatments. A number of surgical methods have been advocated for routine myxomas of the jaws including excision, enucleation and curettage, curettage with and without electrical or chemical cautery, en-block resection and wide resection with and without immediate grafting. A recurrence rate of 43 percent in myxomas that were treated initially by curettage or local surgical exicision was documented in the series reported by Lo Muzio et al.[129] Several authors have emphasized that the rate of recurrence is generally higher with conservatively treated myxomas within the first 2 years of treatment. However, recurrence have occurred several to many years after the surgery, so follow-up should be indefinite.

ODONTOMA

'Broca' first coined the term 'odontome' in 1866. He defined it as a tumor formed by an overgrowth of complete dental tissue.[130]

In the landmark paper Thoma and Goldman[131] narrowed the term "odontoma" to include tumors that were composed of well-differentiated tooth structure. Shafer and Gorlin defined odontoma as a tumor that has developed and differentiated enough to produce enamel and dentin.[132,133]

The second edition of the WHO histologic typing of odontogenic tumors classifies odontomas under the broad category of tumors containing odontogenic epithelium with odontogenic ectomesenchyme, with or without dental hard tissue formation.

Under this classification, three types of odontomas are listed:

1. Odontoameloblastoma
2. Complex odontoma and
3. Compound odontoma.

The odontomas have become to be known as mixed odontogenic tumors because they are composed of both epithelial and ectomesenchymal components. Both the epithelial and the ectomesenchymal tissues and their respective cells may appear normal morphologically, but they seem to have a deficit in structural arrangement. This deficit has led to the opinion that odontomas are hamartomatous lesions or malformations rather than true neoplasms.

Odontoma, Compound Type

Definition (WHO): A tumor-like malformation (hamartoma) with varying numbers of tooth-like elements (odontoids).

Synonym: Compound composite odontoma.

Epidemiological Data

- **Prevalence, incidence and relative frequency:** The compound odontoma is the most common lesion/malformation of odontogenic origin. Its relative frequency varies between 4.2 and 73.8 percent. Sato et al.[134] recorded odontomas in 47 percent of Japanese patients with benign odontogenic tumors.
- **Age:** Based on the data of the odontoma survey by Philipson et al.[135] the mean age at the time of diagnosis was 17.2 years; 74.3 percent of the cases were diagnosed before the age of 20 years with a marked peak in the second decade of life. The compound odontoma is clearly a lesion of childhood and adolescence.
- **Gender:** The male: female ratio varies between 1.2:1 and 1:1 according to the odontoma survey of Phillipson et al.[135]
- **Localization:** Compound odontomas may occur in any tooth bearing area of the jaws. The anterior maxilla is most frequently affected.

Etiology

The etiology is unknown. Several theories have been proposed, including trauma and infection. It seems that these conditions are more likely to result in a hypoplastic tooth germ rather than an odontoma.

Lopez-Areal[136] documented a case in which a child developed multiple odontomas after experiencing trauma with intrusion of the incisor teeth at the age of 10 months.

Hitchin[137] has postulated that odontomas are inherited or developed as a result of a genetic mutation.

Pathogenesis

As with the complex odontoma, the compound odontoma is of odontogenic origin. The theory that the compound odontomas develop from the ameloblastic fibroma if the later is left untreated is questionable but still a matter of debate. The compound odontoma is more differentiated and its pathogenesis is more closely related to the creation of supernumerary teeth, especially mesiodens.

Features

Clinical Features

These are painless, slowly growing lesions. When fully matured, development ceases. The size usually varies between 1 and 2 cm in diameter, but a diameter of up to 6 cm has been reported. Swelling of the jaw is seen in less than 10 percent of the cases. Many are located close to the incisal/occlusal part of an impacted tooth, thus impeding eruption. Displacement of erupted teeth is seen in some cases. Some occur in a site where the permanent tooth is missing. Multiple compound odontomas have been reported and they may be part of Gardner syndrome. Peripheral lesions developing entirely within the gingival soft tissues are rare.

Radiographic Features

Radiographically, the compound odontomas appear as a collection of tooth-like structures surrounded by a radiolucent zone. Adjacent teeth may be displaced but are never resorbed (Figs 28.34A and B).

Pathology

- **Macroscopy:** The specimen consists of a number of teeth-like structures enclosed in a fibrous capsule, which is thin if the lesion has matured. In most cases, the final diagnosis can be made on the basis of macroscopic examination.
- **Histopathology:**
  - **Histopathological findings:** Due to a higher degree of morphodifferentiation than that of complex odontoma, compound odontomas are easily recognizable even macroscopically. Compound odontomas are usually small, but large lesions containing up to 100 denticles have been reported. Denticles are composed of enamel, dentin, cementum and pulp tissues with a more or less regular arrangement. Morphodifferentiation and histodifferentiation of the dental hard tissues in compound odontomas has been studied in detail by Piatelli and Trishi.[138] Three percent of the odontomas may contain *ghost* cells (Fig. 28.35).[139]
  - **Histochemical/immunohistochemistrical findings:** Along with the other odontogenic tumors, Gao et al.[140] studied compound odontomas using immunohistochemistry. The aim of their study was to describe the expression and distribution of the bone morphologic proteins (BMPs) in odontogenic tumors. BMPs, members of the transforming growth factor-beta (TGF-β) superfamily, play a role not only in the bone formation, but also in the epitheliomesenchymal interations, tumors and lesions of epithelial and/or ectomesenchymal origin, including the compound odontoma

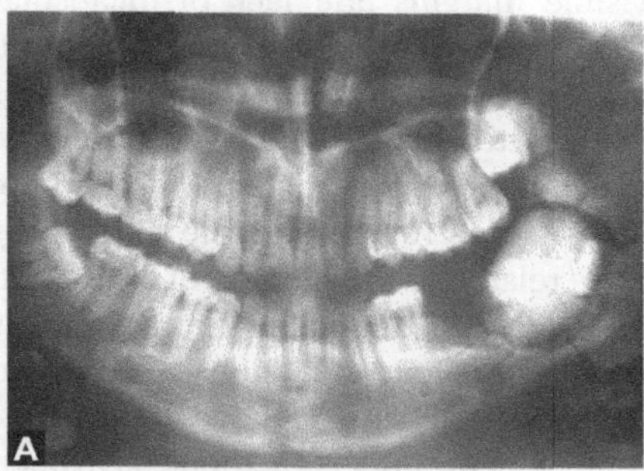

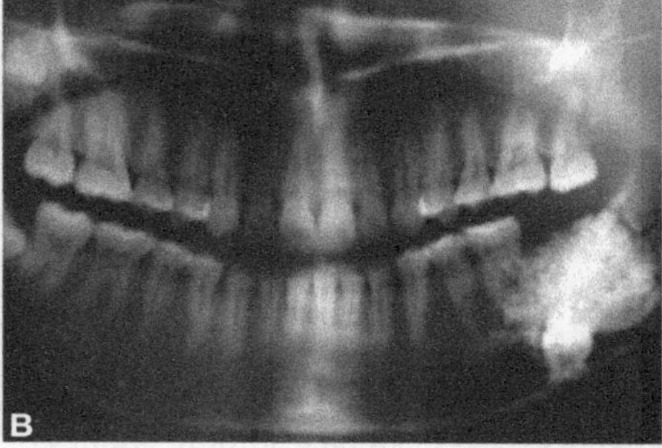

Figs 28.34A and B: Complex compound odontomas involving the posterior mandible

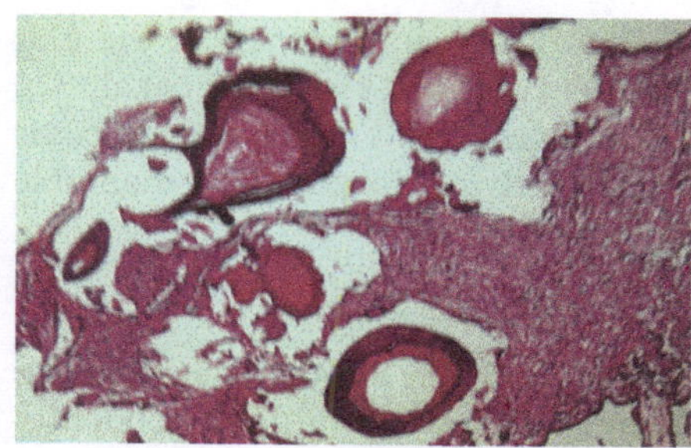

Fig. 28.35: Compound odontoma with tooth like structures composed of dentin and enamel matrix supported by dense fibrous connective tissue

demonstrated positive reactions while epithelial odontogenic tumors were negative.

Complex Odontoma

Definition: Odontoma, complex type (OC) is a tumor-like malformation (hamartoma) in which enamel and dentin and sometimes cementum is present (WHO).

Synonym: Complex composite odontoma.

Epidemiology

Complex odontomas are one of the most common odontogenic tumors. These are primarily diagnosed in children, adolescents and young adults. Based on 137 cases from the odontoma survey the mean age at the time of diagnosis was 19.9 years[141] (*range 2 to 74 years*). About 83.9 percent of cases occurred before the age of 30 with a peak in the 2nd decade of life. The male:female ratio varies from 1.5:1 to 1.6:6 to 0.8:1 according to different studies.

Etiology

The etiology is unknown. Several theories[142] have been proposed including local trauma, infection, family history and genetic mutation. It has also been suggested that odontomas are inherited from a mutant gene or interference, possibly postnataly with the genetic control of tooth development.

Localization

Complex odontomas occur in tooth bearing regions, mostly in the posterior part of the mandible and the second most common site is the anterior maxilla.

Clinical Features

Complex odontomas are painless slowly growing lesions. The growth stops when they are fully matured some reaching upto 6 cm in diameter, the majority measures less than 3 cm. Mild swelling of the jaw may be evident. But, when they become large, produces expansion of the bone and facial symmetry.[143] The adjacent teeth may be displaced and impaction of a permanent tooth is a common finding.

Pathogenesis

The odontogenic origin of the complex odontoma has never been questioned. It is considered a self-limiting developmental anomaly or hamartomatous malformation, characterized by non-descript masses of dental tissues. Recently, it has been suggested that odontomas tend to incease in size with the age of the patient suggesting continous growth.[144]

Several factors may cause anomalous tissue development in odontomas. These include unsuccessful or an altered ectomesenchymal interaction in the earliest phase of dental germ development and/or alterations in the subsequent phases of the development of these tissues. It has also been assumed that alterations in the mineralization mechanisms with modifications of the mineral component in the enamel may lead to incomplete maturation.[145]

Radiographic Features

Complex odontomas appear as a spherical or ovoid radiopacity with a fine radiating periphery, surrounded by a radiolucent zone, which may be broader in a developing complex odontoma (Figs 28.34, 28.36 and 28.37).

Histopathology

In mature complex odontomas, the soft tissue capsule consists of a loose connective tissue containing strands or islands of odontogenic epithelium. In developing complex odontomes, the outer part of the odontoma consists of a cell rich zone of soft tissue with formation of enamel and dentin, not resembling tooth morphology. The lesion appears as a mass of primarily tubular dentin, which encloses

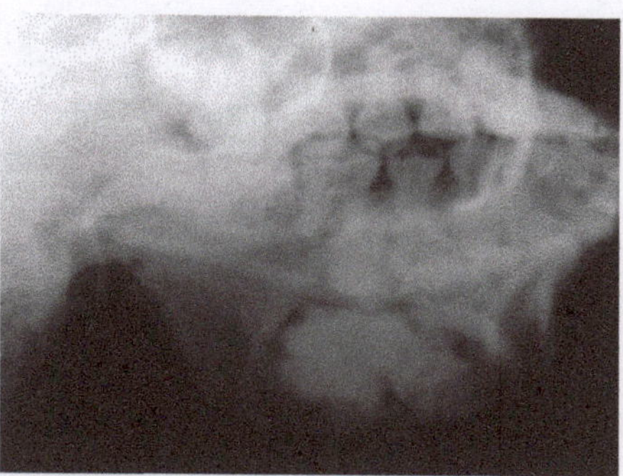

Fig. 28.36: Complex odontoma

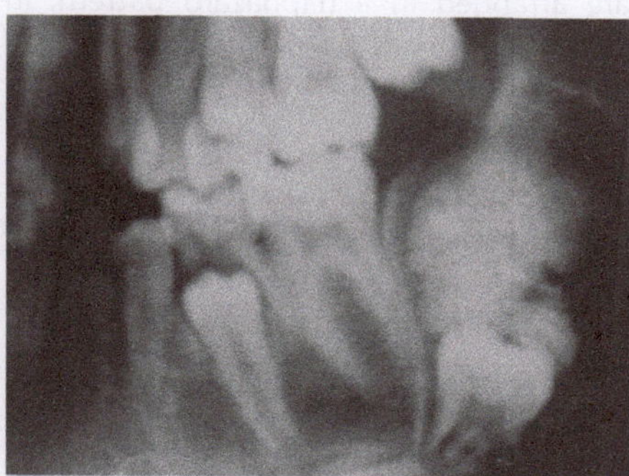

Fig. 28.37: Odontoma, complex type with a dense radiopacity and retained molar

hollow circular or oval structures with empty spaces from decalcified mature enamel, enamel matrix producing epithelium and connective tissue. The structure of hard dental tissue may vary. The lesion consists mainly of wavy and plicated walls of tubular or dysplastic dentin covered by enamel. Between these walls are irregular curvilinear clefts that contain enamel matrix producing epithelium and connective tissue. Cementum is scarce except on the 'root' surfaces of tooth—like structures. Scattered ghost cells may be present (Fig. 28.38).

The distinction between complex and compound odontoma is mainly based on the presence of tooth-like structures in compound odontomas. The differential diagnosis between a developing complex odontomas and an ameloblastic fibro-odontoma is sometimes impossible.

In 1946, Thoma and Goldman[146] first described ghost cells in complex odontomas, but Levy[147] often is given credit for extensively studying this phenomenon.

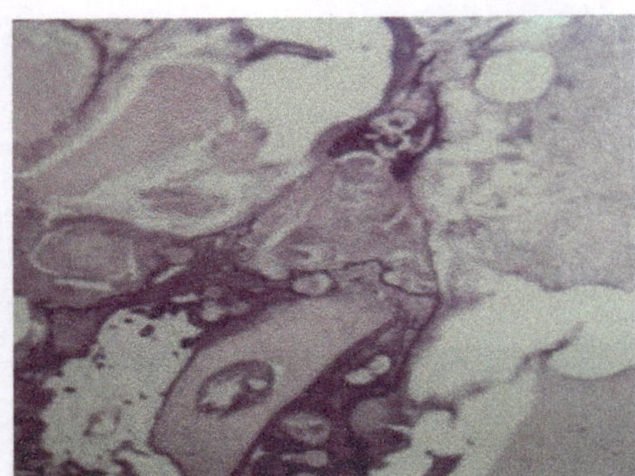

Fig. 28.38: Odontoma, complex type. Enamel, dentin and cementum-like tissue are arranged in a haphazard pattern, in contrast to the regular structures encountered in compound odontoma

Treatment and Prognosis

Conservative surgical excision is the treatment of choice for odontomas, because such treatment results in little to no chance of recurrence. There have been noble approaches to the removal odontomas. In the study of large mandibular odontomas, Blender et al. described a lingual approach to the removal of these large lesions. Because the lingual cortex is thinner than the buccal, it is logical that this approach should be considered to avoid unwanted mandibular fractures.

Kamakura et al.[148] described an interesting treatment approach to a large compound dontoma. The lesion caused intrusion of the maxillary central and lateral incisor teeth. They were able to remove odontoma and with combined orthodontic and surgical therapy, bring the incisor teeth into the proper occlusion.

Odontoameloblastoma

Thoma[149] introduced the term odontoameloblastoma (OA) in 1944. It was considered by some to be yet another member of the odontoma group, together with the ameloblastic fibro-odontoma (AFO), until Hooker[150] showed that they are two separate tumors with different clinical behavior, though previously grouped together under the term ameloblastic odontoma.

Wächter et al.[151] made a critical attempt to differentiate between the odontoameloblastoma and the AFO by means of histologic criteria from 29 cases referred to the DOSAK bone tumor register.

According to the 1992 WHO criteria, 4 cases of OAs and 14 AFOs were classified. Kaugars and Zussmann[152] described a case of odontoameloblastoma in 1991 and critically reviewed the English literature of reported cases, bringing the total to 12. All these studies highlight the rare occurrence of this tumor.

Definition: Odontoameloblastoma (OA) combines features of ameloblastoma with those of an odontoma (WHO).

Synonyms: Ameloblastic odontoma, Odontoblastomas and adamanto-odontoma. Soft and calcified odontoma, Calcified mixed odontogenic tumor.

Epidemiology

- **Prevalence, incidence and relative frequency:** Odontoameloblastoma appear to be extremely rare and figures on incidence, prevalence or relative frequency are available. The situation is complicated even further by the fact that a number of cases published under the names ameloblastic odontoma or odontoameloblastoma do not meet the strict histologic criteria of the lesion and represent instead examples of the ameloblastic fibro-odotoma.
- **Age:** The mean age is 18.8 years (range 3–50 years).
- **Gender:** The male : female ratio 2:1 in the cases reviewed by Kaugars and Zussmann and 1:3 in the four cases reported by Wachter et al.[152]
- **Localization:** The majority of cases located in the posterior mandible region.

Pathogenesis

The OA is clearly of odontogenic origin; however, its relationship to other odontogenic tumors—the ameloblastoma on the one hand and the odontomas on the other—is not well understood.

Features

Clinical features

Presenting signs may include bone expansion (Fig. 28.39A), root resorption, tooth displacement and occasional pain, changes in occlusion and delayed eruption of teeth.

Radiographic features

Odontoameloblastoma appears as a well-defined unilocular or multilocular radiolucent lesion in which varying amounts of radiopaque material may be identified (Fig. 28.39B). Most cases are associated with displaced unerupted teeth.

Macroscopy

Most odontoameloblastoma are unencapsulated. On the cut section, the lesion has a multinodular architecture with soft and hard tissue components. The amount of mineralized tissue may appear as large

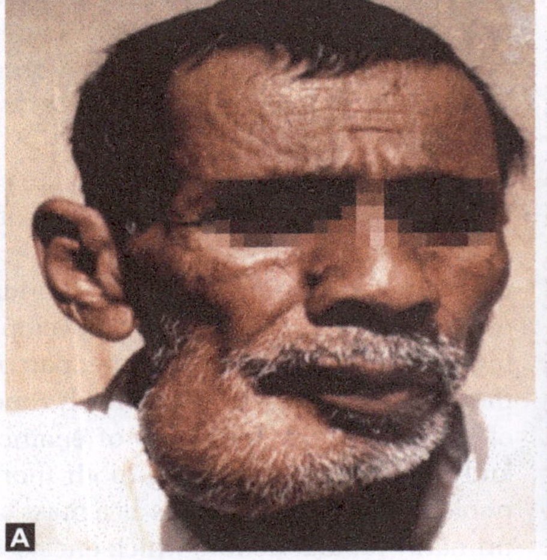

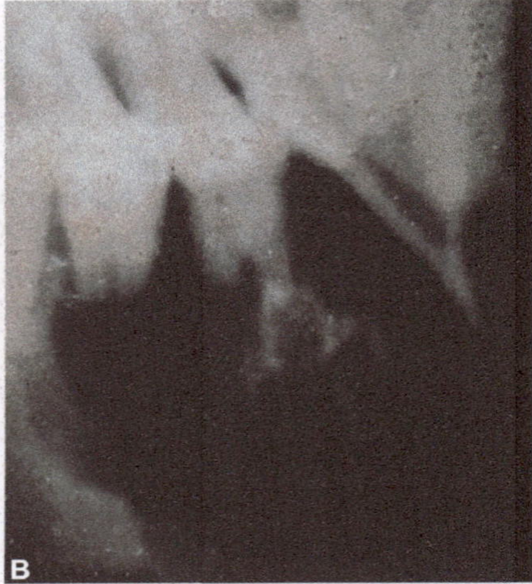

Figs 28.39A and B: Odontoameloblastoma involving mandible in a 45-year-old male

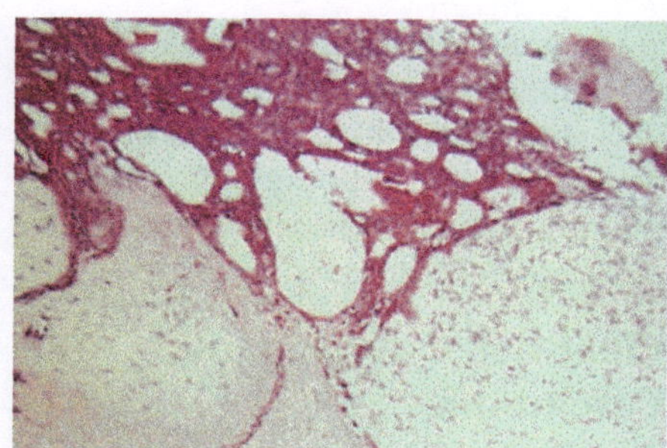

Fig. 28.40: Nodular masses of odontogenic mesenchyme adjacent to a proliferating epithelium that exhibits a plexiform ameloblastoma pattern

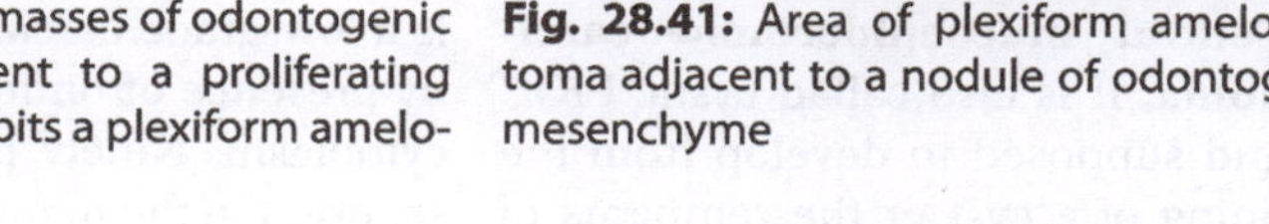

Fig. 28.41: Area of plexiform ameloblastoma adjacent to a nodule of odontogenic mesenchyme

lobulated masses or as rudimentary teeth scattered within the soft tissues.

Histopathology

The epithelial component consists of islands and cords of odontogenic epithelium demonstrating follicular and plexiform patterns, typical of ameloblastoma. In addition to the fibrous stroma, this tumor shows a variable amount of cellular myxoid tissue adjacent to the epithelium, where mineralized dental tissues are formed as in odontomas. Isolated small foci of ghost cells may occasionally be found (Figs 28.40 and 28.41).

Treatment and Recurrence Rate

Since the OA has been considered an aggressive lesion, most authors recommend a radical treatment as applied for ameloblastomas. In the series reviewed by Kaugars and Zussman, three recurrences were noted, including one case in which the OA recurred twice. Wachter et al. did not record any recurrences among their cases.

Kaugars and Zussmann discussed the similarity of OAs with both ameloblastomas and odontomas. While the location, expansion and recurrence rate appear to be similar to those of the SMA, the age at the time of diagnosis is more comparable to that of complex odontoma. Wachter et al. considered the OA and the ameloblastic fibro-odontoma to be one entity because of similar biologic behavior and prognosis. Also, they considered the OA (and ameloblastic fibro-odontoma) to be more of a hamartomatous lesion than a true neoplasm. They recommended the performance of regular follow-up in order to detect 'recurrences' early.

MALIGNANT ODONTOGENIC TUMORS

Metastasizing Ameloblastoma

Traditionally, the ameloblastoma is regarded as a benign, locally aggressive tumor and does not metastasize, occasionally it can metastasize and could be fatal. This triggers the thinking that ameloblastoma could be a low grade malignant tumor. The term metastatic ameloblastoma is used to describe the metastatic tumor that shows histologic features of classic ameloblastoma of jaw.

Clinical Features

The primary ameloblastoma arises in the mandible of a young adult and after the mean latency of 10 to 11 years metastatic nodules develop in the lung (80%), cervical lymph nodes (15%) and other extragnathic bones. The pulmonary nodules are typically bilateral and multifocal. The mean survival rate after detection of the pulmonary metastasis is two years. The pulmonary nodules present as innocuous lung granulomas on routine radiographs. The pulmonary metastasis is thought to be due to aggressive primary tumor or due to tumor embolization in the lymphatics or blood vessels during the surgery. The metastatic ameloblastomas are ambiguously termed as malignant ameloblastoma due to its biological behavior of low-grade, well-differentiated, low-grade carcinoma.

Management

The metastatic ameloblastoma are primarily managed by surgery. However, the survival rate does not improve. The cervical lymph node metastasis is managed by appropriate neck dissection. The pulmonary metastasis is managed by lobectomy, if adequate pulmonary function can be preserved postoperatively. The chemotherapy is usually ineffective but, shows early short-term relief.

Ameloblastic Carcinoma

Ameloblastic carcinoma represents malignant epithelial proliferation associated with the ameloblastoma (carcinoma ex-ameloblastoma) or histologically resembles the ameloblastoma (*de novo* ameloblastic carcinoma). The pronounced cytologic atypia and mitotic activity is demonstrable in ameloblastic carcinoma. Some tumors show basilar hyperplasia and increased mitotic activity and are designated as atypical ameloblastoma or proliferative ameloblastoma, but these findings are not adequate to diagnose the ameloblastic carcinoma. The presence of the criteria-like nuclear pleomorphism, perineural invasion and other histologic evidence of malignancy are needed to diagnose the ameloblastic carcinoma. The ameloblastic carcinoma is locally invasive and metastasizes to the cervical lymph nodes, lungs and long bones. It is managed on similar lines that for squamous cell carcinoma.

Primary Intraosseous Carcinoma

The primary intraosseous carcinoma (PIOC) is the central jaw bone carcinoma. It is called primary because it is not the metastatic secondary deposit from other sites and to call it as a primary intraosseous carcinoma, the metastasis from distant primary to the jaw bones must be ruled out. Similarly, its origin from the oral squamous epithelium and the sinonasal linings must be ruled out.

The PIOC produces diffuse enlargement of the jaw. In the presence of mucosal ulceration the diagnosis of PIOC is doubtful. Similarly, once the tumor fungates through the bone to involve overlying soft tissue then the diagnosis of PIOC is often difficult to make.

The origin of the PIOC is thought to be secondary to remnants of the odontogenic epithelium or from the incisive canal epithelium. Few varieties of PIOC have been described:

- **Solid primary intraosseous carcinoma:** It is rare tumor which presents a painful swelling in the posterior mandible. The mean age of occurrence is 52 years. The patient presents with the complaints of pain, swelling and paresthesia in the distribution of the inferior alveolar nerve. The radiological picture is cup-shaped radiolucent lesion (42%), irregular moth eaten radiolucency (26%) and well-circumscribed radiolucent lesion (10%). The incidence of cervical lymph node metastasis is reported to be 31 percent. The lesion is treated with surgical excision, neck dissection and postoperative radiotherapy. The overall 5 year survival rate is 38 percent.
- **Cystic primary intraosseous carcinoma:** The cystic PIOC (PIOC ex-odontogenic cyst) is a squamous cell carcinoma that demonstrates a cystic component with a lumen that contains keratin of fluid and the lining that shows dysplasia. If the cystic lining does not demonstrate the atypia, then the possibility of gingival carcinoma eroding the bone and colliding with the cystic lining or the development of the carcinoma adjacent to the cyst can be considered. These tumors may mimic odontogenic cysts radiologically.
- **Carcinoma ex-dentigerous cyst:** The most common odontogenic cyst undergoing transformation into the PIOC is dentigerous cyst. It often presents as an asymptomatic or painful radiolucent lesion surrounding the crown of an impacted/unerupted mandibular third molar. Occasionally, they are associated with impacted canines. The mean age of occurrence is 59 years with distinct male predominance. The lesion may become destructive. The lesion is treated by surgery.
- **Carcinoma exodontogenic keratocyst:** The PIOC is reported to develop from the lining of the OKC by Mokwasi et al. (2001).
- **Central mucoepidermoid carcinoma:** It is also called cystic PIOC and supposed to develop from the lining of a cyst or the remnants of the odontogenic epithelium. The central mucoepidermoid carcinoma arises from the sequestrated salivary gland tissue during the development. They are low-grade malignancies and demonstrate well-circumscribed uniloculated or multilocuted radiolucent lesions. The high-grade lesions show destructive pattern and have metastatic potential. The prognosis in low-grade lesions have fair prognosis. The death is usually due to uncontrolled local growth rather than the metastatic disease.

A variety of treatment modalities have been used which comprise of curettage, segmental resection, hemimandibulectomy.

Ghost Cell Odontogenic Carcinoma

Ghost cell odontogenic carcinoma is considered as a variant of malignant ameloblastoma and shows evidence of ghost cell keratinization. The ghost cells are immunoreactive to amelogenin, a protein that is unique to enamel matrix and therefore represent evidence of ameloblastic differentiation. The ghost cell odontogenic carcinoma is more commonly seen in the maxilla and has male predilection. The mean age of presentation being 38 years (range 13–72 years). Radiological picture is not characteristic, but may show multiloculated to poorly delineated radioluscent lesions. The tumor is locally aggressive and behaves like ameloblastoma or low-grade ameloblastic carcinoma and has no significant potential to metastasize. It is treated with wide surgical excision and postoperative radiotherapy. Chemotherapy may be chosen for extensive non-resectable tumors.

Clear Cell Odontogenic Carcinoma

The clear cell odontogenic carcinoma is a low-grade carcinoma characterized by presence of uniform cells with clear cytoplasm. Ninety percent tumors are reported in the mandible and have a female predilection. The radiological picture is variable ranging from unilocular radiolucency with indistinct borders to multiloculated lesions having well-circumscribed borders.

The tumor has high recurrence rate (48%) after resection. It is refractory to curettage. About 20 percent tumors show cervical lymph node metastasis and 17 percent show pulmonary metastasis. The mortality rate is 20 percent in extensive extraosseous tumors postoperative radiotherapy may be useful.

Ameloblastic Fibrosarcoma (Odontogenic Sarcoma, Ameloblastic Sarcoma)

The ameloblastic fibrosarcoma is a malignant connective tissue of odontogenic origin that contains benign odontogenic epithelium similar to that of the ameloblastic fibroma. The tumor commonly (80%) occurs in the mandibular posterior region and has a male predilection. The clinical presentation is an expansile lesion showing a radiolucency with indistinct margins. The lesion may be unilocular or multilocular and may be associated with an impacted molar. The tumor extends to the adjoining soft tissue. The tumor originates in a pre-existing ameloblastic fibroma in 35 percent cases. The mean age of occurrence is 33 years but, the *de novo* ameloblastic fibrosarcoma at a younger age (Average 28 years). The reported recurrence rate is approximately 37 to 40 percent after surgical excision and 20 percent patients die of the disease within 5 years of diagnosis. The mortality is not due to the metastatic disease, but due to the locally aggressive tumor. The tumor is treated with wide local excision and postoperative radiotherapy. Neck dissections are not recommended as the tumor is not known to metastasize.

REFERENCES

1. Sawyer DR, Mosadomi A, Page DG, et al. Racial predilection of ameloblastoma? A probable answer from Lagos (Nigeria) and Richmond. J Oral Med. 1985;40(1): 27-31.
2. Assael LA. Surgical management of odontogenic cysts and tumors. Principles of Oral and Maxillofacial Surgery. Philadelphia: Lippincott; 1992. pp. 692-711.
3. Broca P. Gaz Leb de Med et de Chir (Paris). 1868;5:19,70,113.
4. Malassez L. Archives de Physiologie Normale et Pathologique [in French] 1885;6:379.
5. Bland-Sutton JB. Odontomes. Trans Odontol Soc Great. Brit. 1888;20:32-87.
6. Thoma KH, Goldman HM. Odontogenic tumors: Classification based on observations of epithelial, mesenchymal and mixed varieties. Amer J Pathol. 1946;28:433.
7. Spouge JD, Spruyt CL. Odontogenic tumors. Histochemical comparison of the adenoameloblastoma and developing tooth. Oral Surg. 1968;25:447-456.
8. Pindborg JJ, Kramer IRH, Tortoni H. Histological typing of odontogenic tumors, jaw cyst and allied lesions. Geneva, World Health Organization, 1971.
9. Kramer IRH, Pindborg JJ, Shear M. WHO histological typing of odontogenic tumours (2nd edn), Springer-Verlag, Geneva (1992).
10. Bares Leveson JW, Reichart P, Sidransky D (Eds). Pathology and Genetics. Head and Neck Tumors. WHO, Geneva 2005.
11. Robinson HB. Ameloblastoma: a survey of 379 cases from the literature, Arch. Pathol. 1937;23:831-43.
12. Churchill HR. Histologic Differentiation Between Certain Dentigerous Cysts and Ameloblastoma. Dental Cosmos. 1934;74:1173.
13. Reichart PA, Philipsen HP, Sonner S. Ameloblastoma: biological profile of 3677 cases. Eur J Cancer B Oral Oncol. 1995;31B(2):86-99
14. Neville BW, Damm DD, Allen CM, Bouquot JE. Oral and maxillofacial pathology. 2nd edn. Philadelphia: WB Saunders; 2002.pp.611-9.
15. Joseph BK, Savage NW. Maxillary ameloblastoma—case report and review of the literature. Aust Dent J. 1992;37:98.
16. Small IA, Waldron CA. Ameloblastoma of the jaws. Oral Surg. 1955;8:281.
17. Schafer DR, Thompson LDR, Smith BC, Weing BM. Primary ameloblastoma of the sinonasal tract: a clinicopathologic study 24 cases. Cancer. 1998;82(4): 667-74.
18. Kessler HP, Schwartz-Dabney C, Ellis III E. Reccurent left mandibular enlargement. J Contemp Dent Pract. 2003;3(4):127-37.
19. Infante-Cossio P, Hernandez-Guisado JM, Fernandez-Machin P, Garcia-Perla A, Rollon-Mayordomo A, Gutierrez-Perez JL. Ameloblastic carcinoma of the maxilla: a report of 3 cases. J Craniomaxillofac Surg. 1998;26(3):159-62.
20. Philipsen HP, Reichart PA. Unicystic ameloblastoma: a review of 193 cases from the literature. Oral Oncol. 1998: 34(5): 317-25.
21. Eversole LR, Leider AS, Hansen LS. Ameloblastomas with pronounced desmoplasia. J Oral Maxillofac Surg. 1984;42(11):735-40.
22. Willis RA. Pathology of tumours. Butterworth, London; 1948.
23. Tsakins PJ, Nelson JF. The maxillary ameloblastoma: an analysis of 24 cases. J Oral Surg. 1980;38(5):336-42.
24. Raymond J Fonseca, Michael P Powers. Oral and Maxillofacial Surgery. vol.5. Saunders; 1st edition.
25. David G Gardner. Radiotherapy in the treatment of ameloblastoma. IJOMS. 1988;17(3):201-5.
26. Stanley HRJ, Krogh HW, Peripheral ameloblastoma: report of a case. Oral Surg Oral Med Oral Pathol. 1959;12: 760-5.
27. Kuru H. Ueber das Adamantinom. Zentralbl Allg Pathol. 1911;22:291-5.
28. Mintz S, Anavi Y, Sabes WR. Peripheral ameloblastoma of the gingiva. A case report. Journal of Periodontology. 1999;61:649-52.
29. Robert S Redman. Peripheral ameloblastoma with unusual mitotic activity and conflicting evidence regarding histogenesis. JOMS. 1994: 52(2):192-7.
30. Moskow BS, Baden E. The peripheral ameloblastoma of the gingiva: case report and literature review. J Periodontol. 1982;53:736-42.
31. Kaneko Y, Ueno S. Peripheral ameloblastoma resembling a papilloma: report of case. J Oral Maxillofac Surg. 1986;44:737-9.
32. Horowitz I, Hirshberg A, Dayan D, Peripheral ameloblastoma. A clinical dilemma in gingival lesions. J Clin Periodontol. 1987;14:366-9.
33. Gurol M, Burkes EJ Jr. Peripheral ameloblastoma, J Periodontol. 1995;66: 1065-8.
34. Buchner A, Sciuba J. Peripheral epithelial odontogenic tumors: A review. Oral Surg Oral Med Oral Pathol. 1987; 63(7):688-97.
35. Gardner DG. Some current concepts on the pathology of ameloblastomas. Oral Surg Oral Med Oral Pathol Oral Radiol Endod. 1996;82(6):660-9.
36. Philipsen HP, Reichart PA, Nikai H, Takata T, Kudo Y. Peripheral ameloblastoma: biological profile based on 160 cases from literature. Oral Oncol. 2001;37(1):17-27.
37. Guralnick W, Chuong R, Goodman M. Peripheral ameloblastoma of gingiva. J Oral Maxillofac Surg. 1983;41:536.
38. Stevenson AR, Austin BW. A case of ameloblastoma presenting as an exophytic gingival lesion. J Periodontol. 1990;61:378-81.
39. Redman RS, Keegan BP, Spector CJ, Patterson RH. Peripheral ameloblastoma with unusual mitotic activity and conflicting evidence regarding histogenesis. J Oral Maxillofac Surg. 1994; 52:192-7.
40. Robinson L, Martinez MG. Unicystic ameloblastoma: a prognostically distinct entity. Cancer. 1977;40(5):2278-85.
41. Ackermann GL, Altini M, Shear M. The unicystic ameloblastoma: A clinicopathological study of 57 cases. J Oral Pathol. 1988;17:541-6.

42. Gardner DG, Corio RL. Plexiform unicystic ameloblastoma. A variant of ameloblastoma with a low-recurrence rate after enucleation. Cancer. 1984;53: 1730-5.
43. Leider AS, Eversole LR, Barkin ME. Cystic ameloblastoma: A clinicopathologic analysis, Oral Surg. 1985;60: 624–30.
44. Li TJ, Wu YT, Yu SF, Yu GY. Unicystic ameloblastoma: a clinicopathologic study of 33 Chinese patients. Am J Surg Pathol. 2000;24:1385-92.
45. Philipsen HP, Reichart PA. Unicystic ameloblastoma. A review of 193 cases from the literature. Oral Oncol. 1998; 34:317-25.
46. Eversole LR, Leider AS, Strub D. Radiographic characteristics of cystogenic ameloblastoma.Oral Surg Oral Med Oral Pathol. 1984;57:572-7.
47. Reichart PA, Philipsen HP, Sonner S. Ameloblastoma:biological profile of 3677 cases. Eur J Cancer B Oral Oncol. 1995;31B:86-99.
48. Waldron CA, El-Mofty SK. A histopathologic study of 116 ameloblastomas with special reference to the desmoplastic variant. Oral Surg. 1987; 63: 441-51.
49. Ashman SG, Corio RL, Eisele DW, et al. Desmoplastic ameloblastoma: A case report and literature review. Oral Surg Oral Med Oral Pathol. 1993;75:479.
50. Thompson IO, Van Rensburg LJ, Phillips VM. Desmoplastic ameloblastoma: correlative histopathology, radiology and CT-MR imaging. J Oral Pathol Med. 1996;25:405-10.
51. Philipsen HP, Reichart PA, Takata T. Desmoplastic ameloblastoma (including "hybrid" lesion of ameloblastoma). Biological profile based on 100 cases from literature and own files. Oral Oncol. 2001;37:455-60.
52. Gardner DG. A Pathologist's approach to the treatment of ameloblastoma. J Oral Maxillofac Surg. 1984;42:161-6.
53. Mehlisch DR, Dahlin DC, Masson JK. Ameloblastoma. A clinicopathologic report. J Oral Surg. 1972;30:9-22
54. Holland PS, Mellor WC. The conservative treatment of ameloblastoma, using diathermy or cryosurgery. A 29-year review. Int J Oral Surg. 1981;10:32-6.
55. Gardner DG, Pecak AM. The treatment of ameloblastoma based on pathologic and anatomic principles. Cancer. 1980; 46: 2514-9.
56. Ueno S, Mushimoto K, Shirasu R. Prognostic evaluation of ameloblastoma based on histologic and radiographic typing. J Oral Maxillofac Surg. 1989;47:11–5.
57. Feinberg SE, Steinberg B. Surgical management of ameloblastoma: current status of the literature. Oral Surg Oral Med Oral Pathol. 1996;81:383-8.
58. Bredenkamp JK, Zimmerman MC, Mickel RA. Maxillary Ameloblastoma: A potentially lethal neoplasm. Arch Otolaryngol Head Neck Surg. 1989; 115:99-104.
59. Lee PK, Samman N, Ng IO. Unicystic ameloblastoma—use of Carnoy's solution after enucleation. Int J Oral Maxillofac Surg. 2004;33(3):263-7.
60. Stoelinga PJ, Bronkhorst FB. The incidence, multiple presentation and recurrence of aggressive cysts of the jaws. J Craniomaxfac Surg. 1988;16.
61. Pindborg JJ. A calcifying epithelial odontogenic tumor. Cancer. 1958;11: 838-43.
62. Pindborg JJ. Calcifying epithelial odontogenic tumors. Acta Pathol Microbiol Scand. 1955;Suppl 11:71.
63. Philipsen HP, Reichart PA. Calcifying epithelial odontogenic tumor: biological profile based on 181 cases from the literature. Oral Oncol. 2000;36:17-26.
64. Peter A Reichart, Hans P Philipsen. Odontogenic tumors and allied lesions. Quintessence, London; 2004.
65. Houston GD, Flower CB. Extraosseous calcifying epithelial odontogenic tumor. A review and analysis of 113 cases. Oral Surg Oral Med Oral Pathol Oral Radiol Endol. 1997;83:577-83.
66. Mesquita RA, Lotufo MA, Sugaya NN, De Araujo NS, D Araujo VC. Peripheral clear cell variant of calcifying epithelial odontogenic tumor:report of a case and immunohistochemical investigation. Oral Surg Oral Med Oral Pathol Oral Radiol Endod. 2003;95:198-204.
67. Kaplan I, Buchner A, Calderon S, Kaffe I. Radiologic and clinical features of calcifying epithelial odontogenic tumor. Dentomaxillofac Radiol. 2001; 30:22-8.
68. Chaudhary AP, Holte NO, Vickers RA. Calcifying epithelial odontogenic tumor. Report of a case .Oral Surg Oral Med Oral Pathol. 1962;15:843-8.
69. Robert K Goode. Calcifying epithelial odontogenic tumours. Oral Maxillofacial Surg Clin N Am. 2004;16:323-31.
70. Goode RK. Calcifying epithelial odontogenic tumor. Oral Maxillofac Surg Clin North Am. 2004;16(3):323-31.
71. Houston GD, Fowler CB. Extraosseous calcifying epithelial odontogenic tumor: Report of two cases and review of the literature, Oral Surg Oral Med Oral Pathol Oral Radiol Endod. 1997; 83:577.
72. Bouckaert MMR, Raubenheimer EJ, Jacobs FJ. Calcifying epithelial odontogenic tumor with intracranial extension: report of a case and review of the literature. Oral Surg Oral Med Oral Pathol Oral Radiol Endod. 2000;90:656-62.
73. Pullon, et al. Squamous odontogenic tumor: report of six cases of a previously undescribed lesion. Oral Surg Oral Med Oral Pathol Oral Radiol Endol. 1975;40:616-3.
74. Unal T, Gomel M, Gumel O, squamous odontogenic tumor like islands in a radicular cyst; report of a case. JOMS 1987;45: 346-9.
75. Goldblatt LI, et al. Squamous odontogenic tumour. Report of five cases and review of the literature. Oral Surg Oral Med Oral Pathol. 1982; 54:187-96.
76. Wright Jr JM. Squamous odontogenic tumor like proliferations in odontogenic cysts. Oral Surg Oral Med Oral Pathol. 1979;47:354-8.
77. Melrose RJ. Benign epithelial odontogenic tumors. Semin. Diagn Pathol. 1999;16:271-87.
78. Ide F, Shimoyama T, Horie N, Shimizu S. Intraosseous squamous cell carcinoma arising in association with a squamous odontogenic tumor of the mandible. Oral Oncol. 1999;35(4):431-4.
79. Norris LH, Baghaei-Rad M, Maloney PL, Simpson G and Guinta J. Bilateral maxillary squamous odontogenic tumors and the malignant transformation of a mandibular radiolucent lesion. J Oral Maxillofac Surg. 1984;42(12):827-34.
80. Baden E, Doyle J, Mesa M, Fabie M, Lederman D and Eichen M. Squamous odontogenic tumor: report of three cases

including the first extraosseous case. Oral Surg Oral Med Oral Pathol 1993;75:733-8.

81. Philipsen HE Birn H. The adenomatoid odontogenic tumor, ameloblastic adenomatoid tumor or adenoameloblastoma. Acta Pathol Microbiol Scand. 1969;75:375.

82. Gardner DG. The concept of hamartomas: its relevance to the pathogenesis of odontogenic lesions.Oral Surg. 1978; 45(6): 884-6.

83. Philipsen HP, Reichart PA, Zang KH, Nikai H, Yu QX. Adenomatoid odontogenic tumor: biologic profile based on 499 cases.J Oral Pathol Med. 1991; 20:149-58.

84. Philipsen HP, Reichart PA. Adenomatoid odontogenic tumor: facts and figures.Oral Oncol. 1998;35:125-31.

85. Takahashi K, Yashino T, Hashimoto S.Unusually large cystic adenomatoid odontogenic tumor of the maxilla: case report. Int J Oral Maxillofac Surg. 2001; 30(2):173-5.

86. Kruse A. Uber die Entwicklung cystischer Geschwlste im unterkiefer.Arch Pathol Anat. 1891;124:137-89.

87. Cahn LR, Blum T: Ameloblastic odontoma: Case report critically analyzed. J Oral Surg. 1952;10:169.

88. Philipsen HP, Reichart PA, Praetoius F. Mixed odontogenic tumors and odontomas. Considerations on interrelationship. Review of the literature and presentation of 134 new cases of odontomas.Oral Oncol. 1997;33:86-99.

89. Mosby EL, Russell D, Noren S, Barker BF. Ameloblastic fibroma in a 7-week-old infant: a case report and review of the literature. J Oral Maxillofac Surg. 1998;56(3):368-72.

90. Trodahl JN. Ameloblastic fibroma. A survey of cases from the Armed Forces Institute of Pathology. Oral Surg Oral Med Oral Pathol. 1972;33(4):547-58.

91. Kusama K, Miyake M, Moro I. Peripheral ameloblastic fibroma of the mandible, report of a case. J Oral Maxillofac Surg. 1998;56:399-401.

92. Couch RD, Morris EE, Vellios F. Granular cell ameloblastic fibroma. Report of 2 cases in adults, with observations of its similarity to congenital epulis. Am J Clin Pathol. 1962;37:398-404.

93. Philipsen HP, Thosaporn W, Reichart PA, Grundt G. Odontogenic lesions in opercula of permanent molars delayed in eruption .J Oral Pathol Med. 1992;21:38-41.

94. White DK, Chen SY, Hartman KS, Miller AS, Gomez LF. Central granular-cell tumor of the jaws (the so-call granular-cell ameloblastic fibroma). Oral Surg Oral Med Oral Pathol. 1978;45(3):396-405.

95. Vincent SD, Hammond HL, Ellis GL, Juhlin JP. Central granular cell odontogenic fibroma. Oral Surg Oral Med Oral Pathol. 1987;63(6):715-21.

96. Shiro BC, Jacoway JR, Mirmiran SA, McGuirt WF Jr, Siegal GP. Central odontogenic fibroma, granular cell variant. A case report with S-100 immunohistochemistry and a review of the literature. Oral Surg Oral Med Oral Pathol. 1989;67(6):725-30.

97. Takeda Y. Review: Ameloblastic Fibroma and related lesions: Current Pathologic concept. Oral Oncology. 1999;35:535-40.

98. Abughazaleh K, Andrus KM, Katsnelson A, White DK. Peripheral ameloblastic fibroma of the maxilla: report of a case and review of the literature. Oral Surg Oral Med Oral Pathol Oral Radiol Endod. 2008;105(5):e46-8. Epub 2008 Mar 4.

99. Darling MR, Daley TD. Peripheral ameloblastic fibroma. J Oral Pathol Med. 2006;35(3):190-2.

100. Hooker SP. Ameloblastoma odontoma an analysis of twenty six cases. Oral Surgery. 1967;24:275.

101. Slootweg PJ, et al. An analysis of the inter-relationship of the mixed odontogenic tumors-ameloblastic fibroma, ameloblastic fibro-odontoma, and the odontomas. Oral Surg Oral Med Oral Pahto. 1981;51:266-76.

102. Gardner DG. Central odontogenic fibroma current concepts. J Oral Pathol Med. 1996;25:556-61.

103. Slootweg PJ, Muller H. Central Fibroma of the jaw, odontogenic or desmoplastic. A report of five cases with reference to differential diagnosis. Oral Surg Med Oral Pathol. 1983;56:61-70.

104. Janssen JH, Blijdorp PA. Central odontogenic fibroma :a case report .J Maxillofac Surg. 1985;43:666-74.

105. Allen CM, Hammond HL, Stimson PG. Central odontogenic fibroma, WHO type. A report of three cases with an unusual associated giant cell reaction. Oral Surg Oral Med Oral Pathol. 1992;73:62-6.

106. Odell EW, Lombardi T, Barret AW, Morgan PR, Speight PM. Hybrid central giant cell granuloma and central odontogenic fibroma-like lesions of the jaws. Histopathology. 1997;30:165-71.

107. Norberg O. Zur kenntnis der dysodontogeneschen Geschwülste der Kieferknochen. Wschr zahnheikd. 1930;46: 321-55.

108. Brannon RB, Fowler CB, Carpenter WM, Cario RL. Cementoblastoma: an innocuous neoplasm? A clinicopathological study of 25 cases and review of literature with special emphysis on recurrence. Oral Surg Oral Med Oral Patho Oral Radiol Endod. 2002;93:311-320.

109. Piatelli A, Di Albertti L, Scarano A, Piatelli M. benign cementoblastoma associated with an unerupted third molar. Oral Oncol. 1998;34:229-31.

110. Ulmansky M, Hjørting-Hansen E, Praetorius F, Haque MF. Benign cementoblastoma. A review and five new cases. Oral Surg Oral Med Oral Patho. 1994; 77:48-55.

111. JS Jelic, MJ Loftus, AS Miller, et al. Benign cementoblastoma: Report of an unusual case and analysis of 14 additional cases, J Oral Maxillofac Surg. 1993;51:1033.

112. Slootweg PJ. Cementoblastoma and osteoblastoma: A comparison of hiostological features. J Oral Pathol Med. 1992;21:385-9.

113. Wenig BM. Atlas of head and neck pathology. Philadelphia: WB Saunders; 1993:29-95.

114. Kramer IRH, Pindborg JJ, Shear M. Histological typing of odontogenic tumors. 2nd edn. New York: Springer-Verlag; 1992.

115. Slootweg PJ, Van den Bos T, Straks W. Glycosaminoglycans in the myxoma of the jaw: a biochemical study. J Oral Pathol. 1985;14:299-306.

116. Zachariades N, Papanicolaou S. Treatment of odontogenic myxoma: review of the literature and report of three cases. Ann Dent. 1987;46:34-7,40.

117. Barker BF. Odontogenic myxoma. Semin Diagn Pathol. 1999;16:297-301.

118. Halfpenny W, Verey A, Bardsley V. Myxoma of the mandibular condyle: a case report and review of the literature.

Oral Surg Oral Pathol Oral Radiol Endod. 2000;90:348-53.

119. Goldblatt LI. Ultrastructural study of an odontogenic myxoma. Oral Surg Oral Med Oral Pathol. 1976;42:206-20.
120. Slootweg PJ, Van Den Bos T, Straks W: Glycosaminoglycans in myxoma of jaw: A biochemical study. J Oral Pathol. 1985;14:299.
121. McClure DK, Dahlin DC. Myxoma of bone: report of 3 cases. Mayo Clin Proc. 1977;52:249-53.
122. Heffner DK. Problems in pediatric otorhinolaryngic pathology: I. Sinonasal and nasopharyngeal tumors and masses with myxoid features. Int J Peditr Otorhinolaryngol. 1983;5:77-91.
123. Johnson LC, Yousefi M, Vinh TN, Heffner DK, Hyams VJ, Hartman KS.
124. Heffner DK. Sinonasal myxomas and fibromyxomas in children. Ear Nose Throat J. 1993;72:365-8.
125. Landa LE, Hedrick MH, Nepomuceno-Perez MC, Sotereanos GC. Recurrant myxoma of the zygoma: a case report. J Oral Maxillofac Surg. 2002;60:704-8.
126. Kaffe I, Naor H, Buchner A. Clinical and radiological features of odontogenic myxomas of jaws. Dentomaxillofacial Radiol. 1997;26:299-303.
127. Slootweg PJ, Wittkampf AR. Myxoma of the jaws: an analysis of 15 cases. J Maxillofac Surg. 1986;14:46-52.
128. Pahl S, Henn W, Binger T, Stein U, Remberger K. Malignant odontogenic myxomas of the maxilla: case with cytologic confirmation. J Largyngol Otol. 2000;114:533-5.
129. Lo Muzio L, Nocini PF, Favia G, et al. Odontogenic myxoma of the jaws. Oral Surg Oral Med Oral Pathol Oral Radiol. 1996;82:426-33.
130. Broka P. Traité des tumeurs, vol 1. France: P. Asselin;1866;(1):350.
131. Thoma KH, Goldman HM. A classification based on the observation of the epithelial, mesenchymal, and mixed varities. Am J Pathol. 1946;12:433-71.
132. Shafer WG, Hine MK, Levy BM. Cysts and tumors of odontogenic origin. In: A textbook of oral pathology. 4th edn, Philadelphia: WB Saunders; 1983;258-317.
133. Gorlin RJ, Chaudrey AP, Pindborg JJ. Odontogenic tumors: classification, histopathology and clinical behavior of man and domestic animals. Cancer 1961;14:73-98.
134. Sato M, Tanaka N, Sato T, Amagasa T. Oral and maxillofacial tumors in children: a review. Br J Oral Maxillofac. 1997;35:92-5.
135. Philipson HP, Reichart PA, Praetorius F. Mixed odontogenic tumors and odontomas. Considerations on interrelationship. Review of literature and presentation of 134 new cases of odontomas. Oral oncol. 1997;33:86-99.
136. Lopez-Areal L, Silvestre DF, Gil LJ. Compound odotoma erupting in the mouth: 4-year follow-up of a clinical case. J Oral pathol Med. 1992;21:285-8.
137. Hitchin AD. The aetiology of the calcified composite odontoma. Br Dent J. 1971;130:475-82.
138. Piattelli A, Trisi P. Ghost cells in compound odontoma: a study of undemineralized material. Bull Group Int Rech Sci. Stomatol Odontol. 1991; 34:145-9.
139. Sedano H, Pindborg JJ. Ghost cell epithelium in odontomas. J Oral Pathol. 1975;4:27-30.
140. Gao YH, Yang LJ, Yamaguchi A. Immunohistochemical demonstration of bone morphogenetic proyein in odontogenic tumors. J Oral Pathol Med. 1997;26:273-77.
141. Philipsen HP, Reichart PA, Praetorius F. Mixed odontogenic tumours and odontomas. Considerations on interrelationship. Review of the literature and presentation of 134 new cases of odontomas. Oral Oncol. 1997;33: 86-99.
142. Owen BM, Schumann NJ, Mincer HH, et al. Dental odontomas; A retrospective epidemiological study of 104 cases J Clin Pediatr Dent. 1997;21:261-4.
143. Blinder D, Peleg M, Taicher S. Surgical considerations in case of large mandibular odontomas located in the mandibular angle. Int J Oral Maxillofac Surg. 1993;22:163-5.
144. MacDonald–Jankowski DS, Odontomas in a chinese population. Dentomaxillofac Radiol. 1996;25:186-92.
145. Marchetti C, Piacentini C, Menghini P, Reguzzoni M. Observations on the enamel of odontomas. Scanning Microsc. 1993;7:999-1007.
146. KH Thoma, HM Goldman. Odontogenic Tumors. Amer J Path. 1946;22:433-71.
147. Levy BA. Ghost cell and odontomas. Oral Surg Oral Med. Oral Pathol. 1973; 36:851-5.
148. Kamakura S, Matusi K, Katou F, Shirai N, Kochi S, Motegi K. Surgical and orthodontic management of compound odontoma without removal of the impacted tooth. Oral Surg Oral Med Oral Pathol Radiol Endod. 2002;94:540-2.
149. Thoma KH, Johnson GJ, Ascario N. Case 43: Adamanto-odontoma. Am J Orthod Oral Surg. 1944;30:244.
150. Hooker SP. Ameloblastic odontoma: An analysis of twenty-six cases. Oral Surg. 1967;24:375-6.
151. Wächter R, Remagen W, Stoll P. Is it possible to differentiate between odontoameloblastoma and fibro-odontoma? Critical position on basis of 18 cases in DOSAK list. Dtsch Zahnarztl Z. 1991;46(1):74-7.
152. Kaugars GE and Zussmann HW. Ameloblastic odontoma (odonto-ameloblastoma). Oral Surg Oral Med. Oral Pathol. 1991;71:371-3.

29 Potentially Malignant Disorders of the Oral Cavity

Borle Rajiv M, Gadbail Amol

INTRODUCTION

Although the oral cavity is accessible for clinical examination by the clinician and the self examination by the patient, the irony is that the early detection of the oral malignant lesions is still far from desired. Although majority of cases of OSCC are preceded by precancerous/potentially malignant lesions and conditions which stay in place for the long time, early recognition and treatment of such lesions to prevent their conversion in the malignancy or detecting the malignancy in an early stage is still elusive. A majority of the patients with oral cancer report at a very late stage and thus, the management of such advanced lesions are often difficult and lead to great morbidity and unfavorable prognosis. The oral squamous cell carcinoma is the commonest oral cancer, which in majority of cases are preceded by potentially malignant lesions and conditions like leukoplakia, erythroplakia, oral submucous fibrosis, or sideropenic dysphagia particularly in Asian countries. These are the potentially dangerous lesions and can transform into frank squamous cell carcinoma. The identification of potentially malignant lesions of the upper aero-digestive tract can be possible through proper personal history, clinical examination. Recently, the molecular methods help in to detect the malignant potential, the prevention, early detection and treatment of head and neck carcinomas.

CONCEPT OF PRECANCER

Cancer being a genetic disorder involves multiple alterations of the genome progressively accumulated during a protracted period, the overall effect of which surpasses the inherent reparative ability of the cell. In the course of its progression, visible physical changes are taking place at the cellular level (atypia) and at the tissue level (dysplasia). These changes include genetic changes, epigenetic changes, surface alterations and alterations in intercellular interactions. The sum total of these physical and morphological alterations are of diagnostic and prognostic relevance and is designated as '*precancerous*' changes.

The concept of denoting some lesions or disorders of the oral mucosa as precancerous are based on the evidenced that:[1]

- In the longitudinal studies, areas of tissue with certain alterations in clinical appearances identified at the first assessment as precancerous have undergone malignant change during follow-up.
- Some of these alterations particularly red and white patches are seen to co-exist at the margins of overt oral squamous cell carcinomas.
- A proportion of these may share morphological and cytological changes observed in epithelial malignancies, but without frank invasion.
- Some of the chromosomal, genomic and molecular alterations found in clearly invasive oral cancers are detected in these presumptive 'precancer' or 'Premalignant' phase.

The terms 'precancer', 'precursor lesions', 'premalignant', 'intra epithelial neoplasia' and 'potentially malignant' have been used in the international literature to broadly describe clinical presentation that may have a potential to become cancer. They all convey the concept of a two-step or multi step process of cancer development.

POTENTIALLY MALIGNANT DISORDERS

In the past the potentially malignant disorders were often described as premalignant lesions and conditions and the gradually the nomenclature changed from Precancer—'Precursor lesions', 'Premalignant', 'Intra epithelial neoplasia' and 'Potentially malignant lesion'.

Recently the term '*potentially malignant disorders*' was recommended as it conveys that not all lesions and conditions described under this term may transform to cancer, rather that there is a family of morphological alterations amongst, which some may have an increased potential for malignant transformation.[1] Potentially malignant disorders of the oral mucosa are also indicators of risk of likely future malignancies elsewhere in (clinically normal appearing) oral mucosa and not only site-specific predictors.[1,2]

The Premalignant lesion was defined as *"A morphologically altered tissue in which cancer is more likely to occur than its apparently normal counterpart."* The examples are:

- Leukoplakia
- Erythroplakia
- Palatal changes associated with reverse smoking
- Actinic chelitis
- Bowen's disease.

Premalignant Condition

It was defined as *"A generalized state or condition associated with significantly increased risk for cancer development."* The examples are:

- Oral submucous fibrosis
- Sideropenic dysphagia
- Oral lichen planus
- Syphilis
- Discoid lupus erythematosus
- Dyskeratosis congenita
- Xeroderma pigmentosum
- Epidermolysis bullosa.

As per the recent concept the premalignant lesions and conditions are now called as potentially malignant lesions. The potentially malignant lesions can be described as under:

It conveys that not all lesions and conditions described under this term may transform to cancer, rather that there is a family of morphological alterations amongst, which some may have an increased potential for malignant transformation.[1]

Potentially malignant disorders of the oral mucosa are also indicators of risk of likely future malignancies elsewhere in (clinically normal appearing) oral mucosa and not only site-specific predictors.[2]

Risk Factors for Oral Potentially Malignant Disorders and Oropharyngeal Squamous Cell Carcinoma

- Age older than 45 years. However, the OSCC is detected at much younger patients.
- Combined tobacco and alcohol use or abuse
- Nutritional deficiencies like vitamin deficiency, iron deficiency
- Betel nut use
- Immunosuppression (disease or therapy related)
- Genetic susceptibility
- Prior upper aerodigestive tract cancer
- Sun exposure (lip vermilion)
- Oral human papillomavirus infection
- HIV infection might be associated with increased risk of oral potentially malignant lesions and oropharyngeal squamous cell carcinoma.

The Concept of 'Field Cancerization'

The concept of *"field cancerization"* was first introduced by Slaughter et al. in 1953[3] when studying the presence of histologically abnormal tissue surrounding oral squamous cell carcinoma. It was proposed to explain the development of multiple primary tumors and locally recurrent cancer. Organ systems in which field cancerization has been described since then are: head and neck (oral cavity, oropharynx and larynx), lung, vulva, esophagus, cervix, breast, skin, colon and bladder.[3]

Recent molecular findings support the carcinogenesis model in which the development of a field with genetically altered cells plays a central role. In the initial phase, a stem cell acquires genetic alterations and forms a "patch," a clonal unit of altered daughter cells. These patches can be recognized on the basis of mutations in *TP53* and have been reported for head and neck, lung, skin and breast cancer. The conversion of a patch into an expanding field is the next logical and critical step in epithelial carcinogenesis. Additional genetic alterations are required for this step, and by virtue of its growth advantage, a proliferating field gradually displaces the normal mucosa.

In the mucosa of the head and neck, as well as the esophagus, such fields have been detected with dimensions of greater than 7 cm in diameter, whereas they are usually not detected by routine diagnostic techniques. Ultimately, clonal divergence leads to the development of one or more tumors within a contiguous field of preneoplastic cells. An important clinical implication is that fields often remain after surgery of the primary tumor and may lead to new cancers, designated presently by clinicians as "a second primary tumor" or "local recurrence," depending on the exact site and time interval.[3,4]

This phrase has been used to describe three phenomena:[4]

- A wide field of aerodigestive mucosa that tends to be affected by premalignant disease
- The frequent occurrence of multiple primary tumors in epithelial areas affected by widespread pre-malignant disease, and
- The possibility of distant related primary tumors in the upper aerodigestive tract.

On the basis of recent molecular findings, Braakhuis et al. (2003)[5] proposed the definition of field cancerization: "The presence of one or more areas consisting of epithelial cells that have genetic alterations. A field lesion (or shortly 'field') has a monoclonal origin, and does not show invasive growth and metastatic behavior, the hallmark criteria of cancer."

These clinical expressions of a "field cancerization" phenotype could come about as a result of:

- Either independent molecular events affecting multiple cells separately.
- Or as a molecular event in a single clonal progenitor that gives rise to this phenomenon, *via* mechanisms of widespread clonal expansion or an alternative means of undergoing lateral spread across the mucosa of the upper aerodigestive tract.

Implications for Therapy

- The care providers to be more diligent about screening and directed biopsies in these patients.
- Frequent examination should be done for high-risk patients.
- Molecular techniques may aid in the analysis of surgical margins. In the future, the presence of altered clones at mucosal margins may be an indication for more aggressive therapy, including chemopreventive or radiotherapy, to treat altered clonal patches that are unable to be detected grossly and are beyond the initial scope of surgical excision.
- Screening studies that take advantage of the known genetic alterations may also become routine, especially for those people in a high-risk group (smokers and drinkers).
- The concept of field cancerization, or a mucosa rendered more susceptible to tumor formation, has led to the notion of chemoprevention, whereby a compound could be given to prevent tumor recurrence, prevent the progression of pre-malignant disease into malignancy, or retard tumor progression. Because surgical excision of the entire affected mucosa is not feasible, chemical compounds delivered systemically or topically can provide a wider range of coverage. Retinoids and other compounds such as cyclooxygenase-2 have been studied extensively with promising results, but the side effects and efficacy are still being studied. Newer, promising agents are being tested, but the persistent genetic alterations found in clonal patches that give rise to the clinical appearance of widespread mucosal alteration may ultimately be successfully treated by elimination of genetic alterations or the cells that carry them.[4]

The clinical observations also support the theory of field cancerization as more than one primary at the time of first diagnosis, appearance of second primary at different location, after successful excision of the first primary are reported.

Dysplasia

Epithelial dysplasia is the sum of various disturbances of epithelial proliferation and differentiation as seen microscopically.

When architectural disturbance is accompanied by cytological atypia (variaions in the size and shape of the keratinocytes), the term epithelial dysplasia applies. The combination of cellular and architectural changes observed in the gradual transition to malignancy. Dysplasia is a histopathological diagnosis made on the basis of presence of certain histological and cytological features in premalignant lesions and conditions. The magnitude of surface keratinization (keratosis or hyperkeratosis) is not of significant importance in the assessment of dysplasia.

WHO Criteria

Collaborating Centre for Oral Cancer and Precancer, the Working Group discussed the 2005 WHO classification and recommended its adaptation for wider use. The architecture and cytology criteria used for grading epithelial dysplasia in the WHO classification 2005[6] (Box 29.1).

Grading of Epithelial Dysplasia

The histopathological interpretation of potentially malignant lesions show a presence of dysplastic features of epithelium. In spite of numerous suggested prognostic molecular markers, the presence of epithelial dysplasia as assessed by light microscopic examination is still the strongest predictor of future malignant transformation in an oral potential malignant disorder. Epithelial dysplasia is usually divided into three categories (Box 29. 2):

Recently Warnakulasuriya S. et al. (2008)[7] classified epithelial dysplasia in to:

- Low risk dyspalasia (No/Questionable/Mild)
- High risk dysplasia (moderate or severe).

Box 29.1: Architecture and cytology criteria used for grading epithelial dysplasia in the WHO classification 2005

Architecture criteria	Cytology criteria
Irregular epithelial stratification	Abnormal variation in the nuclear size (anisoneucleosis)
Loss of polarity of basal cells	Abnormal variations in nuclear shape (nuclear pleomorphism)
Basal cell hyperplasia	Abnormal variations in cell size (anisocytosis)
Drop shaped rete pegs	Abnormal variations in cell shape (cellular pleomorphism)
Increased number of mitotic figures	Increased nuclear cytoplasmic ratio
Abnormally superficial mitosis	Increased nuclear size
Premature keratinization in single cells (dyskeratosis)	Atypical mitotic figures
Keratin pearls within the rete ridges	Increase in the number and size of nucleoli
	Hyperchromatism

Box 29.2: Grading of epithelial dysplasia

Mild: Cellular atypia and architectural disturbance limited to basal and parabasal layer (Fig. 29.1 to 29.3)
Moderate: Involvement from the basal layer to the midportion of the spinous layer (Fig. 29.4)
Severe: Alterations from the basal layer to a level above the midpoint of the epithelium. (Fig. 29.5)
Carcinoma in situ: The theoretical concept of carcinoma *in situ* is that malignant transformation has occurred, but invasion is not present. It is the most severe form of epithelial dysplasia and involves the entire thickness of the epithelium (top to bottom change). It is cytologically similar to Squamous cell carcinoma but architecturally the epithelial basement membrane remains intact and no invasion in to connective tissue has occurred (Fig. 29.6)

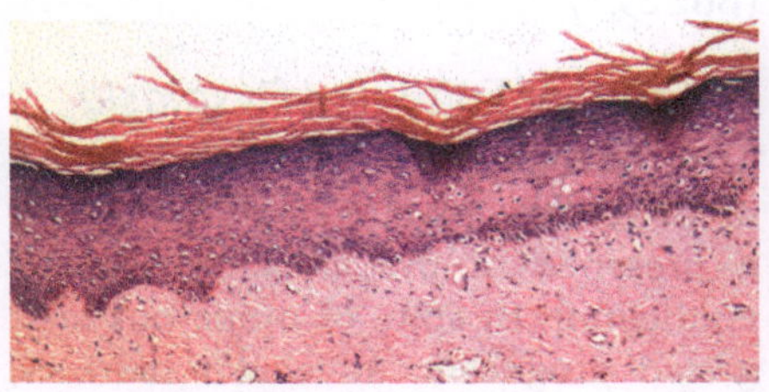

Fig. 29.1: No dysplasia/hyperkeratosis: Keratosis, acanthosis, no cellular atypia, no changes in architectural

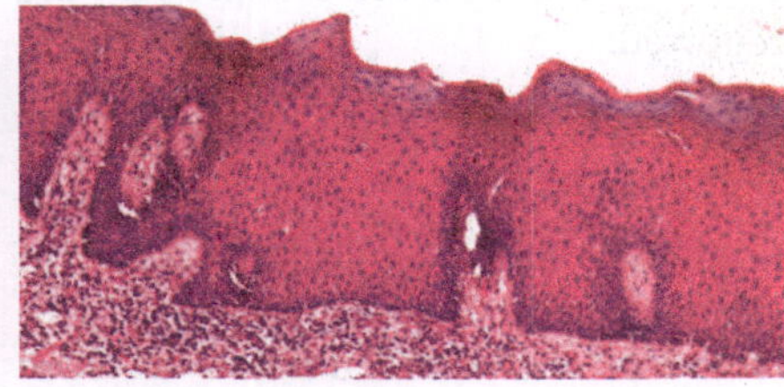

Fig. 29.2: Keratosis, acanthosis, no cellular atypia, basal cell hyperplasia, no changes in architectural

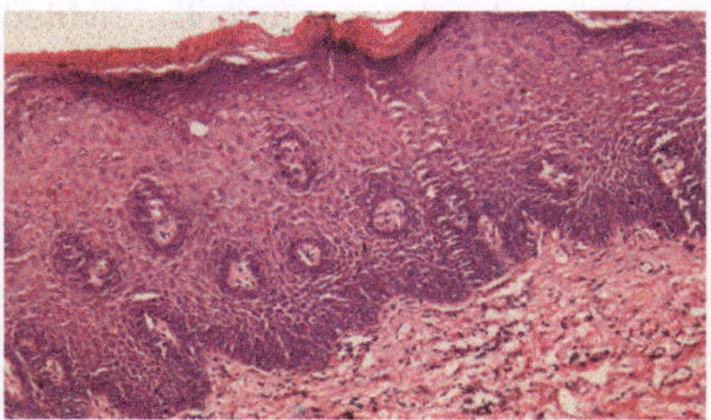

Fig. 29.3: Mild epithelial dysplasia: Keratosis, acanthosis, mild cellular atypia, architectural changes (lower 1/3 rd of epithelium)

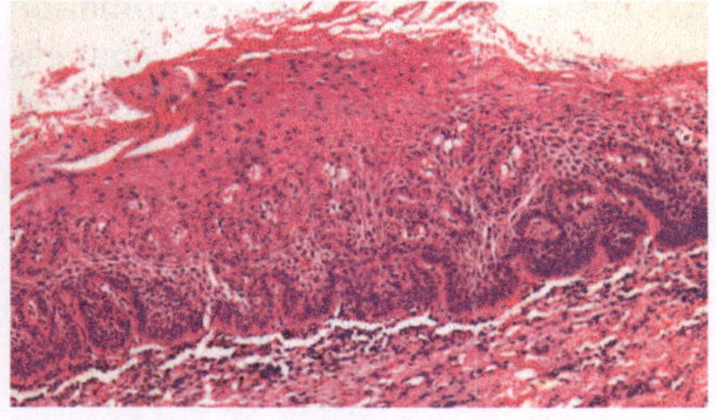

Fig. 29.4: Moderate epithelial dysplasia: Architectural changes extend to middle third of epithelium. Cellular atypia is moderate

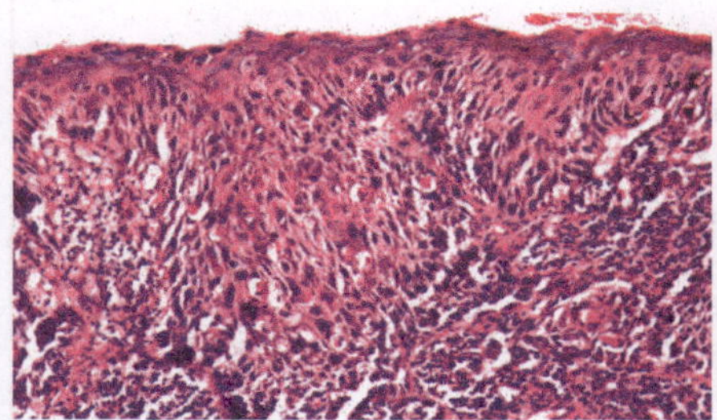

Fig. 29.5: Severe epithelial dysplasia: Architectural changes extend to upper third of epithelium. Cellular atypia is marked

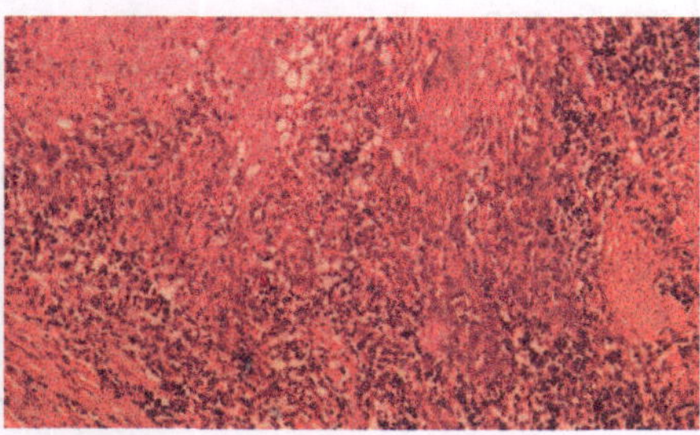

Fig. 29.6: Irregular interface between epithelium and connective tissue with pointed projections of epithelium indicated early invasive carcinoma

Leukoplakia

Definitions of Oral Leukoplakia proposed in the past decades:

WHO[8] (1978): A white patch or plaque that cannot be characterized clinically or pathologically as any other disease.

First International Conference on Oral Leukoplakia Malmo, Sweden[9] (1984): A white patch or plaque that cannot be characterized clinically or pathologically as any other disease and is not associated with any physical or chemical causative agent except use of tobacco.

International Symposium, Uppsala, Sweden[10] (1994): A predominantly white lesion of the oral mucosa that cannot be characterized as any other definable disease.

WHO[11] (1997): A predominantly white lesion of the oral mucosa that cannot be characterized as any other definable lesion.

WHO[12] (2005): Not defined–no distinction is made from other white patches.

Warnakulasuriya et al.[1] (2008): Leukoplakia should be used to recognize white plaques of questionable risk having excluded (other) known diseases or disorders that carry no increased risk for cancer.

Leukoplakia is a clinical term and the lesion has no specific histology. It may show atrophy or hyperplasia (acanthosis) and may or may not demonstrate epithelial dysplasia. It has a variable behavioral pattern but with an assessable tendency to malignant transformation. It must be noted that oral epithelial dysplasia has no specific clinical appearance and the term should not be used as a clinical descriptor of a white lesion.

The following conditions/disorders need exclusion to diagnose leukoplakia[1,9] (Table 29.1).

Etiology

Tobacco: It refers to dried leaves of nicotina tobaccum. Tobacco widely used in two forms.

Table 29.1: Lesions to be considered in the differential diagnosis of leukoplakia

Disorder	Diagnostic features	Biopsy
White sponge nevus	Noted in early life, family history, large areas involved, genital mucosa may be affected	Biopsy not indicated
Frictional keratosis	History of trauma, mostly along the occlusal plane, an etiological cause apparent, mostly reversible on removing the cause	Biopsy if persistent after elimination of cause particularly in a tobacco user
Morsicatio buccarum	Habitual cheek lip biting known, irregular whitish flakes with jagged out line	Biopsy not indicated
Chemical injury	Known history, site of lesion corresponds to chemical injury, painful, resoles rapidly	Biopsy not indicated
Acute pseudo-membranous candidosis	The membrane can be scraped off leaving an erythematous/raw surface	Swab for culture
Leukoedema	Bilateral on buccal mucosa, could be made to disappear on stretching, racial	Biopsy not indicated
Lichen planus (plaque type)	Other forms of lichen planus (reticular) found in association	Biopsy consistent with lichen planus
Lichenoid reaction	Drug history, e.g. close to an amalgam restoration	Biopsy consistent with lichen planus or lichenoid reaction
Discoid lupus erythematosus	Circumscribed lesion with central erythema, white lines radiating	Biopsy consistent with DLE supported by immunofloresence and other investigations
Skin graft	Known history	Not indicated
Hairy Leukoplakia	Bilateral tongue keratosis	Specific histopathology with koilocytosis EBV demonstrable on ISH
Leukokeratosis nicotina palate	Smoking history, grayish white palate	Not indicated

1. **Smokeless tobacco:** Chewable tobacco and snuff. When tobacco is chewed, various chemical constituents leach out such as nitrosonornicotine, nicotine, pyridine and picoline. Alkaline ph: 8.2–9.3 acts as local irritants and leads to alterations of mucosa.
2. **Smoked tobacco:** Cigar, cigarette, beedi and pipe. Smoking tobacco is harmful as this smoke contains polycyclic hydrocarbons, beta naphthalamine, nitrosoamines, CO, nicotine, all of which acts as source of irritation. Heat also plays a major role. Heat induces alterations in tissues increasing reddening and stippling of mucosal surface.

Alcohol: Whether the use of alcohol itself is an independent etiological factor in the development of leukoplakia is still questionable. Its effect, at best, may be synergistic to other well-known etiological factors (physical irritants).

- It causes irritation and burning sensation of oral mucosa.
- It facilitates the entry of carcinogen into exposed cells and thus, alters the oral epithelium and its metabolism.

Chronic irritation: Continuous trauma or local irritation in the oral cavity is suspected as a causative agent for leukoplakia. The source of irritation or trauma may be malocclusion, ill-fitting dentures, sharp broken teeth, hot spicy food or root piece.

Candida albicans: As a possible etiological factor in leukoplakia and its possible role in malignant transformation is still unclear. About 10 percent of oral leukoplakias satisfy the clinical and histological criteria for chronic hyperplastic candidiasis (candidal leukoplakia). Epithelial dysplasia is reported to occur four to five times more frequently in candidal leukoplakia than in leukoplakia general. Various evidences have been presented to justify an aetiological role for candida in neoplastic transformation, which includes among others the catalytic transformation *in vitro* of the carcinogenic nitrosamine, N-nitrosobenzyl-methylamine, by strains of candida albicans demonstrated to be selectively associated with leukoplakia.

Viruses: The possible contributory role of viral agents (such as HPV 16 and 18) in the pathogenesis of oral Leukoplakia particularly with regard to exophytic verrucous leukoplakia.

Vitamin deficiency: Serum levels of vitamin A, B_{12}, C, beta-carotene and folic acid were significantly decreased in patients with oral Leukoplakia than normal control.

Genetic factor: Relatively little is known yet with regard to possible genetic factors in the development of Leukoplakia.

Age and gender: The onset of leukoplakia usually takes place after the age of 30 years resulting in peak incidence above the age of 50 years. The gender distribution in most studies varies, ranging from a strong male predominance in different parts of India to almost 1:1 in the western world.

Clinical Features

Leukoplakia may occur either as a single, localized change of the oral mucosa or as diffuse, often multiple lesions. The site distribution shows worldwide differences, that are partly related to gender and tobacco habits. In fact, any oral site may be affected. In general two clinical variants of leukoplakia are being recognized, the *homogeneous* and the *nonhomogeneous* type. Transition or changes among the different clinical variants of oral leukoplakia may occur.

Homogeneous leukoplakia: It has been defined as a predominantly white lesion of uniform flat, thin appearance that may exhibit shallow cracks and a smooth wrinkled or corrugated surface with a constant texture throughout. The adjective homogeneous not only applies to the homogeneous whitish color of the lesion, but also above all to a flat thin and rather smooth surface. A more elaborate sub-division may be used such as[13-16]

- Homogeneous Smooth (Figs 29.7 and 29.8)
- Homogeneous Furrowed (fissured)
- Homogeneous Ulcerated

Non-homogeneous leukoplakia: It has been defined as predominantly white or white-red lesions that may be irregularly flat, nodular or exophytic. (Figs 29.9 and 29.10). The nodular lesions are characterized by white patches or nodules on erythematosus base, while the exophytic lesions have irregular blunt or sharp projections. The adjective nonhomogeneous is applicable both to the aspect of color, i.e. a mixture of white and red changes and to the aspect of texture, i.e. exophytic, papillary or verrucous.

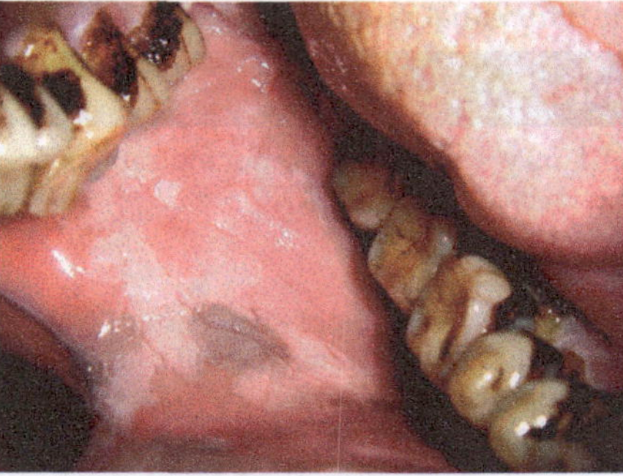

Fig. 29.7: Preleukoplakia ('mild or thin leukoplakia')

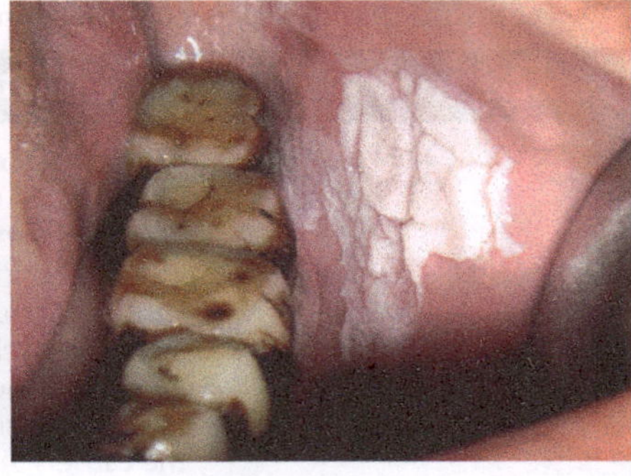

Fig. 29.8: 'Homogeneous or thick leukoplakia'

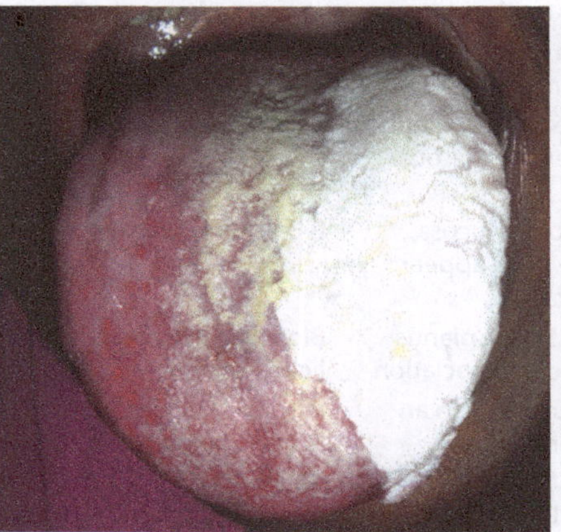

Fig. 29.9: Homogeneous to slightly nodular leukoplakia

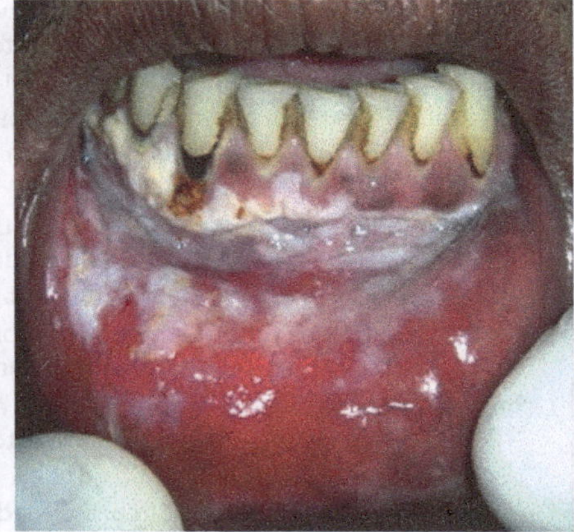

Fig. 29.10: Speckled leukoplakia, or nonhomogeneous leukoplakia

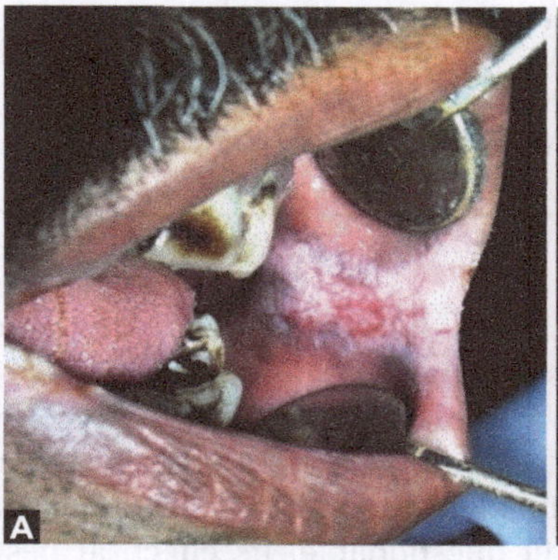

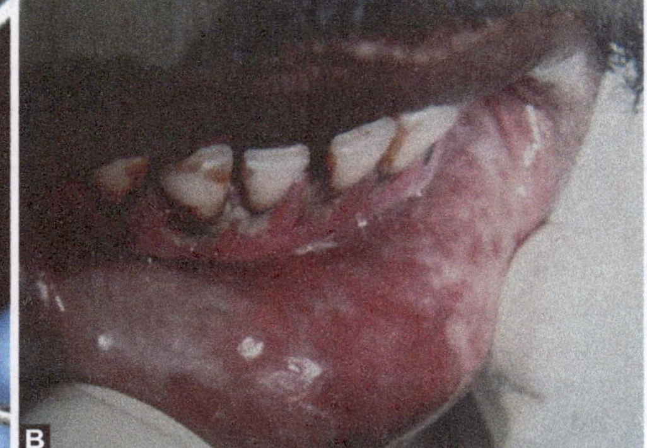

Figs 29.11A and B: (A) Nodular; (B) Speckled leukoplakia

Leukoplakia begins as thin, gray, or gray-white plaques that may appear somewhat translucent, are sometimes fissured or wrinkled, and are typically soft and flat. They usually have sharply demarcated borders but occasionally blend gradually into normal mucosa. This early stage is sometimes referred as *'preleukoplakia'* but preferable designated *'mild or thin leukoplakia'* (Fig. 29.7).

Thin leukoplakia may disappear or continue unchanged but as time progresses as many as two thirds of such plaques slowly extend laterally and acquire a distinctly white appearance from a thickened keratinized layer. They may become leathery to palpation and fissures may deepen, but there should be only a few, if any, localized nodules or surface projections. At this stage the lesions is severe often called *'homogeneous or thick leukoplakia'* (Fig. 29.8).

Most thick, smooth lesions remain indefinitely at this stage, as many as one-third regress or disappear and a few become even more severe. The latter lesions begin to develop surface irregularities of a nodular or granular nature, and hence are referred to as *'granular or nodular leukoplakia'* (Fig. 29.11A). Occasionally, pointed projections develop on the surface and may be so numerous that the resulting lesions are called *'verruciform leukoplakia'*.

An additional change can occur over a time however, multiple circular or oval patches of non-blanching redness or erythroplakia begin appearing in scattered areas. Such areas represent sites in which epithelial cells are so immature that they are no longer able to produce keratin. These intermixed red and white lesions are called *'erythroplakia, speckled leukoplakia, or nonhomogeneous leukoplakia'*. (Fig. 29.11B). These are the most worrisome form of the lesions and carry an extremely high risk of malignant transformation.[17]

A special high-risk form of leukoplakia, ***'proliferative verrucous leukoplakia'***[18] (PVL) is characterized by the development of multiple keratotic plaques with roughened surface projections (Fig. 29.12). The relationship of PVL to cases described as verrucous leukoplakia is uncertain. The multiple PVL plaque tends to spread slowly and involve additional oral mucosal sites. Although the lesions typically begin as simple, flat hyperkeratosis that are indistinguishable from ordinary leukoplakic lesions, PVL exhibits persistent growth, eventually becoming exophytic and verrucous in nature. As the lesions progress, they may go through a stage indistinguishable from verrucous carcinoma, but they later usually develop dysplastic changes and transform into full fledged squamous cell carcinoma usually within 8 years of initial PVL diagnosis. These lesions rarely regress despite therapy. PVL is unusual among the leukoplakia variants in having a strong female predilection (1:4 male to female ratio) and minimal association with tobacco use.[19]

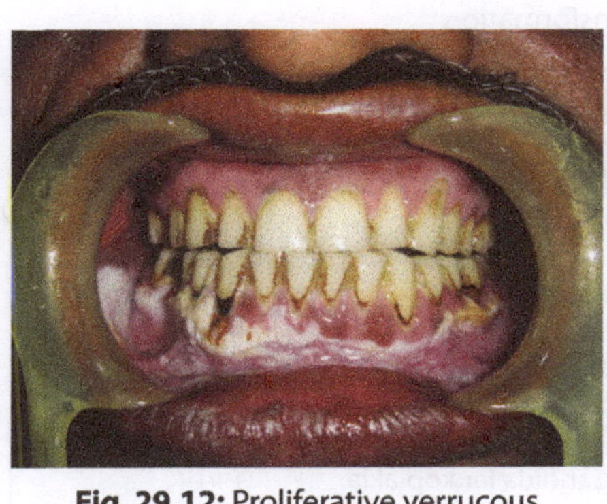

Fig. 29.12: Proliferative verrucous leukoplakia

Diagnostic Procedure (Flow chart 29.1)

Elimination of possible causes: In a patient with a white lesion of the oral mucosa, the clinician should first try to rule out any of the definable white lesion listed in the above table before accepting the definative diagnosis of leukoplakia.

The biopsy: In homogeneous leukoplkia, the taking of a biopsy should be the standard rule. The biopsy may be incisional or a conservative excisional biopsy, if feasible.

In non-homogeneous leukoplakia, that are usually symptomatic, epithelial dysplasia or even carcinoma *in situ* or early squamous cell carcinoma is rather common. The biopsy should be taken at the site of symptoms, if present, and or at a site of redness or induration. Biopsy of exophytic, verrucous or papillary lesions should be taken deep enough to include a sufficient amount of underlying connective tissue and preferably from the margins.

Identification of apppropriate biopsy site

- To improve the sensitivity and specificity of lesion identification and appropiate biopsy site showing maximum dysplastic changes, vital tissue staining is often used.
- Toludine blue is most commmonly used and the intensly stained areas should be considered for biopsy site. Toludene blue is an acidophilic metachromatic thiazin dye which selectively stains tissue acids and particularly DNA and RNA. The rationale for use of this vital stain is that dysplastic cells usually contain more nucleic acid than normal cells.
- Lugol's iodine solution is also used. It produces the brown black stain by reaction of the iodine with the glycogen, which is inversly related to the degree of keratosis.
- The use of vital stains with good measure of clinical experience is of value in accurate diagnosis and deciding where to perform biopsy.
- **Oral brush biopsy:** Computer assisted analysis of oral brush biopsy is an aid to the oral examination which helps to determine the significance of oral lesions with an epithelial abnormality. Its utility is limited as it doesnot provide desired details beyond dysplasia and may be non conclusive in border line cases. It is

Flow chart 29.1: Schematic representation of the steps in the diagnosis of oral leukoplakia

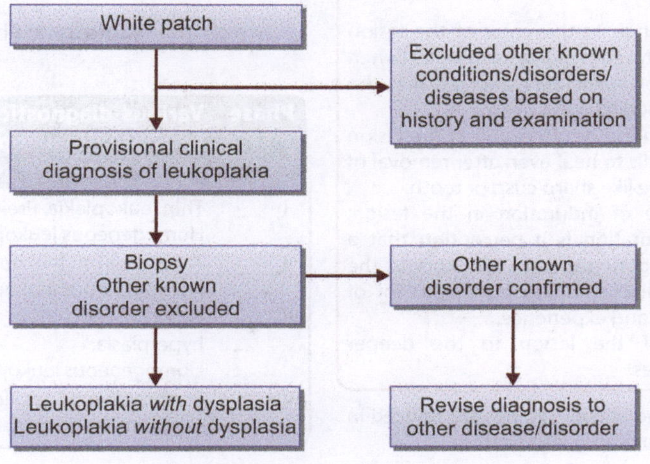

expensive technique and hence, not affordable to majority of population who need it more.
- The exfoliative cytology are of limited value when dealing with leukoplakia.

Identifying malignant change

The advanced molecular investigation like DNA ploid, p53 mutation and chromosome 3 and 9 changes can indicate significantly increased chances of malignancy.

More than the investigations it is very important to identify the clinical changes in the long standing oral precancerous lesion which warrants biopsy for making early diagnosis of malignant transformations in the lesion so that the treatment can be given at a very early stage to ensure good out come and prognosis. By and large too much dependence is shown by the clinicians on the investigations and in the bargain the clinical findings are often ignored. There is no doubt that biopsy still remains the gold standard in making the diagnosis but when to suspect a malignant change and to take a biopsy is purely clinical judgment. The rough guidelines for clinical diagnosis are shown in Box 29.3.

Box 29.3: Routine guidelines for diagnosis of leukoplakia

- Every case should be kept under periodic follow up and during every follow up thorough clinical examination is required.
- Any change in the color of the lesion especially red is highly suspicious (when the lesion turns fiery and red it is the time to scratch your head!).
- Any fissuring or ulceration in the lesion which fails to heal even after removal of the cause like sharp cusp or tooth.
- Presence of induration in the lesion. The induration is a perception that a palpating finger gets and this is the most reliable finding but needs lot of practice and experience.
- Fixity of the lesion to the deeper structures.

*If any of the above changes are noticed in the lesion a biopsy is indicated.

Histo-pathological Features

The histopathological aspects of leukoplakia may vary from atrophy of the epithelium to hyperplasia with or without hyperkeratosis. Epithelial dysplasia, if present, may range from mild to severe. In some instances, carcinoma *in situ* and even squamous cell carcinoma are encountered histologically. A histopathological report of exophytic, verrucous or papillomatous lesions, in spite of the absence of epithelial dysplasia may in time progress to squamous cell carcinoma and that long-term follow up should be considered. The histological report of a leukoplakia should include a statement on the absence or presence of epithelial dysplasia and an assessment of its severity.

Malignant Potential of Leukoplakia

Certain features have been reported to be associated with increased risk of malignant transformation.
- Gender, particularly women seem to be at risk
- Long duration of the leukoplakia
- Leukoplakia in non smokers (idiopathic leukoplakia)
- Location in the floor of the mouth, retro molar area or/and on the tongue
- Non-homogeneous type
- Presence of *Candida albicans*
- Presence of epithelial dysplasia

Of the above-mentioned factors the malignant potential depends on mainly depends upon clinical appearance, site and etiological factors.[15,20]

The incidence of malignant transformation of 07 to 13 percent was reported by Lee et al.[20] while Angadi et al.[21] reported the incidence of 11.6 percent.

Warnakulasuriya[22] reported incidence of malignant transformation in the leukoplakia is 0.3 to 5.6 percent while other workers[23-26] reported it to be between reported 15.6 to 39.2 percent.

- **Clinical appearance:** The homogeneous leukoplakia has low malignant potential. The presence of dysplasia more or less correlating with a clinical non-homogeneous, erythroleukoplakia subtype seems to be more important indicator of malignant potential (Table 29.2). Dysplastic lesions carry a 5-fold greater risk than non-dysplastic ones. Seven percent of the dysplastic lesions progressed to cancer in a mean observation period of 7 years. In two studies from India (Gupta PC et al. 1980,[27] Silverman S[28] et al. 1976) low malignant transformation rate of oral leukoplakia have been reported, 0.3 percent and 0.06 percent, respectively. In reports from western country (Axell T 1987[29]) reported somewhat higher figure.
  - Around 2 to 5 percent of leukoplakia becomes malignant in 10 years.
  - 5 to 20 percent of leukoplakias are dysplastic.
  - 10 to 35 percent of dysplastic leukoplakia proceed to carcinoma.

Table 29.2: Phase I to IV leukoplakia subtype and risk of malignant transformation

Phase	Various diagnostic descriptive terms used for phase I to phase IV leukoplakia subtype and risk of malignant transformation[12]	Risk of malignant transformation
I	Thin leukoplakia, Preleukoplakia, Homogeneous leukoplakia	+/–
II	Thick, smooth leukoplakia, fissured leukoplakia Homogeneous leukoplakia	++
III	Granular, verruciform, rough leukoplakia, Candidial epithelial hyperplasia, Homogeneous leukoplakia	+++
IV	Erythroplakia, Speckled leukoplakia, Candida leukoplakia, Nonhomogeneous leukoplakia	++++

- **Site:** The soft palate complex, ventrolateral surface of tongue, retro molar area and floor of mouth has the high-risk malignant potential. Sublingual keratosis is more common in women.
- **Etiological factors:** Proliferative leukoplakia associated with human papilloma virus, which have an inexorably slow progression over one or two decades to verrucous or squamous cell carcinoma.
  - Idiopathic leukoplakias where there is no obvious etiological factor have noted to have a significantly increased risk of malignant transformation in comparison with leukoplakias where there are associated causative agents. While tobacco is the most important risk factor associated with leukoplakia, lesions in non-tobacco users seem to be at increased risk of developing oral squamous cell carcinoma.
  - Candidal leukoplakia has increase risk of malignant potential. Chronic candidal infection is common in speckled leukoplakia and *Candida albicans* can cause or colonies on keratosis, particularly smokers and is especially likely to form speckled leukoplakia at lip commissures. They may be dysplastic and have high malignant potential than some other keratosis. Candidal leukoplakia responds to antifungal therapy and smoking cessation.
  - Syphilitic leukoplakia has high malignant potential especially seen on the dorsal surface of tongue.
  - Hairy leukoplakia caused by Epstein bar virus usually has a corrugated surface and affects margins of the tongue almost exclusively. This is associated with HIV infections. The condition appears benign and is self-limiting.

The staging of the oral leukoplakia is depicted in Box 29.4.

Treatment

Every leukoplakia does not necessarily transform into a malignancy. The leukoplakias, which are induced by the smokeless tobacco, are more dangerous and tend to resist the conservative treatment. Those, which are precipitated secondary to chronic irritation (sharp tooth, chronic trauma from occlusion), respond, and are reversible on removing the cause and with conservative treatment (Flow chart 29.2).

Box 29.4: Staging system for oral leukoplakia[30]

L (Size of the lesion)
- L1–size of leukoplakia < 2 cm.
- L2–size of leukoplakia 2–4 cm.
- L3–size of leukoplakia > 4 cm.
- Lx–size not specified.

P (Pathology i.e. Presence or absence of dysplasia)
- P0–No epithelial; dysplasia.
- P1–Distinct epithelial dysplasia.
- Px–Dysplasia not specified in the pathology report.

OLEP staging system
- Stage I–L1P0
- Stage II–L2P0
- Stage III–L3P0 or L1L2P1
- Stage IV–L3P1

- The leukoplakia can be treated with conservative treatment comprising of removing the cause and medicines. The other modality being excision. The leukoplakias that are diffuse and involve large area are often difficult to excise.
- The conservative line of treatment comprises of removing the cause by smoothening the sharp cusps, correcting overhanging edges of the restoration/prosthesis or discontinuation of the habits.
- The medicinal treatment comprises of prescription of vitamin A, B complex, and iron preparations as imperical therapy. The vitamin A is epithelial conditioner and helps in healing. The preparations like topical anesthetists (Lidocaine, benocaine) can be prescribed to alleviate the burning sensation while taking the food. Topical steroid preparations are also used. The patients are often prescribed antioxidants like alpha tocopherol, beta-carotene, ascorbic acid, and selenium, Zinc in an

Flow chart 29.2: Management of leukoplakia

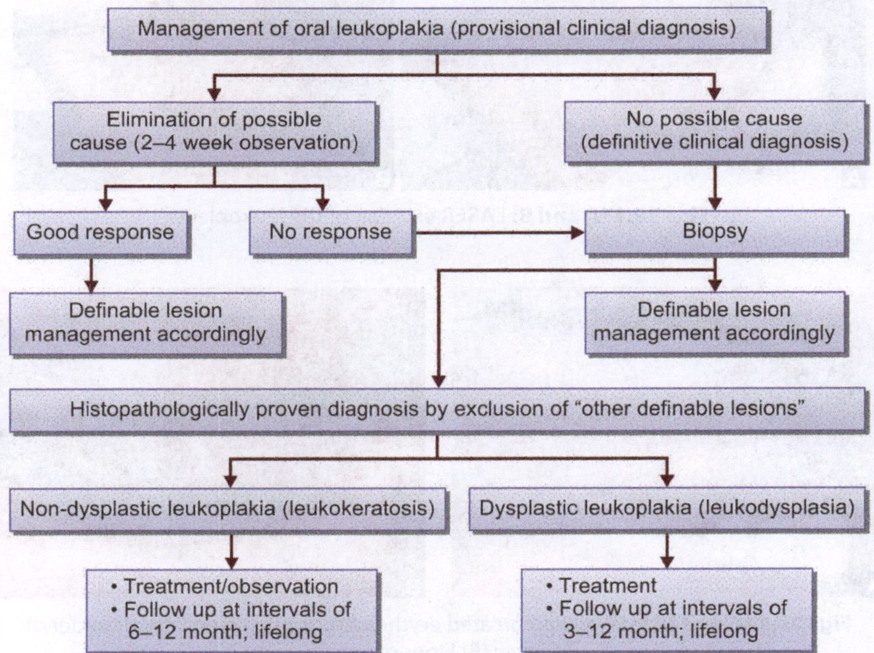

attempt to scavenge free radicals and prevent carcinogenesis. The patients are concealed to discontinue the habits and are kept under long term, periodic follow-up.

- The surgical treatment comprises of excision of the patch. The criteria for deciding surgery are:
  a. Lesions which fail to respond to the conservative treatment
  b. Fast growth
  c. Development of ulceration
  d. Color change
  e. Indurations in the lesion
  f. The moderate and severe epithelial dysplasia considered as *Risky dysplasia* and should be removed surgically.

The lesion should be biopsied from the suspected areas (hot areas) and any malignant transformation, degree, severity of dysplasia should be ascertained, and the potentially dangerous lesions should be excised.

The modalities of excision comprises of excision with electrocautery, LASER excision, (Figs 29.13A and B) cryoexcision and surgical excision. The smaller defects are allowed to granulate and heal by secondary epithelization while as the larger defects recovered with split thickness skin grafts. The entire excised patch is subjected for the histopathologically examination and screened thoroughly to rule out malignancy including carcinoma *in situ.*

Erythroplakia

Erythroplakia is rare condition, while leukoplakia is a relatively common condition. In contrast to leukoplakia, erythroplakia is almost always associated with premalignant changes histologically and is therefore a most important precancerous lesion. The term 'erythroplakia' is used analogously to leukoplakia to designate lesions of the oral mucosa that present as "a bright red velvety plaque or patch which cannot be characterized clinically or pathologically as being due to any other condition".

Described originally as "erythroplasia" by Queyrat[31] in 1911, as a lesion occurring on glans penis of an elderly syphilitic patient with a comparable pre-malignant tendency. Oral erythroplakia is clinically and histopathologically similar to the genital patches. Erythroplakia may also occur in conjunction with leukoplakia and has been found concurrently with a large proportion of early invasive oral carcinoma.[16-17]

The malignant potential of erythroplakia is much higher than the leukoplakia and the red color if often attributed to tall rete pegs and increased vascularity, suggestive of high metabolic lesion. It is therefore said that "*when the lesion appears fiery and red, it is the time to scratch your head*" meaning that the erythroplakia should be more carefully dealt.

Etiology

The etiology of erythroplakia is unknown, although same as for leukoplakia smoking and alcohol abuse are important etiological factors.

Clinical Features

Erythroplakia is predominantly a disease of older men, with peak prevalence at 65 to 74 years. Predilection for sites: Floor of the mouth, retromolar area, followed by tongue, soft palate and especially in Indian, population mandibular sulcus (Figs 29.14 and 29.15).

The altered mucosa appears as a well-demarcated erythematosus macule or plaque with a soft, velvety texture. Many of these lesions are irregular in outline, and some contain islands of normal mucosa within areas of erythroplakia, a

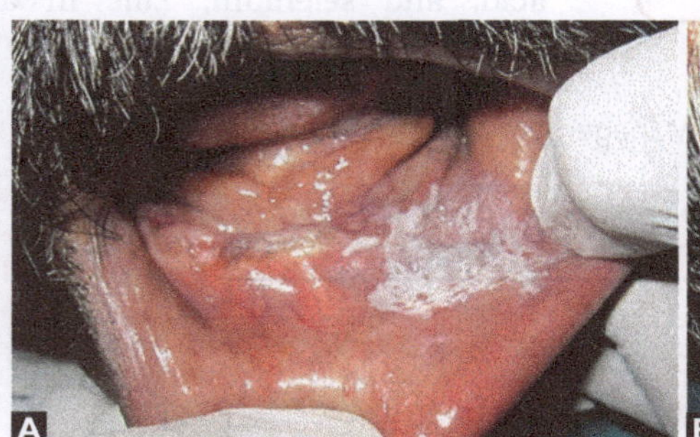

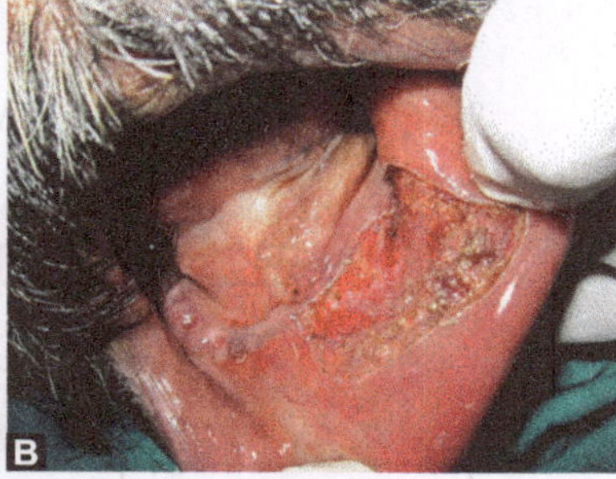

Figs 29.13A and B: LASER excision of the leukoplakia

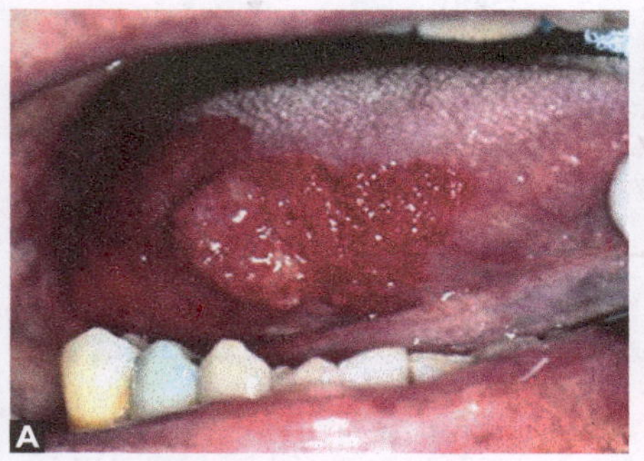

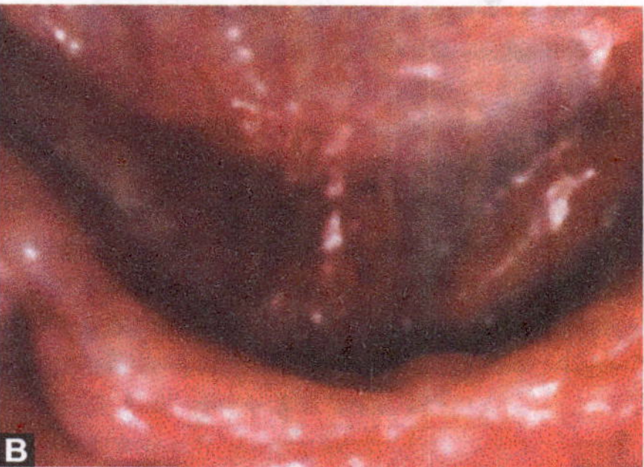

Figs 29.14A and B: (A) Well demarcated erythematous plaque on lateral border of tongue; (B) Floor of mouth

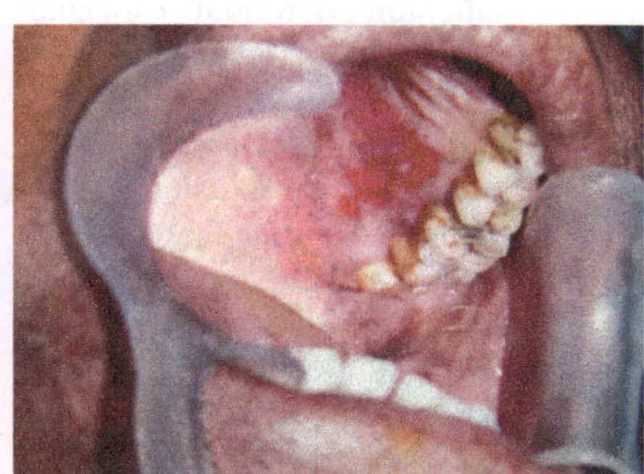

Fig. 29.15: Case of erythroplakia in a patient with SMF of palate

Box 29.5: Differential diagnosis of erythroplakia[1]

Nature of condition	Diagnostic category
Inflammatory/immune disorders	Nonspecific mucositis, Desquamative gingivitis, Erythematous lichen planus, Dyscoid lupus erythematosus, pemphigoids, hypersensitivity reactions, Reither's disease
Infections	Erythematosus candidiasis, histoplasmosis
Hamartomas/neoplasms	Hemangioma, Kaposi's sarcoma

phenomenon that has been attributed to coalescence of a number or precancerous foci. It is usually asymptomatic and may be associated with an adjacent leukoplakia. Clinically erythroplakia can mimic conditions shown in (Box 29.5) and biopsy often required to distinguish between them.

Several clinical variants of erythroplakia have been described by different investigators, but there is no general agreement on classification. Shear,[32] in 1972, described:

- Homogenous form
- Erythroplakia interspersed with patches of leukoplakia, and
- Granular or Speckled erythroplakia (identical to speckled leukoplakia).

Homogeneous erythroplakia has more malignant transformation rate than speckled erythroplakia. The carcinogenic potential of erythroplakia is considered to be higher (14–50%)[33,34] than leukoplakia and SMF.

Histopathological Features

Different studies have demonstrated that 80 to 90 percent of erythroplakia are histologically either severe epithelial dysplasia, carcinoma *in situ*, or superficially invasive squamous cell carcinoma. The epithelium shows a lack of keratin production and is often atrophic, but it may be hyperplastic. This lack of keratinization especially combined with dropped pushing rete pegs along with deep long connective tissue papillae with overlying thin epithelium allows the visibility of underlying microvasculature. This explains the red color of the lesion. The underlying connective tissue often demonstrates chronic inflammation.

Treatment

- Red lesions of the oral mucosa, especially those of the oral floor and ventral or lateral tongue, and in Indian populations should be viewed with suspicion and a biopsy should be performed.
- If a source of irritation can be identified and removed, biopsy of such lesions may be delayed for two weeks to allow a clinically similar inflammatory lesion time to regress.
- As with leukoplakia, the treatment of erythroplakia is guided by the definitive diagnosis obtained by biopsy.
- Lesions exhibiting moderate dysplasia or worse must be removed completely or destroyed by the methods used for leukoplakia.
- The excised specimen must send for microscopic examination because of the possibility that a focal invasive carcinoma might be missed in the initial biopsy material.
- Recurrence and multifocal oral mucosal involvement are common with erythroplakia; hence, long-term follow up is suggested for treated patient.[17]

Palatal Changes Associated with Reverse Smoking

A diffuse thickening of the palatal mucosa occurs in reverse smokers. In several countries, cigars or cigarettes are smoked with the glowing end inside the mouth. The largest numbers of reverse smokers is found in certain areas of India, but the habit is also practiced in some Latin American countries, in Sardinia and in the Philippines. Reverse chutta (crude form of cigar) smoking practiced among females of Srikakulam district of Andhra Pradesh, recorded a prevalence of 8.8 percent of leukoplakia, 4.6 percent of preleukoplakia and 17.9 percent leukokeratosis nicotine palate (Daftary, et al. 1992[35]). Palatal changes associated with reverse smoking thus, exhibited a spectrum of clinical changes, and it was not satisfactory to group under leukoplakia, preleukoplakia, or leukokeratosis nicotina palate.[16-17,36]

Clinical Features

According to Daftary et al. 1992, the incidence of palatal changes (encompassing all components) was 24.9/1000 among men and 39.6/1000 among women and the peak incidence was in the 55 to 64 year age group.

The regression rate was higher, when habit was discontinued or reduced substantially (Gupta PC et al. 1980[21]). Malignant transformation was observed for 0.3 percent of the palatal lesions. In 10-year intervention study in the same area, the malignant potential of various components of palatal changes was evaluated: red patches were found to exhibit a high potential for malignant transformation (Fig. 29.16).

Palatal changes comprise several components[16]:

- **Keratosis:** Diffuse whitening of entire palatal mucosa.
- **Excrescences:** 1 to 3 mm elevated nodules, often with central red spots.
- **Patches:** Well defined, elevated white plaques.

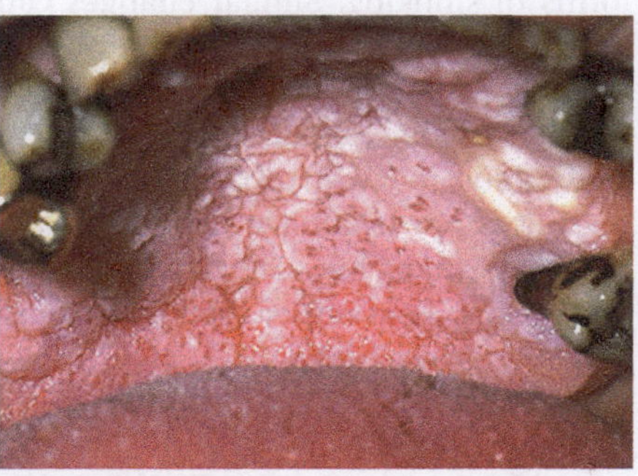

Fig. 29.16: Diffuse whitening of palatal mucosa with small elevated nodules with central red spots

- **Red areas:** Well defined reddening of the palatal mucosa.
- **Ulcerated areas:** Crater like areas covered by fibrin, and
- **Non-pigmented areas:** Areas of palatal mucosa that are devoid of pigmentation.

Histological Features

Histopathologically hyperkeratosis and epithelial dysplasia is noted. Epithelial dysplasia was observed in 52 percent of red areas, 25 percent of excrescences, 20 percent ulcerations, 10 percent of patches and in 19 percent of non-pigmented areas. (Comprises data from only one study i.e. by Daftary et al.).

Palatal changes associated with reverse smoking are characterized by hyperorthokeratosis, epithelial dysplasia and inflammatory cells in the connective tissue. Melanin deposits is seen in the lamina propria of most of them. The epithelium is either atrophic or shows epithelial dysplasia in red areas.

Treatment

The treatment comprises of discontinuation of habit and follow-up of the patient. If suspicious red areas, ulcerations, patches persist, then biopsy should be carried out. If possible, conservative excisional biopsy is the treatment of choice.

Nicotina Stomatitis (Pipe Smoker's Palate)

It is a specific mucosal change of palate, which is frequently seen in heavy pipe smokers. Because pipe smoking generates more heat on the palate than other forms of smoking. Similar changes can also be produced by the long term use of extremly hot beverages. Although this lesion is a white keratotic change, obviously associated with tobacco smoking, it does not appear to have a premalignant nature, perhaps because it developes in response to heat rather than the chemicals in tobacco smoke.[16-17, 27]

Clinical Features

Nicotine stomatitis most commonly is found in men older than 45 years of age. It is first manifested as redness and inflammation of the palate. Later, grayish-white, thickened, multinodular, or papular appearance with a small red spot in the center of each tiny nodule is representing the dilated and sometimes partially occluded orifice of an accessory palatal salivary gland duct. The mucosa that covers the papules frequently appears whiter than the surrounding epithelium. The palatal keratin may become so thickened that fissured or dried mud appearance is imparted.

It is histopathologically characterized by hyperkeratosis and acanthosis of ductal and palatal epithelium. Epithelial dysplasia is very rarely seen. The ducts of minor salivary glands show dilatation and inflammation around them.

Treatment

It is completely reversible even when it has been present for many decades. Although this is not a precancerous lesion, the patient should be encouraged to stop habit and any suspicious area should be examined closely by biopsy. Any white lesions or the palatal mucosa that persist after one month of habit cessation should be considered a true leukoplakia and managed accordingly.

Bowen's Disease

Bowen's disease is a special form of intraepithelial carcinoma occurring with some frequency on skin, particularly in patients who have had arsenical therapy.

Clinical Features

It is often associated with the internal and extracutaneous cancer. On rare occasion as reported by Gorlin[37] Bowen's disease may occur in the oral cavity. It may be seen as leukoplakia or a combination of leukoplakia and erythroplakia or as an ulcerated lesion intraorally. It is usually seen in elderly persons and somewhat more common in males than women.

Actinic Cheilosis (Actinic Chelitis)

Actinic cheilosis is a common premalignant alteration of the lower lip vermilion that results from long term or excessive exposure to the ultraviolet component of sunlight. It is problem confined predominantly to light complexioned people with a tendency to sunburn easily. Outdoor occupation obviously is associated with this problem, leading to the popular use of terms such as '*Farmers lip*' and '*Sailor's lip*'. A person with chronic sunlight exposure and compromised immunity, especially a transplant recipient, has an elevated risk of developing a cancer of the lower lip vermilion.

Pathogenesis

Cumulative ultraviolet radiation can produce mutations in the p53 tumor suppressor gene,[38] an alteration frequently found in this and other precancers and cancers of the head and neck region.

Clinical Features

Actinic cheilosis seldom occurs in person with 45 years and above. It has strong male predilection (male : female = 10 : 1 in some studies).

- The earliest clinical changes include atrophy of the lower lip vermilion border, characterized by a smooth surface and blotchy pale areas.
- Typical blurring of margin between the vermilion zone and cutaneous portion of lip is seen.
- As the lesion progresses, rough scaly areas develop on the drier portions of the vermilion. These areas thicken and may appear as leukoplakic lesions especially when they extend near the wet line of the lip. The patient may report the scaly material can be peeled off with some difficulty.
- With further progression, chronic focal ulceration may develop in one or more sites, especially at places of mild trauma from cigarettes or pipe stems. Such ulcerations may last for months and often suggest progression to early squamous cell carcinoma.

Usually well-differentiated squamous cell carcinoma develops over a time in 6 to 10 percent of actinic cheilosis cases. Such malignant transformation seldom occurs before 60 years of age, with the resulting carcinoma typically enlarging slowly and metastasizing only at late stage.[10]

Histopathological Features

It is usually characterized by an atrophic stratified squamous epithelium, often demonstrating marked keratin production. Varying degrees of dysplasia may be encountered.

It is usually associated with increased degree of epithelial change: acanthosis, basophilic change within the connective tissue, the presence of inflammation within the connective tissue, perivascular inflammation, and thickness of the keratin layer.[39]

Treatment and Prognosis

- Many of the changes associated with actinic cheilosis are probably irreversible, but patient should be encouraged to use lip balms with sunscreens to prevent further damaged.
- Areas of indurations, thickening, ulceration, are leukoplakia/erythroplakia should be submitted for biopsy to rule out carcinoma.
- In clinically severe cases without malignancy; a lip shave procedure (vemilionectomy) may be performed. The vermilion mucosa is removed, and portion of the intraoral labial mucosa is pulled forward or the wound lip allowed healed by secondary intentions.
- Alternative treatments include CO_2 laser ablations and electrodessication. Long-term follow up is recommended.
- If a squamous cell carcinoma is identified, the involved lip is treated accordingly.
- Focal actinic cheilitis is easily treated with cryosurgery or electrosurgery. Extensive actinic cheilitis requires 5-fluorouracil, carbon dioxide laser, or scalpel vermilionectomy for adequate treatment. The carbon dioxide laser offers some advantages over scalpel vermilionectomy.[40]
- Cryosurgery, electrocautery, 5-fluorouracil, carbon dioxide laser, and scalpel verimilionectomy were all clinically effective. All therapies, with the exception of chemical peeling, appear to have a low clinical failure rate. Histological clearance of disease was demonstrated in carbon dioxide laser-treated patients. 5-Fluorouracil failed to achieve complete removal of histologic dysplasia. The carbon dioxide laser may be associated with less scarring and an improved cosmetic outcome in comparison with the scalpel vermilionectomy.

ORAL SUBMUCOUS FIBROSIS

Oral submucous fibrosis (OSF) has been well established in Indian medical literature since the time of *Sushruta as vidari.*[41] In modern literature, Schwartz[42] first described this condition in 1952 while examining five Indian women from Kenya, to which he ascribed the descriptive term "atrophia idiopathica mucosa oris'. Later in 1953, Joshi[43] from Bombay redesignated the condition as 'oral submucous fibrosis' implying predominantly its histologic nature. Its precancerous nature was reported by Paymaster[44] in 1956. *Pindborg* et al.[45] reported a prevalence of OSF in India to be about 0.2 to 0.5 percent with an estimate of no fewer than 2.5 million cases and demonstrated a malignant transformation rate of 4.5 percent. The reported incidence of malignant transformation is 7 to 13 percent in the literature.[46,47]

This condition is predominantly seen in the Indian subcontinent and people of this origin settled elsewhere in the world. There has been an increase in the use of areca nut, particularly pan masala in the younger group in India, due to easy access, effective price changes, and marketing strategies leading to increasing incidence of OSF.

In 1966, *Pindborg*[48] defined OSF as *"an insidious chronic disease affecting any part of the oral cavity and sometimes the pharynx; occasionally preceded by and/or associated with vesicle formation, it is always associated with juxta-epithelial inflammatory reaction followed by a fibro elastic change of the lamina propria, with epithelial atrophy leading to stiffness of the oral mucosa causing trismus and inability to eat."*

Etiology

The pathogenesis of the disease is believed to be multifactorial. Present evidence indicates that chewing areca nut, tobacco, slaked lime or other spices is an important risk factor for OSF. Many etiologic factors,[37,49] hypothesized to trigger the disease process include:

- Betel nut/Areca nut with or without tobacco
- Excessive consumption of chilies (capsaicin) or spices
- Vitamin B deficiency
- Protein deficiency
- Iron deficiency
- Trace element deficiency such as iron, zinc and essential vitamins
- Genetic susceptibility
- Autoimmunity and hypersensitivity states.

It is apparent that fibrosis and hyalinization of sub epithelial tissues account for most of the clinical features encountered. Since the increased collagen synthesis or reduced collagen degradation as possible mechanisms in the development of the disease. It is likely that the normal regulatory mechanisms are either down regulated or up regulated at different stages of disease.

Various Mechanisms Suggested for the Etiopathogenesis of OSF

- Stimulation of fibroblast proliferation and collagen synthesis by areca nut alkaloids (Harvey W et al.[50] 1986)
- Clonal selection of fibroblast with a high amount of collagen production during the long term exposure to arecanut ingredients (Meghji S et al.[51] 1987)
- Stabilization of collagen structure by catechin and tannins from arecanut (Scutt A et al.[52] 1987)
- Decreased secretion of collagenase (Shieh TY et al.[53] 1992)

- Production of stable collagen (type I trimmer) by OSF fibroblasts (Kuo MYP et al.[54] 1995)
- Increase in collagen cross linking by up regulation of lysyl oxidase (Ma RH et al.[55] 1995)
- Deficiency in collagen phagocytosis (Tsai CC et al.[56] 1999) and
- Effect of fibrogenic cytokines secreted by activated macrophages and T lymphocytes on fibroblasts (Haque MF et al.[57] 2000).

Clinical Features

The onset is insidious, over two to five years.

Early OSF

- Burning sensation of the mouth, particularly while eating spicy foods.
- Followed by the formation of vesicles (often on the palate), ulcerations, or recurrent generalized stomatitis, with excessive salivation, defective gustatory sensation, and xerostomia.
- There are periods of exacerbation manifested by the appearance of small vesicles in the cheek and palate with intervals of three months to one year. The vesicles heal within few days and the burning sensation diminishes. The healing of the vesicles is characterized by blanching, indication induction of fibrosis. Borle (1991) proposed two distinct cyclic phases in OSF, an erruptive phase, characterized by increased burning sensation and formation of vesicles (Fig 29.17D) and a fibrosis induction phase, characterized by diminished acute symptoms and blanching as the vesicles heal and fibrous tissue is formed.
- Focal vascular dilatations manifest clinically as petechiae in the early stages of the disease. This may be the part of vascular response due to hypersensitivity of the oral mucosa towards some external irritant like areca nut products.
- Pain in areas where submucosal fibrotic band are developing when palpated is a useful clinical test.

Advanced OSF

- As the disease progresses, the oral mucosa become blanched and slightly opaque, and white fibrous bands appear. In patients, who spit the areca nut, tobacco and lime, the buccal mucosa and lips may be affected at an early stage where as in patients who swallow the areca nut, tobacco, lime and quid the palate and the faucial pillars are the areas involved first.
- The buccal mucosa is involved symmetrically and the fibrous bands in the buccal mucosa run in a vertical direction.
- The fibrosis varies from a slight whitish area of the soft palate, causing no symptoms, to a dense fibrosis resulting in fixation and shortening or even deviation of the uvula and soft palate (Fig. 29.17 B and C).
- The fibrosis in the faucial pillars varies from slight submucosal to a dense fibrosis extending deep into the pillars with strangulation of the tonsils.
- Difficulty in mouth opening, inability to whistle or blow out a candle and difficulty in swallowing due to dense fibrosis involving the tissues around the pterygomandibular raphae, with progressive fibrosis and the stiffening of certain area of mucosa (Fig. 29.17A).
- Impairment of tongue movement with atrophy of the tongue papillae and some times loss of gustatory sensation.
- Involvement of esophagus can lead to progressive dysphagia and reduced oesophageal mobility.
- In extensive cases throat pain, ear pain and losses of auditory acuity due to stenosis of the eustachian tube are noted.
- The fibrosis of nasopharynx leads to referred pain to the ear and a nasal voice as one of the later signs in some patient.

Precancerous Nature and Malignant Transformation

Paymaster[35] first described the precancerous nature of OSF in 1956 by observing the slow growing squamous cell carcinoma in one third of the patient with the disease. Various groups confirmed this and Pindborg[58] in 1972 put forward five criteria to prove that the disease is precancerous.

1. High occurrence of OSF in oral cancer patient

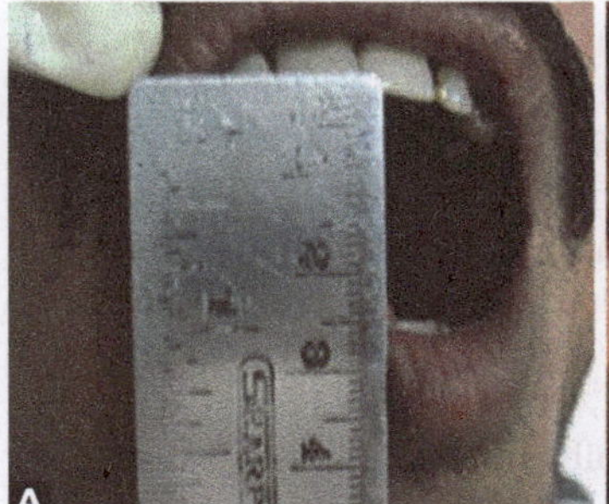
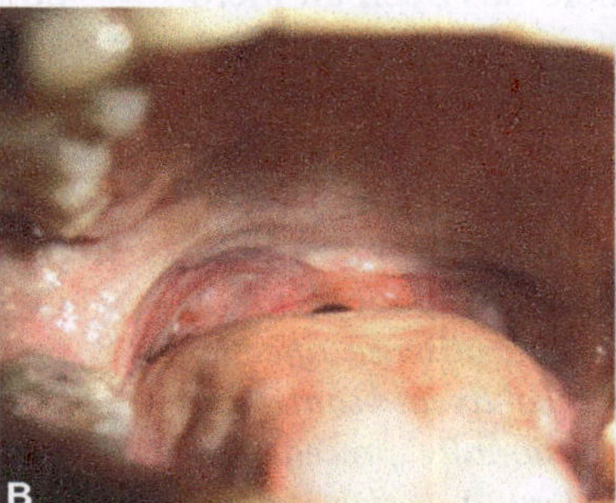
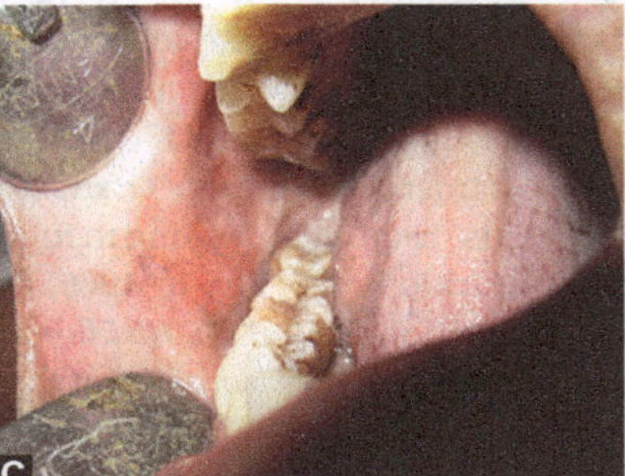
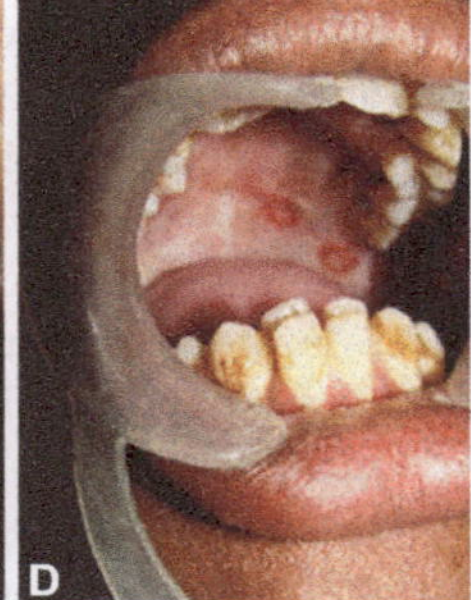

Figs 29.17A to D: (A) Interincisal opening of 22 mm; (B and C) Blanching on the buccal mucosa and palate with atrophic uvula; (D) Vesicles on the palate

2. Higher incidence of SCC in-patient with OSF
3. Histological diagnosis of cancer without any clinical suspicion in OSF
4. High frequency of epithelial dysplasia, and
5. Higher prevalence of leukoplakia among OSF cases.

Malignant transformation rate of OSF was found to be in the range of 7 to 13 percent.[59] According to long term, follow up studies a transformation rate of 7.6 percent over a period of 17 years was reported by Murti PR et al. in 1985.[48]

The dense fibrosis and less vascularity of the corium, in the presence of an altered cytokine activity create a unique environment for carcinogens from both tobacco and areca nut to act on the epithelium. So that carcinogens from areca nut accumulate over a long period either on or immediately below the epithelium, allowing the carcinogens to act for longer duration before it diffuses in to deeper tissues. Less vascularity may deny the quick absorption of carcinogens in to the systemic circulation. This possible mechanism of carcinogenesis in OSF was hypothesized by Tilakaratne WM et al.[60] 2000.

- **OSF and coexistent leukoplakia:** Leukoplakia is precancerous lesion; its coexistence with OSF implies the high risk for oral cancer. More frequently homogeneous and nodular leukoplakias occur.
- **OSF and coexistent oral cancer:** The coexistence of the oral squamous cell carcinoma and the OSF is well documented in the literature and various studies have shown it to be between 5 to 42 percent.[61] Of late in the clinical practice more and more cases of OSCC are seen to be associated with pre existing, long standing OSF. As OSF is generally of a long duration the presence of oral cancer implies that it is a later development i.e. a consequences of the malignant transformation of OSF. The peculiarity of such association is that it is seen in relatively younger patients, and the youngest patient reported at our center (SPDC, Wardha, India) was 18 years of age (mean age 31.3 years). The OSCC secondary to SMF is generally seen in the retromolar areas (probably due to chronic irritation from the buccally tilted and malposed maxillary third molars), tongue and the floor of the mouth and always makes the identification and assessment very difficult due to presence of severe trismus (Figs 29.18A to D). Majority of the cases are diagnosed at stage III or IV making the prognosis very poor. The disease is usually resistant to treatment and early recurrence is a common occurrence. In some cases second primary after the treatment of the first carcinomatous lesion or at the time of first diagnosis more than one primary are seen suggesting the phenomenon of field cancerization (Fig. 29.18E).

Histopathological Features

The excessive fibrosis in the mucosa seems to be the primary pathology in OSF. The atrophic changes in the epithelium are secondary.

Epithelial changes: In the different stages of OSF are predominantly

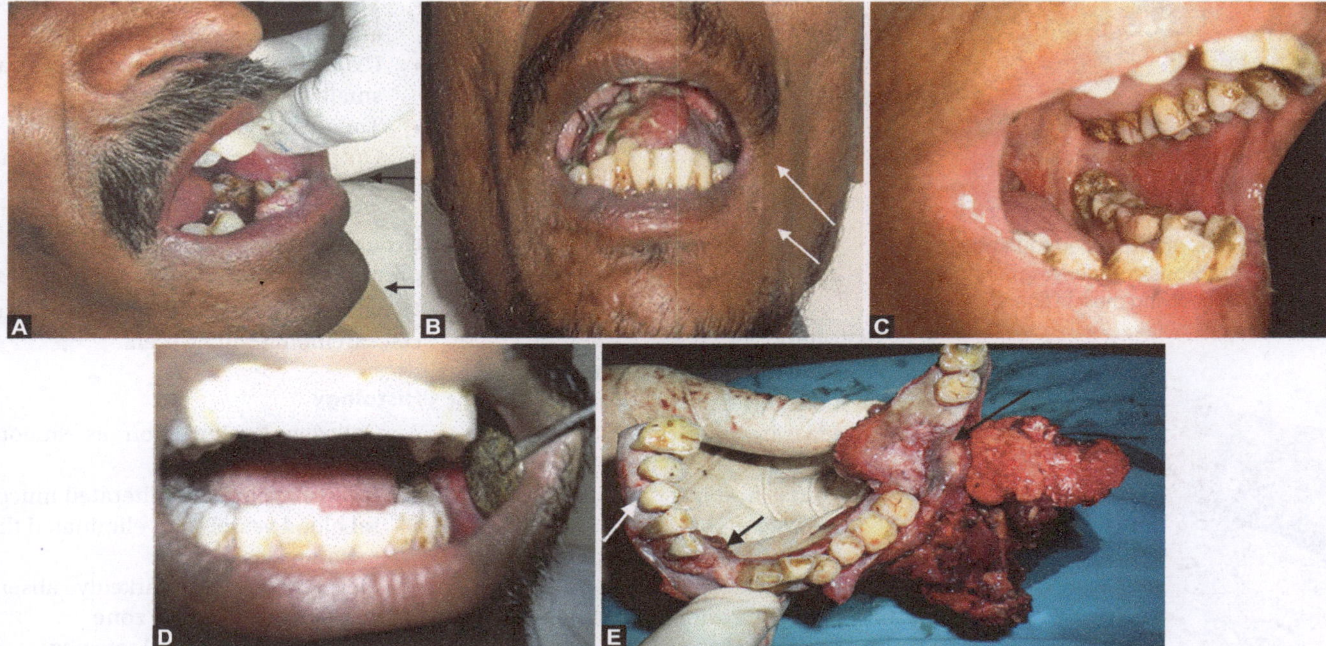

Figs 29.18A to E: (A) SMF with OSCC of retromolar area and lower lip (two primaries); (B) Tongue and retromolar area; (C) Red patch on buccal mucosa in SMF is warning sign of malignant transformation; (D) Malignant growth in the retromolar area due to cronic trauma from occlusion in a case of SMF; (E) Multiple primaries in a case of SMF shown in a ressected specimen of wedge mandibulectomy and SOHD on left side

hyperplasia (early), atrophy (advanced), and loss of rete pegs of epithelium, associated with an increasing tendency for keratinizing metaplasia. The epithelial dysplasia without carcinoma is found in 10 to 15 percent of cases and carcinoma is found in at least five percent of cases. However, the concomitant association of OSCC and SMF was found in 28 percent cases at our center (SPDC, Wardha, India).

Subepithelial changes: In early stages juxtaepithelial chronic inflammatory cell infiltrate with dilated blood vessels and rise in mast cells. In advanced cases submucosal deposition of extremely dense and avascular collagenous tissues with variable numbers of chronic inflammatory cells is seen (Figs 29.19 and 29.20).

Several classification have been put forth by various researchers, based on different aspect of Borle R M and Borle S R have suggested two clinical stages in the SMF (1) An eruptive phase—characterized by vesiculation and increased burning sensation and (2) A fibrosis induction phase characterized by diminished burning sensation and blanching due to healing of vesicles by fibrosis. They claimed that these phases come in cyclic manner and the stage 1 is induced by irritants like betel nut, lime and tobacco.[62]

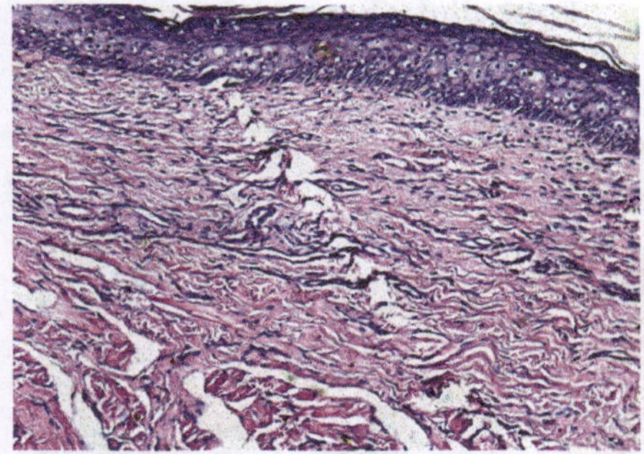

Fig. 29.19: Atrophic stratified squamous epithelium with fibrosis in underlying connective tissue stoma involving muscle fibers

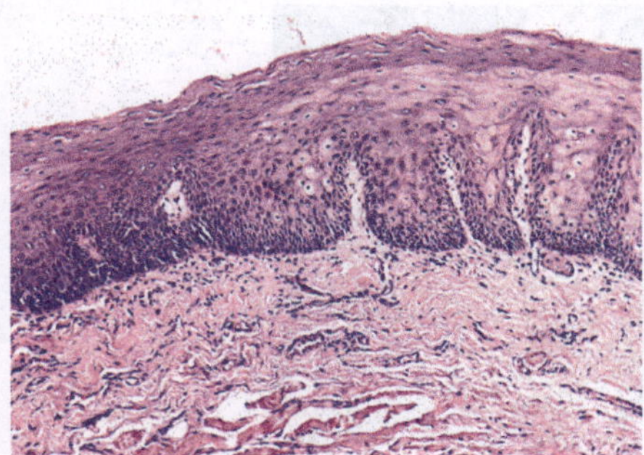

Fig. 29.20: Mild epithelial dysplasia with fibrosis in underlying connective tissue stoma involving muscle fibers

Recently Khanna JN and Andrade NN[63] (1995) developed a group classification system for the surgical management of OSF.

Group I: Very early cases

- Common symptom is burning sensation in mouth
- Acute ulceration and recurrent stomatitis.

Histology

- Fine fibrillar collagen network interspersed with marked edema
- Dilated and congested blood vessels
- Large aggregate of plump, young fibroblasts present with abundant cytoplasm
- Inflammatory cells mainly consist of polymorphonuclear leukocytes with few eosinophils
- Normal Epithelium.

Group II: Early cases

- Buccal mucosa appears mottled and marble-like
- Widespread whets of fibrosis palpable
- Patient is with an interincisal distance of 26 to 35 mm.

Histology

- Juxtaepithelial hyalinization present
- Collagen present as thickened but separate bundles
- Blood vessels dilated and congested
- Young fibroblast seen in moderate number
- Inflammatory cell mainly consists of polymorphonuclear leukocytes with few eosinophils and occasional plasma cells
- Flattening or shortening of epithelial rete pegs evident with varying degree of keratinization.

Group III: Moderately advanced cases

- Trismus evident, with an interincisal distance of 15 to 25 mm
- Buccal mucosa appears pale and firmly attached to underlying tissues
- Atrophy of vermilion border
- Vertical fibrosis bands palpable at the soft palate, pterygomandibular raphe, and anterior faucial pillars.

Histology

- Juxtaepithelial hyalinization present
- Thickened collagen bundles faintly discernible, separated by very slight, residual edema
- Blood vessels mostly constricted
- Mature fibroblast with scanty cytoplasm and spindle shaped nuclei
- Inflammatory exudates consist mainly of lymphocytes and plasma cell
- Epithelium markedly atrophy with loss of rete pegs
- Muscle fibers seen interspersed with thickened and dense collagen fibers.

Group IVA: Advance cases

- Trismus is sever with interincisal distance of less than 15 mm
- The fauces thickened, shortened and firmed on palpation
- Uvula is shrunken and appears as small, fibrous bud
- Tongue movement limited
- On palpation of lips, circular band felt around entire moth.

Group IVB: Advance cases with premalignant and malignant changes

Hyperkeratosis leukoplakia, squamous cell carcinoma can be seen.

Histology

- Collagen hyalinization as smooth sheet
- Extensive fibrosis obliterated mucosal blood vessels and eliminated the melanocytes
- Fibroblast were markedly absent within the hyalinized zone
- Total loss of epithelial rete pegs
- Mild to moderate atypia present
- Extensive degeneration of muscle fibers evident.

Differential Diagnosis

OSF has a characteristic clinical appearance and there are few conditions that need to be differentiated from it. One is oral manifestation of scleroderma. More often pale mucosa coupled with pigmentation seen in anemic conditions, may be mistaken for blanching in OSF.

Treatment modalities

- The reduction or even elimination of the habit of areca nut chewing is an important preventive measure. In the early stage of OSF it could probably slow the progress of the disease.
- **Nutrition support:** Mainly for high proteins and calories and for vitamin B complex and other vitamins and mineral.
- **Immunomodulatory drugs:** Local and systemic applications of glucocorticoids and placental extracts are commonly used. These also prevent or suppress inflammatory reaction, thereby preventing fibrosis by decreasing fibroblastic proliferation and deposition of collagen.
- **Local drug delivery:** Local injections of corticosteroids and placental extract have been tried in addition to hyaluronidase, collagenase and similar substance which break down intercellular cement substance and also decrease collagen formation.
- **Physiotherapy:** This includes measures such as forceful mouth opening and heat therapy. Heat has been commonly used and the results have been described as satisfactory.
- **Combined therapy:** Medical line of treatment includes usage of Gold, Iodides, Hyaluronidase, Hydrocortisone, Placental extracts, Triamcinolone, Vitamins, and Iron supplements. Peripheral vasodilators like Buflomedial hydrochloride and Nylhydrin hydrochloride. They are useful in early stages of OSF. They are of temporary benefit in advanced stages of OSF and do not offer any long-term relief to the patients, also have no role in advanced stages in OSF.
- **Surgical treatment:** Modalities include excision of fibrous bands with or without grafting. Grafts included, split thickness grafts, placental grafts,[64] tongue flaps,[65] buccal fat pad[66] (Fig. 29.21A). They also have been largely unsuccessful due to graft rejections and development of secondary scar contracture in the raw buccal mucosa and pterygomandibular raphae areas. The involvement of tongue and palatal mucosa in advanced cases of OSF precludes its use as a flap to reconstruct the defect in buccal mucosa.

Advanced cases of OSF require apart from surgical release of fibrosis, bilateral temporalis myotomy and coronoidectomy. Reconstruction of the defect can be performed by the application of the nasolabial skin island flap[67] to provide supple skin and subcutaneous tissue to interpose in the defect (Fig. 29.21B).

The advantages of this technique is that the donor site is in the same operating field, reliable, and rich vascularity, versatility in design, proximity to defect, ease of flap elevation, supple skin thus aiding in increased mouth opening, the donor site can easily be undermined and closed linearly with minimal deformity.

LICHEN PLANUS

Lichen planus (LP) is a relatively common, chronic immunologic inflammatory mucocutaneous disorder that varies in appearance from keratotic (reticular or plaque like) to erythematous and ulcerative. The British physician Erasmus Wilson[68] provided the strange name of the condition in 1869. The disease is relatively common affecting approximately 1 to 2 percent of the population. In the majority of instances cutaneous lesion of LP are self limiting and cause inching, oral lesions in LP are chronic, rarely undergo spontaneous remission, are potentially malignant and are often source of morbidity.[10]

Etiopathogenesis

The OLP is a T-cell mediated autoimmune disease in which cytotoxic CD8+ T cells trigger the apoptosis of oral epithelial cells.[69] The CD8+ lesional T-cells may recognize an antigen associated with the major histocompatibility complex (MHC) class I on keratinocytes. After antigen recognition activation, CD8+ cytotoxic T-cells may trigger keratinocyte apoptosis. Activated CD8+ T-cells (and possibly keratinocyte) may release cytokines that attract additional lymphocytes into the developing lesion. The lichen planus antigen unknown, although it may be self-peptide. The over expression or unmasking of the OLP antigen may be induced by drugs, contact allergens in dental restorative materials or toothpastes, mechanical trauma (Koebner phenomenon[70]), viral infections specially hepatitis C virus or unidentified agents. Patient with OLP exhibit the higher levels of anxiety, greater depression and increased vulnerability to psychic disorder. Other causes suggested include malnutrition and infection.

Grinspan has described an interesting association of lichen planus, diabetes mellitus, and vascular hypertension. The triad being described as "Grinspan

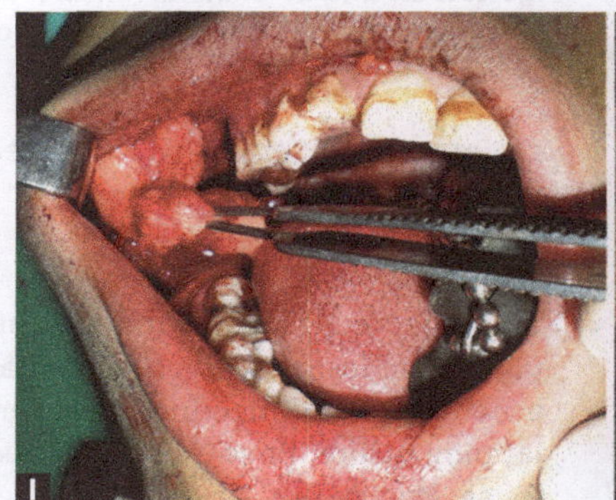

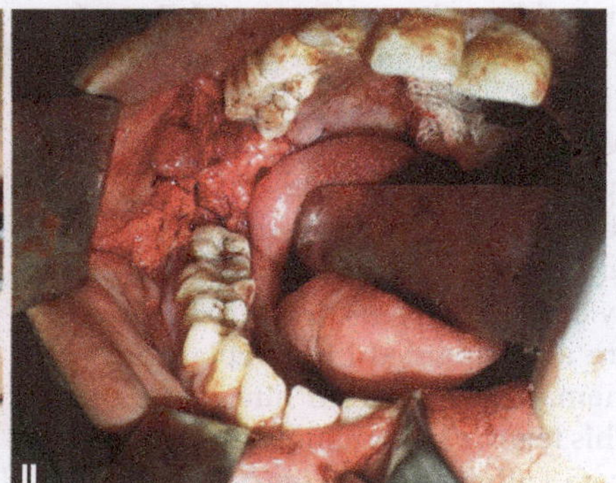

Fig. 29.21A: Case of SMF treated with Buccal flap pad grafting.

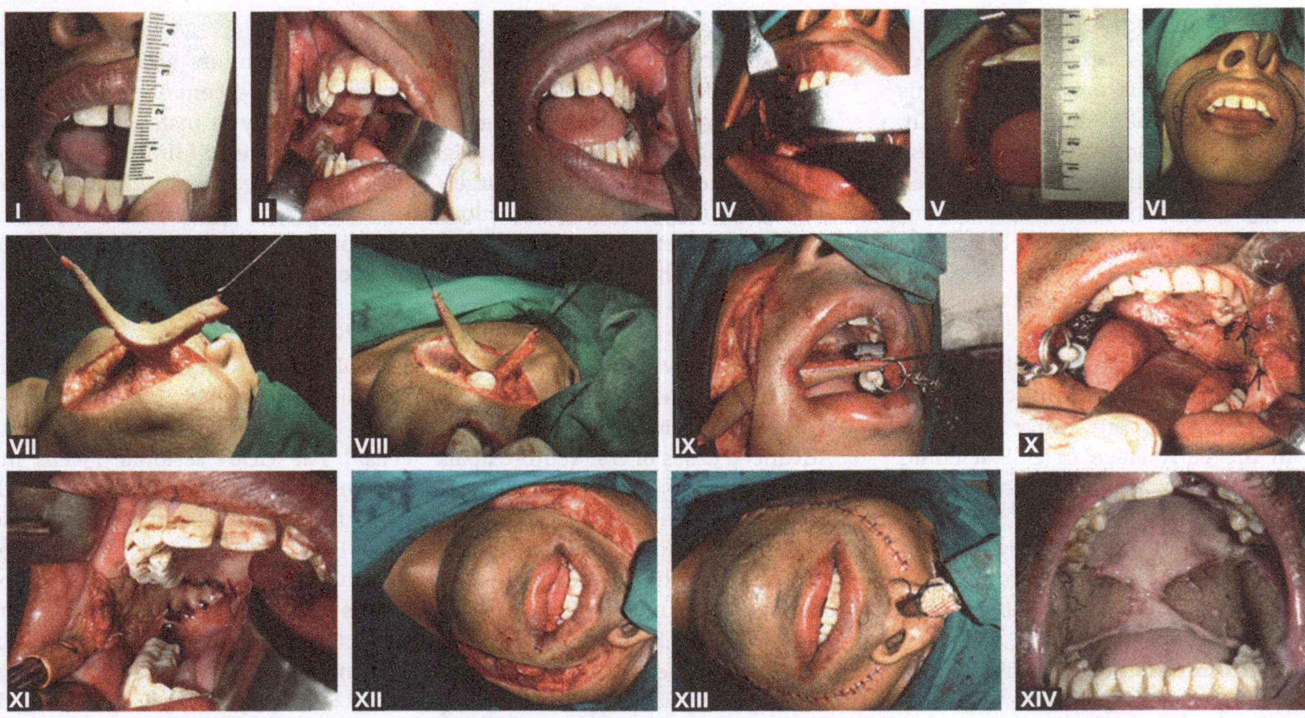

Fig. 29.21B: Bilateral fibrotomy and reconstruction by bipedaled nasolabial flap (Sawangi protocol)

syndrome"[71] by Grapper. The oral lichenoid lesions develops as an adverse reaction to the drugs used for the treatment of hypertension and diabetes mellitus.[72]

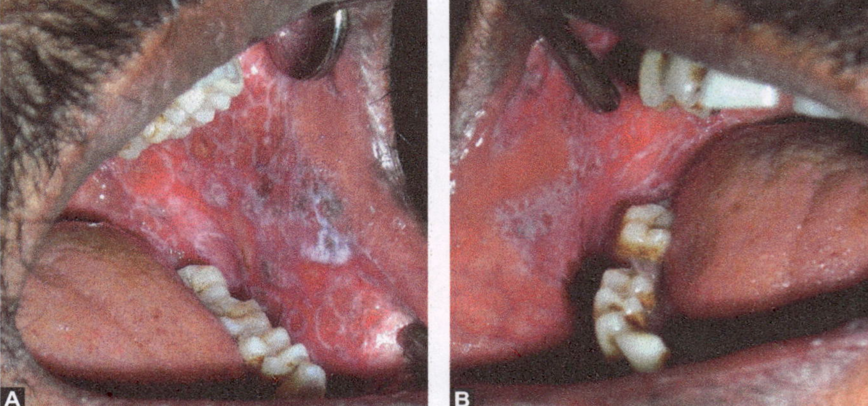

Figs 29.22A and B: Bilateral reticular lichen planus: The network of connecting and overlapping thin white lines on both right and left side of buccal mucosa

Clinical Features

Oral lichen planus develops most commonly in the fifth to sixth decade of life and in women more than twice as often as men. It is rarely affected in children. Oral lichen planus lesions usually have recognizable and distinctive clinical features and a characteristic distribution. OLP may manifests in one of four clinical forms: (a) Reticular, (b) Erythematous (atrophic) (c) Erosive (ulcerated) and (d) Bullous forms.[73] Where as reticular lesions occur as isolated lesions and are often the only clinical manifestations of the disease, erythematous lesions are accompanied by reticular lesions, and erosive lesions are accompanied by reticular and erythematous lesions in almost all cases. This feature helps clinically differentiate from other vesiculo-erosive diseases such as pemphigus and pemphigoid, which are characterized by isolated areas of erythema and/or erosions.

The Reticular Lesions

- The most recognized form, encompass white lesions, which appear as a network of connecting and overlapping white lines (also referred to as *Wickham's striae*,[74] however the white lesions may appear as papules, or plaques in some instances (Figs 29.22A and B).
- The patients with reticulate lesions rarely complain of symptoms and often, are unaware of their presence.
- These lesions are typically not static, but wax and wane over weeks or months.
- The reticular form usually involves the posterior buccal mucosa

bilaterally. Other oral mucosal surfaces may also be involved concurrently such as the lateral and dorsal tongue, the gingiva, the palate, and vermilion border of lip.

Erythematous and Erosive OLP

- Although not as common as reticular form, are more significant for the patient because the lesions are usually symptomatic.
- Clinically there are atrophic, erythematous areas with central ulcerations of varying degrees. The periphery of the lesions is usually bordered by fine, white radiating striae.
- Sometimes the atrophy and ulceration are confined to the gingival mucosa, producing the reaction pattern called desquamative gingivitis. In such cases, biopsy specimens should be obtained for light microscopic and immunofluorescent studies of perilesional tissues, because cicatricial pemphigoid and pemphigus vulgaris may appear in a similar fashion.
- If erosive component is severe, epithelial separation may occur. This results in relatively rare presentation of bullous OLP.

Cutaneous Manifestations

- Approximately 15 percent of patient with OLP develop cutaneous lesions.
- The classic appearance of skin lesions consists of erythematous to violaceous papule that are flat topped and occasionally polygonal in form. A network of fine lines often overlies many of the papules.
- The lesions are distributed in a bilaterally symmetrical pattern, most often on flexor surfaces of wrist, forearms, inner aspect of knees, thighs, trunk and sacral area.
- Typically, cutaneous lesions develop within several months after the appearance of the oral lesions, and the severity of the oral lesions does not seem to correlate with the extent of cutaneous involvement.
- Other sites of extraoral involvement include the glans penis, the vulvar mucosa, and the nails.

Histopathological Features

The histopathological features of OLP are characteristics but may not be specific, because other conditions such as lichenoid drug reaction, lichenoid amalgam reaction, lupus erythematosus, and chronic ulcerative stomatitis may also show a similar histopathological pattern.

- Varying degrees of orthokeratosis and parakeratosis and sometimes-atrophic epithelium depending on biopsy taken from erosive or reticular lesion.
- The rete ridges may be absent or hyperplastic but they classically have a pointed or "saw toothed" shape.
- Destruction of the Basal cell layer of the epithelium (hydrophic degeneration) is also present.
- This is accompanied by juxtaepithelial intense band of chronic inflammatory cell infiltrate predominantly of T lymphocytes.
- Degenerating keratinocytes may be seen in the area of the epithelium and connective tissue interface and have been termed colloid, cytoid, hyaline, or civatte bodies (Figs 29.23A and B).
- Dysplastic changes are sometimes seen.

Immunofluorescence of Perilesional Mucosa

- Fibrin and shaggy fibrinogen in a linear pattern at the basement membrane zone
- Cytoids deposition in the absence of deposition of fibrinogen.

Diagnosis

The characteristic clinical aspects of OLP may be sufficient to make a correct diagnosis if classic skin lesions are present. It is important that other lesions, which bear superficial resemblance to OLP, include lichenoid reaction, leukoplakia, erythroplakia, candidiasis, pemphigus, cicatricial pemphigoid, erythema multiforme, syphilis, recurrent aphthae and lupus erythematosus. An oral biopsy with histopathological study is recommended to confirm the clinical diagnosis and mainly to exclude dysplasia and malignancy. The diagnosis of OLP is based on clinicohistopathological correlation. Sometimes immunofluorescence can be used as an important diagnostic tool.

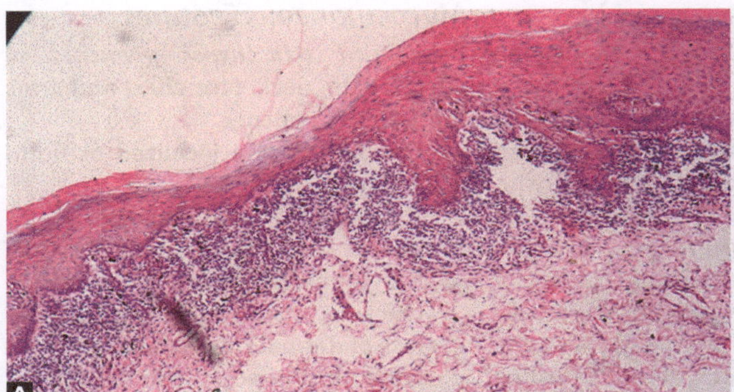

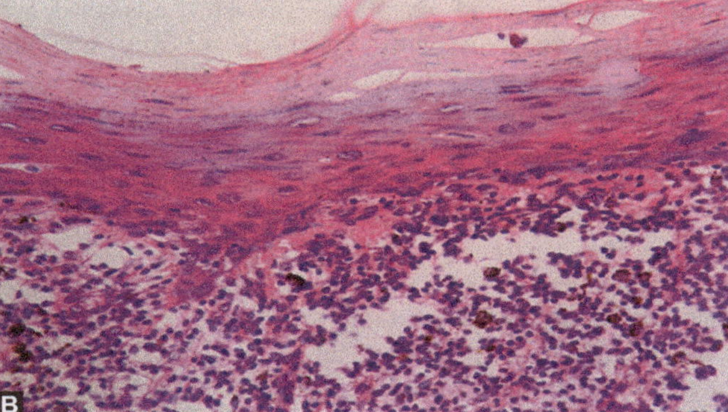

Figs 29.23A and B: Hyperparakeratotic stratified squamous epithelium with degeneration of basal cell layer and subepithelial band of chronic inflammatory cell infiltrate

Oral Lichenoid Reactions

The concept of oral lichenoid reactions or lesions, eruptions in the oral cavity that have an identifiable etiology and that clinically and histologically resemble OLP, is well recognized but controversial. Other authors use the term oral lichenoid reaction when several clinical and histological features are present but the diagnosis remains inconclusive.

Dental restorative materials including amalgams, composite resins, cobalt, gold and even flavoring and plastics can be important in the pathogenesis. Drug induced oral lichenoid reactions have been reported most commonly to non-steroidal, anti-inflammatory, the angiotensin-converting enzyme inhibitors, beta-blockers, methyldopa, and penicillamine.

Clinically the oral lichenoid lesions are unilateral and erosive. Histologically shows more diffuse lymphocytic infiltrate and contain eosinophils and plasma cell and there may be more colloid bodies than in classical OLP.[19]

Malignant Potential

The reported frequency of malignant transformation varies greatly between 0.4 percent to over 5 percent over periods of observation from 0.5 to over 20 years.[75-78] There is considerable controversy regarding the malignant transformation of OLP. Many investigators have questioned the criteria utilized for diagnosing OLP in published reports. Some published cases of OLP associated with malignant transformation, diagnosed clinically as OLP may actually have been lichenoid dysplasia, premalignant condition with lichenoid features. The patient with lichenoid dysplasia often displays erythematous and erosive lesions clinically to identical to OLP lesions. Where as other studies with strict diagnostic criteria for the disease demonstrated significant risk for OLP patient to develop squamous cell carcinoma. The uncertainty of the premalignant nature of OLP and the fact that early detection of oral cancer results in improved survival, so that it is important to monitor all patients with OLP carefully over the long term.[79]

Possible Risk Factors for Malignant Transformation in OLP

- Habit of tobacco and betel nut, smoking and alcohol consumption.
- Atrophic-erosive forms of OLP predisposed to cancer development as it enhance the action of carcinogens on epithelium.
- OLP lesions on tongue has increased risk for cancer.
- Gender and age risk is higher in women than in men frequently develop between sixth and seventh decade of life.
- After OLP diagnosis, the increased malignant transformation risk after 3 to 6 years duration.
- Modification in diet (less fresh vegetables and fruit especially citrus fruit) imposed by symptoms especially in erosive and atrophic forms.
- Infections:
  - *Candida albicans* may be an important factor in OLP malignant transformation.
  - Hepatitis C virus infection may increases the risk of cancer.

Treatment

- Reticular lesions that are asymptomatic generally require no therapy but only observation for change. Occasionally patient may have superimposed candidiasis in which patient may complain of burning sensation of the oral mucosa. Antifungal therapy necessary in such cases.
- Any etiological agent should be removed or stopped.
- Psychological counseling of patient.
- An optimal oral hygiene program should be instituted in-patient with gingival disease.
- Topical corticosteroids (e.g. fluocinonide, betamethasone, clobetasol gel) applied several times per day to the most symptomatic areas is usually sufficient to induce healing within 1 or 2 weeks.
- Other topical agent such as topical retinoids or cyclosporine has occasionally been advocated for erosive/atrophic lichen planus.
- For intractable erosive OLP lesions intralesional steroids such as triamcinolone acetonide (10–20 mg/mL) injections can be effective and repeated every 2-4 weeks.
- Systemic steroids should be reserved for recalcitrant erosive or erythematous OLP, where topical approaches have failed, or for widespread OLP with concomitant skin, genital, esophageal or scalp involvement.
- Surgical excision is usually not indicated except in cases where concomitant dysplasia is identified.

Dyskeratosis Congenita

Dyskeratosis congenita is a rare, inherited disorder, with premature aging, bone marrow failure, and malignancy:

It consists of Triad of:

- Nail dystrophy
- Skin pigmentation and
- Mucosal Leukoplakia

The syndrome often proves fatal due to Bone marrow failure or Malignant changes within areas of mucosal leukoplakia.[80]

Clinical Presentation

Nail dystrophy, Leukoplakia and skin hyper pigmentation tend to appear in the first decade of life with medial ages of onset of six, seven and eight years respectively.

Mucocutaneous Features

Reticulated skin hyper pigmentation affecting the neck, face chest and arms (app. 90% of patient)

- Can be either a localized or florid generalized form.
- A variety of other changes: Cutaneous atrophy, hyperhidrosis of the palms and soles, telagiectasia, cracking, fissuring, bulla formation, loss of dermal ridges, hair tufts with keratotic plugs on the limbs and keratinized basal cell papillomas.

Dystrophic changes in the nails (90% of patient)

- More severed in fingers than toes
- Begin with longitudinal ridging and splitting and may progress to nail loss.

Leukoplakia (80% of patient) occurs any mucosal surface

- Most frequently reported on oral mucosa, tongue being the most frequently affected other include lingual mucosa, buccal mucosa and the palate.
- Increased risk of malignant transformation app. 35 percent with peak in third decade of life.

Malignant disease reported include, solid tumors of the tongue, buccal mucosa, nasopharynx, rectum, cervix, vagina, skin, oesophagus and pancreas.Hematological malignancies include myelodysplasia and Hodgkin's lymphoma.

The Non-mucocutaneous Features

- *Bone marrow failure (BMF)* resulting in peripheral cytopenias of one or more lineages (85%). Pancytopenia 75 percent, onset in less than 20 years of age (80%), with half develop before 10 years.
- Principle cause of death in 70 percent of cases is as a consequence of bleeding or opportunistic infections with cytomegalovirus, pneumonia.
- Some times it is initially diagnosed as idiopathic aplastic anemia. The clinical features also overlap with Fanconi's anemia characterized by BMF and predisposition to malignancy.
- Pulmonary complication in 20 percent of patients are reduced diffusion capacity with or without a restrictive defect. Abnormalities of pulmonary vasculature and abnormally high levels of pulmonary fibrosis.
- Ophthalmic abnormalities epiphoria secondary to nasolacrimal duct obstruction, conjuctivitis, blepharitis, pterygium formation, ectropion, loss of eyelashes, strabismus, cataracts and optic atrophy.
- Skeletal anomalies in 20 percent of cases include mandibular hypoplasia, osteoporosis, abnormal bone trabeculation, avascular necrosis, and scoliosis.
- Other manifestations of oral cavity are hyperpigmentation of buccal mucosa, severe periodontal disease, hypo calcified teeth and taurodontism.
- Genitourinary abnormalities include hypoplastic testes, hypospadias, phimosis, urethral stenosis and horseshoe kidneys.
- Gastrointestinal abnormalities include, developmental oesophageal webs in the postcricoid region resulting in dysphagia which have been associated with malignant transformation, hepatomegally and cirrhosis.
- Other abnormalities include altered mental status and learning difficulties, microcephaly, intracranial calcifications, alopecia, hair greying, deafness and amyloidosis, peripheral neuropathy and choanal atresia.[21]

The Diagnosis of Dyskeratosis Congenital

- Diagnosis may not be so easy, for example with the presentation of aplastic anaemia without any mucocutaneous features.
- Screen for the DKC1 gene if the patient is male with two of the following features of the disease: abnormal skin pigmentation, nail dystrophy, leukoplakia, and bone marrow failure.
- Any patient presenting with idiopathic aplastic anaemia should undergo chromosomal breakage analysis with mitomycin-C or diepoxybutane to exclude Fanconi's anaemia.
- If this chromosomal breakage analysis is normal (i.e., negative for Fanconi's anaemia) then progression to analyse hTERC gene is appropriate.
- Although rare, *Dyskeratosis congenita should be considered and excluded whenever a child presents with oral leukoplakia.*
- Identification of the gene responsible offers the potential for
  - Improving diagnosis
  - Monitoring progression of the disease once diagnosed and
  - Novel forms of therapy for this inherited disorder.[68]

Syphilis

Syphilitic leukoplakia was a characteristic complication of tertiary syphilis but is now rare due to the early and intensive treatment of the disease with antibiotics since 1940. Leukoplakic lesions may develop in the atrophic epithelium associated with the glossitis often seen in tertiary syphilis. In later stages, the prediction for syphilitic glossitis associated with leukoplakic changes to undergo carcinomatous transformation has been recognized for many years. The incidence of such malignant transformation has been as high as 30 percent in various reported series.[20]

Clinical Features

Syphilitic leukoplakias have no distinctive features but typically affect the dorsum of the tongue and spare the margins. Lesions have an irregular outline and surface and are usually regarded as having a high risk of malignant change. Carcinoma developing near the center of the dorsum of the tongue may be a sequel to syphilitic leukoplakia. Cracks, small erosions or nodules may prove on histology to be foci of invasive carcinoma.

Pathology

In addition to hyperkeratosis, acanthosis with dysplasia is the characteristics features. Of late syphilitic chronic inflammatory changes with plasma cell predominantly may be seen. Giant cells and rarely granulomas may be present. Endarteritis of small arteries is particularly characteristic. However, distinctive features of a syphilitic tissue reaction may be lacking.

Behavior and Management

The diagnosis is confirmed mainly by the serological findings. However, even if positive, biopsy is still essential, as minute areas of malignant change may be found and the management is affected accordingly. In particular, the presence of syphilitic endarteritis may be a contradiction to the radiotherapy. Antibiotic treatment of syphilis does not cure the leukoplakia, which permits and can undergo malignant change even after serology has become negative.[16,20]

Sideropenic Dysphagia

Sideropenic dysphagia (Paterson-Brown-Kelly or Plummer[81]-Vinson[82] syndrome) mainly affects middle-aged women,[83] with iron deficiency being the underlying cause. Iron deficiency is endemic in many tropical countries where oral cancer is also common. The iron deficiency is due to chronic blood loss as result of hookworm infestation and nutritional deficiencies.

Patient suffering from sideropenic dysphagia generally complain of fatigue and difficulty in swallowing. The dysphagia is due to the formation of an esophageal web (the presence of abnormal band of tissue). The common oral mucosal changes seen in this syndrome are angular cheilosis, mucosal pallor, and atrophy which gives tongue a smooth glossy appearance. Histologically, the mucosa of the whole aerodigestive tract is often atrophic with varying degree of submucosal chronic inflammation. In advanced cases, evidence of epithelial atypia and dysplasia may be seen.

The relationship between sideropenic dysphagia and the subsequent development of carcinoma of upper alimentary tract is well documented. Five to fifty percent prevalence of upper aerodigestive tract malignancy has been reported in affected persons.[84] The carcinoma of buccal mucosa and tongue is well recognized. Iron deficiency, whether it is sever enough to cause anemia or not leads to mucosal atrophy. Iron deficiency leads to changes in the cell kinetics and increases the susceptibility to topically applied carcinogens. It has been suggested that mucosal atrophy, increased mitotic activity, and diminished repair capacity are among the major common underlying predisposing factors in oral cancer. The entire oral mucosa is red, shiny, and atrophic. Leukoplakias as well as multiple oral carcinomas may develop, predominantly in the posterior part of the mouth and in the oropharynx.

Treatment

- Dietary iron supplementation for the correction of iron deficiency anemia. This therapy resolves the anemia, relives the glossodynia, and may reduce the severity of the esophageal symptoms.
- Occasionally, esophageal dilation is necessary to help improve the symptoms of dysphagia.
- The patient should be evaluated periodically for oral hypopharyngeal, and esophageal carcinoma.

Discoid Lupus Erythematosus

Oral lesions in discoid lupus erythematosus may show pseudoepitheliomatous hyperplasia and consequently are described in classification with other precancerous conditions is necessary because a few cases of squamous cell carcinoma developing in discoid lupus erythematosus have been reported, especially in atrophied epithelium on the vermilion border of lower lip.

Xeroderma Pigmentosum

Xeroderma pigmentosum is a rare genodermatosis in which cutaneous malignancies develop at an early age with a recessive mode of inheritance. One of several defects in the excision repair and/or post replication repair mechanism of DNA causes the disease. As result of the inability of the epithelial cells to repair ultraviolet light induced damage mutation in the epithelial cells occur, leading to the development of skin cancer at a rate 1000 to 4000 times what would normally be expected in people under 20 years of age. The lips are mainly affected. Epithelial atrophy, telangiectasia and hyperpigmentation, which may occasionally also be observed on the oral mucosa. Squamous cell carcinoma of the oral mucosa had been observed in some affected individuals.

Epidermolysis Bullosa

Epidermolysis bullosa, particularly the dystrophic type, is an inherited disorder of either autosomal or recessive pattern. The disease is characterized by formation of bullae of the skin and oral mucosa. Oral scarring results in loss of the oral vestibule, ankyloglossia and microstomia. Carcinoma of the tongue has been described in cases of dystrophic epidermolysis bullosa.

REFERENCES

1. Warnakaulasuriya S, Newell, Johnson W, et al. Nomenclature and Classification of Potentially Malignant Disorders of The Oral Mucosa. J Oral Pathol Med. 2007; 36:575-80.
2. Napier SS, Speight PM. Natural History of Potentially Malignant Oral Lesions and Conditions: An Overview of the Literature. J Oral Pathol Med. 2008;37: 1-10.
3. Slaughter D, Southwick H, Smejkal W. "Field cancerization" in oral stratifide squamous epithelium: clinical implications of multicentric origin. Cancer. 1953;6:963-8.
4. Ha PK, Califano JA. The Molecular Biology of Mucosal Field Cancerization of the Head And Neck. Crit Rev Oral Biol Med. 2003;14(5):363-9.
5. Braakhuis BJ, Tabor MP, Leemans CR, et al. Second primary tumors and field cancerization in oral and oropharyngeal cancer: molecular techniques provide new insights and definitions. Head Neck. 2002;24:198-206.
6. Kujan O, Oliver RJ, Khattab A, et al. Evaluation of a new binary system of grading oral epithelial dysplasia for prediction of malignant transformation. Oral Oncology. 2006;42:987-93.
7. Warnakaulasuriya S, Reibel J, Bouquot J. et al. Oral epithelial dyspalsia classification systems: predictive value, utility, weakness and scope for improvement. J Oral Pathol Med. 2008;37:127-33.
8. WHO Collaborating Centre for Oral Precancerous Lesions. Definition of leukoplakia and related lesions: An aid to studies on oral precancer. Oral Surgery, Oral Medicine, Oral Pathology. 1978;46(4):518-39.

9. Axéll T, Holmstrup P, Kramer IRH, et al. International seminar on oral leukoplakia and associated lesions related to tobacco habits. Community Dent Oral Epidemiol. 1984;12:145-54.
10. Axéll T, Pindborg JJ, Smith CJ, et al. and an International Collaborative Group on OralWhite Lesions. Oral white lesions with special reference to precancerous and tobacco-related lesions: conclusions of an international symposium held in Uppsala, Sweden, May 18–21, 1994. J Oral Pathol Med. 1996;25:49-54.
11. Pindborg JJ, Reichart PA, Smith CJ, et al. World Health Organization International Histological Classification of Tumours. Histological typing of cancer and precancer of the oral mucosa. Berlin: Springer, 1997.
12. World Health Organization. World Health Organization Classification of Tumours. In: Barnes L, Eveson JW, Reichart P, Sidransky D, eds. Pathology and Genetics. Head and Neck Tumours. Lyon: International Agency for Research on Cancer (IARC) IARC Press. 2005;177-9.
13. Vander Waal I, Schepman KP, Vander Meij EH, et al. Oral leukoplakia: a clinicopathological Review. 1997;33 (5):291-301.
14. Rajendran R. Oral leukoplakia (leukokeratosis): complication of facts and figures. J Oral And Maxillo Facs Patho. 2004;6(2):58-68.
15. Shafer WG, Hine MK, Levy BM. Benign and malignant tumors of the oral cavity. In textbook of oral pathology. Fourth edition. 1993. Saunders. 92-109.
16. Neville BW, Damm DD, Allen CM, et al. Epithelial pathology. In oral and maxillofacial pathology. Second Edition. 2009. WB Saunders and Co. NY. 337-53.
17. Bouquot BE, Whitaker SB. Oral leukoplakia—rationale for diagnosis and prognosis of its clinical subtypes or "phases". Quintessence Int 1994;25: 133-40.
18. Hansen LS, Olson JA, Silverman S. Proliferative verrucous leukoplakia. A longterm study of thirty patients. Oral Surg Oral Med Oral Pathol. 1985;60: 285-9.
19. Cawson RA, Odell EW. Oral premalignancy. In essentials of oral pathology and oral medicine. Sixth edition. 2002. Churchil Livingstone. pp. 216-27.
20. Lee Koyc CH, Huang HL, Chao YY, et al. Precancer risk of betel chewing, tobacco use and alcohol consumption in oral leukoplakia and OSMF in southern Taiwan, Br J Cancer. 2003; 88:366-72.
21. Angadi Punya V, Rekha KP. Oral submucous fibrosis, a clinicopathologic review of 205 cases in Indians. Oral and Maxfac Surg. 2011;15:15-19.
22. Warnakulasuriya S, Kovacevic T, Madden P, et al. Factors predicting malignant transformations in oral potentially malignant disorders among patients accrued over ten year period in south eastern England. J Oral Path and Med. 2011;40:677-83.
23. Shafer WB, Waldron CA. A clinical and histopathologic study of oral leukoplakia. Surg Gynecol and Obst. 1961;112:411-20.
24. Waldron CA, Shafer WG. Leukoplakia revisited: A clinicopathologic study of 3256 oral leukoplakias. Cancer 1975; 36:1386-92.
25. Pindborg JJ, Ranstrup G, Poulsen HE, et al. Studies in oral leukoplakia. V. Clinical ansd histologic science of malignancy. Acta Odontol Scand. 1963;21:407-14.
26. Feller L, Altini M, Slabbert H. Premalignant lesions of the oral mucosa in a south African sample: A clinicopathologic study. J Dent Assoc South Africa. 1991;46:261-5.
27. Gupta PC, Mehta FS, Daftary DK, et al. Incidence rates of oral cancer and natural history of oral precancerous lesions in a 10-year follow-up study of Indian villagers. Community Dentistry and Oral Epidemiology. 1980;8:287-33.
28. Silverman Sol jr, Bhargava K, Mani NJ, et al. Malignant transformation and natural history of oral leukoplakia in 57,518 industrial workers of Gujarat, India. 1976;38(4):1790-5.
29. Axell T. Occurrence of leukoplakia and some other oral white lesions among 20333 adult Swedish people. Community Dent Oral Epidemiol 1987;15:46-51.
30. Vander Waal I, Axell T. Oral leukoplakia: A proposal for uniform reporting. Oral Onco. 2002;38:521-6.
31. Queyrat L, Erythroplasia du gland, Bull Soc Fr Dermatol Syphiligr. 1911;22: 378-82.
32. Shear M, Erythroplakia of the mouth. Int Dent J. 1972;22(4):460-73.
33. Bouquet JE, Ephros H. Erythroplakia the dangerous red mucosa. Pract Periodontics Aesthet Dent. 1995;7:59-67.
34. Shafer WG, Waldron CA. Erythroplakia of the oral cavity. Cancer. 1975;36: 1021-8.
35. Daftary DK, et al. Primary prevention trial of oral cancer in India: A 10-year follow-up study. J Oral Pathol Med. 1992;21:433-9.
36. Prabhu SR, Wilson DF, Daftary DH, et al. Oral precancerous lesions and condition of topical interest. In oral diseases in the tropics. Oxford University Press. 1992;402-24.
37. Robert J. Gorlin. Bowen's disease of the mucous membrane of the mouth: A review of the literature and a presentation of six cases. Oral Surgery, Oral Medicine, Oral Pathology. 1950; 3(1):35-51.
38. Dalva R, Neto P, et al. Actinic cheilitis: Histopathology and p53. Journal of Cutane Path. 2006:33(8):539-44.
39. George E. Kaugars. Actinic cheilitis: A review of 152 cases. Oral Surg Oral Med Oral Pathol Oral Radiol Endod. 1999;88:181-6.
40. Raymond G. Dufresne. Actinic cheilitis: A treatment review. Dermatologic surgery. 1997:23(1);15-21.
41. Mukherjee AL. Oral submucosal fibrosis. A search for aetiology. Ind J Otolaryngol. 1972;24:1:11-5.
42. Schwartz J. Atrophia idiopathica mucosa oris. Presented at the 11th International Dental Congress, London; 1952.
43. Joshi SG. Submucous fibrosis of the palate and pillars. Ind J Otolaryngo. 1953;4:1.
44. Paymaster JC. Cancer of the buccal mucosa: A clinical study of 650 cases in Indian patients. Cancer 1956;9:431-5.
45. Pindborg JJ, Mehta FS, Gupta PC, et al. Prevalence of oral submucous fibrosis

among 50915 Indian villagers. Br J Cancer. 1968;22(4):646-54.
46. Paymaster JC. Cancer of buccal mucosa: A clinical study of 650 patients. Cancer, 1956;9:431-5.
47. Angadi Punya V, Rekha KP. Oral submucous fibrosis: A clinicopathologic review of 205 cases in Indians. Oral and Maxfac Surg. 2011;15:15-19.
48. Pindborg JJ, Sirsat SM. Oral submucous fibrosis. Oral Surg Oral Med Oral Pathol. 1966;22(6):764-79.
49. Canniff JP, Harvey W. The aetiology of oral submucous fibrosis: The stimulation of collagen synthesis by extrats of areca nut. Int J Oral Surg. 1981;10: 163-7.
50. Canniff JP, Harvey W, Harris M. Oral submucous fibrosis: Its pathogenesis and management. Br Dent J. 1986;160: 429-34.
51. Meghji S, et al. An in-vitro comparison of human fibroblasts from normal and oral submucous fibrosis tissue. Arch Oral Biol. 1987;32:213-15.
52. Scutt A, et al. Stabilisation of collagen by betel nut polyphenols as a mechanism in oral submucous fibrosis. Cellular and Molecular Life Sciences. Volume 1987;43:(4).
53. Shieh TY, Yang JF. Collagenase activity in oral submucous fibrosis. Proc Natl Sci Counc Repub China B. 1992; 16(2):106-10.
54. Kuo MYP, Chen HM, Hahn LJ, et al. Collagen biosynthesis in human oral submucous fibrosis fibroblast cultures. J Dent Res. 1995;74:1783-8.
55. Ma RH, Tsai CC, Shieh TY. Increased lysyl oxidase activity in fibroblasts cultured from oral submucous fibrosis associated with betel nut chewing in Taiwan. J Oral Pathol Med. 1995.
56. Tsai CC, Ma RH, Shieh TY. Deficiency in collagen and fibronectin phagocytosis by human buccal mucosa fibroblasts in vitro as a possible mechanism for oral submucous fibrosis. J Oral Pathol Med. 1999;28:59-63.
57. Haque MF, et al. Oral submucous fibrosis patients have altered levels of cytokine production. J Oral Pathol Med. 2000;29(3):123-8.
58. Pindborg JJ. Is submucous fibrosis a pre-cancerous condition in the oral cavity? Int Den J. 1972;22:472-80.
59. Murti PR, Bhonsle RB, Pindborg JJ, et al. Malignant transformation rate in oral submucous fibrosis over a 17-year period. Community Dent Oral Epidemiol. 1985;13:340-1.
60. Tilakratne WM, Klinikowski Saku T, Peters TJ, et al. Oral Submucous Fibrosis: Review on Aetology and Pathogenesis. Oral Oncology. 2006;42: 561-8.
61. Mehta, James E. Hamner. Tobacco-related oral mucosal lesions and conditions in India: Basic Dental Research Unittata Institute of Fundamental Research Bombay. 1993.
62. Borle RM, Borle SR. Management of Oral sub mucous fibrosis - A conservative approach. J Oral Maxillofac Surg. (USA). 1991;49(8):788-91.
63. Khanna JN, Andrade NN. Oral Submucous Fibrosis: A New Concept In Surgical Management: Report of 100 Cases. Int J Oral Maxillofac Surg. 1995;24(6):433-9.
64. Gupta D. Oral submucous fibrosis—A new treatment regimen. J Oral Maxillofac Surg. 1988;46(10):830-3.
65. Tepan MG, Use of tongue flap in submucous palatal fibrosis. The Journal of Laryngology and Otology. Cambridge University Press. 1986;100:455-60.
66. Chin-Jyh Yeh. Application of the buccal fat pad to the surgical treatment of oral submucous fibrosis. Int J Oral Maxillofac Surg. 1996;25(2):130-3.
67. Borle RM, Nimonkar PV, Rajan R. Extended nasolabial flaps in the management of oral submucous fibrosis. Br J Oral Maxillofac Surg. 2009;47(5):382-5.
68. Wilson, E. On lichen planus. J Cutan Med Dis Skin. 1869;3:117-32.
69. Sugerman P. Oral lichen planus. Clinics in Dermatology. 2000;18(5):533-9.
70. Joshi A. Koebner Phenomenon Due to Sacred Thread in Lichen Planus. J Dermatol. 2000;27(2):129-30.
71. Grinspan D, Diaz J, Villapol LO, et al. Lichen ruber planus of the buccal mucosa. Its association with diabetes. Bull Soc Fr Dermatol Syphiligr. 1966; 73(6):898-9.
72. Lodhi G, Scully C, Carrozzo M, et al. Current Controversies In Oral Lichen Planus: Report of An International Consensus Meeting. Part 1. Viral Infections And Etiopathogenesis. Oral Surg Oral Med Oral Pathol Oral Radiol Endod. 2005;100:40-51.
73. Eisen D, Carrozzo M, Bagan Sebastian JV, et al. Number V Oral lichen planus: Clinical features and management. Oral Dis. 2005;11:338-49.
74. Wickham LF. Sur un signe pathognomonique delichen du Wilson (lichen plan) stries et punctuations grisatres. Ann Dermatol Syph. 1895;6:17-20.
75. Kaz RW, Brahim JS, Travis WD. Oral squamous cell carcinoma arising in a patient with long-standing lichen planus. Oral Surg Oral Med Oral Pathol. 1990;70:282-5.
76. Lozada-Nur F, Miranda C. Oral lichen planus: Epidemiology, clinical characteristics, and associated diseases. Sem Cutan Med Surg 1997;16:273-7.
77. Krutchkoff DJ, Eisenberg, E. Lichenoid dysplasia: A distinct histopathologic entity. Oral Surg Oral Med Oral Pathol. 1985;30:308-15.
78. Onofre MA, Sposto MR, Navarro CM, et al. Potentially malignant epithelial oral lesions: Discrepancies between clinical and histological diagnosis. Oral Dis. 1997;3:148-52.
79. Scully et al. OLP and malignant transformation. Oral diseases. 2008;14; 229-43.
80. Handley TPB, McCaul JA, Ogden GR. Dyskeratosis Congenita. Oral Oncology. 2006;42:331-6.
81. Plummer S: Diffuse dilatation of the esophagus without anatomic stenosis (cardiospasm). A report of ninety-one cases. J Am Med Assoc. 1912;58:2013-2015.
82. Vinson PP. A case of cardiospasm with dilatation and angulation of the esophagus. Med Clinics North Am. 1919;3:623-7.
83. Vinson PP. Hysterical dysphagia. Minnesota Med. 1922;5:107-8.
84. Larsson LG, Sandström A, Westling P. Relationship of Plummer-Vinson disease to cancer of the upper alimentary tract in Sweden. Cancer Res. 1975;35(11 Pt. 2):3308-16.

30 Oral Cancer

Borle Rajiv M, Arora Aakash, Bhola Nitin

The oral cancer is one of the common cancers in the Indian subcontinent due to rampant abuse of tobacco. Oral cancer is the sixth most common cancer in the world.[1] It accounts for about 4 percent of all cancers and 2 percent of cancer deaths worldwide.[2]

There is a wide geographical variation (approximately 20-fold) in the incidence of this cancer. The areas characterized by high incidence rates for oral cancer (excluding lip) are found in the South and Southeast Asia (Sri Lanka, India, Pakistan and Taiwan), parts of Western (France) and Eastern Europe (Hungary, Slovakia and Slovenia), parts of Latin America and the Caribbean (Brazil, Uruguay and Puerto Rico) and in Pacific regions.[3]

In the United States, Europe and Australia it accounts for 0.6 to 5 percent of all cancers, but it accounts for up to 30 to 50 percent of all cancers in India. However, it ranks number one among men and number three among women in India. Usually 91 percent of the cases occur after the age of 40 years and highest incidence is found between ages 60 and 70 years. Langdon[4,5] (1977) stated that ninety five percent of patients with oral cancer are over 40 years of age at first diagnosis and the mean age at diagnosis is 60 years (males 63.5 years, females 60.6 years) with the male: female ratio between 1.3:1 and 2:1.

Oral cancer constitutes 12 percent of all cancers in men and 8 percent of all cancers among women.[6] In Indian population incidence rate of oral squamous cell carcinoma is slightly high because of greater exposure to its known predisposing factors and is most common of all cancers. About 94 percent of all oral malignancies are squamous cell carcinomas.[7]

Gingivobuccal sulcus malignancies accounts for about 80 percent of oral cancers in Indian population. Tongue is the most common site for intraoral cancer among European and the US populations, amounting to 40 to 50 percent of oral cancers.[3] Buccal mucosa cancer is more common among Asian populations due to betel quid/tobacco chewing habits.[8] In Sri Lanka, 40 percent of oral cancers are found on buccal mucosa.[9] Other intraoral sites for mouth cancer include floor of mouth, gingiva and palate.

Although the oral cavity is readily accessible for self-examination, the early detection of the oral cancer is still illusive. Most of the cases report with advanced disease, thus the management becomes very challenging and difficult. The OSCC of the gingivobuccal sulcus is commonest due to use of smokeless tobacco in the form of ghutka, pan, khaini, kharra, pan masala, etc. which is consumed not only frequently, but also kept in the buccal vestibule for prolonged periods of time. In the western countries, the habit of smoked tobacco is more common, thus the cancers of the tongue and pharynx are more common.

Although the understanding regarding the oral cancer has improved significantly and the management modalities have evolved and are available widely, still the prognosis of oral cancer has not improved significantly in India. The basic reason for the same is that although the mouth is accessible for the self-examination and the clinical examination and the fact it does not require any sophisticated facilities, the early diagnosis of oral cancer is still a dream. In the west, the early detection of the breast cancer has improved significantly following awareness towards the self-examination. Most of the patients with oral cancer report in stage III or IV with wide spread cervical nodal metastasis making the prognosis poor. This is due to ignorance and illiteracy. Although the government and social organizations have launched a massive awareness drive and the hazards of tobacco have been widely publicized, it has not achieved the desired results. In the rural set up there is paucity of trained clinicians who are able to diagnose a precancerous lesion or an early malignancy and thus, the patient does not get proper advice and is not referred to the specialist on time. The testimony to this fact is that in the clinical practice, it is observed that the teeth, which are involved in a malignant growth and become mobile are extracted without detecting the cancerous growth.

The oral submucous fibrosis is a commonly encountered clinical condition in India and it has chronic course.

The patients and clinicians tend to take it lightly and patient continues with the habits. Clinicians tend to treat this condition conservatively and whenever the malignant transformation takes place, it is invariably missed and the patients often report very late with advanced malignancy.

ETIOLOGY

Tobacco

The tobacco still remains the major etiological factor for the oral squamous cell carcinoma. The tobacco is consumed in various forms such as:

- Smoked form—bidi, cigarette, pipe, cigar, hukka, chutta, out of which cigar and pipe is uncommon in India.
- Non-smoked tobacco
  - As chewable tobacco in the form of tobacco lime mixture, kharra, khaini, ghutka, pan, kimam, cakes, pan masala, jarda, etc.
  - Inhaled form—tobacco snuff.
  - As dentifrice—tobacco snuff.

Out of the smoked forms, bidi is the most common cause of oral cancer in India due to its affordability to poor and rural population as compared to the cigarettes and other forms like cigars and pipe, which are seen to be more popular in urban areas. The bidi not only has the smoke, but invariably the heat generated during smoking also produces burns on the vermilion and palate. The chutta (reverse smoking) habit is seen in Andhra Pradesh,[10] a south Indian state, where even females smoke the bidi keeping the burning end inside the mouth. The palatal lesions like *nicotina palatini* are commonly associated with this habit. The smoked tobacco generally leads to precancerous lesions like leukoplakia and erythroplakia commonly on sites like cheek mucosa, palate, tongue, anterior mandibular gingiva, tongue and the floor of mouth and subsequently leads to oral squamous cell carcinoma (OSCC) of one of these sites (Figs 30.1A to D). The smoked tobacco additionally carries a risk of developing the carcinoma of pharynx, posterior one third of the tongue, larynx and broncogenic carcinoma. It is important to know the duration of the habit, frequency and quantity of the bidi or cigarette smoking as it has the direct bearing on the development of precancerous or cancerous lesions.

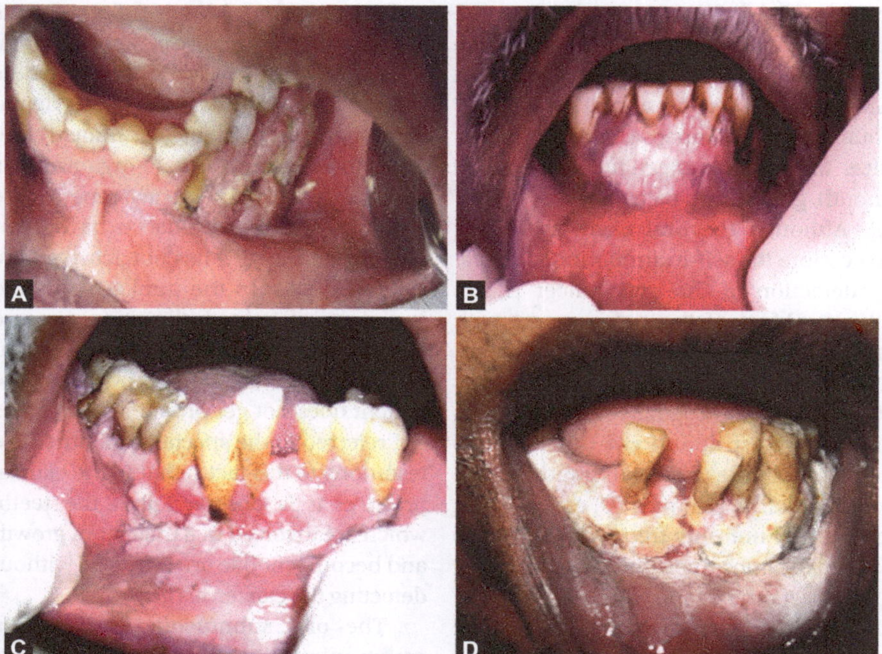

Figs 30.1A to D: (A) OSCC of posterior GB sulcus due to kharra/mawa; (B) At gingivo labial sulcus tobacco/lime chewing habits; (C and D) At the labial sulcus with extensive leukoplakia

The smokeless tobacco is the preferred form of tobacco use in India. Smoking is considered a taboo and there are statutes banning it in public places and thus, people resort to tobacco chewing habits. The tobacco is still offered to guests as a social custom. The use of tobacco in this form is common throughout the country, but more commonly in Maharashtra, Madhya Pradesh, UP, Bihar and most northern states. The habit of ghutka or kharra is common amongst the youngsters including the school going children as this habit is picked up quite early in life and is not considered as bad as smoking. Even women are addicted to tobacco in a smokeless form. The habituated individual often keeps the tobacco lime mixture in the anterior gingivobuccal sulcus of the mandible, leading to precancerous or cancerous lesions of this site (Figs 30.1B to D) and the kharra or khaini is kept in the mandibular buccal vestibule in the posterior area for a long period (Fig. 30.1A). Sometimes the kharra chewers sleep at night keeping the tobacco in the buccal vestibule. These habits facilitate the contact of tobacco and other materials used in the kharra/ghutka to remain in contact with the mucosa for a long time, causing chronic irritation. Some of the ingredients like lime are caustic and in addition to irritation induce chemical burns on the mucosa. Thus, this habit produces precancerous or cancerous lesions of posterior gingivobuccal sulcus. The habituated individual consumes the tobacco as many as 20 to 30 times a day, posing a greater risk of inducing precancerous or cancerous lesions.

Betel Nut Chewing

The betel nut is a major cash crop of the tropical region. The betel nut chewing in various forms is a social custom in India and not considered dangerous or hazardous. It is consumed by males, females, children, adults, rich and poor alike. The betel nut alkaloids (arecoline, arecolidine, arecaidine, guvacine and guvacoline) have been investigated by various authors[11,12] to establish their role in the etiology of submucos fibrosis (SMF) and oral cancer. The betel nut is consumed unripe, processed and processed forms with addition of various flavoring and sweetening agents. It is consumed alone or with tobacco and pan. Although the carcinogenic potential of betel nut is disputed,[13] but still it remains a fact that majority of the patients who have SMF are habituated to betel nut chewing in some form or other and some of the patients with OSCC give history of betel nut chewing alone, without tobacco. The fact remains is that the SMF is an established precancerous condition and the association of OSCC with SMF is increasing. Thus, the carcinogenic potential of betel nut can not be denied.

Alcoholism

Most of the chronic alcoholics are often heavy smokers, too. The alcoholics derive energy from the alcohol and eat poorly leading to nutritional deficiencies, which could be a predisposition to development of chronic stomatitis and OSCC. Alcohol may influence the proliferative cells by both intracellular (e.g. endocytosis) and intercellular (permeability) pathways. The carcinogenic exposure of the proliferating stem cells in the basal layer may be regulated through these pathways.[14]

Chronic Irritation

The chronic irritation from sharp or malposed teeth (Trauma from occlusion), over hanging restorations and ill fitting dentures, etc. leads to frequent mucosal ulceration. The chronic irritation brings about the dysplastic changes in the epithelium, which initially are reactionary dysplasia, but subsequently become irreversible and may change into leukoplakia or OSCC.

Nutritional Deficiencies

Malnourishment, secondary to poor intake, lack of balanced diet, malabsorption syndromes, chronic GI infections or due to parasites such as worm infestations, amoebiasis/giardiasis are common causes of nutritional deficiencies in India. Apart from this the chronic blood loss due to menorrhagia, piles and hemorrhoids leads to iron deficiency anemia, sideropenic dysphagia and Plummer-Vinson's syndrome. The deficiency of vitamins especially the vitamin A, B complex and iron leads to inflammatory changes, dysplasia and transformation into malignancy.

Oral syphilis[15] and lichen planus[16] are also implicated in the etiology of OSCC.

Exposure to the UV Rays[17]

The exposure to UV rays induces the carcinoma of the vermilion of the lower lip (Figs 30.2A to C). It is commonly seen in the farm laborers who work in the sun for long times. The basal cell carcinomas have also been implicated to sun exposure (UV rays). It is more commonly seen on skin above the ala-tragus line, however the lesions have been reported from the skin of the upper lip. It is more common in Caucasian population due to less melanin pigment.

PATHOGENESIS

The etiology, clinical behavior, incidence of malignant transformation behavior and malignant potential, concept of field cancerization and oxidative damage, etc. are discussed in the previous chapter on the premalignant lesions and conditions.

CARCINOGENESIS

Carcinogenesis is a multistep process at both phenotypic and genotypic levels, where the tumor progression occurs in a step wise fashion (Flow chart 30.1).

Goldhaber and Berenbaum studied development of cancer in animal skin and mucosa and suggested two stage mechanism hypothesis for carcinogenesis

- Initiation
- Promotion.
  - **Initiation phase:** Normal cells are changed into dormant tumor cells by some carcinogenic influences in a short period of time. Tissue may appear clinically and histologically, normal.
  - **Promotion phase:** Subsequent exposure of the initiated tissue to cocarcinogens changes the dormant tumor cells to visible tumor mass in longer period.

Recent advances in oral mucosa research suggest the modified concept of carcinogenesis. The conventional two stage theory was expanded to three stages.

- **Progression phase:** It is a process whereby a neoplasm develops by one or more permanent qualitative irreversible changes into its constituent cells. The progression phase once initiated continues to progress even if the cause, which had initiated the same, has been eliminated. Once the changes in the cells are progressive, they can not be reversed even if the stimulus that has promoted the changes has been withdrawn.
- **Oncogenes:** They are the genes that promote cell growth in cancer cells. They are characterized by the ability to promote cell growth in the absence of normal mitogenic signals.
- **Proto-oncogenes:** They are the normal counter part of oncogenes. They are physiologic regulators of cell proliferation and differentiation. They may be converted to cellular oncogenes by a process known as insertional mutagenesis, where the mutated proviral DNA is inserted near the proto-oncogene.

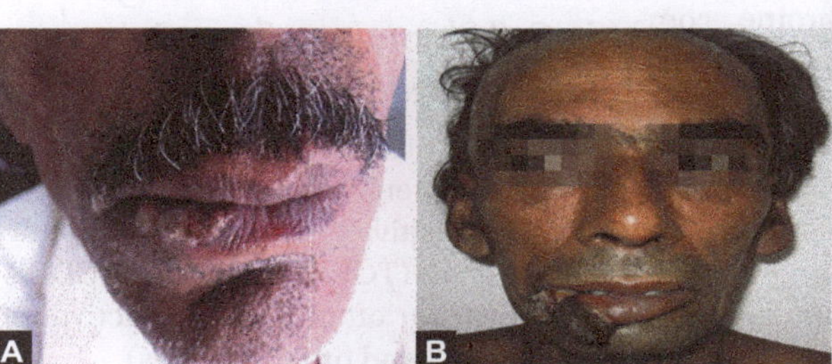
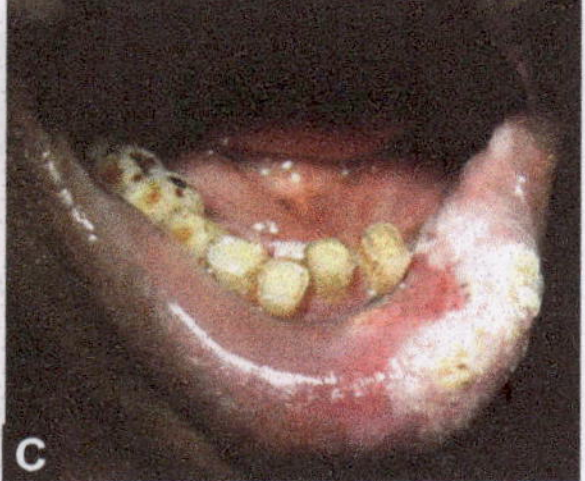

Figs 30.2A to C: Carcinoma of the vermilion border of the lower lip

Flow chart 30.1: Carcinogenesis

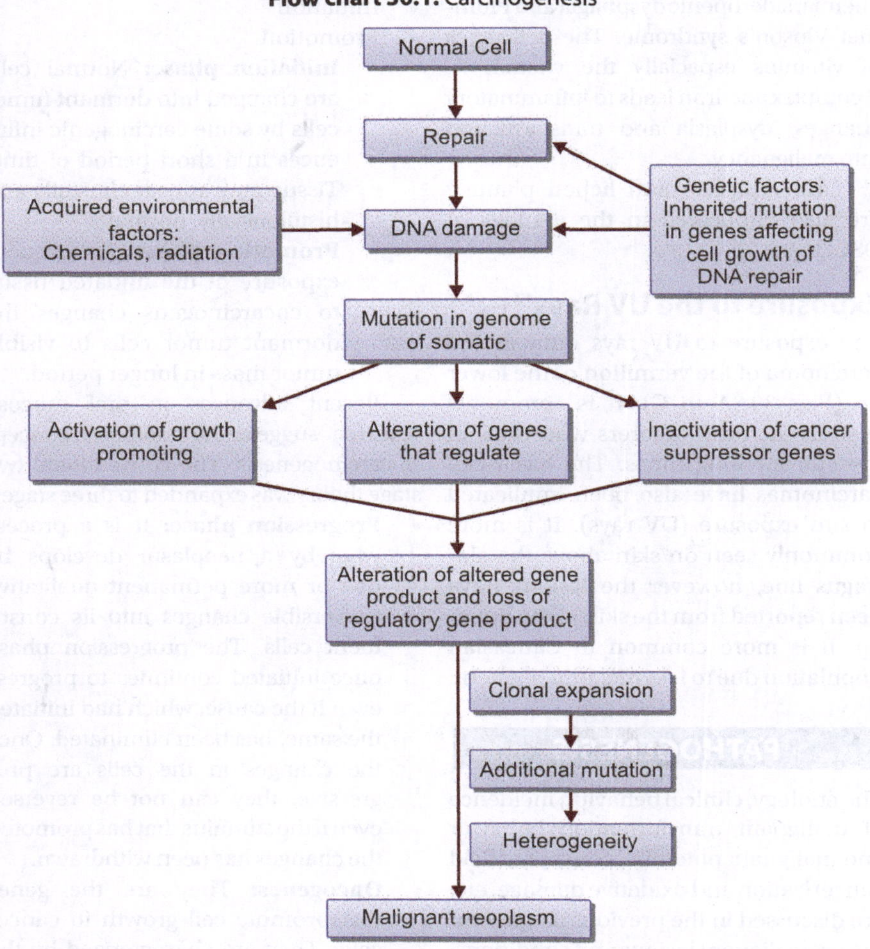

Oncoproteins—are the products of oncogenes and proto-oncogenes.

Carcinogens[18]

Carcinogens are the factors which initiate conversion of normal cells into tumor cells or cause initiation of the carcinoma. They include various chemical, physical and viral carcinogens.

- **Chemical carcinogens:** Most of oral neoplasms are caused by chemical carcinogens. Nickel chrome compound, cigarette smoke, betel nut, tobacco quid, asbestos, benzene, certain tars, soots, oils and arsenic compounds.
- **Physical carcinogens:** Actinic radiation, ionizing radiation.
- **Viral carcinogens:** Human T-lymphotropic virus type I (HTLV I), Human papilloma virus (HPV), Epstein-Barr virus (EBV), Hepatitis B virus, have been implicated in the etiopathogenesis of oral cancer.

Cocarcinogens

Cocarcinogens are the factors which convert altered cells to visible mass, e.g. chronic irritation, trauma, vitamin deficiency and poor oral hygiene.

Seven Fundamental Changes in Cell Physiology Essential for Malignant Transformation

i. Self-sufficiency in growth signals (oncogene activation)
ii. Insensitivity to growth-inhibitory signals (TGF-β, inhibitors of CDK's)
iii. Evasion of apoptosis (inactivation of p53 and other changes)
iv. Defects in DNA repair
v. Limitless replicative potential
vi. Sustained angiogenesis (vascular endothelial growth factor, VEGF)
vii. Ability to invade and metastatize.

CLINICAL PRESENTATION OF ORAL CANCER

- **A red indurated patch:** A red indurated patch is usually the preexisting erythroplakia or leukoplakia, which changes into malignancy (Figs 30.3A to E). There may not be any exuberant growth or an ulcer, but a perceptible change in color (white to red), fissuring, change in size and the most important; presence of induration. The lesions are slightly raised from the surface and may have slightly granular appearance on its surface. The most important finding is presence of induration and fixity and hence, the lesions cannot be suspected or detected without palpation. The lesions require being biopsied to establish the final diagnosis. These lesions could be early malignant transformation and subsequently change into an ulcerated or exophytic growth, which is a classical presentation of OSCC. The malignant potential of these growths should not be underestimated as they may have widespread lymph node metastasis.
- **An ulcerated growth:** The OSCC presents mostly as an ulcerated growth. The malignant ulcer has classical everted or rolled out edges (Figs 30.4A and B). This is due to rapid division of the cells at the periphery, where the tumor grows optimally and excessive cellular bulk leads to compaction of the cell mass, which produces elevation or evertion of the edges. The ulcer is irregular in shape and the floor is covered with whitish materia alba composed of desquamated cells and food debris with projecting red granulomatous areas. The palpatory findings are indurated edges due to compaction of the cell mass, indurated and friable base and bleeding on provocation. The ulcer has fixity to the deeper structure. The ulcerated growths are

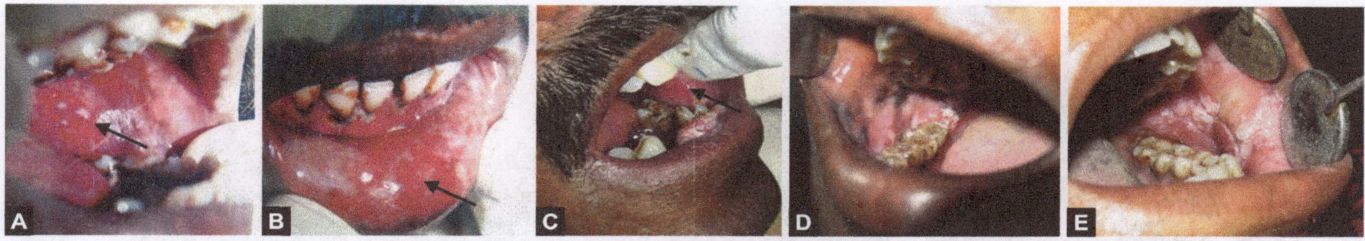

Figs 30.3A to E: Leukoplakia changing into a red lesions, on biopsy they were found to be well differentiated squamous cell carcinoma

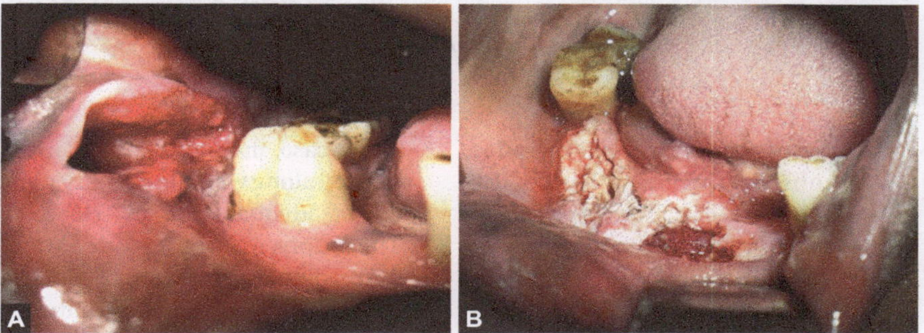

Figs 30.4A and B: (A) Classical malignant ulcer with everted/rolled out edges; (B) Infilterative character

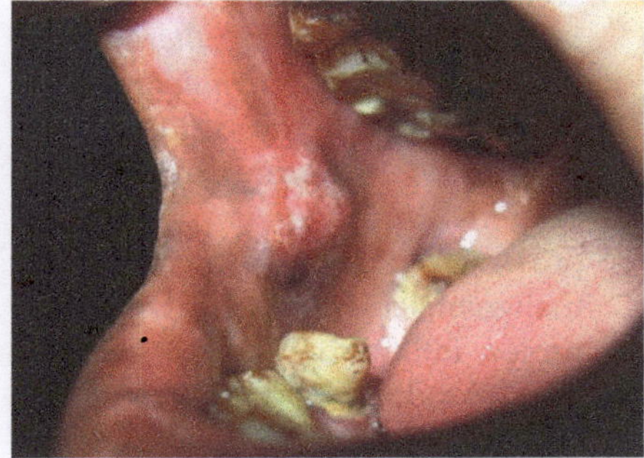

Fig. 30.5: Early exophytic growth

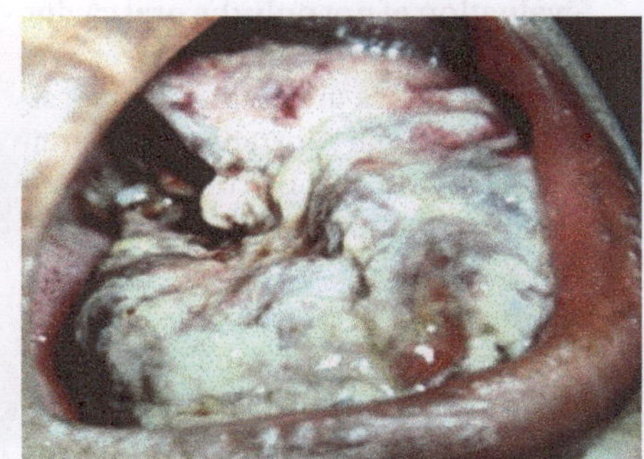

Fig. 30.6: Advanced exophytic growth

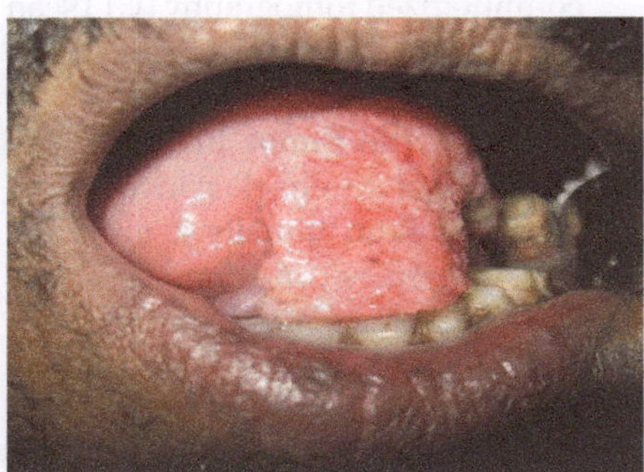

Fig. 30.7: Advanced exophytic growth on tongue

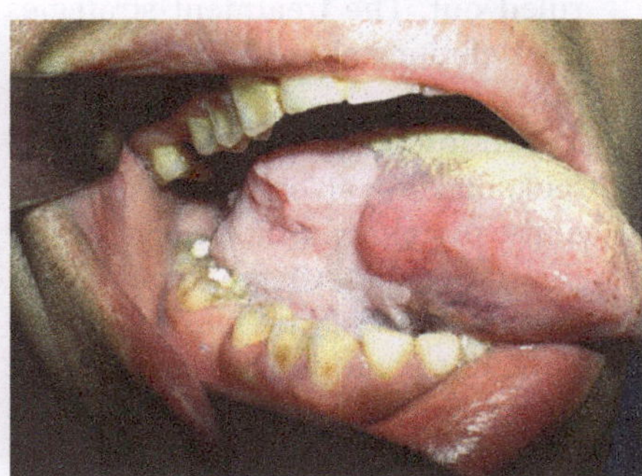

Fig. 30.8: Exophytic growth on tongue

more aggressive as compared to the exophytic growths in their behavior and as they readily infiltrate into the deeper tissue, the bulk (i.e. depth of infiltration) of the tumor is greater with early and widespread cervical metastasis. It is being said that whenever the tumor bulk increases beyond 2 mm, the chances of lymph node metastasis increase significantly.

- **Exophytic growth:** The third picture is an exophytic growth, which is often described as *'cauliflower'*—like growth. The tumor grows more outwards and although the outward growth is more the relative deeper infiltration is less (Figs 30.5, 30.6, 30.7 and 30.8). Such growths are less aggressive and also metastasize to regional nodes. The metastasis is late as compared to the ulcerative growths. The tumor has a multilobulated, with granular appearance, firm in consistency and friable causing bleeding on provocation or trauma from occlusion during mastication. It also infiltrates into the deeper tissue, but to a lesser extent than the ulcerated growths.

The verrucous carcinomas also present as exophytic cauliflower-like growths (Figs 30.9 and 30.10). The verrucous carcinomas do not metastasize as the basement membrane is intact. The verrucous carcinoma is characterized by acanthosis. The behavior of the tumor is not very aggressive and usually wide local excision, without addressing the neck is adequate. However, although the tumor is labeled as verrucous carcinoma histopathologically, a

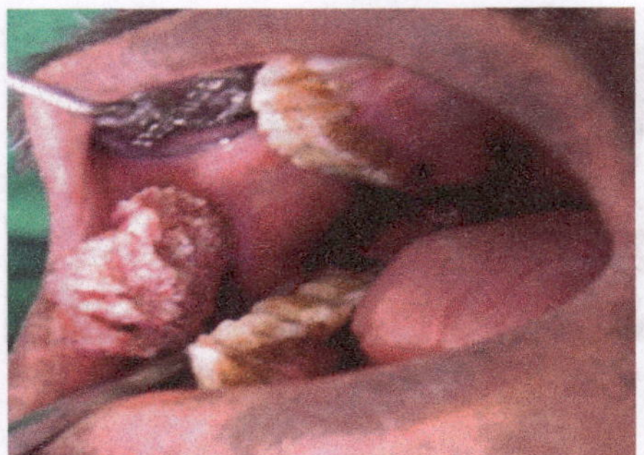

Fig. 30.9: Early exophytic growth, verrucous carcinoma

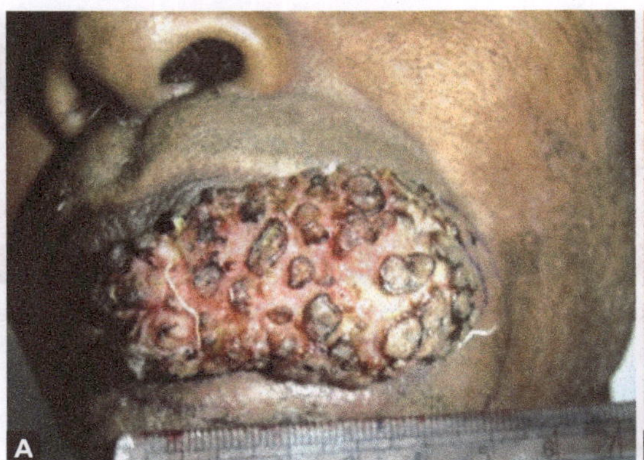

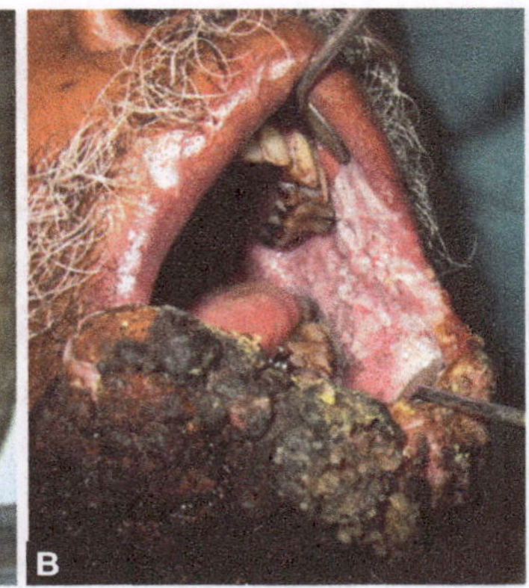

Figs 30.10A and B: Verrucous carcinoma

transitional change to invasive squamous cell carcinoma may be present in some parts of a large lesion, which will be often missed if the biopsied tissue does not include this part of the lesion. The same is applicable to the *in situ* carcinomas, as both these lesions are border line and have a threshold to change into an invasive squamous cell carcinoma. Hence, it is imperative that these lesions be evaluated thoroughly for regional metastasis and the entire excised lesion be thoroughly screened histopathologically to find out any area of invasive changes in the lesion. The cases of verrucous carcinomas should be kept under long term follow-up to detect any locoregional recurrence.

- **A mixed growth with both ulcerated and exophytic areas:** Some tumors present with such a mixed picture. The behavior in spite of the dual presentation is aggressive similar to the ulcerated growth.
- **As a nodule:** It is not a very usual presentation of the OSCC except in some cases of the carcinoma of the tongue. It may present as a small ulcer on the venterolateral margin of the tongue, but when palpated, a nodular lump may be felt in the substance of the tongue, which could be appreciably large involving large area of the tongue. It is the reason why evaluation of tongue is done with a magnetic resonance imaging (MRI), in addition to the clinical examination (*see* Figs 30.27A to D).
- **Metastatic tumor in neck nodes with obscure primary:** Rarely, the squamous cell carcinomas primarily present as a metastatic mass in the cervical nodes and the primary is not detectable in the oral cavity. The fine needle aspiration cytology (FNAC) of the involved lymph nodes shows deposits of squamous cell carcinoma. A thorough clinical evaluation of not only the oral cavity, but of nasal cavity, nasopharynx and oropharynx is needed. The possibility of primary intraosseous carcinoma should also be ruled out. Four quadrant incisional biopsy from most common sites of development of OSCC like tongue, floor of mouth, cheek and tonsils is taken in an attempt to locate the obscure primary, which is rarely productive. The chances of distant lymphatic metastasis from viscera like upper GI tract are there and warrant to be ruled out. The treatment strategies are definitely altered, if the primary is obscure.

The tumor may be associated with leukoplakic or an erythroplakic patch at the periphery, which suggests that the tumor might have originated in the pre-existing premalignant lesions, but some tumors are without such picture. Whenever such patches are present, they should also be biopsied and evaluated. Sometimes they may show severe dysplasia or frank invasive carcinoma and in either case, the patch should also be excised along with the primary tumor to get adequate surgical clearance. The lesions associated with SMF are more difficult to evaluate clinically due to the presence of trismus and altered tissue consistency due to which the induration is difficult to elicit. The common sites of OSCC secondary to SMF are retromolar area (probably *due to trauma from occlusion [TFO] from the buccally placed maxillary third molars and loss of elasticity of the cheek mucosa*) and tongue and both cannot be evaluated properly, if trismus is present. The presence of trismus in the retromolar malignancies could also be due to tumor infiltration in the muscles, but this cannot be ascertained if the patient has trismus due to SMF and invariably the growths are extensive, involving the infratemporal fossa and surgical clearance is difficult. A computerized tomography (CT) scan with contrast is ideal to assess the tumor extent in such cases.

When the tumor infiltrates full thickness of the cheek, it invades the overlying skin. Initially it produces '*peau d'orange*' or orange peel appearance. Then the skin becomes eroded and finally the tumor fungates extraorally (Figs 30.11A to C). Such open growths get infected secondarily, leading to formation of orocutaneous fistulas and foul smell. The growths can get infected

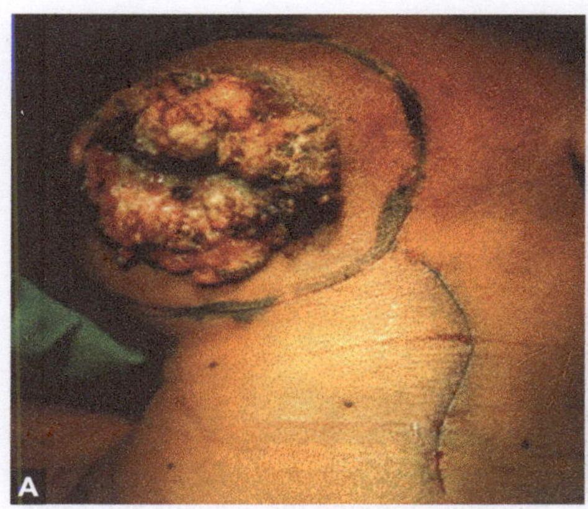

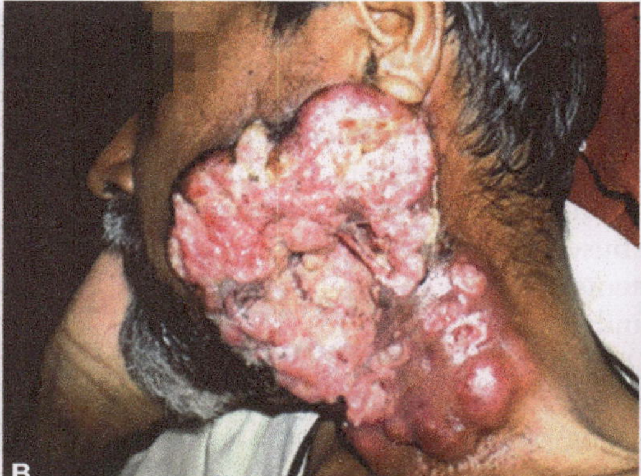

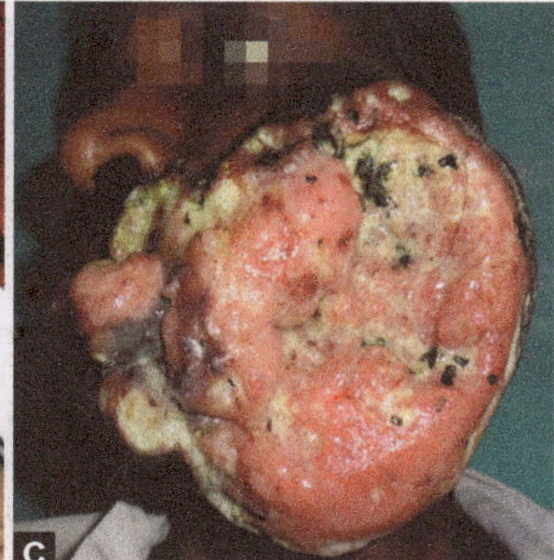

Figs 30.11A to C: Extraoral fungation

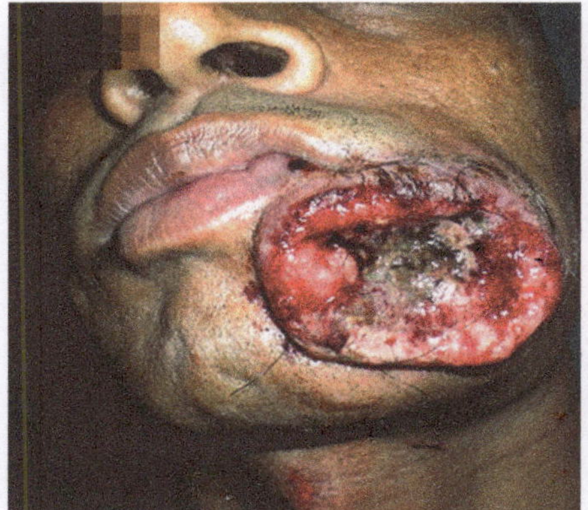

Fig. 30.12: Extraoral fungation with maggots

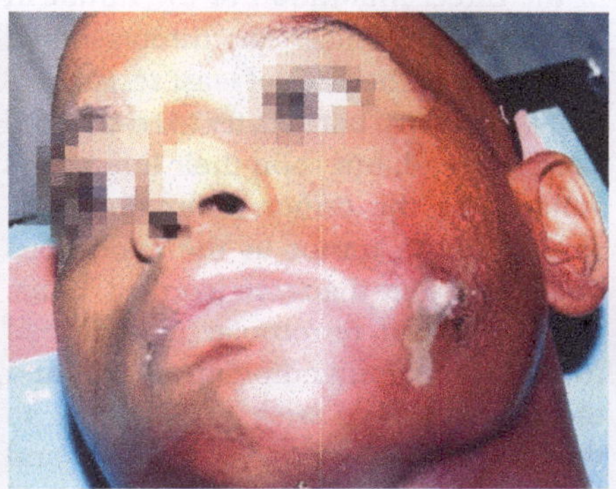

Fig. 30.13: Extraoral fungation of the OSCC with secondary infection, presenting as a cutaneous sinus like osteomyelitis

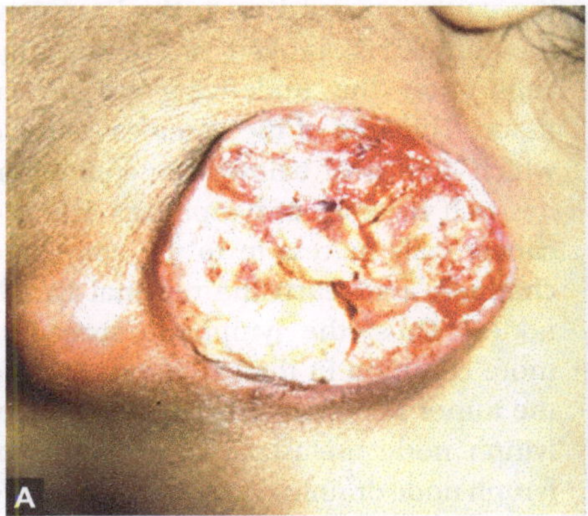

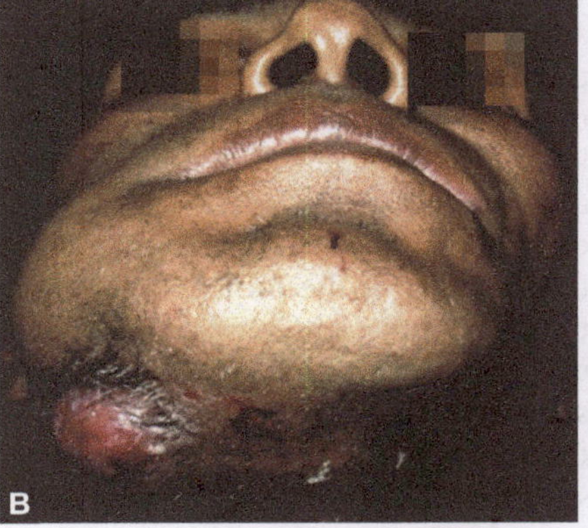

Figs 30.14A and B: External fungation of the metastatic lymph nodes

with myasis, which is a common presentation in such growths in rural India (Fig. 30.12). The fungation with pus discharge due to the secondary infection often mimics the presentation of chronic suppurative osteomyelitis (Fig. 30.13) and needs careful clinical evaluation and histopathological examination for correct diagnosis. Similarly, the metastatic cervical lymph nodes can also fungate on the skin surface (Figs 30.14A and B). Such lymph nodes also infiltrate the deeper vital structures such as carotid artery making them unresectable and the chances of major vessel blow outs and life threatening hemorrhage during the surgery are increased.

PRIMARY INTRAOSSEOUS CARCINOMA

Primary intraosseous carcinoma (PIOC) is an uncommon neoplasm. According to the most recent edition of the World Health Organization (WHO) classification for histological typing of odontogenic tumors, it is defined as a squamous cell carcinoma arising within the jawbone without connection to the oral mucosa, probably from odontogenic epithelial residues. This tumor was first described by Loos in 1913. Pindborg coined the term PIOC in the first edition of the WHO classification for histological typing of odontogenic tumors. Affecting more males than females (M:F, 3:2), PIOC is more frequent in the 6th and 7th decades of life. It occurs more frequently in the mandible (especially the posterior section) than in the maxilla.

Since PIOC essentially occurs only in the tooth bearing areas of the jawbone, the hypothesis of odontogenic epithelial origin is theoretically acceptable, except in the maxillary incisive canal. At termination of the odontogenesis, remnants of the odontogenic epithelium, derived from different origins such as the tooth germ, remain in the oral tissues as epithelial rests. Occasionally, owing to some unknown stimuli, these epithelial rests are activated and, either alone or in conjunction with mesodermal tissues, they then proliferate and develop into odontogenic cysts or carcinomas. In contrast to the classic oral mucosa squamous cell carcinomas, the risk factors of alcohol, tobacco or betel quid abuse are usually not present in PIOC patients. The most common risk factor for inducing neoplastic formation of PIOC is assumed to be a reactive inflammatory stimulus, with/without a predisposing genetic cofactor.

The WHO has published criteria to differentiate PIOC from other primary and metastatic squamous cell carcinomas of the jaw bone such as:

- Intact oral mucosa before diagnosis.
- Microscopic evidence of squamous cell carcinoma without a cystic component or other odontogenic tumor cells.
- Absence of another primary tumor on chest radiographs obtained at the time of diagnosis and during a follow-up period of more than 6 months.

Therefore, exclusion of the possibility of metastatic lesion from a distant primary tumor is always necessary for the final diagnosis of PIOC.

Although the clinical features of PIOCs are non-specific, still most of them are associated with complaints of sensory disturbances like paresthesia and numbness, mimicking facial neurological problems. When solely neurological disturbances are present and there is absence of any obvious mucosal abnormalities within the oral cavity, especially in case of the early lesion, increases the probability of delayed diagnosis. Delay in correct diagnosis will worsen the prognosis; hence, it is important to consider intraosseous carcinoma in the jawbone in the differential diagnosis for all cases of facial paresthesia and numbness to facilitate the early identification of PIOC and enabling prompt institution of suitable treatment.

Radiographic examination is one of the most effective methods for detecting PIOCs. A lesion that is completely surrounded by bone can be regarded as of intraosseous origin. CT scan can also facilitate correct diagnosis.

Once the diagnosis is made, the PIOC should be treated as any other squamous cell carcinoma and treated in the similar fashion. Due to its intraosseous nature, radiotherapy as primary modality of its treatment is not recommended.

Modalities of Spread of the Oral Squamous Cell Carcinoma

The modes of spread of the oral squamous cell carcinoma are:

Local Spread

The local spread of the OSCC is as a result of the direct infiltration of the tumor in the adjacent tissues. The tumor spread occurs along the path of least resistance. The anatomical barriers try to restrict the tumor spread, but soon their integrity is violated by the tumor infiltration. The spread of the tumor in the cancellous bone is faster than the cortical bone. The tumors of retromolar area spread to the pterygomandibular space and the infratemporal area rapidly due to the potential spaces present there and infiltrate the muscle like medial pterygoid resulting in trismus. Similarly, due to the presence of more spongy bone, the tumors of the maxillary sinus or those originating in the maxillary gingivobuccal vestibule, spread rapidly involving large areas. The tumor rapidly extends to the paranasal sinuses and the involvement of ethmoidal and sphenoidal sinuses leads to the involvement of the base of anterior cranial fossa. The involvement of the posterior wall of maxilla leads to extension of the tumor in the infratemporal fossa and renders it virtually unresectable. The tumors of the maxillary sinus involving the inferior wall, fungate through the alveolar bone and the extension of such tumors on to the buccal mucosa after crossing the buccal vestibule changes the clinical behavior of the tumor (Fig. 30.15). The maxillary sinus malignancies do not frequently metastasize in the regional lymph nodes, but extension of this tumor on the buccal mucosa causes lymph node metastasis, which warrants neck dissection along with the maxillectomy thus, changing the treatment requirements.

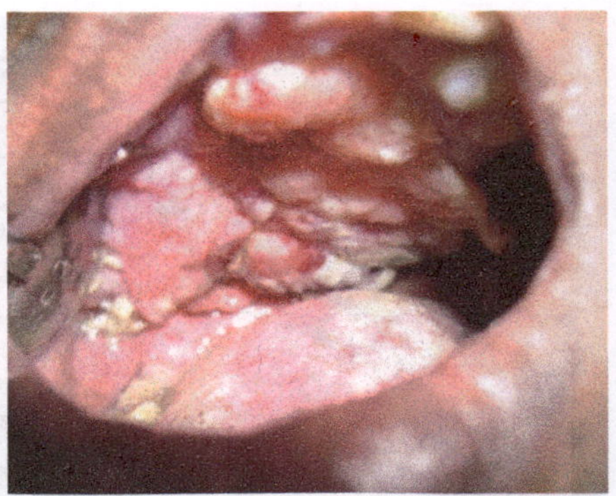

Fig. 30.15: Carcinoma of maxillary sinus fungating through the alveolus and extending to the buccal mucosa

The OSCC of lower gingivobuccal sulcus infiltrates the alveolar bone and extends to the lingual gingiva and thereon involves the floor of the mouth causing widespread lymph node metastasis bilaterally, changing the clinical course and management of the malignancy (Figs 30.16A and B).

Regional Lymph Node Spread

The OSCC are known to metastasize to the regional lymph nodes quite early necessitating the management of the metastatic nodes imperative for the effective locoregional control of the disease. The carcinomas originate from the epithelium and once the basement membrane is broken the cancerous cells enter the underlying connective tissue. The area of the connective tissue which lies just below the epithelium has rich network of lymphatics and the cancer cells ingress in to the lymphatic channels and reach the regional lymph nodes. Thus, the lymphatic spread is more common in the carcinomas. More the tumor bulk, more are the chances of lymph node metastasis. The groups of lymph node draining a particular area are most likely to be involved in metastasis. The carcinomas of the tongue and floor of the mouth have optimum tendency for widespread lymphatic metastasis, and in the latter case they could be bilateral. This is because both these sites have rich lymphatic networks and there is crisscrossing of the lymphatics from the contralateral side. Similarly, the malignancies of the midline tend to

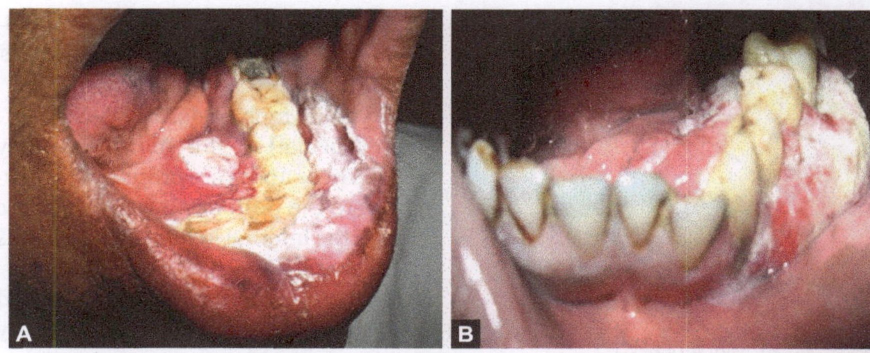

Figs 30.16A and B: Gingivobuccal carcinoma extending on to the floor of mouth by direct infiltration, changes the behavior of the tumor

metastasize bilaterally. The retromolar area malignancies are also known to metastasize in deep cervical nodes more often than the gingivobuccal or buccal mucosa carcinomas. Thus, the carcinomas of the tongue, floor of the mouth and the retromolar area are often treated by elective neck dissection along with the excision of the primary. The other indications for the elective neck dissection being, the anaplastic carcinoma and malignant melanoma.

The metastatic lymph nodes are firm to hard in consistency as the metastatic cells reach the cortex of the lymph node through the afferent lymphatics. The tumor cells proliferate in the lymphatic nodules present in the subcortical area and compaction of the cell mass takes place. As a result of this, the lymph node becomes round in shape and the node becomes non-compressible and stony hard in consistency (Fig. 30.17).

The cervical lymphatics are located along the major veins of the neck. The lymphoid sinuses roughly around 80 to 90 in number develop around the developing venous channels in the neck. Over a period of time they reduce in number and form aggregates, which develop in the nodes, which have different locations around the veins in the neck. The various locations at which the cervicofacial lymph nodes are present are (Fig. 30.18):

- Occipital
- Retroauricular (mastoid)
- Parotid

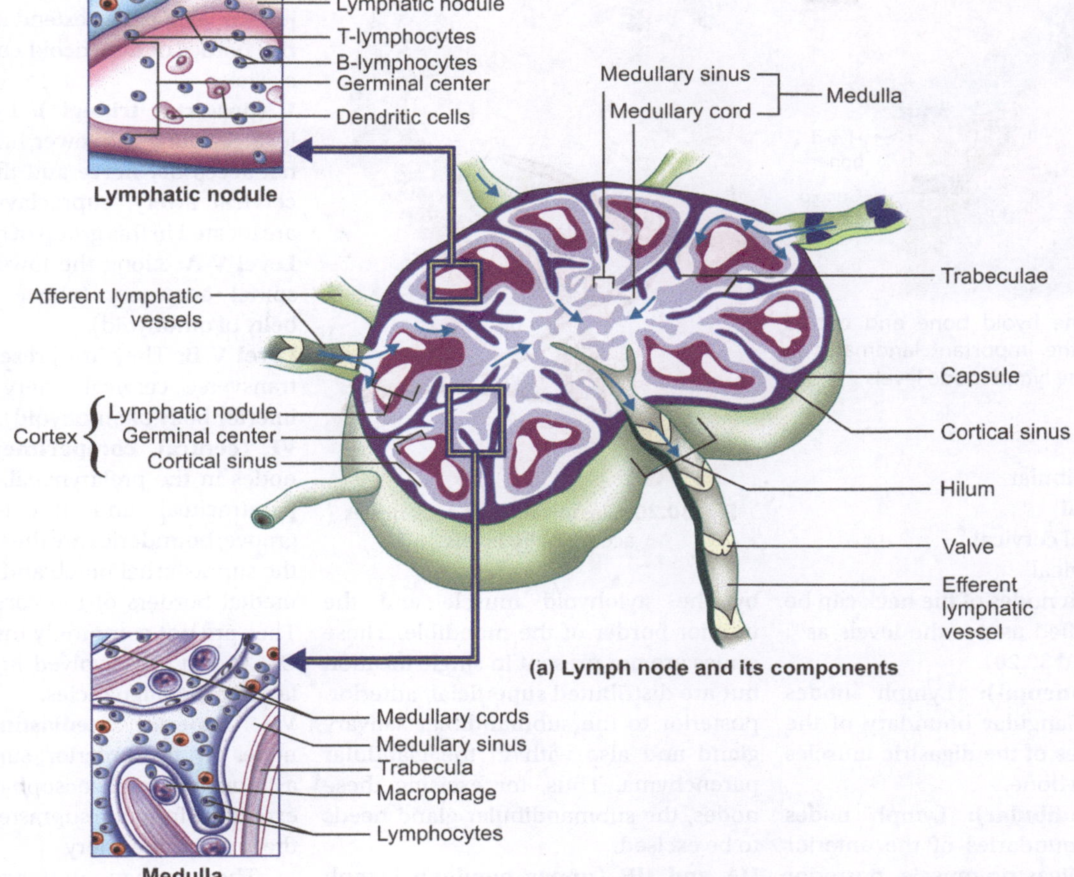

Fig. 30.17: Structure of the lymph node. The metastatic cells reach the lymph node through the afferent lymphatic to get lodged in the subcortical area, making the node hard in consistency and round earlier

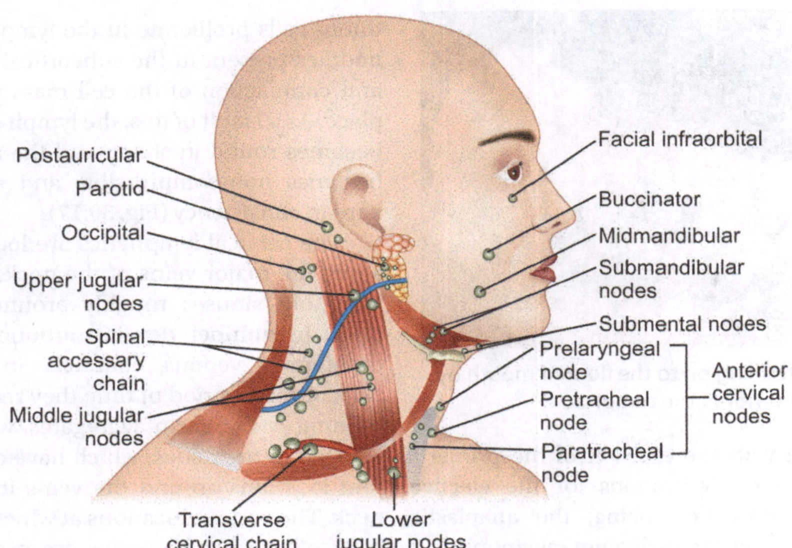

Fig. 30.18: Various groups of cervical lymph nodes[19]

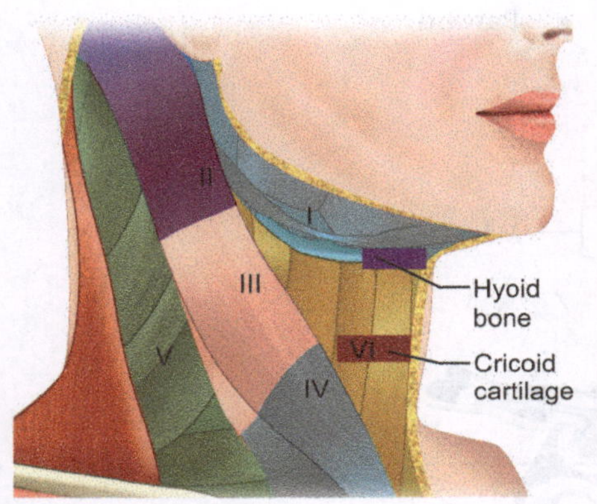

Fig. 30.19: The hyoid bone and cricoid cartilage are the important landmarks in determining the lymph node levels

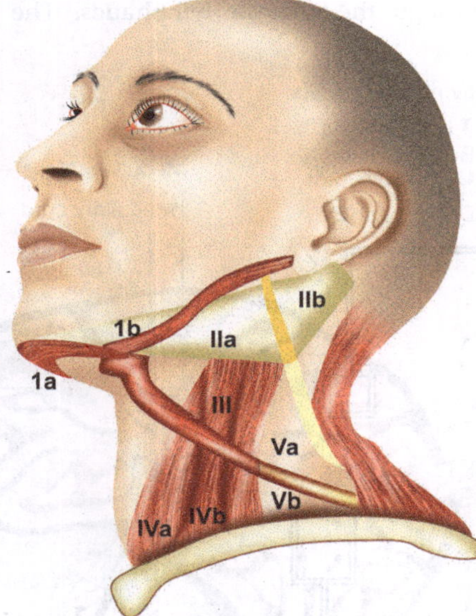

Fig. 30.20: Classification of neck nodes according to levels

- Facial
- Submandibular
- Submental
- Superficial cervical
- Deep cervical.

The lymph nodes of the neck can be further classified as per the levels as[19]: (Figs 30.19 and 30.20)

IA (submental): Lymph nodes within the triangular boundary of the anterior bellies of the digastric muscles and the hyoid bone.

IB (Submandibular): Lymph nodes within the boundaries of the anterior belly of the digastric muscle, posterior belly of digastic muscle, complemented by the stylohyoid muscle and the inferior border of the mandible. These nodes are not present in single location but are distributed superficial, anterior, posterior to the submandiblar salivary gland and also with in the glandular parenchyma. Thus, for excising these nodes, the submandibular gland needs to be excised.

IIA and IIB (upper jugular): Lymph nodes located around the upper third of the internal jugular vein (Jugulo-diagastric) and the adjacent spinal accessory nerve.

Level IIA: Lymph nodes are located anterior (medial) to the spinal accessory nerve. These nodes are present at the level, where the posterior belly of digastric crosses the internal jugular vein and thus are referred to as *jugulo digastric nodes.*

Level IIB: Lymph nodes are located posterior (lateral) to the spinal accessory nerve.

III (middle jugular): Lymph nodes located around the middle third of the internal jugular vein; nodes are located between the inferior border of the hyoid bone and the inferior border of the cricoid cartilage. They are present at the level, where the superior belly of the omohyoid crosses the internal jugular vein and are also designated as *jugulo-omohyoid group of nodes or midjugular nodes.*

IV (lower jugular): Lymph nodes located around the lower third of the internal jugular vein; nodes extend from the inferior border of the cricoid cartilage to the clavicle.

V (posterior triangle): Lymph nodes located along the lower half of the spinal accessory nerve and the transverse cervical artery; supraclavicular nodes are located in this group of lymph nodes.

Level V A: Along the lower half of the spinal accessory (above the inferior belly of omohyoid).

Level V B: They are present along the transverse cervical artery (below the inferior belly of omohyoid).

VI (central compartment): Lymph nodes in the prelaryngeal, pretracheal, paratracheal and tracheoesophageal groove; boundaries are the hyoid bone to the suprasternal notch and between the medial borders of the carotid sheaths. They are not commonly involved in the OSCC, but are involved in thyroid and laryngeal malignancies.

VII (superior mediastinal): Lymph nodes in the anterior superior mediastinum and tracheoesophageal grooves, extending from the suprasternal notch to the innominate artery.

The lymphatic drainage of the oral structures is primarily in the particular

Box 30.1: Lymphatic drainage of oral structures

Floor of mouth	Anterior part—upper deep cervical nodes, either directly or via submental nodes Remaining part—submandibular and upper deep cervical nodes
Maxillary sinus	Drains in the submandibular nodes Paranasal sinuses—upper deep cervical nodes, directly or through retropharyngeal nodes
Teeth	Lower incisors—submental and therefore to submandibular or lower deep cervical nodes Rest lower teeth and all upper teeth—submandibular lymph nodes and upper deep cervical nodes Occasionally upper and lower teeth also drain into the buccal and mandibular lymph nodes
Tonsil	Do not possess afferent lymphatics or lymph sinuses Dense plexus of fine lymphatic vessels surround each follicle, forming efferent lymphatic, which drain to upper deep cervical lymph nodes, especially the jugulodigastric nodes
Hard palate	Anterior part—submandibular lymph nodes Posterior part—upper deep cervical nodes and to the retropharyngeal nodes
Soft palate	Lymphatics drain partly to the retropharyngeal and partly to the upper deep cervical nodes
Tongue	Tip of tongue—bilaterally to submental nodes Anterior 2/3rd—unilaterally to submandibular nodes Central vessels—jugulodigastric or jugulo-omohyoid nodes

groups of lymph nodes as mentioned above (Box 30.1). However, there can be variations due to crisscrossing of the lymphatics, aberrant lymphatic channels, anastomosis and due to a phenomenon called skip metastasis.

Hematogenous Spread

The hematogenous spread of OSCC is a rare and late occurrence. The tumor cell seeding in the bloodstream can occur if a tooth involved in the malignant growth is extracted. The cells can invade the blood vessels during surgery. In cases of advanced disease, the tumor cells involve deeper connective tissue and spread hematogenously. The other causes of the hematogenous spread could be that the lymph nodes are located along the venous channels right from their development. This proximity can make a metastatic node involve the adjacent vein and the tumor cells can spread via the bloodstream. Lastly the lymph drains in to the venous compartment through the efferent channels or finally through the ductus *chylus* and the tumor cells present in these channels can spread along the bloodstream in this way also. The cellular emboli can get lodged at distant sites and start proliferating there, producing metastatic disease. Usually the richly vascular visceral organs like lungs, liver, kidneys and the brain are involved in hematogenous metastasis (Fig. 30.21). The metastasis can occur to the bones as well like the vertebra, cranial bones, or long bones. The distant hematogenous spread of the disease is a poor prognostic sign (Fig. 30.22).

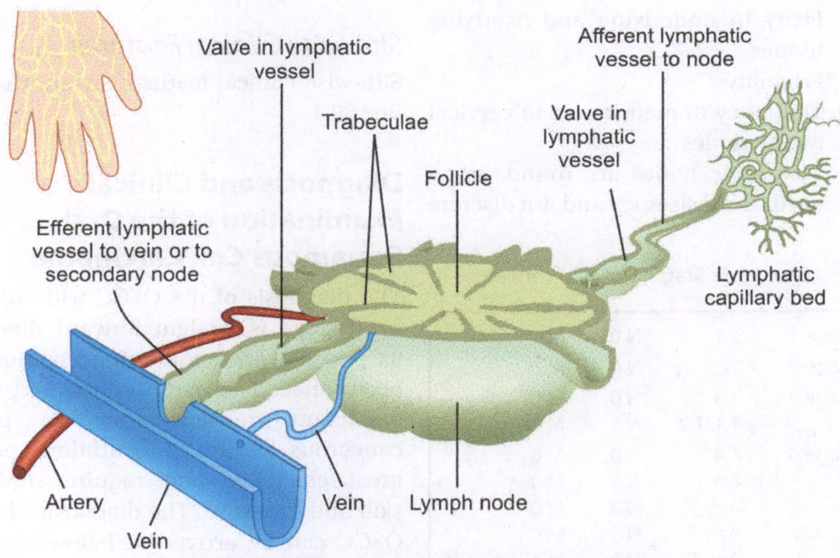

Fig. 30.21: Drainage of lymph in the veinous system

Contact Spread

Contact spread is a rare type of spread of OSCC. It is more common in the malignancies of vulva. In the oral cavity contact spread could take place in the malignancies involving vermilion, where the tumor can spread to the opposing lip or occasionally from gingiva to the buccal mucosa.

TNM Classification of Oral Squamous Cell Carcinoma (Box 30.2)

The TNM system for the classification of malignant tumors was developed by Pierre Denoix[20] in France between 1943 and 1952 and eventually was adapted by the International Union against Cancer.[21]

The objectives of such classification are as follows:

- To aid the clinician in treatment planning.
- To provide prognostic value.
- To evaluate the results of treatment.
- To facilitate exchange of information between surgical teams.

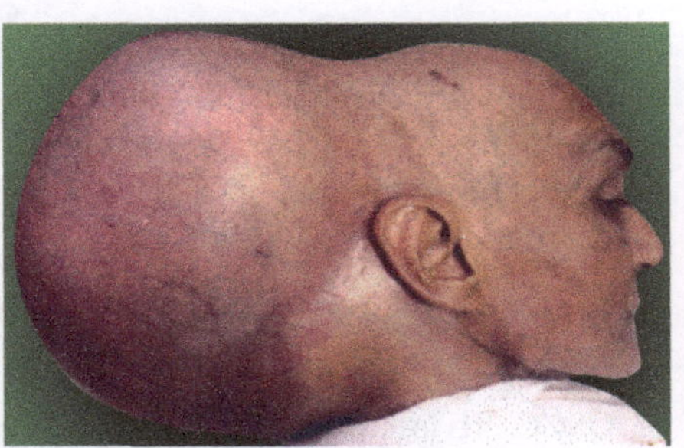

Fig. 30.22: An advanced case of OSCC with secondaries in the brain

- To contribute to the continuing investigation of human cancer.[22]

Staging of OSCC

The staging of the tumor is as shown in Box 30.3.

Clinical Features of the Oral Squamous Cell Carcinoma as per the Site of Involvement

Although the general presentation of the OSCC is common to all the sites, there are site wise clinical features, which are described below.

General Clinical Features

- An ulcerated growth with rolled out edges or an exophytic growth, (cauliflower like) details are given above
- Rapid growth
- Infiltrative nature
- Fixity to underlying and overlying tissues
- Friability
- Tendency to metastasize to cervical lymph nodes
- Metastatic nodes are round, stony hard in consistency and are discrete in the earlier stage, but get fixed to adjacent structures in the advanced disease
- Weight loss, cachexia in the advanced stages.

Box 30.2: TNM classification

T staging for tumors of the lip and oral cavity
- TX: Primary tumor cannot be assessed
- T0: No evidence of primary tumor
- Tis: Carcinoma *in situ*
- T1: Tumor 2 cm or less in greatest dimension
- T2: Tumor >2 cm but not >4 cm in greatest dimension
- T3: Tumor >4 cm in greatest dimension
- T4a: Lip Tumor invades through cortical bone, inferior alveolar nerve, floor of mouth, or skin of face (i.e. chin or nose). Oral tumor invades through cortical bone, into deep [extrinsic]. Cavity muscle of tongue (genioglossus, hyoglossus, palatoglossus, and styloglossus), maxillary sinus, or skin of face
- T4b: Tumor involves masticator space, pterygoid plates, or skull base and/or encases internal carotid artery

N staging for all head and neck sites except the nasopharynx and larynx
- Nx: Regional lymph nodes cannot be assessed
- N0: No regional lymph node metastasis
- N1: Metastasis in a single ipsilateral lymph node, 3 cm or less in greatest dimension
- N2: Metastasis in a single ipsilateral lymph node, >3 cm but not >6 cm in greatest dimension; or in multiple ipsilateral lymph nodes, none >6 cm in greatest dimension; or in bilateral or contralateral lymph nodes, none >6 cm in greatest dimension
- N2a: Metastasis in a single ipsilateral lymph node >3 cm but not >6 cm in greatest dimension
- N2b: Metastasis in multiple ipsilateral lymph nodes, none >6 cm in greatest dimension
- N2c: Metastasis in bilateral or contralateral lymph nodes, none >6 cm in greatest dimension
- N3: Metastasis in a lymph >6 cm in greatest dimension

M staging for head and neck tumors
- Mx: Distant metastasis cannot be assessed
- M0: No distant metastasis
- M1: Distant metastasis

Box 30.3: Staging of oral cancer

Stage 1	T 1	N 0	M 0
Stage 2	T2	N 0	M 0
Stage 3	T 3	N 0	M 0
	T 1/T 2	N 1	M 0
Stage 4	T 4	N 0	M 0
	T 4	N 1	M 0
	Any T	N 2	M 0
	Any T	N 3	M 0
	Any T	N 0	M 1

Site-wise Clinical Features

Site-wise clinical features are shown in Box 30.4.

Diagnosis and Clinical Examination of the Oral Squamous Cell Carcinoma

The diagnosis of the OSCC with advanced stage is straight forward due to its peculiar presentation and common occurrence. The early lesions and the malignant transformations in precancerous lesions or conditions pose great challenge and require clinical skill and expertise. The diagnosis of the OSCC can be arrived at following the steps mentioned below.

Detailed History

In the clinical practice, arriving at a diagnosis is always a sequential process. It requires a methodology. The history taking is an essential step for leading to a proper diagnosis. The relevant findings in the history pertaining to the OSCC are:

- **Age:** Commonly seen in 40 to 60 years of age. However, of late the patients developing the OSCC as early as 20 to 30 years of age, secondary to SMF have been seen.
- **Sex:** More commonly seen in males.
- Signs of malnourishment, iron deficiency, vitamin deficiency.
- **Habits:** Tobacco, betel nut, alcoholism are commonly associated with the OSCC. The duration of the habits, frequency and quantity are also noted. The carcinomas of the tongue have been reported in females without associated habits, but having chronic iron deficiency anemia, perimenopausal age or having sharp

Box 30.4: Site-wise clinical features

Gingivobuccal sulcus	Loosening of the teeth/exfoliation Inability to masticate Involvement of the bone and inferior alveolar nerve producing numbness
Tongue	Commonly involving the venterolateral surface and rarely the dorsum Salivation Hypomobility of tongue Inability to swallow Fixity of the tongue (ankyloglossia), which is poor prognostic sign (Fig. 30.23) Lump in the tongue Bilateral and widespread lymph node metastasis
Floor of mouth	Inability to swallow Involvement of tongue leading to hypomobility Bilateral and widespread lymph node metastasis
Cheek	Inability to chew Fixity to the skin Extraoral fungation
Posterior one third of the tongue	Inability to swallow Fixity of the tongue, lack of protrusion Microaspiration leading to chest infections Spread to adjacent structures like larynx which can lead to change in speech Late detection
Maxillary sinus	Details given in the chapter no. 14
Retromolar trigone	Trismus due to involvement of muscles of mastication Spread to the infratemporal fossa Deep cervical lymph node metastasis Poor prognosis
Primary intraosseous carcinoma	Rare Absence of other primary Irregular, oesteolytic lesion in the bone Mobility of the teeth Involvement of nerve leading to paresthesia Metastatic disease from other sites must be ruled out.

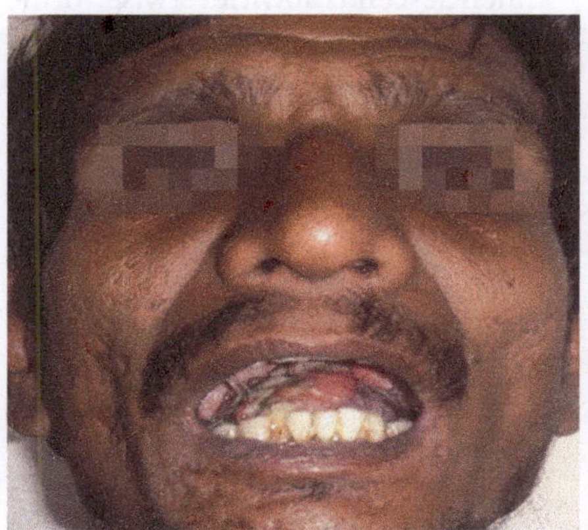

Fig. 30.23: Carcinoma anterior 2/3rd of tongue with ankyloglossia

teeth or over hanging restorations, or chronic TFO.

- Lack of pain and tenderness, unless signs of secondary infection are present.
- **Nature of growth:** Whether it is an ulcerated or exophytic growth. If it is an ulcerated growth it has indurated everted or rolled out edges indurated base, fixity to deeper structures, friability. The exophytic growths are sessile and friable. They are rapidly growing and develop fixity to the underlying structures.
- Short history and rapid growth or long standing precancerous lesion or condition such as leukoplakia, lichen planus or SMF, etc.
- Color and size change in the precancerous lesion.
- Development of *induration* and fixity. The induration is hall mark of malignancy. The elicitation of this sign needs practice. A palpating finger can tell the nature of lesion accurately. Due to the infiltrative nature of the lesion fixity to the adjacent structures develops.
- **Neurological deficit:** When a gingivobuccal growth infiltrates the mandible, the inferior alveolar nerve gets involved leading to paresthesia of the inferior alveolar nerve. This sign is absent in large benign lesions like ameloblastoma, which tend to displace the neurovascular bundle than involving it.
- Signs of involvement of paranasal sinuses like epistaxis and foul smelling discharge.
- Presence of trismus due to involvement of muscles of mastication, especially in the retromolar trigone and maxillary sinus malignancies.
- *Peau d'orange* of the skin and extraoral fungation.
- ***Presence of cervical lymph node metastasis:*** The OSCC are open growths in oral cavity and are liable to get secondarily infected and also tend to metastasize in the regional cervical lymph nodes depending upon their anatomical location. A careful clinical evaluation of the lymph nodes is required.

Assessment of Cervical Lymph Nodes

The OSCC often metastasize to the cervical lymph nodes. The secondaries in the neck, i.e. metastatic disease in the cervical lymph nodes need to be evaluated carefully. If the primary disease is present in the oral cavity and the examination of the neck nodes reveals that the lymph nodes are either not palpable or insignificant, the neck is then labeled as N_0 neck. However, the N_0 neck

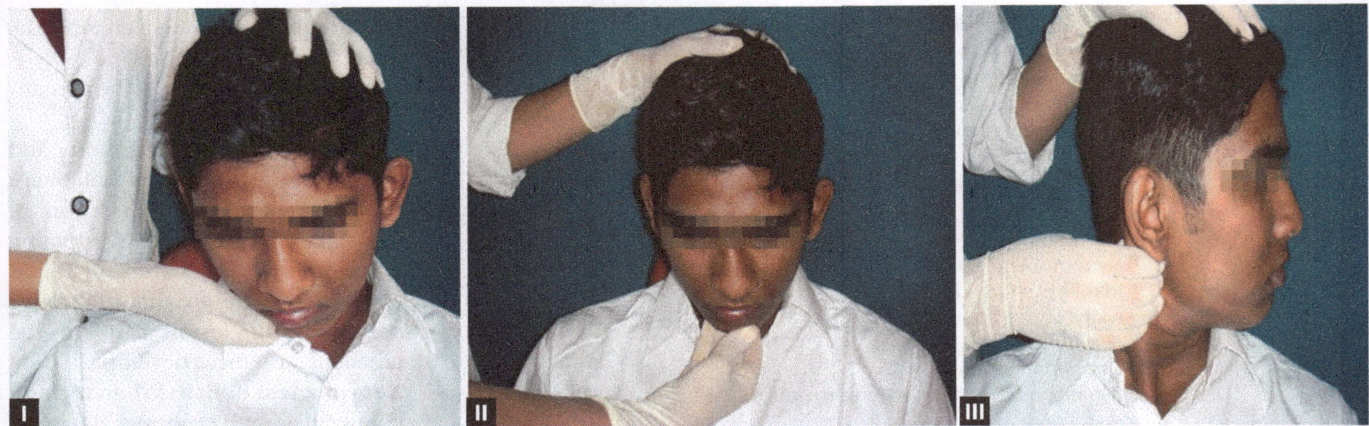

Fig. 30. 24A: Clinical examination of the nodes

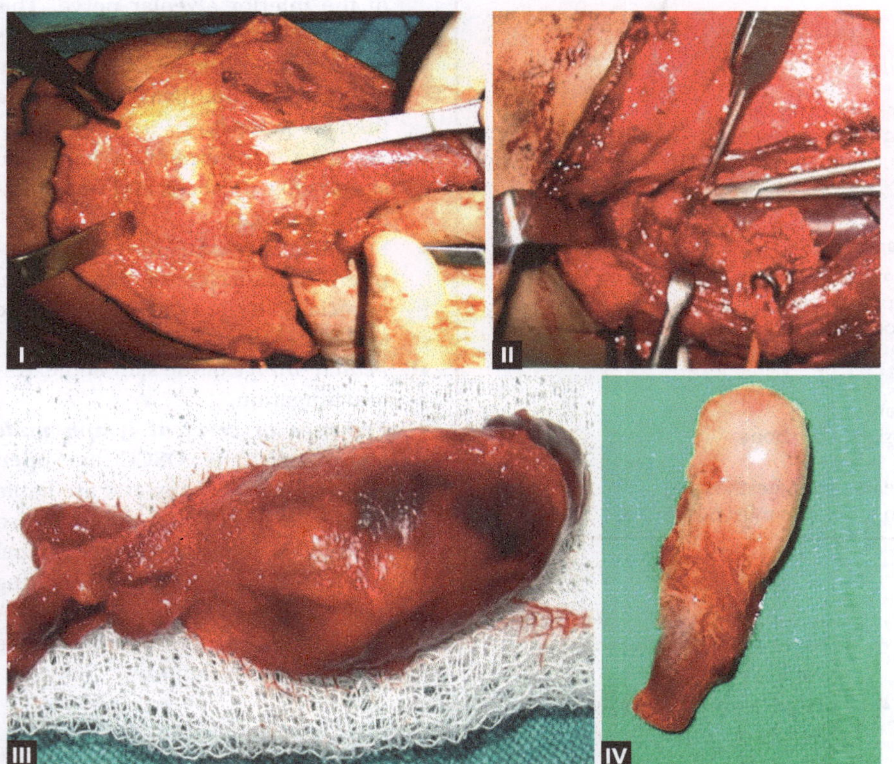

Fig. 30.24B: Intra operative photographs: (I and II) Note the submandibular LN are smaller but rounded and hard in consistency and turned out to be metastatic, while as the upper jugular nodes are larger, soft and oval and were found to be negative for metastasis; (III) Specimen of round, hard lymph node highly suspicious of secondaries; (IV) Oval node mostly inflammatory

does not necessarily mean that the tumor has not metastasized in the neck nodes as micrometastasis cannot be ascertained clinically and in such cases additional evaluation of the neck nodes using other modalities as mentioned below, may be required to ascertain the nodal metastasis. Similarly, some times the metastatic disease may not be present in the group of nodes draining that site, but may be present in the subsequent group of nodes due to skip metastasis. The metastasis in transit implies when the cancer cells are present in the lymphatics and not yet lodged in the recipient lymph node. Thus, the examination of the neck has to be methodical and comprehensive. With the advancement in techniques and technology, the accuracy, sensitivity and specificity has increased significantly, but still the assessment is not cent percent accurate. Thus, in some cases the surgeon has to make a decision of undertaking an elective neck dissection (electing to perform the neck dissection in presence of N_0 neck) or advising the postoperative radiotherapy to take care of occult metastasis or to do a second surgery, if the metastatic nodes are detected during the follow-up.

- **Clinical evaluation:** The neck is flexed to relax the muscles and the lymph nodes are carefully palpated. The palpation starts from level one, i.e. from the submental group and then descends down level wise. All the groups should be palpated, bilaterally and any lymphadenopathy should be noticed along with the characteristics of the nodes. Simultaneous bilateral palpation facilitates the comparison of findings (Fig. 30.24A). The inflammatory nodes are enlarged, soft, oval and tender. The metastatic nodes are often round, stony hard, initially discrete, but subsequently become adherent (Fig. 30.24B). The tubercular lymph nodes are often matted.

  The findings that are required to be noted on the clinical examination are:
  - Site/level
  - Size

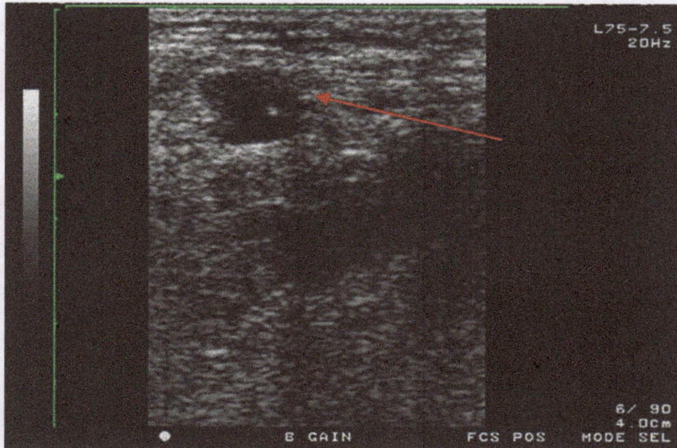

Fig. 30.25: USG of malignant lymph node

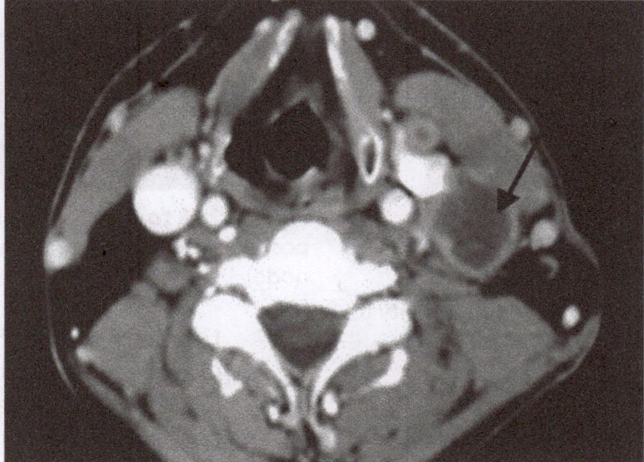
Fig. 30.26: Axial computerized tomography (CT) scan showing central necrosis within a left cervical lymph node metastasis contrast enhanced axial CT image showing enlarged jugulodigastric lymph node

- Shape
- Extent
- Number
- Consistency
- Fixity
- Tenderness
- Matting.

- **Ultrasonography**[23,24]**:** It is an effective method for evaluation of the deep cervical nodes, lying below the sternocleidomastoid muscle (Fig. 30.25). The USG criteria for iden tifying the metastatic node are:
  - Size—more than 1 cm
  - Shape—round
  - Number
  - Echogenicity—hypoechogenic
  - Intactness of phylum—it is distorted
  - Central necrosis—present in advanced disease
  - Perinodal infilteration (extracapsular spread)
  - Fixity to vessels.
- **Fine needle aspiration cytology**[25] **(FNAC):** The lymph nodes which are 1 cm plus in size and have clinical or USG features suspicious of metastasis are further evaluated by FNAC. The cytology may not be always be confirmatory and accurate, but is effective in most cases to determine type of the neck dissection required in a particular case. The FNAC could be USG guided or CT guided to enhance its sensitivity and accuracy.
- Computed tomogram scan[26] (CT) and magnetic resonance imaging[27,28] (MRI) (Figs 30.26 and 30.27).

  These are more effective not only in determining the extent of primary, but also in assessing the deep cervical nodes than the UGC. The MRI scans are particularly more useful in the assessment of the carcinomas of the tongue (Figs 30.28A to C).
- **Sentinel node biopsy (SNB):** It is the first euchlion lymph node that is most likely to drain a part. If this lymph node is biopsied there are optimum chances of detecting the nodal metastasis. The first successful SNB in a head and neck SCC was performed, in 1996, by Alex[29] and Krag on a patient with a laryngeal supraglottic carcinoma.

  Rationale:
  - Cervical metastasis is the single most important prognostic factor in patients with oral cancer, with the presence of nodal spread decreasing the 5-year disease-free survival rate by approximately 50 percent.
  - SNB is a staging tool.
  - Improved the accuracy of staging, while reducing the morbidity caused by unnecessary lymphadenectomy in melanomas and breast cancers.

  Preoperative technique: Lymphoscintigraphy (SPECT) and gamma probe-guided localization have emerged as useful techniques for identification of the sentimental lymph node (SLN). Lymphoscintigraphy[30] is typically performed in the nuclear medicine suite. A radiotracer is injected at several sites around the tumor and gamma camera images depict the laterality and approximate anatomic location of the SLN(s).

  The nuclear medicine physician marks the area(s) that corresponds to the SLN(s) on the patient's skin. In the operating room, the surgeon uses a gamma probe transcutaneously to confirm the location of the SLN(s). Next, blue dye is injected intradermally and the SLN exposed.[31]

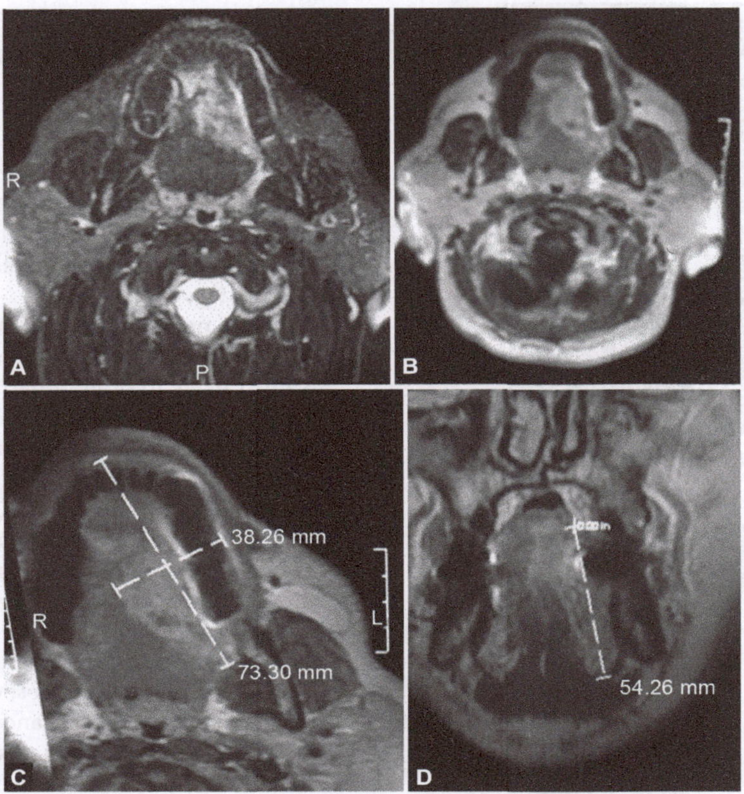

Figs 30.27A to D: MRI of the tongue for the carcinoma of tongue is a good modality to see tumor infiltration in the tongue

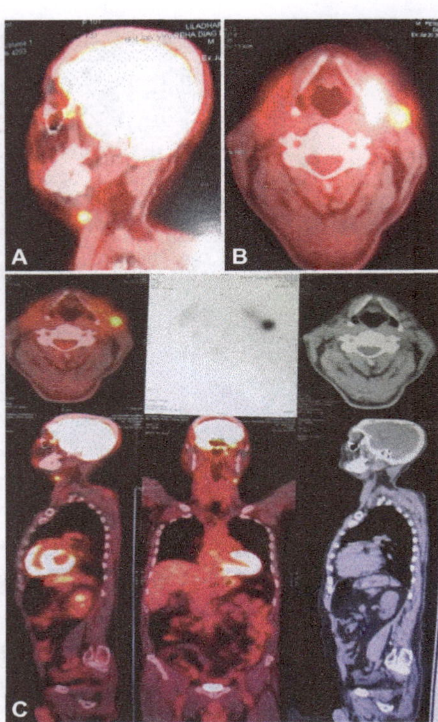

Figs 30.28A to C: PET scan of neck showing positive node (the yellow node is postive node)

SLNs are identified by the presence of blue staining and/or radiotracer uptake, as detected by the gamma probe. Concurrent use of blue dye and radiotracer is currently recommended; in view of the fact that many studies suggest that the SLNs are not always blue, or always radioactive.

Having two methods to identify the SLN intraoperatively increase the identification rate and probably account for the sensitivity and specificity reported in recent studies. The SLNs are removed and sent to the pathologist for histologic and immunohistochemical analysis. Therapeutic node dissection is performed only in patients whose SLN is positive.

Silent features:

- Sentinel nodes found in more than 90 percent of cases.[32]
  - 56 percent success in SLNB (*data in relation to breast cancer)
  - In June 2001, the conclusions of the 1st International Conference on SNB of head and neck SCC, held in Glasgow, underlined that results were significantly better in those centers that performed more than 10 cases a year: overall sentinel node identification was 98 percent, and sensitivity of the procedure was 90 percent.[33] Reliability of SNB was confirmed 2 years later, at the 2nd International Conference held in Zurich. Pooled data on 397 cN0 head and neck patients from 20 centers have been presented: the identification rate was 97 percent (range 90–100%), with a 96 percent (range 88–100%) negative predictive value of a negative sentinel node for the remainder of the neck using both preoperative lymphoscintigraphy and intraoperative hand-held gamma probe.[32]
  - Lymphoscintigraphy revealed unexpected bilateral or contralateral disease in about 14 percent of patients.[34]
  - Up to 46 percent of SLN harbor metastases (data for breast cancer metastasis)
    - i Fine section frozen analysis increases sensitivity to about 95 percent
    - ii. Immunohistochemical staining.
  - False negative rate is roughly 10 percent and the grossly involved nodes less likely to take up tracer.
  - Better sensitivity for T1/T2 lesions: Most false negative results associated with larger T3 lesions.
- **Positron emission tomography (PET) scan:** The positron emission tomography with flurodeoxyglucose is functional imaging modality that used abnormal tissue metabolism to detect neoplasms and metastatic node. The radioactive glucose analogue FDG is metabolized in normal tissue and neoplastic tissues in

proportion to the rate of tissue glucose metabolism. FDG is metabolically trapped in the intracellular space, this occurs more in the tumors than in normal tissues and can be used to identify tumors based on accelerated glycolytic rates (hypermetabolic lesions) using PET (Figs 30.28A to C).

- **Radiographic examination:** The malignant lesions produce typical radiological appearance on X-ray, the irregular, mouth-eaten radiolucency. The destruction of the periodonitium leads to a typical floating teeth appearance (Figs 30.29A and B).
- **Biopsy:** The biopsy still remains the gold standard in the final diagnosis of the OSCC. The oral cavity tumors are readily accessible and the biopsy is easy to obtain. It is economical and most importantly confirmatory. The types of the biopsy are:
  1. Punch biopsy
  2. Incisional biopsy
  3. Excisional biopsy
  4. Fine needle aspiration cytology/biopsy (FNAC/FNAB).

The incisional biopsy is obtained from the lesion, mostly under local anesthesia as an out door procedure. The guidelines for the biopsy are:

- As far as possible take a piece of 1 cm × 1 cm × 1 cm, as the wide representation of the tumor is available and the depth of the biopsy should also be adequate for ascertaining the depth of penetration of the tumor.
- The biopsy should be taken from the periphery of the lesion and certain amount of normal tissue should also be included for the comparative purposes. The lesion grows at the periphery and has optimum mitotic activity and is more representative rather than the center, where the exfoliated, necrotic cells are present.
- The representative area is one where the optimum induration is present and it should be biopsied. Hence, out of the edge of the ulcer, the area which is more indurated should be included in the biopsy.
- The biopsy specimen should be fixed in 10 percent formaldehyde solution for transporting in the laboratory for further processing.

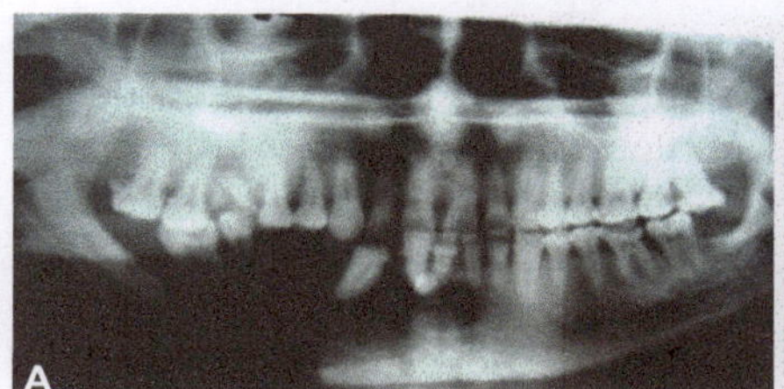

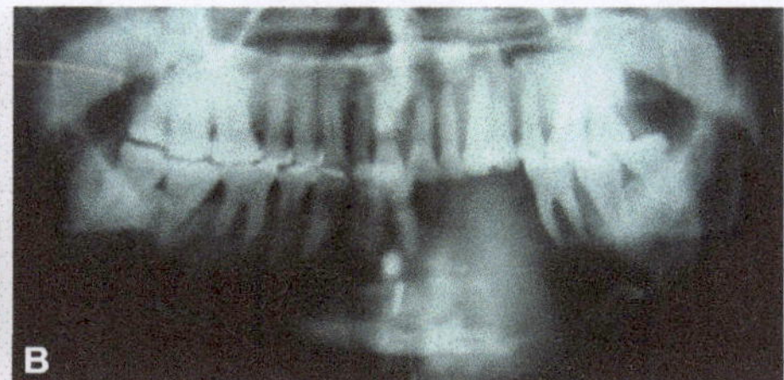

Figs 30.29A and B: Mouth eaten, irregular radioluscency with floating teeth and pathological fracture

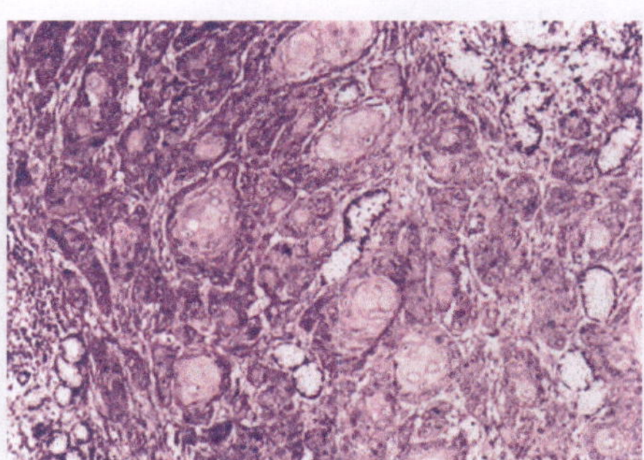

Fig. 30.30: Well differentiated SCC

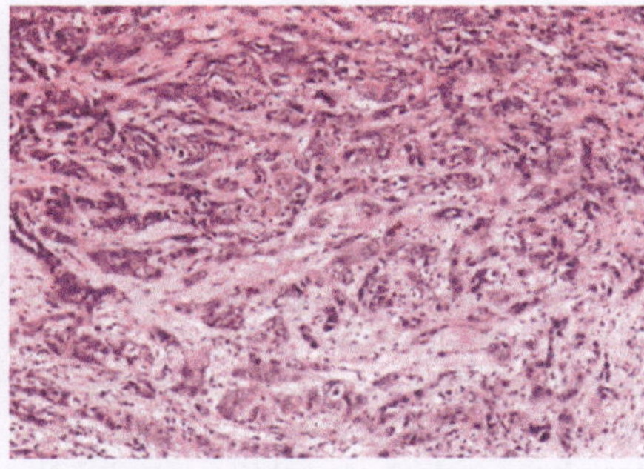

Fig. 30.31: Moderately differentiated SCC

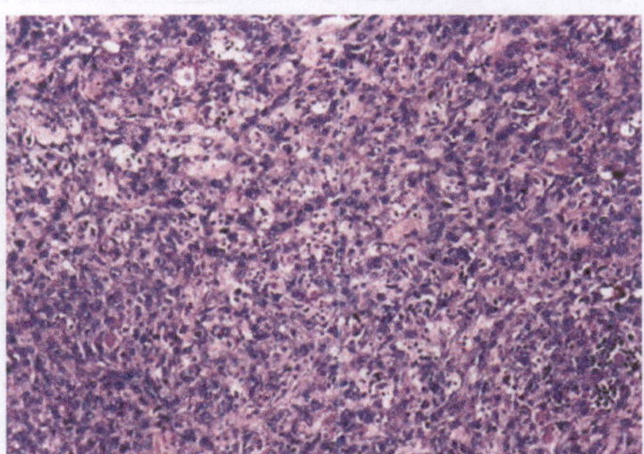

Fig. 30.32: Poorly differentiated SCC

Histopathological Grading of OSCC and its Clinical Relevance

The histopathological diagnosis alone is not adequate in the management of the OSCC, but the histopathological grading of the lesion is important to know its biological behavior. Generally the well differentiated squamous cell carcinomas are less aggressive than the poorly differentiated and highly anaplastic growths.[35]

The histopathological grading of OSCC can be done as:

- Well differentiated (Fig. 30.30)
- Moderately differentiated (Fig. 30.31)
- Poorly differentiated, based on the degree of differentiation of the cells (Fig. 30.32).

Apart from the degree of *differentiation,* the depth of involvement or the bulk of the tumor is also important. As the depth increases beyond 2 mm in the connective tissue, the chances of the regional lymph node metastasis are enhanced and the lymph node metastasis compromises the prognosis.

General Examination

Although OSCC originates in the oral cavity, it has systemic ramifications as it tends to spread to regional lymph nodes and occasionally to the distant sites by hematogenous metastasis. Thus, the clinical examination is necessary to detect the distant metastasis. The examination of the chest and X-ray of the chest is required to rule out pulmonary metastasis. The clinical examination of the abdominal viscera to rule out organomegaly and in suspected cases USG or CT scan may be useful. The biochemical assessment like renal function test or liver function test could be of value. The neurological examination to detect any neurological deficit is done in cases suspected to have cerebral metastasis followed by a CT scan or MRI.

MANAGEMENT OF OSCC

The modalities for the management of oral squamous cell carcinoma are:

- Surgery
- Radiation therapy
- Chemotherapy
- Combination of above.

Surgery

The surgery is still the most preferred primary treatment modality of all resectable cancers. The wide surgical excision of the growth along with the 2 cm margins of normal tissue all around is recommended for adequate surgical clearance. The surgical clearance has to be three dimensional, i.e. apart from periphery adequate clearance in the depth should also be achieved. The tumor excision not only removes the primary, but also abolishes the chances of further spread and metastasis. Surgical management of the cancer not only revolves around the excision of the primary, but a comprehensive surgical management comprising of excising the metastatic lymph nodes with block dissection and reconstruction of the defect.

The purpose of the cancer surgery is not only to eradicate the disease, but also to ensure the quality of life postoperatively. The surgery is intended to establish the locoregional control and the term *cure* may not be always applicable. The locoregional control is better in the early malignancies, i.e. the stage I and stage II rather than the advanced malignancies with wide spread regional lymph node metastasis. The presence of regional lymph node metastasis itself is taken as a sign of guarded or poor prognosis. Rather than the term 'cure' the disease free period or locoregional control with minimum 5 years life expectancy is realistic.

Management of Primary

The primary growth is treated surgically by wide local excision keeping ideally 2 cm margins—into the normal tissue all around (Figs 30.33 and 30.34). The frozen sections are of immense value in determining adequacy of the surgical resection. The malignancies involving the mandibular bone are also treated with a segmental resection of the involved segment keeping two centimeter margins as the tumor can extend beyond the radiological margins through the cancellous bone. The cortical bone offers more resistance to the tumor spread than the cancellous bone and hence in selected, early cases the wedge madibulectomy could be adequate and avoid morbidity in the patients (Figs 30.35A and B). The growths involving the anterior region and the body of the mandible can be treated with segmental mandibulectomy with adequate soft tissue clearance (Fig. 30.36). The malignancies involving the retromolar area

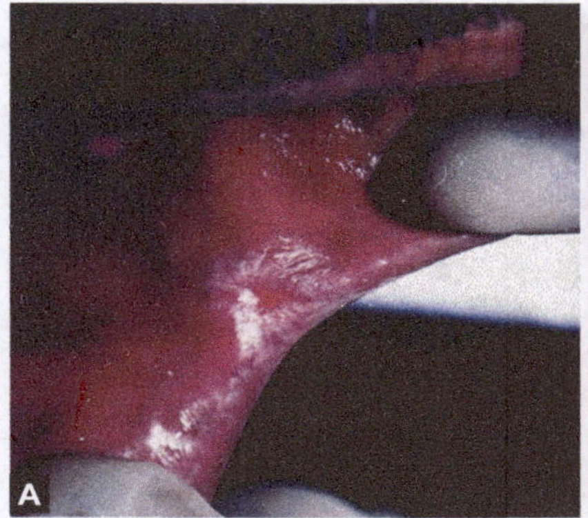

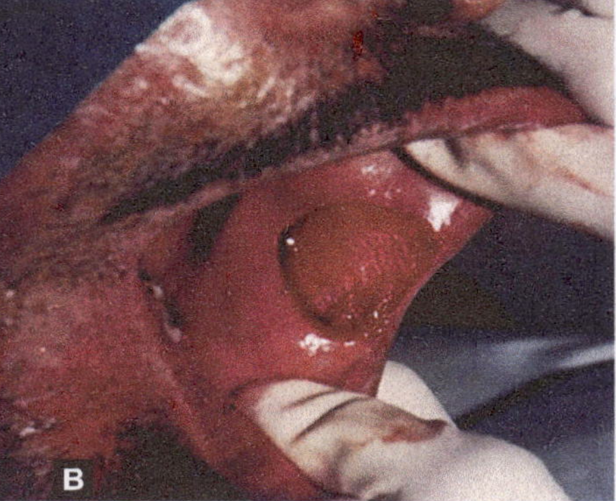

Figs 30.33A and B: Wide local excision of a very early (T1) growth

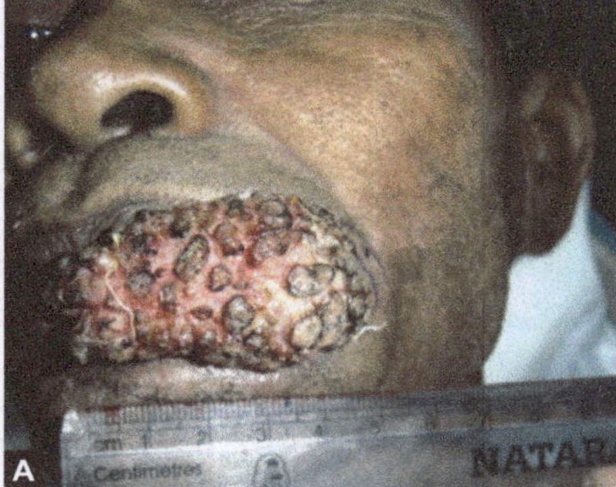

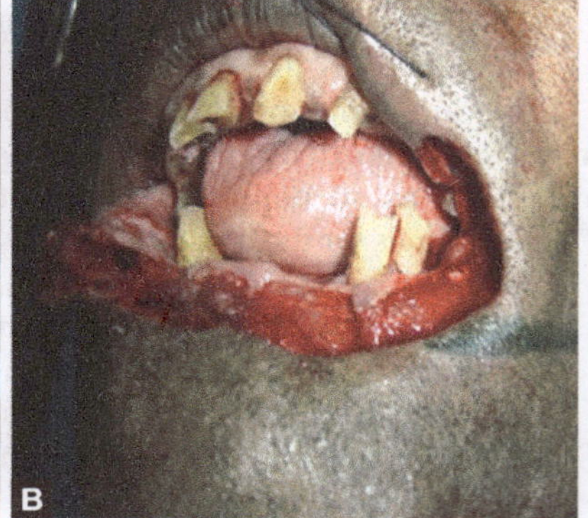

Figs 30.34A and B: (A) Preoperative photograph of a case of verrucous carcinoma of lower lip; (B) Wide local excision

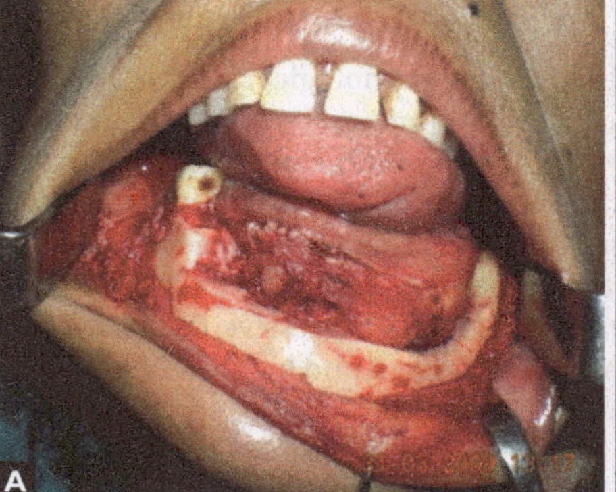

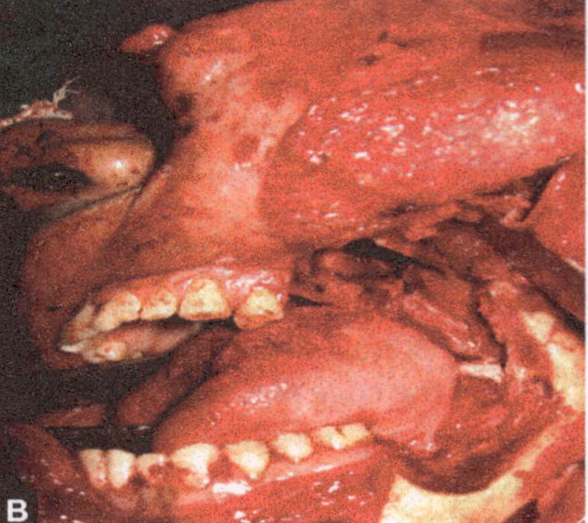

Figs 30.35A and B: Wedge mandibulectomy

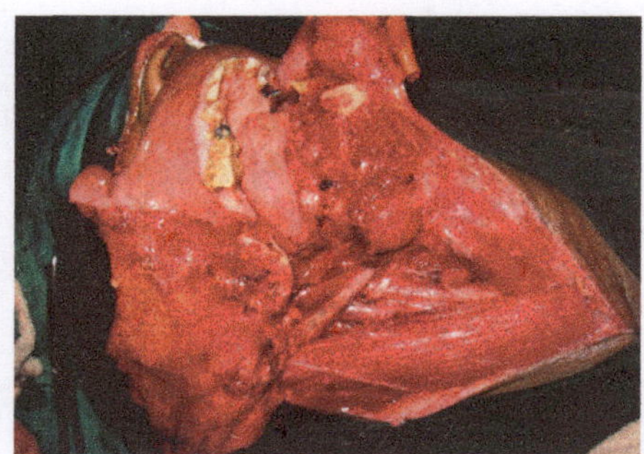

Fig. 30.36: Segmental mandibulectomy

are treated by resecting the mandible along with disarticulation of the condyle. The condylar stump preservation could be helpful in reconstruction for fixing the screws for a reconstruction plate; however, it should not be at the cost of adequate surgical clearance. '*There is no scope of conservative surgery, while treating the malignancy*' and '*the first chance is the best chance for the surgical resection*'. The recurrence will always be unplanned and the salvage surgery may not be possible. A thorough presurgical evaluation of the case to ascertain the resectability is mandatory. It is desirable to have the facilities of frozen section biopsy to determine adequate surgical margins of the ressected tumor. While obtaining the specimen for the frozen section, it should be taken from edge of the surgical defect rather than the specimen to ascertain that what is left *in situ* is disease free.

Those growths where the doubts pertaining to safe surgical margins exist preoperatively are relatively unresectable. In such cases, the surgery is not free of risk of early recurrence and have guarded prognosis. They may require postoperative chemoradiations. The preoperative chemotherapy or radiotherapy certainly reduces the tumor bulk, but their ability to shrink the surgical margins is doubtful and hence the surgical margins do not shrink is the dictum. Hence, the surgery could serve only debulking purpose and residual tumor mass can be managed with chemoradiation as a palliative resort. The debulking surgeries tend to recur fast, but serve the purpose of reducing tumor load for subsequent therapy. In cases of extraoral fungation, gross unhygienic conditions due to secondary infection, the debulking of the tumor is indicated.

If the excision of the primary tumor is planned with the neck dissection as is the case in majority of the patients, it is desirable to excise the neck block along with the primary enblock (i.e. in continuity) to ensure that all the intervening lymphatic channels are removed, so that any metastasis in transit is not left behind.

Regional Lymph Node Metastasis Management

The OSCC metastasize to the cervical lymph nodes. The incidence of nodal metastasis also depends upon the site of tumor, the nature of the tumor, the histopathological grading of the tumor and the clinical stage of the tumor.

Site

The tumors of the floor of mouth tend to metastasize early and bilaterally due to rich lymphatic supply and crisscrossing of the contralateral lymphatics. The tongue is also lymphatic rich organ and wide spread cervical lymph node metastasis is commonly seen upto deep cervical nodes and level IV and V also. The tumors in midline tend to metastasize bilaterally and the tumors of the retromolar region also metastasize to the lymph nodes of deep cervical chain. The incidence of lymph node metastasis amongst the cases of OSCC in relation to the site of the primary as depicted in the table given below (Table 30.1).

Table 30.1: Co-relation between site of primary tumor and percentage of cases having nodal metastasis

Site of primary	Percentage of cases having nodal metastasis
Lip	12%
Floor of mouth	72%
Buccal mucosa	32%
Gingivobuccal sulcus buccal vestibule	43%
Gingivobuccal sulcus linual vestibule	67%
Tongue	71%
Maxillary sinus	8%
Retromolar area	63%

Clinical Stage

The stage III and IV tumors have more incidence of cervical lymph node metastasis as compared to the stage I and II tumors as observed in a study carried out at our center (Box 30.5).

Box 30.5: Incidence of lymph node metastasis as per the clinical stage of OSCC (statistics at SPDC, Wardha, India)

Stage	Percentage
Stage I	2%
Stage II	2%
Stage III	13%
Stage IV	83%

Clinical Presentation

The ulcerative growths tend to metastasize to the neck nodes faster than the exophytic growths due to their deeper invasion. The tumor bulk also plays a major role in the nodal metastasis. The more the bulk of the tumor, the more are the chances of the lymph node metastasis (Table 30.2).

Histopathological Grading

The poorly differentiated lesions are highly anaplastic and tend to have more incidence of nodal metastasis than the well differentiated growths (Box 30.6).

The surgery for excising the cervical lymph nodes is termed as the neck dissection or cervical block dissection as the entire block of the fibrofatty tissue along with the lymph nodes is excised in continuity. The concept of block dissection was introduced by Sir George Crile[36] who demonstrated classical radical neck dissection under local anesthesia (LA) for a case of oral cancer in 1906. However, the history of cervical lymphadenectomy prevailed from the year 1839 when Warren,[37] removal of submandibular lymph node in a case of

Table 30.2: Incidence of lymph node metastasis as per the clinical presentation of OSCC (statistics at SPDC, Wardha, India)

Lesion	No of cases/100	Node positive	Percentage
Ulcer	82/100	31	37.80%
Exophytic growth	18/100	5	27.78%
Total	100	36	36%

Box 30.6: Incidence of L N metastasis according to grade of biopsy (statistics at SPDC, Wardha, India)

Incidence of L N metastasis according to grade of biopsy	
Well differentiated SCC	18%
Moderately differentiated SCC	53%
Poorly differentiated SCC	100%

carcinoma of the tongue. M von Chelius,[38] 1847 gave the first systematic description of cervical lymph nodes in HNF cancers. Subsequent to demonstration of the classical neck dissection by George Crile, many authors did research in the field of neck dissection and the technique, understanding and practices evolved. Hayes Martin,[39] 1951 considered the prophylactic neck dissection to be illogical in the cases of HNF cancers, whereas Bocca and Pignataro,[40] 1967 introduced a concept of '*functional neck dissection*' to avoid morbidity secondary to neck dissection. Initially the concept of 'commando *operation*' was very popular in which the primary and neck node block were excised in continuity without much emphasis on the postoperative morbidity and quality of life. But, with the better understanding of neck node levels and their involvement, the biological behavior of the cancer it was felt that the neck dissection can be selective and functional without compromising the outcome. The structures like sternomastoid muscle, internal jugular vein (IJV) and spinal accessory nerve are excised in a classical radical neck dissection are now preserved, unless their excision is indicated as they may be involved in the disease or come in the way of adequate surgical clearance. The excision of the sternomastoid muscle leads to neck morbidity, while the excision/sacrifice of the spinal accessory nerve lead to shoulder dysfunction, which is ill afforded by the patients, especially in the subcontinent who are poor and do physical labor to earn their livelihood. The excision of the IJV leads to facial edema and raised intracranial pressure especially in bilateral neck dissections as it is one of the major veins draining the cranial cavity and the face, it is more pronounced as the other draining channels, i.e. the lymphatics are also excised.

The types of the neck dissections that are commonly undertaken are:

- **Suprahyoid neck dissection:** It is the excision of the lymph node groups, which are present above the hyoid bone, i.e. the level I and IIA nodes along with the submandibular salivary gland. It is often considered to be inadequate and the supra omohyoid neck dissection is more preferred.
- **Selective neck dissection:** When one or more lymphoid groups are preserved. The examples are:
  - Supraomohyoid neck dissection
  - Lateral neck dissection
  - Postereolateral neck dissection
  - Anterior neck dissection.
- **Radical neck dissection:** Excision of fibrofatty tissue along with level I to V lymph nodes along with the SCM, IJV and spinal accessory nerve (Fig. 30.37).
- **Modified radical neck dissection:** One or more of the above mentioned structures are preserved, while doing clearance from level I to level V nodes.
  - **Modification I:** Selectively preserves only spinal accessory nerve (Fig. 30.38).
  - **Modification II:** Selectively preserves IJV and spinal accessory nerve (Figs 30.39A and B).
  - **Modification III:** Selectively preserves SCM, IJV and spinal accessory nerve (Fig. 30.40).

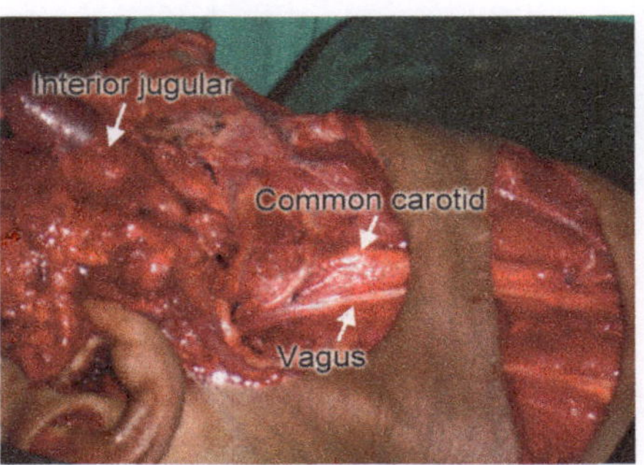

Fig. 30.37: Radical neck dissection (RND) the SCM, IJV and spinal accessory are sacrificed

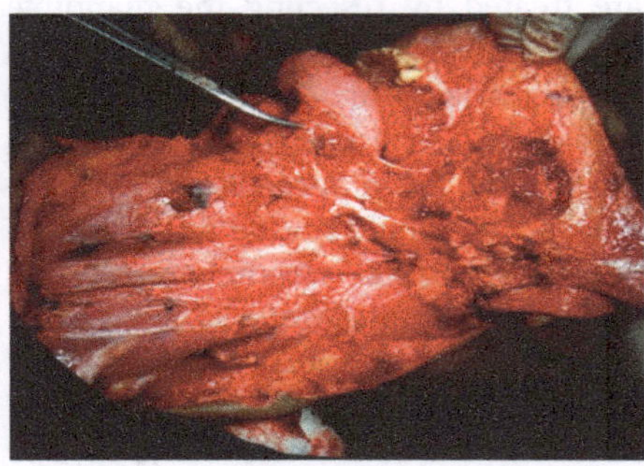
Fig. 30.38: Modified radical neck dissection, type I (MRND-I) preserving the spinal accessory nerve

Extended neck dissection: When the procedure removes other lymph node groups or non-lymphoid structures different from those removed in the radical neck dissection.

The neck dissections can be further categorized as

- **Therapeutic:** When the positive nodes exist and are excised.
- **Elective or prophylactic:** In the N_0 neck the surgeon elects to perform the prophylactic neck dissection (for carcinoma of tongue, floor of mouth, retromolar trigone or where the patient compliance is poor and he/she is unlikely to come for follow-up as seen in Indian conditions, which is due to illiteracy, poverty and ignorance).

Incisions for the Neck Dissection

Various incisions for the neck dissection have been described in the literature.

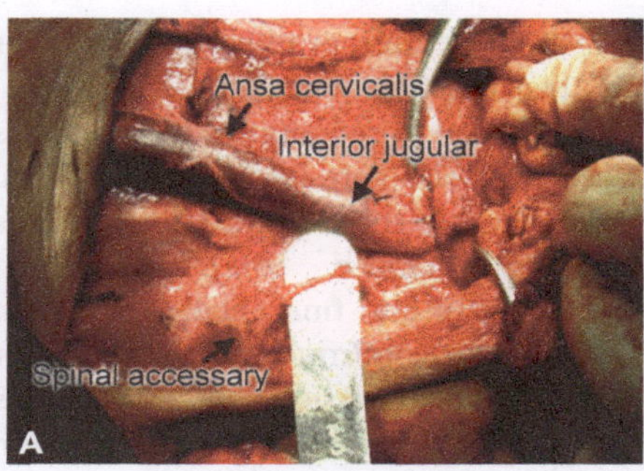

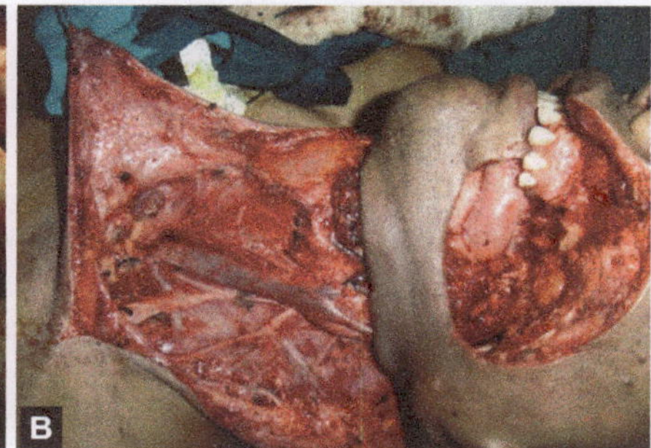

Fig. 30.39: MRND-II, preserving the IJV and spinal accessory nerve

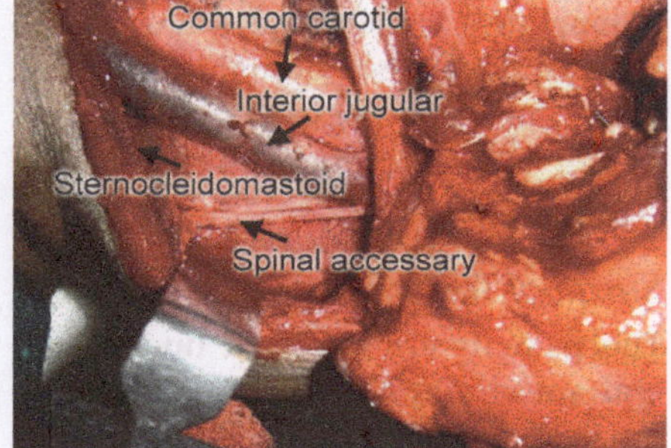

Fig. 30.40: MRND-III, preserving the SCM, IJV and the spinal accessory nerve

The ideal requirements of an incision are:

- It should provide good, liberal access to the deeper structures of neck.
- The flaps should have good vascularity to avoid ischemic necrosis.
- As far as possible the triangular edges in the flaps should be avoided as they are liable to undergo ischemic necrosis. Similarly, the sharp edges and curves should be avoided. (*Nature does not like sharp edges and curves, if you make them sharp nature makes them round by inducing ischemic necrosis at the edges*).
- The vertical legs in the incision should be avoided as they produce unsightly scars and contractures, which produce neck morbidity.
- The triangular edges of the incision lines should not fall on the major vessels as dehiscence can lead to major vessel exposure (Figs 30.41 and 30.42).

The other incisions taken for neck dissection are Schobinger's incision (Fig. 30.43), modified Conley's incision (Fig. 30.44), Hay-Martin's double 'Y' incision (Fig. 30.42) and McFee's incision (Fig. 30.45) which are taken when the dissection is to be carried out upto level IV and V. The McFee's ladder incision produces very good cosmetic results and the chances of marginal necrosis are also very less as the incision falls in skin creases and there are no

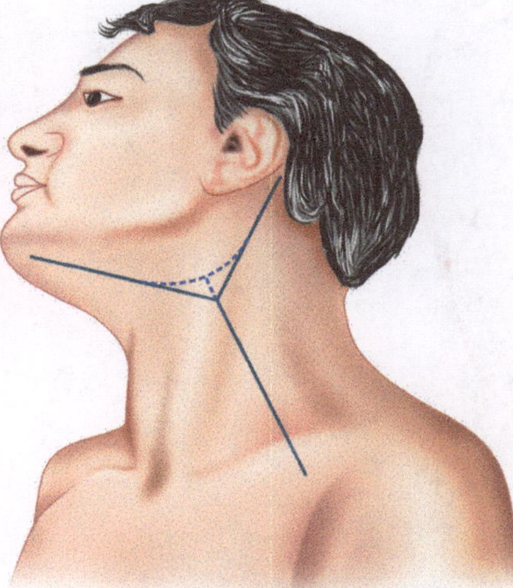

Fig. 30.41: Crile's 'Y' incision

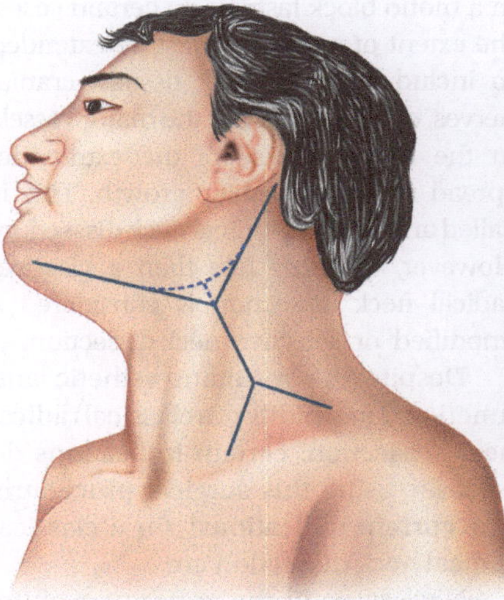

Fig. 30.42: Hay-Martin's double 'Y' incision

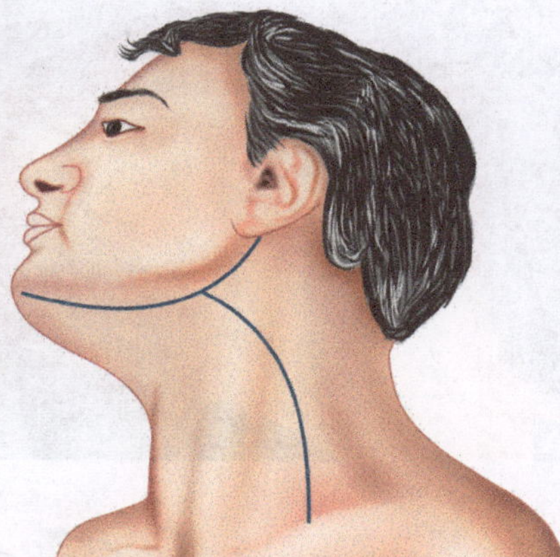

Fig. 30.43: Schobinger's incision

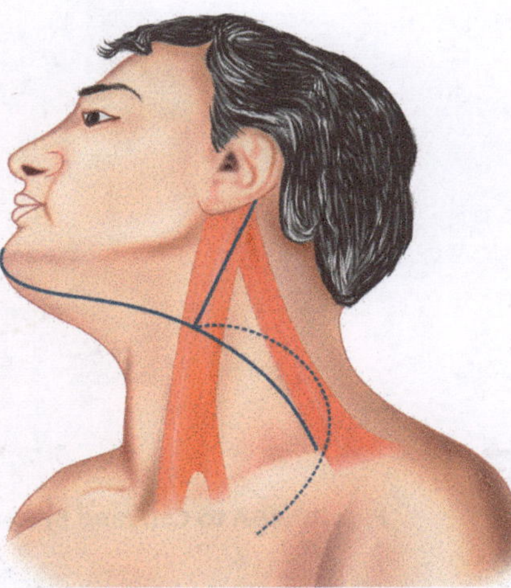

Fig. 30.44: Modified Conley's incision

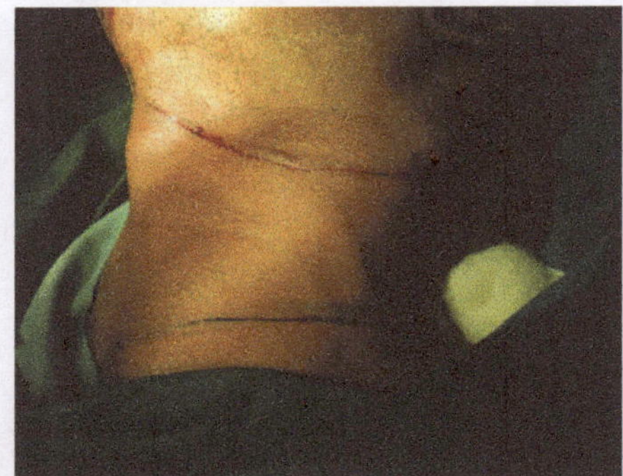

Fig. 30.45: McFee's incision

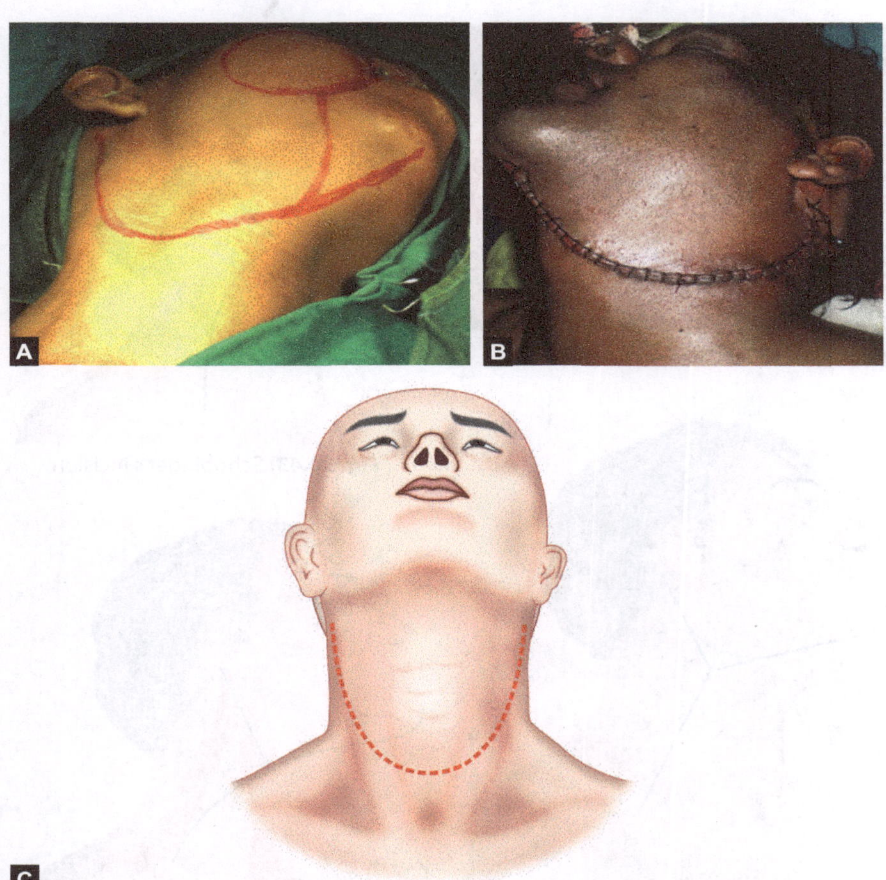

Figs 30.46A to C: (A and B) Apron for unilateral; (C) Bilateral SOHD

triangular areas. However, the neck dissection through this incision demands greater skills. The apron incision is good for the Supraomohyoid neck dissection (dissection upto level III) and produces good cosmetic results and has negligible chances of marginal necrosis (Figs 30.46 A to C).

Radical Neck Dissection

Radical neck dissection is a technique of monoblock removal of regional cervical lymph nodes from the lateral neck for malignant tumors involving the upper aerodigestive tract. This technique was first described by Sir George Crile in 1906. The classical radical neck dissection includes excision of cervical lymph nodes at all the five levels of the lateral neck. This entails clearance of essentially all of the fibrofatty and lymphatic tissue in the lateral neck, as well as resection of the spinal accessory nerve, the sternocleidomastoid muscle, the internal jugular vein and the submandibular salivary gland in a mono block fashion. In certain cases, the extent of resection must be extended to include adjacent soft tissues, cranial nerves, overlying skin, or the major vessels in the neck because of the extranodal spread of the metastatic growth. This is called an extended radical neck dissection. However, anything less than a classical radical neck dissection is considered a 'modified' or 'selective' neck dissection.

Despite the resultant esthetic and functional morbidity of a classical radical neck dissection, certain indications do exist for using this surgical procedure. The current indications[41] for a classical radical neck dissection are:

- N3 disease in the upper part of the neck.
- Gross invasion of the spinal accessory nerve by metastatic lymph nodes at level II in the neck.
- Recurrent or persistent metastatic carcinoma after previous radiation therapy, chemoradiation therapy, or previous selective neck dissection.

Relevant preoperative evaluations are essential before performing classical radical neck dissection. This includes contrast-enhanced computed tomography scan and fine needle aspiration cytology for confirmation of tissue diagnosis. Frank invasion or encasements of the internal carotid artery or invasion of the deep prevertebral musculature by metastatic cancer are contraindications to radical neck dissection. Thus, preoperative radiological evaluation to assess these areas is desirable; however, often the extent of such involvement is only apparent during intraoperative exploration.

Surgical Technique

The patients are operated under General anesthesia through suitable endotracheal intubation with adequate muscle relaxation. The patient typically is in the supine position, and neck is hyperextended by placing sand bag under the shoulder to make the structures prominent. The head is turned to the opposite side. The head and chest are elevated to 30° to prevent excessive blood loss. Hypotensive anesthesia is preferable to avoid blood loss (Fig. 30.47). Although the skin incision is influenced by the planned resection of the primary tumor and subsequent reconstruction, adequate exposure and preservation of cutaneous vascular supply must be ensured. Most commonly, a single trifurcate incision is used, extending

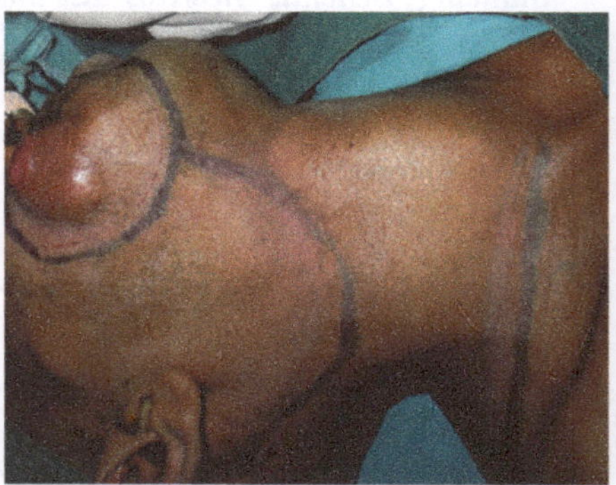

Fig. 30.47: The extension of the neck by providing a sand bag below the shoulder for performing the neck dissection

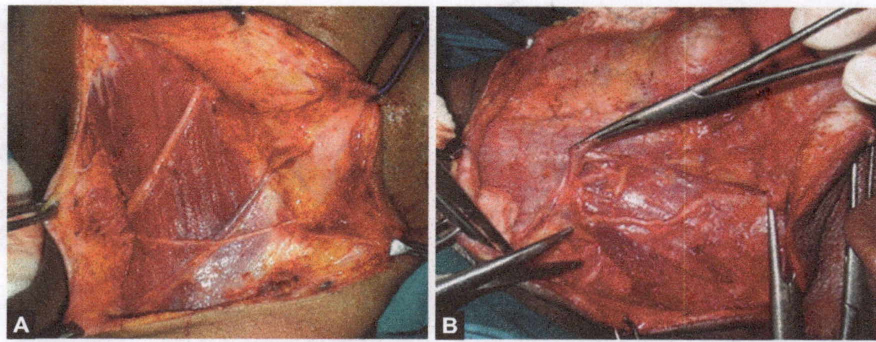

Figs 30.48A and B: (A) Sub platysmal dissection exposing SCM, EJV and greater auricular nerve; (B) Identification of spinal accessory nerve using greater auricular N as a guide. The spinal accessory N lies deep to SCM and within 1 cm superior to the greater auricular nerve

from the ipsilateral mastoid tip along an upper neck skin crease up to the midline at the level of the thyrohyoid membrane, approximately two fingers breadths below the mandible.

The descending limb of the incision begins at the posterior border of the ipsilateral sternocleidomastoid muscle and travels in a curvilinear fashion to the midclavicular point. The skin incision is made with a scalpel and the dissection proceeds thereafter with electrocautery. At the beginning of the procedure, only the posterior half of the transverse incision and the descending limb are incised; the remaining incision is made after the posterior triangle dissection has been completed.

Posterior Triangle Dissection

The posterior skin flap is elevated initially, in the subplatysmal plane, up to the anterior border of the trapezius muscle, which should be exposed from the mastoid to the clavicle and represents the posterior limit of dissection. If the platysma is invaded by metastasis, it is resected and dissection therefore proceeds superficial to the platysma in a subcutaneous plane (Figs 30.48A and B). Countertraction is applied and the soft tissue is divided from the anterior border of the trapezius muscle and elevated off of the floor of the posterior triangle of the neck, with sequential exposure of the splenius capitis, levator scapulae and scalene muscles. During this dissection the peripheral cutaneous branches of the cervical plexus and the spinal accessory nerve are divided. The external jugular vein which is superficial in location and runs superior-inferiorly, and gently curls posteriorly, is also divided between the two clamps and ligated. The transverse cervical artery and vein are identified, divided between clamps and ligated inferiorly. Care is taken to identify the brachial plexus between the middle and anterior scalene muscles, and the phrenic nerve on the surface of the anterior scalene muscle. The thin fascia covering the scalenious table may be preserved as it ensures preservation of these important structures. The identification of the phrenic nerve is made due to its unique anatomical feature that it is the only nerve in the neck which runs from the lateral to the medial direction (Figs 30.49A and 30.50).

This is facilitated by division of the inferior belly of the omohyoid and its retraction medially. Cutaneous cervical nerve branches are identified coming off of the cervical roots as dissection proceeds cephalad. (Erb's point) (Figs 30.49A and B). The cutaneous branches are divided, carefully preserving the motor branches to the posterior compartment muscles and the phrenic nerve (Fig. 30.51). The cutaneous roots are legated along with their accompanying small blood vessels (veina commitance). The superior attachment of the sternocleidomastoid muscle to the mastoid tip is divided and the specimen is allowed to rest *in situ*.

Anterior Triangle Dissection

The remaining transverse skin incision is then completed and attention is turned anteriorly. The anterior flap is elevated in the subplatysmal plane

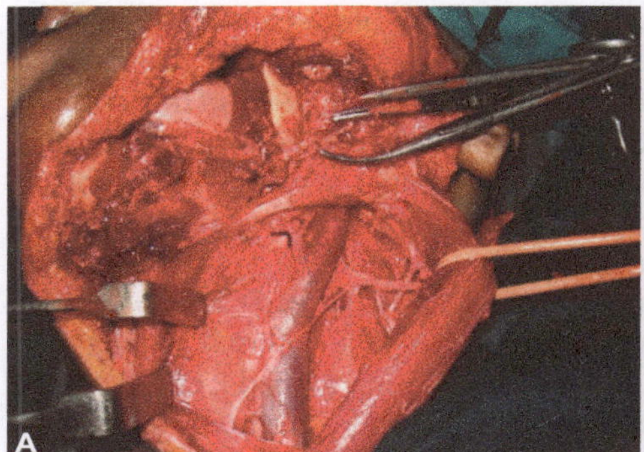

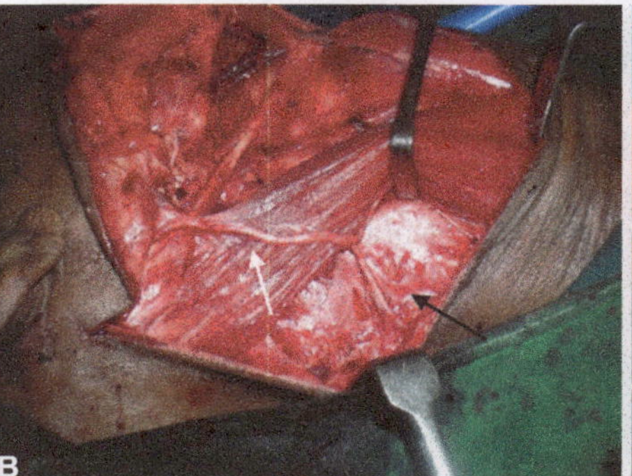

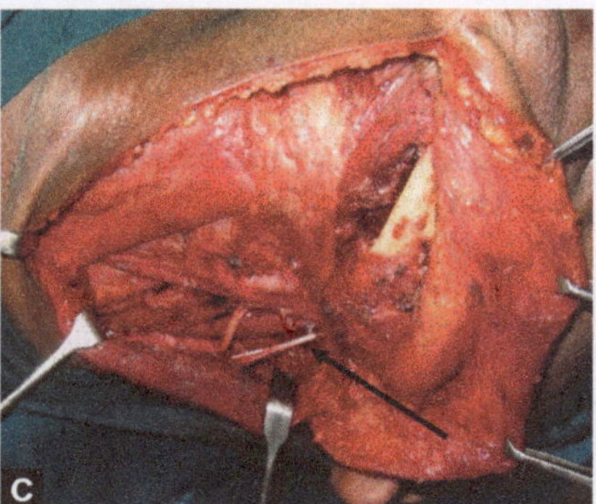

Figs 30.49A to C: (A and B) Descendens hypoglossi, *Ansa cervicalis* and branches of C3 and C4 cervical roots, (black arrow) and greater auricular nerve (white arrow), (C) Spinal accessory nerve running deep (black arrow) to SCM

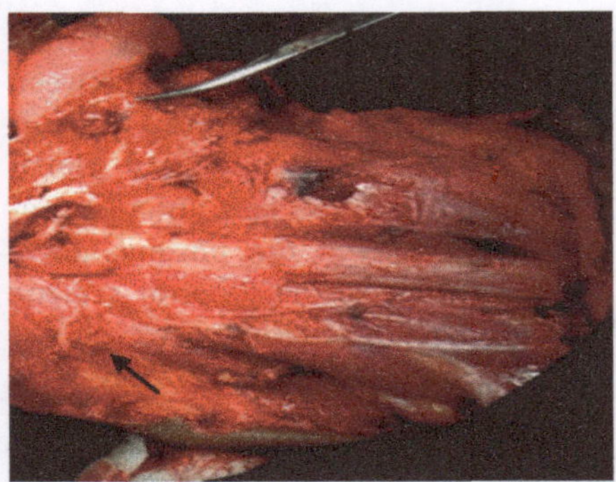

Fig. 30.50: Spinal accessory nerve (black arrow), phrenic nerve running over the anterior scalene muscle and the branches of the brachial plexus running in the groove between anterior and middle scalene muscles

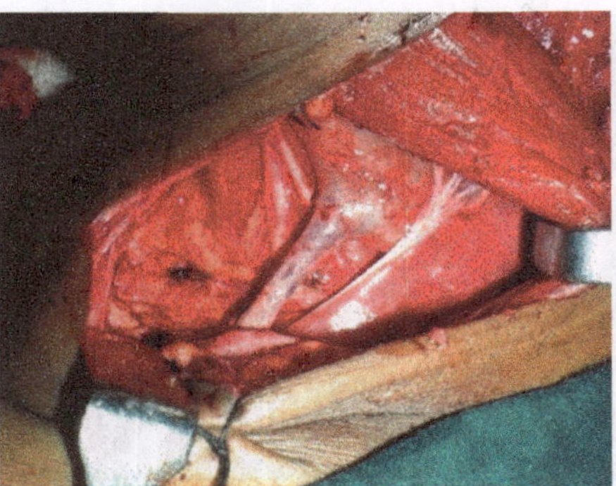

Fig. 30.51: Elevation of the fibrofatty and lymphatic tissue of the floor of the reveals the inferior belly of the omohyoid, transverse cervical vein and brachial plexus between the middle and anterior scalene muscles

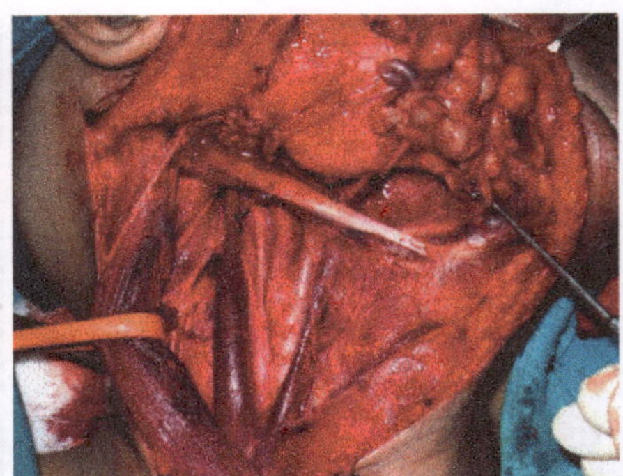

Fig. 30.52: Dissection of the carotid triangle, carotid sheath, apex of the posterior triangle. The submandibular triangle dissection above the digastricus is started with mobilization of the submandibular salivary gland

until the sternal and clavicular heads of the sternocleidomastoid muscle are exposed and divided. Retraction of this detached muscle superiorly allows identification of the carotid sheath (Fig. 30.52). Meticulous sharp and blunt dissection exposes the contents of carotid sheath, the common carotid artery and the vagus nerve, which are preserved, and the internal jugular vein, which is divided at its lower end and doubly ligated.

Care is taken to identify and ligate lymphatic vessels on either side of the neck, with particular attention to controlling the thoracic duct on the left side of the neck. The thoracic duct lies posterior to and passes deep to the IJV and at times there are multiple ducts which are thin and fragile. They should be identified and ligated. In case of the doubt about its adequate ligation the anesthetist is asked to ventilate the patient, during the inspiration as the intrathoracic pressure increases, milky white chyle leak can be observed which facilitates the ligation. The proximal stumps of the transverse cervical artery and vein are divided and ligated. The entire block of ligated IJV and divided sternomastoid muscle is raised cephalad.

Dissection of Carotid Triangle

The dissection reaches the midpoint of the neck and the common tendon of the omohyoid is identified. The dissection anterior to the common Carotid artery and superiorly, leads to dissection of the carotid triangle. The fibrofatty tissue in the carotid triangle is raised and the bifurcation of the carotid is identified. This area is susceptible to handling as there are baroreceptors in this area and thus, needs careful handling to prevent bradicardia. The external and internal carotid arteries are identified, the former lies superiorly and anteriorly to the former. The superior thyroid artery is preserved as it runs deep to the block. The middle thyroid vein is ligated. At the level of the greater cornue of hyoid bone, the common facial vein which runs deep to the posterior belly of the digastricus and is seen merging with IJV. It is identified and ligated. Along with the common facial vein and several pharyngeal veins crossing the digastric muscle are divided to expose the posterior belly and tendon of the digastric up to the hyoid bone. The hypoglossal nerve after crossing the carotid bifurcation may loop around the occipital branch of the external carotid artery (Fig. 30.53). The descendens hypoglossi to the strap muscles is often a good guide, leading up to the hypoglossal nerve (Fig. 30.49A).

The upper border of carotid triangle dissection ends at the level of the common tendon of digastric muscle, superiorly and at the superior belly of omohyoid, anteriomedialy. Once the lower border of the digastric muscle is exposed completely, the specimen is allowed to rest in the surgical field. All the major vessels run deep to the digastric.

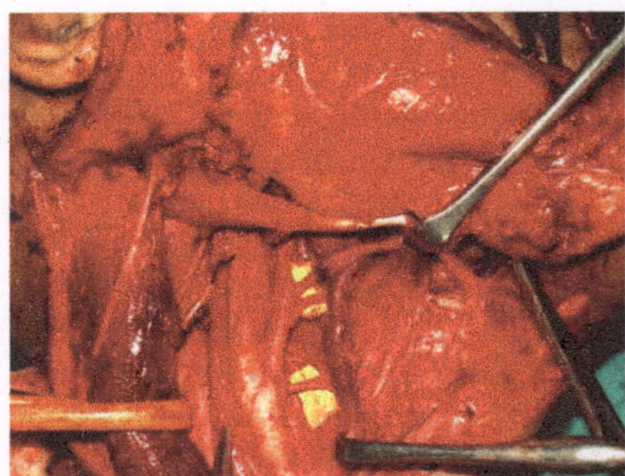

Fig. 30.53: Branches of the ECA, from inferior to superior, superior thyroid, lingual and facial arteries

The attention is turned to the posterior triangle block elevated previously. The block is raised from the mastoid, along the posterior belly of digastric and the fibrofatty contents of the Bocca's triangle (spinal accessory chain of Lymph nodes, i.e. 2B nodes) are cleared and the root of the spinal accessory, (*see* Fig. 30.49C) greater auricular nerve are divided. The internal jugular vein is clamped and divided 2 cm below the skull base before it enters the jugular foramen and double ligation of the cephalic end is done to prevent slipping of ligature, bleeding and retraction of

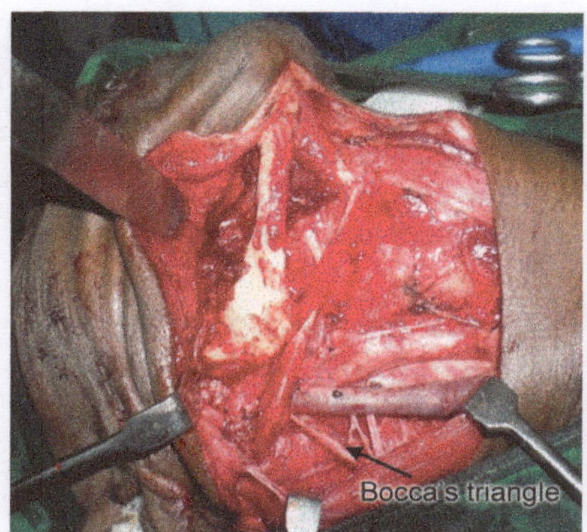

Fig. 30.54: Bocca's triangle, the posterior belly of the digastricus, spinal accessory nerve running deep to IJV (black arrow)

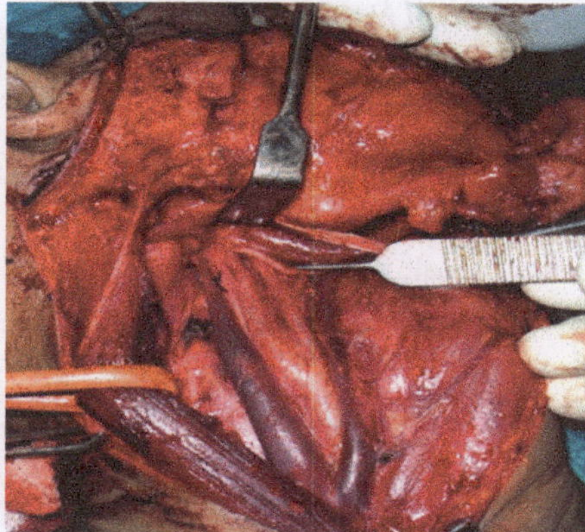

Fig. 30.56: Identification of the hypoglossal nerve below the posterior belly of digastric

the vein intracranially (Fig. 30.54). Some surgeons prefer to divide the posterior belly of digastric to visualize the IJV and some retract the muscle superiorly. The block is now raised anteriorly and the dissection of the tissue at the tail of parotid is done. The retromandibular vein is ligated.

Digastric and Submental Triangle Dissection

Attention is then turned to the superior flap, which is also elevated in the subplatysmal plane with care taken to identify and preserve the marginal mandibular branch of the facial nerve as it crosses the facial artery and vein. Retraction of the superior stumps of these vessels after their division further protects the nerve (Fig. 30.55).

Dissection continues anteriorly along the inferior border of the mandible. The superomedial limit of dissection is the anterior belly of the contralateral digastric muscle. The submandibular gland is mobilized. The hypoglossal nerve lies deep to the posterior belly of digastric and inferiomedial to the submandibular gland, after it crosses the external carotid artery and runs medially and superiorly, it should be identified and protected (Fig. 30.56). The facial artery and common facial vein are present deep to the submandibular salivary gland and after lifting the gland, blunt dissection is carried out to identify these vessels. They are identified and ligated. The facial artery originates from the external carotid artery at the level of greater cornu of hyoid bone and runs deep to posterior belly of digastic muscle (Figs 30.57A and B). If cut accidentally it gets retracted below the posterior belly of diagnostic and bleeds sizably. It is difficult to clamp and ligate it, in such cases the posterior belly of digastric is divided to visualize the cut end of the artery.

As the submandibular gland is lifted from the mylohyoid and hyoglossus curtain, the deep part leading into the Wharton's duct is identified. The lingual nerve and submandibular ganglion lie close to the deep part near the origin of the duct. The lingual nerve is identi fied, and its postganglionic secretomotor fibers are divided, as is Wharton's duct (Fig. 30.58). Any remaining veins of the pharyngeal venous plexus accompanying the hypoglossal nerve must be divided between claps and ligated. The dissection is then carried out anteriorly in the sunbmental trangle and the submental block between the two anterior bellies of the digastric muscles upto the body of the hyoid bone, is ressected. The terminal branch of anterior jugular vein and the submental branch of the facial artery are ligated.

Meticulous hemostasis is achieved and the wound is closed over two suction drains. One drain is tacked posteriorly along the trapezius muscle with a loop of catgut suture. The anterior drain lies along the strap muscles. These drains are brought out through separate stab incisions inferiorly.

The platysma is closed with 3-0 chromic catgut interrupted sutures and the skin with 3 or 4 '0' proline or silk suture. Care is taken to achieve an airtight closure and to initiate suction on the drains during closure to prevent

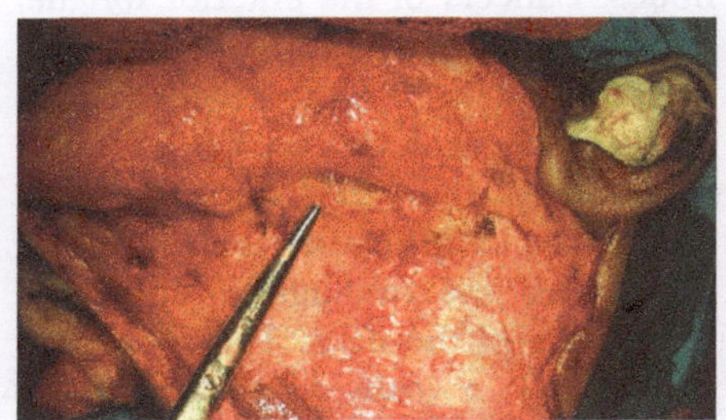

Fig. 30.55: Identification of the marginal mandibular nerve

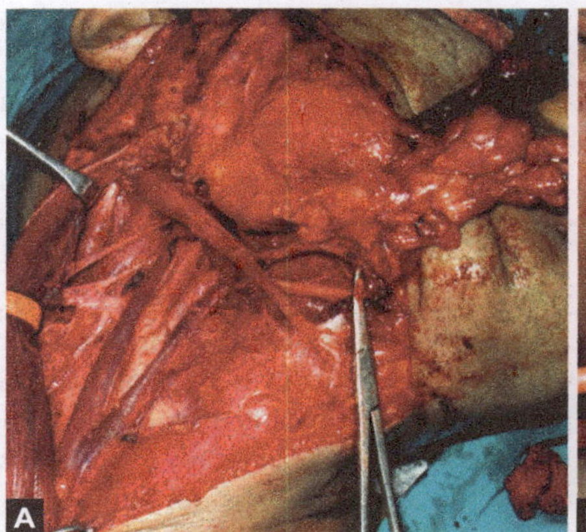

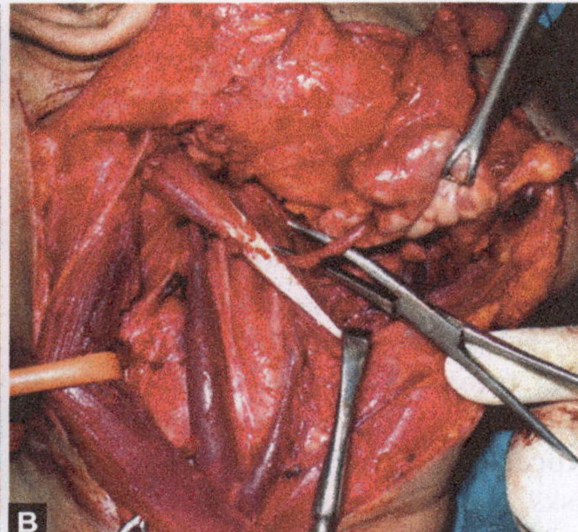

Figs 30.57A and B: The lower pole of the submandibular salivary gland, posterior belly of digastric and facial artery and vein identified

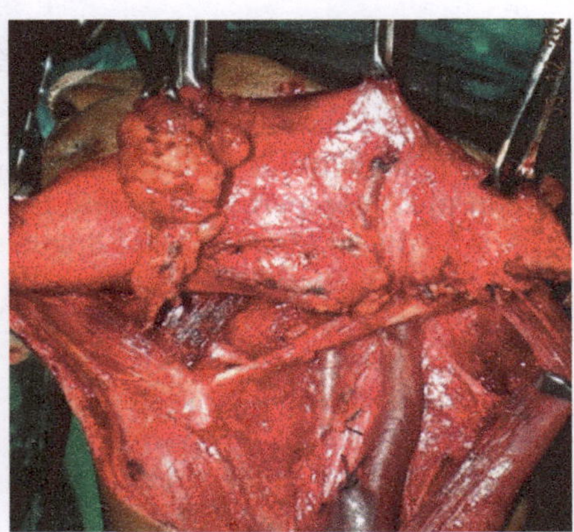

Fig. 30.58: The submandibular salivary gland is lifted from the submandibular triangle. The Wharton's duct is ligated before excising the gland. The lingual nerve is often identified deep to the mylohyoid, inferior to the duct

clots from forming within the drains. Postoperatively, the drains are removed when there is minimal serous drainage.

Complications unique to radical neck dissection are related to the sacrifice of the sternocleidomastoid muscle and the spinal accessory nerve. This may result in shoulder dysfunction and the resultant "Frozen shoulder syndrome" can be debilitating and requires diligent physical therapy.

Bilateral radical neck dissection can result in significant facial lymphedema, which dissipates only slowly.

If combined with laryngectomy, simultaneous bilateral resection of the internal jugular veins can result in acute obstruction to both intra- and extracranial venous drainage and massive venous edema. The extent of resection of soft tissue in a radical neck dissection can leave the carotid artery relatively exposed and subsequent radiation therapy increases the risk of hemorrhage.

A regional musculocutaneous flap can provide some protection from this. Current indications for radical neck dissection are such that only patients with extensive disease, or disease that has failed prior treatment, undergo the procedure. Thus, their postoperative risks, both of complication and recurrence, are significant.

Functional Neck Dissection

Functional neck dissection is not a technique, but it is a concept wherein the neck dissection is carried out preserving certain structures, preserving the optimum function and preventing postsurgical morbidity, without compromising the surgical clearance.

Origin of Functional Neck Dissection

The main goal of the 'functional' approach to neck dissection proposed by Suárez[42] in 1963 and popularized by Bocca[43] is the removal of all lymphatic tissue in the neck, preserving the remaining neck structures. This is achieved by using the fascial planes of the neck that surround most cervical structures and separating them from the adjacent lymphatic tissue. As long as the tumor cells remain confined within the lymphatic system of the neck, they can be safely removed by carefully stripping the neck structures from their fascial covering. There is no oncological benefit from removing the sternocleidomastoid muscle, internal jugular vein, or any other important neck structure, when cancer is locked up inside a partially isolated lymphatic space. The situation changes when the lesion invades the walls of this anatomical container, fixing the nodes to surrounding structures. Then, the tumor is no longer a 'nodal cancer' but becomes a 'neck cancer.' This situation invalidates the 'functional' spirit and justifies the use of a classic radial approach with removal of the involved neck structures.

Therefore, the spirit of functional neck dissection is to take advantage of the particular anatomy of the neck to remove all or part of the lymphatic system, with preservation of the remaining neck structures.

It may be argued that preservation of some nodal groups requires cutting through the fibrofatty tissue that contains the lymphatic system of the neck, something that seems to be in contradiction with the basic principle of fascial dissection, but it was justified as nodal groups are only a schematic representation of the lymphatic system of the neck, which is really configured in different chains that follow the course of the major cervical vessels and nerves.

Rationale and Anatomical Basis for Functional and Selective Neck Dissection

Functional neck dissection, as described by Osvaldo Suárez,[42] is based on the existence of a fascial barrier between the lymphatic tissue and the muscular, glandular, neural and vascular structures of the neck. This anatomical separation allows the creation of a surgical plane of dissection. The fascial layer invests muscles and organs in the neck, forming planes and spaces, where many important structures are crowded together. This fact, known as fascial compartmentalization, holds the rationale for functional neck dissection.

Fascial compartmentalization allows the removal of cervical lymphatic tissue by separating and removing the fascial walls of these "containers" along with their contents from the underlying vascular, glandular, neural and muscular structures.

Selective Neck Dissections: Types and Indications

The anatomical studies of Rouviere[44] demonstrated that the lymphatic drainage from normal head and neck mucosal sites is relatively predictable. Later clinical studies concluded that oral cavity cancers mostly metastasized to the jugular digastric and midjugular nodes. Cancers of the anterior tongue, floor of the mouth and buccal mucosa metastasize first to the nodes in the submandibular triangle. Some metastasis may skip the submandibular and upper deep jugular nodes and go directly to the midjugular nodes on either side of the neck. The Lindberg[45] study and a subsequent study by Skolnik,[46] observed that oral cavity and oropharynx tumors rarely metastasize to posterior or lower deep jugular nodes in the absence of metastases in the upper jugular and submaxillary nodal groups. Shah's[47] (1990) retrospective review of radical neck dissection specimens from patients with oral, laryngeal and pharyngeal cancers concluded that oral cavity cancers metastasize most often to levels I, II and III, whereas oropharynx cancers most often go to levels II, III and IV (Table 30.3).

Based on these findings, several selective neck dissections have been proposed.

Table 30.3: Nodal groups at greatest risk of developing metastases according to location of the primary tumor

Nodal region	Location of the primary tumor
Area I: Submental nodes	Floor of mouth, anterior oral tongue, anterior mandibular alveolar ridge, lower lip
Submandibular nodes	Oral cavity, anterior nasal cavity, soft tissue structures of the midface, submandibular gland
Area II: Upper jugular nodes	Oral cavity, nasal cavity, nasopharynx, oropharynx, hypopharynx, larynx, parotid gland
Area III: Middle jugular nodes	Oral cavity, nasopharynx, oropharynx, hypopharynx, larynx
Area IV: Lower jugular nodes	Hypopharynx, larynx, cervical esophagus
Area V: Posterior triangle	Nasopharynx, oropharynx
Area VI: Anterior compartment	Thyroid gland, larynx (glottic and subglottic), apex of the piriform sinus, cervical esophagus
Area VII: Upper mediastinal group	Thyroid, larynx (glottic and subglottic), lung

Supraomohyoid Selective Neck Dissection

This procedure is used for oral cavity cancers. The submental, submandibular, upper and midjugular groups of nodes are the usual sites of metastases from the oral cancers (Figs 30.59 to 30.61). Supraomohyoid neck dissection removes levels I, II, III (Figs 30.62A and B) and at times (oral tongue cancer) level IV. The level V is excluded. Bilateral dissection is recommended for midline, floor of the mouth, ventral surface of the tongue tumors, provided that there is clinical evidence of lymph node metastasis on the either side of neck. In patients with significant (N2) nodal metastases in the ipsilateral neck, bilateral dissection or contralateral neck radiation is crucial. It is suggested that if there are metastases in level II, then the level IV and V should be dissected.

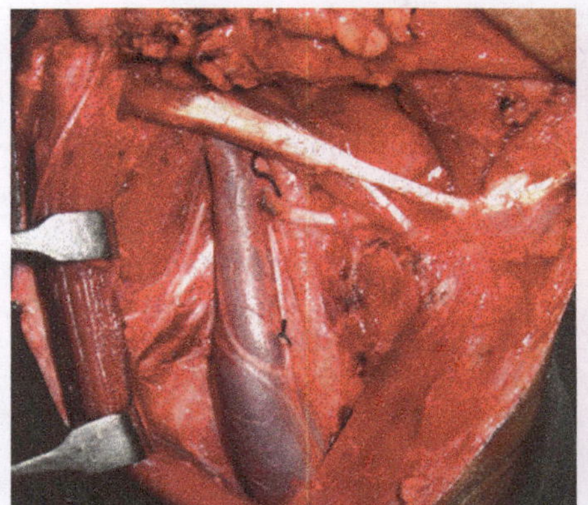

Fig. 30.59: Clearance of Bocca's triangle with sparing the spinal accessary nerve, notice the hypoglossal nerve running deep to IJV and crossing the carotid artery. Notice the descending hypoglossi and *Ansa cervicalis*

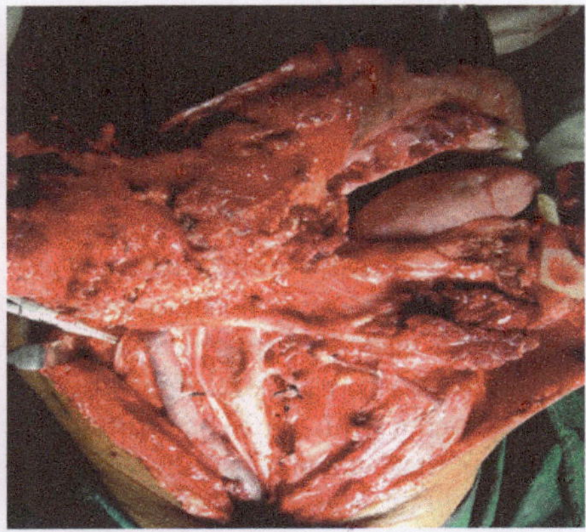

Fig. 30.60: Exposure of spinal accessory, vagus, branches of ext. carotid artery

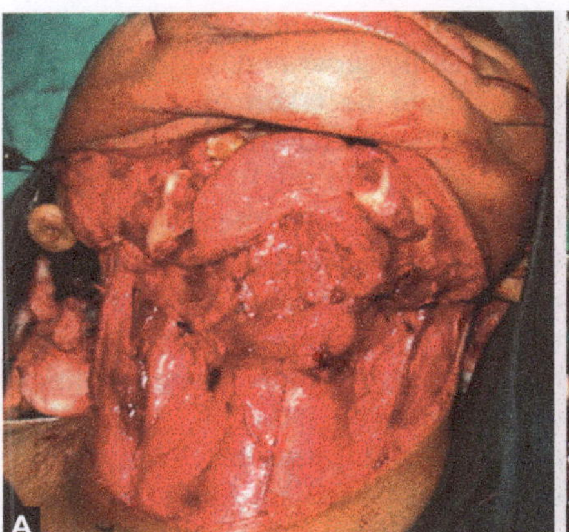

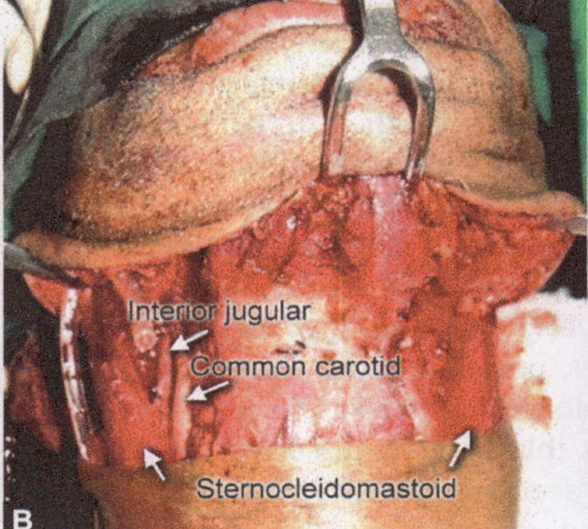

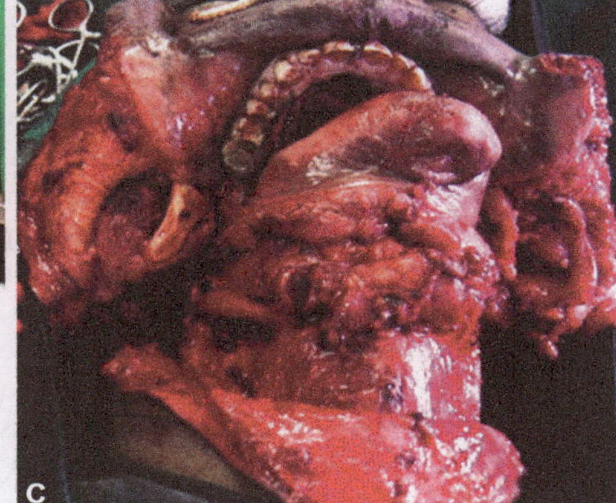

Figs 30.61A to C: Bilateral supraomohyoid neck dissection

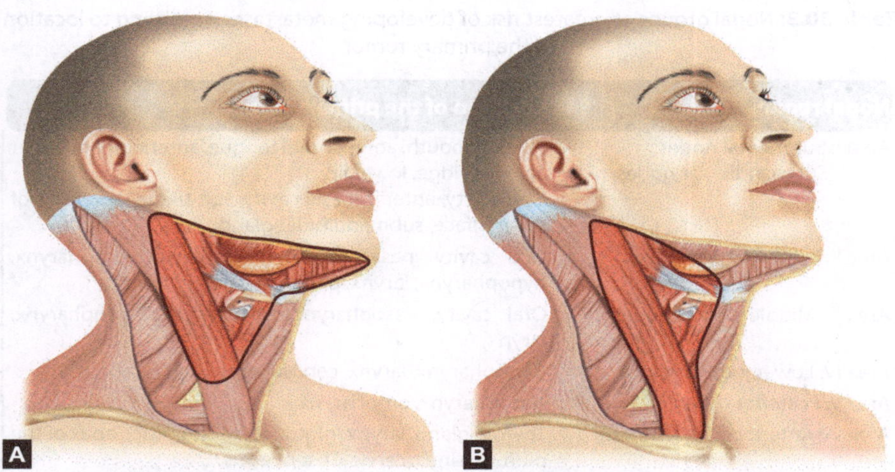

Figs 30.62A and B: (A) Supraomohyoid; (B) Anterolateral neck dissection

Most of the squamous cell carcinomas of oral cavity in India are due to smokeless tobacco and manifest in the gingivobuccal sulcus. The common lymphatic metastasis pattern is involvement of level I and II nodes, except where the tumor is originating from tongue or floor of mouth, where the tumor may have metastasis in deep cervical chain and contralaterally also. The involvement of 2B nodes is also rare in the gingivobuccal malignancies and hence, supraomohyoid neck dissection is usually adequate in majority of cases. The dissection may be extended to level IV or V if there is evidence of involvement of level III or obvious metastasis in level IV or V nodes. In cases of midline tumor, crossing the midline, supraomohyoid dissection is very useful and avoids morbidity. The post surgical radiotherapy can take care of micrometastasis, if any at Level IV and V.

The supraomohyoid neck dissection is very acceptable method. As all the structures like sternocleidomastoid muscle, IJV, spinal accessory including the *Ansa cervicalis* and greater auricular (*see* Fig. 30.59) can be preserved, without compromising the outcomes. The patient has negligible morbidity and the quality of life after surgery is acceptable.

Supraomohyoid Neck Dissection (SOHD)

The supraomohyoid neck dissection is a type of selective neck dissection, commonly practiced while treating the gingivobuccal SCC. It is indicated when the metastasis is restricted to upper cervical nodes up to level I and II. It is shown to be equally effective as the RND or MND, while treating Stage I to III SSC of the gingivobuccal sulcus. It comprises of excising the lymph nodes at level IA, IB, IIA, IIB, level III and the occasionally the dissection is extended up to level IV for the SSC involving tongue and floor of mouth. Although the apex of the posterior triangle is cleared during the SOHD, the VA nodes may not be completely removed. Usually an apron incision is taken (*see* Figs 30.46A to C). The skin flap is raised in the subplatysmal layer up to the inferior border of the mandible anteriorly and up to the tip of the mastoid process in the posterior region. As the flap is raised the platysma ends just posterior to the sternocleidomastoid muscle and the tissue is more adherent and tenacious in this region. While reflecting the flap over the SCM, the external jugular vein is seen running anteriosuperiorly over the SCM, which is dissected superiorly up to the tail of the parotid as it enters the parotid. The greater auricular nerve is also seen entering the parotid and lies posterior to the external jugular vein, which is also dissected carefully. As this nerve is dissected inferiorly, it is seen running over the SCM muscle and it curls around the posterior border of the SCM and goes deep to it (*see* Fig. 30.48). The greater auricular nerve is a very important landmark for the identification of the spinal accessory nerve. The spinal accessory nerve lies within 1 cm distance superior to the greater auricular nerve at the point where it curls around the posterior border the SCM (*see* Fig. 30.48B). Careful blunt dissection in this area shows the spinal accessory nerve which lies deep and superiorly to the greater auricular nerve (*see* Fig. 30.49B). The inferior flap is also raised in the subplatysmal plane for its entire length taking care not to damage the anterior jugular vein or the external jugular vein. The venous perforators going to the platysma are cauterized. The lower level of the dissection ends inferior to the intersection of the SCM and the superior belly of the omohyoid muscle. The latter runs obliquely, deep to the SCM and superiorly to the IJV. The posterior border of the SCM is dissected free from the adjoining fibrofatty tissue from its superior aspect going inferiorly up to the inferior extent of the flap. As the spinal accessory nerve is already identified earlier, the chances of the damage to it are minimum during the sharp dissection. The external jugular vein is ligated at the level of the inferior extent of the dissection. The spinal accessory nerve is carefully dissected inferiorly as it runs posterioinferiorly towards the anterior border of the trapezius muscle. The attention is then shifted to the anterior border of the SCM. The anterior border of the SCM is carefully dissected for its entire exposed length. The SCM is then lifted and all the fascial attachments inferior to it are carefully separated. While doing so care should be taken to stay close to the inferior surface of the muscle to avoid damage to the IJV. Minor venous perforators are seen inferior to the SCM which are cauterized and the entire SCM muscle is mobilized. Once an access is created the mobilization of the entire muscle can be done by gentle finger dissection. The SCM is skeletalized and retracted posteriorly, the carotid sheath is opened by blunt dissection and the next step is skeletalization of the IJV. The middle thyroid branch and the common facial veins are identified and ligated. The veins are fragile and thus, should be handled carefully to prevent their avulsion. The end of the vein towards the IJV should be ligated and smaller peripheral branches can be cauterized with bipolar cautery. There are no branches originating from the common carotid artery. The carotid bifurcation (carotid bulb) area has baroreceptors, and handling during the dissection in this area can lead to bradycardia and hypotension. Spraying two percent lidocaine solution in this area can reduce the chances of bradiacardia. The branches of the external carotid (superior thyroid, lingual, facial arteries) are given at the level and superior to the greater cornue of the hyoid bone but, unlike the branches of the IJV they lie deeper and should be preserved. Hypoglossal nerve is seen running horizontally, deep to the IJV at its intersection with the posterior belly of the digastricus and should be preserved. The descending hypoglossi (*Ansa cervicalis*) is seen originating from the hypoglossal nerve at this point and it runs inferiorly, anterior to the IJV and it should also be preserved (*see* Fig. 30.59). After the entire fibro-fatty tissue along with the embedded lymph nodes is freed from the anterior aspect of the IJV and the carotid artery, the superior belly of the omohyoid is identified as it crosses the IJV in the mid portion of the neck. This point marks the lower limit of the supra omohyoid neck dissection. The dissection is carried superiorly along this muscle and all the fibro-fatty tissue and lymph nodes between the superior belly of the omohyoid and the anterior aspect of the IJV are mobilized enblock from the base of the carotid triangle up to the level of digastricus muscle and its common tendon. The block is left *in situ* and the attention is shifted to the posterior side of the IJV.

The inferior level of the posterior triangle dissection also ends at the level of the superior belly of the omohyoid. The SCM is retracted anteriorly with L retractor or by passing a red rubber catheter around it (*see* Figs 30.49A and C). The fibro-fatty tissue is mobilized superiorly over the scalenus table, preserving the fascia covering the anterior, midius, posterior scalenus muscles and the levator scapulae muscle. This is very important to prevent damage to the phrenic nerve and the branches of the brachial plexus as they lie deep to this fascia. The phrenic nerve runs from lateral to medial side over the scalenus anterior muscle.

The dissection is carried cephald in the posterior triangle. The skeletalized spinal accessory nerve is retracted and protected. The IJV and common carotid artery are retracted and guarded using the vessel guard to protect them while dissecting the lymph nodes and fibro-fatty tissue below them. The carotid artery does not give any branches, posteriorly. The IJV also seldom gives branches posteriorly and even if they are present, they should be either ligated or cauterized. The cutaneous branch of the C3 and C4 roots are seen entering into the lifted block and are divided. The greater auricular nerve can be easily protected. The spinal accessory nerve is dissected deep to the SCM, after it emerges deep to the IJV at the level of the posterior belly of the digastrics (*see* Fig. 30.49C). It runs clinging to the deep surface of the SCM. It gives a branch to the SCM and gets a twig from the cervical plexus all these braches can be easily protected by proper retraction while dissecting around them. The dissection is carried superiorly into the Bocca's triangle. All the fibro-fatty tissue around the spinal accessory nerve is carefully dissected taking care not to damage the IJV, which is protected by retraction with vessel retractor and the posterior belly of digastrics is also retracted superiorly to facilitate proper dissection in this area (*see* Figs 30.54 and 30.59). A branch of occipital artery is often encountered in this area which can be coagulated using bipolar cautery. The entire block is lifted as the lower border of the deep lobe of parotid is reached. The dissection then goes superiorly to the posterior belly of the digastrics muscle. The tail of the parotid gland should be carefully palpated and if the lymph nodes are present they should be excised as they are known to produce recurrence in some cases due to metastatic growth, which remains unaddressed. Some surgeons deliberately excise the portion of the tail of the parotid to excise the lymph nodes in this region. The dissection is then carried anteriorly, the retromandibular vein is ligated. The rest of the dissection for clearing the submandibular triangle and the submental triangle remains the same as described under the radical neck dissection.

Lateral selective neck dissection: The lateral dissection (Fig. 30.63) removes nodal groups II, III and IV, leaving levels I and V undissected. The lateral operation is recommended for oropharyngeal,

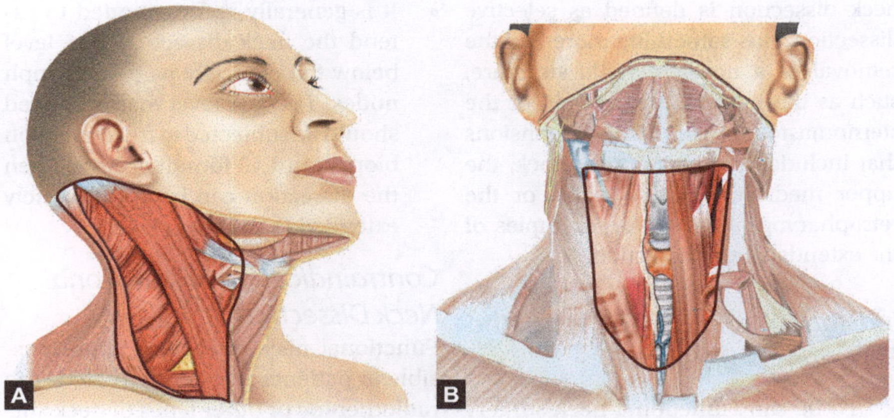

Figs 30.63A and B: (A) Lateral; (B) Anterior neck dissection

hypopharyngeal and laryngeal cancers and should be done bilaterally if there are proven metastases to one side of the neck.

Posterolateral neck dissection: This operation removes the nodes of levels II, III, IV and V, the suboccipital and the postauricular nodal groups. It is recommended for metastases from skin malignancies of the posterior scalp, posterior neck and some parotid salivary gland cancers that have metastasized posteriorly. The dissection differs from the dissections favored for aerodigestive system metastases. It removes the lymph nodes and lymphatics containing fibrofatty tissue of the posterior neck, the subdermal fat and fascia between the primary site and nodal compartments, where there are no distinct fascial compartments.

Anterior neck dissection: This dissection removes only area VI, which includes the paratracheal nodes, perithyroid and precricoid (Delphian) groups (Figs 30.63A and B). The procedure is favored for thyroid cancer, cervical trachea, subglottic laryngeal cancer (subglottic or transglottic), cervical esophagus and hypopharynx cancer. The procedure is usually bilateral for cervical esophageal and large hypopharyngeal cancer. It can be combined with a lateral dissection and occasionally needs to be extended to the upper mediastinum.

Extended neck dissection: There are situations where none of these selective operations will fit a clinical scenario. This requires another category called the extended neck dissection. The extended neck dissection is defined as selective dissection plus something more like the removal of a non-lymphatic structure, such as the internal jugular vein or the sternomastoid muscle. Other extensions that include, in a descriptive block, the upper mediastinum, the axilla, or the retropharyngeal space, are examples of the extended neck dissection.

Indications and Limitations of the Functional Approach

- To be safe, functional neck surgery requires all metastatic disease to be confined within the lymphatic tissue. Thus, this approach is ideal for N_0 cases with a high risk of occult metastasis. An additional advantage of functional neck dissection is that it may be performed simultaneously on both sides of the neck without increasing morbidity. In all midline head and neck lesions with high risk of cervical metastasis (floor of the mouth, base of the tongue, supraglottic larynx and gingivolabial malignancies crossing the midline) functional neck dissection is the best surgical option for N_0 cases.
- In patients with small palpable nodes functional neck dissection is still a valid option as long as some principles are carefully observed. The nodes should not be greater than 2.5 to 3.0 cm in greatest diameter. This is justified by the need to have all metastatic disease confined within the lymph node capsule. Although extracapsular spread is possible in lymph nodes of all sizes, it is well known that chances of extracapsular spread increase with increasing lymph node size.[48] Gross extracapsular extension results in lymph node fixation to contiguous structures. In no instance should functional neck dissection be attempted in patients with fixed nodes.
- The number of palpable nodes and location of primary tumor is not a contraindication for functional neck dissection as long as all nodes fulfill the previously mentioned criteria.
- It is generally recommended to extend the neck dissection one level below the clinically palpable lymph nodes. The last level that is excised should be subjected to frozen section biopsy and if found positive then the dissection can be appropriately extended to the lower levels.

Contraindication of Functional Neck Dissection

Functional neck dissection is not possible in patients previously treated with radiotherapy or other types of neck surgery. In these patients the fascial planes have disappeared as a consequence of the previous treatment. Thus, fascial dissection is not possible anymore. In these cases, modified radical neck dissection appears as an alternative to radical neck dissection as a means to preserve structures not involved by the tumor. The dissection will be made according to the basic principles of radical neck dissection, but preservation of uninvolved neck structures will be accomplished according to the surgical scenario. This is a clear example that illustrates the difference between functional and modified radical neck dissection.

Reconstruction of Surgical Defects

The ablative cancer surgeries produce large surgical defects. The defects cannot be planned as the wide excision of the lesion with safe margins is the goal of the surgery and the surgeon does not have many options. The reconstruction of the defect needs to be planned prior to the surgery with an appropriate flap. The reconstruction should not only plug the effect with the tissue, but also serve the cosmetic needs and help in the restoration of the function. The lack of reconstruction leads to lot of morbidity and cosmetic compromises. The small defects which are seen only in early malignancies can be closed primarily by mobilizing the local tissue. However, too much tension across the suture line invariably leads to dehiscence and orocutaneous fistula. The dribbling saliva, secondary infection, foul smell and unhygienic conditions lead to poor social acceptance of such patients. The osseous defects and large soft tissue resections leads to microstomia, inability to masticate and swallow making the overall nutritional status severely compromised and the patient becomes malnourished and cachexic. Thus, the resection of the tumor should not be the only goal, but to provide adequate reconstruction and quality of life by restoring function and esthetic should also be kept in high priorities.

The surgical defects could be osseous and soft tissue and both require to be addressed.

The modalities for the osseous reconstruction are:

- **Implants:** Reconstruction plates made up of stainless steel or titanium, titanium mesh, custom made titanium prosthesis using CAD/CAM technology, etc.

  The problem with the cancer surgery is that due to the loss of large portion of the soft tissue, the implants do not get adequately covered by soft tissue and the tight closure might lead to wound dehiscence, exposure and infection of the implant. The reconstruction of the midline defect of the mandible, which is reconstructed with the reconstruction plate invariably fails and the plate dehiscence through the mucosa or skin takes place due to the erosion of these structures due to the friction from the plate during the movements (Figs 30.64A and B). Thus, if the cortical bone at the inferior border is not involved, a wedge mandibulectomy should be performed for the midline malignancies of the mandible as far as possible. If the patient is required to be subjected to the postoperative irradiations, the metallic implants interfere with the radiation therapy by either scattering the radiations or absorbing the radiations and inducing tissue necrosis around the implant. Hence, either they are avoided or removed prior to the radiation therapy.
- **Grafts:**
  - Free bone grafts—rib graft, iliac crest bone grafts. As the water tight cover of the wound cannot be always achieved due to the loss of the soft tissue, there is high risk of graft rejection due to infection and thus its not a good option.
  - **Vascularized bone grafts (free tissue transfer, microvascular free grafts):** The popular options for the osseous reconstruction are microvascular fibular grafts based on the peroneal vessels, iliac crest graft based on the circumflex iliac artery and vein and the lateral scapular graft. Out of these, the free fibular graft is the most popular and widely used graft (Figs 30.65A to D). The graft is harvested along with a vascular pedicle of regional artery and the vein and anastomosed to the neck artery and vein (Figs 30.66A and B) (e.g. facial artery, external carotid artery, common facial vein or jugular vein by either end-to-end or end-to-side anastomosis technique). The advantage with the free tissue transfer is that it provides good reconstruction, healing and contour. The survival of the graft is predictable

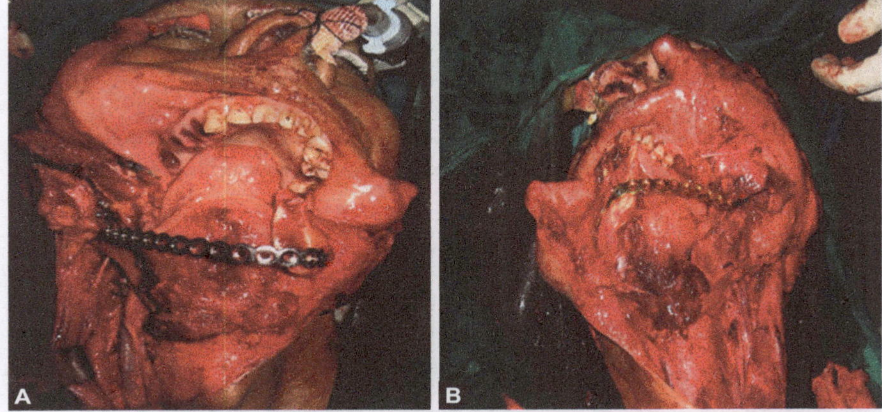

Figs 30.64A and B: Reconstruction of the mandibular osseous defect with the SS and titanium recon plates

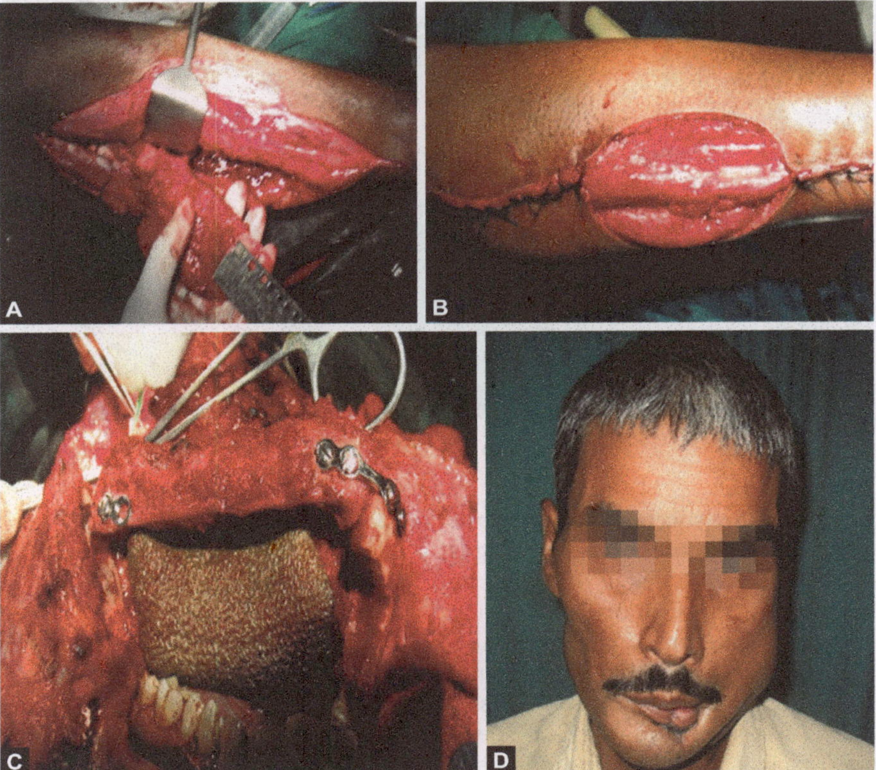

Figs 30.65A to D: Free fibular graft with skin pearl used for mandibular reconstruction

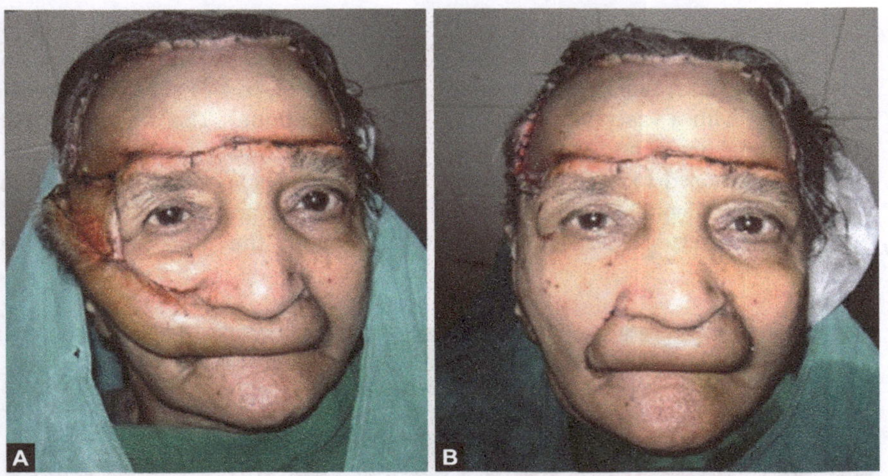

Figs 30.66A and B: Forehead flap used to reconstruction of surgical defect of upper lip

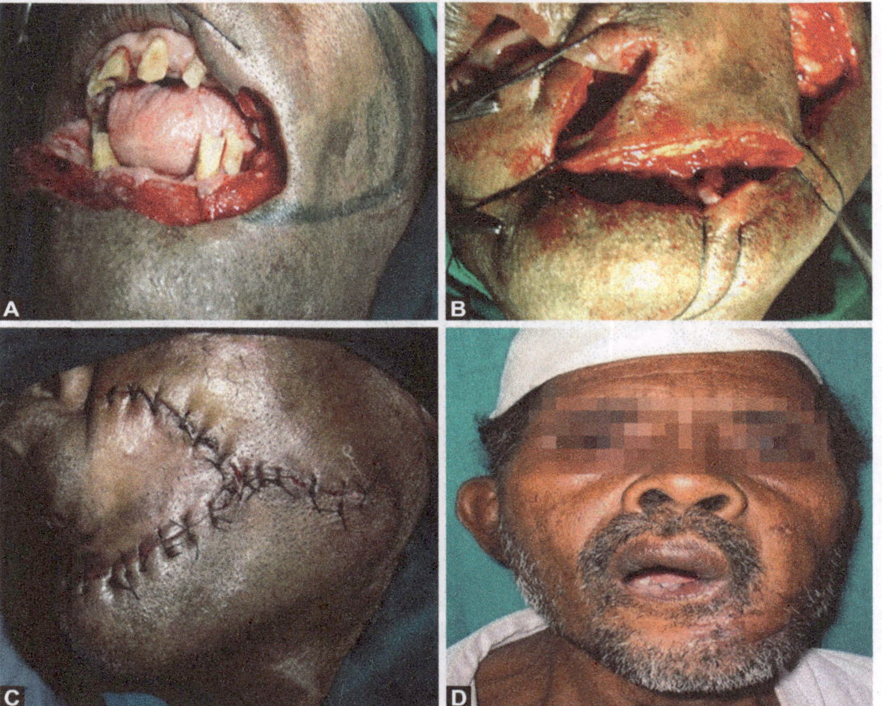

Figs 30.67A to D: Local eastlander flap

after the successful anastomosis and the most important thing is that such a stable bone can be used for dental rehabilitation by placement of implants in this transferred bone, which is not possible with other modalities.

The free tissue transfer is a specialized facility, which is not universally and widely available.

Soft Tissue Reconstruction

The soft tissue reconstruction can be done in:

- Local tissue advancement (Figs 30.67A to D), local pedicled flaps like myomucosal tongue flaps, nasolabial flaps, (Figs 30.68A and B) temoralis muscle fascia flap and forehead flap (*see* Fig. 30.66).
- **Distant flaps:** Deltopectoral flap (Fig. 30.69A), pectoralis major myocutaneous flap (Fig. 30.69B), pectoralis major myocutaneous-osseous composite flap, latissimus dorsi myocutaneous flap, sternomastoid myocutaneous flap, platysmal flap, etc.
- **Free tissue transfer:** Radial forearm flap (thin flap very good for the floor of mouth, tongue, for lining and covering of other moderate defects) (Figs 30.70A to E), rectus abdominous flap, fibular flap with the skin pedal, etc.

Complications

- **Wound infections and wound breakdown:** Incidence higher in irradiated tissue; soilage of wound by saliva, tracheal aspirates, or gastric secretions; tight wound closure; immunocompromised and malnourished states and presence of a foreign body, hematoma, or seroma.

  Treatment: Aggressive antibiotic regimen, monitor for fistula, control diabetes, maximize nourishment, meticulous wound care (debridement, wet to dry dressings), evaluate potential for carotid blow out.
- **Flap necrosis:** Poorly planned incision that compromises vascular supply may result in tissue loss, wound infection, fistulas, or vessel exposure (Figs 30.71A to C).

  To avoid the same, properly designed neck incisions are recommended (e.g. curvilinear, MacFee, modified Schobinger incision and the trifurcation should begin at right angles from the main incision). The posterior leg of the flap should be smaller than the anterior and linear incisions should be avoided and gentle curvatures should be incorporated to ensure tension free approximation.
- **Shoulder syndrome:** Injury or sacrifice of spinal accessory nerve leads to shoulder dysfunction and pain. The shrugging and abduction is hampers and the winged scapulas are seen (Figs 30.72A and B).

  The treatment comprises of physical therapy, may also consider early

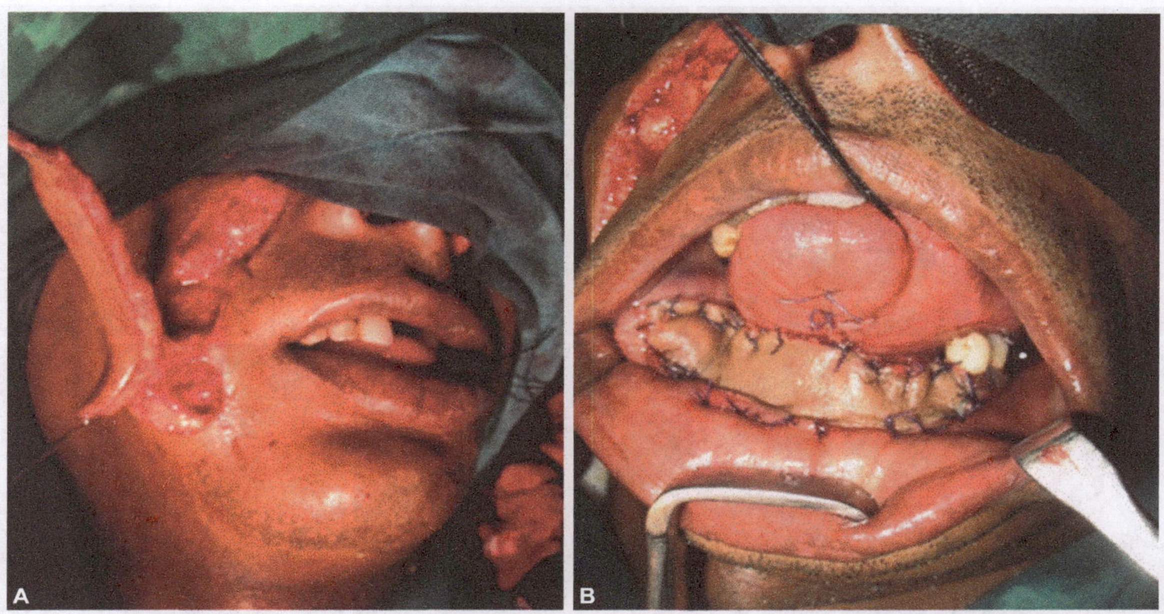

Figs 30.68A and B: Bipedaled nasolabial flap for the reconstruction of anterior alveolar defect

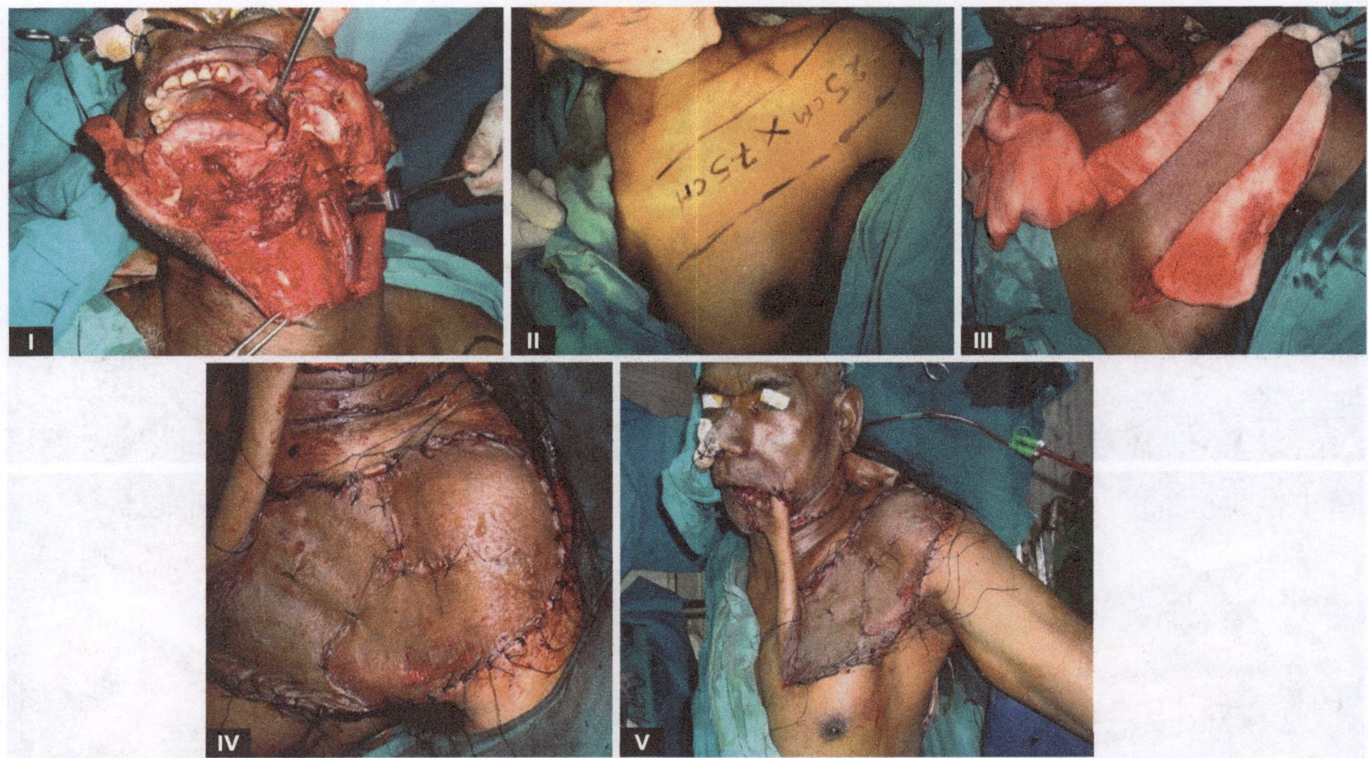

Fig. 30.69A: DP flap used for the reconstruction of the surgical defect of anterior region. The raw area on the chest is skin grafted

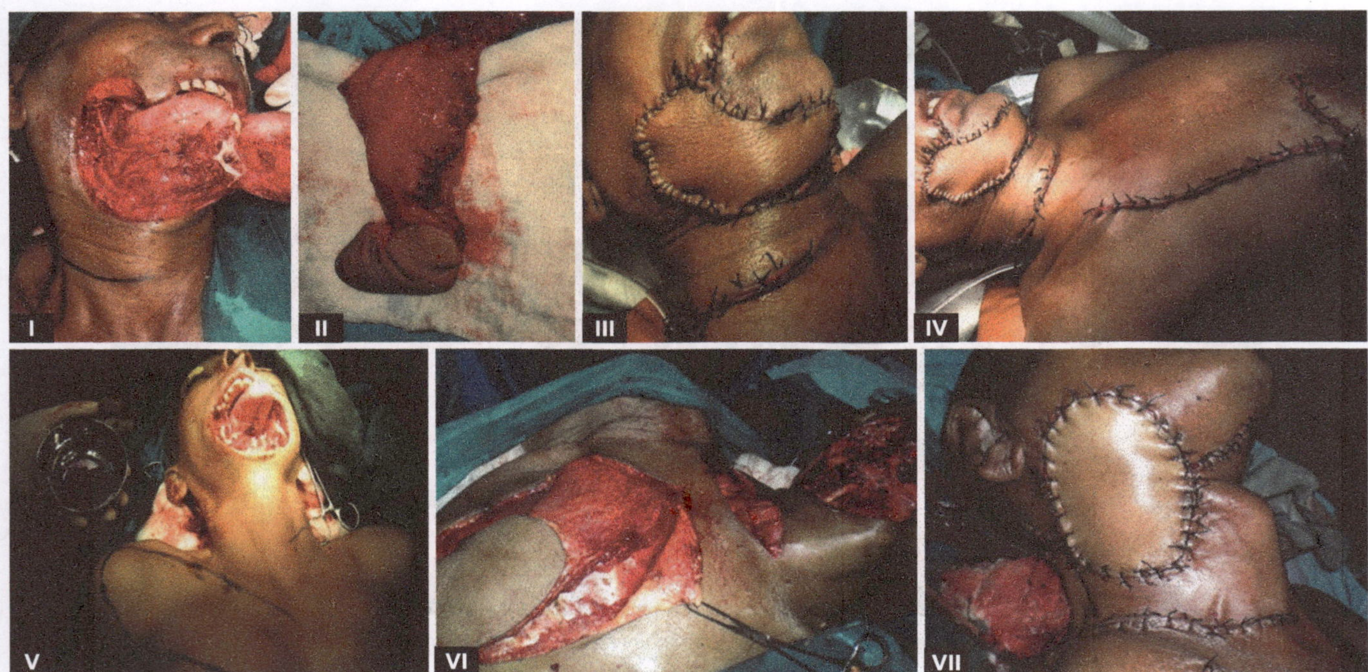

Fig. 30.69B: PMMC flap used for the reconstruction

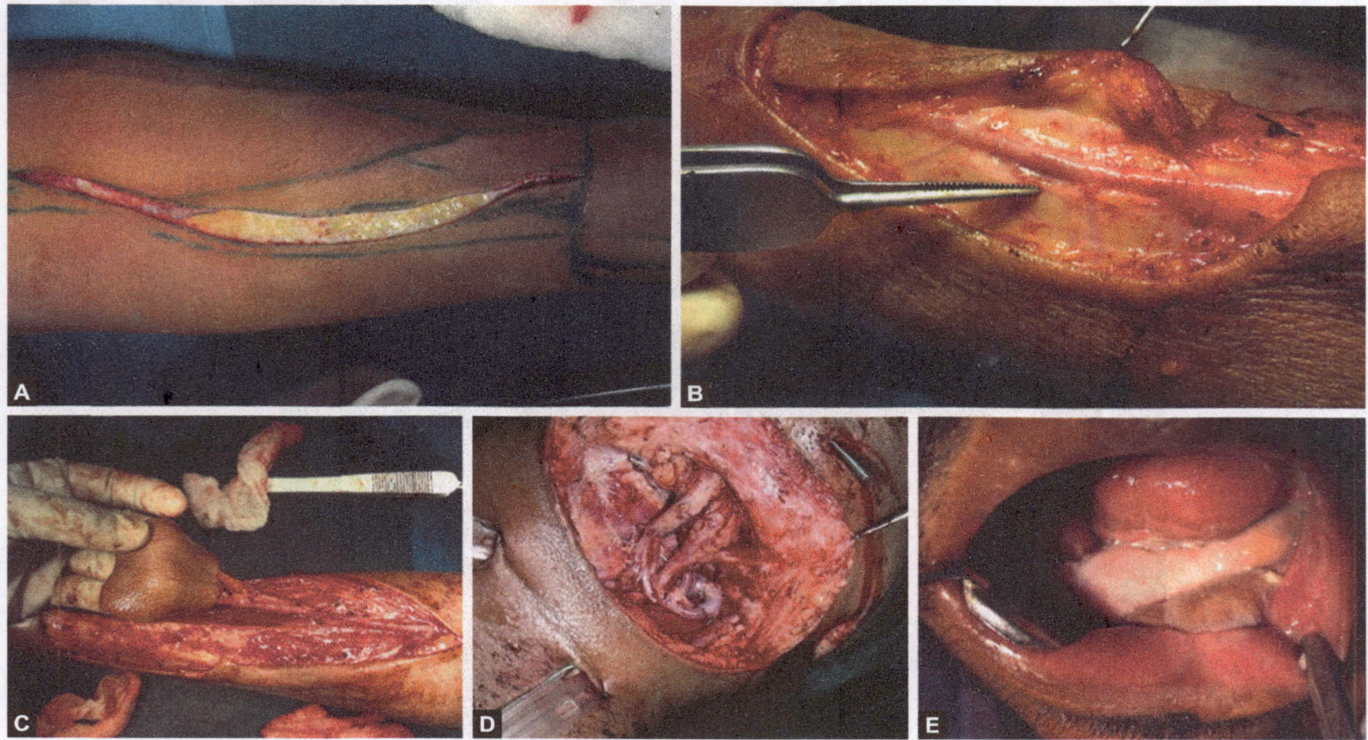

Figs 30.70A to E: Radial forearm bases on radial artery and vein used for the reconstruction of the floor of mouth

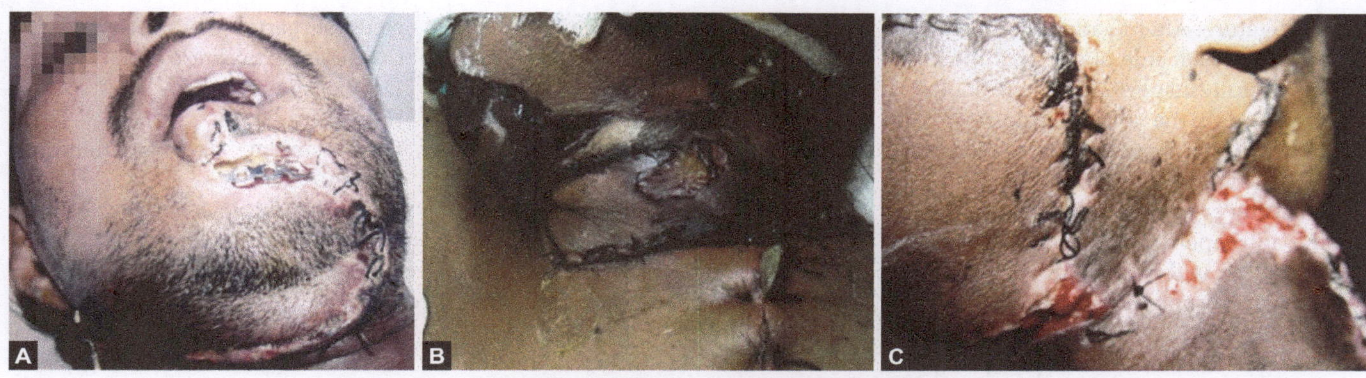

Figs 30.71A to C: Flap necrosis and dehiscence

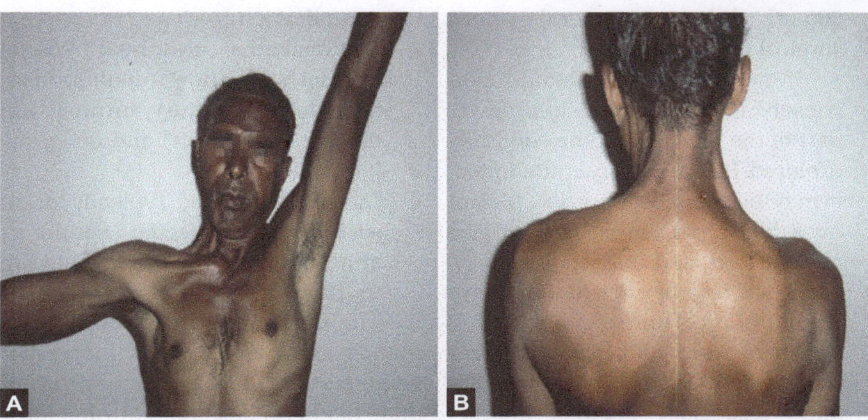

Figs 30.72A and B: Shoulder morbidity

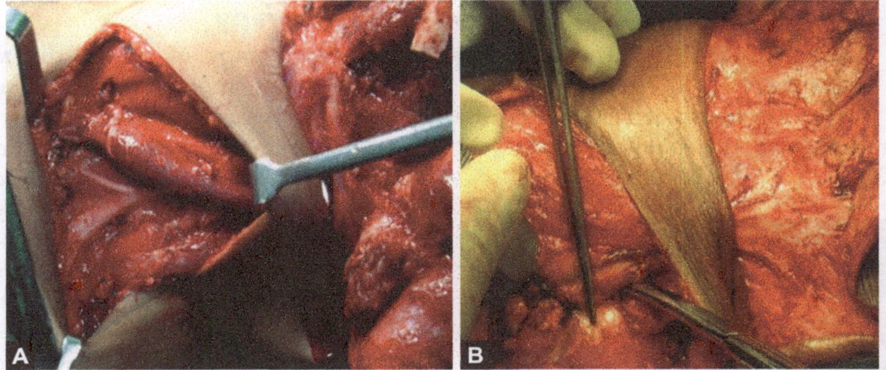

Figs 30.73A and B: Identifying the branches of the brachial plexus

cable grafting or orthopedic reconstruction.

- **Injury to the vagus nerve:** Injury results in varying presentations depending on level and branch of injury; superior laryngeal nerve injury typically may present with only subtle voice changes, recurrent laryngeal nerve injury may result in hoarseness, aspiration, or airway compromise.

Treatment: The treatment may require tracheotomy for airway management (especially for bilateral vocal fold paralysis), management of aspiration and vocal fold paralysis.

- **Injury to the marginal mandibular branch of the facial nerve:** At risk during elevation of the cervical flap, should be identified and protected (*see* Fig. 30.55), bilateral injury may result in oral incompetence.

Treatment: The best treatment is careful dissection and avoiding the damage during the surgery. If it is discovered intraoperatively immediate neurorrhaphy should be performed and may consider facial reanimation procedures.

- **Hematoma/Seroma:** Prevented with meticulous hemostasis and placement of suction drains.

Treatment: Consider reopening for major hematomas with removal of clot and controlling bleeding; for minor hematomas may wait 7 to 10 days to allow for liquification then aspirate; may also consider pressure dressings and prophylactic antibiotics; seromas may also be aspirated.

- **Injury to the brachial plexus:** While dissecting the fibrofatty tissue over the sceleneal table at the base of the posterior triangle, the dissection should be carried out carefully to avoid the damage to the branches of the brachial plexus. The phrenic nerve should be identified and preserved (Figs 30.73A and B). The damage to the phrenic nerve leads to paralysis of the diaphragm. The phrenic nerve is the only nerve in the neck, which runs from lateral to medial side.

Chylous fistula: Chylous leakage is an uncommon complication, with a reported incidence of 1 to 2.5 percent. It is much more frequent on the left side of the neck. When the thoracic duct is to be ligated during surgery, it should be surrounded by muscle, fascia, or adipose tissue to avoid sectioning its thin wall with the ligature. After ligation, the lower part of the left side of the neck must be carefully inspected for chyle pooling. Asking the anesthesiologist to increase the intrathoracic pressure and placing the patient in the Trendelenburg position are helpful in the intraoperative identification of chyle leak in the area of the thoracic duct. It is important to note that in most patients developing postoperative chyle fistula, this was previously identified and apparently controlled intraoperatively. In the postoperative period, chylous fistula is recognized by the appearance of a milky fluid in the drains. This is usually evident within the first 5 days of surgery. The chylous origin of the fluid can be confirmed by measuring the content of triglycerides, usually over 100 mg/dL. When chylous leak is suspected, dietary modifications can be prescribed. Low fat diet, either enteral or parenteral, is usually recommended, because medium-chain triglycerides are absorbed directly into the portal venous circulation, avoiding the thoracic duct. The patient should be given parenteral feeding rather than gastric feeding. Elevation of the head, repeated aspiration, and pressure dressing are also recommended. However, use of indwelling vacuum drains should be avoided. It is important to note that preservation of the sternocleidomastoid muscle in functional and selective neck dissection constitutes an important obstacle for successful compression. Insertion of a pressure packing impregnated with irritant solution, like Betadine or tetracycline, into the area of the thoracic duct has also been recommended as a nonsurgical method to stop chylous leak. The daily volume of the leak has been reported to range from 80 to 4500 mL. When more than 500 mL of chyle drain per day, nonsurgical stop is unlikely.[49]

If no response is found upon conservative treatment, the lower part of the neck should be surgically explored. Before surgery is attempted, it may be helpful to put the patient on a high lipid enteral diet to give chyle a thick and milky consistency, which will improve the intraoperative identification of the leak.

- **Cerebral and facial edema:** Higher risk with internal jugular vein ligation (especially bilateral internal jugular vein ligation), (Figs 30.74A and B) may present with syndrome of inappropriate antidiuretic hormone secretion (SIADH) or mental status changes.

The treatment of cerebral edema must be undertaken urgently:

- Neurosurgery consultation
- Consider corticosteroids
- Lumbar drainage
- Hyperventilation
- Hyperosmolar agents (mannitol) and diuretics.

The bilateral IJV ligation can be avoided by choosing modified radical neck dissection on at least one side and preservation of the IJV there in.

- **Blindness:** Caused by optic nerve infarction (uncertain etiology, may be from hypotension and increased intracranial pressure) and is a rare complication.
- **Postoperative dyspnea:** Possible etiologies include pneumothorax, phrenic nerve injury, intrinsic lung disease (atelectasis) and congestive heart failure.
- **Carotid blowout:** Typically occurs secondary to infected wound site and wound breakdown and has high mortality rate (approximately 10%).

The treatment comprises of airway management, compression, large-bore catheters with fluid replacement, immediate blood replacement, intraoperative ligation and venous grafts for repair.

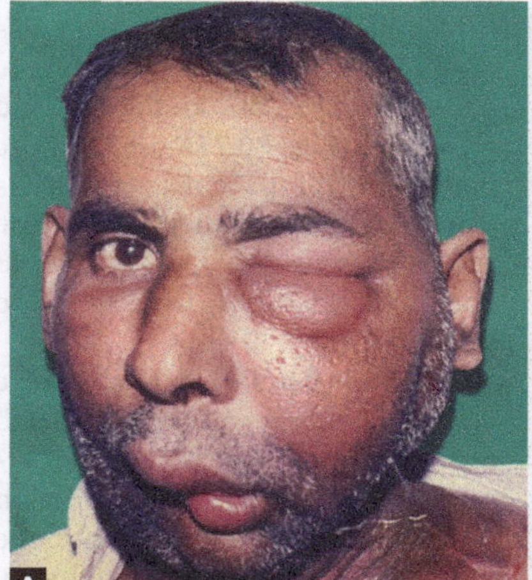

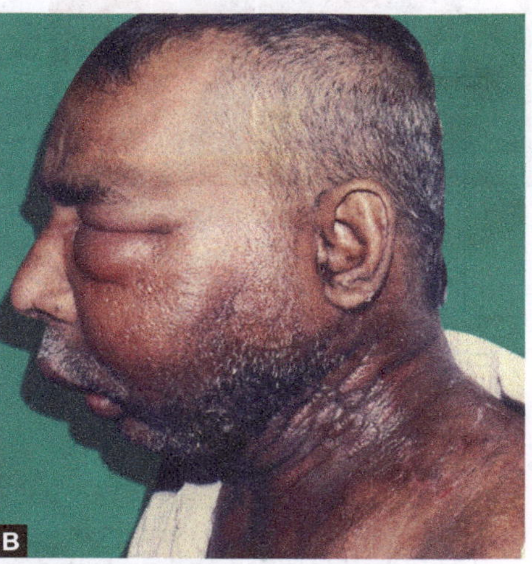

Figs 30.74A and B: Lymphedema of face following RND due to ligation of veins and lymphadenectomy

Chemotherapy

The chemotherapy of cancer differs from the chemotherapy of infection. The microorganisms have distinct metabolic pathways as compared to the human cells and thus, they can be selectively targeted and eliminated by the antibiotics. However, the metabolic pathway of the malignant cells is similar to that of normal cells and thus, this specificity is not present. Hence, the chemotherapeutic agent affects the malignant cells and normal cells alike and induces high toxicity. The division rate of the malignant cells is very high as compared to the normal cell and thus, this rapidity of the cell cycle renders the malignant cell more vulnerable to the chemotherapeutic agents. The hematological malignancies respond well to the chemotherapy, but in the management of the OSCC, the role of the chemotherapy as a primary modality is questionable. It is often used as an

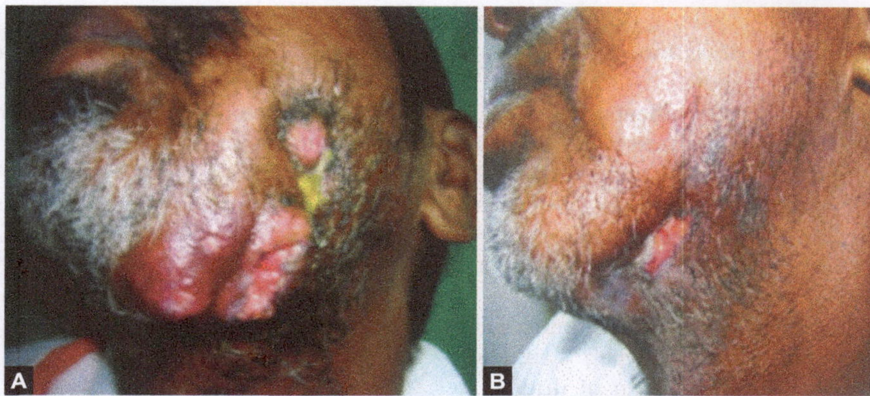

Figs 30.75A and B: (A) Clinical photograph prior to neoadjuvant chemotherapy; (B) Post treatment photograph showing reduction of tumor size

adjuvant therapy with other modalities like radiation therapy or surgery or as a palliative therapy in the management of advanced, unresectable cancers.

A chemotherapeutic agent affects a cell in its dividing cycle and induces irreparable damage to the DNA to induce cell death.

Indications for Chemotherapy

- Nasopharyngeal cancer
- Unresectable head and neck cancer
- Laryngeal organ preservation
- Pyriform sinus cancer organ preservation
- **Recurrent and distant metastatic disease:** Original traditional role in head and neck cancer, essentially provides palliation for recurrent unresectable disease or incurable cancer with distant metastatic disease.

Chemotherapy Strategies

Neoadjuvant (induction)

Definition: Sequential chemotherapy before local treatment modality (surgery or radiation).

Advantages: Initial chemotherapy may allow better drug penetration prior to impaired vascularity secondary to radiation effects, initial chemotherapy may also reduce tumor bulk or 'cure' patient of disease (organ preservation or organ salvage). The neoadjuvant chemotherapy in the management of the oral SSC is not very popular modality. It is practiced with variable success. The tumor shrinks significantly with the neoadjuvant chemotherapy (Figs 30.75A and B). The reduction in size of the tumor certainly improves the tumor handling, reduces blood loss during the surgery and also facilitates the endotracheal intubation. However, whether the tumor margins also shrink or not is not certain. Second disadvantage is that the texture of the tissue in the shrunken area of the tumor gets altered following the chemotherapy, which makes clinical decision of the safe surgical margins difficult. The frozen section biopsy can be of great help in such cases.

The concept of organ salvage was primarily induced to salvage the visceral organs by reducing the tumor bulk and reducing the quantum of resection. The same concept is not applicable to OSCC as the tumor bulk may shrink with the preoperative chemotherapy, but the resection margins do not and the quantum of resection remains the same.

Disadvantages: Postchemotherapy patients are often more debilitated, which may increase complications of surgical intervention or radiotherapy and the margins are difficult to access.

Concominant (Radiation Therapy and Chemotherapy)

Definition: Concurrent chemotherapy and radiation (chemotherapy may be given continuously or interrupted [split course]).

Advantages: Simultaneous therapies may synergistically maximize therapeutic effect (chemotherapy sensitizes cells to radiation and simultaneously kills micrometastatic disease).

Disadvantages: Results in increased side effects from concurrent therapies (mucositis, infection, malnutrition, hematopoetic depression).

Radiation and Chemotherapies

- Chemotherapy inhibits the repair of cells that may otherwise recover from radiation
- Concomitant radiation and chemotherapies result in synchronization of cell cycles increasing the effectiveness of both therapies
- Resistant cells of one mode of therapy may be susceptible to the other mode of therapy thus, producing synergistic action
- Shrinking the tumor with radiation improves drug delivery for increased effectiveness of chemotherapy
- Combined therapy may initiate cells from G0 phase to active phases rendering the cells more susceptible to therapy
- Concomitant modalities damage cells in different ways and increase chances of cells' death.

Adjunctive

Definition: Chemotherapy after primary treatment modality to control microscopic disease.

Indications: Locally advanced disease, multiple positive regional neck nodes, nodal extracapsular spread, positive margins, recurrence.

Advantages: May improve survival.

Disadvantages: Exposes patient to side effects of chemotherapeutic agents. If it is given after the surgery, the penetration of the drug in the operated area is questionable due to disturbed vascularity and fibrosis in the operated area. It will have more side effects than the therapeutic effects. However, the distant metastasis and nodal micrometastasis may be treated with this modality, which is away from the primary surgical site.

Chemoprevention[50]

- Retinoids (analogues of vitamin A) have been shown to reduce malignant potential of premalignant oral lesions[51] (54% reversal of dysplasia with retinoids versus 10% for controls, P = 0.01) and prevent the development of second primaries in a single-institution phase III trials (4% developed second primaries with retinoids versus 24% in controls, P = 0.005)[52]; the effect, however, is not sustained once treatment is stopped.
- **Mechanism of action:** Regulate cellular differentiation and proliferation in epithelial tissue (via retinoic acid receptors) and modulate neoplastic cell growth differentiation and apoptosis.

Common Side Effects of Chemotherapy

- Mucous membrane and skin dryness
- Alopecia
- Conjunctivitis
- Transitory elevated transaminases
- Hyperlipidemia
- Myalgia
- Teratogenicity
- Skeletal effects
- Hematopoetic depression
- Leucopenia
- Immunosupression
- Superinfections
- GI bleeding due to erosive changes.

Common Chemotherapeutic Agents and Combinations in Head and Neck Cancer

Cisplatin

Mechanism of action: Heavy metal that acts as an alkylating agent, covalently binding with DNA and RNA.

Common side effects: Nausea, nephrotoxicity, peripheral neuropathy, ototoxicity, electrolyte disturbances, anorexia.

Indications: Best single-agent against squamous cell carcinoma of the head and neck in recurrent disease; common combination agent for neoadjuvant, adjuvant and concomitant chemotherapy of the head and neck; radiation sensitizer.

Carboplatin

Mechanism of action: Similar to cisplatin (less reactive).

Common side effects: Better tolerated than cisplatin (less nephrotoxicity, nausea, neurotoxicity and ototoxicity).

Indications: Not been fully investigated in head and neck cancer, often used in combination with taxol 5-fluorouracil (5-FU).

Mechanism of action: Antimetabolite that binds to thymidylate synthetase blocking the conversion of uridine to thymidine preventing DNA synthesis in S-phase.

Common side effects: Anorexia and nausea, mucositis, diarrhea, alopecia, myelosuppression, cardiac toxicity.

Indications: Similar to cisplatin (cisplatin and 5-FU is the most studied combination chemotherapy regimen in head and neck cancer).

Methotrexate

Mechanism of action: Antimetabolite that binds to dihydrofolate reductase preventing DNA synthesis in S-phase. Its action is similar to the action of the ionizing radiations and thus reffered to as radiomimetic drug and it potentiates the action of the radiations.

Common side effects: Bone marrow suppression, gastrointestinal disturbances, mucositis, alopecia, dermatitis, nephrotoxicity, teratogenicity, interstitial pneumonitis.

Indications: 'Standard' palliative therapy for recurrent or metastatic disease.

Leucovorin (tetrahydrofolic acid): Utilized as a 'rescue' agent, competitively overcomes increases intracellular pools of dUMP (also used with 5-Fluorouracil).

Taxanes (paclitaxel and docetaxel)

Mechanism of action: Prevent normal microtubular reorganization.

Common side effects: Neutropenia, alopecia, mucositis.

Indications: Currently being investigated for recurrent disease and as a potential radiation sensitizer.

Bleomycin

It is an antibiotic having antineoplastic properties. It is a mixture of glycopeptides. It acts on a cell specifically in G2 and mitotic phase.

Mechanism of action: Causes DNA breakage in susceptible malignant cells through an activated free radical mechanism.

Dose: 10 to 15 mg/m2 IV daily for 3 to 4 days every 3 to 4 weeks.

Vinca alkaloids

They are the vinca alkoloids, derived from the plant and include vincristine, vinblastine, vindesine.

Mechanism of action: Bind to the protein tubulin, preventing polymerization to form microtubules and is M-phase specific.

Dose: 1-2 mg/m2 weekly IV.

Disadvantages

- No selectivity
- Hematopoetic depression
- Immunosuppression.

Radiation Therapy

The ionizing radiations are known to induce damage to the nucleotide chains of DNA and induce cell death. When a single chain is damaged, the damage is repairable, but when the double stranded damage occurs the cell death results.

Mechanism of Injury

- **Direct mechanism of radiation injury:** Direct damage of radiation with critical elements in a cell (e.g. DNA, cell membranes).
- **Indirect mechanism of radiation injury:** Secondary damage from direct radiation effects on other cell moieties; primary mechanism of cell death (e.g. DNA injury from production of free radicals).

Determinants of Sensitivity of Radiation Therapy

Radiotherapy is not considered to be the first line of treatment yet it can be quite useful if following principles are understood before instituting the patient for radiotherapy.

- Larger tumors have a more hypoxic center, therefore, are less sensitive to radiation because less free radicals are generated (1 cm tumor = 109 cells; 3 cm tumor = 1,010).
- Oxygenated cells are more susceptible to radiation than hypoxic cells (exophytic tumors are typically well vascularized and therefore, more susceptible to radiation injury, ulcerative and infiltrative tumors are less vascularized and therefore, more resistant to radiation).
- Cell death occurs with proliferation (usually 4–5 times before lysis), therefore, rapidly growing tumors are more susceptible to injury.
- Cells tend to be more radiosensitive in mitosis and late G1 and early S-phases.
- The intrabony tumors are relatively radioresistant than the soft tissue tumors. The term radioresistant is little misnomer as all the tissues are affected by the radiations with a variable degree. Those tissue or tumors which are affected to a greater extent by radiations are termed as radiosensitive and those which are not affected significantly are termed as radioinsensitive due to various factors mentioned above.

Types of Radiation

- Electromagnetic radiation
  For example, radiowaves, heat waves, light waves, UV waves, X-rays and gamma-rays.
- Particulate radiation
  For example, electrons, protons, alpha-rays, neutrons, negative pi-mesons.

Types of Radiotherapy

Radical radiotherapy

- Radiotherapy given at high dose with curative intent.
- Dose delivered is the highest that can be delivered without undue functional consequences.
- **Palliative therapy:** Seeks to control symptoms in which the cancer is deemed incurable or in which the patient is not sufficiently fit to withstand.

External beam radiotherapy (teletherapy)

It is usually cobalt-60 radiations given in a dose of 2 Gy/day for 5 days in a week total of 30 cycles (total dose of 60–70 Gy).

Disadvantage: Since beam directed through skin, it causes skin reactions, ORN and thus, the incidence of adverse reactions is very high.

Neutron beam therapy

It is a heavy particle therapy, which was popular for its penetration in the tissue. However, this therapy is most damaging to normal cells, as well as tumor cells leading to ORN. It is rarely used today because of its complications of significant muscle and deep tissue fibrosis.

Interstitial radiotherapy (brachytherapy)

The word brachytherapy is derived from a Greek word, brachy meaning 'short range'. This term is used to describe the treatment of malignant disease by interstitial, intracavitary and surface application of sealed radioisotopes.

Sources

- Radium-226
- Caesium-137
- Cobalt-60
- Iridium.

Advantage: Maximum radiation dose is delivered to selectively targeted tumor tissue with sparing of surrounding vital structures.

Disadvantage: ORN.

Hyperfractionated radiation therapy

- **Rationale:** To allow normal cells to proliferate and to suppress the tumor cells in between the fractions.
- **Dose:** 1 Gy twice daily, for total dose of 60 to 70 Gy over a period of 7 weeks.

Intensity modulated radiotherapy (IMRT)

It is a type of CT-CRT (CT guided conformal radiotherapy). The delineation of target tissue by CT and MRI is better and the computer controlled delivery of radiation is ensured. It is a conformal radiotherapy: it conforms to the tumor tissue in 3 dimensions. The maximum dose can be given to target tumor tissue with precision avoiding radiation to surrounding vital structures.

Fractionation

Conventional fractionation: In fractionation, radiotherapy is given in small interval doses rather than the whole dose at once. It allows cells to proceed in their cycle to more radiosensitive stages in their cell cycle and allows for reoxygenation of previously more hypoxic cells (more susceptible), prolonged waiting between fractions results in regrowth of tumor cells from sublethal damage. Furthermore, normal tissue tends to have better repair than tumor cells, therefore, recovery more quickly from sublethal damage.

Fractionation results in total less biological injury due to the greater opportunity for repair, therefore, requires a higher total dose than single or hypofractionated dosing, hypofractionization (less fractions) are used for tumors with good reparation of sublethal injury (malignant melanoma).

Methods of fractionation

- **Conventional fractionation:** Typically uses one treatment per day (generally 1.8–2.2 Gy) for 5 days a week
- **Pure hyperfractionation:** Increases rate of treatment (e.g. 2-times a day dosing), smaller dose per fraction, same duration of therapy, higher total dose than conventional fractionation; decreases late side effects.
- **Accelerated (standard) fractionation:** Decreases duration of therapy, increases rate, higher dose per fraction, with same decreased total dose as conventional fractionation; increases acute side effects, decreases late side effects, increases tumor cell kill (prevents tumor cell proliferation)
- **Accelerated hyperfractionation:** Increases rate of treatments, decreases duration of therapy, increases total dose.
- **Concomitant boost accelerated fractionation:** Changes rate to twice a day dosing in the last 2 weeks of therapy.

Radiation Strategies

- **Shrinking fields:** Selective radiation dosing to varying region depending on primary size and shape (e.g. 7,000 cGy to primary site as primary therapy, 5,000–5,500 cGy to N0 neck or adjuvant treatment)
- **Brachytherapy:** Delivery of radiation to malignant tissue by placement of permanent radioisotopes intraoperatively via a temporarily placed radioactive source within tumor bulk
- **Three-dimensional multiple treatment beam therapy:** Utilizes CT and MRI imaging, multiple treatment fields arranged to maximize radiation dose to target area yet achieve maximum normal tissue sparing
- Concomitant radiation therapy and chemotherapy (Chemoradiation)
- **Hyperfractionation**
- **Neutron beam therapy:** 'Heavy' neutron particle that result in greater direct mechanisms of injury, less dependence on cell cycling and proliferation; however, less repair of sublethal damage by normal tissue.

Preoperative Radiation Therapy

Advantages: May reduce tumor bulk, which may cause inoperable lesions to become operable, reduce surgical excision area, or cure (organ preservation); requires smaller portals than postoperative radiation therapy; microscopic tumor is more sensitive than postoperative residual tumor (microscopic disease may be in scar tissue, therefore, more hypoxic).

Disadvantages: Increased difficulty in operating in irradiated tissue due to fibrosis, which makes the clinical assessment more difficult and the tissue planes are lost, which makes the dissection more difficult, increased postoperative complications (wound infections, carotid blowout).

Postoperative Radiation Therapy

Advantages: Allows for adequate postoperative healing prior to beginning adjuvant therapy, accurate assessment of pathologic staging and factors for recurrence.

Disadvantages: Requires higher dose of radiation due to hypoxia in operated tissue, microscopic disease may be within scar tissue resulting in decreased radiosensitivity, requires larger fields than preoperative radiation therapy.

Advantages of Radiotherapy

- No tissue defect causing final or cosmetic problem
- Mortality rate less than in surgery
- Both local and regional diseases are taken care simultaneously.

Side Effects

Cutaneous reactions: May result in dryness, erythema, hyperpigmentation, desquamation, telangiectasias, or subcutaneous fibrosis; Rx: skin moisturizers, mild skin cleaning, oral diphenhydramine (pruritis), corticosteroid creams.

Mucositis: Presents as tender, erythematous and swollen mucous membranes; increased risk of coexisting infections with *Candida*, herpes simplex virus and other bacteria; may result in sepsis for severe cases; Rx: aggressive oral hygiene (oral irrigations), adjust dental appliances, smoking and alcohol cessation, cool food, nutritional supplements, oral and topical anesthetics (viscous lidocaine, diphenhydramine, aluminum hydroxide-magnesium hydroxide-simethicone mixture).

- **Alopecia:** Temporary hair loss may occur in radiation field, may be permanent at higher doses.
- **Xerostomia/dental caries:** Salivary acinar cells are extremely sensitive to radiation therapy causing irreversible xerostomia, increased risk of dental caries, change in taste and tenacious oral secretions; Rx: fluids with meals, artificial saliva, pilocarpine, fluoride treatment, aggressive oral hygiene (prevent with preoperative dental evaluation).
- **Osteoradionecrosis of the mandible/cartilage radionecrosis of the larynx:** Hypocellularity, hypovascularity, and ischemia of tissue (not infectious); Rx: initially should treat conservatively with antibiotics, analgesics, meticulous oral hygiene and soft diet; debridement may be required; may also consider hyperbaric oxygen therapy.
- **Radiation induced cancer:** Increased risk of thyroid, salivary gland cancer, leukemia, sarcomas (may have lag period of 20 years).
- **Otologic sequelae:** Increased incidence of otitis externa, sterile otitis media and auricular chondritis.

CACHEXIA IN MALIGNANCY

Cancer cachexia occurs most frequently in malignancy and accounts for more than 20 percent of cancer deaths. Patients with cancers of oral cavity and upper aerodigestive tract are most likely to suffer from substantial weight loss (Figs 30.76 and 30.77). The word *'cachexia'* comes from the Greek words *'kakos'* and *'hexis'*, meaning 'bad conditions'. Cachexia is a complex metabolic status with progressive weight loss and depletion of host reserves of adipose tissue and skeletal muscle. Cachexia should be suspected if involuntary weight loss greater than 5 percent of premorbid weight occurs within a

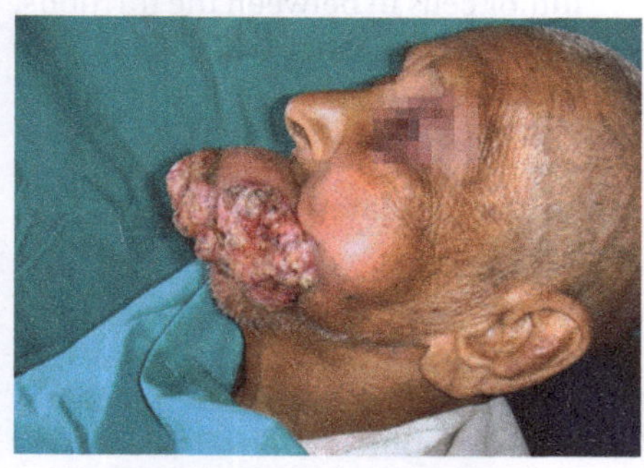

Fig. 30.76: Cachexia of malignancy

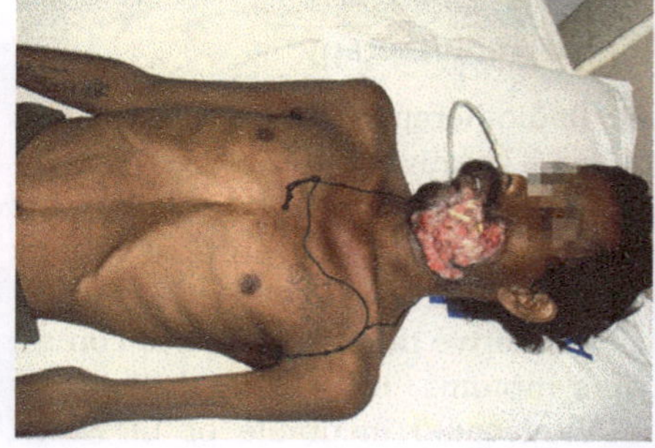

Fig. 30.77: Severe cachexia of malignancy

6-month period. Cachexia represents the clinical consequence of a chronic, systemic inflammatory response, with high hepatic synthesis of acute-phase proteins resulting in depletion of essential amino acids. In contrast, in starvation only fat metabolism is increased, while the organism tries to conserve lean body mass. In addition to metabolic changes, cachexia is often associated with anorexia. In cancer patients there can be mechanical interference such as obstructions, as well as treatment-related toxicity. In patients receiving chemotherapy or radiation, subsequent nausea, vomiting and diarrhea can contribute to weight loss. But the lack of nutrients alone cannot explain the metabolic changes seen in cachexia.

Theories Related to Pathophysiology of Cachexia

The first theory is the pathological alteration of control cycles. Food intake is regulated through a complex system of hormones and neuropeptides. Inui et al. demonstrated that *neuropeptide Y (NPY)*, the most potent feeding stimulatory peptide in this cycle, is deregulated in the hypothalamic orexigenic network, leading to decreased energy intake but high metabolic demand for nutrients. High levels of leptin, a hormone secreted by adipocytes, block the release of NPY. In cachexia the leptin feedback loop seems to become out of control, altering the neuropeptidergic control cycles.[53]

The second theory is based on the idea that tumor-derived factors maintain the cachectic syndrome. Tisdale et al.[54] postulated a factor that was extracted from the urine of cachectic patients and which induces protein degradation in skeletal muscle by upregulation of the ubiquitin-proteasome pathway. This proteolysis-inducing factor (PIF) is closely related to weight loss in cachexia and in a recent study, it was shown that PIF is produced in human colon cancer.

A second factor extracted from the urine of cachectic patients is the lipid mobilizing factor (LMF). It is closely related to weight loss and induces lipolysis in murine adipocytes. A recent study showed that this lipolytic process is mediated through the β-3 adrenoceptors. LMF produces a significant increase in the mitochondrial uncoupling proteins (UCPs) in brown adipose tissue, skeletal muscle and liver.

Despite the controversial discussion of cachexia-inducing mechanisms uncertainty over what causes cachexia, it is quite clear that proinflammatory cytokines are linked to all pathways that induce cachexia. As mentioned, cachexia is associated with a chronic systemic inflammatory response and the elevation of acute phase proteins. High serum levels of IL-1, IL-6 and INF gamma are present in many cancer patients and the levels of these cytokines seem to correlate with tumor progression.

These cytokines stimulate the expression of leptin and/or mimic the hypothalamic effect of negative feedback from leptin by disarranging the signaling pathway of NPY, resulting in long-term inhibition of food intake. IL-1 antagonizes NPY-induced feeding in rats and disrupts the orexigenic pathway of NPY. On the other hand, central corticotropin-releasing factor (CRF), which is upregulated by IL-1, seems to influence satiety and is a potent anorexigenic signal.

Treatment

Supportive Care

In clinical trials, nutritional supplementation and dietary counselling failed to increase body weight. Several appetite-stimulating drugs have been tested in an attempt to increase the food intake of cachexia patients, but most of them had little or no effect on body weight.

Patients with anorexia from decreased physical activity, concomitant infection and toxicities from chemotherapy and radiotherapy are managed symptomatically for maintenance of nutritional status and quality of life. Such management includes the use of mouthwash for stomatitis, frequent small volume feedings, antiemetics, antibiotics, transfusions of blood components and/or oral, and parenteral nutritional supplement.

For the correction of cancer related malnutrition, enteral and parenteral administration of nutrient solutions has been widely used. In patients with oropharyngeal dysfunction from head and neck neoplasm or esophageal obstruction, blenderized food and liquid supplement can often achieve an adequate level of nutritional repletion, although percutaneous gastrostomy or jejunostomy offer bypass-feeding methodology when necessary. For patients who cannot tolerate the use of the gastrointestinal tract because of nausea, vomiting, obstruction, malabsorption, or absence, it may be necessary to begin total parenteral nutrition (TPN, *hyperalimentation*).

Parenteral nutritional support is an intensive method of clinical care, requiring physicians, pharmacists, dieticians and experienced nurses who, as a team, must make daily rounds to evaluate nutritional status and check for complications. Complications from parenteral nutrition can be multiple. Among them, the complications from infection are the most problematic when long-term nutritional support is used. In addition, the costs of nutrient solutions, prolonged hospitalization, and/or frequent visits to a special clinic or office are formidable medical and financial burdens.

Newer Pharmacotherapy

Many trials have been performed in the search for a treatment for cachexia, but most therapies have not fulfilled expectations. Currently, eicosapentaenoic acid is being tested in cachectic patients.[55] Eicosapentaenoic acid seems to interfere with the signaling pathway of PIF and first results are promising. Future therapies may consist of anticatabolic and anabolic drugs in combination with appetite stimulants.

BASAL CELL CARCINOMA

Basal cell carcinoma is a nonmelanocytic, low grade, slow growing and locally invasive carcinoma of the basal layer of the epidermis. Basal cell carcinoma is particularly liable to occur in fair and dry skinned people and it typically appears on sun-exposed skin and rarely metastasize.

Basal cell carcinomas have a typical body distribution: 70 percent on head (most frequently on face), 25 percent on trunk, and 5 percent on penis, vulva, or perianal skin.[56]

Etiology

The exact cause of basal cell carcinoma is unknown. Environmental and genetic factors that are believed to predispose patients to basal cell carcinoma skin cancer. Basal cell carcinoma has a high frequency in older men who have a long history of unprotected exposure to ultraviolet (UV) light. In a few patients, the contributing factors are contact with arsenic,[57] tar, coal, paraffin,[58] certain types of industrial oil, radiation exposure, scars (i.e. burn complications), xeroderma pigmentosum,[59] vaccinations, or even tattoos.

- **Exposure to sunlight:** The sunlight is the most frequent association and risk is associated with the amount and nature of accumulated sun exposure over a lifetime, especially during childhood. UVB, 290 to 320 nm, which causes sunburn, is believed to play a greater role in the development of basal cell carcinoma than UVA.
- **Gene mutations:** Recent studies demonstrate a high incidence of p53 gene mutations in basal cell carcinoma. Researchers speculate that UV sunlight may play an important role in the genesis of this mutation; however, genetic involvement has been demonstrated on chromosome 9 only in patients with familial basal cell nevus syndrome.
- **Exposure to artificial ultraviolet light** (e.g. tanning booths, ultraviolet light therapy).
- **Ionizing radiation exposure** (e.g. X-ray therapy for acne).
- **Arsenic exposure through ingestion:** Arsenic was used as a medicinal agent, predominantly Fowler's solution of potassium arsenite, which was used to treat many disorders, including asthma and psoriasis. A contaminated water source has been the most common source of arsenic ingestion.
- **Immunosuppression:** A modest increase in the lifetime risk of basal cell carcinoma has been noted in chronically immunosuppressed patients, such as recipients of organ or stem cell transplants.
- **Xeroderma pigmentosum:** This autosomal recessive disease results in the inability to repair UV-induced DNA damage. Pigmentary changes are seen early in life followed by the development of basal cell carcinoma, squamous cell carcinoma and malignant melanoma. Other features include corneal opacities, eventual blindness and neurological deficits.

Basal cell carcinoma can be divided into three groups, based on location and difficulty of therapy:

1. *Superficial basal cell carcinoma*, or some might consider to be equivalent to *in situ*. Very responsive to topical chemotherapy such as Aldara, or fluorouracil. It is the only type of basal cell cancer that can be effectively treated with topical chemotherapy.
2. *Infiltrative basal cell carcinoma*, which often encompasses morpheaform and micronodular basal cell cancer. More difficult to treat with conservative treatment methods such as electrodessiccation and currettage, or with currettage alone.
3. *Nodular basal cell carcinoma*, which essentially include most the remaining categories of basal cell cancer. It is not unusual to encounter morphologic features of several variants of basal cell cancer in the same tumor.

Clinical Features

- Elderly people are usually affected, especially in middle or late age.
- Males are more affected than females.
- Particulary seen in whites residing in tropical countries.
- Grow slowly over a course of years.
- It is particularly prevelant in Australia and is confined to white people of the labor class whose skin is exposed to bright sunlight of high actinic value.
- Frequently multiple and multiple growth may be confined to one area or may occur in different areas.
- 90 percent of the basal cell carcinoma is seen in the face above a line from corner of the mouth to the lobule of the ear, the commonest site being around the inner canthus of the eye (Figs 30.78A and B). The common sites are:
  - Inner canthus of the eye
  - Outer canthus of the eye
  - Nose
  - On and around nasolabial fold
  - On the forehead—more common in females.

Rodent ulcer is seen more commonly in places of the face over where tear roll down. That is why it is often called 'tear cancer'.

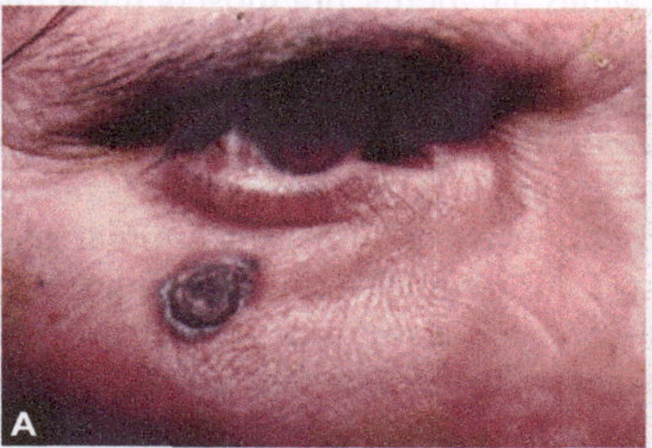

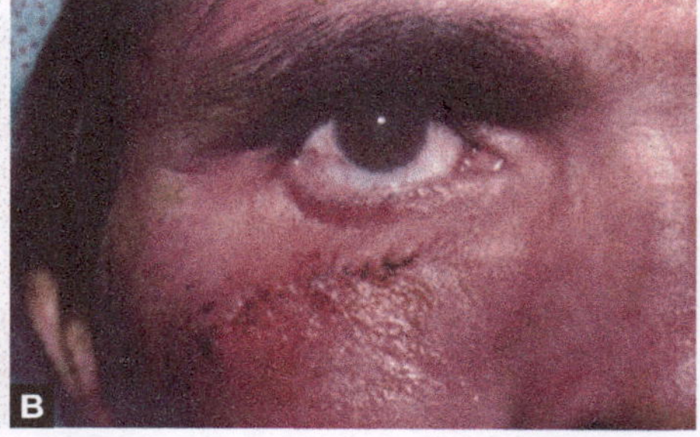

Figs 30.78A and B: Basal cell carcinoma in the infraorbital area treated by wide local excision

- Principle complaint is persisting lesion—either as a nodule or an ulcer. It is not painful in the beginning, though it may itch. The lesion grow slowly and show little bleeding. If untreated, it may become big and deep. It may then cause pain and bleeding and become infected.
- The tumor always starts as nodule. Gradually, the center of the nodule dies and an ulcer results. Such a ulcer has rolled edges, i.e. raised and rounded. As the growth spreads, the shape of the ulcer becomes irregular. An irregular raised edge around a flat white scar is sometimes called field fire BCC.
- Appears as deeply eroding ulcer with typical rolled edges, often beaded and floor shows scabbing over some areas and breaking at the others and is covered with coat of dried serum and epithelial cells.
- Regional lymph nodes are usually not involved.
- Although it is called rodent ulcer, many of the lesions are non-ulcerated. Clinical presentation of basal cell carcinoma varies by type:
  - **Nodular basal cell carcinoma:** Nodular basal cell carcinoma is the most common type of basal cell carcinoma and usually presents as a round, pearly, flesh-colored papule with telangiectases. As it enlarges, it frequently ulcerates centrally, leaving a raised, pearly border with telangiectases.
  - **Cystic basal cell carcinoma:** An uncommon variant of nodular basal cell carcinoma, cystic basal cell carcinoma is often indistinguishable from nodular basal cell carcinoma clinically, although it might have a polypoid appearance. Typically, a bluish-gray cyst-like lesion is observed. The cystic center of these tumors is filled with clear mucin that has a gelatin-like consistency.
  - **Pigmented basal cell carcinoma:** Pigmented basal cell carcinoma is an uncommon variant of nodular basal cell carcinoma that has brown-black macules in some or all areas, often making it difficult to differentiate from melanoma. Typically, some areas of these tumors do not retain pigment; pearly, raised borders with telangiectases that are typical of a nodular basal cell carcinoma can be observed. This aids clinically in differentiating this tumor from a melanoma.
  - **Morpheaform (sclerosing) basal cell carcinoma:** It is an uncommon variant in which tumor cells induce a proliferation of fibroblasts within the dermis and an increased collagen deposition (sclerosis) that clinically resembles a scar. The tumor appears as a white or yellow, waxy, sclerotic plaque that rarely ulcerates. The morpheaform subtype is the most difficult subtype to diagnose. Because the tumor infiltrates in thin strands between collagen fibers, treatment is difficult and the clinical margins are difficult to distinguish. Mohs micrographic surgery is the treatment of choice for this type of basal cell carcinoma.
  - **Superficial basal cell carcinoma:** It is often multiple, most often developing on the upper trunk or shoulders. It grows slowly and appears clinically as an erythematous, well-circumscribed patch or plaque, often with a whitish scale. Occasionally, minute eschars may appear within the patch or plaque. The tumor appears multicentric, with areas of clinically normal skin intervening among clinically involved areas.
  - **Field fire or forest fire or geographic variety:** With advancing edges and healing center. It has irregular raised edge around flat white scar.

About two-thirds of basal cell carcinomas occur on sun-exposed areas of the body. One-third occurs on areas of the body that are not exposed to sunlight, emphasizing the genetic susceptibility of basal cell cancer patients.

Pathophysiology

Although the exact etiology of basal cell carcinoma is unknown, a well-established relationship exists between basal cell carcinoma and the pilosebaceous units, as tumors are most often discovered on hair-bearing areas. Tumors are currently believed to arise from pluripotent cells (which have the capacity to form hair), sebaceous glands and apocrine glands, Tumors usually arise from the epidermis or the outer root sheath of a hair follicle.

Sun light exposure leads to the formation of thymine dimers, a form of DNA damage. While DNA repair removes most UV-induced damage, not all crosslinks are excised. There is, therefore, cumulative DNA damage leading to mutations. Apart from the mutagenesis, sunlight depresses the local immune system, possibly decreasing immune surveillance for new tumor cells.

Basal-cell carcinoma also develops as a result of basal-cell nevus syndrome, or Gorlin syndrome.

Histologic Findings

Usually, basal cell carcinomas are well differentiated and cells appear histologically similar to basal cells of epidermis. It consists of densely packed islands of darkly stained cells, which extend down from the epidermis, although no connection with the epidermis may be seen. The cells on the periphery of the islands are more deeply stained and have 'palisade' arrangement. There are no cell rests or keratinization. Prickle cells are also absent. Mitotic figures are usually absent. Stromal component is composed of benign fibrovascular tissue and chronic inflammatory cells.

Histologically, basal cell carcinoma is divided into two categories: Undifferentiated and differentiated. Basal cell carcinoma with little or no differentiation is referred to as solid basal cell carcinoma and includes pigmented basal cell carcinoma, superficial basal cell carcinoma, sclerosing basal cell carcinoma and infiltrative basal cell carcinoma (a histologic subtype). Differentiated basal cell carcinoma often has slight differentiation toward cutaneous appendages, including hair (keratotic basal cell carcinoma), sebaceous glands (basal cell carcinoma with sebaceous differentiation), or tubular glands (adenoid basal cell carcinoma). Noduloulcerative (nodular) basal cell carcinoma is usually differentiated. Histologic types can be summarized as follows:[60]

- Nodular or noduloulcerative basal cell carcinoma, which is the most common type, generally consists of large, round or oval tumor islands within the dermis, often with an epidermal attachment. Artificial retraction of the tumor islands from the surrounding stroma is commonly seen.
- Micronodular basal cell carcinoma is similar to the noduloulcerative type, although the tumor islands are small (often < 15 cells in diameter).
- Pigmented basal cell carcinoma consists of large, round or oval tumor islands containing large amounts of melanin within melanocytes and melanophages.
- Cystic basal cell carcinoma consists of large, round or oval tumor islands within the dermis with mucin present within the center of the island.
- Infiltrative basal cell carcinoma is a common type of basal cell carcinoma in which strands of basaloid tumor cells are seen infiltrating between collagen bundles.
- Morpheaform or sclerosing basal cell carcinoma consists of elongated strands of basaloid cells that lead to the adjacent formation of a dense fibrous stroma.
- Superficial basal cell carcinoma consists of buds of basophilic cells within the papillary and occasionally superficial reticular dermis, but they are attached to the epidermis.

Clinical Staging

- **Stage 0:** Cancer involves only the epidermis and has not spread to the dermis.
- **Stage I:** Cancer is not large (i.e. < 2 cm) and has not spread to the lymph nodes or other organs.
- **Stage II:** The cancer is large (i.e. > 2 cm), but has not spread to lymph nodes or other organs.
- **Stage III:** The cancer has spread to tissues beneath the skin (e.g. muscle, bone, cartilage) and/or has spread to regional lymph nodes, but has not spread to other organs.
- **Stage IV:** The cancer can be any size and has spread to other organs.

Treatment

Standard surgical excision with either frozen section histology, or parafin embedded fixed tissue pathology. This is the preferred method for removal of most BCCs. The cure rate for this method is totally dependent on the surgical margin. Unlike the SCC, when standard surgical margin of 4 mm or more[61] is taken, a high cure rate can be achieved with excision.[62] A weakness with standard surgical excision is the high recurrence rate of basal cell cancers of the face, especially around eyelids, nose and facial structures[63] (Figs 30.79 and 30.80). On the face, or on recurrent basal cell cancer after previous surgery, complete circumferential peripheral and deep margin assessment using

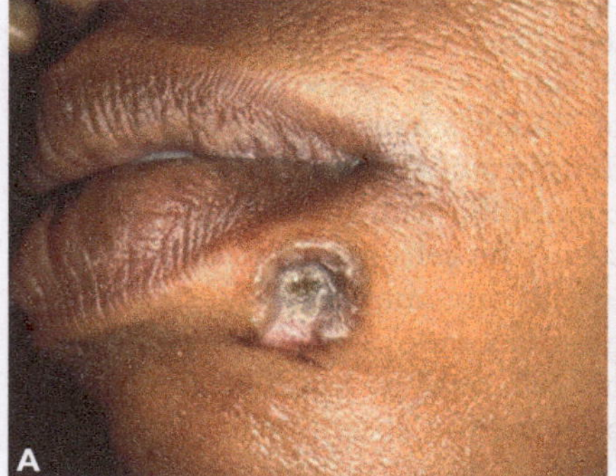

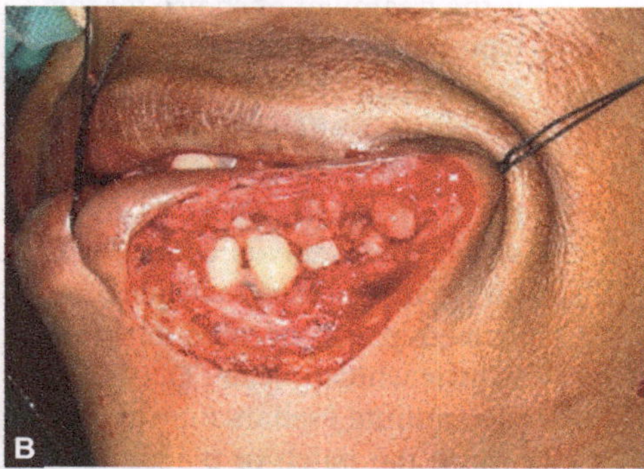

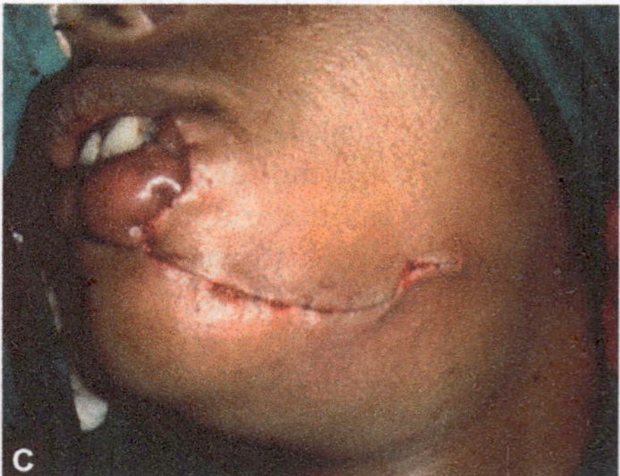

Figs 30.79A to C: Surgical excision of basal cell carcinoma of lower lip and reconstruction with local flap

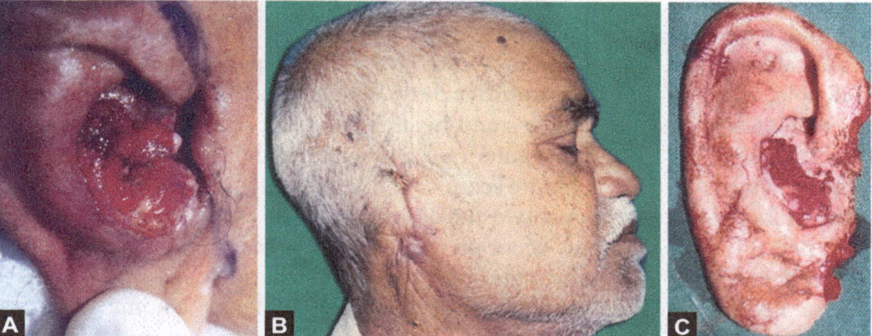

Figs 30.80A to C: Basal cell carcinoma of pinna

frozen section histology is employed[64] (Figs 30.79A to C and 30.80A to C).

Moh's Surgery

Moh's surgery[65] (or Moh's micrographic surgery) is an outpatient procedure in which the tumor is surgically excised and then immediately examined under a microscope. It is claimed to have the highest cure rate of 97 to 99.8 percent by some individuals.[66] The base and edges are microscopically examined to verify sufficient margins before the surgical repair of the site. If the margins are insufficient, more is removed from the patient, until the margins are sufficient.

Chemotherapy

Some superficial cancers respond to local therapy with 5-fluorouracil, a chemotherapy agent. Topical treatment with 5 percent imiquimod cream, with five applications per week for 6 weeks has a reported 70 to 90 percent success rate at reducing, even removing, the BCC (basal cell carcinoma). Chemotherapy often follows Mohs surgery to eliminate the residual superficial basal cell carcinoma after the invasive portion is removed.

Immunotherapy

Immunotherapy research suggests that treatment using *Euphorbia peplus*, may be effective.

Radiation

Radiation therapy is appropriate for all forms of BCC as adequate doses will eradicate the disease. Although radiotherapy is generally used in older patients who are not candidates for surgery.

Photodynamic Therapy

Photodynamic therapy is a new modality for treatment of basal cell carcinoma, which is administrated by application of photosensitizers to the target area. When these molecules are activated by light, they become toxic; therefore, destroy the target cells, e.g. methyl aminolevulinate.

Cryosurgery

Cryosurgery is an old modality for the treatment of many skin cancers. When accurately utilized with a temperature probe and cryotherapy instruments, it can result in very good cure rate. Disadvantages include lack of margin control, tissue necrosis, over or under treatment of the tumor and long recovery time.

Electrodessication and Curettage

Electrodessication and curettage (EDC) is accomplished by using a round knife, or curette, to scrape away the soft cancer. The skin is then burned with an electric current. This further softens the skin, allowing for the knife to cut more deeply with the next layer of curettage. The cycle is repeated, with a safety margin of curettage of normal skin around the visible tumor. This cycle is repeated 3 to 5 times and the free skin margin treated is usually 4 to 6 mm. Cure rate is very much user dependent and depends on the size and type of tumor. Infiltrative or morpheaform BCCs can be difficult to eradicate with EDC. Generally, this method is used on cosmetically unimportant areas like the trunk.

Malignant Melanoma

Oral melanomas are uncommon and they are thought to arise primarily from melanocytes in the basal layer of the squamous mucosa. Melanocytic density has a regional variation. Facial skin has the greatest number of melanocytes. In the oral mucosa, melanocytes are observed in a ratio of about 1 melanocyte to 10 basal cells. Pigmented entities are relatively common in the oral mucosa and arise from intrinsic and extrinsic sources. Conditions such as melanotic macules, smoker's melanosis, amalgam and graphite tattoos, racial pigmentation, and vascular blood-related pigments occur with some frequency. Addison disease and Peutz-Jeghers syndrome also appear in perioral and oral locations as pigmented macules. Oral pigmentations may range from light brown to blue-black, red, or purple. The color depends on the source of the pigment and the depth of the pigment from which the color is derived. Melanin is brown, yet it imparts a blue, green, or brown color to the eye. This effect is due to the physical properties of light absorption and reflection described by the Tyndall light phenomenon or effect. Oral conditions with increased melanin pigmentation are common; however, melanocytic hyperplasias are rare.

In contrast to cutaneous melanomas, which are etiologically linked to sun exposure, risk factors for mucosal melanomas are unknown. These melanomas have no apparent relationship to chemical, thermal, or physical events (e.g. smoking; alcohol intake; poor oral hygiene; irritation from teeth, dentures, or other oral appliances) to which the oral mucosa constantly is exposed. Although benign, intraoral melanocytic proliferations (nevi) occur and are potential sources of some oral melanomas; the sequence of events is poorly understood in the oral cavity. Currently, most oral melanomas are thought to arise *de novo*.

Although most melanomas occur on skin, they may develop at any site where melanocytes are present.[67] Malignant-melanoma is a neoplasm of epidermal melanocytes in that OMM has a more aggressive course, because tumors tend to metastasize or locally invade tissue more readily than other malignant tumors in oral region.[68]

In oral cavity, the most common site is palate (32%), followed by maxillary gingiva (16%) (Fig. 30.79A and B); mandibular gingiva (7%), buccal mucosa (7%), lips (7%), and alveolar gingiva (5%).[69,70] In one-third of cases, melanosis precedes the tumor, thus pigmented oral lesions should be viewed with suspicion and biopsy is mandatory when clinical diagnosis is uncertain. Oral melanoma reportedly occurs more commonly in the Japanese than in other groups. Oral malignant melanoma, although rare in whites, is still more common in whites than in the pigmented races. The incidence of primary OMM has been between 0.2 to 8 percent of all melanomas. Oral melanoma occurs more often in males (2.8:1) in all ages.[71] Oral malignant melanoma is largely a disease of those older than 40 years, and it is rare in patients younger than 20 years. The average patient age at diagnosis is 56 years. Oral malignant melanoma is commonly diagnosed in men aged 51 to 60 years, whereas it is commonly diagnosed in females aged 61 to 70 years.

Clinical Features

- Because oral malignant melanomas are often clinically silent, they can be confused with a number of asymptomatic, benign, pigmented lesions.
- Oral melanomas are largely macular, but nodular and even pedunculated lesions occur.
- Pain, ulceration, and bleeding are rare in oral melanoma until late in the disease.
- The pigmentation varies from dark brown to blue-black; however, mucosa-colored and white lesions are occasionally noted, and erythema is observed when the lesions are inflamed.
- The palate and maxillary gingiva are involved in approximately 80 percent of patients, but buccal mucosa, mandibular gingiva, and tongue lesions are also identified.
- The oral mucosa is primarily involved in fewer than 1 percent of melanomas.
- Metastatic melanoma most frequently affects the mandible, tongue, and buccal mucosa.
- Features of long-standing lesions include elevation, color variegation, ulceration, and satellite lesions that may have the appearance of physiologic pigmentation.
- A neck mass may be present, indicating regional metastasis; however, this is rare unless the primary tumor is extensive.

Evaluation

The evaluation is done following imaging techniques:

- Imaging studies, such as computed tomography (CT), may be of benefit in determining the extent of the tumor when contrast enhancement is used.
- Contrast-enhanced CT can be used to determine the extent of the melanoma and whether local, regional, or lymph node metastasis is present.
- Studies such as bone scanning with a gadolinium-based agent and chest radiography can be beneficial in assessing metastasis.
- Magnetic resonance imaging (MRI) is used to diagnose melanoma in soft tissue.

Biopsy is mandatory for establishing the diagnosis.

Histologically, primary OMM is indistinguishable from cutaneous-melanoma; as its pathogenesis differs from latter which causes them to be more aggressive, and may permit blood vessel invasion, hematogenous dissemination early in the course of the disease. Malignant-melanoma metastasizes via lymphatic and vascular channels, while cutaneous-melanoma spreads to four main lymph nodes intraparotid, cervical, axillary, and ilioinguinal.[72] Primary OMM has marked propensity to metastasize locally to submucosa and to regional lymph nodes.[73] However, distant metastases occur to lungs, brain, liver, kidneys, and bones. Mucosal-melanoma may be primary or metastatic from other locations in the body, it is therefore important to rule out the possibility of a primary malignant-melanotic lesion. The criteria for diagnosis of a primary OMM are following:

- Demonstration of clinical and microscopic tumor in the oral mucosa,
- Presence of junctional activity in lesion, and
- Inability to show any other primary site.

The difficulty of applying cutaneous-melanoma classification to oral-melanomas has been noted by several investigators.[74] The use of Clark's criteria for degree-of-invasion and prognosis are not applicable to oral-melanomas as there is no intraoral counterpart for reticular and papillary dermis.[75] OMM were classified as:

- Pigmented-nodular
- Non-pigmented nodular
- Pigmented-macular
- Pigmented-mixed and
- Non-pigmented mixed type.

Staging

The American Joint Committee on Cancer does not have published guidelines for the staging of oral malignant melanomas. Most practitioners use general clinical stages in the assessment of oral mucosal melanoma as follows:

- **Stage I:** Localized disease
- **Stage II:** Regional lymph node metastasis
- **Stage III:** Distant metastasis
- Tumor thickness and lymph node metastasis are reliable prognostic indicators
- Lesions thinner than 0.75 mm rarely metastasize, but they do have the potential to do so. On occasion, a small primary lesion is discovered after a symptomatic lymph node is harvested.

Histologic Findings

Although any of the features of cutaneous malignancy can be found, most oral melanomas have characteristics of the acral lentiginous (mucosal lentiginous) and, occasionally, superficial spreading types.

The malignant cells often nest or cluster in groups in an organoid fashion; however, single cells can predominate. The melanoma cells have large nuclei, often with prominent nucleoli, and show nuclear pseudoinclusions due to nuclear membrane irregularity. The abundant cytoplasm may be uniformly eosinophilic or optically clear. Occasionally, the cells become spindled or neurotize in areas. This finding is interpreted as a more aggressive feature, compared with findings of the round or polygonal cell varieties. In the oral mucosa, the prognosis is dismal for patients with any type of malignant cell.

Melanomas have a number of histopathologic mimics, including poorly differentiated carcinomas and anaplastic large-cell lymphomas. Differentiation requires the use of immunohistochemical techniques to highlight intermediate filaments or antigens specific for a particular cell line.

Leukocyte common antigen and Ki-1 are used to identify the lymphocytic lesions. Cytokeratin markers, often cocktails of high- and low-molecular-weight cytokeratins, can be used to help in the identification of epithelial malignancies.

S-100 protein and homatropine methylbromide (HMB-45) antigen positivity are characteristic of, although not specific for, melanoma. S-100 protein is frequently used to highlight the spindled, more neural-appearing melanocytes, whereas HMB-45 is used to identify the round cells. Melanomas, unlike epithelial lesions, are identified by using vimentin, a marker of mesenchymal cells. Recently, microphthalmic transcription factor, tyrosinase, and melano-A immunostains have been used to highlight melanocytes. The inclusion of these stains in a panel of stains for melanoma may be beneficial.

In the test named "rubbing-with-gauze" the surface of lesion was rubbed with a piece of gauze and was considered positive if gauze stained brown/black due to presence of melanin-laden cells on epithelial surfaces; however, a negative result does not exclude this neoplasm. The metastatic disease also show brown of black discoloration of the lymph nodes and the visceral organs at the site of metastasis (Fig 30.82B).

In one-third of cases, melanosis precedes the tumor, thus pigmented oral lesions should be viewed with suspicion and biopsy is mandatory when clinical diagnosis is uncertain. The mainstay of treatment is wide surgical resection aiming at complete resection of primary tumor and any positive cervical lymph nodes; however, this could also be in combination with chemo-radiotherapy or radiotherapy alone in inoperable tumors or in the elderly. The management of clinically negative nodes still remains controversial. Inspite of aggressive treatment modalities, survival in patients with advanced-stage-disease remains poor. Because of lack of data, the biological behavior of these lesions still remains unpredictable and its outcome is dismal, probably due to its long, 'silent' course.

The prognosis is generally poor, with a 3-year mortality rate higher than 50 percent. The survival of patients with mucosal-melanoma is less than cutaneous-melanomas.[69] Negative surgical margins and size of primary lesion do not appear to be predictive of outcome. The only clinical finding that appears to have definitive prognostic significance is presence of distant metastasis at the time of diagnosis.[75] In the case of primary oralmalignant melanoma arising from the maxillary gingiva, shown in Figures 30.81 and 30.82, a solitary metastatic lesion was detected within 2 months of surgery. The patient was administered chemotherapy but he died due to widespread distant metastasis, within one year of surgery, depicting the aggressive behavior of the tumor.

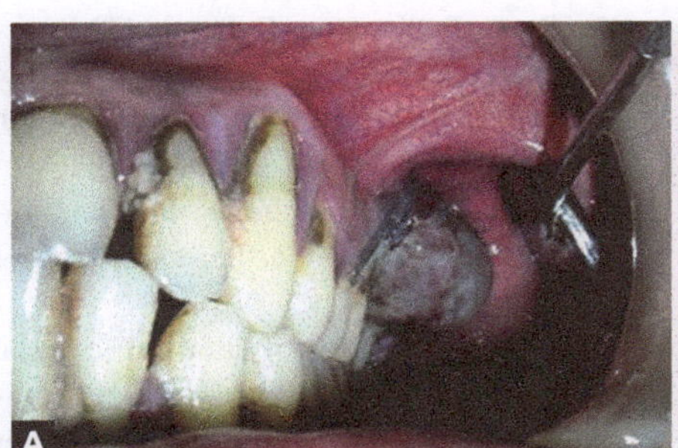

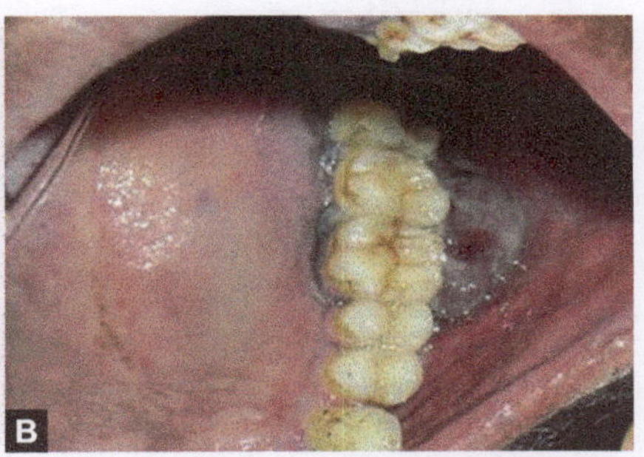

Figs 30.81A and B: (A) Primay oral malignant melanoma arising from maxillary gingiva; (B) Mirror image

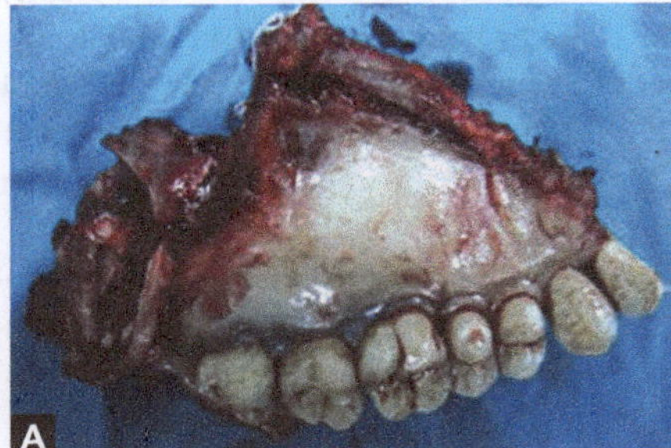

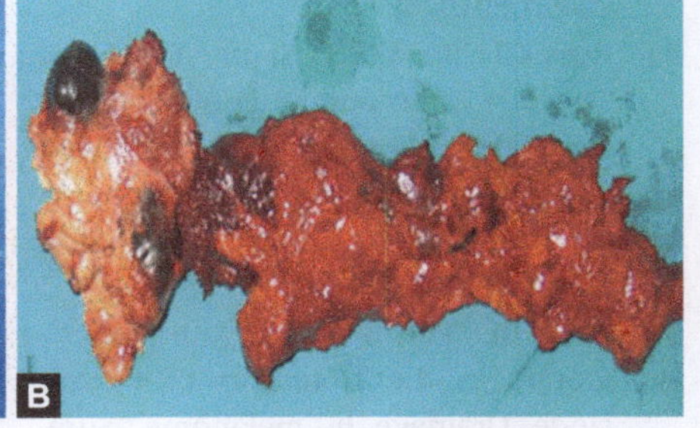

Figs 30.82A and B: (A) Resected specimen of maxilla; (B) Neck dissection block showing black lymph nodes due to metastatic disease.

REFERENCES

1. Shah JP, Singh B. Keynote comment: why the lack of progress for oral cancer? Lancet Oncol. 2006;7(5): 356-7.
2. Hawkins RJ, Wang EEL, Leake JL. Preventive health care, 1999 update: prevention of oral cancer mortality. J Can Dent Assoc. 1999;65.
3. Warnakulasuriya S. Global epidemiology of oral and oropharyngeal cancer. Oral Oncol. 2009;45(4):309-16.
4. Langdon JD, Rapidis AD, Harvey PW, et al. STNMP-a new classification for oral cancer. Br J Oral Surg. 1977;15(1): 49-54.
5. Langdon JD, Harvey PW, Rapidis AD, et al. Oral cancer: The behaviour and response to treatment of 194 cases. J Maxillo Fac Surg. 1977;51227-37.
6. Hamada GS, et al. Comparative epiderniology of oral cancer in Brazil and India. Tokai J Exp. Clin Med. 1991; 16(1):63-72.
7. Abdul Wahid. Pattern of carcinoma of oral cavity reporting at dental department of Ayub medical college. J Ayub Med Coll Abbottabad. 2005; 17(1):65-6.
8. Pathak KA, Nason R, Talole S, et al. Cancer of the buccal mucosa: a tale of two continents. Int J Oral Maxillafac Surg. 2009;38(2):146-50.
9. Siriwardena B. Demographic, aetiological and survival differences of oral squamous cell carcinoma in the young and the old in Sri Lanka. Oral Oncol. 2006;42(8):831-6.

10. Gupta PC, Mehta FS, Pindborg JJ. Mortality among reverse chutta smokers in south India. Br Med J (Clin Res Ed). 1984;289(6449):865-6.
11. Bhavana J Dave. Role of areca nut consumption in the cause of oral cancers. A cytogenetic assessment. Cancer. 1992;70(5):1017-23.
12. Yi-Shan Tsai. Arecoline, a major alkaloid of areca nut, inhibits p53, represses DNA repair, and triggers DNA damage response in human epithelial cells. Toxicology. 2008;249(2-3):230-7.
13. Ramesha Rao A, Padma Das. Evaluation of the carcinogenicity of different preparations of areca nut in mice. Int J Cancer. 2006;43(4):728-32.
14. Graham R. Ogden. Alcohol and oral cancer. Alcohol. 2005;35(3):169-73.
15. Lund CL. Syphilis in relation to cancer of the buccal mucosa. J Med. 1933; 209:131-4.
16. Lozada-Nur F. Oral lichen planus and oral cancer: Is there enough epidemiologic evidence? Oral Surg Oral Med Oral Pathol Oral Radiol Endod. 2000; 89(3):265-6.
17. IARC monographs on the evaluation of carcinogenic risks to humans: Solar and ultraviolet radiation. IARC Monogr Eval Carcinog Risks hum. 1992;55:01-316.
18. Ramzi S Cotran, Stanley L Robbins. Basic Pathology, 6th edition. W.B. Saunders Company, New York, 1997.
19. Lindberg R. Distribution of cervical lymph node metastases from squamous cell carcinoma of the upper respiratory and digestive tracts. Cancer. 1972;29(6): 1446-9.
20. Denoix PF. The TNM staging system. Bull Inst Nat Hyg (Paris). 1952;7:743.
21. Sobin LH, Wittekind C. TNM Classification of Malignant Tumours, 6th edition. Hoboken, New Jersey: John Wiley and Sons; 2002.
22. Marx RE, Stern D. Oral and maxillofacial pathology: a rationale for diagnosis and treatment. Hanover Park (IL): Quintessence Publishing; 2003.pp.284-9.
23. Lawrence E. Ginsberg. The Role of Diagnostic Imaging in Identifying Cervical Metastases in Oral Cavity Cancer. Oral Cancer Metastasis. New York: Springer. 2010:pp.33-48.
24. Hodder SC, Evans RM, Patton DW, et al. Ultrasound and fine needle aspiration cytology in the staging of neck lymph nodes in oral squamous cell carcinoma. Br J Oral Maxillofacial Surg. 2000;38(5):430-36.
25. Lee RE, et al. Lymph node examination by FNA in patients with known or suspected malignancy. Acta cytological. 1987;31:563-71.
26. Sarvanan Y. Computed tomography and ultrasonographic evaluation of metastatic cervical lymph nodes with surgicoclinicopathologic correlation. J Laryngol Otol. 2002;116(3):194-9.
27. Miwako Oomori. Dynamic magnetic resonance imaging of cervical lymph nodes in patients with oral cancer: utility of the small region of interest method in evaluating the architecture of cervical lymph nodes. Oral Radiol. 2008;24(1).
28. Ding ZX, Liang BL, Shen J, et al. Magnetic resonance imaging diagnosis of cervical lymph node metastasis from lingual squamous cell carcinoma. Ai Zheng. 2005;24(2):199-203.
29. Alex JC, Krag DN. The gamma-probe-guided resection of radiolabeled primary lymph nodes. Surg Oncol Clin N Am. 1996;5(1):33-41.
30. Vigili MG, Tartaglione G, Rahimi S, et al. Lymphoscintigraphy and radioguided sentinel node biopsy in oral cavity squamous cell carcinoma: same day protocol. Eur Arch Otorhinolaryngol. 2007;264(2):163-7.
31. KT Pitman. Sentinel lymph node biopsy in head and neck cancer. Oral Oncol. 2003;39(4):343.
32. Stoeckli SJ, Pfaltz M, Ross G, et al. The second international conference on sentinel node biopsy in mucosal head and neck cancer. Ann Surg Oncol. 2005;12:919-24.
33. Ross GL, Shoaib T, Soutar DS, et al. The first international conference on sentinel node biopsy in mucosal head and neck cancer and adoption of a multicenter trial protocol. Ann Surg Oncol. 2002;9:406-10.
34. Uren RF. The Role of Lymphoscintigraphy in the Detection of Lymph Node Drainage in melanoma. Surg. Oncol Clin N Am. 2006;15(2):285-300.
35. Nakazawa Mitsuhiro. The significance of histological malignancy grading and its clinical use in oral squamous cell carcinoma. Head and Neck Cancer. 2004;30(1):25-32.
36. Crile, George. Excision of cancer of the head and neck. J Am Med Assoc. 1906;47:1780-6.
37. Warren JC. Surgical Observations on Tumours, With Cases and Operations. London, England: John Churchill; 1839.
38. Chelius JM. A System of Surgery. Translated by John F. South, Volume 3. (Philadelphia: Lea and Blanchard. 1847.
39. Martin H. The case for prophylactic neck dissection. Cancer. 1951;4:92-7.
40. Bocca E, Pignataro O. A conservation technique in radical neck dissection. Ann Otol Rhinol Laryngol. 1967;76:975-87.
41. Shah JP (Ed). Cervical lymph nodes, in Color Atlas of Operative Techniques in Head and Neck Surgery: Face, Skull, and Neck. Orlando, FL. Grune & Stratton. 1987.pp.353-94
42. Suárez O, El problema de las metastasis linfáticas y alejadas del cáncer de laringe e hipofaringe. Rev Otorrinolaringol. 1963;23:83-99.
43. Bocca E, Pignataro O, Sasaki CT. Functional neck dissection: a description of operative technique. Arch Otolaryngol. 1980;106:524-7.
44. Rouviere H. Anatomie des lymphatiques de l'homme. Paris: Masson et Cie; 1932.
45. Lindberg R. Distribution of cervical lymph node metastases from squamous cell carcinoma of the upper respiratory and digestive tracts. Cancer. 1972;29:1446.
46. Skolnik E. Metastatic neck disease: Evaluation by computed tomography. Arch Otolaryngol. 1984;110:443-7.
47. Shah JP. Patterns of cervical lymph node metastasis from squamous carcinomas of the upper aerodigestive tract. Am J Surg. 1990;160(4):405-9.
48. Kadir Imre. Predictors of extracapsular spread in lymph node metastasis. European Archives of Oto-Rhino-Laryngology. 2008;265(3).
49. Scorza LB, Goldstein BJ, Mahraj RP. Modern management of chylous leak

following head and neck surgery: a discussion of percutaneous lymph-angiography-guided cannulation and embolization of the thoracic duct. Otolaryngol Clin North Am. 2008;41(6): 1231-40.

50. Takuji Tanaka. Chemoprevention of oral carcinogenesis. Eur J Cancer B Oral Oncol. 1995;31B(1):03-15.
51. Hong WK, Endicott J, Itri LM, et al. 13-cis-retinoic acid in the treatment of oral leukoplakia. N Engl J Med. 1986; 315:1501-05.
52. Hong WK, et al. Prevention of second primary tumors with isotretinoin in squamous-cell carcinoma of the head and neck. N Engl J Med. 1990; 23(323): 795-801.
53. Inui A. Neuropeptide Y: a key molecule in anorexia and cachexia in wasting disorders? Mol Med Today. 1999;5:79-85.
54. Tisdale MJ. Cachexia in cancer patients. Nat Rev Cancer. 2002;2:862-71.
55. Zuijdgeest-Van Leeuwen SD. Eicosapentaenoic acid ethyl ester supplementation in cachectic cancer patients and healthy subjects: effects on lipolysis and lipid oxidation. Clin Nutr, 2000;19(6):417-23.
56. Mulvany NJ, Allen DG. Differentiated intraepithelial neoplasia of the vulva. Int J Gynecol Pathol. 2008;27(1):125-35.
57. Cabrera HN, Gómez ML. Skin cancer induced by arsenic in the water. J Cutan Med Surg. 2003;7(2):106-11.
58. Romao-Correa RF, Maria DA, Soma M, et al. Nucleolar organizer region staining patterns in paraffin-embedded tissue cells from human skin cancers. J Cutan Pathol. 2005;32(5):323-8.
59. Mohanty P, Mohanty L, Devi BP. Multiple cutaneous malignancies in xeroderma pigmentosum. Indian J Dermatol Venereol Leprol. 2001;67(2):96-7.
60. James, William D, Berger. Timothy G, Andrews' Diseases of the Skin: Clinical Dermatology. 11th Ed. W.B. Saunders Co Elsevier. 2005.
61. Wolf DJ, Zitelli JA. 'Surgical margins for basal cell carcinoma'. Arch Dermatol. 1987;123(3):340–4.
62. Silverman MK, Kopf AW, Bart RS. 'Recurrence rates of treated basal cell carcinomas. Part 3: Surgical excision'. J Dermatol Surg Oncol. 1992;18(6): 471-6.
63. Sigurdsson H, Agnarsson BA. 'Basal cell carcinoma of the eyelid. Risk of recurrence according to adequacy of surgical margins'. Acta Ophthalmol Scand. 1998;76 (4):477-80.
64. Dhingra N, Gajdasty A, Neal JW. 'Confident complete excision of lid-margin BCCs using a marginal strip: an alternative to Mohs' surgery'. Br J Ophthalmol. 2007;91(6):794-6.
65. Mohs. Frederic Edward. Chemosurgery: microscopically controlled surgery for skin cancer. Springfield, Ill: Thomas. 1978.pp.3-6.
66. Bene NI, Healy C, Coldiron BM. 'Mohs micrographic surgery is accurate 95.1% of the time for melanoma *in situ*: a prospective study of 167 cases'. Dermatol Surg. 2008;34(5):660-4.
67. Neville, Damm, Allen, Bouquot. Oral and Maxillofac Path. 2nd ed. W.B. Sounders Co; 2004. pp.377-80.
68. Midion Mapfumo Chidzonga, Leonard Mahomva, Rudo Makunike-Mutasa. Primary Malignant Melanoma of the Oral mucosa. J Oral Maxillofac Surg. 2007;65:1117-20.
69. Pandey, Mathew, Iype, Sebastian, Abraham, Nair. Primary malignant mucosal melanoma of the head and neck region: pooled analysis of 60 published cases from India and review of literature. European Journal of Cancer Prevention. 2002;11:3-10.
70. Gao Man Gu, Epstein JB, Morton TH. Intraoral melanoma: Long-term follow-up and implication for dental clinicians. A case report and literature review. Oral Surg Oral Med Oral Pathol. 2003; 96:404-13.
71. Barker BF, Carpenter WM, Daniels TE. Oral mucosal melanomas: The WESTOP Banff proceedings. Oral Surg Oral Med Oral Pathol 1997;83:672-9.
72. Patton LL, Brahim JS, Baker AR, et al. Metastatic malignant melanoma of the oral cavity. Oral Surg Oral Med Oral Pathol. 1994;78:51-6.
73. Rapidis AD, Apostolidis C, Vilos G, et al. Primary Malignant Melanoma of the Oral Mucosa. J Oral Maxillofac Surg. 2003;61:1132-9.
74. Patton LL, Brahim JS, Baker AR, et al. Metastatic malignant melanoma of the oral cavity. Oral Surg Oral Med Oral Pathol. 1994;78:51-6.
75. Jeevan Lata, Satya Narain. Primary mucosal melanoma of oral mucous membrane—A report of two cases. J Maxillofac Oral Surg. 2005;4:28-30.

Section 11

Important Tips for Postgraduate Students

- Thesis Writing
- Seminar and Journal Club Presentation

31 Thesis Writing

Gaidhane Abhay, Quazi Syed Zahiruddin

> ***It is science alone that can solve the problems of hunger and poverty, insanitation and illiteracy, of superstition and deadening custom and tradition, of vast resources' running to waste, of a rich country inhabited by starving people.***
>
> **—Jawaharlal Nehru**

One of the major components of the Postgraduate curriculum is writing thesis. Work for writing the thesis is aimed at contributing to the development of a spirit of enquiry, besides exposing the candidate to the techniques of research, critical analysis, acquaintance with the latest advances in medical science and the manner of identifying and consulting available literature. A postgraduate student is required to carry out work on an assigned short-term research project under the guidance of a recognized postgraduate teacher, the result of which shall be written up and submitted in the form of a thesis. Thesis should be submitted at least six months before the theory and clinical/practical examination. A candidate shall be allowed to appear for the theory and practical/clinical examination only after the acceptance of the thesis by the examiners.

PREPARING SYNOPSIS

As per the existing statute, a postgraduate student is assigned to a recognized postgraduate teacher. Within first 6 months from the date of commencement of the academic term, the postgraduate student has to prepare synopsis and submit for approval of the thesis. The synopsis initially has to be submitted to the Institutional Ethical Committee and/or Animal Ethical Committee as applicable, for the approval. After clearance from the Institutional Ethical Committee, the synopsis is communicated to the concerned university for approval of the thesis. The work on any research project can be started only upon the ethical committee clearance. The purpose of this exercise is to allow the next 18 months to the students to undertake the study according to the protocol (data collection). As the study is completed in the 18 months, over the next 6 months the collected data can be compiled, processed and interpreted and finally the text is prepared in the form of thesis. This allows the student complete 2 years for the thesis work after the ethical committee clearance.

OUTLINE OF THE STUDY PROTOCOL

At the postgraduate level the concerned postgraduate teacher is expected to allot a suitable and feasible research topic to the postgraduate student. The viability of the study must be ascertained in terms of:

- Feasibility
- Availability of relevant infrastructure and facilities
- Availability of adequate clinical material to constitute a sample size, which can be processed statistically to generate cognigible data
- Possibility of completing the work in the prescribed time frame
- Considering ethical aspects
- Considering financial feasibility.

It is not feasible to fix the sole responsibility on the postgraduate student to search for the topic of research as he/she has no insight in the speciality nor he/she is acquainted to the facilities and other protocols. The role of the postgraduate student should be facilitative. The research topic is often selected by the student, while doing a doctoral research (PhD) and not during the postgraduation. Once the topic is finalized the student is entrusted a responsibility of making a synopsis under the due guidance and supervision of the postgraduate teacher.

The ideal way for starting on thesis is working on study protocol. This approach gives clarity and guide to select the research work for the thesis. The candidate can work on the study protocol as given in Table 31.1.

Table 31.1: Study protocol designing

Sr. No.	Element	Purpose
1.	Research question	What question will the study address?
2.	Background and significance	Why are these questions important?
3.	Design a. Time frame b. Epidemiological approach	How the study is structured?
4.	Subjects a. Selection criteria b. Sampling design	Who are the subject and how they will be selected?
5.	Variables a. Predictor variables b. Confounding variables c. Outcome variables	What measurement will be made?
6.	Statistical issues a. Hypothesis testing b. Sample size c. Analysis approach	How large will be the study? How it will be analyzed?

START WITH RESEARCH QUESTION

> *A question well stated is half answered; but a question that is poorly stated or unstated is not likely to be answered at all.*
>
> —**Charles Franklin Kettering**

Remember the most important task is to identify and clearly define the research question (RQ) of the study. To decide the research question the student should consult teachers, discuss with colleagues, go through literature review, identify problems that are faced in clinical practice, identify researchable area, look at your personal interest, go for divergent thinking. Try to think..... outside the box.

A RQ should have sound biologic rationale and plausibility. The RQ should be feasible, have adequate number of subjects, technical expertise, affordable in time and money and manageable in scope. The research question should be novel, confirms or refutes previous findings, extends previous findings and provide new findings. Research question should be ethical and should be relevant to scientific knowledge, clinical and health policy, and should be able to provide future research direction.

Once you are ready with your RQ and sub research question, you will be able to write research objectives, hypothesis, define key variables and select study design, make dummy tables and what statistics to apply.

A POORLY FRAMED RESEARCH QUESTION

Example of poorly framed RQ, it only describes *type of intervention* (anticoagulant agent) and on what *type of target population* (patient who had stroke) but does not explain what is the outcome which needs to be studied and whether there is any comparison in the study with another group (Flow chart 31.1).

A Nicely Framed Research Question

One way of making research question is by seeing whether the RQ contains PICO (P–Population/person/thing; I–Intervention/exposure if any; C–Comparison; O–Outcome).

Flow chart 31.1: Example of poorly framed research question

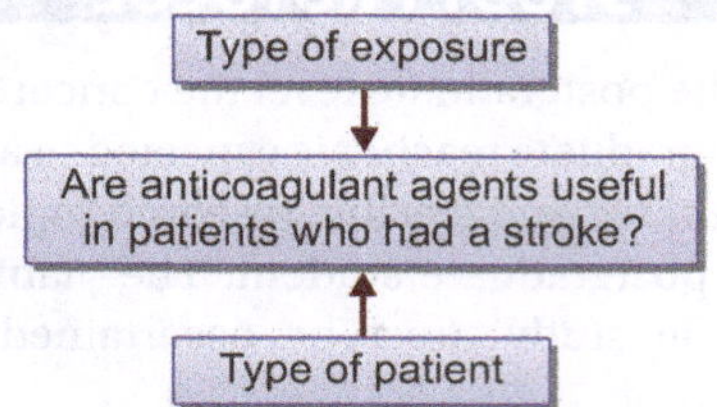

Do anticoagulant agents improve outcomes in patients with acute ischemic stroke compared with no treatment?

In this example, the *type of target person/population* on whom study is being conducted is patients with acute ischemic stroke. It should be during the process of making type of target person/population in the RQ decided, what you meant by acute ischemic stroke, what age, sex, severity of patients you will include, by what means will be your clinical diagnosis for acute ischemic stroke, whether you will include Outpatient/Inpatient; and within 48 hours of stroke onset (Flow chart 31.2).

The *type of exposure* (anticoagulant agents) whether it will be unfractionated heparin, low-molecular-weight heparin, heparinoids, oral anticoagulants, etc. It should be very clear initially when making a research question of what type of exposure/intervention is being given in the study or should be known that there is no exposure nor any intervention is given.

The *type of comparison* what type of control or comparison is in the study. In this example there is control group, i.e. no anti-coagulation is given to the study group.

The *type of outcome* anticipated in the study is to be described. In this example, outcome can be death, disability, major hemorrhage, recurrent stroke or deep vein thrombosis (DVT).

Flow chart 31.2: An example of nicely framed research question

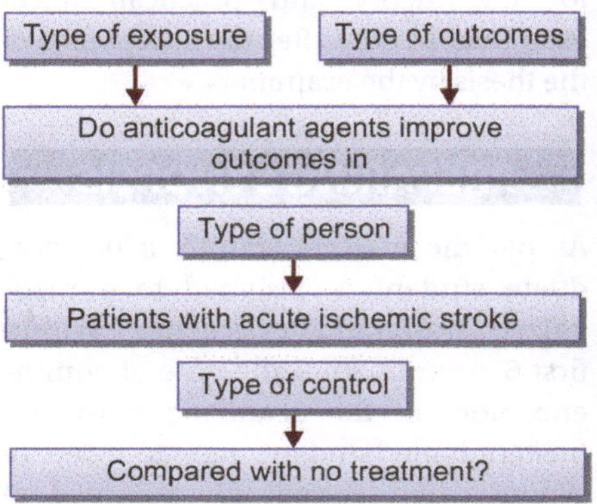

HYPOTHESIS

The great tragedy of Science—the slaying of a beautiful hypothesis by an ugly fact.
—Thomas Henry Huxley

Once the research question or research problem is identified, the next step would be to make guess/guesses (based on review of literature and experience survey) about the possible answer. These guesses are *hypothesis*, which either solve problem or guide for further investigation. Thus, hypothesis is a provisional formulation, a tentative solution to the problem facing the researcher. In other words, hypothesis is a statement about an expected relationship between two or more variables that permits empirical testing. While ultimate objectives identify the anticipated contributions arising from a study and immediate objectives (stated in behavioral terms) specify what will be done or measured in the study, hypotheses specify the expected relationship among the variables. Hypothesis statements are most appropriate for field intervention or evaluative studies. Diagnostic or exploratory studies do not normally require hypothesis statements because they generally do not test relationships between variables.

Descriptive studies can formulate hypothesis, but for testing it if is true or false, we need to undertake the analytical studies. Descriptive and analytical studies are discussed subsequently in detail.

A well formulated hypothesis of analytical studies can:

- Help researcher proceed in correct direction.
- Guide the researcher for order among facts.
- Give points to the inquiry (helps researcher to know specifically, what he has to find out).
- Help in selection of pertinent or relevant facts.
- Help in drawing conclusion.

To formulate a good hypothesis, extensive literature search on related topics is most essential, because the facts established by previous investigation in the related area are essential to conceptualize the logical outcome/answer of our research question. Other things that could add up to this understanding is our experience, observation (Intuitions), reasoning, insight and logical derivation from the theory.

Research hypothesis are of two types:

1. *Null hypothesis:* Denoted by the symbol HO.
2. *Alternative hypothesis:* Denoted by the symbol HA.

Null hypothesis (HO) is the hypothesis in which the sample or populations being compared in a study or test are similar. If there is any difference, it is due to chance, not due to measurable factor. HO is initially accepted and considered true for analytical comparison. An *Alternative hypothesis (HA)* is the hypothesis to be tested and must be stated, before the study is designed (Table 31.2).

HO is used to define significant difference. A significant difference occurs, if HO is disproved and HA is accepted.

Table 31.2: Sampling error

Null hypothesis	Decision	
	Accepted	Rejected
True	Correct conclusion	Type I or (α) error
False	Type II or (β) error	Correct conclusion

Testing of Hypothesis

It means accepting or rejecting HO. This is usually done on statistical analysis. For testing the level of confidence for rejecting HO is arbitrary, usually fixed at 5 percent. Type of statistical test used for testing and its interpretation is also different for unidirectional (one tailed) hypothesis and bidirectional (two tailed) hypothesis. There could be three situations on hypothesis testing:

1. If HO is rejected and HA is accepted, the two population, sample are significantly different.
2. If HO in not rejected, the two population, sample are similar (no difference).
3. If HO is not rejected, even if the two population, sample are different—an error is committed.

An error that occurs in hypothesis testing is called as *'sampling error'*. These can be of two types:

Type I Error

Type I error also called α error: When HO is rejected even if it is true, then type I error is committed. The α error is defined as 5 percent.

Type II Error

Type II error also called β error: When HO is accepted even if it is false, then type II error is committed. The β error is usually defined as 20 percent and is linked to power of the study (1-β = power of study; 100 - 28 = 80 Power of study).

For ease of understanding refer the following example and figure.

Sampling Error

Sampling is done to determine the characteristics of a whole population, the difference between the population values and the sample is considered as sampling error. Statistics on the samples differ from the parameters on the entire population since the sample does not include all the members of the population.

Example:

A study to estimate the hemoglobin level in high-school students was conducted. The results showed that the mean Hb level in one school was 14 g/dL and in other school 13 g/dL. On analysis it was observed that the probability that it is due to chance alone is 15 percent. The *Interpretation* would be that the difference is not significant. Therefore; the null hypothesis is not rejected, as α error (also called as level of significance) is defined as 5 percent. If the same study is repeated 100 times and 5 out of 100 studies showed significant difference. This means that the probability, that it is due to chance alone is less than 5 percent and HO is rejected. The type I error is made in these five studies.

To understand type II error, consider this, if there is a difference between Hb level of students, the probability of the study detecting the difference is 80 percent whereas not detecting the difference is 20 percent.

OBJECTIVES

> *"The successful man is the average man, focused."*
>
> **—Anonymous**

Objective indicates the accomplishment of the study. Just by reading an objective, other persons must get a sense of what you are doing (even if they do not understand technical terms). Thus, objectives must be clearly linked to problem and question and framed in clinical/epidemiological terms that measure outcome, rates, incidence, mortality, morbidity etc. This will allow us to evaluate the *success* of the research project. The study objective also influences the study design, data collection and interpretation.

Hint: While, reading the research paper in any journal, the objective(s) is usually the last sentence of the 'introduction' section.

To formulate a good objective, use no more or less than one verb each, (i.e. an objective is an action and must clearly and strongly reflect that). The objective should be clear about whether they call for testing a hypothesis (e.g. 'we are going to compare....') or they call for measuring a quantity (e.g. we are going to describe....')

Be careful not to get too broad or you can lose focus. Too general formulations, "e.g. to study the health status of ------" will not be useful at all. To make good quality study objectives we can make use of pneumonic '***SMART***':

- **Specific:** Specify what you want to achieve. Describe a precise outcome that is linked to measurement (rate, prevalence, frequency, etc.)
- **Measurable:** Objective unit that can indicate achievement
- **Achievable:** With a reasonable amount of effort, can this be done?
- **Relevant:** Appropriate impact, output, products?
- **Time-bound:** Indicates target dates and study context.

Examples to Understand Objectives More Clearly

Example 1: A Survey of Diabetes to be Conducted in the Community

Objective 1: To establish the exact number of diabetics in the community.

Comment: Statement is clear, but formulation is incomplete (prevalence rate, age, gender, etc).

Objective 2: To discover the undiagnosed cases of diabetes.

Comment: Not a complete statement (--- and to compare their age and sex distribution with that of known cases).

Objective 3: To investigate the possible hereditary factors.

Comment: Too non-specific for blue print for study planning. Did the investigator want to—study a familial clustering of cases, association with an occurrence of genetic markers, compare the frequency of the positive family histories of diabetes among diabetic, newly detected, or non-diabetics.

Example 2: A Report on National Study of Cerebral Palsy in Adolescent and Adulthood

Objective 1: To learn about the extent and nature (of the problem) and specific need of the cerebral palsied youngster and adult through socio-medical study.

Objective 2: Collect an epidemiological data of cerebral palsied individuals.

Objective 3: To evoke the interest of public agencies and local communities in the program.

Comments: These formulations may be OK as a starting point, but much specification is needed as a blue print of the study planning.

PLANNING THE RESEARCH

After deciding the research question/thesis topic formulation of hypothesis and objectives, the next step is to plan for the research. In planning, the researcher needs to consider the different options available to investigate the research question/hypothesis/objectives. In other words, the investigator needs to finalize the suitable research design. The various issues that need to be looked into for planning the research are:

- Selecting the suitable study design
- Calculating sample size and defining the sampling methodology (random error and level of significance and power of study)
- Data collection: Tools and techniques (methods)
- Data quality
- Data analysis.

SELECTING THE SUITABLE STUDY DESIGN

The study objective can be achieved by number of alternative designs. Researcher has to select the most appropriate and feasible design. Selection of the study design may depend upon the following issues:

- What is the research question/hypothesis/objective.
- Time available for study.
- Resources available for the study.
- Common/rare disease or production problem.
- Type of outcome of interest.
- Quality of data from various sources.
- Often there are multiple approaches, which will all work.
- Choosing an established design gives you a huge head start in design, analysis and eliminating biases.

Broadly the research designs can be classified as observational and interventional/experimental. Observational studies could be either descriptive or analytical.

Descriptive Studies

These studies describe the patterns of diseases with regards to person, place and time. Descriptive studies are a necessary antecedent of analytic studies and are less expensive than analytic studies. Descriptive studies help in formulating research questions or hypothesis, but they cannot be used for testing hypotheses. They can also be used to assess the associations between putative risk factor and disease, but cannot comment on causation by doing descriptive studies. The different types of descriptive studies are—case reports, case series, cross-sectional surveys, correlation studies.

Case Reports

The most basic descriptive study with no control group. They describe the experience of a single patient. Case reports are used for documenting the unusual medical occurrence and may lead to identification of new disease. They can be done quickly with little money.

Case Series

Descriptive studies, which focus on individuals. They examine the experience of a group of individuals sharing a common experience. This may be a shared exposure (or risk factor) or a shared outcome (perhaps symptoms, or a disease). A key characteristic of case series is that there is no comparison group. Case series are common in clinical medicine, where they are often used to highlight unusual or interesting findings. They may be used to describe a new disease or a rare manifestation of an existing disease. Case studies can also be used to help detect the effects (adverse or beneficial) of a new treatment. Case series can be particularly useful for generating hypotheses, which can then be explored in larger, well-designed studies. Case series are attractive as they can usually be conducted quickly and cheaply. However, despite their popularity in clinical medicine, case series are less commonly used in epidemiology. This is largely because they are considered to be weak in terms of empirical evidence. The lack of a comparability can lead to misleading conclusions. In addition, the number of individuals involved in case series is often small.

Case report and case series studies may describe:

- A previously described disorder involving a new population or subgroup
- A known disorder with unusual clinical presentation or clinical course
- A condition in which novel treatment methods are used
- A previously unknown condition
- A index case in an epidemic situation.

Example of case report: *Thalidomide tragedy* in 1957, thalidomide was created by West German company Cheme Gruenthal to treat hyperemesis gravidarum. Developmental deformities possibly due to thalidomide. A Case Report Ihno Y. Russell WJ, May 1963.

Example of case series: 'Human Immunodeficiency Virus (HIV) and PCP pneumonia' Gottlieb, Michael et al, "Pneumocystis carinii pneumonia (PCP.) and mucosal candidiasis in previously healthy homosexual men," NEJM, 1981:305:1425-31.

Cross-sectional Surveys

Cross-sectional surveys are also called *Prevalence Surveys.* Exposure and disease are measured simultaneously. These surveys provide a 'snapshot' of the population.

In a cross-sectional study, measure the frequency of a particular exposure(s) and/or outcome(s) in a defined population at a particular point in time. Cross-sectional studies can either be descriptive or analytical.

In a descriptive cross-sectional study, simply describe the frequency of the exposure(s) and/or outcome(s) in a defined population.

In an analytic cross-sectional study, the information is simultaneously collected on both the outcome of interest and exposure to potential risk factor(s). The frequency of the outcome in the people exposed to each risk factor is then compared with the frequency in those not exposed.

Cross-sectional studies are especially useful for defining the health needs of a population at a particular point in time, and as the first step in more detailed etiological investigations. However, as they are based on prevalent (existing) cases rather than incident (new) cases, they are of limited value for investigating etiological relationships.

Correlation studies are also called as ecological studies. In these studies we consider populations as unit of analysis and use database from entire populations to compare frequency of a particular disease. In other words, we look to see whether the outcome is more frequent in groups where the exposure is more frequent. For each group, the exposures and outcomes are measured for the group as a whole. So, it is not possible to link the exposure of any particular individual to his or her outcome. Ecological studies can be done quickly and inexpensively using existing data such as, vital statistics, hospital discharge data, product consumption data, environmental data, etc. Because of this, correlation study are often used as a first step in the investigation of a possible exposure-outcome relationship. However, it can be difficult to interpret the results of an ecological study.

Analytical Studies

The analytical studies are conducted to test the hypothesis and to find out the association between the risk factors or predictors and disease or outcome. The most commonly used analytical study designs in health research are case control studies, cohort studies and nested case control studies. Interventional/experimental studies are also type of analytical studies.

Cohort Study

This study is started by selecting a study population or cohort of people who do not initially have the outcome of interest. The members of the cohort are then according to whether they have been exposed to the potential risk factor or not. The entire cohort is then over time followed and comparison is made between the incidence of the outcome(s) in the exposed individuals with the incidence in those not exposed. The cohort studies are particularly useful for investigating the rare exposures or rare risk factor or rare cause and in situations, where we are interested in studying more than one outcome. The limitation of cohort study is that they are time consuming and expensive to carry out. They are also inefficient for investigating rare outcomes.

Design of Cohort Study

Cohort study can be prospective, retrospective or ambidirectional. This is given in the flow chart below (Flow chart 31.3 and 31.4). For more information readers are requested to refer the suggested reading.

Flow chart 31.3: Design of cohort study

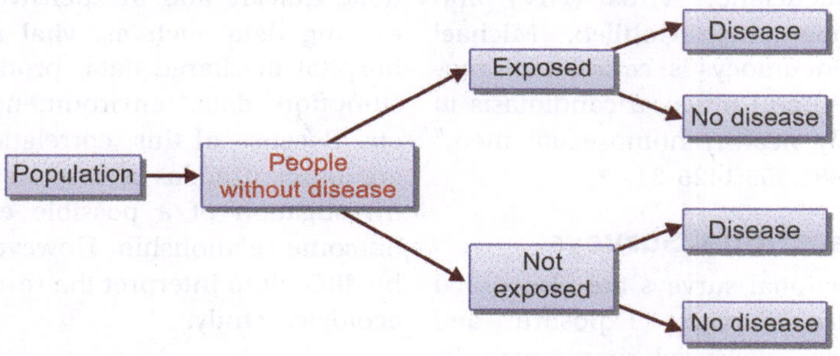

Flow chart 31.4: Schematic representation of concurrent, retrospective and ambidirectional cohort studies

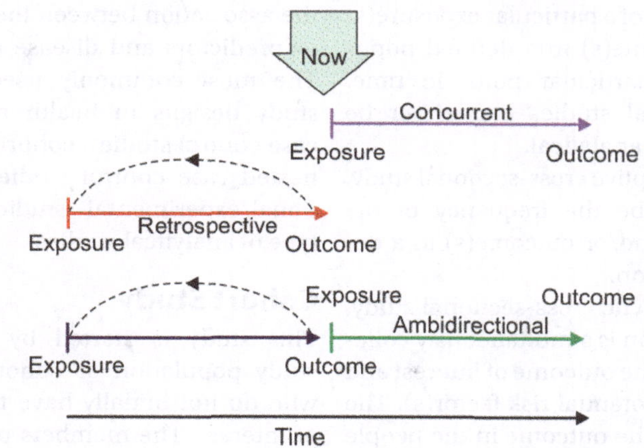

Examples of cohort studies (to give the source for these studies)

- Framingham Heart Study
- National Health and Nutrition Examination Surgery (NHANES) Studies
- Physicians' Health Study
- Nurses' Health Study
- Ndoll R, Peto R, Boreham J, Sutherland I. Smoking and dementia in male British doctors: prospective study. BMJ 2000;320:1097-1102.

Case-control Studies

Case-control studies are retrospective studies. The case-control study is started by identifying individual cases of the outcome of interest. A representative group of individuals is then identified who do not have the outcome. These individuals act as controls. Cases and controls are compared to assess whether there were any differences in their past exposure to one or more possible risk factors. These studies can measure the association between the risk factor and outcome. The case control studies are useful, if the disease is rare. The big advantage of case-control studies is that past exposures and outcomes are measured at the same time. Because of this, these studies can be done quickly, without the need to wait for the outcome to occur. Another advantage of case-control studies is that they are a good way to study rare outcomes and outcomes with a long induction period. This is because the starting point is the identification of people with the outcome in question.

The major difference between case-control studies and cohort studies is the way that the study subjects are chosen. In a cohort study, subjects are selected before they have had a chance to develop the outcome of interest. They are classified according to their exposure or non-exposure to the possible risk factor. We then follow them over time to see, if they develop the outcome. In contrast, in a case-control study we select subjects on the basis of the presence or absence of the outcome. We then look to see if they were exposed or not to the possible risk factor (Flow chart 31.5).

Nested Case Control Study

In cohort study when enough individuals have developed the outcome of interest, they can be compared to controls. In other words a case-control study is inserted into a cohort study. This type of design is called as nested case control study. Such design allows interim evaluation of the association between the variables (Fig. 31.1).

Flow chart 31.5: Case control study design

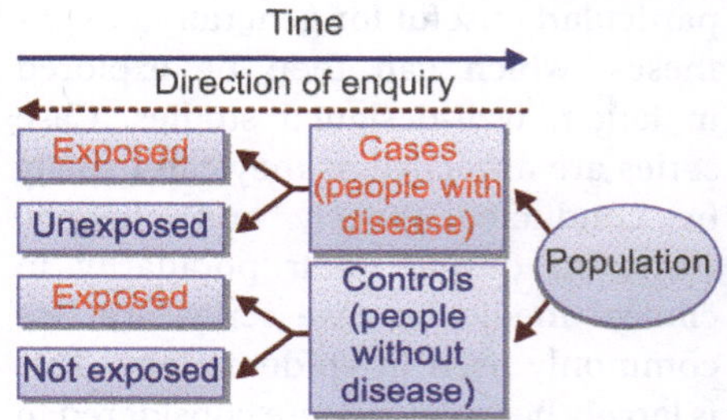

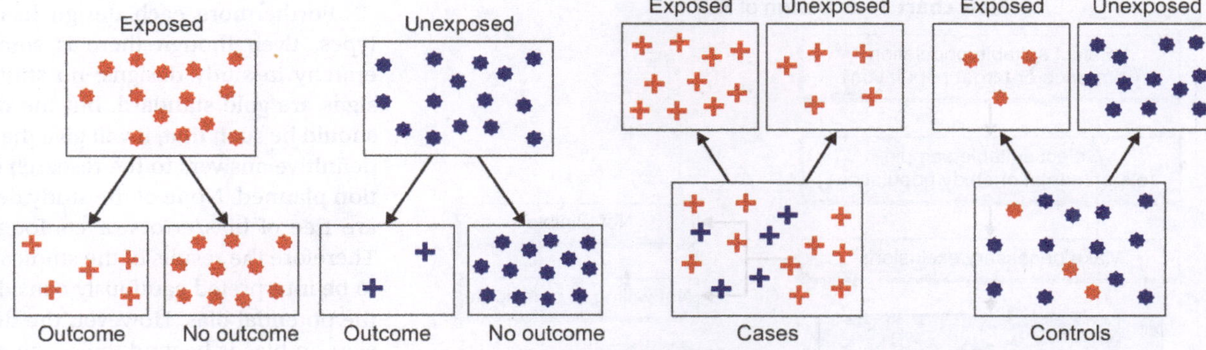

Fig. 31.1: Cohort study design

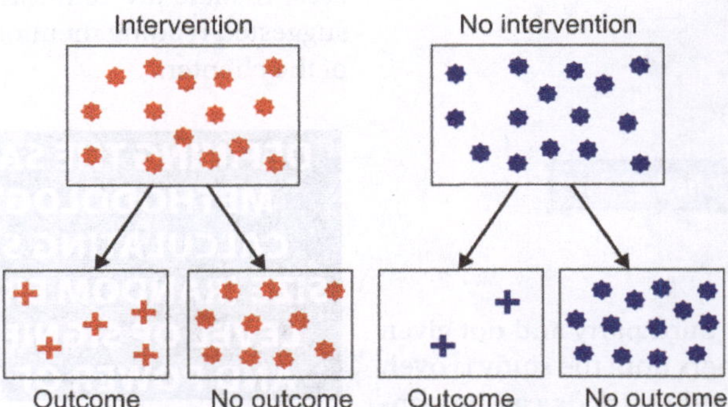

Fig. 31.2: Intervention study design

Interventional/Experimental Studies

In an interventional study, the distribution of the exposure and outcome in a population is observed. The exposure (or intervention) to one of the study groups is then actively allocated. The group that is allocated not to receive the intervention acts as a control group. If the intervention is a type of treatment, the control group can be described as receiving standard treatment. The groups are then followed over a period of time. The frequency of the outcome in the group allocated to receive the intervention is compared with the frequency of the outcome in the group who were allocated not to receive the intervention (Fig. 31.2).

Intervention studies provide strong evidence about causation, because when designed well (with random allocation) they minimize the possibility of selection bias and confounding. However, for ethical reasons we can only use them to study interventions that are of potential benefit to patients, such as preventive or therapeutic measures.

Most commonly used experimental studies are the randomized clinical trial or randomized trial or randomized control trial (*RCT*). These are similar to a cohort study as individuals are studied on the basis of exposure. However the main difference between observational and intervention studies are that individuals in the intervention study have no control over the exposure they receive. In RCT study participants are assigned treatment group and control group by randomization. This ensures that the allocation of the intervention is determined by chance alone.

RCT can be used to:

- Evaluate new drugs.
- Evaluate new treatment procedures.
- Testing efficacy of new health care program.
- Assess preventive measures.
- Assess new program for screening.
- Assess new ways to deliver health services.

Clinical Trials

These are experimental studies (RCTs) (Flow chart 31.6). Clinical trials are conducted in different phases:

- **Phase I:** Initial testing in healthy human volunteers following animal studies. In this phase the dose limiting toxicities, tolerated doses etc. are studied.
- **Phase II:** Testing in subjects with disease to determine activity and therapeutic efficacy. In this toxicity and dosage data of the drug is validated.
- **Phase III:** Randomized trials for comparison. In this phase the efficacy of the drug on patients is measured.
- **Phase IV:** Post marketing trials. These are post-marketing surveillance for monitoring the long-term adverse effect of drugs, if any.

Single Blind Trials

Single-blind describes *experiments*, where information that could introduce bias or otherwise skew the result is withheld from the participants, but the experimenter will be in full possession of the facts.

In a single-blind experiment, the individual subjects do not know whether they are so-called 'test' subjects or members of an *experimental control* group. Single-blind experimental design is used, where the experimenters either must know the full facts (for example, when comparing sham to real surgery) and so the experimenters *cannot* themselves be blind, or where the experimenters will not introduce further bias and so the experimenters *need not* be

Flow chart 31.6: Design of RCT

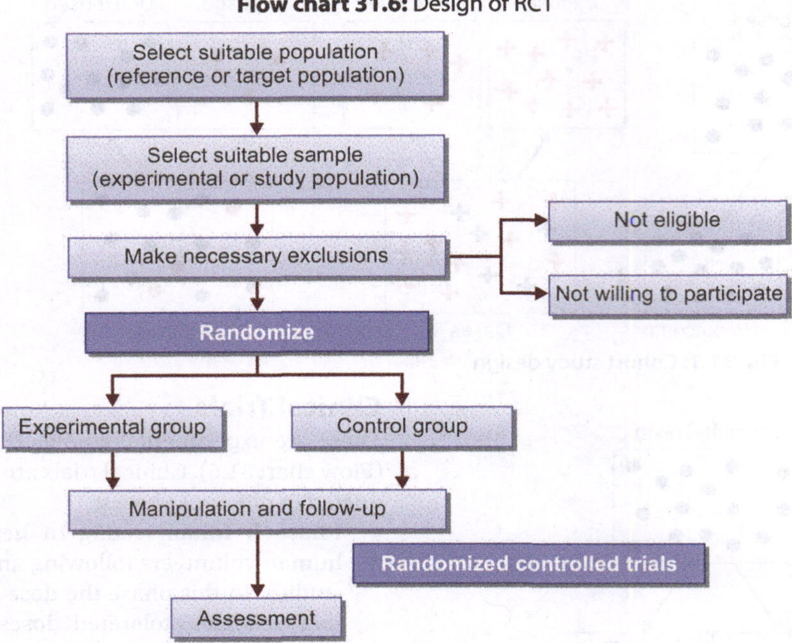

blind. However, there is a risk that subjects are influenced by interaction with the researchers—known as the *experimenter's bias.*

Double-blind Trials

Double-blind describes an especially stringent way of conducting an *experiment,* usually on human subjects, in an attempt to eliminate subjective bias on the part of both experimental subjects and the experimenters. In most cases, double-blind experiments are held to achieve a higher standard of scientific rigor.

In a double-blind experiment, neither the individuals nor the researchers know which subject belongs to the control group and the experimental group. Only after all the data have been recorded (and in some cases, analyzed) do the researchers learn, which individuals belong to which group. Performing an experiment in double-blind fashion is a way to lessen the influence of the prejudices and unintentional physical cues on the results (the placebo effect, observer bias, and experimenter's bias). Random assignment of the subject to the experimental or control group is a critical part of double-blind research design. The key that identifies the subjects and which group they belonged to is kept by a third party and not given to the researchers until the study is over.

Double-blind methods can be applied to any experimental situation where there is the possibility that the results will be affected by conscious or unconscious bias on the part of the experimenter.

Design of RCT

In health research, various study design options available, with regards to their hierarchy, from weakest to strongest design, can be arranged as under:

- Case Report
- Case Series
- Correlational Study
- Cross-Sectional Study
- Opinion/KAP Study (health social sciences)
- Longitudinal Study
- Case-control study–observational analytical retrospective studies
- Cohort Study
- Ecologic Study
- Research on Diagnostic Tests
- Economic Evaluation
- Program Evaluation
- Health System Research
- Experimental Study (trials)
- Systematic Reviews (meta-analysis)
- Methodologic Research
- Hybrid Designs.

Furthermore each design has subtypes. Even though there is some hierarchy in study designs; no study designs are gold standard, but the design should be such that, it will give the most definitive answers to the research question planned. None of the study designs are free of bias/errors or confounding. Therefore the results of the studies need to be interpreted cautiously considering the potential bias. However, the discussion on bias is beyond the scope of this chapter. For more information on biases, readers are requested to refer the suggested reading mentioned at the end of the chapter.

DEFINING THE SAMPLING METHODOLOGY AND CALCULATING SAMPLE SIZE (RANDOM ERROR AND LEVEL OF SIGNIFICANCE AND POWER OF STUDY)

Sampling Methodology

Sampling methodology is that part of statistical practice concerned with the selection of individual observations intended to yield some knowledge about a population of concern, especially for the purpose of statistical inference.

Population, Sample and Sampling Frame (Fig. 31.3)

Population: Population means people from whom the sample is drawn. There are five dimensions of population:

- Size, could be infinite or finite
- Geographic area
- Structure that could be either homogenous or heterogeneous
- Nature that could be static or dynamic
- The time frame.

Sampling frame: Sampling frame is the list of ultimate sampling entities, which may be people, households, organizations or other units of analysis. For example, the list of registered students may be the sampling frame for a survey of the student body at a university. To

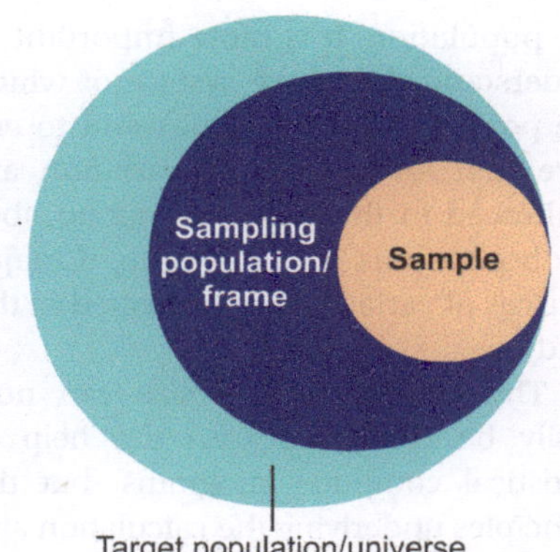

Fig. 31.3: Concept of target population or universe, sampling population/frame and sample

select the representative sample, first the sampling frame should be prepared from the population of interest.

Sample: Sample is a proportion of population selected by a pre-decided and scientific method (different types of sampling methods). In other words sample is a drawn from a population of interest so that by studying the sample the results may fairly be generalized back to the population from which they were chosen.

Sampling Methods

Sampling methods can be categorized as:

- Probability or random sampling:
  - Simple random
  - Stratified
  - Systematic
  - Multi-stage/multi-phase
  - Cluster
  - PPS (population proportional to size).
- Non-probability or non-random sampling:
  - Accidental/haphazard
  - Convenience
  - Purposive—modal instance, expert, quota, heterogeneity, snowball.

Probability sampling

A probability sampling method is any method of sampling that utilizes some form of random selection. In order to have a random selection method, some process or procedure must be set that assures that the different units in population have equal probabilities of being chosen. Humans have long practiced various forms of random selection, such as picking a name out of a hat, or choosing the short straw. These days, computers are used as the mechanism for generating random numbers as the basis for random selection.

Simple random sampling: The simplest form of random sampling is called simple random sampling. In a simple random sample of a given size, all such subsets of the frame are given an equal probability. Each element of the frame, thus has an equal probability of selection—the frame is not subdivided or partitioned.

Stratified sampling: Where the population embraces a number of distinct categories, the frame can be organized by these categories into separate 'strata.' A sample is then selected from each 'stratum' separately, producing a stratified sample. The two main reasons for using a stratified sampling design are:

1. To ensure that particular groups within a population are adequately represented in the sample.
2. To improve efficiency by gaining greater control on the composition of the sample. In the second case, major gains in efficiency (either lower sample sizes or higher precision) can be achieved by varying the sampling fraction from stratum to stratum. The sample size is usually proportional to the relative size of the strata.

Systematic sampling: Selecting (say) every 10th name from the telephone directory is called an every 10th sample, which is an example of systematic sampling. It is easy to implement and the stratification induced can make it efficient, but it is especially vulnerable to periodicities in the list. If periodicity is present and the period is a multiple of 10, then bias will result. It is important that the first name chosen is not simply the first in the list, but is chosen to be (say) the 7th, where 7 is a random integer in the range 1–10-1. Every 10th sampling is especially useful for efficient sampling from databases.

Multi-stage or cluster sampling: It is where the researcher divides the population into strata, samples the strata, then stratifies the samples and then resamples, repeating the process until the ultimate sampling units are selected at the last of the hierarchical levels. When the strata are geographic units, this method is sometimes called area sampling. For instance, at the top level, states may be sampled (with sampling proportionate to state population size); then cities may be sampled; then schools; then classes; and finally students.

Nonprobability sampling

The difference between non-probability and probability sampling is that non-probability sampling does not involve random selection and probability sampling does. Does that mean that non-probability samples are not representative of the population? Not necessarily. But it does mean that nonprobability samples cannot depend upon the rationale of probability theory. At least with a probabilistic sample, we know the odds or probability that we have represented the population well. Nonprobability sampling methods can be divided into two broad types—accidental or purposive. Most sampling methods are purposive in nature because we usually approach the sampling problem with a specific plan in mind. The most important distinctions among these types of sampling methods are the ones between the different types of purposive sampling approaches.

Accidental, haphazard or convenience sampling: One of the most common methods of sampling goes under the various titles listed here. The traditional 'man on the street' (of course, now it is probably the 'person on the street') interviews conducted frequently by television news programs to get a quick (although non-representative) reading of public opinion can be included in this category.

Purposive sampling: In purposive sampling, sampling is done with a purpose in mind. Usually would have one or more specific predefined groups that we are seeking. For instance, run into people in a mall or on the street who are carrying a clipboard and who are stopping various people and asking if they could interview them? Most likely they are conducting a purposive sample (and most likely they are engaged in market research).

Modal instance sampling: In statistics, the *mode* is the most frequently occurring value in a distribution. The most frequent case, or the 'typical' case is sampled. In a lot of informal public opinion polls, for instance, they interview a 'typical' voter. There are a number of problems with this sampling approach. First, is to identify the 'typical' or 'modal' case? The modal voter can be a person who is of average age, educational level and income in the population. But, it is not clear that using the averages of these is the fairest (consider the skewed distribution of income, for instance). And, how do we know that those three variables—age, education, income—are the only or event the most relevant for classifying the typical voter? What if religion or ethnicity is an important discriminator? Clearly, modal instance sampling is only sensible for informal sampling.

Expert sampling: Expert sampling involves the assembling of a sample of persons with known or demonstrable experience and expertise in some area. Often, we convene such a sample under the auspices of a 'panel of experts'. There are actually two reasons you might do expert sampling. First, because it would be the best way to elicit the views of persons who have specific expertise. In this case, expert sampling is essentially just a specific sub-case of purposive sampling.

Quota sampling: In quota sampling, you select people nonrandomly according to some fixed quota. There are two types of quota sampling:

1. Proportional
2. Nonproportional.

In *proportional quota sampling* you want to represent the major characteristics of the population by sampling a proportional amount of each. For instance, if you know the population has 40 percent women and 60 percent men and that you want a total sample size of 100, you will continue sampling until you get those percentages and then you will stop. So, if you've already got the 40 women for your sample, but not the 60 men, you will continue to sample men, but even if legitimate women respondents come along, you will not sample them because you have already 'met your quota.'

Heterogeneity sampling: We sample for heterogeneity, when we want to include all opinions or views and we are not concerned about representing these views proportionately. Another term for this is sampling for *diversity*. In many brainstorming or nominal group processes (including concept mapping), we would use some form of heterogeneity sampling because our primary interest is in getting broad spectrum of ideas, not identifying the 'average' or 'modal instance' ones. In effect, what we would like to be sampling is not people, but ideas.

Snowball sampling: In snowball sampling, you begin by identifying someone who meets the criteria for inclusion in your study. You then ask them to recommend others who they may know meeting the criteria. Although this method would hardly lead to representative samples, there are times when it may be the best method available. Snowball sampling is especially useful when you are trying to reach populations that are inaccessible or hard to find. For instance, if you are studying the homeless, you are not likely to find good lists of homeless people within a specific geographical area. However, if you go to that area and identify one or two, you may find that they know very well who the other homeless people in their vicinity are and how we can find them.

Calculating Sample Size (How Much Sample is Needed?)

Where the frame and population are identical, statistical theory yields exact recommendations on sample size. However, where it is not straightforward to define a frame representative of the population, it is more important to understand the cause system of which the population is outcomes and to ensure that all sources of variation are embraced in the frame. Large number of observations is of no value, if major sources of variation are neglected in the study.

The desired sample size can now easily be calculated with the help of statistical computer programs, but the principles underlying the calculation and the limitation must be clearly understood by the researcher. To put this in simple way, if the sample is too small, even the most rigorously executed study may fail to answer its research question. Study may fail to detect important effects or associations, or may estimate those effects or associations too imprecisely. If the sample is too large, the study will be more difficult and costly than necessary, it will be waste of resources and may even lead to a loss in accuracy, as it is often more difficult to maintain high data quality. Thus, calculating the precise sample size is important in any health research.

For calculating the desired sample size before beginning the study, we need to do exercise in reverse. We have to decide beforehand the level of probability or uncertainly (allowable error) that we are willing to accept for the study and then we find the desired sample size to provide that level of statistical significance. For most studies, the level of significance is set at 0.05 or 5 percent, it means that accepting the chance of 5 percent of an association that is not actually there. In general the researcher should aim for a lower probability of error, when it is particularly important to avoid making a false positive statement about the findings.

As discussed earlier in section of sampling error, the power of study (1β) also depends upon the sample size. Larger the sample size, higher will be the statistical power of the study. For most studies, the power is set at 80 percent, means that accepting 20 percent chance of missing a difference or an association that is actually there.

The other issue that needs consideration for calculating the sample size is a prior estimate of the frequency of the condition under study and the degree of variation in the data. Some information may be available from the previous studies to guide the estimates. If not, it is up to the researcher to come up with a tentative estimate that statistician can use.

The other term we need to understand, particularly for calculating sample size of analytical studies, is *Effect Size.* It refers to the actual size of the difference observed between the groups or the strength of relationship between the variables. The likelihood that a study will be able to detect an association between predictor and outcome variable depends upon the magnitude of the association we decided to look for. Larger sample size is needed to detect smaller differences. The choice of effect size is difficult and arbitrary, but it must be set beforehand and must make a meaningful difference.

In making final estimation of the sample size, factors such as drop outs, attrition and loss to follow-up should also be accounted. If the calculated sample size is larger than that can be practically obtained, then we may consider increasing effect size or decrease the power of study (increase allowable error) or change the design or give up the study. For calculating the sample size readers are requested to consult statistician or refer the WHO manual (Lwanga) after considering the entire perquisite as discussed above.

Ethical Issues in Thesis

Various ethical guidelines are available to which strict adherence is required. Main guidelines are:

- Guidelines for Institutional Ethics Committee (ICMR)
- Guidelines for Care and Use of Animals in Scientific Research (Indian National Science Academy, New Delhi)
- Guidelines for Exchange of Human Biological Material for Biomedical Purpose (MOH and FW, GOI)
- GCP-ICH Guidelines
- Nuremberg Code (ethical issues)
- Helsinki Declaration (ethical issues)
- World Medical Assembly Declaration (ethical issues)
- Guidelines for Clinical Trials on Pharmaceutical Products in India (MOH, GOI, 2001)

We have to apply to the *Institutional Ethical Committee* for Clearance and only after the approval we can proceed to data collection.

DATA COLLECTION: TOOLS AND TECHNIQUES (METHODS)

Tools

Much of the data in clinical research is gathered using *questionnaires or interviews.* A questionnaire or the interview schedule is a document designed for the purpose of seeking specific information from the respondents. The term questionnaire is mainly used for self-administered document, whereas the interviews schedules are usually administered by interviewer. The self-administered questionnaire approach is cheap, less susceptible interviewer bias and can be administered by mail, but there may be high non-response or some incomplete responses.

There are two major formats for developing the questionnaire/interview schedule—the open ended and closed response types. In closed response questions, the respondent is provided with the pre-determined response options. Closed ended questions can enhance the participant recall. Open ended questions elicit more elaborate responses, but the researcher required much effort to encode it for data analysis. The open ended questions can pick up unanticipated situations. A data collection tools can include the both types of questions formats.

Example

Open ended question: What physical activities/sports you undertake daily on regular basis (at least 30 minutes) since last episode of chest pain?

Closed ended question: For each of the following physical activity/sports, check the box, if you spend more than 30 minutes daily, since the last episode of chest pain?

- Walking
- Cycling
- Jogging
- Swimming
- Racket sports
- Yoga
- Other (specify-----------------------).

If we wish to study attitude of the respondent to a certain statement, we may use either *Likert Scale* (strongly agree, undecided, disagree or strongly disagree) or *Forced Choice Format* (strongly agree, agree, disagree, strongly disagree). This format does not allow an undecided answer (Plogar and Thomas 2000).

If questionnaire or interview schedule has to be in local language, then first prepare it in English, translate it into local language and then again translated it into English. This is usually done to ensure correct translation. A questionnaire must be pre-tested in a pilot study, before using it in a main study.

For many studies, the validity of the results depends on the quality of these instruments, therefore is important to develop the questionnaire or interview schedule correctly to address the research question or hypothesis. To develop a good data collection instrument, we need to consider the following issues:

Ask one question at a time: A double-barrelled question asks more than one question, making it difficult to know which part of the question is answered.

Example: Is the water in your community contaminated or does it smell? This question is asking two different things, contamination of water and odor and do not lead us anywhere. The better way of asking the same thing could be—can you drink the water coming out of your faucets without getting diarrhea?

Use accessible language: Avoid questions with prolonged jargon that may be unfamiliar to the respondents.

Example: Do you take any of the following drugs?

- Pain killer
- Anti dyspeptic
- Diuretics.

The respondent may not understand the medical terms, in such cases it is better to ask open ended question to list names of the current medication.

Keep questions simple: Use synonyms for longer words.

Example: What is your current occupation, if not currently employed, please put your most recent job? This question is too vague concerning the amount of detail required. The question needs to be very specific, requesting the organization/firm and exact job title.

Avoid using biased questions: Biased or leading questions can indicate to the respondent that they are expected to answer in certain way. Leading questions are different from the probe, which we used most of the time in in-depth interview for qualitative research.

Example: Since last episode of chest pain, you undertake walking (at least 30 minutes) daily, didn't you?

Yes/No

This question hint's the respondent to answer "Yes".

Be specific in wording question: The more concrete and specific your wording, the more confident you can be that the question will be answered in the way you intended.

Example: Is consumption of Iodine salt useful? This is less specific question. The appropriate one would be—has consumption of iodine salt been useful in reducing the number of new goitre patients in your community?

Pick up an appropriate number of response choices: The options/choice should be appropriately given. Too few can lead to over simplification of the issue; whereas too many choices can lead to confusion about and minimize the difference between responses. Usually aim for four to five choice and offer 'do not know' or 'can not remember' or 'Not applicable', as it may be needed sometime to avoid inaccurate responses.

Example: What was your height at age 25 years? In such questions there may be difficulty in recalling the height. No option for 'Can not remember' and the respondent may be forced into inaccurate responses.

A typical questionnaire or interview schedule include following section:

- An introductory statement by the interviewer to introduce herself/ himself and explain the purpose of the study (study objectives).
- The respondents should also be informed about the confidentiality of their responses.
- Sociodemographic questions to collect the relevant information about the background of the respondents.
- Factual questions.
- Opinion questions—answering the opinion questions require a reflection; it is generally easier for the respondents to answer factual questions. Putting the factual questions first serve as a warm up to the opinion questions.
- Closing statement by the interviewer to thank respondents and wherever appropriate if she/he wants to provide any additional information.

Reliability of the results obtained by the questionnaire can be studied by looking for the internal consistency, which is the extent to which the different questions related with each others. Nowadays this can be done using the computer programs.

DATA QUALITY (FIG. 31.4)

In any health research the accountability for results reported is increasingly important as it may have implications on either clinical care of patients, or designing the preventive intervention and influence on the health policy and programs. Therefore the quality of collected data is of utmost important. To ensure the quality data, following issues needs to be looked into:

Validity/Accuracy

Refers to the extent to which a measure actually measures what it is meant to measure (accuracy). Valid data are considered accurate. For data to be valid/accurate we need to check for measurement, transcription and non-sampling errors.

Reliability

Refers to the degree of similarity of information obtained when the measurement is repeated in the same subject (consistency), i.e. the data are measured and collected consistently.

Precision (Precise)

The data have sufficient detail and are at the appropriate level of detail. The expected change being measured is greater than the margin of error.

Timeliness

Data are up-to-date (current) and information is available on time. Performance data are available on a frequent enough basis to regularly inform program management decisions.

Integrity

The data are protected from deliberate bias or manipulation for political or personal reasons.

Confidentiality

Study subjects/participants are assured that their data will be maintained according to national and/or international standards for data.

Good data are valid as well as reliable

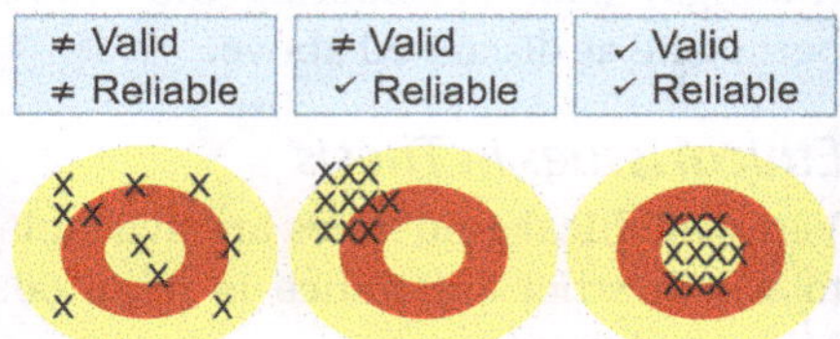

Fig. 31.4: Valid and reliability of data due to good quality

DATA ANALYSIS AND BASIC BIOSTATISTICS PRINCIPLES

Some measures used in research for analysis of the health data are:

The list below is not exclusive. There are many measures that can be used in epidemiology and health research for data analysis. The measures to be used depend upon the research question, objectives, hypothesis, study design and type of data collected. Therefore, it is essential that in the planning stage itself, one should define what measure to be used for analysis. In other words, we have to plan the study depending upon the measures that we will be using in analysis stage.

- Numbers of cases
- Proportional mortality
- Proportional mortality ratio
- Prevalence rates
- Incidence rates
- Specific prevalence and incidence rates
- Standardized rates
- Standardized ratios
- Relative risk
- Odds ratio
- Attributable risks and population attributable risk
- Numbers needed to treat and prevent
- Number needed to harm
- Relative risk reduction
- Absolute risk reduction
- Life years lost
- Disability adjusted life year (DALY)
- Quality adjusted life year (QALY).

Discussion on each study measures are beyond the scope of this chapter. Readers are requested to refer the suggested reading at the end of this chapter.

Basic Biostatistics

Statistics is fundamental to epidemiology and contributes to the majority of studies published in the medical literature. It is essential for anyone studying epidemiology to have an understanding of the key statistical principles and methods. Statistics are most essential to move data (crude information) to knowledge in three steps. First the data becomes information when they become relevant to decision problem. In second stage information become facts when the data is summarized into different characteristics or measures and finally in third step facts become knowledge when they are used in the successful completion of the decision process. Broadly two types of statistics can be used for analyzing the health data:

Descriptive Statistics

It summarizes the data by describing what was observed in the sample numerically or graphically.

Inferential Statistics

Uses patterns in the data to draw inferences about the population represented, accounting for randomness.

Before moving on the actual data analysis, let us have a look at various types to study variables and scales of measurement, because the choice of statistics depends on the type of the variables studied and scale used for measuring these variables.

Analytic Procedures I

The purpose of data analysis is to provide answers to the research questions being studied. The research question also dictates the type of data to be collected during a study and the type of analyses to be performed. For almost all studies, we want to describe what is typical of the group studied and how the cases differ from each other. Our measure of what is typical is called the *Central Tendency.* Our measure of how the cases differ is called the *Variance or Dispersion* in the data.

Before examining the central tendency and variance of data, you must first decide on the type of measurement that you will use. For example, is it more appropriate to use a median or a mean? Can you calculate the variance in the data? The type of analytic procedure or measurement that you can apply to a variable depends on the characteristics of the variable.

Central Tendency or Characteristic of the Data

A measure of central tendency is a central value, which describes the distribution of a particular variable in terms of its location. It is the aggregate measure of the values of a variable:

- Mean
- Median
- Mode.

The mean, the median, and the mode are measures of central tendency. The mean is simply an arithmetic average. It is the sum of individual scores divided by the number of individuals. The median is the midpoint measure in a group of measures—half of the observations fall above the median and half below. The mode is the most frequently occurring figure in a set of figures. Each of these statistical measures describes the typical characteristic or tendency of a group in a slightly different way.

Variance in the Data

Measures of dispersion refer to those measures, which describes the spread or dispersion of data points. These are as follows:

- *Range*
- *Variance*—average squared distance of any value from its mean
- *Standard deviation*—square root of variance.

Often a researcher is interested not only in the average characteristic of a group, but also in the variance or dispersion within the group, i.e. how individuals in a group differ from the average or central tendency of the group. For example, if the mean age of first voluntary HIV testing is 28, what is the age range of the group? What is the age of the youngest person tested and the oldest person tested? A group with a mean of 28 years, but with a range of 24 to 30 years at first testing is probably quite different from another group with a mean of 28 years, but with age at first testing that range from 15 to 59. The term *variance* is used when researchers measure dispersion around a *mean.* A common statistical measure of variation within a group is the *standard deviation.* This measure gives the average distance of individual measurement observations from the group mean. The larger the standard deviation, the greater the variation in the individual observations. The formulas of some commonly used statistical tests of differences between means such as the *t* test and the *F* test, also called the analysis of variance (ANOVA), use variance estimates to establish whether differences are statistically significant.

Other Measures of Dispersion

You can obtain other measures of dispersion in the data by counting the number of cases in each category. The resulting count is called *frequency distribution.*

Variables can be of two types:

I. Categorical:
   a. Records, such as several groups or categories to which an individual belongs. If there are two possible categories we called it as a binary variable.
   b. Example: Gender, marital status, socioeconomic status (SES), etc.

II. Quantitative:
   a. Numeric values
   b. Example: Age, height, income, etc.

Classification of Variables

Although variables can be characterized in many ways, for the purposes of data analysis we classify variables by a *measurement scale.* A scale is a rule for assigning numbers to objects or events. The type of scale that characterizes a variable also determines the types of analyses or measurements that can or cannot be performed on that variable. The four levels of variable measurement are *nominal, ordinal, interval* and *ratio.*

Nominal Scale

In nominal measurements, the categories of variables differ from one another *in name only.* In other words, one category of a variable is not necessarily higher or lower, or greater or smaller than another category; it is just different in name. For example, gender, race, blood types, etc.

A special type of nominal variable is a *dichotomous variable,* which can take only one of two values. Examples of dichotomous variables include sero-positive status (positive or negative) or sex (male or female).

Only very limited statistical manipulations are possible with nominal variables. While examining central tendency, we can calculate the mode (the most frequently occurring number). In looking at dispersion, we can calculate a percentage or frequency distribution. But we cannot calculate a mean or a standard deviation. It makes no sense to speak of the 'mean sexually transmitted disease,' or the average distance from 'female.'

Ordinal Scale

Numbers represent the rank order of the variable being measured. However these numbers do not represent the magnitude of the difference between two subjects, only which one is higher or lower. For examples, disease stages (stage I, stage II, stage III and stage IV).

With ordinal variables, you can use all the statistical manipulations appropriate for nominal variables (such as the mode and the frequency distribution). Because there is a rank order to the numbers, you can also use the median and the percentile. But you cannot use a mean, or a standard deviation. It makes no sense to speak about the mean attitude of respondents to condom advertising. The reason is that the distance or interval between the categories is not known.

Interval Scale

Numbers indicate relative amounts of the attribute, also, equal distances between numbers assigned to subjects, reflect equal differences in the amounts of the attribute measured. Temperature and calendar dates are examples of interval variables. For example, the difference between the beginning of day 1 and the beginning of day 2 is 24 hours, just as it is between day 3 and day 4. With interval variables such as temperature, you can say that a temperature of 80°F is 40°F warmer than a temperature of 40°F. However, an important point is that 80°F cannot be said to be twice as warm as 40°F because interval variables do not have a true zero point. At best, they have zero points that are set by convention or convenience.

The lack of a true zero point means that you cannot calculate ratios with interval data. However, you can calculate all of the measures of central tendency and dispersion that are allowed with nominal and ordinal variables plus the mean and standard deviation.

Ratio Scale

Numbers represent magnitude, equal interval and an absolute zero point, For example, number of living children, number of sexual partners, etc.

As you can see, the characteristics of the four measurement scales are cumulative. All the statistics that we can use in analyzing nominal data can be used in analyzing ordinal data, plus we can use additional analyses that cannot be used with nominal data. Similarly, all the analyses that you can use with nominal, ordinal and interval data can also be used with ratio data. In addition, ratio data permits use of additional analyses that the lower level of scales does not.

Analytic Procedures II

Descriptive Statistics

All studies should describe the characteristics of the group being studied. Basic descriptive statistics include frequency distributions, percentages and percentiles, means and standard deviations, and contingency tables (cross-tabulations) (Flow chart 31.7).

Differences within the Data

Most often, you want to know whether the differences between groups or observations can be attributed to the intervention or whether they could have occurred by chance alone. The three common significance tests that we will discuss are the chi-square (χ^2) test, *t* test and analysis of variance (ANOVA or *F* test).

All statistical tests of significance assume that differences are produced

Flow chart 31.7: Various statistical tests used for data processing

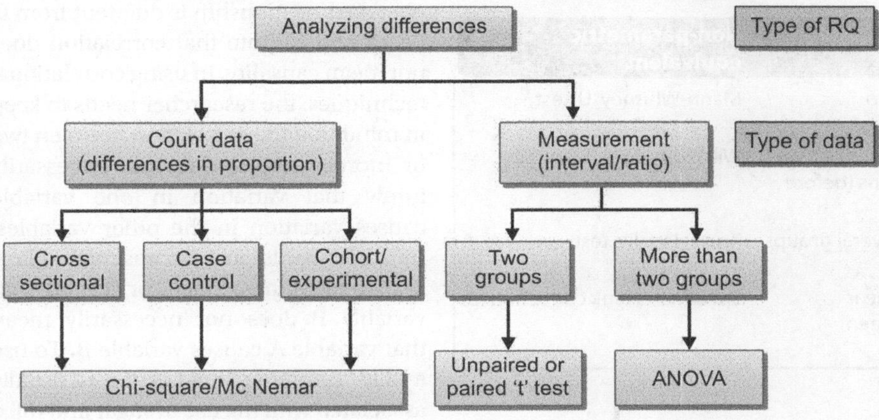

Flow chart 31.8: Correlations between variables

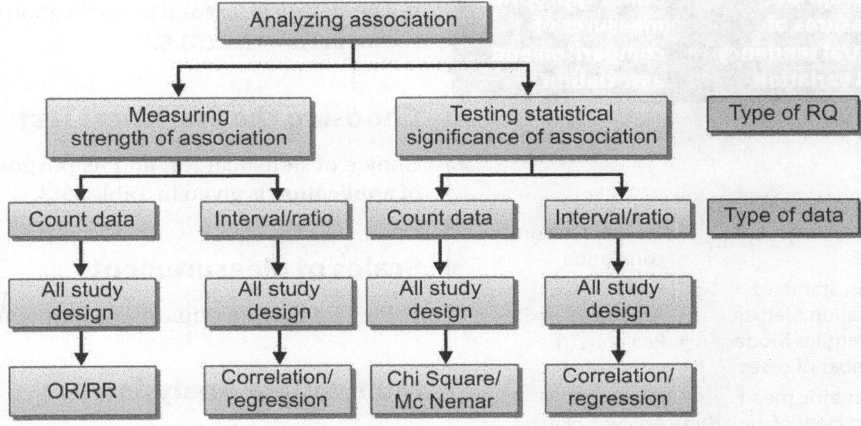

by chance alone. This assumption is called the *null hypothesis.* The statistical tests tell us the probability that the observed differences could have occurred by chance. This number is called *significance level.* The convention for writing the significance level is p < followed by the probability that the result could have occurred by chance. Thus, $p < 0.05$ means that the probability that the result is due to chance alone is less than 1 in 20. By convention, researchers do not usually reject the null hypothesis unless they find $p < 0.05$. Obviously, if you choose a very small p value for your significance level, you decrease the probability of rejecting the null hypothesis. The statistical test also tells you how often you will be wrong in rejecting the null hypothesis. If $p < 0.05$, you will be wrong 5 percent of the time. If $p < 0.75$, you will be wrong three-fourths of the time. You will be committing a *Type I error* when the results of the test lead you to reject the null hypothesis, when in fact the result was due to chance. You commit a *Type II error*, when you accept the null hypothesis, when in fact the intervention did affect the results. A small significance level decreases the probability of making a *Type I error*, but increases the probability of making a *Type II error.* A common way to decrease the probability of making a *Type II error* is to hold the significance level constant and increase your sample size.

A common misconception is that statistically significant also means important. This is not true.

Chi-Square (χ^2) Test

The chi-square (χ^2) test is the *only significance test that can be used with nominal data.* It is also frequently used with ordinal data and can be used with ratio data, but it is less powerful than statistics that make use of the mean and variance of the data. The chi-square test is used to determine whether frequency distributions differ significantly. When using χ^2 you first prepare a cross-tabulation of the variables. The chi-square test can then be applied to the cross-tabulation to determine whether there is a significant difference between distributions.

t Test of Means

The *t* test is used to determine whether the difference between two means is statistically Significant. A *t test* can be used only with interval or ratio data.

F Test (Analysis of Variance)

The *F* test, or analysis of variance (ANOVA) is usually used to determine whether the difference between three or more means is significant. We can use an ANOVA test whenever we do a multiple group experiment. For example, will peer educators perform better, if they are given one, two or three days of retraining? Both *t* tests and *F* tests require interval or ratio data because they use variance estimates in calculating statistical significance.

The statistical test and its application is shown in Flow chart 31.7.

Correlations between Variables (See Flow chart 31.8)

In a descriptive study (a design that does not include an experimental treatment), researchers often look for 'correlations' between variables to determine whether there is an underlying relationship between them or whether one factor (for example, age of positive HIV test) is related to another (such as years of survival) factor. If you have interval or ratio data, you can use *Pearson's correlation coefficient* to measure the degree of association between the variables. When you have ordinal data, *Spearman's and Kendall's rank correlation tests* are appropriate for measuring association.

Table 31.3: Choice of statistical test and its purpose

Parametric test	Purpose of application	Non-parametric equivalent
't' test for independent samples	Comparison of two independent groups	Mann-Whitney 'U' test
't' test for paired samples	To test the difference between paired observations (before and after)	Wilcoxon signed rank test
Analysis of variance	Comparison of several groups	Kruskal Wallis test
Pearson's correlation (r)	To quantify the linear relationship between variables	Spearman's rank correction (p)

Table 31.4: Sample measurement

Measurement scale	Examples	Appropriate measures of central tendency and variation	Some appropriate measures of comparison and association
Nominal	Assigning classes like 'HIV-negative' or 'HIV-positive' to numbers	Number of cases Mode	Chi-square
Ordinal		Median Percentiles Mode Number of cases	Chi-square Tests of rank order correlation
Interval		Mean Standard deviation Median Percentiles Mode Number of cases	*t* test Analysis of variance Pearsons'(r)
Ratio		Geometric mean Coefficient of variation Mean Standard deviation Median Percentiles Mode Number of cases	*t* test Analysis of variance Pearson's(r)

The tests produce numbers called *correlation coefficients* that range from −1.0 to +1.0. When the correlation coefficient is negative (i.e. preceded by a minus sign), it means that the relationship is such that one variable decreases as the other increases. In the example above, a negative correlation would mean that the older people are at age of HIV diagnosis, the shorter their survival time and vice versa. If the correlation coefficient is positive (preceded by a + sign), it means that when one variable is high, so is the other and that when one variable is low, so is the other. The closer the correlation coefficient is to +1.0 (or to −1.0), the stronger the relationship or association between the two variables (for example, a correlation of 0.2 implies a weaker relationship than a correlation of 0.7). A correlation coefficient of 0 means that no relationship between the two variables exists and a coefficient of 1.0 means that the two variables are perfectly related or correlated. Tests of significance can be applied to the correlation coefficient. However, instead of testing the probability that differences between groups could have been the result of chance, as is the case in making comparisons between experimental groups, measures of association test the probability that the degree of the observed relationship is different from 0. Be careful to note that correlation does not mean causality. In using correlational techniques, the researcher needs to keep in mind that the correlation between two or more variables does not necessarily imply that variation in one variable causes variation in the other variables. In other words, just because variable A is correlated, associated, or related with variable B does not necessarily mean that variable A causes variable B. To use a silly example, drinking tea is usually associated with the use of sugar and milk. But tea drinking does not cause sugar and milk use; rather, it is only associated with it. The statistical test and its application is shown in Flow chart 31.8.

Choosing the Statistical Test

Choice of statistical test and its purpose of application is given in Table 31.3.

Scales of Measurement

Table 31.4 shows sample measurements.

Multivariate Analysis

Unlike the *bivariate* (only two variables) statistical measurements described above, *multivariate analysis* is used to examine the relationship between more than two variables.

Typically, we are concerned with the relationships between multiple independent variables and a single dependent variable. But this is not always the case. Multivariate techniques also exist for examining the relationship between multiple dependent variables and a single independent variable, as well as multiple independent and multiple dependent variables. Multivariate analysis is sometimes used with quasi-experiments and is often used in descriptive, diagnostic studies. For example, suppose you complete a quasi-experiment to determine whether a training intervention to improve provider competence results in better patient adherence to antiretroviral drug treatment regimens. You perform a *t* test and discover that the patients of providers in the training intervention group have significantly better adherence than did the comparison group. In selecting the intervention and comparison groups, you matched the clinics on the type of antiretroviral treatment regime most often used by patients. However, you did not match the clinics on patient age or education. When you analyze the data, you find that age and education differences between groups are statistically significant. Our provider training intervention is confounded with patient age and education, which means that the difference in groups may be due to the age or education differences rather than to the training intervention. In this situation, you might be able to separate the effects of client age, education and provider training by doing a multivariate analysis. If the relationship between the intervention and adherence continues to be undiminished (statistically significant), even when the other two factors are held constant, you could conclude that age and education have little or no influence on adherence and you may attribute the differences between groups to provider training. However, if the relationship between provider training and adherence disappears (is no longer statistically significant), when you control for the other two variables, you must conclude that your intervention was not successful in improving patient compliance. In addition to determining, which independent variables are significantly related to a dependent variable, multivariate techniques, like simple correlations, may also allow you to measure the strength of the relationship. There are several multivariate techniques. The one you should use depends, just as with bivariate techniques, on the measurement scale of the variables.

The five of the more commonly used multivariate procedures for different combinations of independent and dependent variables.

Table 31.5 shows multivariate procedures.

Graphical Presentation of Data

Graphical presentation of data gives the reader immediate and overall view/perspective without having to read each column/row in a table.

Some common forms of graphical presentation are given in Figure 31.5.

Plan of Analysis

- Describe in detail each of the analytical techniques and statistical measures you plan to use, indicating how each technique and measure will help you meet your study objectives. What variables will be involved? Why have you selected a particular technique for the analysis of the data?
- Provide examples of important dummy tables.
- Be sure that your plan of analysis clearly explains how you will meet all your study objectives, use all your study variables, and test all your study hypotheses.

WRITING THE THESIS/ DISSERTATION REPORT

Research Spiral

Title

Indicate the study's design with a commonly used term in the title.

Table 31.5: Multivariate procedures

Measurement scale of independent variables	Measurement scale of dependent variables			
	Dichotomous (two categories)	Nominal (more than two categories)	Ordinal (more than two categories)	Interval and ratio
Dichotomous, nominal and ordinal	Logistic regression	Multinomial logistic regression	Multinomial logistic regression ordered	Multiple regression with dummy independent variables
Interval and ratio	Logistic regression	Multinomial logistic regression	Multinomial logistic regression ordered	Multiple regression
Mixed (any combination of measurement scales)	Logistic regression	Multinomial logistic regression	Multinomial logistic regression ordered	Multiple regression

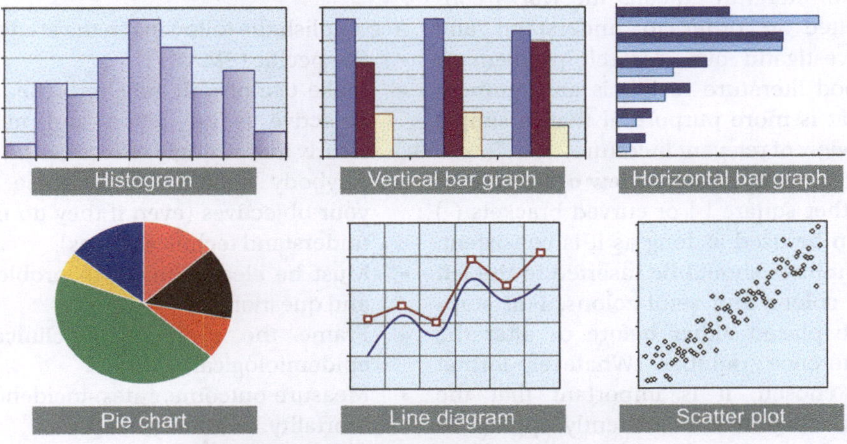

Fig. 31.5: Various graphical depictions of data

Concise titles are easier to read than long, convoluted ones. Titles that are too short may, however, lack important information. Readers should be able to easily identify the design that was used from the title. An explicit, commonly used term for the study design also helps ensure correct indexing of articles in electronic databases. Title should be specific, but comprehensive. Should be short, but should be sufficiently descriptive. No abbreviations should be used.

Introduction

The Introduction section should describe, why the study was done and what questions and hypotheses it addresses. It should allow others to understand the study's context and judge its potential contribution to current knowledge.

Background/Rationale

Explaining the scientific background of the study provides important context for readers. It sets the stage for the study and describes its focus. It gives an overview of what is known on a topic and what gaps in current knowledge are addressed by the study. Background material should note recent pertinent studies and any systematic reviews of pertinent studies. It does not include review and history of the subject. Does not identify all the other gaps in knowledge. Does not include methods, results and discussion.

Literature Review

The 'literature' means the works consulted in order to understand and investigatin our research problem. A good literature review is an argument that is more purposeful than a simple review of relevant literature.

How to quote review of literature: Either square [ ] or curved brackets ( ) can be used as long as it is consistent. Numbers should be inserted to the left of colons and semi-colons. Full stops are placed either before or after the reference number. Whatever format is chosen, it is important that the punctuation is consistently applied to the whole document. A number is allocated to a source in the order in which it is cited in the text. If the source is referred to again, the same number is used.

Example:...as one author has put it 'the darkest days were still ahead' [1]: which is well documented in the literature. [2-5] This proves that 'the darkest days were still ahead'. [1] The author's name can also be integrated into the text, e.g. Scholtz [2] has argued that...

Objectives

State specific objectives, including any prespecified hypotheses. Objectives are the detailed aims of the study. Well-crafted objectives specify populations, exposures and outcomes and parameters that will be estimated. They may be formulated as specific hypotheses or as questions that the study was designed to address. In some situations, objectives may be less specific, e.g. in early discovery phases. Regardless, the thesis should clearly reflect the investigator's intentions. For example, if important subgroups or additional analyses were not the original aim of the study, but arose during data analysis, they should be described accordingly. Both the main and secondary objectives should be clear and any prespecified subgroup analyses should be described.

How to Make and Write Objectives

Accomplish the following in the study:

- Be specific (SMART).
- Make use of only one verb (i.e. an objective is an action and must clearly and strongly reflect that).
- Anybody should get a sense of your objectives (even if they do not understand technical terms).
- Must be clearly linked to problem and question.
- Frame the problem in clinical/ epidemiological terms.
- Measure outcome, rates, incidence, mortality, morbidity, etc.
- Evaluate the 'success' of your project.
- Influences your study design, data collection and interpretation.
- **Hint:** this is usually the last sentence of the 'introduction' section of a journal article.
- Should be clear about whether:
  - They call for testing a hypothesis (e.g. 'we are going to compare....').
  - They call for measuring a quantity (e.g. we are going to describe....').
  - Can be created to measure process, impact, outcome.
  - May be sorted out as primary and secondary.
  - Be careful not to get too broad or you can lose focus.
- M-A/R-S-T is often the best way.
  - Measurable is the most important consideration. You will know that you have achieved your objective.
  - A non-'A' non-'R' objective will not get beyond paper (has it been done before?, other resources?) or will have little use.
  - The devil is in the 'S' details—avoid assumptions and jargon, define terms, use appropriate and understandable language.
  - T relates to S, M, and R—provides a frame-work.

Example Objectives

Study Objectives Examples

- Estimating a quantity or burden:
  - To determine the prevalence of diabetes among South Indian children from 2000 to 2005
- Testing a hypothesis/association:
  - To estimate the relative frequency of iodine deficiency among poorer people
  - To estimate the effect of vitamin A supplementation on cure rates of tuberculosis patients in Peru.

The Objective should be *SMART/ RUMBA* (Box 31.1).

Box 31.1: SMART/RUMBA objective

S-Specific	R-Relevant
M-Measurable	U-Understandable
A-Achievable	M-Measurable
R-Relevant/Reliable	B-Behavioral
T-Time Bound	A-Achievable

SMART Objective:

- **Specific:** Specify what you want to achieve. Describe a precise outcome that is linked to an epi measurement (rate, prevalence, frequency, etc.)
- **Measurable:** Objective unit that can indicate achievement
- **Achievable:** With a reasonable amount of effort, can this be done?
- **Relevant:** Appropriate impact, output, products
- **Time-bound:** Indicates target dates and study context.

Methodology

The methods section should describe what was planned and what was done in sufficient detail to allow others to understand the essential aspects of the study, to judge whether the methods were adequate to provide reliable and valid answers and to assess whether any deviations from the original plan were reasonable.

Study Design

Present key elements of study design early in the paper.

We advise presenting key elements of study design early in the methods section so that readers can understand the basics of the study. For example, authors should indicate that the study was a cohort study, which followed people over a particular time period and describe the group of persons that comprised the cohort and their exposure status. Similarly, if the investigation used a case-control design, the cases and controls and their source population should be described. If the study was a cross-sectional survey, the population and the point in time at which the cross-section was taken should be mentioned. When a study is a variant of the three main study types, there is an additional need for clarity. For instance, for a case-crossover study, 1 of the variants of the case-control design, a succinct description of the principles should be given.

We recommend that investigators refrain from simply calling a study 'prospective' or 'retrospective', because these terms are ill defined. We recommend that, whenever investigators use these words, they define what they mean. Most importantly, we recommend that investigators describe exactly how and when data collection took place.

Setting

Describe the setting, locations and relevant dates, including periods of recruitment, exposure, follow-up and data collection.

Examiner or reader needs information on setting and locations to assess the context and generalizability of a study's results. Exposures, such as environmental factors and therapies, can change over time. Also, study methods may evolve over time. Knowing when a study took place and over what period participants were recruited and followed up places the study in historical context and is important for the interpretation of results.

Information about setting includes recruitment sites or sources (for example, electoral roll, outpatient clinic, cancer registry or tertiary care center). Information about location may refer to the hospitals or practices where the investigation took place. We advise stating dates rather than only describing the length of time periods. There may be different sets of dates for exposure, disease occurrence, recruitment beginning and end of follow-up and data collection.

Participants

Cohort study participants: Give the eligibility criteria and the sources and methods of selection of participants. Describe methods of follow-up.

Case–control study participants: Give the eligibility criteria and the sources and methods of case ascertainment and control selection. Give the rationale for the choice of cases and controls.

Cross-sectional study participants: Give the eligibility criteria and the sources and methods of selection of participants.

Detailed descriptions of the study participants help examiner/readers understand the applicability of the results. Investigators usually restrict a study population by defining clinical, demographic and other characteristics of eligible participants. Typical eligibility criteria relate to age, gender, diagnosis and comorbid conditions. Despite their importance, eligibility criteria often are not reported adequately.

Eligibility criteria may be presented as inclusion and exclusion criteria, although this distinction is not always necessary or useful. Regardless, we advise authors to report all eligibility criteria and also to describe the group from which the study population was selected (for example, the general population of a region or country) and the method of recruitment (for example, referral or self-selection through advertisements).

Knowing details about follow-up procedures, including whether procedures minimized non-response and loss to follow-up and whether the procedures were similar for all participants, informs judgments about the validity of results.

Variables

Clearly define all outcomes, exposures, predictors, potential confounders and effect modifiers. Give diagnostic criteria, if applicable.

Disease outcomes require adequately detailed description of the diagnostic criteria. This applies to criteria for cases in a case-control study, disease events during follow-up in a cohort study, and prevalent disease in a cross-sectional study. Clear definitions and steps taken to adhere to them are particularly important for any disease condition of primary interest in the study.

Data sources/measurement: For each variable of interest, give sources of data and details of methods of assessment (measurement). Describe comparability of assessment methods, if there is more than one group.

Bias

Describe any efforts to address potential sources of bias.

Biased studies produce results that differ systematically from the truth. It is important for a reader to know what measures were taken during the conduct of a study to reduce the potential of bias. Ideally, investigators carefully consider potential sources of bias when they plan their study. At the stage of reporting, we recommend that authors always assess the likelihood of relevant biases. Specifically, the direction and magnitude of bias should be discussed and if possible, estimated. For instance, in case-control studies, information bias can occur, but may be reduced by selecting an appropriate control group.

Study Size

Explain how the study size was arrived at.

A study should be large enough to obtain a point estimate with a sufficiently narrow confidence interval to meaningfully answer a research question. Large samples are needed to distinguish a small association from no association. Small studies often provide valuable information, but wide confidence intervals may indicate that they contribute less to current knowledge in comparison with studies providing estimates with narrower confidence intervals. Also, small studies that show 'interesting' or 'statistically significant' associations are published more frequently than small studies that do not have 'significant' findings. While, these studies may provide an early signal in the context of discovery, readers should be informed of their potential weaknesses.

While Writing Methodology—Common Mistakes

- Grammar not consistent
- Do not follow a logical order
- No reference of standard methods
- No reference of manufacturer's instructions
- No approval of Institutional Ethical Committee
- Not taking consent
- Not using corrective abbreviations and SI units
- Missing essential details
- Use of lab jargon
- Incorrect word usage
- No mechanism of data quality checks
- No confidentiality of the information.

Statistical Methods

Describe statistical methods with enough detail to enable a knowledgeable reader with access to the original data to verify the reported results. When possible, quantify findings and present them with appropriate indicators of measurement error or uncertainty (such as confidence intervals). Avoid relying solely on statistical hypothesis testing, such as *p* values, which fail to convey important information about effect size. References for the design of the study and statistical methods should be to standard works when possible (with pages stated). Define statistical terms, abbreviations and most symbols. Specify the computer software used.

Results

The Results section should give a factual account of what was found, from the recruitment of study participants, the description of the study population, to the main results and ancillary analyses. It should be free of interpretations and discursive text reflecting the author's views and opinions.

Participants

Report the numbers of individuals at each stage of the study, e.g. numbers potentially eligible, examined for eligibility, confirmed eligible, included in the study, completing follow-up and analyzed.

Give reasons for non-participation at each stage.

Consider use of a flow diagram.

An informative and well-structured flow diagram can readily and transparently convey information that might otherwise require a lengthy description, as in the example above. The diagram may usefully include the main results, such as the number of events for the primary outcome. While, we recommend the use of a flow diagram, particularly for complex observational studies, we do not propose a specific format for the diagram.

Discussion

The discussion section addresses the central issues of validity and meaning of the study. Surveys have found that discussion sections are often dominated by incomplete or biased assessments of the study's results and their implications and rhetoric supporting the authors' findings. Structuring the discussion may help authors avoid unwarranted speculation and over interpretation of results, while guiding readers through the text. *Investigators structure the discussion section by presenting the following:*

- A brief synopsis of the key findings
- Consideration of possible mechanisms and explanations
- Comparison with relevant findings from other published studies
- Limitations of the study
- Brief section that summarizes the implications of the work for practice and research.

Key Points

- Past tense
- Focus, then discuss the bigger picture
- Be critical of the literature
- Be specific in pointing out where further gaps in knowledge can be fulfilled instead of just writing 'further research is needed'
- What gaps in knowledge remain to be filled?
- Only mention previous results or comments, which illuminate or which are illuminated by the present results.
- Final paragraph in which the message of the article is firmly stated.

Discussion—Common Mistakes

- Repetition—introduction and results.
- Lack of organization, no logical flow
- Not addressing the key points.

Summary

Summarize key results with reference to study objectives.

It is good practice to begin the discussion with a short summary of the main findings of the study. The short summary reminds readers of the main findings and may help them assess whether the subsequent interpretation and implications offered by the authors are supported by the findings.

Limitations

Discuss limitations of the study, taking into account sources of potential bias or imprecision. Discuss both direction and magnitude of any potential bias.

The identification and discussion of the limitations of a study are an essential part of scientific reporting. It is important not only to identify the sources of bias and confounding that could have affected results, but also to discuss the relative importance of different biases, including the likely direction and magnitude of any potential bias.

Interpretation

Give a cautious overall interpretation considering objectives, limitations, multiplicity of analyses, results from similar studies and other relevant evidence.

The heart of the discussion section is the interpretation of a study's results. Overinterpretation is common and human; even when we try hard to give an objective assessment, reviewers often rightly point out that we went too far in some respects. When interpreting results, authors should consider the nature of the study on the discovery to verification continuum and potential sources of bias, including loss to follow-up and nonparticipation.

Generalizability

Discuss the generalizability (external validity) of the study results.

Generalizability, also called external validity or applicability, is the extent to which the results of a study can be applied to other circumstances. There is no external validity *per se*; the term is meaningful only with regard to clearly specified conditions. Can results be applied to an individual, groups, or populations that differ from those enrolled in the study with regard to age, sex, ethnicity, severity of disease and comorbid conditions? Are the nature and level of exposures comparable and the definitions of outcomes relevant to another setting or population? Are data that were collected in longitudinal studies many years ago still relevant today? Are results from health services research in one country applicable to health systems in other countries?

The question of whether the results of a study have external validity is often a matter of judgment that depends on the study setting, the characteristics of the participants, the exposures examined and the outcomes assessed. Thus, it is crucial that authors provide readers with adequate information about the setting and locations, eligibility criteria, the exposures and how they were measured, the definition of outcomes and the period of recruitment and follow-up. The degree of non-participation and the proportion of unexposed participants in whom the outcome develops are also relevant. Knowledge of the absolute risk and prevalence of the exposure, which will often vary across populations, are helpful when applying results to other settings and populations.

Conclusion

Refer back to Research Question posed and describe the conclusions that you reached from carrying out this investigation. Stress the importance of the thesis statement? Leave a final impression on the reader. Summarize new observations, new interpretations and new insights that have resulted from the present work. Include the broader implications of your results. Do not repeat word for word from introduction or discussion.

Recommendations

Remedial action to solve the problem. Write in brief of further research to fill in gaps in our understanding and specify in which directions for future investigations on the topic or related topics is needed. Investigators should suggest ways in which subsequent research can improve on their studies rather than blandly stating 'more research is needed'.

Bibliography

It should be written as per the guidelines set by the university. Follow the mentioned order. Authors (use et al. after 6 authors, if there are more than six authors, complete names should not be written). Article title (should be exact as existing). Journal name (should be in standard PubMed abbreviations, full journal name should not be written). Year, Volume, Page numbers (325–327 to be written as 325–27) (Fig. 31.6).

Example: As shown in Fig. 31.6.

Use full internet resources for how to write references:

- http://www.nlm.nih.gov/bsd/uniform_requirements.html
- http://www.icmje.org/

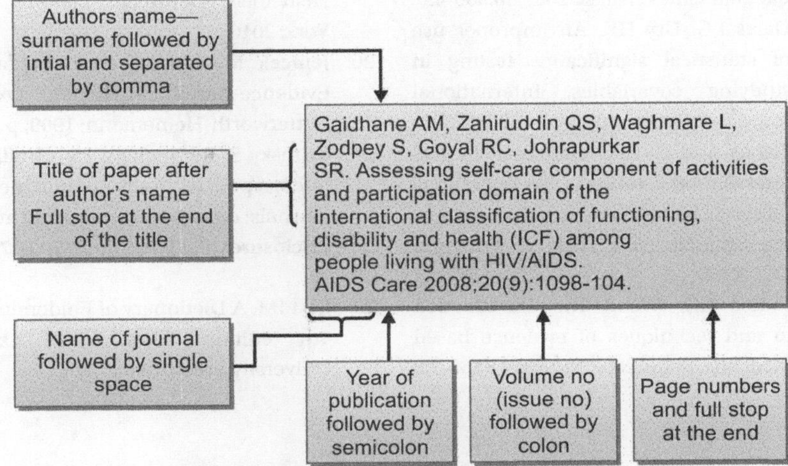

Fig. 31.6: Bibliographic method for journal article

Appendices

- The study questionnaire
- The informed consent form
- A copy of the approval from the Institutional Review Board.

Dissemination and Utilization of Research Findings

- The utilization of research results is the goal of every research.

BIBLIOGRAPHY

1. Als-Nielsen B, Chen W, Gluud C, Kjaergard LL. Association of funding and conclusions in randomized drug trials: a reflection of treatment effect or adverse events? JAMA. 2003;290:921-8.
2. Altman DG, De Stavola BL, Love SB, Stepniewska KA. Review of survival analyses published in cancer journals. Br J Cancer. 1995;72:511-8.
3. Altman DG. Categorizing continuous variables. In: Armitage P, Colton T, editors. Encyclopedia of biostatistics. 2nd ed. Chichester: John Wiley; 2005.
4. Black N, Brazier J, Fitzpatrick R, and Reeve B. (Eds). Health Services Research Methods. A Guide to Best Practice. London: BMJ Publishing; 1998.
5. Bland JM, Altman DG. One and two sided tests of significance. BMJ 1994; 309:248.
6. Brian Haynes R. Forming research questions. J Clin Epidemiol. 2006;59: 881-6.
7. Carlin JB, Doyle LW. Sample size. J Paediatr Child Health. 2002;38:300-4.
8. Dales LG, Ury HK. An improper use of statistical significance testing in studying covariables. International Journal of Epidemiology. 1978;7:373-5.
9. Fisher, Andrew A. Designing HIV/AIDS intervention studies: an operations research handbook/Andrew. Populat-ion Council. New York, Washington, DC; 2002.
10. Fisher CG, Wood KB. Introduction to and techniques of evidence based medicine. Spine 2007;32(Suppl): S66-72.
11. Freedman B. Equipoise and the ethics of clinical research. N Engl J Med. 1987;317:141-5.
12. Greenland S, Neutra R. Control of confounding in the assessment of medical technology. International Journal of Epidemiology. 1980;9:361-7.
13. Greenland S. Randomization, statistics, and causal inference. Epidemiology. 1990;1:421-9.
14. Guyatt G, Rennie D. User's guide to medical research: a manual for evidence based clinical practice. 3rd ed. Chicago (IL): AMA Press Printing; 2002.
15. Hanson BP. Designing, conducting and reporting clinical research. A step by step approach. Injury 2006;37:583-94.
16. Haynes RB, Sackett DL, Guyatt GH, et al. Clinical epidemiology: how to do clinical practice research. 3rd ed. New York (NY): Lippincott Williams and Wilkins; 2007.
17. Hulley S, Cummings S, Browner W, et al. Designing clinical research. 3rd ed. Philadelphia (PA): Lippincott Williams and Wilkins; 2007.
18. International Committee of Medical Journal Editors (ICMJE). Uniform req-uirements for manuscripts submit-ted to biomedical journals. Electronic version updated February 2006, avail-able at http://www.icmje.org. The New England Journal of Medicine 1997;336: 309-15.
19. Jan Jonker, Bartjan Pennink. The Ess-ence of Research Methodology A Con-cise Guide for Master and PhD Stud-ents in Management Science. Springer Heidelberg Dordrecht London, New York; 2010.
20. Jenicek M. Clinical Case Reporting. Evidence-Based Medicine. Oxford: Butterworth-Heinemann; 1999; p. 117.
21. Krimsky S, Rothenberg LS. Conflict of interest policies in science and medical journals: editorial practices and author disclosures. Sci Eng Ethics. 2001;7:205-18.
22. Last JM. A Dictionary of Epidemiology. 4th edition. New York: Oxford University Press; 2000.
23. Leon Gordis. Epidemiology. 5th edition. Philadelphia: Pennsylvania; 2013.
24. Lilienfeld AM. Foundations of Epide-miology. New York: Oxford University Press; 1976.
25. Lohr SL. Design Effects (Chapter 7.5). Sampling: Design and Analysis. Pacific Grove: Duxbury Press. 1999.
26. MacMahon B, Trichopoulos D. Epid-emiology, principles and methods. 2nd ed. Boston: Little, Brown and Co.; 1996. p. 81.
27. Maldonado G, Greenland S. Simul-ation study of confounder-selection strategies. American Journal of Epide-miology. 1993;138:923-36.
28. Miettinen OS. Theoretical Epidemio-logy: principles of occurrence research in medicine. New York: Wiley; 1985.
29. Mullner M, Matthews H, Altman DG. Reporting on statistical methods to adjust for confounding: a cross-sectional survey. Ann Intern Med. 2002;136:122-6.
30. Olson SH, Voigt LF, Begg CB, Weiss NS. Reporting participation in case-control studies. Epidemiology. 2002;13:123-6.
31. Pocock SJ, Collier TJ, Dandreo KJ, et al. Issues in the reporting of epide-miological studies: a survey of recent practice. BMJ. 2004;329:883.
32. Rigby AS, Vail A. Statistical methods in epidemiology. II: A commonsense approach to sample size estimation. Disabil Rehabil. 1998;20:405-10.
33. Robins JM. Data, design, and back-ground knowledge in etiologic infer-ence. Epidemiology. 2001;12:313-20.
34. Rothman KJ, Greenland S, Lash TL. Modern Epidemiology, 3rd edition. Philadelphia, PA: Lippincott, Williams and Wilkins; 2008.
35. Rothman KJ, Greenland S. Precision and Validity in Epidemiologic Studies. In: Rothman KJ, Greenland S (Eds). Modern epidemiology, 2nd edition. Lippincott Raven; 1998.pp. 120-5.
36. Rothman KJ, Greenland S. Types of Epidemiologic Studies. In: Rothman KJ, Greenland S (Eds). Modern Epi-demiology. 2nd edition. Lippincott Raven; 1998. pp. 74-5.

37. Sackett D, Strauss S, Richardson W, et al. Evidence-based medicine: how to practice and teach evidence-based medicine. 2nd ed. Edinburgh (UK): Churchill Livingstone; 2000.
38. Schulz KF, Grimes DA. Case-control studies: research in reverse. Lancet. 2002;359:431-4.
39. Schulz KF, Grimes DA. Sample size calculations in randomised trials: mandatory and mystical. Lancet. 2005; 365:1348-53.
40. Taubes G. Epidemiology faces its limits. Science. 1995;269:164-9.
41. Temple R. Meta-analysis and epidemiologic studies in drug development and postmarketing surveillance. JAMA. 1999; 281:841-4.
42. Vandenbroucke JP. In defense of case reports and case series. Annals of Internal Medicine. 2001;134:330-4.
43. Vandenbroucke JP. Prospective or retrospective: what's in a name? BMJ. 1991;302:249-50.
44. Von Elm E, Altman D, Egger M, Pocock S, Gøtzsche PC, Vandenbroucke JP. The Strengthening the Reporting of Observational Studies in Epidemiology (STROBE) Statement: guidelines for reporting observational studies. Epidemiology. 2007;18:800-804.

32 Seminar and Journal Club Presentation

Borle Rajiv M

INTRODUCTION

There is a significant difference between the level of the undergraduate (UG) and postgraduate (PG) training. Although most of the topics that are covered in the curriculum are same, the length and depth at which they are required to be studied at the postgraduate level are different. The topics taught in a didactic manner at the undergraduate level are required to be studied by the postgraduate student himself in greater depth. As the postgraduate student is already sensitized to these topics during the undergraduate level, and it is expected that the knowledge should get consolidated. The student should understand the subject rather than reading it only as the things which are understood are seldom forgotten. It means that the learner should not only gather information or should get structured training, but he should know the reasoning, should be able to analyze on the basis of evidence, think and articulate the subject. He should develop ability to take decision and make appropriate alterations in the treatment plan as per the situation and condition of patient. He should develop ability for lifelong learning. In nutshell the student should be "Educated" and not only trained. The training at the postgraduate level is guided or supervised learning. It requires initiative on part of the student. The didactic component of training at the postgraduate level is marginal. The incidental learning and allied reading is very important at the postgraduate level for better understanding. For example, if a patient is admitted in the ward and it is presented by the postgraduate student during the clinical case discussion or if the case is to be operated all the details of the presenting pathology along with treatment modalities and operative procedure must be read. While performing any bedside procedure or even during the monitoring of the cases postoperatively all details pertaining to procedures and allied literature must read and understood. If a drug is prescribed to the patient the pharmacological properties, actions, indications, adverse reactions, and precautions must be read. This is a very sound habit of augmenting the knowledge as simultaneously the clinical exposure is also gained, which provides better insight in the subject and consolidates the knowledge. The UG student is expected to acquire the basic understanding through the textbooks, but the objective of postgraduate training is not served until the other sources of information like journals, internet, attending continuing medical education programs and workshops are also utilized. After acquiring the information the postgraduate student should be able to interpret, organize, apply and present the same information in a systematic manner. There can be two ways of evaluating the theoretical acumen of the postgraduate student, the first is through the formative and summative examinations and the second is through the ability to present. The goal of the two modalities are different. The presentation apart from the depth of the reading done by the presenter, will also test his communication skill, ability to condense a vast topic in to a small time bound presentation without missing out the key points, understanding of the basics, capability to organize the presentation for better understanding and effectiveness for audience and skill of being able to summarize the topic. The ability to answer the accrued questions out of the presentation is another aspect, which highlights the presenter's understanding of the subject. This aspect is vital as the current postgraduate student is the teacher of the future and thus, inculcating these skills in the student is imperative. The postgraduate training is not restricted to just acquiring information, but, the student should be able to implement this knowledge in clinical practice and for the same should acquire matchable skills and he should be able to communicate the acquired knowledge in the most effective way.

The good presentation is not always a result of individual brilliance nor it is accidental. A scientific planning, repeated practice and learning by imitating the good presenters can enhance the average skills of the beginner, to make him/her more accomplished presenter in due course of time. The purpose of this chapter is to give few important tips to the budding postgraduate students, to enhance their abilities to make an effective scientific presentation.

SEMINAR

Definitions

A seminar can be defined as:

"Any meeting for exchanging *information and holding discussions*".

Or

"A course or subject of advanced students".

Or

"A small group of students, engaged in advanced study and original research under a member of faculty and meeting regularly to *exchange information and hold discussions*".

Or

"A class held for advanced studies in which students meet regularly to discuss original research, under the *guidance of a professor*".

Or

"A meeting held for the *exchange of useful information* by members of a common business community'.

If we look at the definition of the seminar a few key words catch our attention like '*exchange of information*', '*discussion*', '*guidance of professor*'. These terms are self-explanatory and it can be easily gathered that it is not a mere speech or a didactic activity, it has a dimension of interactiveness. It means that both the presenter and audience must be equally prepared for free flowing discussion and interaction to give completeness to this activity. The other dimension is '*guided*' by the teacher. The teacher has a vital role to play. He should ensure that the set objectives of the seminar are met with; the student is not missing vital points and not deviating from the objectives. A beginner will always require this guidance until he gains that maturity.

Guidance for Seminar

Topic Selection

The selection of the topic is essential for a meaningful activity. It should be based on the relevance of the topic to the presenter and the audience. At a postgraduate level step by step grooming of the students is required. The topic should be based on the level of the training the postgraduate student is going through (i.e. whether he/she is junior, senior or the chief resident). For example, if the presenter is the junior resident he should be given topics based on the basic sciences. It is irrelevant for the junior resident to straight away talk on the treatment modalities, alternative techniques of management or the current advances. It is also desirable to distribute the topic amongst 2 to 3 postgraduate students, according to the level of training of the residents so that the junior resident talks about basic sciences, senior resident talks about the clinical features and management and the chief resident talks about complications and their management along with recent advances to make the presentation complete.

It is desirable to talk about common topics first than talking about rare, but important topics. Look at the phrase '*bread and butter*' or '*cake and icing*', it means bread or the cake (common) has to be first and then the luxury of butter or icing (rarities). This is a practical approach, as the common topics are not only routinely required in the clinical practice, but are also commonly asked in the examination by majority of the examiners. Hence, it also serves the purpose of preparing the student for the examination.

However, advances are equally important. The common topics fall in the category of '*must know*' and the advanced topics fall in the category of '*desirable to know*' or '*nice to know*' category. Hence, any presentation should be a good blend of basics and advances, however the degree of emphasis may vary depending upon the level of the training of the presenter and the level of the audience.

While selecting the topics for the seminars, it must be ensured that wider coverage of topics is made, so as to complete the entire curriculum in a phased manner rather than sticking to the same areas.

Apart from the standard topics some innovative, thought provoking topics should be selected. For example, rather than selecting straight forward topics like odontogenic cyst or tumors, topic like differential diagnosis of multiloculated lesions of the jaw be given to make it more interesting. As it is not straightforward, the presenter will have to refer wider literature to search for such pathologies, their salient features so as to discuss differential diagnosis. In case of topics that require multidisciplinary approach, the concerned specialties should also be involved. One must remember that the horizons of the knowledge are so wide, that they cannot be restricted in small water tight compartments. As the knowledge has no barriers, the student and teacher also do not have any barrier. Any input from any body if enhances, the quality must be accepted with open mind. There should be a good example of horizontal and vertical integration.

Purpose

The purpose of the seminar activities at the postgraduate level have already been discussed earlier. They can be summarized as:

- No didactic teaching at the postgraduate level
- Requires own efforts under guidance
- To know the topic in a broader sense
- To learn to search literature
- To compile the literature
- To analyze the literature
- To develop understanding and concept.

Topic Elaboration

Once the topic is identified for the presentation/seminar, it needs to be elaborated in the systematic way. Haphazard presentations may cover lot of things, but loose its impact as the communication value is poor and generate negative impact. It must be remembered that all the aspects pertaining to the topic must be covered. The degree of emphasis on certain areas may be more or less, depending upon the purpose of presentation, time limits, level of audience. Any presentation that is too lengthy, loses its impact. An ideal seminar should be constructed under the following headings:

- **Introduction:** Should spell out the outline of the topic and the objectives of presentation
- Historical aspects
- Brief review covering wider areas
- Controversies
- Current advances
- Summary
- Bibliography.

Contents

The contents of the seminars should be enriched using wider sources of literature such as:

- Books (lesser)
- Journals
- Internet.

The bibliography given at the end of the seminar should be able to depict the quantum of efforts done by the presenter in preparation of the seminar. It also validates the information incorporated in the seminar. The seminar would never be capable of causing cognigible impact, unless it is prepared with lot of involvement and effort. It is simply governed by the old quote '*no pain no gain*'.

Presentation

- **To discuss with the concerned teacher:** Once the topic is allotted it must be discussed with the concerned teacher, so as to formulate the objectives and make the outline of the presentation. The information can be searched, compiled and organized under appropriate heads. Once the rough draft is made it should be again discussed with the concerned teacher and then the necessary editing (additions, deletions be made). The final draft should be approved by the teacher before it is taken up for the presentation.
- **To be prepared well in advance:** It is a good practice to prepare the seminar well in advance, so that you get plenty of time for practice and refinement. Rushing at the eleventh hour reflects poor practice, lack of commitment/involvement and a casual attitude. Anything done half-heartedly is never going to be effective.
- **To practice:** As the final draft is made it is necessary to practice the presentation. '*Practice makes a man perfect*' holds true. The practice should be done as follows:
  - First practice yourself with time limit and audit.
  - Then in front of friendly audience.
  - Then again yourself.

  The practice will make the presenter well versed with the topic, contents of the presentation, sequence of points and provide insight as to what to speak for each slide. It also brings about fluency in presentation and facilitates *time auditing*. It is always better if the slides have only key points and the elaboration is done by the presenter in his own words in an extempore manner. Practice will facilitate this, as every individual may not be good at extempore manner and may struggle to find effective and appropriate words on time.
- **Emphasis on important areas:** A presenter must identify important or key areas of the presentation and lay more emphasis on them rather than wasting time on discussing the issues, which are not so vital.
- **Tell the objectives first:**
  - *A talk is not a mystery novel*

  Before starting the presentation always spell out the contents and objectives rather than starting and ending abruptly.
- **One major point per slide—you can always add the points verbally:** Do not flood your slides with too much information and many important points on a single slide. It looses the focus of the audience and the presenter as well. The information may be added verbally.
- **Amount of information per slide—less the better:** The large amount of information on single slide has the same drawbacks as the preceding point. In addition to that more the lines and more the words per line, smaller becomes the font. The slide appears staggering due to packed information and the focus is lost. It is better that each slide has 4 to 6 lines and each line has 4 to 6 words. The best way is to elaborate the points by speaking (Fig. 32.1).
- **Number of slides, less minutes you speak:** The time frame of the presentation must be taken into account. Too lengthy presentations are often less effective and unable to generate the desired impact. It is an established fact that the audience rapport cannot be obtained beyond 45 minutes. On an average in 1 minute not more than two slides can be presented by an experienced and established speaker and for a beginner, this ratio is even more critical and he/she may require more than 1 minute and hence the slides should be less in number than the minutes for which you speak.
- **Slides with best contrast (light foreground and dark background):** The color scheme and contrast is very important. What appears good on the screen of the computer may not look good on projection. The

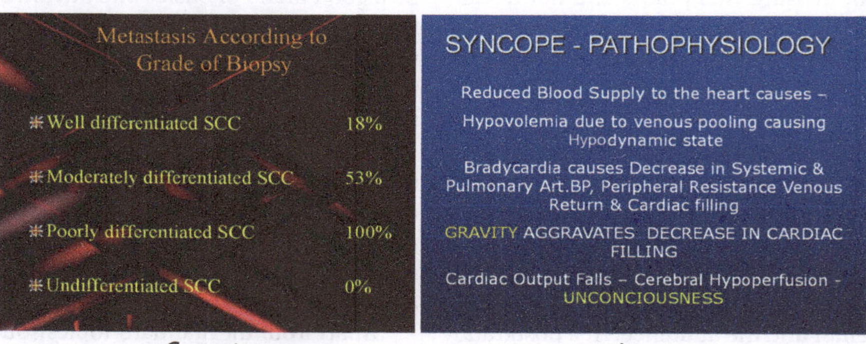

Fig. 32.1: Correct and incorrect way of making a powerpoint slide

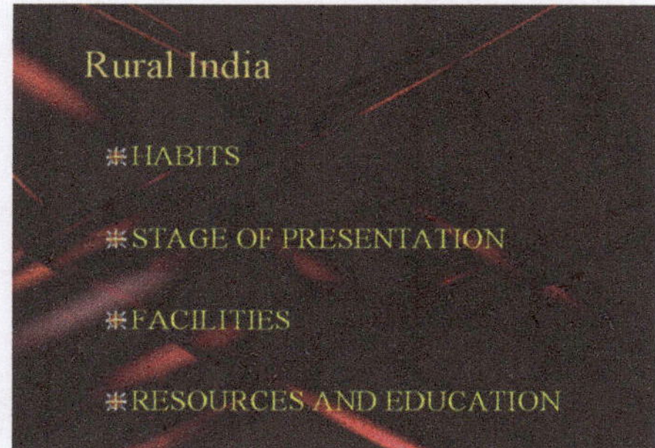

Fig. 32.2: Dark background and faint foreground is easy to read

Diagnostic Difficulties In Rural Setting
⌘Lack Of Trained Clinicians
⌘Lethargy Towards Comprehensive Clinical Examination
⌘No Sound Histopathological/ Cytological Backing

OKC
❖High rate of recurrence
• Thin &Fragile lining
• Invasive Nature
❖Needs more radical treatment
❖Carbolization of the base

Fig. 32.3: Dot not make slides unnecessarily colorful. Only matter to be highlighted can be of separate color

scientific presentation should be sober. The impact is created by contents and quality of presentation and not by the flashy slides devoid of substance. The slides should be soothening to eyes and easy to read. Usually the dark backgrounds and faint foreground (letters) is preferred (Fig. 32.2).

- **Do not use more colors than is needed to be effective:** Flashy color schemes and designs do not add to the value of the presentation. It should have minimum required color scheme. The colors are very effective means of communication provided that they are used judiciously. Rather than making the entire presentation use different colors to highlight the salient features of key points, only it will create more impact. Red, pink and other shades of the red appear clear on the computer screen, but are hard to see when projected (Fig. 32.3).
- **Font size preferably more than 24 pt:** Too small font size is not easily visible especially when it is presented before large gathering. It is desirable to have a font size of greater than 24. Similarly the font pattern should be simple and easy to read for establishing an effective communication (Fig. 32.4).

Diagrams

The illustrations and diagrams should be liberally used in the presentation provided, that they are relevant and able to simplify and explain the subject. There is no upper limit for use of diagrams or illustrations as-long-as they serve the desired purpose. The general guidelines for use of diagrams and illustrations are:

- No imitation for use
- Preferably self-designed through your own imagination rather than copied
- Use sketches along with the photographs or book diagrams
- Maintain originality
- Use of computer animations.

Audience Rapport

The involvement of the audience is equally important as is the involvement of the presenter. It is an art to involve the audience in your presentation. Presenters would appreciate undivided attention and less interruptions. Primarily the presentation should be rich in contents. Secondly the effective communication skill should be demonstrated by way of body language, command over the language and speed of presentation, accent and clarity of pronunciation. Rushed speed of presentation is not well conceived by the audience and similarly monotony should be avoided. A pause at the right place, when important diagrams or clinical photographs are projected and ability to brush through less important points is real test of the skill. Some people are gifted, but those who are not can always acquire these skills by practice. The positive body language is generally an out come of confidence generated within you as a result of thorough knowledge of the subject. Few important tips to engage the audience are as follows:

- Engage the audience—make eye contact, but do not linger on one person
- Use humor, but do not force it
- Be spontaneous in your humor punch and talk
- Be a good story teller.

Conclusions

After the presentation the presenter should be able to generate a summary or conclusion of the presentation in the condensed manner. Similarly the

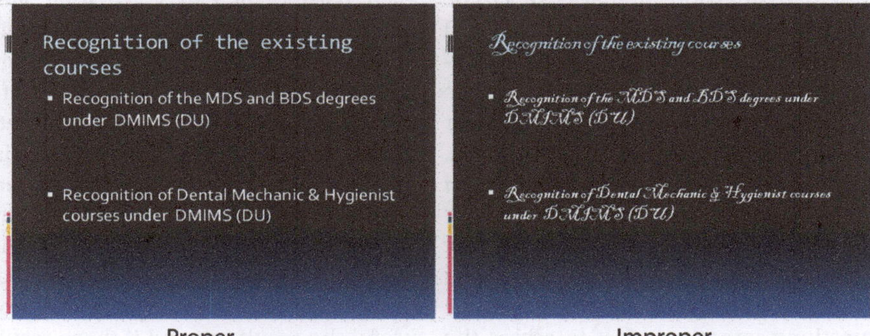

Proper Improper

Fig. 32.4: Font type should be easy to read

presenter should be able to deliver the take home message out of the presentation.

Role of Audience

The seminar activity should be interactive in nature and not like monologue. The role of audience is also very important, they should not be only passive listeners, but their active participation in the seminar is very important. The seminars are always mutually beneficial. The presenter gets an opportunity to study the topic in depth and the audience gets readymade information. The topic needs to be discussed threadbare, which is not possible without active involvement of the audience. It is therefore necessary for the audience also to come prepared with the given topic. The topic for presentation must be informed to other participants well in advance to facilitate them to prepare the topic. The audience should not ask questions just for the sake of asking, but the quality of questions should be such that they should throw light on the unaddressed, unexplained areas or should help in bringing completeness to the discussion. The audience can share any added information if the presenter has missed that during the presentation. The criticism if any must be constructive and logical. The levels of the audience are variable, some are beginners and some are established and accomplished people.

Anticipate Questions

While preparing for the seminar, think if you were on the other side of the table, anticipate questions that are likely to be asked by the audience and be prepared with the answers. The testimony of completeness of preparation of the topic lies in the ability of the presenter to answer the questions asked by the audience. The level of the questions asked by them is also variable for example the beginners tend to either keep quiet or ask very basic things, but the more accomplished people like teachers may ask advanced questions sometimes just to assess the preparation of the presenter. When ever a question is asked take a pause, think and compose your answer, so that you are to the point and precise.

JOURNAL CLUB PRESENTATION

Another important aspect of the postgraduate training is a journal club activity. The purpose of this activity is 'critical appraisal' and 'analysis of an article'. The primary goal of journal club is to improve the resident's ability to critically evaluate the medical literature and how it applies to clinical practice.

The earliest references to a journal club is found in a book of memoirs and letters by the late Sir James Paget, a British surgeon, who describes a group at St. Bartholomew's hospital in London in the mid-19th century as "a kind of club—a small room over a baker's shop near the Hospital-gate where we could sit and read the journals."[1]

Sir William Osler established the first formalized journal club at McGill University in Montreal in 1875. The original purpose of Osler's journal club was 'for the purchase and distribution of periodicals to which he could ill afford to subscribe.'[2]

A journal club is a group of individuals who meet regularly to critically evaluate recent articles in scientific literature. Journal clubs are usually organized around a defined subject in basic or applied research. For example, the application of evidence-based medicine to some area of medical practice can be facilitated by a journal club. Typically, each participant can voice their view relating to several questions such as the appropriateness of the research design, the statistics employed, the appropriateness of the controls that were used, etc. There might be an attempt to synthesize together the results of several papers, even if some of these results might first appear to contradict each other. Even if the results of the study are seen as valid, there might be a discussion of how useful the result are and if these results might lead to new research or to new applications.

Journal clubs are also used in the education of graduate or professional students. These help make the student become more familiar with the advanced literature in their new field of study. In addition, these journal clubs help improve the student's skills of understanding and debating current topics of active interest in their field. This type of journal club may sometimes be taken for credit. Research laboratories may also organize journals clubs for all researchers in the lab to help them keep up with the literature produced by others who work in their field.

Selection of Article for Journal Club

The article that are selected for the journal club must not be routine case reports, rather they should be the articles generated out of:

- Structured scientific studies
- Innovative ideas
- Modification of techniques
- Thought provoking
- Topics, which are rare and not included in routine curricular activities.

Presentation of the Journal Club

The journal club activity is not a *group reading* of an article, but it is the *critical appraisal* of a study. The entire text of the article must not be projected on the screen, but the article should be presented in the form of a condensed powerpoint presentation. This approach enhances the ability of the trainee to critically read, summarize, pickup important key areas of the study. The hard copy of the article may be kept handy for any reference, if needed. There should be a structured, chronological, analytical approach in the presentation.

The presentation of the article should include:

- Brief background of the study
  - Explain the rationale for undertaking the study.

  - What is the context for the study?
  - What previous work has led up to experiments done in the study?
  - Focus on key studies leading to this set of experiments and explain the importance of the problem in a wider context.
- Research question asked and main outcome of interest in the present study.
- Methodology used—case-control study, case series, randomized trial, etc.
- Subjects used including inclusion and exclusion criteria.
- How the study was done and how the outcome of interest was measured?
- Describe the results of the study and statistical tests used.
- What conclusions were drawn by the authors?
- Comparison of results with other studies—It means the resident cannot present a journal club by referring only one article, but has to widely search articles on the similar subject and compare the current study with other studies to discuss the merits and demerits, differences in results and reasons thereof.

Critique the Study

This component of the presentation will define the success of your journal club. A useful and widely accepted approach to this analysis has been published in Journal of American Medical Association series "User's guide to the medical literature." The Centre for Health Evidence in Canada has made the complete full-text set of these user's guides available online. The important areas that are addressed, while one critiques the study are:

a. Remember to critique (critically discuss) the study. Strengths and weaknesses.
b. Are there alternative interpretations for the data presented?
c. Can you think of additional controls that should have been done?
d. What other approaches could be undertaken to improve on the study?

Summary and Conclusion of Journal Club Presentation

Restate the author's take-home message followed by your own interpretation of the study. Provide a personal perspective, detailing why you find this paper interesting or important. Then, look forward and use this opportunity to "think outside the box". Do you envision these study results changing the landscape of clinical practice or redirecting research in this field? If so, how? Or do you find the results of this study to be counterproductive or inapplicable in your clinical practice? If yes, why?

Good journal club discussions are integral to the educational experience of postgraduate trainees. Following the above approach, while utilizing the resources available, will lay the ground work for an outstanding presentation.

REFERENCES

1. Esisi, Martina. "Journal clubs." BMJ Careers. 13 Oct. 2007. Web. 09 Jan. 2010. <http://careers.bmj.com/careers/advice/view-article.html?id=2631#ref2>
2. Milbrandt Eric B, Jean-Louis Vincent. "Evidence-based medicine journal club." Critical Care (2004): 401-02. PubMed. U.S. National Library of Medicine, 3 Nov. 2004. Web. 10 Jan. 2010. <http://www.ncbi.nlm.nih.gov/pmc/articles/PMC1065082/.

Section 12

Appendices

Commonly Prescribed Investigations in Surgical Practices, their Values and Interpretation

Borle Rajiv M

APPENDIX-I: HEMATOLOGY

Common Hematological Investigations

Sr. No.	Name of investigation	Sample collection	Normal values	Interpretation
1.	Hemoglobin	2 mL of blood sample is taken by method of venous puncture in bulb containing 0.2 mL of EDTA	*Male:* 12–14 g% *Female:* 10–12 g%	*A decreased* value is indicative of anemia. The most common cause of anemia is iron deficiency due to decreased intake of essential compounds, like vitamin B_1, B_6, B_{12}, iron, vitamin C. Bone marrow depression, acute blood loss, chronic blood loss as in bleeding piles, gastric/duodenal ulcers, heavy menstrual flow, hemoptysis and postpartum bleeding are also other causes.
2.	Complete blood count	2 mL of blood sample is taken by method of venous puncture in bulb containing 0.2 mL of EDTA	**RBC:** *Male:* 4.5–6.2 million/cumm *Female:* 4.5–5.5 million/cumm	*A decrease* in the RBC count is seen in anemia, pellagra, hemorrhage, liver disease. *An increase* is seen polycythemia and extreme dehydration. *A physiologic increase* in the RBC count is seen in high altitude, hypoxia, emotional stress, pregnancy.
			WBC: 5000–10000/cumm	WBC is *increased* in acute infections, uremia, leukemia and with steroid therapy. WBC is *decreased* in aplastic anemia, radiation therapy, infectious mononucleosis, malaria, AIDS, enteric fever, and drug poisoning.
			DLC: *Neutrophils*—50–62%	*Increase* in infection, granulocytic, leukemia, postsurgery, severe hemorrhage and burns. *Decrease* in aplastic anemia, viral infection and in patient undergoing radiation or dialysis.
			DLC: *Eosinophil*—2–8%	*Increase* in allergies, parasitic infection, collagen vascular diseases, Addison's disease and malignancy. *Decreased* in stress, steroid therapy, ACTH excess and Cushing's syndrome.
			Monocytes—1–3%	*Increased* in tuberculosis, chronic inflammation, collagen diseases, malaria, typhoid, kala azar and protozoal infections.

Contd...

Contd...

Sr. No.	Name of investigation	Sample collection	Normal values	Interpretation
			Lymphocytes—25–30%	*Increased* in viral infection, tuberculosis, syphilis, whopping cough. *Decreased* in stress, uremia and steroid therapy.
			Basophils—0–1%	*Increased* in polycythemia and chronic myeloid leukemia. *Decreased* in stress, steroid therapy and thyrotoxicosis.
			Platelet count: 1,50,000–4,00,000/cumm	*Increased* in allergic conditions, asphyxia, hemorrhage, bone fractures, surgical operations, splenectomy, rheumatic fever and trauma. *Decreased* in acute infections, acute leukemia, aplastic and pernicious anemia, chicken pox, small pox, splenomegaly, scarlet fever, typhoid and tuberculosis.
3.	Erythrocyte sedimentation rate (ESR)	2 mL of blood sample is taken by method of venous puncture in bulb containing 0.2 mL of EDTA	*Males:* 17–50 years 10 mm >50 years 12–14 mm *Females:* > 50 years 19–20 mm (Westergren's method at 1 hour)	*Increased* in tuberculosis, malignant tumors, rheumatoid arthritis, rheumatic fever and liver disease. *Decreased* in allergic conditions, sickle cell anemia, peptone shock, polycythemia.
4.	MCV (Mean corpuscular volume)	2 mL of blood sample is taken by method of venous puncture in bulb containing 0.2 mL of EDTA	85 ± 8 fl	*Lesser than lower limit of normal:* Microcytic anemia *Within normal range:* Normocytic anemia *Greater than normal:* Macrocytic anemia
5.	MCH (Mean corpuscular hemoglobin)	2 mL of blood sample is taken by method of venous puncture in bulb containing 0.2 mL of EDTA	29.5 ± 2.5 pg	*Lesser than normal:* Hypochromic anemia *Within normal range:* Normochromic anemia *Greater than normal:* Hyperchromic anemia
6.	MCHC (Mean corpuscular hemoglobin concentration)	2 mL of blood sample is taken by method of venous puncture in bulb containing 0.2 mL of EDTA	32.5 ± 2.5 g/dL	Since MCHC is independent of RBC count and size, it is considered to be of greater clinical significance, compared to absolute values. It is low in iron deficiency anemia but is usually normal in macrocytic anemia.

Peripheral Smear

Name of investigation	Sample collection	Indications	
Peripheral smear	2 mL of blood sample is taken by method of venous puncture in bulb containing 0.2 mL of EDTA or finger puncture	Platelet count, TLC, DLC, anemia typing, septicemia, parasitic infections like malaria or filiriasis, sickling in sickle cell anemia	• Platelet count in parasitic and viral infections. Decrease in count < 70,000 is suggestive of thrombocytopenia, patient has spontaneous bleeding tendency when the count is < 30,000–40,000. • Normochromic, hypochromic, microcytic, macrocytic character of the RBCs help in typing the anemia. • The morphological anomalies of the RBCs can be detected. • On addition of the reducing agent, classical sickling of RBCs can be seen in sickle cell disorders. • PS in a patient with septicemia shows immature WBCs in the form of band cells and intracellular eosinophilic granules termed as septic granules. • Peripheral smear detects malarial parasite in the RBCs when the sample is taken during the spike of fever and chills as the parasites come in the peripheral circulation. The filarial parasite can be seen if the sample is taken at the night as the parasites are present in the peripheral blood during night.

Peripheral Blood Smear Cell Picture

Cells	Interpretation
Target cells	Decreased osmotic fragility Deficiency of an enzyme called lecithin cholesterol acyl transferase Hemoglobin abnormalities (hemoglobinopathies) Iron deficiency Liver disease Spleen removal Thalassemia
Spherocytes	Autoimmune hemolytic anemia Hereditary spherocytosis Increased osmotic fragility
Elliptocytes	Hereditary elliptocytosis or hereditary ovalocytosis
Schistocytes	Artificial heart valve Disseminated intravascular coagulation Hemolytic uremic syndrome (HUS) Microangiopathic hemolytic anemia Thrombotic thrombocytopenic purpura (TTP)
Normoblast	Cancer that has spread to bone marrow Erythroblastosis fetalis Leukoerythroblastic anemia (myelophthisis process) Miliary tuberculosis Myelofibrosis Removal of spleen Severe hemolysis Thalassemia
Echinocytes (Burr cells)	Uremia
Acanthocytes (Spur cells)	Abetalipoproteinemia Severe liver disease
Teardrop-shaped cells	Leukoerythroblastic anemia Myelofibrosis Severe iron deficiency Thalassemia major
Howell–Jolly bodies	Myelodysplasia Post splenectomy Sickle cell anemia
Heinz bodies	Alpha thalassemia Congenital hemolytic anemia G6PD deficiency Unstable form of hemoglobin
Few reticulocytes (immature RBCs)	Anemia with bone marrow recovery Hemolytic anemia Hemorrhage
Basophilic stippling	Lead poisoning Myelofibrosis Myelophthisic process
Neutrophilic hypergranulation (toxic granulation)	Severe inflammation, septicemia, burns, trauma, and upon exposure to hematopoietic growth factors such as granulocyte-colony stimulating factor (G-CSF)
Döhle bodies	Infection, burns, uncomplicated pregnancy, toxic states, or during treatment with hematologic growth factors such as G-CSF

APPENDIX-II: BIOCHEMICAL INVESTIGATIONS

Liver Function Test

Sr. No.	Name of investigation	Sample collection	Normal values	Interpretation
1.	Alanine aminotransferase (ALT) Serum glutamic pyruvic transaminase (SGPT)	*Plain Bulb:* Blood samples are allowed to clot at 15–24°C for minimally 30 minutes and maximally one hour. For serum samples—specimens should be centrifuged at a temperature 15–24°C for 10 minutes at 1500 gravity within 1 hour after blood collection.	*Normal Adult* *Range:* 0–48 I.U./L Optimal Adult *Reading:* 24 I.U./L *Male:* 0–40 I.U./L *Female:* 0–36 I.U./L	*Increased levels* • Hepatocellular disease • Active cirrhosis (mild increase) • Metastatic liver tumor • Obstructive jaundice or biliary obstruction (mild to moderate increase) • Bone metastasis • Congestive heart failure • Muscle inflammation • Shock, trauma • Viral, infectious or toxic hepatitis (30–50x normal) • Infectious mononucleosis *Drugs that increase* ACE inhibitors, acetaminophen, anticonvulsants, antibiotics, heparin, NSAID's
2.	Aspartate aminotransferase (AST) Serum glutamic oxalaoacetic transaminase (SGOT)		*Male:* (10–55 I.U./L) *Female:* (7–30 I.U./L) *Children:* 2–3 times adult normal values. SGPT:SGOT = 1:1	Reflects damage to the hepatic cell Less specific for liver disease Elevated in viral hepatitis, mononucleosis, and acute hepatotoxicity, ischemia. SGOT > x 2 higher than SGPT characteristic of alcoholic liver disease; also in cirrhosis, hepatitis, pancreatitis, liver CA SGPT > SGOT viral or drug induced hepatitis and hepatic obstruction other than malignancy
3.	Bilirubin–Total		*Male:* (0.3–1) mg% *Female:* (0.3–1) mg%	• Hepatogenous/obstructive jaundice (increased total and conjugated bilirubin) • Hemolytic jaundice (increased total bilirubin but conjugated bilirubin does not rise) • Not a sensitive indicator of hepatic dysfunction • Must exceed >2.5 mg/dL to produce clinical jaundice • >10 mg/dL hepatocellular jaundice • >20 mg/dL in obstructive jaundice (neoplastic/intrahepatic) • <30 mg/dL in extrahepatic jaundice after which there is a plateau due its renal excretion • >50 mg/dL in severe heptaocellular jaundice
	Unconjugated bilirubin		*Male:* (0.2–0.7) mg% *Female:* (0.2–0.7) mg%	Increased unconjugated bilirubin: increased hemolysis, decreased hepatic uptake/conjugated (e.g. Gilbert's syndrome), cirrhosis, erythroblastosis fetalis, malaria
	Conjugated bilirubin		*Male:* (0.1–0.3) mg% *Female:* (0.1–0.3) mg%	Elevated conjugated bilirubin: biliary obstruction, cirrhosis, pregnancy.
4.	Alkaline phosphatase		*Adults:* 65–306 I.U/L *Children:* Less than 645 I.U/L	*Increased* • Cholestasis, biliary obstruction, bone metastasis, calcium deficiency, cirrhosis, high fat intake, hyperparathyroidism, infectious mononucleosis, leukemia, osteogenic carcinoma, vitamin D deficiency, fibrous dysplasia, Paget's disease. • Infiltrative diseases of liver

Contd...

Contd...

Sr. No.	Name of investigation	Sample collection	Normal values	Interpretation
				• Serum ALP by osteoblast-rapid growth of bone (growth, healing of fracture, osteosarcoma, bone metastasis, Paget's disease, fibrous dysplasia, multiple myeloma, rickets). *Decreased in*—Cystic fibrosis, excessive vitamin D intake, hypophosphatemia, pernicious anemia, celiac disease, chronic nephritis, scurvy. *Drugs that increase*—ACE inhibitors, anticonvulsant, heparin, NSAID's, estrogens *Drugs that decrease*—Fluorides, propranolol.
5.	Gamma glutamyl transferase (GGT) Enzyme		*Female:* 5–29 U/L *Male:* 5–38 U/L *Child:* 3–30 U/L *Newborn:* 5 times child's normal value	*Elevated levels (> 10–30 IU/L) are observed in:* Chronic alcoholism, acute pancreatic disease, myocardial infarction, renal failure, chronic obstructive pulmonary disease and in diabetes mellitus, biliary obstruction, cholecystitis, cholelithiasis, renal cancer, SLE. *Drugs that increase:* Aminoglycosides, Barbiturates, NSAID's, Phenobarbital, Phenytoin. *Drugs that decrease:* Oral contraceptive.
6.	Serum protein		*Male:* (6–8) g% *Female:* (6–8) g%	• Proteins levels are nonspecific for liver disease • No changes in protein levels in acute liver disease but evident changes in chronic liver disease like cirrhosis, hepatocellular damage.
	Serum globulin		*Male:* (2.5–3.5) g% *Female*: (2.5–3.5) g%	Decreased in malnutrition, severe illness, nephritic losses and protein losing enteropathies.
	Serum albumin		4.0 to 5.7 g/dL	*Hypoprotienamia:* Decreased serum protein decreases the osmotic pressure of the blood, leading to loss of fluid from the intravascular compartment, or the blood vessels, to the interstitial tissues, resulting in edema. This is termed as hypoproteinemia.

RA Factor

Name of test	Collection of blood samples	Normal values	Interpretation
RA factor	Venous blood in plain sterile bulb	• Less than 40–60 u/mL or • Less than 1:80 (1 to 80) titre	High levels of rheumatoid factor occur in rheumatoid arthritis and Sjögren's syndrome. The higher the level of RF the greater the probability of destructive articular disease. It elevates in chronic hepatitis, primary biliary cirrhosis, any chronic viral infection, bacterial endocarditis, leukemia, dermatomyositis, infectious mononucleosis, systemic sclerosis, and systemic lupus erythematosus (SLE)

Kidney Function Test

Sr. No.	Name of investigation	Sample collection	Normal values	Interpretation
1.	Serum creatinine	*Plain sterile bulb* • Blood samples are allowed to clot at 15–24°C for minimally 30 minutes and maximally one hour. • For serum samples—specimens should be centrifuged at a temperature 15–24°C for 10 minutes at 1500 g within 1 hour after blood collection	*Male:* (0.7–1.5) mg% *Female:* (0.5–1.2) mg%	*Increased* • Renal parenchymal damage and catabolic disorders muscle • More sensitive indicator of GFR than blood urea nitrogen
2.	Serum potassium		*Male:* (3–5) mEq/L *Female:* (3–5) mEq/L	*Hyperkalemia:* Urine potassium level above 40 mEq/L suggest intact renal excretory mechanism. Implying that high intake or failure of cell uptake is the major mechanism for hyperkalemia. Seen in dehydration, kidney failure, acidic blood pH, burns, diabetes, drugs like ACEI (Angiotensin converting enzyme inhibitor) *Hypokalemia:* Is a metabolic disorder that occurs when the level of potassium in the blood drops too low. Seen in severe burns, cystic fibrosis, alcoholism, Cushing's syndrome, dehydration, malnutrition, vomiting, diarrhea and certain kidney diseases, such as Bartter's syndrome.
3.	Serum sodium		*Male:* (136–145) mEq/L *Female:* (136–145) mEq/L	*Increased:* (Hypernatremia) Hypotonic fluid loss—diarrhea, vomiting, Chronic renal failure *Decreased:* < 135 mEq/L (Hyponatatremia) Hypothyroidism, Addisons disease, prolonged vomiting, decreased oral intake, severe diarrhea, SIADH (Syndrome of inappropriate antidiuretic hormone secretion)
4.	Serum urea		*Male:* (18–40) mg% *Female:* (18–40) mg%	*Increased* Renal parenchymal disorder Decreased GFR *Decreased* Advanced liver disease Low protein diets

Other Biochemical Investigations

Name of the investigation	Method of sample collection	Normal values	Interpretation
Serum calcium	For total and ionic serum calcium, blood collected in RA tubes, centrifuged to draw serum	*Total:* 9–11 mg/dL	*Hypercalcemia:* Malignancy, hyperparathyroidism, hyperthyroidism, osteomyalacia, pagets disease. *Hypocalcemia:* Hypoparathyroidism, vitamin D deficiency, excess of fluid loss from body.
Ionized Ca^{++}		Ionized calcium of 1.1–1.4 mmol/L or (4.5–5.6 mg/dL)	An ionized calcium value within the reference range implies adequate calcium homeostasis, as this is a direct measure of calcium in its active form. *Decreased levels:* Hyperparathyroidism, multiple myeloma, sarcoidosis *Increased levels:* Hypoparathyroidism, acidosis, hypoalbuminemia, malignant neoplasm.
Serum phosphorus		*Adults:* 3.0–4.5 mg/dL *Children:* 4.5–6.5 mg/dL	*Hyperphosphatemia:* Liver disease, renal failure, excess of vitamin D, hypocalcemia, and hypoparathyroidism. *Hypophosphatemia:* Malnutrition, low intake of vitamin D, hypercalcemia, and hyperparathyroidism
Acid phosphatase		*Male:* 0–0.8 U/L	It is a type of enzyme used to free attached phosphate groups from other molecules during digestion. It is stored in lysosomes. Different forms of acid phosphates are found in different organs, their levels are used to evaluate the success of the surgical treatment of prostate cancer.
Alkaline phosphatase			Discussed earlier in liver function tests

Blood Glucose Test

Name of investigation	Normal values (range)	Sample	Interpretation
Random blood sugar (RBS)	80–140 mg/dL	1 mL venous blood sample in fluoride bulb	*Increased* in diabetes *Decreases* in states of hypoglycemia
Fasting blood sugar (FBS)	70–110 mg/dL	1 mL venous blood sample in fluoride bulb	Increased in diabetes
Post prandial blood sugar or post meal blood sugar (PPDS/PMBS)	<140 mg/dL	1 mL venous blood sample in fluoride bulb	Increased in diabetes

Glycosylated Hemoglobin (HbA1c)

Glycosylated hemoglobin testing is recommended for both

i. Checking the blood sugar control in people who might be prediabetic.
ii. Monitoring blood sugar control in patients with more elevated levels, termed diabetes mellitus. It provides accurate assessment of glucose control of past four months, thus helps in titrating anti diabetic medications.

Glycosylated hemoglobin measurement is not appropriate when there has been a change in diet or treatment within 6 weeks. Likewise, the test assumes a normal red blood cell aging process and mix of hemoglobin subtypes (predominantly HbA in normal adults). Hence, people with recent blood loss, hemolytic anemia, or genetic differences in the hemoglobin molecule (hemoglobinopathy) such as sickle-cell disease and other conditions, as well as those that have donated blood recently, are not suitable for this test.

Investigation	Reading	Type of sample	Interpretation
HbA1c Test	<7%	Venous blood sample	Good diabetic control
	10%	Venous blood sample	Fair control
	13–20%	Venous blood sample	Poor control

Oral Glucose Tolerance Test

The test is usually used to test for diabetes, insulin resistance, and sometimes reactive hypoglycemia and acromegaly or rare disorders of carbohydrate metabolism.

FBS (For >8 hours)	<100 mg/dL	Venous blood and urine sample	Increased in diabetes mellitus
FBS (Two hours after 75 g oral glucose load)	<140 mg/dL	Venous blood and urine sample	Increased in diabetes mellitus
RBS	>200 mg/dL	Venous blood and urine sample	Diabetes mellitus

Thyroid Function Test

Test	Method	Normal range	Interpretation
"TSH" test—thyroid stimulating hormone/serum thyrotropin	2 mL venous blood in plain sterile bulb	0.4–6 μIU/mL 0.3–3.0 μIU/mL (as of 2003)	< 0.4 μIU/mL can indicate possible hyperthyroidism. Over 6 μIU/mL is considered indicative of hypothyroidism. *Note:* The American Association of Clinical Endocrinologists has revised these guidelines as of early 2003, narrowing the range to .3–3 μIU/mL.
Total T4/serum thyroxine		4.5–12.5 μIU/mL	< 4.5 μIU/mL can be indicative of an under functioning thyroid when TSH is also elevated. > 12.5 μIU/mL can indicate hyperthyroidism. Low T4 with low TSH can sometimes indicate a pituitary problem.
Free T4/free thyroxine-FT4		0.7–2.0 ng/L	< 0.7 ng/L is considered indicative of possible hypothyroidism.
T3/serum triiodothyronine		*1–9 years*: 94–269 ng/dL *10–19 years*: 102–220 ng/dL *> 20 years old*: 80–220 ng/dL	< 80 pg/mL can indicate hypothyroidism.

APPENDIX-III: COAGULATION

Coagulation Profile

Sr. No	Investigations	Method of sample collection	Normal values	Interpretations
1.	Bleeding time Duke's method Ivy method	Finger prick (Blotting paper) Capillary blood	3–8 min	Prolonged in Aspirin therapy Thrombocytopenia Disorders of platelet function von Willebrand disease Vascular abnormalities (Ehlers Danlos syndrome) Severe deficiency of factor V and IX
2.	Clotting time	Finger prick Capillary blood	9–14 min	Prolonged in cases of Hemophilia A and B vitamin K deficiency Coagulation disorders in liver disease
3.	Prothrombin time (PT) Quick's one stage PT	Venous blood in the ratio of (blood: anticoagulant) 9:1 Oxalate bulb	12–15 sec	Evaluation of extrinsic and common pathway (deficiency of Factors I, V, VII and X) Prolonged in cases of Oral anticoagulant therapy DIC, liver diseases
4.	Partial thromboplastin time (PTT)	Venous blood in oxalate bulb	30–40 sec	Evaluation of intrinsic and common pathway (deficiency of Factors I, II, V, VIII, IX, X, XI and XII) Prolonged in cases of Prolonged parenteral heparin therapy DIC, liver diseases
5.	aPTT + PT			**aPTT prolonged, PT normal** Deficiencies of intrinsic pathway Factor(s) VIII, IX, XI or XII **PT prolonged, aPTT normal** Deficiency of extrinsic pathway Factor VII Occasionally, mild to moderate deficiency of common pathway factor(s) fibrinogen, II, V or X **Both PT and aPTT prolonged** Deficiency of common pathway Factor(s) fibrinogen, II, V, or X Multiple factor deficiencies
6.	Thrombin time (TT)	Venous blood in the ratio of (blood: anticoagulant) 9:1 oxalate bulb	8–12 sec	Evaluation of common coagulation pathway Prolonged in • Afibrinogenemia • DIC • Parenteral anticoagulant therapy
7.	D–Dimer test (Latex agglutination test)	1 mL of platelet poor plasma incubated with 3.2% sodium citrate in plastic vial	110–250 ng/mL	D-dimers are not normally present in human blood plasma, except when the coagulation system has been activated, for instance because of the presence of thrombosis or disseminated intravascular coagulation. The D-dimer assay depends on the binding of a monoclonal antibody to a particular epitope on the D-dimer fragment. It is useful in diagnosis of DVT, pulmonary embolism and DIC.
8.	INR (international normalized ratio) to express the intensity of anticoagulant therapy. INR = patient PT/lab PT			Maintaining an INR of 2.0 to 3.0 is advised for prophylaxis/treatment of venous thrombosis and thromboembolic complication associated with atrial fibrillation, for pulmonary embolism, for prophylaxis of systemic embolism after myocardial infarction and for prosthetic cardiac valves. A higher INR of 2.5 to 3.5 is recommended for cardiac valve replacement which involves mechanical valves and anti-phospholipid antibody syndrome. Range of INR > 2.0 can cause serious bleeding sequences.
9.	Clot retraction time	3 mL in sterile plain bulb	0–2 hrs	A normal value means that outside-in signaling through integrin αIIbB3 in the clotting process is normal. This generalizes that overall platelet function is normal, although it does not test every factor.

Contd...

Contd...

Sr. No	Investigations	Method of sample collection	Normal values	Interpretations
				A long clot retraction time is abnormal and suggests an abnormality somewhere in the coagulation cascade after integrin αIIbB3 interacts with fibrin. This suggests a prolonged bleeding time and abnormal platelet thrombus formation, such as can be seen with acquired or hereditary platelet disorders. Integrin αIIbB3 receptor dysfunction is specifically implicated in Glanzmann thrombasthenia. Low platelets or fibrinogen as well as high RBC concentrations prolong clot retraction time. Anitplatelet medications can also prolong clot retraction time. A low value, or short clot retraction time, may suggest tendencies toward thrombosis and other pathologies. This could also be due to nonstandardized conditions for the test.

Individual Factor Assay

Sr. No.	Test performed	Sample collection	Normal range	Inference
1.	Factor I assay	Coagulation citrated samples obtained by clean venipuncture	Normal range 1.5–4.0 g/L	*Fibrinogen levels are reduced in:* DIC due to the consumption of clotting factors. Liver disease due to decreased synthesis. An abnormal fibrinogen may also be found in patients with liver disease due to an abnormal (increased) sialic acid content. Massive transfusion leading to a dilutional coagulopathy. Inherited deficiencies e.g. hypofibrinogenemia, afibrinogenemia and dysfibrinogenemia [the latter is often associated with reduced fibrinogen levels as well as activity]. Following thrombolytic therapy. In some patients following treatment with asparaginase. *Fibrinogen levels are increased in:* Increasing age. Female sex, pregnancy, oral contraception. In postmenopausal women. Acute phase reaction. Disseminated malignancy [but may also be decreased if this is associated with DIC].
2.	Factor II assay	Coagulation citrated samples obtained by clean venipuncture	Normal range 50–150 u/dL	Intracranial hemorrhage, disseminated intravascular coagulation (DIC) both PT and PTT prolonged, to evaluate a prolonged PT (with normal PTT), vitamin K deficiency
3.	Factor V assay	Coagulation citrated samples obtained by clean venipuncture	Normal range 50–150 u/dL	Both PT and PTT prolonged, to evaluate a prolonged PT (with normal PTT)
4.	Factor VII assay	Coagulation citrated samples obtained by clean venipuncture	Normal range 50–150 u/dL	To evaluate a prolonged PT (with normal PTT), liver dysfunction vitamin K deficiency, thrombosis
5.	Factor VIII assay	Coagulation citrated samples obtained by clean venipuncture	Normal range 50–150 u/dL	von Willebrand disease evaluation, hemophilia A (Factor VIII deficiency), PTT prolonged, PT normal, thrombosis, increase during pregnancy
6.	Factor IX assay	Coagulation citrated samples obtained by clean venipuncture	Normal range 50–150 u/dL	Hemophilia B, to evaluate a prolonged PTT (with normal PT), Warfarin or vitamin K deficiency
7.	Factor X assay	Coagulation citrated samples obtained by clean venipuncture	Normal range 50–150 u/dL	Both PT and PTT prolonged, to evaluate a prolonged PT (with normal PTT), Warfarin or vitamin K deficiency
8.	Factor XI assay	Coagulation citrated samples obtained by clean venipuncture	Normal range 60–150 u/dL	PTT prolonged, PT normal, thrombosis, decrease during pregnancy, liver dysfunction, proteinuria
9.	Factor XII assay	Coagulation citrated samples obtained by clean venipuncture	Normal range 40–150 u/dL	PTT prolonged, PT normal, liver dysfunction, proteinuria

APPENDIX-IV: ARTERIAL GAS ANALYSIS

Arterial Blood Gases

Blood gas analysis, also called arterial blood gas (ABG) analysis, is a test which measures the amount of oxygen (O_2) and carbon dioxide (CO_2) in the blood, as well as the acidity (pH) of the blood.

Blood gas studies are usually done to assess respiratory disease and other conditions that may affect the lungs, and to manage patients receiving oxygen therapy (respiratory therapy) and the patients on assisted ventilation.

In addition, the acid-base component of the test provides information on kidney function too.

Indications

There is no single method for deciding the ABG to be done. It needs to be determined after proper evaluation of individual patient.

When ABG is Needed

a. In emergency critical and unstable patients where significant acid base disorder is suspected, ABG is needed immediately.
b. If history examination and serum electrolytes suggests severe or progressive acid base disorders.
c. Sick patient with significant respiratory distress secondary to acute respiratory diseases or exacerbation of chronic respiratory diseases.

How to Collect Blood for ABG

Technique for radial artery puncture:

1. Perform modified Allen's test.
2. Under proper asepsis 21 gauge needle heparin flushed syringe is used.
3. Palpate artery with one hand and enter the skin at 45° angle
4. Obtain 2–4 mL of blood without aspiration.

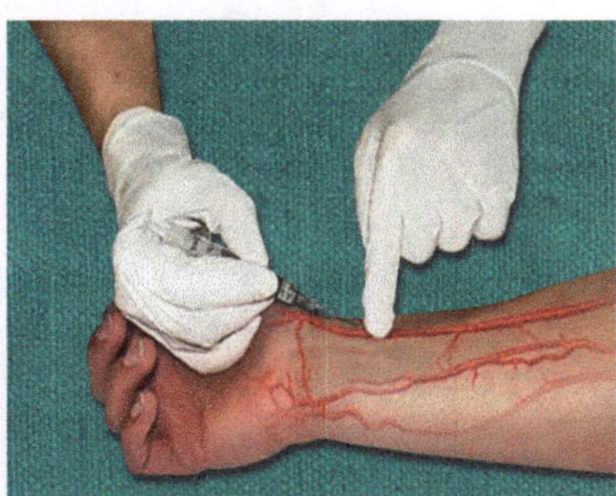

After a pulse is found, a blood sample is taken from the artery

Information Provided by an ABG

Parameter	Significance	Normal value	Interpretation
$PaCO_2$	This is the partial pressure of carbon dioxide dissolved within the arterial blood. It is used to assess the effectiveness of ventilation.	The normal range for a healthy person is 4.7–6.0 kPa or 35–45 mm Hg although in chronic pulmonary diseases it may be considerably higher and still normal for that patient.	A high $PaCO_2$ (respiratory acidosis) indicates underventilation, a low $PaCO_2$ (respiratory alkalosis) indicates hyper- or overventilation.
PaO_2	This is the partial pressure of oxygen dissolved within the arterial blood and will determine oxygen binding to hemoglobin (SaO_2).	The normal range is 9.3–13.3 kPa or 80–100 mm Hg.	It is of vital importance but is not used in determining patients' acid base status and normally low readings indicate hypoxemia.

Contd...

Contd...

Parameter	Significance	Normal value	Interpretation
SaO_2 Oxygen saturation	Oxygen saturation measures how much of the hemoglobin (Hb) in the red blood cells is carrying oxygen (O_2). Although similar to SpO_2 (measured by a pulse oximeter), it is more accurate.	The normal levels are 97% and above, although levels above 90% are often acceptable in critically ill patients.	Reduced in hypoxia
pH	The pH measures hydrogen ions (H^+) in blood.	The pH of blood usually between 7.35 to 7.45.	A pH of less than 7.0 indicates acidosis and pH greater than 7.4 indicates alkalosis.
HCO_3 (Bicarbonate)	Bicarbonate is a chemical (buffer) that keeps the pH of blood from becoming too acidic or too basic and indicates whether a metabolic problem is present (such as ketoacidosis).	Normal range is 22–26 mmol/L.	A low HCO_3^- indicates metabolic acidosis, a high HCO_3^- indicates metabolic alkalosis. HCO_3^- levels can also become abnormal when the kidneys are working to compensate for a respiratory issue so as to normalize the blood pH.
Base excess (BE)	The base excess is used for the assessment of the metabolic component of acid-base disorders.	Normal range is –3 to +3 mmol/L.	Low value indicates metabolic acidosis and high value indicates metabolic alkalosis.
Anion gap (AP)	The charge difference between unmeasured anion and cation is termed the anion gap (AP).	Anion gap (AP) = Na (Cl + HCO_3) = 12 ± 2 mEq/L	AG in metabolic acidosis: anion gap is most useful to establish etiological diagnosis of (hyperchloremic) acidosis is diarrhea. While important cause of increased anion gap acidosis are lactic acidosis, ketoacidosis and CRF. Increased anion gap acidosis is characterized by two factors: 1. Low HCO_3 and 2. Increased anion gap. It is important to remember that fall in HCO_3 = Rise in anion gap.

APPENDIX-V: URINE EXAMINATION

Gross and Biochemical Examination

Name of investigation	Sample collection	Normal values	Interpretations
Color	In human medicine, 4–10 mL of urine is used as the standard volume in sterile plain bulb. Early morning, mid stream urine sample is collected.		Many things affect urine color, including fluid balance, diet, medicines, and diseases. Vitamin B supplements can turn urine bright yellow. Some medicines, blackberries, beets or blood in the urine (hematuria) can turn urine red-brown.
Turbidity		Urine is normally clear	Turbidity or cloudiness may be caused by excessive cellular material or protein in the urine (proteinurea) or may develop from crystallization or precipitation of salts upon standing at room temperature or in the refrigerator. Clearing of the specimen after addition of a small amount of acid indicates that precipitation of salts is the probable cause of turbidity.
Odor		Nutty odor	Some diseases cause a change in the odor of urine. For example, an infection with *E. coli* bacteria can cause a bad odor, while diabetes or starvation can cause a sweet, fruity odor.
Specific gravity	Specific gravity between 1.002 and 1.035 on a random sample should be considered normal if kidney function is normal		This test detects the ion concentration of urine. Small amounts of protein or ketoacidosis tend to elevate the urine's specific gravity (SG). This value is measured using a urinometer and indicates hydration or dehydration. If the SG is under 1.010, the patient is hydrated; an SG value above 1.020 indicates dehydration.
pH of urine		The pH of urine can vary between 4.6 and 8, with neutral 7 being normal	A diet high in meat can decrease urine pH (more acidic). Cranberries, popularly thought to decrease the pH of urine, have actually been shown not to acidify urine. Drugs that can decrease urine pH include ammonium chloride, chlorothiazide diuretics, and methenamine mandelate
Bence-Jones protein (BJ proteins)	They are the light chain gamma globulins (kappa and lambda)		This protein is precipitated at 40° and at 50–60°C redissolves. It precipitates again on cooling. It is pathognomonic of multiple myeloma. It is also seen in leukemia, hypergammaglobulinemia, lymphoma and carcinomatous metastasis in bones, injured glomerular membrane. Bence Jones proteins are particularly diagnostic of multiple myeloma in the context of end-organ manifestations such as renal failure, lytic (or "punched out") bone lesions, anemia, or large numbers of plasma cells in the bone marrow of patients. Bence Jones proteins are present in 2/3 of multiple myeloma cases. Certain nonmalignant diseases, such as rheumatoid arthritis, systemic lupus erythematosus, and chronic renal insufficiency, can have Bence Jones proteins in the urine. High doses of penicillin or aspirin before collecting the urine can give a false positive result.
Ketone bodies		Ketone bodies are normally absent	*When Ketone bodies are present in urine it is termed as 'Ketoneuria'* With carbohydrate deprivation, such as starvation or high-protein diets, the body relies increasingly on the metabolism of fats for energy. This pattern is also seen in people with diabetes mellitus, when a lack of the hormone insulin prevents the body cells from using the large amounts of glucose available in the blood. This happens because insulin is necessary for the transport of glucose from the blood into the body cells. The metabolism of fat proceeds in a series of steps. First, triglycerides are hydrolyzed to fatty acids and glycerol. Second, the fatty acids are hydrolyzed into smaller intermediate compounds (acetoacetic acid, betahydroxybutyric acid, and acetone). Thirdly, the intermediate products are used

Contd...

Contd...

Name of investigation	Sample collection	Normal values	Interpretations
			in aerobic cellular respiration. When the production of the intermediate products of fatty acid metabolism (collectively known as ketone bodies) exceeds the ability of the body to metabolize these compounds, they accumulate in the blood and some end up in the urine (ketonuria). Ketone bodies are present in urine in conditions like diabetic ketoacidosis and nondiabetic ketonuria, febrile illness, hyperemesis in pregnancy, cachexia, excessive fatty acid metabolism and failing anesthesia, on exposure to cold, severe exercise and fasting.
Bile pigments		In trace amounts	The fixed phagocytic cells of the spleen and bone marrow destroy old red blood cells and convert the heme groups of hemoglobin to the pigment bilirubin. The bilirubin is secreted into the blood and carried to the liver, where it is bonded to (conjugated with) glucuronic acid, a derivative of glucose. Some of the conjugated bilirubin is secreted into the blood and the rest is excreted in the bile as bile pigment that passes into the small intestine. The blood normally contains a small amount of free and conjugated bilirubin. An abnormally high level of blood bilirubin may result from an increased rate of red blood cell destruction, liver damage (as in hepatitis and cirrhosis), and obstruction of the common bile duct as with gallstones. Increased urobilinogen (conjugated form of bilirubin) in urine is diagnostic of hemolytic jaundice. Urobilinogen is a colorless product of bilirubin reduction. It is formed in the intestines by bacterial action. Some urobilinogen is reabsorbed, taken up into the circulation and excreted by the kidney. This constitutes the normal "enterohepatic urobilinogen cycle." Increased amounts of bilirubin are formed in hemolysis, which generates increased urobilinogen in the gut. In liver disease (such as hepatitis), the intrahepatic urobilinogen cycle is inhibited also increasing urobilinogen levels. Urobilinogen is converted to the yellow pigmented urobilin apparent in urine. The urobilinogen (also known as stercobilinogen) in the intestine is then oxidized to brown stercobilin, which gives the feces their characteristic color. In biliary obstruction, below-normal amounts of conjugated bilirubin reach the intestine for conversion to urobilinogen. With limited urobilinogen available for reabsorption and excretion, the amount of urobilin found in the urine is low. High amounts of the soluble conjugated bilirubin enter the circulation where they are excreted via the kidneys. These mechanisms are responsible for the dark urine and pale stools observed in biliary obstruction. Low urine urobilinogen may result from complete obstructive jaundice or treatment with broad-spectrum antibiotics, which destroy the intestinal bacterial flora. (Obstruction of bilirubin passage into the gut or failure of urobilinogen production in the gut.) Low urine urobilinogen levels may result from congenital enzymatic jaundice (hyperbilirubinemia syndromes) or from treatment with drugs that acidify urine, such as ammonium chloride or ascorbic acid. Elevated levels may indicate hemolytic anemia (excessive breakdown of red blood cells), overburdening of the liver, increased urobilinogen production, reabsorption—a large hematoma, restricted liver function, hepatic infection, poisoning or liver cirrhosis. The most common cause of bilirubinuria is hepatocellular disease. More rare causes include inherited disorders, such as Dubin-Johnson syndrome and Rotor syndrome.

Contd...

Contd...

Name of investigation	Sample collection	Normal values	Interpretations
Proteins	Dipstick method with indicator dye, Bromphenol blue. Heat precipitation test. or Sulfosalicylic acid test	<150 mg/day or 10 mg/100 mL of single specimen	Since proteins are very large molecules (macromolecules), they are not normally present in measurable amounts in the glomerular filtrate or in the urine. More than 150 mg/day is defined as proteinuria, proteinuria >3.5 g/day is severe and known as nephotic syndrome. This may be caused by renal infections or by other diseases that have secondarily affected the kidneys, such as hypertension, diabetes mellitus, jaundice, or hyperthyroidism.
Glucose	Dipstick method Benedict's test	Normally absent or present in traces Normal glucose range in urine: 0–0.8 mmol/L (0–15 mg/dL)	• The renal threshold for glucose is 180 mg/dL. When blood sugar is > the renal threshold the glucose appears in urine (glycosuria). • Glycosuria leads to excessive water loss into the urine with resultant dehydration, a process called osmotic diuresis. • However the glycosuria can be seen in pregnancy (gestational glycosuria), ailimentary glycosuria secondary to transient elevation of blood sugar after ingestion of large quantity of sweets (carbohydrate rich diet), or it could be renal glycosuria, i.e. due to renal pathology the glucose appears in urine inspite of normal blood levels. Glycosuria alone does not mean that the patient is diabetic but it can be a useful screening and monitoring investigation. It is an unreliable indicator.

Microscopic Urine Analysis

Cellular casts	RBC	Normally not present	They may stick together and form red blood cell casts. Such casts are indicative of glomerulonephritis, with leakage of RBC's from glomeruli, or severe tubular damage.
	WBC	Normally not present	They may stick together and form red blood cell casts. Such casts are indicative of glomerulonephritis, with leakage of RBC's from glomeruli, or severe tubular damage.
Cells	RBC	Normally not present or 1–2 /HPF is considered normal	Hematuria is the presence of abnormal numbers of red cells in urine. Indicating damage to renal parenchyma and urinary tract. It may be due to a generalized bleeding diathesis or a urinary tract-specific problem (trauma, stone, infection, malignancy, etc.) or artifact of catheterization in case the sample is taken from a collection bag, in which case a fresh urine sample should be sent for a repeat test. If the RBCs are of renal or glomerular origin (due to glomerulonephritis), the RBCs incur mechanical damage during the glomerular passage, and then osmotic damage along the tubules, so get dysmorphic features.
	WBC	Less than 5 WBC/HPF is commonly accepted as normal	Pyuria refers to the presence of abnormal numbers of leukocytes that may appear with infection in either the upper or lower urinary tract or with acute glomerulo nephritis. Nonseptic causes on inflammation such as uroliths and tumors, also must be considered. It is an indication for urine culture.
	Epithelial cells	Normally not present or < 2/HPF considered normal	Indicator of normal tubular cell renewal or regeneration. Renal tubular epithelial cells, usually larger than granulocytes, contain a large round or oval nucleus and normally slough into the urine in small numbers.
	Squamous cells	≤ 15–20 squamous epithelial cells/HPF	Squamous epithelial cells: Squamous epithelial cells from the skin surface or from the outer urethra can appear in urine. It indicates improper method of urine collection and possible contamination with perigenital skin.
Bacteria		Bacterial species which are commensals to urinary tract are present	Bacteria are common in urine specimens because of the abundant normal microbial flora of the vagina or external urethral meatus. Bacteriuria can be confirmed if a single bacterial species is isolated in a concentration greater than 100,000 CFU/mL of urine in clean-catch midstream urine specimens (one for men, two consecutive specimens with the same bacterium for women).

Contd...

Contd...

Yeast	Normally not present	Yeast cells may be contaminants or represent a true yeast infection. Most often they are *Candida*, which may colonize in bladder, urethra, or vagina.
Crystals	Common crystals may be seen in healthy individuals. Uncommon crystals are present in cases of nephrolithiasis	Crystalluria indicates that the urine is supersaturated with the compounds that comprise the crystals. Common crystals seen even in healthy patients include calcium oxalate, triple phosphate crystals and amorphous phosphates. Uncommon crystals such as calcium oxalate are present in cases of nephrolithiasis

BIBLIOGRAPHY

1. Dacie and Lewis, Practical hematology; 7th Ed, 1991, Churchill Livingstone Elsevier.
2. De Gruchy, Clinical hematology in medical practice; 3rd Ed, 1970, Blackwell Willey.
3. June and Cella Junaitha Watson, Manual of laboratory tests; 1st Ed, 2006, AITBS.
4. Pagana, Kathleen Deska. Mosby's Manual of Diagnostic and Laboratory Tests, 1998, St. Louis: Mosby, Inc.
5. Todd, Sanford Davidsohn, Clinical diagnosis and management by Laboratory investigation; 17th Ed, 1989, W B Saunders Philadelphia Inc.

Index

Page numbers followed by *f* refer to figure and *t* refer to table, respectively.

B

C

G

M

Q

R

S

T

U

V